Eat4Earth Online Event
Transcripts

Copyright 2018-2021
Printed and Bound in the USA

NOTICE OF RIGHTS:

DISCLAIMER:

ISBN 9798640736991 paperback

Table of Contents

The Experts

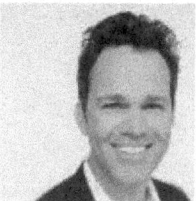
Zach Bush, MD
Physician, Medical Researcher, Founder of ION Biome

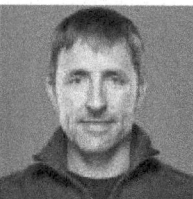
Dave Asprey
Biohacker, Author, Founder of Bulletproof 360

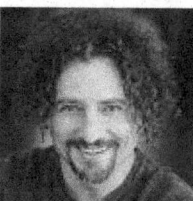
David Wolfe
Author, Educator, Farmer, Founder of Longevity Now

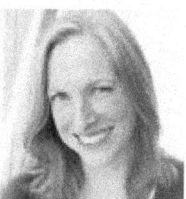
Alexis Baden-Myer, Esq.
Organic Consumers Association

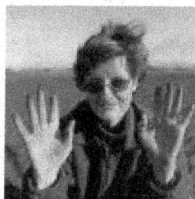
Elaine Ingam, PhD
Soil Scientist and Consultant

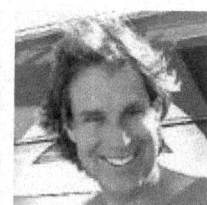
Reese Halter, PhD
Eco-Stress Physiologist, Author

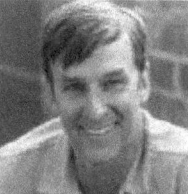
John Roulace
Author, Activist, Founder of Nutiva,

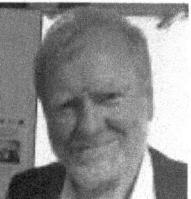
Walter Jehne
Soil and Climate Expert

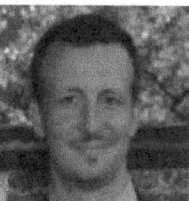
Eric Toensmeier
Author, Trainer, Research Fellow for Project Drawdown

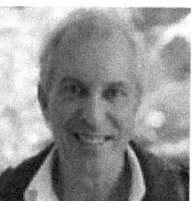
Graeme Sait
CEO, Nutri-Tech Solutions, Educator

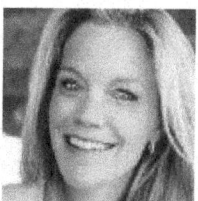
Robyn O'Brien
Author, Lecturer, Founder of Allergy Kids

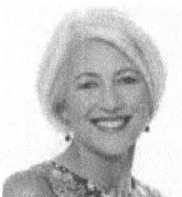
Véronique Desaulniers
Author, Educator, Cancer Conqueror

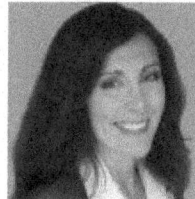
Manuela Boyle, PhD, NMD
Oncologist, Scholar

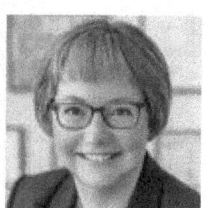
Linda Isaacs, MD
Internal Medicine, Cancer Specialist

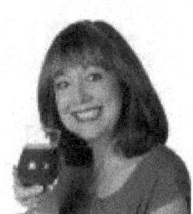
Cherie Calbom, MS
"The Juice Lady", Nutrition Educator

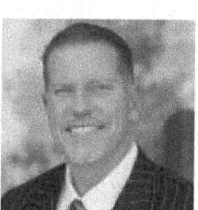
Ty Bollinger
Founder of The Truth About Cancer

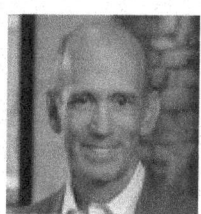
Joseph Mercola, DO
Author, Lecturer, Founder of Mercola.com

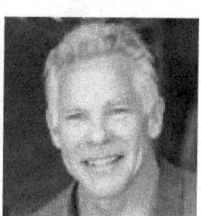
Mark Sisson
Author, Athlete, Entrepreneur, Founder of Primal Blueprint

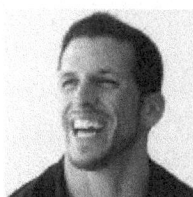
Drew Manning
Author, Trainer, Host of A&E TV show *Fit2Fat2Fit*

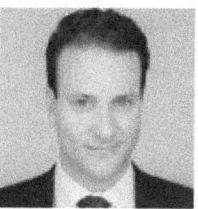
Greg D. Wells, PhD
Author, Researcher, Professor

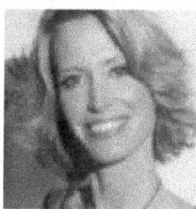
Erin Elizabeth
Journalist, Founder HealthNutNews.com

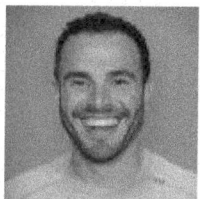
Alex Charfen
Entrepreneur, Coach

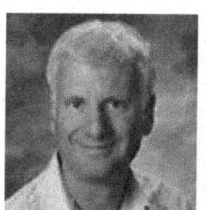
Joseph Pizzorno, ND
Founder, Bastyr University

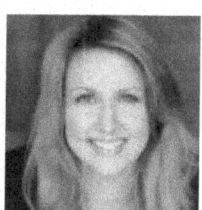
Wendy Myers, FDN-P, NC
Detox Expert, MyersDetox.com

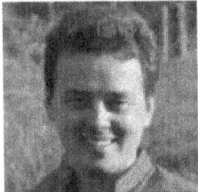

Dan Kittredge
Organic Farmer, Bio Nutrient Food Association

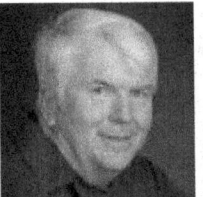

Robert Van Risseghem
Minerals Researcher, NaturallyNoble.com

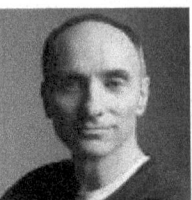

Jeffrey M. Smith
Author, Filmmaker, Institute for Responsible Technology

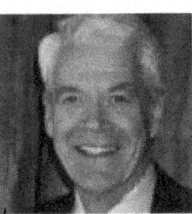

Caldwell Esselstyn, MD
Heart Disease Reversal Program, Cleveland Clinic

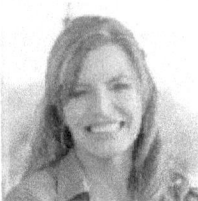

Michelle Norris
CEO, Paleo f(x)

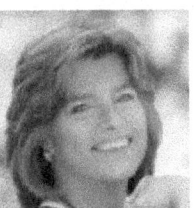

Nora Gedgaudas, CNS, CNT
Author, Clinical Nutritionist

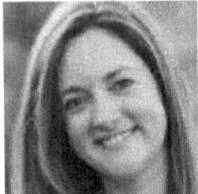

Diana Rodgers, RD, LDN
Author, Coach, Filmmaker

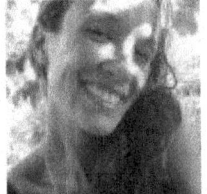

Sarah Wu
Herbalist, Trainer, Coach

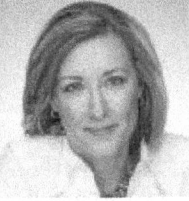

Victoria Keziah
Biomimicry Specialist, Marketing Strategist

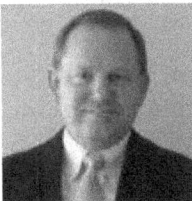

Allen Williams, PhD
Geneticist, Rancher, Consultant

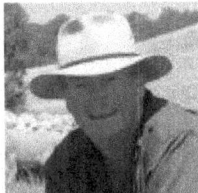

Colin Seis
Farmer, Rancher, Consultant

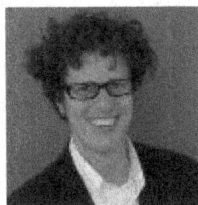

Peter Byck
Author, Filmmaker, Professor, Arizona State University

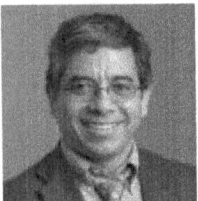

Reginaldo Haslett-Marroquin
Agronomist

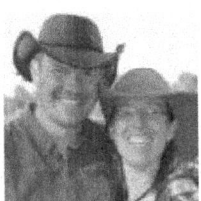

Elizabeth Kaiser
Organic Famer, Singing Frogs Farm

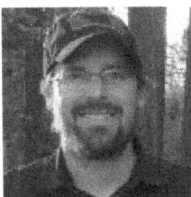

Erik Ohlsen
Permaculture Trainer, Entrepreneur

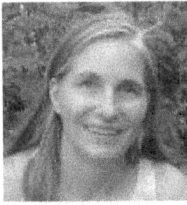

Marjory Wildcraft
The Grow Network

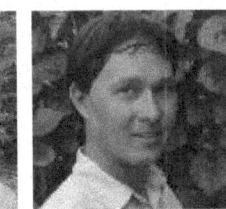

John Kohler
Raw Food Enthusiast, YouTuber

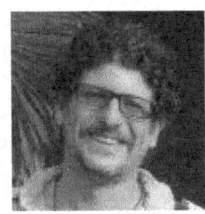

Stephen Brooks
Permaculture Trainer

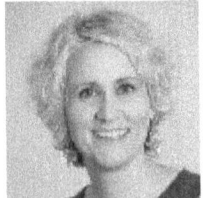

Kelly Kennedy
Biological Holistic Nutritionist

Some of What You Will Discover in This Book

- **How to instantly raise levels of glutathione** (your body's important antioxidant in the body) in your gut-associated immune complex by 10x (Zach Bush, Day 1)
- **The deeper truth about "leaky gut syndrome"** and how you can start healing it in minutes (Zach Bush, Day 1)
- **Which common mineral deficiencies put you at higher risk** of cancer (Veronique Desaulniers and Manuela Boyle, Day 3)
- **Which mineral is associated with the lowest incidence of cancer** in populations around the world, and why turmeric grown in India has high levels of phytonutrients like curcumin (Robert Van Risseghem, Day 5)
- **How to protect yourself from surprising sources of arsenic** and cadmium, two of the most dangerous heavy metals, including the "health food" that carries arsenic into your body, even from organic sources (Dr. Joseph Pizzorno and Walter Jehne, Day 5 and Day 9 bonus interviews).
- **Little-known binders for removing heavy metals from your body**, one of which also removes radioactive isotopes like cesium 137 from Fukushima (Joseph Mercola, Day 4 and Wendy Myers, Day 5)
- **A new technology that neutralizes heavy metals virtually instantly** (Wendy Myers, Day 5)
- **The rare potentially cancer-fighting mineral** you've never heard of that is deficient in American soils (Robert Van Risseghem, Day 5)
- **The crucial role of molybdenum for liver health and blood sugar** regulation (Robert Van Risseghem, Day 5)
- **Which mineral to add more of to your soil** to increase the levels of 22 other minerals by as much as 10x in plants grown there (Robert Van Risseghem, Day 5)
- **The four key practices** that enable Elizabeth Kaiser to produce $105,000 in revenue per acre on her vegetable farm (Elizabeth Kaiser, Day 7)
- **What you need to do to grow nutrient-rich foods anywhere** starting with any kind of soil, even beginning with dead dirt (Elaine Ingham, Day 1 and Graeme Sait, Day 9 bonus interview).
- **A delicious formula for opening congested arteries in the heart** and blocking the formation of a certain carcinogen in your gut (Caldwell Esselstyn, Day 6).
- **The enzyme some people lack for converting plant-based omega-3** fats to the form used in our bodies, and why people lacking this enzyme can probably only get enough of these essential fats from animal sources (Nora Gedgaudas, Day 6 and bonus interviews)
- **The phenomenon of "paramagnetism"** for powerful growing conditions in your soils (David Wolfe, Day 1)
- **How to 12x the delivery of nutrients directly to your plants** (Graeme Sait, Day 9 bonus interview)
- **How your body's response to caffeine provides a clue** about the bio-individuality of your detoxification pathways (Joseph Pizzorno, Day 9 bonus interview).
- **How Phase 1 and Phase II detoxification enzymes can get out of balance** and what you need to do to correct this (Joseph Pizzorno, Day 5 and Day 9 bonus interview)
- **"Phase III" detoxification**, and how this is affected by the mix of bacterial species in your microbiome (Joseph Pizzorno)
- **The type of gut bacteria that correlate with better health** (Day 9 bonus interview with Zach Bush).
- **What happens in your body when you eat too much meat** (Joseph Mercola, Day 4)

- **The little-known secret of soil** that determines whether the plants you eat accumulate heavy metals, or have been protected to deliver safe nutrient-rich food (Day 9 bonus interview with Walter Jehne)
- **Why each type of cancer requires a different type of anti-cancer diet** (fascinating!), and why the best anti-cancer diet for a person also depends on their unique metabolism (Manuela Boyle and Linda Isaacs, Day 3)
- **Key tips for an easier transition to a ketogenic metabolism** (Mark Sisson, Day 4).
- What John Kohler adds to compost to **grow "beyond organic" food**(John Kohler, Day 8)
- **Why friends don't let friends eat beef fed "dried distillers' grains"**(nutritional nightmare), and why beef raised in a very different way may actually be one of our best hopes for regenerating a healthy planet (Allen Williams, Day 7)
- **The exciting, fresh look at climate change** that Walter Jehne provides as he overturns mainstream assumptions and gives us more hope and power to turn things around (Walter Jehne, Day 2 and Day 9 bonus interview).
- **The new GMO technology that could be the most dangerous yet** and why it's vital that you understand it (Jeffrey M. Smith, Day 5)
- Two new artificial sweeteners 10,000x stronger than Aspartame that don't have to be disclosed on food labels and how to avoid them (Alex Charfen, Day 5).
- How a regenerative chicken production system designed in collaboration with the chickens themselves captures "free" ecological energy to **out-produce conventional agriculture 4 to 8 times while reducing consumer cost** per unit of nutrition (Reginaldo Haslett Marroquin, Day 7).
- Colin Seis' story of **how a devastating fire and drinking too much beer turned out to be a good thing** for food and agriculture all around the world, inspiring a crazy idea that enabled Colin to revive a natural grassland ecosystem that also produces grains, animals, and native plant seeds ... while never again having to spend $80,000 a year on chemical fertilizers or pesticides (Colin Seis, Day 7).
- **The vegetable that is _supposedly safe_ to eat non-organic** but is actually \sprayed with RoundUp / glyphosate (Jeffrey Smith, Day 5)

Day 1: A New Paradigm of Health

Heal Your Body from Your Membranes to Your Mitochondria: Food Sensitivities, Allergies, Glyphosate, Gluten, Your Microbiome, the Extracellular Communication Network, Gene Regulation, and the Shikimate Pathway
Zach Bush, MD makes it all easy to understand while he blows your mind and warms your heart.
<u>What You Will Discover</u>

- The deeper truth about glyphosate and chronic illnesses from "leaky gut" to autism and Alzheimers
- How to prevent and reverse "leaky gut" even if you are still being exposed to glyphosate
- How to instantly raise the level of glutathione (your body's important antioxidant) in your gut by 10x.

Food, "Kryptonite", and the Survival of Humanity
Dave Asprey tells it like it is about Nature's 500-million-year-old secret that keeps our bodies and our oceans healthy. You've probably never heard him talk about some of what he covers in this interview.
<u>What You Will Discover</u>

- The #1 thing to stop eating that's more harmful than smoking
- How the bacteria in your gut and the mitochondria in your cells are influencing your behavior
- Why healthy soil is vital to your health and your entire future

Forest Superfoods That Heal Your Body and the Planet
David Wolfe shows you a side of himself that most of his fans have never seen. A really fun interview.
<u>What You Will Discover</u>

- The "pioneering" power of avocado trees to start a rainforest
- Surprising uses for sand and saltwater in your garden or farm
- The little-known power of paramagnetic soils to grow healthy plants and food

Regenerative Agriculture to Reverse Climate Change
Alexis Baden-Myer, Esq. from the Organic Consumers Association provides a *tour de force* of our food system landscape and glimpses of the next food food revolution.
<u>What You Will Discover</u>

- How GMOs and glyphosate are contributing to climate change and chronic illness
- The difference between cows that accelerate climate change and cows that help reverse climate change
- Why the Farm Bill is one of the biggest influences on your health and our future on Earth

How Healthy Soil Provides Unlimited Mineral Nutrition and the Ultimate Solution to Climate Change
Elaine Ingham, PhD explains how regenerating the Soil Food Web restores high nutrient levels to your food,

makes gardening and farming easier and more productive without fertilizers or pesticides, and helps reverse climate change by drawing carbon dioxide out of the atmosphere and storing it in soil.

<u>What You Will Discover</u>

- Which plants need bacteria-dominated soil, which plants need fungal-dominant soil, and how to "balance the biology" of soil for your needs
- How Elaine turned a farmer's sandy soil into a "loamy" soil that produced 3x the county average crop yield in one growing season
- Why most scientists have vastly underestimated the power of soil to capture and store atmospheric carbon and potentially reverse climate change

Zach Bush, MD Interview 1

Heal Your Body from Your Membranes to Your Mitochondria: Food Sensitivities, Allergies, Glyphosate, Gluten, Your Microbiome, the Extracellular Communication Network, Gene Regulation, and the Shikimate Pathway

Brendan [00:02]: Welcome to the Eat4Earth event. We're exploring how you can heal yourself, your loved ones and the Earth with food. This is Brendan Moorehead and I am very excited to be speaking with Dr Zach Bush. Dr. Bush is a medical doctor and researcher, and he's one of the few triple board-certified physicians in the country with expertise in internal medicine, endocrinology and metabolism, and hospice palliative care. The breakthrough science that Dr. Bush and his colleagues have developed offers profound new insights into human health and longevity. In 2012, he discovered a family of carbon- based redox molecules made by bacteria. He and his team subsequently demonstrated that this cellular communication network functions to compensate for glyphosate and many other dietary, chemical and pharmaceutical toxins that disrupt our body's natural defense systems. This science has resulted in a revolutionary class of dietary supplements including the product RESTORE™ (now called "ION* Gut Health"). Dr. Bush's education efforts provided grassroots foundation from which we can launch change in our legislative decisions, ultimately upshifting and consumer behavior to bring about a radical change in the mega- industries of Big Farming, Big Pharma and Western medicine at large. Dr. Bush, I'm really excited to have you here.

Dr. Bush [01:21]: Thank you so much for having me, Brendan, I'm really excited to be here.

Brendan [01:24]: Awesome. So you've made a series of discoveries that have changed the course of your career, and it's changing the lives—are changing the lives—of many people around the world. What exactly did you discover, and how did you discover it?

Dr. Bush [01:39]: What we were really trying to untangle, and I guess to answer that in order to … what we discovered is that there's methodology in the single celled organisms to communicate amongst one another and unbeknownst to us at the time, but what's untangled over last few years, is the realization that as the bacteria and fungi begin their journey into a cooperative community and that huge communication network they make, they actually have the ability to communicate across human cell systems to the mitochondria within us and actually right down into our own nuclei to change the genetics of our own makeup. And so they really modify which genes in our body are turning on and off, which proteins we produce, an extraordinary story of just this cooperative living within our ecosystem. The way in which we came upon that discovery was in my nutrition clinic. And so I had previously been in academia for about 17 years, first at the University of Colorado and then at the University of Virginia. And I had gotten through a lot of training and education and research, and my research had really moved from mental health disorders and neuroplasticity in the late 1990's to, by the time I left in 2010 I was studying tumor genesis and how cancer cells grow and how nutritional aspects can function as chemotherapy to kill cancer cells. So I'd really had a broad journey through my educational background, and much of that was because I wasn't being satiated by my experience. I was really feeling like at each step of my education I was lacking any real tools that were having a meaningful impact on my patients' quality of life, et cetera. And so I finally left in 2010, the academic environment, to start just basic nutrition clinic in rural Virginia, a town of 550 people. I really believed at that time that my career had just taken a really drastic turn, and I'd probably never get the chance to do my research and teach again. And I just … academia was actually collapsing with the recession; our department of endocrinology at fallen from 70 faculty down to 25 and you know, everything was kind of in free fall in academic medicine. So, I said I'll just to kind of reengage in my life as a physician, and I was suddenly all alone in a primary care practice teaching people how to eat food. But really what I was doing is I was suturing up farmers, and I was treating head injuries, and I just kind of front lines doc again, and I hadn't done that a long time. And it was a great experience just to get really re-acquainted to my patients and find out that I was capable of being in community with patients. And unfortunately, that's really lacking from medical experience. And so 17 years of training and three board specialties, you would think that I was just steeped in that. But we're so isolated in academia, and we're so isolated in hospital systems and through insurance models. And all this stuff that gets in the way of real patient provider relationships. And so I got that experience out there, and ironically that kind of human experience of communication community was a macrocosm of what we were about to discover on the microcosm level {which} was that our patients who were not thriving on nutrition were really starting to fail on the healthiest foods out there. They were—the inflammation was going up, not down. All kinds of unexpected things were happening. And so it made us drill down into what's wrong with the food, or has the food changed, or what is the secret of food even because as you start to really get into nutrition you realize nobody actually really knows what they're talking about. And that's why there can be 32 opinions on what you should even eat today. And everybody seems to have the same firmly held beliefs about what you should or shouldn't be eating. And they're all at opposition to one another. So it's really amazing how little we understand about nutrition. And that's what I was kind of humbly realizing in my own journey is like, I don't even know what I'm talking about anymore when I was talking about nutrition. So in that journey we started to ask, well, "What about the soil?" Because it's where the plants come from, and that was the moment we discovered this family of molecules that you referred to and that discovery really uncovered this beautiful truth of the single-celled organisms are trying to really create the foundation for communication all of life to spring from, which I guess makes it a lot of sense since we probably all spring out of the soil at some point.

Brendan [06:04]: Yeah. And you developed a product. I'd like to kind of summarize—I don't know if you agree with this—but it's … you're healing our body with ancient soil. Tell us more about that. What is this communication network that derives from ancient soil extracts, I guess, that you've modified to make them … to bring them back to life physio-chemically.

Dr. Bush [06:29]: Yeah, that's pretty good description actually. It's a hard topic, and you did a good job with that. So the discovery of these molecules is largely because of the similarities that I had seen with my biochemical research and in the pharmaceutical industry, and what I recognized was that there was some arms off these central carbon rings that were … had the potential to release and absorb hydrogen molecules really easily because of their three-dimensional structure. And when you get something, a molecule that's able to release and absorb hydrogen, you get what's called a redox phenomenon, and this is a reduction and oxidation of that where you're able to donate or absorbs electron exchange very quickly. And that seems to be the magic on a lot of levels of the cellular environment. The departure from anything I'd ever experienced before was that there was this huge carbon backbone on this thing. Because previous to that I'd been studying mitochondria and the mitochondria live inside of ourselves and they look a lot like bacteria. Their DNA actually looks like a virus. It's a ring DNA, and so it's very much a primordial structure, these mitochondria. But human life is impossible, in fact, not just human, but any multi-cellular organism's life is impossible without the mitochondria, and the reason is these eukaryotes, these multicellular organisms, which could be an earth worm or human. We are incapable of creating fuel on our own. We have to be fed, and so at the cell level the mitochondria are responsible for taking the protein that's now converted by your liver to glucose and sugar, and then the fatty acids that are coming out of the fat sources in your diet. So you've got basically sugar and fat that are being derived from either carbohydrates or protein, and then you've got your fat. Those are being burned by the mitochondria, and the mitochondria in turn are fueling the human cell or the multicellular organism with ATP or adenosine triphosphate, one molecule which is really the fuel for the whole system. It doesn't matter if you're a brain, a muscle, a liver cell, all of it's running on ATP. Well, I knew—and my research had really been in the in the cancer environment around the fact that if the mitochondria are damaged—they can't make enough of these redox, and as well that kind of decreased mitochondrial threshold or our capacity. This is a real hallmark of just the natural aging process. And so I knew that this was a critical piece of health. If we were going to re-engineer a healthy body, we were going to have to have a huge signaling system, and at the time I and all of the researchers in the world, we were really thinking that redox signaling was really coming from these tiny little ethereal oxygen-based molecules that were being made through the Krebs cycle and then subsequently actually the electrons from Krebs cycle through what's called the respiratory chain in the mitochondria. And so that's a lot of complicated pathways you don't need to know about, but basically think of it as compost. And so the mitochondria making this compost-type waste product that we literally thought was waste for many, many decades and we thought that was harmful waste that needs to be cleared or else it would kill something. But it turns out that that waste is critical. There is no such thing as waste in biology. In the end, biology's always reutilizing and uses every part of the buffalo as the Indians would say there. So you've got this phenomenon where every piece of fuel is being used and all of the exhaust that's coming out of that fuel production is making a communication network down in cellular level. The aha moment of 2012 when we discovered the carbon molecules that would become RESTORE™ (now called "ION* Gut Health") and other dietary supplement lines would be that the bacteria and fungi that are in the soil don't have mitochondria. And so for that reason, they would have to make a unique subset of their own ion exchange. And we've recently untangled this - not me, but we as a science community. UCLA and UCSD for example, are doing some great work on this right now. But they've shown that the ion channels in the surface of bacteria are identical to the ion channels in human neurons. And so the bacteria have this capacity to communicate much like your brain is. And so ... but they're not communicating with self. They're communicating with the larger organism of many, many bacteria living in community. And so that ion exchange they're capable {of} has to have a carrier, and this is much different than the human inside of the cell system where the mitochondria dwell. Inside the cells, it's like the holy of holies. There's ... it's so protected; it's so regulated; it's so carefully guided as to what the osmolality is, what the pH is, what this environment is is strongly governed.

And so the mitochondria have the luxury of living in the Hilton Hotel where nothing's ever off. You know, like room service is always perfect. And that those mitochondria don't have to worry about those redox molecules being lost in the mix because the environment is so controlled. So these ethereal little molecules that are redox molecules, oxygen-based, last about a millionth of a second in the cell. One millionth of a second is the lifespan of these communication molecules. That's a very long time in quantum physics. And so millionths of seconds energy is a huge signal when you're talking quantum physics land, and they're using these signals to go out and pulse across a whole cytoplasm of a cell, which is, you know, like a galaxy in and of itself when you're down at this molecular level. But it can also shoot into other cells because the cells are tied together by gap junctions, which are like fiber optic cables that run between each other. And so you can send these redox signals of oxygen ethereal molecules from a single mitochondria and get a regional response. Now think about the bacteria and fungi. There is no control around that, their environment, and so the pH may be changing from an acidic environment to an alkaline environment in a single day in the life of a bacteria. Or think about the bacteria that are in your mouth, and you swallow and then they might end up in your colon. The pH just went from seven to three to eight to seven just in, you know, a few inches of space. So that bacteria is seeing a huge stress environment from a pH standpoint. pH of course is acid. Acid is hydrogen ions, and so that's gonna really change the ability of a redox signaling molecule to survive. So there's no way an oxygen-based high redox signaling molecule is going to be able to really survive and do a communication network in these adverse environments of your gut or the soil. You take a shovel into the soil, and you flip it over. You just changed, the entire environment; pH has changed; sunlight's on it, you know, just diversity all over the place. So the bacteria and fungi had to create a communication network that would have stability to it, and that's what we found in 2012—this eloquent carbon backbone chain. And I'm talking too, like I discovered this personally. Nature discovered this billions of years ago. I just got to witness it and say, oh my gosh, I think I know what that might do. You know, there's no such thing as discovered, really, there's nothing new under the sun as King Solomon said. And so the reality is Nature figured out how to communicate in these adverse environments, in the bacteria and the fungi. This is a really interesting timing in our understanding of human biology for this discovery to happen, and the reason is is because we knew that redox molecules somehow were kinda governing the inside of the cell environment. They were helping govern everything from internal metabolism, genetic production, and all this stuff at the human gene level, but we hadn't been paying attention to the importance of this extracellular matrix, the outside of the cell environment. And I think this is, my suspicion is, we aren't quite there yet. I think it's going to be 2020 to 2030. That decade I think will be the decade of the extra cellular environment. That's when we will know more about the extracellular environment in that decade than we ever have in all biologic history, and the reason is going to come down to the fact that we're starting to see the truth that bacteria and fungi are governing so much of human genomics and human health. You can't pick up a peer reviewed journal anymore without … it doesn't matter if it's endocrinology, neurology, pulmonology, every journal is saying there is some link to bacteria. And right now all they're doing is correlating this species of bacteria with this organ system or this disease. It's cooler than that I believe. I believe that it's so much cooler than that because it's not the bacteria, essentially; it's what the bacteria are saying to each other]. And we've seen this, and this isn't just in our lab. There's many labs around the world now that are starting to realize that if you study what's going on in that kind of soup, when you … in a petri dish when you have a single bacteria growing {it} changes radically if you put two bacteria into that environment. And so now they're doing cross-species communication. They're changing each other's genomics. They're changing what each other are making. So we're starting to realize that when you start putting multiple species together, the whole thing changes and that's what we're seeing now because our lab is taking that bacterial environment and putting in the context of human cells and we're watching human biology be redefined every day. So really exciting time where we're starting to realize the mitochondria are taking care of the inside the cell, bacteria and fungi are taking care of the outside of the cell environment.

Brendan [15:55]: And I've heard you ground this in very clear ways as far as how this impacts us personally because you've got the tight cell junctions … so many people are becoming aware of gut dysfunction, so-called "leaky gut syndrome". The tight junctions between the single … the cells of the single layer of cells that line our gut … they get pried open by certain things, and glyphosate and gluten are two of those things. And you've done tests to demonstrate that these stabilized redox molecules created by bacteria in ancient soil—and I guess you went to the ancient soil for a reason, because you couldn't find good soil today, and that's the whole reason for this conference, this summit, is we've got to rebuild soils. You've got to rebuild biodiversity in the soil of the planet and in our guts. And like you're pointing to when you put two bacteria and then more bacteria together a whole new universe erupts, and the signaling goes to a different level. And we're … I guess we're completely, almost completely—we'll see how much in coming decades—governed by this. We think it's our genes that are controlling us, but … (laughs)

Dr. Bush [17:12]: We need to get some serious humility going. We are so outnumbered.

Brendan [17:17]: Yeah, it's quite interesting. So now we're going to realize that at the biological level we are not separate from Nature in the least. And we've been making ourselves so. And I love how you've said in another context that antibiotics followed by maybe a little bit of yogurt, probiotics, we're kind of creating a monoculture in our gut. We're losing the signaling, I guess. Is that what you're saying? The signaling from the biodiverse organisms in our gut when we do that?

Dr. Bush [17:53]: You just presented a lot of great topics that we didn't hit on. So maybe I'll spin back to your tight junctions real quick, and we'll just give a picture to the audience of that. So tight junctions are the Velcro-like proteins that hold the carpets of membranes together. So the biggest membrane in your body is the sinu-nasal system that goes into your gut, so it starts in the nose (and) runs all the way to the rectum. So that huge gut membrane covers about two tennis courts in surface area. It's made of over trillion cells. That massive membrane is all knitted, knitted together by these Velcro-like proteins. And so they're intelligent too; they're not just not structural. They actually are gatekeepers. And so they're sensing what's on the luminal side, where your food is passaging and all the bacteria are living and everything else. They're sensing that, and when it's time to open up and let large macromolecules through, they unzipper, allow stuff to come in, and then zip right back up. So these intelligent gatekeepers that are moving a lot of the large charged particles and macro molecules from your food and intestinal environment into your immune system first and then into your bloodstream. And so that is really the gatekeeper for your body, and it's also really pertinently the gatekeeper for your immune system. Some 70 percent of the immune system lives right behind the tight junction system, and that's called the gastrointestinal-associated lymphatic tissue, and so the reason why we see unbelievable amounts of environmental sensitivities, food sensitivities, food allergies, environmental allergies, all of this in our children right now is because they're being raised in an environment where they are lacking the bacterial biome that would support that extra cellular matrix. And so as you spoke to with the antibiotics, we've shown now really definitively in our group, this is what I lecture on all the time, is that if you look at the CDC, the Centers for Disease Control, maps of chronic disorders in America, you're going to see a huge overlay correlation with the antibiotic prescribing of physicians. And so you don't have to look at infectious disease. Look at things like cancer and things like that. You see this huge overlay between antibiotic prescribing behavior and chronic disease. And so the more sterile we get as humans, the more we are prone to chronic inflammation and disorder of the gut. And so that is a really kind of the background of physiology for you to understand why the bacteria and microbes that are living around you are so critical. The fungi and the bacteria that are living around us are building this communication network to help improve our sensing at this cellular matrix environment of the extra cellular matrix, the gatekeeper between the outside and the inside.

Brendan [20:34]: And how is it that molecules like glyphosate, the main ingredient, one of the main ingredients, in the Roundup branded herbicide, and gluten, which is I guess one of many plant lectins that has become the celebrity of the potentially damaging plant lectin world … how does it actually affect this, these tight junctions? What's the mechanism? I used a word that sounded like a physical action—prying—but that's not accurate. How does it work?

Dr. Bush [21:07]: Yeah. So it's actually really a cooperative relationship with the gut lining. So gluten of course has been, and all the plant lectins have been in our diet for thousands of years without any problem. I mean, we've been living healthy lifestyles, but more importantly, healthy societies have built themselves on these plants as their staple crops. And so it wasn't really until the last couple of decades where we started to see really significant sensitivity to these molecules. Gluten as a molecule isn't … nobody's ever sensitive to that. That's a huge macromolecule that can pass through the gut if it's undigested, (and) never cause you any problems whatsoever. It has 13 peptide structures within it, and so as it passes through the gut and is digested. It breaks down in these 13 structures, and one of those is called gliadin. And gliadin happens to bind a receptor in the intestinal lining. And that receptor, it's not important to remember, but it happens to be called CXCR3, kinda like R2D2 or something like that. But CXCR3 is the guy that will grab gliadin, and when that happens it triggers a chemical to be made in the gut lining, which is a naturally occurring compound, very important for gut regulation called zonulin. And zonulin unzippers the tight junctions to allow stuff through. So regulated zonulin stimulation is really important for letting stuff through. And my guess is, the relatively informed guess, is that the bread and the wheat and all these things have built-in structures, likely gliadin, to allow fiber to get into our bodies. And so large fibers, the soluble fibers that you would find in wheat and things like this that you would find like in the wheat germ, they need to get into the body to be a nutrient source. And to get through they need zonulin to open up the tight junction and go. So I think that gliadin is there in a balanced meal to go through. So like in my clinic we're not gluten-free at all. We are really a fan of naturally occurring gluten balance. And so what you want is something like a sprouted grain bread or something that's really built from these heirloom grains that still have a balance between the amount of gluten in there with the amount of fiber. Very much like the fructose story. So high-fructose corn syrup is, you know, completely artificially derived chemical that's very harmful to the liver, can't actually be processed as well as a sugar. And the apple has a lot of fructose and is the main sugar in an apple. But if you go to the heirloom apples, which of course nobody eats it from a grocery store anymore, but if you pick an heirloom apple off the tree, the fiber is the difference there. So we've bred our apples to be these big giant, you know, Fujis and everything else to be juicy and sweet and everything else. And they're very easy to eat. They're crisp; they snap off in your mouth. If you eat an heirloom apple, if you've ever eaten one from an apple orchard that is making great apple pie or whatever, you'll know that's a very chewy apple, like it doesn't snap off and just melt in your mouth. But the difference is the amount of fiber there. So if you go back to the original nature design of an apple, the fibers were there and the fiber is the antidote to the sugar. So same thing now, if we go to the plant lectins is if you have a heirloom grain and you sprout it and you make a bread out of that, you're going to have a very equal amount and a healthy ratio, I believe, of the fibers in there and the and the gluten which would break down into gliadin. And so I think we've just … we've damned gluten inappropriately. I think that all the plant lectins are probably playing a really important role of nutrient delivery, and we need to go back to the way in which Nature designed those compounds and not fear them. So that gets at gluten. Now Glyphosate is … you know, we should probably do a little bit of history on that. I know your audience is probably completely steeped in science of herbicides and pesticides just because of the topic of your summit here. But I think that, you know, it's worth kind of a quick history of you don't mind is that. It was founded in 1957 by a Japanese researcher, and the Japanese researcher put it on a shelf at that point. It's an organophosphate, very harmful to anything that it touches. And so I think out of just sense of propriety for humanity, he put it on a shelf. Then in 1976, a company that you've probably never heard of called Monsanto came along and said, we'd like to buy that patent on that molecule. The reason being that Monsanto and many of the chemical companies have been engaged in making Agent Orange. And as you remember, Agent Orange was defoliating the jungles of Vietnam and Korea and all that. And so that defoliation or destruction of green stuff was extremely toxic. They knew that the soldiers that were being exposed were getting skin cancer almost immediately and just were being devastated immune systems and all that. So way too toxic of an organophosphate. So they needed a less toxic organophosphate, and they found it in this patent from the Japanese researcher. And so they bought the patents that he had, and they patented in the US, not as a weed killer, but as an antibiotic. And so it's been patented now multiple times as an anti-parasite, antifungal, basically touches any single celled organism it touches, it kills. And so that's, that's the lifespan of this chemical Glyphosate. Well, Glyphosate, it's worth noting, is only one of the horrible things in what we call Roundup today. Roundup has these surfactants and other chemicals that are designed to break apart cell membranes and deliver the chemical in deep into the weed or whatever is trying to kill. And so the Roundup, though, is the carrier for this Glyphosate molecule, and what our lab is publishing right now is the mechanism by which that Glyphosate is interacting with gluten to induce the gluten sensitivity. And we're really excited about the details of it, and it's way down in cellular biochemistry. So I'm not going to go into all those details here. But the take-home is interesting—is that that CXCR3 receptor that I mentioned that gliadin binds to, and which is also the one that unzippers the tight junctions, is radically upregulated by Glyphosate. And so that's why in the last 20 years we've suddenly seen this huge explosion of quote unquote gluten sensitivity. When in reality what's happening is our gut lining is getting hypersensitized to plant lectins because of the CXCR3 receptor rising up in completely abnormal amounts. So now if you eat a piece of bread and the gliadin goes across it, you get this over-hyperstimulation, and all of the tight junctions unzipper, and you get this unregulated gut permeability. And so there's this huge synergy, and we published the paper on the synergy between gluten and Glyphosate almost two years ago now. I think—and you can find that on our science website—but that relationship I think is really telling us something about when you throw a manmade chemical in the environment you're gonna have unexpected impact on how the body is able to handle nutrients and nutrition that it's been handling for thousands of years. So it's a big warning. But the second thing Glyphosate is doing is not just sensitizing the gut lining; it's also of course, as I just said, functioning as an antibiotic. It's destroying the microbiome and your gut. It's destroying the microbiome, unfortunately in the soil and water systems. And so if you now take a look at worldwide impact, it's laughable the impact of physician contributions of antibiotics when you start to think of Glyphosate. For example, if you look at just pounds of antibiotics right now, physicians in the United States are prescribing about 7.7 million pounds of antibiotics a year. That's a disgusting reality, and it's embarrassing, and we shouldn't be doing that. However, 7 million (7,000,000) pounds blushes in comparison to 2 billion (2,000,000,000) kilograms of Glyphosate. And so we are so vastly being dumped on by this antibiotic, which unfortunately is going not just into our bodies but into our food itself. And so we're destroying the soil from which our food is growing at. This has very interesting implications for the nutrition within the plant. I just gave you a picture of the impact on the gut and its ability to handle nutrition. In a moment when the timing is right, we'll move to the food industry.

Brendan [29:19]: So the … also I wonder, is the reduction of biodiversity in our gut also playing a role in our ability to resist things like the gliadin, the imbalance in gliadin? Or is it just primarily the Glyphosate creating this situation in combination or without gluten? Either with gliadin and gluten, or gluten, or not?

Dr. Bush [29:47]: Perfect. Yeah, absolutely true, for a couple of reasons. So when we start to kill the microbiome, there's a number of bacteria that are pretty good at shooting up the Glyphosate, actually Roundup, and we're now we're lacking those. And Roundup's like in competition and is killing the very organisms that could digest it you know. We've got that reality of OK, we're getting less and less good at breaking down Glyphosate. But then on the other side of that equation as if we look back towards gluten for example, there's eight different major protozomes, these huge enzymatic processes that happen in the gut when it comes to plant lectins. And if you have the right sequence of these protozomes that are being made by the microbiome and in cooperation with the human gut lining, then you can break down gluten and gliadin very effectively. And, and if you don't have the right protozome mix, then gliadin ends up getting overexpressed. You got too much of the gliadin break down stuff, so absolutely as the microbiome collapses, we can't detox, we can't metabolize normal food, we can't do our normal composting process. We can't break down the food into that compost that would become the communication network that would then go and affect the human genome to create more protein structures like the tight junctions and all this. So it's like almost at every single layer. And we can't of course deliver nutrients to the mitochondria, so you're losing cell repair at the human level. It's just this cascade of events from the microbiome outside your body, all the way down to the tiny nucleus of the cell, all the way down to the atomic structure of water inside yourself. Like it's just this horrible cascade that's going on, and it's why we're seeing what we're seeing. I mean, from a science standpoint, it should be ... it was unimaginable that we would have the disease burden on the planet that we do today. In 1980, one of the huge successful reports that's ever come out of the government was from the Carter administration. Believe it or not, Carter's administration was amazing. But one of the things they did, and they never got much news about this, but they wrote something called the 2000 Report. And they brought together academicians and scientists and thought leaders from around the world, and they wrote a single report on what would be the challenges that would face the world in the year 2000. And that paper—I think it's probably available publicly online still—the 2000 Report, Carter. That predicted just about everything you know—global warming patterns, water shortages, worse storms, a shift in currents and tides, all kinds of things that were just for most of us, unforeseeable ... fuel changes, fuel shortages, changes in the coal industry ... foresaw everything except it had no inkling that we would have a disease epidemic like we have today. And that's where they missed. And that's why the economic modeling of the 1980's completely collapsed by the end of the 1990's into the 2000's. We were losing any sense of reality because we hadn't predicted that such a huge part of our GDP was going to be pouring into healthcare. And so we really missed on the big kind of forecasting of the economic models and stuff like that. The reason we missed is nobody could understand how human biology could collapse so fast. We went from, you know, one in 5,000 children with autism in 1975, which happens to be the year before we had Roundup ... and so 1975, one in 5,000 children. Today we have one in 40. That's ... that's in such a short period of time. In just 35, 40 years we've developed this epidemic. And we're looking into 2035 now, which is only shockingly 18 years away here. In the next 18, 17 years we expect to see autism rates in the one to three to one to five children. That ... that's unsustainable. How is human life collapsing where our children, which would be the most resilient healers on the planet and always have been, how can they be failing to heal at such a young age? And so it's just an unimaginable thing from a science standpoint, and it doesn't make any sense until you back up to this level that we just talked about. You screw up the microbiome. You have collapse of nutrient in the plant food. You collapse the nutrients in the food. You have collapse of bacterial biome in the human gut. You lose the protective membrane in the gut lining. You overwhelm the immune system. You shift from acute inflammatory capacity to chronic inflammation. You then shift to dehydration within the cell, mitochondrial collapse; the mitochondria can't make redox molecules. You have collapse of hydration within the nucleus. The DNA can't hydrate. You get abnormal micro-RNA signaling there; you get protein collapse there. You can't build a human body! And that's what's happening. We literally are losing the ability to build a normal human body. And so that's happening at the foundation of life which is of course in the soil. And so that's, that's what we're doing as humans, and we're likely not to survive that unless you guys here at Eat4Life (Eat4Earth) and all these summits that are coming out around the world ... and unless we really start to communicate as humans and say we have got to do it completely differently. We've got to change everything right now, if we're gonna survive. Certainly, if we're going to not lose generations of children to really, really unpleasant suffering. And so we really need to correct things like yesterday. And so it's really not time to be looking for ... to our legislation; t's not time to be looking to our politicians. It's time for us to look into our communities and our neighborhoods, into our backyards and say, what can we do to make a radical grass roots change?

Brendan [35:32]: Fortunately, you've at least for us on a personal level, and I really appreciate your comments about the . . . we'll back to it if we have time or that might be for another conversation about what we can do on the grassroots level, but I want to also talk about what we can do for ourselves individually right now. And you've created an amazing product that I've started to enjoy just recently. I'm on my second bottle. It's called RESTORE™ (now called "ION* Gut Health") and you've got this product helping to recreate balance in our intestinal, our internal—it's not just intestinal—our internal soil and microbiome. Can you tell us about what that does and how it … you've talked about kind of how it could work by talking about these redox molecules, but you've got that now in a product. So how does that work individually for us?

Dr. Bush [36:27]: Yeah. So you had mentioned earlier that we were going to fossil soils, and that's exactly accurate. And so we're going to a fossil soil levels there. Did I lose you there?

Brendan [36:39]: No, I still hear you. I heard a system sound, but …

Dr. Bush [36:46]: I just wanna make sure you're still with me. The fossil soils … so we're going into the fossil soil, and what we're doing there is really relying on an ecosystem that really doesn't exist anymore on planet Earth. The amazing thing about the soils that we have today is they are nowhere near resembling what existed around the time of the dinosaurs, for example. And so if you go back to that time period, plant life was massive. We had ferns that were nearly the size of houses. We had animals like the Allosaurus and Brontosaurus, which were many times the size of the modern elephant. And they were plant eaters with a tiny little head at a tiny little jaw, and so they were not consuming massive amounts of food. It looks like they were probably consuming not much more than a than a horse would be consuming today. And yet they were supporting a biologic body that was massive. And so they had a nutrient density in that soil, in that plant life that we just have never experienced in our human lifespan or human history. And so it's interesting that our planet itself has gone through decrements of nutrient diversity and microbial diversity in its history before we even showed up. But now if you look at the last 50 to 60 years is we've really introduced billions and billions of kilograms of a toxin that's destroying nutrients within the soil, and the microbiome there, you start to realize that we're really hard-pressed to find intelligent soil. And so we ducked back into that fossil layer of soil. And we're extracting that from the deserts of southwest United States. And then we go through a catalyst process here in our labs in Virginia to get the hydrogen bonding right. So when we pull it out of the soil, actually none of these carbon molecules are really doing anything, and they're very inert because they've been there for 50 million years. They've lost this ion exchange capacity, so we take it through a catalyst process, which is basically just taking it through an organic kitchen. And so what you're doing is you're exposing it again to micro mineral environments that will help balance out that osmolality, the pH, and the hydrogen oxygen binding capacity of those carbon molecules. And then we get a finished product, and that finished product RESTORE™ (now called "ION* Gut Health") has got this really nice interesting phenomenon where it's maybe one of the first supplements ever to do nothing—like it has no intention of hitting a receptor in your body to do something in particular. It's not like vitamin D or vitamin C or a multivitamin where you're trying to do all these steroid effects. You're trying to hit hormone receptors, your trying to do all this stuff with the vitamins on a normal shelf in your supplement store. RESTORE™ (now called "ION* Gut Health") is vastly different. Instead it's just putting a neutral communication network into play. It's just being present, and then the cells are then utilizing that to send out whatever signal they're trying to manifest to either signal normal natural cell repair, cell turnover, mitochondrial metabolism, protein synthesis, the DNA level, we're basically helping just put the whole system back online. It's very similar to your cell phone down at the cell level. So your cell phone always works. It's got a computer in there that can receive and transmit signal, but it's further than seven miles from the closest cell phone tower, it's pretty much useless. And so it will start to decay. It will start to fragment its software within months of not touching the bigger network. It'll start to not function well. Same thing at the cell level. If it's not tied into that big wireless network, you're going to start to see dysfunction over time. And so as soon as you put the communication network, it's not doing anything particular. It's not healing anything. It's not trying to fix anything, it's just being there to let that whole system come back online and that's where we get to see over and over again. It's become, you know, a major foundational piece in over 2000 clinics across the country now. And it's so interesting for me to travel around to some of these clinics because they're doing vastly different things. You know, physicians are all practicing different areas of medicine and doing all kinds of different things and they all have different reports of what they see it doing. Well of course it's not doing anything. What they're seeing is in their little niche or their prism of what they're looking at human health, things are changing because there's a communication network back in place, and they are through their prism of whether they're looking at the lungs or the heart or whatever they're looking at. They're seeing improvement because the heart is simply starting to do what it does best, which is heal. The blood vessels that they're looking are starting to heal because that's what they do. That's what a kid does. A kid is born, and it starts healing immediately. And it's constantly being damaged by exposure to the sun or a drink of water or drinking breast milk, you know, all of this stuff is doing damage, and the kid's healing, healing, healing. So we're healing machines, and RESTORE™ (now called "ION* Gut Health") has been a fun thing to realize what a miraculous thing that the soil and the microbial life has really got this intelligence that's giving human life its infrastructure. It's giving human life the ability to do what it does best.

Brendan [41:32]: And so, RESTORE™ (now called "ION* Gut Health"), as I understand it re-regulates zonulin. Is that correct? Which is the, our own, our own signaling molecule, I guess, that we use to open the tight junctions but in moderation appropriately.

Dr. Bush [41:52]: Um, yeah. So again, it's not doing anything designed on this directly, it's an indirect effect there where ... so there's four major functions, and there's a video that I think it's downright at the moment, but it'll be a week or so back up on the science website there, restore4life (now IonBiome.com). And I'll take you back through this if you ... don't memorize all this right now, but in a nutshell, there are four major functions that we've proven out in the labs. And so when you put the communication network into play, what happens to the human biology? Number one, you get really huge microbiome shifts. This isn't quite human yet. So you get a shift of the really healthy, genus of bacteria which are called Bacteroides, or previously Bacteriodetes, and Bacteroides is that huge kind of anti-inflammatory family of a bacterial microbiome that is going to help do complex carbohydrate digestion, micronutrient processing, anti-inflammatory, antioxidant production, it's a huge, powerful thing. So in our current clinical trial, we're showing this huge shift within two weeks of being exposed to this communication network, the gut starts making a lot more of these, and it decreases the amount of Firmicutes, which is the other big genus. And those tend to be the fermenters, the acidifiers, and they can ultimately be inflammatory if they're out of balance. So we see this very beneficial shift from the Bacteroides to Firmicutes. So that's kinda step one is get a beneficial shift the microbiome. And let that microbiome start to take care of itself. It'll start cleaning up its own weeds. The typical weeds you see in the garden of the gut are things like Klebsiella, Pseudomonas, Clostridium, Candida. These, if they appear, are not the problem, like we just, we spend way too much time to try to kill Candida for example, things like that. We shouldn't be killing it. We should just be trying to foster a healthy soil so that those weeds become superfluous and they're not needed. And that's what we see happen. So whether it's the Bacteroides goes up, you see the weeds disappear, and you'll see that balance happen. So step one, very different than a probiotic, which again is just giving three or seven species of the same vector over and over again and never gonna create that huge rich, 30,000 species organic garden. So very beneficial shifts there. Number two, it has a direct ability—and we don't know all of the mechanisms yet by which it goes down to the human cell nucleus and does the DNA shift—what we're showing is that the DNA shifts into this very high-speed protein synthesis of the Velcro. And so we see this really strengthening of the tight junction system so that when zonulin is produced, the whole thing doesn't fall apart and makes it very resilient; and you're always making new tight junctions; and it's a very quick response system. And so zonulin still functions. It should still be there, but now we've got a really good response system to that natural zonulin environment. So it's up-regulating the whole zonulin cascade, so it's in balance again. We've also shown that it decreases CXCR3, which is that receptor that grabs gluten, so it's going to counteract that Glyphosate effect of up-regulating that CXCR3. So we're seeing this huge counterregulatory factor antidote type effect to that Roundup touch. So beautiful thing, and you can see those slides where we're showing the gut lining with and without that communication network in play. You can see it resilient or falling apart in the face of small amounts of Glyphosate. And so those are the kinds of pathways that are in the first two. The number one of microbiome, number two … tight junctions, strengthening the zonulin pathway, and number three … a direct effect on the immune system, sitting right behind it. We see almost a 10-fold increase in glutathione, which is the main antioxidant that your body makes. within just minutes of introduction. And so a huge explosion of glutathione is very unique, in biology. You can get glutathione supplements. If you go to a functional medicine clinic, they might give you an IV of glutathione that last seconds to minutes in the bloodstream. At best you're getting a four percent increase in total body glutathione. Here we're seeing this massive endogenous, from within, because there is no glutathione in RESTORE™ (now called "ION* Gut Health") or anything we're doing. From within, the microbial life is telling the immune system, "Rev up. Get the antioxidant going." How fascinating that the bacteria (are) actually preparing the immune system for life itself. And so the huge explosion of glutathione. So that's the third piece, is support the acute inflammatory pathways in that big powerful inflammatory thing that makes you stronger, not weaker. Acute inflammation is very good for you. Chronic inflammation, bad for you. Acute inflammation is really critical, so we're helping modulate and support, a healthy, acute inflammatory immune system. And then the fourth thing that we've shown is that it's talking directly to the mitochondria, and it's helping reduce the stress of mitochondria in healthy cells. And it's up-regulating the ability of damaged cells to get a reactive oxygen species burst out of the mitochondria to say, "Help! I need help. I need help." So it's up-regulating the help signals, and it's down-regulating stress, unhealthy signals, or unhealthy cells. So really exciting four kind of levels that were showing support to through that RESTORE™ (now called "ION* Gut Health") in the human biology.

Brendan [46:54]: Wow. And there's another piece of this whole puzzle that I'm curious about. I wonder if you can say more about the so-called shikimate pathway. What is that, and how does that affect us personally in this matrix of bacteria and these lectins and this toxin Glyphosate.

Dr. Bush [47:11]: And this is a great question to wrap up with. I mean, it's so, so interesting. So here you guys are having a summit on soil. And you know, 2 billion kilograms a year of a chemical are being used that blocks the shikimate pathway. The shikimate pathway is a series of enzymes that exists only in bacteria and plants— (it) doesn't exist in humans. That pathway is responsible for producing the ringed amino acids ... and so the aromatic ring amino acids which are the building blocks for protein in the human body or any multicellular organism. And so think of the amino acid kind of like the alphabet. There's 26 amino acids, and each are kind of like the letters of the alphabet that you could make hundreds of thousands of words out of 26 letters. Well we make hundreds of thousands of proteins out of those 26 letters or amino acids. And so unfortunately, we've got a chemical now, Glyphosate, that's blocking the ability to make some of those essential amino acids that we can't make ourselves. We have to get them from our food. And so we're blocking the ability of soil microbes and the plants themselves to make these critical building blocks for human protein and human life. So that's ridiculous enough on its own. I mean, that's ... that's enough to destroy human health right there. But then while human life is suffering from a lack of building blocks, the shikimate pathway also was supposed to be making our medicines. And so, you know, back to the very beginnings of medicine as we know it, Hippocrates a couple thousand years ago said, "Let thy food be thy medicine." And some 2000 years before him, Chinese medicine said, "Let thy food be thy medicine". So there were 4 or 5 thousand years physicians and scientists have been recognizing that nutrients in the food can heal anything. And the medicinals that are in the food, the anti-cancer effects, the anti-hypertensives, the anti-diabetics, the antidepressants, the anti-anxiety, the neuromodulators that would prevent seizure in autism, things like this. All of those medicinals that are in the food are made by the frickin' shikimate pathway. And so we are blocking the ability of the food to produce medicine. It's the most ludicrous plan. Unless you're a drug company; it's a brilliant plan because now you have a whole society that's living on non-nutrient, non-medicinal food that's obviously going to develop high blood pressure, high cholesterol, diabetes, major depression, insomnia, all of these things because the food doesn't have the nutrients that would've blocked those things from happening. And so now they need drugs. Well, we did the same thing to the plant kingdom. We made the plants weak through the use of this stuff. They have weak immune systems. They started to suffer, and so we made herbicides and pesticides and all this stuff to drugify farming. And so we've drugified farming. We've drugified human life. We have pharmaceuticalized the whole thing from gut to stern, and it's time for us to just take back the revolution here. And we created it. This is not a conspiracy theory. We literally created Monsanto. We as consumers created factory farming. And so this is why the grassroots revolution is so easy. All we have to do is start doing something again about food and about our own soil in our backyard. And so if you're going to do one thing this week, go on your backyard and start planning your spring garden. We're at a perfect time right now for you to have a few months to like learn how to plan a little square foot garden. If you've never planted a garden before grab something like "Square Foot Gardening" or any one of these little books that shows you how to grow, you know, a four by four square and which plants you should put in there for the easiest garden to maintain. Tomato plant, basil, and a couple of peppers and squash plant are a good start. So if you got that going, next spring, you are part of the revolution. In 1945 we were growing 45 percent of our food in our backyard victory gardens. That's amazing because now we're growing less than one thousandth of one percent of our food in our backyards. We have completely checked out of the food production industry, and we've said, "Go for it farmers; go for it Big Farming. You guys produce our food." We would like to go to a Trader Joe's or something like this and buy a zucchini wrapped in plastic and take that home and pretend we're eating vegetables. You know, like we have got to reengage the nutrients, and to do that you actually have to touch the soil. You need to be part of the process. And I guarantee you are going to have a different experience eating a salad that you grew. It's going to taste different. The tomatoes that I just brought to the party the other day, everybody's like, "Are those tomatoes?" I had them chopped up, and they were in olive oil and vinegar with just salt and pepper on. They were so red that nobody could even believe they were tomatoes. And so we aren't used to seeing real food on a plate. And so the confusion that happens when you see real food is exciting. If we get back into the nutrients that are in real food, we're going to heal the world, and we're going to heal our families and most of all our children, and then they get passionate about it. And I'm very excited for my children's generation. My kids are—my son's almost 20, my daughter's 17—and I watched their generation, and they're … they're excited about being engaged at that level. Like they, they are so uninterested in being part of the machine, you know, doing the things with the factory farming and everything else. They're very interested in getting back into kind of a, you know, an agrarian type lifestyle where even though they're engineers and performing arts, they're interested in being a part of eating real food, of watching stuff come into a farmer's market or participated in a CSA, so that their generation is really engaged, and that's really exciting. I think that if they don't heal it, then we're really screwed. So their generation and the generation coming up behind them are going to have to have the answer which is communicate together as humans, start to communicate and trust the microbiome and care for it and not fear it and really nurture that microbiome back into our lives. And this doesn't have to be through your food. Remember that much of the bacteria that is introduced to your body is breathe. And so get outside and breathe fresh air. If you spend all day in a dry, a drywall box that's air-conditioned, and you then go out and get in an air-conditioned, plastic car, drive home, get in another air-conditioned, drywall box. You're not breathing any healthy microbiome, and so you're seeding your sinuses that are then going to seed your gut with a bunch of Fermicutes, abnormal weeds, a really toxic environment. Weird fungi that are growing in the in your air ducts. Get outside, just touch the soil for a few minutes at the end of your workday. Take off your shoes. When was the last time you felt grass between your toes? It's ridiculously fun. I mean you like lose 10 years off your age immediately, like it is something you might actually giggle, this feeling, the feeling of grass between your toes. So kick off your flip flops, kick off your shoes, get into that soil, and touch it, and realize how long it's been since you touched Mother Earth. And then start to think about the billions of ways you could work that into your day. Take a five-minute break at lunch. Get outside, literally wrap your arms around a tree. One crazy thing, and this is probably a really bad public health recommendation to make globally, but in a rainstorm, go and hug a tree. A Native American friend of mine showed me this recently, and it's just ridiculously cool, and it doesn't happen all the time, so don't give up if you don't hear it the first time. But when there's a big storm going on and doesn't have to be pouring or anything like that, but there's a lot of energy and ionic charge in the sky ... if you go to the biggest tree you can find, wrap your arms around it and put your ear to the to the bark of the tree and listen to the tree. The tree can sing. It can actually get an audible vibration going through the tree from that huge ionic environment. Listen to that thing. It gives me goosebumps just to even explain it to you right now, but I mean it's so cool. All this stuff we're missing. You're not getting in your day a touch of Nature, I think. And so you and I have the opportunity to push each other to new experiences of "Did you hear a tree yet? Have you ever heard a tree talk to you or sing to you in a rainstorm? Have you ever felt rain on your, on your shoulders when your toes are in the grass, have you smelled that soil, you know, getting hit by that rain?" So that's what I think we're all here in this summit together to celebrate as we have a Nature that has been gifted to us, we're floating on a little blue marble in the middle of black space. It's ours to help, you know, really be a part of a community that powers to help nursemaid it back into health. And if we do, it's going to welcome us so quickly. The grace that's in the soil from 50,000,000 years ago. What crazy story that I just told you: 50,000,000 years ago, Mother Earth planting an antidote to an insane chemical that we would kill her soils with 50,000,000 years later. I don't understand that kind of grace. I don't understand why the humans had been allowed to survive as long as we've been allowed to survive, but we must be important to something that we've been kept here as long as we have in our insanity, and then our isolation and loneliness. I think Mother Earth is literally just begging and groaning for us to enter back into communication and a celebration with her. So let's do it together, and let's continue to teach each other. Thanks for listening to all my words.

Brendan [56:47]: My goodness, Dr. Bush! You ... it's such a gift to us to have such a brilliant mind in such a ... in a body with such a beautiful heart.

Dr. Bush [56:47]: Thank you.

Brendan [56:59]: Thank you for ... and you're such a gifted communicator, and you just made me cry. So, you know, I love the Earth so much. That's why I'm doing this. And to have somebody who can bring so much together in this science to the, you know, reconnecting with the community of Nature. And you know, maybe that's why we're here is we can actually help Nature thrive even ... it's hard to say ... imagine even more than it would naturally without interference ... but there are ways that we can work with Nature to create such bounty, and you're leading a big part of the way. So thank you. Thank you for your leadership and your contribution to the world at large and to the Eat4Earth community. Thank you for being here.

Dr. Bush [57:49]: Thank you guys for what you're doing. I'm just very excited that there's a community joining around your message and are consuming this education. All of you are going to become an epicenter with the education you're getting from this whole series. So very excited for each of you to go out with all that information wand become your own epicenter of truth and change. So thank you for participating in that revolution.

Brendan [58:09]: Thank you Dr. Bush. I'm looking forward to our next communication, our next conversation for sure!

Dr. Bush [58:14]: Thank you for having me.

Brendan [58:16]: Bye for now.

Dave Asprey Interview
Food, "Kryptonite", Performance, and the Survival of Humanity

Brendan [00:01]: Welcome to the Eat4Earth event. We're exploring how you can heal yourself, your loved ones, and the planet with food. This is Brendan Moorehead and I'm so super psyched to speak with our next guest, Dave Asprey. Dave Asprey is the founder and CEO of Bulletproof 360 a high-performance coffee and food company and creator of the wildly popular Bulletproof Coffee. He is a two-time New York Times best-selling author, host of the Webby Award-winning podcast, Bulletproof Radio, and has been featured on the Today Show, Fox News, Nightline, CNN, and dozens more. Over the last two decades David has worked with world renowned doctors and scientists to uncover the latest, most innovative methods for enhancing mental and physical performance by taking control of his own biology, a process known as bio hacking. His newest book, *Headstrong*, focuses on simple tips to have a smarter, faster and more resilient brain, with information and techniques to take control of your biochemistry, your body, and your mind so that you can reach a state of high performance. Through the Bulletproof Diet Dave has maintained a 100-pound weight loss, improved his sleep, and upgraded his brain, ultimately transforming himself into a better entrepreneur, a better husband and a better father. Dave has helped hundreds of thousands of people perform at levels far beyond what they'd expect and without burning out, getting sick or allowing stress to control decisions. Dave I'm super happy that you've been able to make the time to be with us today.

Dave [1:32]: My pleasure Brendan.

Brendan [01:34]: So, you and I share something in common which is having struggled with serious cognitive dysfunction due to some health issues. And in your books and your blog and in your approach to eating a low-toxin, nutrient-rich diet—*The Bulletproof Diet*, that's helped me a ton with my brain fog and my performance—in that you focus a lot on food quality. What are some of the ways that food quality affects performance and everything that we do?

Dave [02:07]: Well it turns out that if you want to perform really well, it's important to eat the stuff that makes you strong. But a lot of people talk about that in a lot of different diet books, but one of the biggest and easiest things to do is to stop doing the things that make you weak. It's a little bit counter intuitive, but if you're walking around, saying you were carrying a backpack full of bricks, but you've always carried it so you didn't know that. One thing you can do is, "I'm going to work out so I can be really strong." And then one day like, "Actually I'm just going to set the backpack down. Look how strong I am!" We have this going on nutritionally. I'll tell you right now, if you're eating fried foods, even if they're fried in so-called healthy fats, it doesn't really matter. You are completely wrecking your body. One plate of French fries or fried Brussels sprouts, if you want to be more Paleo about it, it doesn't really matter. What that does for 24 hours to your blood vessels, to your brain, to inflammation markers throughout the body, is actually much worse than smoking a cigarette. Now, I don't think cigarettes are particularly good for you. I wouldn't recommend smoking. It's just a nasty habit, but it only causes that kind of damage for four hours. So maybe you could not eat fried stuff. And if you look at the rampant inflammation that's caused by eating grains, including a lot of the so-called gluten free grains, they have these things in them that are called vegetable defense systems. Think about it like this. You don't want anyone to eat your babies. That's why if someone tried to eat your babies, you'd stop them. Well, plants, they don't really have good ways to do that, so they will cover themselves in poison to keep from being over-predated and there's some poisons we know really, really well. Caffeine is a poison to keep insects from eating plants. Nicotine is a poison to keep animals from eating plants. All of the polyphenols that are healthy for us, these, these colored compounds that give oregano or nutmeg or turmeric or any of these herbs and spices their flavors, those are there to keep them from being eaten. And we're in a situation where, well, we can detoxify some of these things naturally in our bodies, and that's why we know those plants are food. And if I eat those plants (gesturing to indicate different plants), I get really sick or I die. Well, it turns out that the plants that we can eat oftentimes come with stuff that makes you weaken them. And grains, even if they're organic and whole and sprouted and blessed by fairies, they still are inherently equipped with chemicals that make you weak when you eat them. They cause changes in blood flow, they cause increases in inflammation, and you're less likely to have a high functioning brain and more likely to have inflammation systemically. So bottom line is yes, there's fiber in whole grains. Unfortunately, there are these compounds that lower your performance. So get rid of fried stuff, get rid of grains, don't eat industrial oils, and don't eat these man-made chemicals that come into our food supply, things like dyes, artificial flavorings, additives, MSG, including natural sources of MSG. You can actually get organic MSG in your organic ranch dressing. It's just called textured vegetable protein or paprika extract. It's 74 percent MSG by volume. And MSG causes your neurons to fire until they cannot fire anymore. It's called an excitatory neurotoxin. Get that stuff out of your diet before you focus on, you know, eating more of the stuff that's going to make you stronger. That's a really big piece of advice, and it's something that's largely missing.

Brendan [05:48]: Yeah that, that's … I like the concept of Kryptonite, that you … you call these these kinds of things Kryptonite because they're debilitating to us. How do they do that?

Dave [05:58]: Well it depends on which of the Kryptonites we're talking about there. Things like food colorings are directly neurotoxic, and you can actually see the studies, and they change behaviors of kids and adults, or they trigger headaches, or they trigger a blood sugar crash. And this is something that MSG does really nicely. So you get these sort of science trolls like, well there's no evidence that MSG is bad for you, blah blah blah. But if you look at the biochemistry, what you find is that it causes hypoglycemia; your blood sugar drops. What happens when your blood sugar drops? Let's see, the stuff your brain is using to make electrons for you to think, it goes down, your body gets a stress response, and two things happen. One is cortisol and adrenaline go up because those raise your blood sugar, which are stress hormones. Your anxiety levels go up, but at least you didn't have a hypoglycemic attack. But also your body sends out a really strong sugar craving. So then the siren call of the chocolate cake or whatever it is, the cookie in front of you, instead of just being like a murmur in the background going, "Eat the cookie, eat the cookie", it becomes a very loud voice going, "EAT THE COOKIE!" and then you eat the cookie. You feel like a bad person, but at least your brain got some sugar, and then that leads to another blood sugar crash. So not eating stuff in food that's going to cause that is a big issue. And that leads also just plain sugar. If you're eating sugar, sugar lowers immune function. It lowers testosterone. And it does give you a quick energy hit, but it comes at a long-term cost of your performance. In the Bulletproof Diet, in fact, people can download the infographic for free ... just go to Bulletproof or search for Bulletproof Diet Roadmap, and it's all of these foods, on a single infographic. And there's Kryptonite foods that are listed, things like trans fats, fried stuff, these grains, these additives. These are things that really you just don't want to eat those. There's also a list of suspect foods, and this is where it gets really interesting. There are basically four classes of naturally occurring compounds that mess up different people in different amounts, and one of them is these plant defense systems called lectins. And these are made by just about every type of vegetable. Our body makes them too, and there's many different kinds of lectins. But the big categories of them are in nuts and legumes and whole grains and in particular nightshade vegetables. These are potatoes, tomatoes, eggplants and peppers. Roughly 25 percent of people or so ... one or more of the foods in that category cause chronic inflammation, weight gain, brain fog and lead to rheumatoid arthritis. So for let's say for you, tomatoes, which are great source of lycopene, which is really good for you, are going to be great. But for someone sitting right next to you, who eats the tomatoes, they're going to cause chronic inflammation, and they're going to cause the energy production units in your cells to make less energy. That's where they're a suspect food. Until you know if they're guilty or innocent for you, you'll never know. So it's your job to find the foods that are biologically compatible with you. So we talked about lectins, and then the next one that's particularly interesting is oxalic acid, and people say, "Oh, you should eat your beet greens or eat some raw kale." Well, a good number of people are sensitive to this, but they don't know it. I run an organic farm. I've got sheep. Try and feed a sheep raw kale, and they'll spit it out. And they do this because it has this bitter tasting compound that turns to tiny crystals inside your body when it comes in contact with calcium, and the crystals can accumulate in your brain where some researchers have tied them to autism. They can go into your joints where they cause a form of gout that isn't caused by uric acid. And even worse, they go into your kidneys and cause kidney stones. This is something you might want to know about. Some people handle it really well, but if you drink a kale juice, and then you have sore feet or sore hands-or your muscles start to hurt, or you get a blood sugar crash, and you just have cravings afterwards. Here's a note: cook your kale and dump the water, and you won't have that problem. It's just a hackable solution. The next category that Mother Nature provides us with is histamines. And there are other things like histamine. They're called biogenic amines that happen when foods are fermented or just when there's a little bit of microbial spoilage. So if you ever had fish that was, you know, sat in the fridge for a couple of days before you cook it and eat it, and then you just get really tired or you get a headache or sugar cravings afterwards. That's a prime example of this, but quite often leftovers are a problem. The two-day old leftovers usually have biogenic amines for them because they've started to have microbial fermentation even though they're not technically spoiled. For a good number of people you do that, you're just not going to feel as good as you could have because histamine is a neurotransmitter. It also triggers hives, rashes and sneezing attacks and things like that. And the final category there would be mycotoxins, not microtoxins, but myco(toxins). And these are mold toxins. These happen during fermentation of foods, where, ah, things like beer, wine, coffee, chocolate and most whole grains during the time they grow in the field or when they're stored or processed, mold grows and the poison the mold makes, which is basically a kind of antibiotic. It's really bad for humans and the reason for this is that our power system is made of a quadrillion ancient bacteria. They're called mitochondria, and we'd like to think, "Oh, they're just part of our cells." They're actually an independent network of cells in the body that decide whether a cell gets cancer, or doesn't get cancer, whether you get Alzheimer's, (or) don't get Alzheimer's. They control inflammation throughout the body. In fact, they control a huge number of our behaviors, and they're a separate consciousness from our thinking brain, yet they provide power and the energy for the brain. From the perspective of a ancient bacteria, mitochondria, your body is a petri dish, and they're trying to make the petri dish behave itself to make sure that the mitochondria get what they need to stay alive. And since they are ancient bacteria, the enemy of bacteria is mold and fungus, like that's where antibiotics come from. So if you're eating these low grade antibiotics that come from Mother Nature, and they're poisoning your power production systems, it's going to really tweak on you, but you might not know that's what's going on. So I talk about the high risk foods, and coffee is a high risk food until the point that I quit drinking coffee for five years until I came up with a new process for making coffee. This is the green coffee process. I ended up doing lab tests on 27 different toxins that come from fermentation and avoiding those, and what you get is coffee without the jittering crash that you probably associate drinking normal coffee. This is such a problem. Most governments around the world have legal protections in place for their population for the high-risk foods. Unfortunately, in the US there are no limits. So I have the President of the Specialty Coffee Association, the former President, on video with me at our plantation in Guatemala and he's like, "Oh yeah, I was in Japan when the trade minister rejected a thousand shipping containers of coffee because it was too moldy for Japanese consumers." And I said, "Well, what'd you do with the coffee?" And he said, "We shipped it to the U.S." So yeah, you can't make that stuff up. But if you recognize that, well, this cup of coffee or this chocolate bar is not the same as this one, this quality of grain, if you're going to be eating grains, is not the same as this one. So quality really matters because the lower-quality stuff tends to have problems. Nuts are another high-risk food. Those discount slivered almonds or ground up nuts or like the very finely chopped ones, they take the discolored ones that are much more likely to have toxins in them, and they chop them up finely because they were too ugly to sell whole. And this is why getting nuts in the shell or whole nuts, even though they're more expensive, they're probably better quality, and you might feel very different if you ate a handful of cheap nuts versus a handful of good quality nuts.

Brendan [14:12]: You know, let's say a person ... so obviously this is about going for fresh food, you know, figuring out what works best for your body, being aware of things like mycotoxins, oxalates and so-forth. Let's say somebody dialed in their diet ... is there anything else they should be aware of as far as, let's say, how agricultural Kryptonites might affect them? You've talked about Glyphosate here and there. I'm just curious how important you feel that that kind of thing is in choosing, let's say, organic over conventional and so forth?

Dave [14:45]: You should always choose organic and grass-fed over conventional produce and the reason is not just glyphosate. It's that when you use non-organic farming techniques, you end up with food that is less nutrient dense. But this glyphosate contamination is a horrible problem right now, and it's creeping into organic food. For instance, they recently found almost all California wines had glyphosate in them, including the organic wines because they're spraying billions of pounds of this toxic chemical that inhibits your mitochondrial function. That stuff we just talked about, the power production. Well, if you're based on bacteria, and this nasty chemical, glyphosate, actually affects bacteria, but they make this strange argument,

"Oh, it can't affect people because we're not bacteria." Sorry guys. You're a quadrillion bacteria and only like a trillion or so you're forty ... ah whatever, I'm going to mix up my numbers. There's a lot more ancient bacteria in you than there are cells in you, but they like to claim that we're not bacterial, not to mention what's going on in our gut, which is all bacteria. So if you eat glyphosate, it causes disruptions in your gut biome. And what's fascinating is that the bacteria in your gut talk to the bacteria that run your power system, and they talk using light. It's called bio photons, and this is actually well established. They make about 5,000 times more bio photons then your body does when it communicates amongst itself, and we communicate with the electricity, with chemistry and with light all at the same time. Which is fascinating and cool, but if you're going to be putting this stuff in your body in the levels, is going to cause a systemic problems. It has no place on our planet in agriculture, and it's completely unacceptable. and I have a pretty strong hopes that the companies who are making these toxins will be held accountable. And 25 years from now, we'll just look at each other and say, "How could we have allowed this to happen? We're still trying to clean up this incredible mess because we've destroyed our soil." You break the soil, everybody dies. And we're in the process of doing that right now.

Brendan [16:53]: What I'm wondering is you're talking about these energy plants that are in our cells that are like bacteria, like ancient bacteria, and our bacteria in our microbiome are communicating with them. We're talking about the mitochondria in our cells. How does it, how does it work? How are the mitochondria affected by these various forms of interference with our natural system?

Dave [17:19]: Well, mitochondria, their job is to take food and air, and convert them into electrons, but they also make chemicals in the body. And a lot of people don't know your mitochondria directly manufactures some of the hormones, things like pregnenolone, which is a precursor hormone for everything. What they also do, which is really fascinating, is they, (on a) microsecond by microsecond basis, monitor the environment around you to make sure that you're making the right kind of energy for the situation that you're in. For instance, they're really keenly interested in knowing is it morning because in morning you're supposed to raise the acid level in the body. You're supposed to raise cortisol and adrenaline, but if they get confused or if it's night time at nighttime, they're supposed to turn down energy production and turn on rest and repair and things like autophagy, which is when they clean out proteins inside your cells. Well, if you're staring at a bright light at night or you've disrupted the bacteria in your guts so you're not getting the environmental signal that comes in from that, they get confused and some of them think it's day time. Some of them think it's night time. So what we're finding is that they're a system. It's almost like if you were to have your own compost pile, and you have to make the right environment for fermentation to happen there. Or your gut bacteria ... you take care of your gut bacteria with probiotics and eating the right foods. Well, I hate to tell you, you have a biome. It's your mitochondrial biome. It's a network of bacteria, and you have to take care of it the same way you take care of all these other things. These plant compounds like lectins, the glyphosate and many prescription drugs are shown in studies to lower mitochondrial function. And what happens is that half of us under age 40, it's actually 48 percent, have early onset mitochondrial dysfunction. And everyone over age 40 has mitochondrial dysfunction, they just make the argument that it's not early onset because that's what happens when you age. My belief is that it's always early onset mitochondrial dysfunction. I'm planning to live to at least a hundred and eighty in my mitochondria. If I do everything right, it should be functioning like those have a 25-year-old when I'm 180 because that's how you live a long time. And it's not like it's an on/off button for these guys. It's that if you take one unit of energy in, you get one unit of energy out, but what happens is you take one unit of energy in and you only get point seven (0.7) units of energy out? Well, what's going on there? All those extra electrons that you should've made, they went somewhere. They went into inflammation, or they went into fat storage. And your job is just make it so your body is incredibly good at knowing when to turn food and air into energy for you. And one of the big signals for that is the environment around you. We're talking the temperature of the environment around you - when you eat, what spectrum of light you're exposed to, and if you get all those things right, and then you dump in some poisons that directly inhibit your ability to make energy, you still did it wrong. So you've got to line up your environment to avoid the toxins and to get the right signal in at the right time. And when you do that, you can tap into this huge amount of power your body can make you're probably not making right now.

Brendan [20:28]: In your first book, *Better Baby*, you talked about, you wrote about, how these things influence the next generation basically, you know a woman's unborn children, when she's a gestating. So I'm just curious ... I actually haven't read the book ... did you cover anything in particular as far as how these influences work, in terms of ... I guess I want to add to that, let's say agricultural toxins since that's my big focus. Agricultural toxins and nutritional content of food and so forth.

Dave [21:06]: We talk a lot about that in a *Better Baby* book, and if you're not doing organic or biodynamic farming, you're just doing it wrong. And there's a reason that I've got an eight-year old and 10-year-old, and we live on an organic farm, and we grow our own food. We follow mostly biodynamic and certainly organic practices and we get incredible food production. The food tastes better, and it's more nutrient dense and we're fortunate to be able to do that. We also moved to a part of the world where land is affordable in order to do it, which is something that you might want to do. And before that, there's always farmers' markets. And do you want to know the people who raise your food? And you can say, "Oh, it's just too much work. I'd rather go to a fast-food joint." I'm like, "Look living a long time and feeling good all the time does take work. But, when you decide to order the grass-fed meat instead of the industrial fed meat, look at what you're doing. When you, when you're doing grass-fed meat, that means there's an animal walking around hopefully on pasture and not eating genetically modified grass, which is another bad trend happening. But, say organic grass fed so you can avoid that, what's going on as the animal is walking around in a bio diverse environment. The sheep that I have here on my farm, they're wandering the property, finding whatever they, whatever is best for their body and eating it. And then they poop. And it's shocking. But plants eat animal poop and the best, most fertile soil has animals involved, not just for micronutrients, but because they have bacteria in their gut that change what's happening in the soil. And you get these sort of radical vegan ideologies that say somehow we're going to eat vegetables with no animals involved, and that's not how soil ecology works. It's not how it's ever worked and operating farms have at least chickens or some sort of animals around because you need it for the cycle of life to continue. And soil is at the very base of doing it right. And if you decide you're going to poison the soil and poison the bacteria in the soil to make it easier so you don't have to pull weeds, which is basically what's going on here, it's like it's just bad math. Because that steak, that hamburger you buy it made acres of land that would have supported bunnies, turtles, rabbits, butterflies, all the good stuff that you associate with farms ... there's nothing ... you drive through the corn fields of Iowa right now no bugs hit your windshield anymore. It is basically sterile land. You put your hands in the soil, and it's 12 inches of basically sawdust. It's not actually sawdust, but it's soil that has no, no fungal web connecting together. It is dead soil that's propping these things up as they pour chemicals on them. This is not sustainable, and it will actually lead to huge amounts of cancer dysfunction. And it's going to take many years to grow that soil back if we even can.

Brendan [24:05]: Agreed. You know you've spend most of your life in technology, and what seems ... when I look at people from technology they seem to want to look for a technical solution for everything, yet you're talking about soil and natural processes. I'm just curious ... why are you different? How has it come about that Dave is talking about soil, talking about natural processes, and if we're running out of soil, why don't we just grow things indoors and you know, hydroponics and aquaponics and aeroponics and so forth?

Dave [24:39]: Well, I am a systems thinker, and the field that I worked in was the very early creation of the Internet as we know it. I ran the Internet engineering program for the University of California in Silicon Valley, Santa Cruz actually, UC Santa Cruz, trained engineers in how to work on this Internet thing. And the Internet's funny because it's such a complex system that you cannot know the state of everything on the Internet. Like we're talking right now over Skype, as you're recording the interview, and our little bits are touching literally tens of thousands of devices that you and I don't know anything about, owned and controlled by many different people, and we don't have control over them, yet we have influence. And the same thing is happening inside our body and inside our ecosystem. So there's interdependencies that we don't understand yet, but we can detect them, and we can manipulate them. And when you look at the system as a whole, the inputs and outputs and all the different levels, it's blindingly obvious that our bodies are plugged in to the environment around us. And if you look at yourself as just a brain with a support system, which is the most limiting, most wrong way of looking at it, you're doing it wrong. And if you look at yourself as just a body, you're also doing it wrong because your body cannot be separated from the environment that it's in. Now we might learn over the course of the next 20 or so years how to create an environment, an artificial environment, that actually supports our body to its fullest extent. We could probably trick ourselves, but what we're going to create is going to look and act and feel an awful lot like Mother Nature. In the meantime ...

Brendan [26:16]: Trying to replicate it, that's what were gonna figure, "Oh we're just trying to replicate something that's already perfect."

Dave [26:20]: And since we haven't figured out how to do that yet, maybe taking care of what we've got is a good idea, and maybe, yeah, maybe throwing away what we've got is a bad idea even if we can replicate it. And I'll tell you right now, as a technologist, I am all in favor of learning how to make everything right in the environment here in my biohacking labs so that when I'm indoors, and I'm not in this horrible Canadian winter where it just rains all the time—I don't particularly enjoy that—but how do I make my indoor environment so that it supports my biology as fully as being outdoors would? That's a really important skill because if we're going to go to Mars, and there's people talking about doing that in the next five years, you're not going to be alive when you get to Mars or if you are alive, you're not going to be functioning very well if you think that humans could live in a metal tube with artificial junk lighting and dehydrated food for that period of time. It just ... we don't work like that, and we haven't figured out how to do it. Maybe we will, but until then the only working system I know of is Mother Nature. I think we had to take really good care of that and do our best to allow the signal from Mother Nature into our bodies so that we can do everything that we're capable of doing. It simply doesn't work to think of yourself as an island. You're plugged into a big system, and you're plugged in with light, magnetism, electricity and chemistry all at the same time and all of them matter.

Brendan [27:41]: And do these influence us in non-obvious ways? I mean, we're talking about health and performance and I think we might have touched on mood. What about spiritual development?

Dave [27:53]: Well, I'm a ... I've spent a huge amount of time on personal development work to the point that I opened a neuroscience facility in Seattle called 40 years of Zen, where you spend five days with electrodes glued to your head using some custom hardware and software to teach yourself how to go to the places that you normally get to after 40 years of daily Zen practice. And the idea is there are spiritual states. You will not access these states of high performance ... By the way, every state of high performance is an altered state because if it wasn't, if it wasn't, if it's an average state, it's not a high-performance state. High performance means above average. It's not normal. So if you want to be able to go to those places, it takes one thing always; it takes energy. And the system in your body that makes energy, it comes from food and air and light. Like if you get that stuff wrong, no matter how much effort you apply to personal development, to developing a meditation practice or a spiritual practice or just feeling a sense of oneness with the universe, it's hard to do that If you don't have enough energy to really feel good. And I made that mistake when I weighed 300 pounds when my brain really stopped working, and I was like, "This is an emergency situation. I'm here in Silicon Valley. I can't remember what was going on in my meetings. Like something's really wrong." And it turns out there that it all comes down to energy production. One of the ... the line of supplements that I make ... I make a bunch of stuff at Bulletproof designed for mitochondrial enhancement ... These are things that cause your cells to make more energy even if they're not getting all this stuff that you wanted them to get. And one of the things is called Keto Prime. And it's called that because it's a rare ketone, different than the ones you get from food that primes the pump for your cells to make more energy. And the interesting thing here is two studies just came out that show it treats the symptoms ... or it treats the emotional symptoms of PMS. Like what the heck is going on? We turned up energy in the mitochondria, and the crankiness that comes with PMS goes down? What's going on there is that whenever your energy levels drop in the brain, then these ancient survival systems that make you cranky, that make you look for threats and make you more anxious and make you feel like you don't have enough, they actually get turned up. And so when your energy levels are high, it's easy to access to spiritual states and feel gratitude. And where your energy levels are low, everyone around you is a jerk, and it's hard to be a spiritual state when everyone's a jerk.

Brendan [30:26]: Right. In terms of technology again I'm curious to know ... you mentioned the geo (genetic) engineering of grass now ... that's scary as heck. What's wrong with genetically engineered organisms in your opinion?

Dave [30:40]: The number one risk for genetically engineered organisms right now is that they do it to spray them with Glyphosate, which is not OK. Glyphosate is out there, but there's more going on. When you look at things and how, especially bacteria and fungus's swap skills. Imagine, uh, one of my favorite movies, X-Men. OK, you have all these mutant x-men, and Wolverine comes along and says, "I've got claws," and Mystique comes along says "I'm blue and I can change what I look like." Well, plasmids are groups of genes that come together, and plants and bacteria are capable of swapping these with each other, like trading cards. Single level mutations, which is what happens when we're doing hybrid development, or just when there's natural selection. They don't make plasmid level changes; these are things that don't transfer between species very easily. The problem is that when we do the engineering the way we've been doing it, we end up with basically the ability to give mutant nasty superpowers to something that it can give to other things. An example of this is they made corn designed to automatically grow a pesticide inside the corn. Like what a terrible idea because they're expecting us to eat this stuff. Anyway, that's just, that's just stupid on its face to be perfectly honest. And what happens there is that this Bt-Toxin; the plasmids that allow that to be made can be taken up by the bacteria in your gut. And they're like, "Oh look, I got a new skill. Why don't I try making Bt-Toxin?" So then because you ate this genetically modified corn, now you've got bacteria in your gut that's capable of making a pesticide onboard as you eat other foods. This is not a cool situation, and it's getting worse. I just saw a study or a proposal out there where scientists found a mold that only eats some sort of fruit fly or some sort of environmental pest like ... well, the mold, it affects these, but it doesn't really kill them. So we added a gene from a, let's see, a deadly tarantula and a deadly snake to the mold toxin there. Now it'll kill these bugs really effectively. Look at that. And I'm like, "Jesus Christ, people what do think is going to happen when that plasmid gets into some other kind of soil fungus and spreads around?" And this is the crap that's going on right now. So I'm actually not philosophically opposed to single gene editing, things like CRISPR. There might be a safe and effective and useful way to do this and certainly heck, I'm kind of interested in modifying some of my own genes, but I'm not going to do it and let it go in the environment without an off switch because like this is the stuff of science fiction horror movies. Like are they really doing that? They are, and I just have a problem with that. I'm, I'm very into the science. I'm very into taking control of our own biology. But one of the things that any systems level thinker knows is if you let something into the system, and you can't turn it off, you better be damn sure that it isn't going to cause harm. And we have abundant evidence that what they're doing now is causing harm.

Brendan [33:48]: You mentioned systems level thinking, which I think is so super important. And one of the things that has struck me about Nature's system is the primacy of, you know, the centrality, in a sense, of polyphenols, because they're communicating something between the plant ... they have an effect on bacteria; they have an effect on the bacteria in our gut, the bacteria in our soils, the bacteria that are our mitochondria. What's interesting in soils is if you have a certain level of biodiversity in the plants, plants from five different families, they suddenly start sending all those phenolic compounds into the soil, and it turbo charges the bacterial activity of beneficial microbes which turbo-charges their processes of making minerals available to the plants, and the whole system goes to another level of productivity and nutrient density and so forth. So I'm curious what you can tell us because you spend a lot of time talking about polyphenols and knowing that they're so important to our health, and of course polyphenols from coffee are way up there as a human source. How, how do they work in terms of our bodies and the bacteria around us and in us?

Dave [35:05]:   Polyphenols are these brightly-colored compounds that you find in vegetables to some extent, but really in herbs and spices and coffee, tea, chocolate, brightly-colored berries and things like that. And they're vitally important for your cellular biology. They're light-modifying and signaling compounds, and your mitochondria are very light-sensitive. They're little semi-conductors that are magnetically sensitive, but they're even more light sensitive. So if you're under the wrong color light, or you don't get sunlight, it changes things. And if there's a shortage of polyphenols, your performance goes down. This is why a lot of the diets they don't eat a lot of white foods. Like well, one of the reasons there is that you're just not getting the polyphenols that are required. The average American gets about one gram of polyphenols in their diet per day, if they're drinking coffee and maybe 0.5 if they're not drinking coffee. Coffee's the number one source. And they act as antioxidants, but more importantly they're signaling molecules. And even more interestingly, they aren't just a food for bacteria in the soil. Your gut bacteria eat polyphenols. Thin people have a predominance of a type of gut bacteria called *Bacteroides*, and those bacteria cannot be taken in a probiotic. They form when they eat polyphenols. You eat polyphenols, you get thin people bacteria, and you're more likely to have a normal weight. You don't eat polyphenols, you get fat people bacteria, and you're more likely to be fat. So this is something that we've known as a species for a very long time. If you look at a map of Asia, there's all these weird jagged borders. Those are the original spice trading routes. The first really long-distance international trade we had was salt traders because salt is required for life. And salt, no, it's not bad for you. Industrial process salts could be bad for you, but actually most people are sodium deficient right now. So we'd solve that problem thousands of years ago with trading and then the roots became spice trading routes. And I asked my teacher in seventh grade, hey, why did they need spices? Why would people die on high mountain tops with, you know, 20 kilos of whatever, oregano or something? And she scratched her head, and she said it's because they didn't have refrigerators, and they needed the meat to taste good when they put spices on it. I'm like, that's the biggest bunch of hoowie ever. The reason they did this is that these are the most dense sources of mitochondria-charging polyphenols out there. So they were trading these because they mattered. Even something as simple as vanilla was a medicinal herb back when it was first used. And we since use them for flavoring agents and to make food taste good. But it's actually about what the food does for you biologically, so you have to eat these things. I just came out literally two months ago with something called Poly Phenomenal, which is a supplement that has 1.7 grams of polyphenols from 10 different sources. So what I do is I eat a plate full of vegetables as my standard meal with a small amount of grass fed protein and tons of the right kinds of fat on it. But I also, in addition to that, take enough polyphenol supplements to get myself now 4 or 5 grams of total polyphenols a day, which is more than most humans could get. You couldn't do this if you're just eating food, and that includes two cups of caffeinated coffee and three cups of DECAF coffee every day. And I use the Bulletproof, lab-tested beans and all that. But the deal is … you want to live a long time, you must get these compounds wherever you get them. Do not go lightly on the spices when you're cooking. Put in three tablespoons of rosemary, not a pinch. It will still taste good. In fact, it'll taste better, but you'll live longer, feel better, and you'll look better along the way.

Brendan [38:44]: Awesome. You know in terms of what you eat on the Bulletproof Diet or what anybody eats, it's a low to moderate protein diet, but it does have animal products and a lot of people feel that animal foods in general are not necessarily the best for the planet. And that's largely based on the assumption that it's coming from this factory farm system and all of that where it's grain-based. And certainly those foods are, I would agree, are not healthy for the planet at all and not healthy for us. And in various parts of your books and blogs and podcasts and so forth, you talk a bit about animal foods in terms of the saturated fat and the cholesterol. I won't dive into that here, but I am curious to know if you have ever looked at the issue of the sugar, the NEU5GC, in the red meats?

Dave [39:42]: There are some people who respond to this, this type of sugar in red meats, and there's the question of how much, how much of it you eat. And I haven't seen the evidence that says this is having a large impact on huge populations. I will tell you that if it's your habit to go out there and eat a, you know, a 12-ounce steak every night, which is pretty common in the Paleo world right now, you're doing it wrong. And you're doing it wrong possibly because of the sugar, but more likely simply because you're getting so much meat that it becomes pro-inflammatory. But if you eat no meat at all, what you end up with is you're not getting enough of the nutrients that you need. You're not getting collagen, and you're not getting some of the fat-soluble compounds that are really precious. In terms of animal fats, that's what we're made out of. But an animal that eats corn and soy, it doesn't make proper animal fat. If you eat corn and soy you don't make proper animal fat either. And fat is what your mitochondria are made out of. The cell membranes for the mitochondria, and your cells themselves, and your hormones, are all made out of fat. They're not made out of vegetables. They're not made out of carbohydrates, and they're not even made out of protein. So for me it's a moderate amount of these proteins seem to work very, very well for the vast majority of people, but there are people who, who don't respond well to them. They tend to be people who've been bitten by a surprisingly, uh, ticks. There's some tick-borne illnesses that can give you a strange allergies to red meat, which is a pretty horrible thing that's happening to people right now as well, that's tied to that same, the same sugar you're talking about.

Brendan [41:12]: Okay, by the way, I misspoke. It's a, I believe it's 5NAUGC. I seem to be dyslexic on this molecule. I can't seem to make up my mind which one it is. I have to keep looking it up and go, "Oh yeah, the 5 goes there." So anyhow, in terms of the Bulletproof Diet, I've actually noticed that it has helped me eat less meat because I'm going into the, you know, ketosis more often and being more keto-adapted. So I'm eating less meat, less grains and so forth, less carbohydrate, more fat, healthy fat. I'm just curious if you've seen that as an effect on other people. I would think the Bulletproof Diet by its nature can shift people from a heavy, an overly meat-intensive diet, to one that's more balanced and getting all this good plant foods in there with the moderation of protein from animals.

Dave [42:04]: We had this weird history where, around the year I was born, in the early seventies, they came around and they said, "Oh, we're going to hypothesize that dietary fat and cholesterol cause heart disease." The guy who hypothesized this had never treated an obese patient. And it was a theory, and it sorta got taken up into the brilliance of the government system with the first food pyramid. And when it turns out that didn't work, like people didn't lose weight, they got fatter, people got unhealthy. They said, "Oh, it's not that the diet doesn't work. It's not that we should go back to eating these things. It's a lack of fiber, so let's include all these whole grains that include these compounds that inhibit mitochondrial function and let's ignore all the stuff that makes you weak because fiber's good." And so they tried that, and it didn't work, and they said, "Oh, well, let's go on a high-protein, low-fat diet?" And for God's sake, a high-protein diet, especially with most of the protein that's available out there, it's inflammatory. Protein is a horrible fuel source. It's a backup emergency fuel source. We are wired to run on carbohydrates and fat. Those are the two things, and if you're going to die, you can run on protein, but if you force somebody to do that, very, very bad things like that happen.

Brendan [43:18]: You know Dave, you've been, you've been disrupting industries for a long time in technology and now in food on the demand side by shifting consumer behaviors and shifting demand towards different types of agriculture, you know, cleaner food, organic and so forth. I'm curious, if you were working on the supply side, how would you disrupt the Monsantos and the Cargills of the world?

Dave [43:45]: Here's the very simple way to put Monsanto out of business, and if you're Monsanto listening to this, I hope that you're paying attention because I'm going to tell you how to save your company. Here's the reason Monsanto's sprays crap on our fields—to kill weeds. Yeah, here's what we can do today. We can make self-driving cars, okay? If we can do that, how hard is it to have a solar-powered little remote-controlled thing that rolls around with optical image recognition and spots weeds as they're sprouting and hits them with the laser or with a little hammer? It doesn't really matter. Humans don't have to bend over to pick weeds anymore. We have robots to do that for us, and the fact that you think it's OK to spray chemicals on the soil that harm us, harm the soil, and are persistent, in order to support your business model, it's crappy. So why don't you just rent little robots that pull weeds and get it over with already? OK? It's not that hard. There, that's how to disrupt those guys.

Brendan [44:44]: Awesome. Dave, one of the last questions here … what would you say is the number one influence on performance? Is it, is it diet? Is it light? Is it sleep? Is it exercise? Is it gratitude? What is it?

Dave [44:59]: The number one impact on performance was the subject of *Headstrong* on my last book, and I gotta plug the book. It hit the New York Times best-selling science list, not just the advisor list, which to me, it was like, holy crap, anyway there's real stuff in there. It's mitochondrial performance. If you kick ass at turning food into energy, you will have almost unlimited energy to do the things that matter to you. And if you suck at turning food into energy, you'll be inflamed. You'll get cancer, Alzheimer's disease, diabetes, or any of the other degenerative diseases. And you'll be cranky; you'll be hypogly-bitchy and hangry, and you won't like your life. It comes down to—how good are you at that? And what are the factors that matter? That's the topic of the whole book. But the light you're exposed to before you go to bed, that's a really big variable. So if you tell your body, oh look, it's day time right before bed by staring at a brightly lit iPhone and turning on the bright bathroom lights with LED lighting that you just got looking at big screen TV, it's going to harm your mitochondrial performance. The evidence is in. If you're eating, you know a huge amount of sugar it's going to impact your mitochondrial performance. If you're eating a bunch of fried stuff, even fried asparagus, it doesn't matter. It's fried; it's bad. And all these things they stack up. So for each person listening, you probably have a different set of things you do that you're more susceptible to than other people, and you probably haven't really factored into. Is this behavior, whatever it is, whether it's a conscious thing or an unconscious thing, is it making my body better at making energy or worse at making energy? Because the more energy you make, the better of a person you're capable of being, and it comes down to that.

Brendan [46:45]: Awesome. Dave, thank you so much for, you know, you're kind of one of my heroes. I have to say I get all giddy when (laugh) … "I'm gonna be talking with Dave!" So I really respect you because you're so willing to explore and experiment and report back, and you take risks, and you report back in and tell us like it is. So, I'm excited that you, that you reference soil health pretty frequently in podcasts and so forth. And so thank you for all that you're doing to help shift the food system. And thank you for being here with us in the Eat4Earth community today.

Dave [47:23]: Brendan thanks very much. And I hope everyone listening to this just takes action. And the one thing that supports every single thing that we're doing today is actually our soil. And when you look at the system, there's a soil, and there's the oceans. They kinda go together. But if those things break, if you don't take care of those things, you will pay the price personally in your lifetime. In fact, you'll pay for it today if you're eating stuff that came from bad soil. So there isn't anything more foundational than that because your body talks to the soil all the time. There's intercommunication, so get that right and everything else on top of it gets better.

Brendan [48:06]: Well said … as usual.

Dave [48:08]: Awesome thanks Brendan.

Brendan [48:10]: Thank you.

That was a fun conversation and another great contribution to the Eat4Earth event. I really love the way Dave puts things, the way he describes how we're plugged into Mother Nature at all levels. Just a very powerful statement of how dependent, how interdependent, we are with everything and how much is at stake and how much power we potentially have if we just seize it. Now if you got any insights or inspirations or have any questions, please do put them in the Facebook comments, and I will enjoy answering them.

David Wolfe Interview

Forest Superfoods That Heal Your Body and the Planet

Brendan [00:00:02]: Welcome to the Eat4Earth event. We're exploring how you can heal yourself, your loved ones, and the planet with food. This is Brendan Moorehead, and I'm super excited about this conversation with our next guest, David Avocado Wolfe. David probably needs no introduction, but I'm going to give one anyway. David is the Rockstar and Indiana Jones of the superfoods and longevity universe. The world's top CEOs, ambassadors, celebrities, athletes, artists, and the real superheroes of this earth realm, Moms, all look to David for expert advice and health, beauty, peak performance, herbalism, nutrition, and of course, chocolate. He is also an organic farmer, beekeeper, a vanilla grower and gourmet chocolatier, with over 22 years of dedicated experience and having hosted over 2,750 live events David has led the, I'll say, environmental charge for radiant health via a positive mental attitude, Eco community buildings, spending time in nature, growing one's own food, living spring water, and the best ever quality organic foods and herbs. David is also the author of many best-selling books and has appeared in numerous breakthrough documentaries and films. He's shared the stage with success and business coaches like Anthony Robbins, Richard Branson, Brian Tracy, John Dimartini, as well as acclaimed doctors and health researchers, including Dr Bruce Lipton, Dr Joseph Mercola, Dr. Sara Gottfried, Dr. Lissa Rankin, Dr. Dave Woynarowski and many, many more. David is a lead educator and presented at the annual Longevity Conference, the Institute of Integrative Nutrition, and The BodyMind Institute where he hosts his own course. David, I have a feeling this is going to be an epic conversation. Thanks for being here.

David Wolfe [00:01:53]: Thanks so much for having me. And thanks for coming up and saying hello in London, which is where we got to spend some time. That was great. And I was very excited about the content of your summit, and this is a very near and dear to my heart subject matter. So I'm excited to share.

Brendan [00:02:11]: Yeah. You know, obviously many people know you as a champion of raw foods and super foods and of course, chocolate, other plant-based foods, but not many people know that you have a lot of experience in farming. So how long have you been farming?

David Wolfe [00:02:27]: It started ... well, geez, I started planting my own trees. I'd started guerilla planting pine trees in my neighborhood in Seaside Park, Seaside Heights, New Jersey when I was five years old. So I think that's where it started for me. And I would plant pine trees in people's backyards and you know, they didn't even know, and nurtured them along. That was something I didn't even realize until years later, looking back. I was like, geez I started as a guerilla planter back then. In 1977 when I was seven years old we came to California, and that's when I really started planting fruit trees in particular, citrus and avocados, pomegranates and mulberries, and grapefruit trees. And that's probably what really got me started. So it's really been since I was seven years old, meaning I've been growing avocados for 40 years.

Brendan [00:03:11]: Well, I guess that makes sense since it's your middle name now. And we'll get into why, probably a little later. But, so a big theme of this event is soil, and when we care for soil it cares for us. You've been an intrepid researcher both in very established science and also more esoteric science, around health. And so we're going to dive into the unseen realm of health that most of us, I guess maybe take for granted, don't really realize how much it's influencing us, and that's the health of the soil or the lack thereof. What do you think is most important for people to understand about soil?

David Wolfe [00:03:52]: Soil is very intimately related to our nervous system and the way, the reason why I say that is because we now know that our skin is formed out of our nervous system tissue, including the same tissue that our brain and eyes are formed out of when we develop as a zygote. So as an embryo and we developed all those tissues, skin, brain, eyes are developed out of the same tissue. Well, what is the soil? It's the ecstatic skin of the Earth. It's part of what makes the Earth amazing and great. And it's that mix up of the glacial till, in combination with the composting microorganisms that build up that black soil that can be found in river valleys. That is really the basis of the complexity, of our potential complexity, of our thoughts and imagination. So to me, the skin is really an exact duplication of the soil, and they're connected.

Brendan [00:04:55]: That is really profound. And I love the word that you used ecstatic. That's something that we could really unpack if we have time, but, you know, life is the expression of ecstasis really, and life's only worth living when we're fully in flow, and that's what ecstasis is—being in flow, being fully present. And so in terms of soil and … what are some practical tips you might have for people who, you know a lot of us are considering growing our food or already are. And so, lay it on us. What are some tips we could use?

David Wolfe [00:05:33]: Back in the early days in the raw food scene, I met a gentleman by the name of Don Weaver. Amazing man. He worked with John Hamaker and John Hamaker's essential hypothesis was that you would use the techniques that glaciers used to grind down a rock into a powder and then essentially use that rock dust or that rock powder as an amendment or as a fertilizer for your trees, your orchard, your gardens. And that's what got me started. Now I started. That's kind of the wrong way to start because, the thing about rock powders, granite powder and calcium powder, you know, lime powder and even sand, which we'll get into, I hope, is that they don't have a lot of carbon. And so I kind a got into it in the wrong way, actually. I put in all this rock dust, but it didn't have the carbon present had to kind of learn that back, the backwards way.

David Wolfe [00:06:26]: So through composting and in particular where there's a major area of focus now in, in traditional science, even bureaucratic science, bio char, when, as soon as I got into using it, bio char or charcoal in the soil, that just brought a whole another … that's where your carbon comes from. Plants are carbon-based life forms. Plants, microbes are carbon-based life forms. So we want to make sure we have enough carbon first, and then we want enough organic material. That's your compost. And then you want that rock dust, which is kind of like the little food that the organisms get to feast on when the carbon chain has been built up.

Brendan [00:07:05]: You know, the way I see all this fitting together and revolving around carbon … you know, many people in this event are talking about how we can draw down massive quantities of carbon through what plants and soil organisms do together. The plants are drawing the carbon out of the atmosphere to build sugar and cellulose and all kinds of carbon molecules. And a lot of that sugar gets sent down to the soil to feed microorganisms that kind of barter with them for the minerals that they make available. They secrete the organic acids and enzymes that effectively mine the soil, the parent materials like sand, silt and clay, of the nutrients. But like you mentioned this bio char, and that brings a whole new realm to it, so much more surface area and home for these microorganisms. And interestingly enough, I just learned that Phil Callahan who talks about a particular type of rock dust, paramagnetic rock dust. And paramagnetism is well understood—I don't know if it's well understood—but it's an established physical property of certain types of certain states have certain elements in the periodic table where they have unbound electrons in the outer valence, the outer shell rather. And so they can, they can respond to magnetic fields. And then something interesting happens that we don't maybe fully understand, but he mentioned that he, or let's say he's been quoted as having hypothesized that burning wood and putting it in soil is a way that paramagnetism can be in induced and enhanced in soil, if I'm recalling correctly. And of course, bio char is that, so it might be another element of bio char's function and source of benefit that we hadn't really realized is this paramagnetism.

David Wolfe [00:09:00]: Yeah, absolutely. Well, one of the things about bio char and charcoal in general is it's very strongly negatively charged, and so therefore it actually … it's a very strong enhancer of growth. And we have this paramagnetic diamagnetic phenomenon going on. So the earth should be paramagnetic; the tree is diamagnetic, and they're perpendicular energies to each other. And that was Philip Callahan's amazing insight and his book, *Paramagnetism*. He also had some incredible insights on the Irish stone towers and the structure of antennae on moths and insects and how they work and how they're related to towers because if you look at them, they have conical cross sections, and there is a parallel or a metaphor that can be made between them. His work is seminal, very interesting and one of the biggest things I learned from, from Callahan's work, I'm trying to see …

David Wolfe [00:09:52]: I have his books on a shelf right? There it is right there. I got it. Can you grab that book for me? It's just right there. I've got Callahan's book in front of me. I, this is, I'm in my office right now, and I do collect books on many, many different subjects. Just on the right, right here it says Giza power plant. Just next to that, down and over … yeah, next shelf over. The textbook case over to the right. Anyway, we'll find it … yes! And then down next to the Giza power plant book, there's a book says, *Paramagnetism*. See that one? I was looking for it. Anyway, one of the things that came out of Callahan's work, and it's also crossed with Viktor Schauberger's work, (shows a book entitled *The Fertile Earth) is* this idea that when you use iron implements instead of diamagnetic substances like copper or wood to dig into the earth, you can discharge that paramagnetic energy.

David Wolfe [00:10:45]: It's like a hymen or a surface charge that exists in the Earth that as soon as you stab iron through it, it dissipates the energy. It can decrease your production of growth—for example, your crop yield—by even as much as 40 percent.

Brendan [00:10:59]: Wow, now is that because the iron is, from what I understand, iron can be diamagnetic or paramagnetic depending on whether it's oxidized. I'm not sure if that's correct.

David Wolfe [00:11:09]: That's a good question. I'd have to reference on that one. Generally, it's paramagnetic, irons are paramagnetic unless you if you take like, iron bearing rock and you put them in a circle, you can get … it can flip and become diamagnetic. You know, strange things like that can occur. But you may be right about that. I have to check, check up on my notes. But the insight there is very interesting. It's like we think that the Egyptians were just behind us, they were less capable than us because they used copper implements and wood, but maybe they were more advanced because they had greater yields over longer periods of time. You know, in our age, everything is so quick fix. "Let's get the answer tomorrow. Let's get this thing going." We don't think about that seventh generation, and when it comes to the, you know, the way that the ancients did it, that's where we can learn something about sustainability.

Brendan [00:12:03]: Absolutely. By the way, it occurs me, maybe we should define the difference between the paramagnetic and diamagnetic because this language is probably foreign to most, and I'm just now myself starting to get familiar with it. What is diamagnetic as opposed to paramagnetic?

David Wolfe [00:12:17]: Diamagnetic reacts perpendicularly or not at all, to magnetic fields. So wood, for example, is a diamagnetic substance, copper is diamagnetic, iron is typically paramagnetic, so it will react to a compass, for example, and will point north. Soils like granite dust, for example, have a paramagnetic quality to it. But if you take limestone or silica they're diamagnetic, so they have an opposite thing going on. And basically they are always perpendicular. So I'd like to think of the easiest way to think about it is we have the level of Earth right here. And then you've got the tree coming out. The tree is diamagnetic, the earth is paramagnetic, should be paramagnetic. The most paramagnetic soils in the world are typically volcanic soils. And that's why volcanic soils have such a strong propensity for growth. And that's what you're always looking for, is try to get that right. Rock dust made of a lava rock is really always the best.

Brendan [00:13:11]: Yeah. And that's what I recall is that a basalt-based, those are the best. Basalt crusher dust is the best if you're trying to introduce a paramagnetism into your soils, or let's say enhance it. I mean, it's, it's there regardless. It's a question of how much.

David Wolfe [00:13:27]: Right. What I did in the beginning was way too much rock dust, not enough carbon, not enough organic material and then realize later, "Oh geez, these trees need … well, you know, basically your typical fruit trees and vegetables and stuff that we're all familiar with -apples and oranges and avocado trees and all the vegetables you can think of, the brassica family, pretty much every single thing that's growing in a garden like, like lovage or celery or carrots, the stuff that we typically think of in the garden really, really like heavy, heavy, black, organic material and, and to some degree, charcoal and then a sprinkling of rock dust. Right? And I kind of did it the opposite. Um, but you know, that's how you learn your lessons. And it's typical of all our major fruit trees that we … you know, they really like everything, like your compost pile, your ash pile, your liming agents and calcium and even sand, to keep the space. You don't want the soil to get clogged up. So I do use a lot of sand in my farming to keep that space open for farming things like tobacco, which likes a sandy loamy type of material in the soil, basically like the river silt. And by the way, rivers silt as an amendment for soil is the best. It's amazing!

Brendan [00:14:46]: Yeah. I guess it's carrying so much off of a soil from above and from rocks that have been weathered. It's just a super dense, concentrated source of various types of nutrients, both organic and inorganic nutrients, inorganic meaning, you know, from just mineral stuff (broken rocks). Yeah. So when we spoke in London, I thought I heard you use the word "purines" as something related to soil. And what was it? Oh, it was the paramagnetism. So I wrote down something that said "purine", but it had nothing to do with purines. OK.

David Wolfe [00:15:22]: Um, purines, Yeah, no, I probably mentioned purines, just in passing. Purines are very interesting group of chemicals. They typically range from white to very soft or dull yellow colors, due to their conjugated bonds. The purines that we're most familiar with are theobromine and of course caffeine, but these were first found to be in a family that later became known as purines, from studying uric acid. And uric acid plays a very important role in farming and urea and urine, right? Which is nitrogen. So basically, let's just talk about some of the basic pieces of the puzzle. Carbon is your neutralizer, and it's your negative battery charge. Nitrogen is what stinks in your compost pile. So whenever you have ... when you ever have a smell coming from your garbage or from a compost pile, that's nitrogen escaping.

David Wolfe [00:16:16]: What you want to do is you want to hold that nitrogen in, and that's where you're going to use your liming agents like calcium, or I use ash, just ash, boom, throw the ash on top and keep that smell in there. Or you can use like silica, for example. You can just put sand on top of the pile or, 'cause that will hold that nitrogen in, or you can use grass clippings and just pile grass clippings which are basically silicaceous in character, and that holds that energy in. So that's, that's nitrogen. Oxygen is very important, which means that you never want that soil to have too much clay. You're always trying to break up the clay, help the tree and the plants break up that clay. So you want that rich loamy aerated earthworm-friendly soil. So that's where I ... that's why I like to use sand. I mean, people use vermiculite, that's just, that's just popped sand, like popcorn. Maybe just take the silica, you popped it like popcorn with heat, and it turns into vermiculite.

Brendan [00:17:10]: I didn't know that's what vermiculite was. I've actually wondered, because I heard somebody mention it recently. I'm like, yeah, I never really did look at what vermiculite really is.

David Wolfe [00:17:19]: It's a silicate!

Brendan [00:17:22]: Another way to, to help the soil breathe as I understand from learning through Graeme Sait's Nutrition Farming Course that I attended in Australia, but he gives it around the world, is making sure that the calcium to magnesium ratio is, is correct for that soil. The ratio is not always exactly the same for each soil. It depends on what else is going on in the soil, but usually it kind of hovers around seven to one, calcium to magnesium. And so calcium tends to flocculate soils, meaning it helps them open. It's got, you know ... it's a larger diameter, and so it helps hold particles apart, whereas magnesium, much smaller diameter and higher ratio of charge to mass, so it pulls tightly to particles. So if you have too much magnesium to calcium, you get a compacted soil and not enough oxygen getting in there versus the opposite, if you have too much calcium to magnesium, then the soil is going to be very loose and easily washed away, let's say in rain events or something, if there's nothing else countering that influence. And so that's another really interesting feature of all the dynamics going on down there under the soil.

David Wolfe [00:18:38]: It's fascinating. What happens typically with a compost pile is you're developing a lot of acids, humic acids, folic acids. It's ... everything's breaking down into a very acidic black soil, which is great for growing vegetables, but they will be incomplete unless that calcium is there, that magnesium is there. And so that's why, you know, when I say these vegetables, the typical stuff we're growing in our gardens want everything. That's what they're used to. That's what they like. It's OK to have all that rich black soil, but you don't want it to be too acidic because these great vegetables that we grow, the grapefruit trees that would grow, like that balanced PH. So they like all that acid and all that black stuff. But they like to have enough calcium there to keep the soil open. You know, we use gypsum a lot actually, we've used gypsum a lot to keep that soil open and also to keep the alkalinity presence so that the soil doesn't go too far one way, and all of a sudden you're only able to grow blueberries and pine trees which liked that acid soil. You need to, you need to make sure if you're doing too much composting and even, even too much, too much fertilization of any kind of like, you know, you're composting, you're using leaf matter, cutting it from your trees and stuff. It can go too far to the acid side.

Brendan [00:19:51]: You know, that reminds me that people, some people that are farming vegetables in their backyard, some people that are farming fruit trees in their backyard and herbs and so forth ... I'm just curious if you have any tips on how to organize all that, given that each type of plant, they want a different type of soil. Do you have to kind of have different zones within your plot in the backyard or ...

David Wolfe [00:20:18]: Well said. Well said. That's a very important point. What we do is we, I got into raised-bed gardening, and so that allows me to do like blueberries and raspberries in their own beds because they need a very acidic soil, and that way that bed doesn't interfere with like the fruit trees next to them. And that works really well. In fact, we've had this year we had blueberries all the way until October 15th in Ontario, Canada. Way, I'm talking way up north too. So we had food. We had so much food this year, and it's because we've gotten smarter about farming and gardening. We've made all the mistakes and now we know. OK instead ... and by the way, the soil there's very granitic and acidic, and it's hard to get into it. So the raised-bed concept is really nice. What we do for raised beds is instead of cutting lumber, we'll just use cut pieces of trees that have died around the house, and we'll cut them to a certain height, you know? So there's, they're circular, right? Like a log and then you just stack them all around and then you fill up the dirt on the inside.

Brendan [00:21:19]: Sounds like a plan. Really like sort of log cabin style.

David Wolfe [00:21:19]: Yes, that's it. You got it!

Brendan [00:21:26]: You know, I suspect that there's, you know, that the resistance to frost and things like that, I don't know if you had any early frost, comes from the soil. I know that there's a soil organism that is actually involved in frost-related events in plants. And I'm just curious if, if there's also any kind of protection against frost from healthy soils. I don't know.

David Wolfe [00:21:51]: Well, one of the things that we pretty much have to do and is very important is what the forest does naturally to protect itself, is it drops all its leaves onto the surface of the forest or you know, we're, we've got around us on all sides of forest, in Ontario. I also farm in Hawaii and in California. So we'll get into all those ecosystems. I want to talk about the differences. But that forest ecosystem dropped so many leaves on to the orchard, plus the orchard leaves themselves, the apple leaves come down and the pear and all that. And that protects the soil or the protects the heart of the tree, which is essentially the locus of action of trees and garden vegetables that are perennial in Ontario, Canada, because of the cold, is in the ground. It's just below the layer of the soil.

David Wolfe [00:22:37]: That's where you have the most biological action. So you have to make sure you protect that biological action by layering leaves up above the ground. It happens naturally anyway, as you go into winter, so that the locus of action is prepared. You don't want to do too much around your tree though, because there might be a vole. Then it'll get it in there and it will nibble around your tree. It'll ring your tree. Oh, so you have to be very careful you don't stack too much on top around the tree because that'll be a nice little warm spot for a little animal. And then they'll, they'll start gnawing on your apple tree and eventually they can ring your tree and kill your tree, in a cold winter from eating the bark.

Brendan [00:23:15]: Interesting! You know, and also with all that dry organic matter from the leaves and twigs and so forth, what is that going to do? It's going to feed the cellulose-digesting bacteria and fungal organisms like the mycorrhizal fungi, which we can't leave a conversation about soil without talking about that character in the soil food web.

David Wolfe [00:23:39]: That, that's such an important piece of the puzzle. And mycorrhizal fungi, essentially my experiments have shown that it beats bacteria in the soil every time. So grassy land and long meadows, those are bacterially-dominated in the soil. When you get into forest ecosystem, you have a fungal domination. Now you would think that some of these vegetables that we're eating, or even fruit trees, they should have some bacteria in the soil. But my experiments have shown that they always do better with mycorrhizal fungi. It's interesting.

Brendan [00:24:11]: Well, Elaine Ingham and others have shown that there's a relationship between the fungal to bacterial ratio and plant succession. So at the lower end where you have weeds and the grasses and more complex grasslands, the ratio of fungal organisms to bacterial organisms is going up until you got to the whatever the climax ecosystem is, which in many areas of the world is some kind of forest. And so that forest has the, especially in old growth forest, has much more fungally dominant soils, which also tend to be a little more acidic, and that's where you grow your berries and so forth more naturally.

David Wolfe [00:24:49]: Yes. And that's what we do actually. Our hill is actually, it's a raspberry hill naturally. So we found our thrill not on a blueberry hill but on a raspberry hill. Although we do now, we grow really good black raspberries, lots of wild raspberries, really good blueberries. Our blueberries this year are just amazing. But the main thing that we're really always looking at is to try to make sure that each year we are supplementing what that orchard needs. And I wanted to say something I thought was very important for this conversation … we found just from experience living next to a great forest, that the forest provides everything you need. Unique carbon. Forest has it. You need, um, cellulose. The forest has it. You need fungus. The forest has it. You need black dirt. The forest has it. You need poop. Like people go get their poop from … and I have done this …

David Wolfe [00:25:39]: An organic farmer lives down the road and I've gotten his manure, but it always has nettle seeds in it. It always has motherwort seeds in it, which can develop a little prickle on it. And it's not the best for, for what we're doing because I like to walk around barefoot, and I don't want to be hitting nettles and motherwort. So we've found just, it's just the simplest thing we just got through the forest, we get moose, deer and porcupine poop. And then we use that as a fertilizer and it's perfect. There are no seeds in it, nothing. It's amazing. And I just keep coming back to this. And I want to repeat it because I've just found it's the truest thing about farming ever. You know, when we lost our forest, we lost a lot. And one of the things we lost Is everything that we need, right? You need amendments for your soil. No problem. It's all there in the forest. You need leaves to cover your soil, it's all there in the forest. The forest provides everything. And I say that also with, you know, a little bit of tongue in cheek. It's a little bit metaphorical because if you're having a bad day, walk in the forest, right? The forest does provide everything. You need inspiration? Take a walk in the forest. The fractal patterns of the forest and natural patterns of the forest relate something to us that is important, and it's connected to fulfillment.

Brendan [00:26:54]: Yes. Forests bring us so many things from the physical to the spiritual. I mean, walking in a forest is like, you know, it's like church for many of us. And then you know, brings us all kinds of biodiversity. You can find unique species that you don't find outside of a forest. A lot of your favorite foods, I think, come from forests. You get some really unique properties in the edible fungus, you know mushrooms and so forth, and the types of berries and other fruits that grow in forests both tropical and temperate. And interestingly enough, there's a soil researcher named David C. Johnson at New Mexico State University— he's really exposing some serious secrets of the soil with what he's doing—and how he creates his soil in part is he grabs some leaf litter from a forest to inoculate his compost. So that's where he's getting all of the various bacteria and the fungal species and so forth. And so it's … anyway, I just thought it mentioned it, a little piece of trivia there as far as like, he's got this magic compost and part of the sourcing of that is the leaf litter from a forest.

David Wolfe [00:28:05]: He's got the bio reactors, right? That's it. That's the same guy.

Brendan [00:28:09]: Yes, exactly.

David Wolfe [00:28:10]: I've checked him out. A very interesting character, and what he's really doing is he's teaching us how to make better and better compost and also how to make incredible compost just out of what's there, what's available to you, and that's an important consideration is you always want to start where you're at. And you don't have to take on everything all at once. You just start. You make the right moves and the wrong moves, and you learn as you go. And one of the things I can definitely say is the most important to start with is start composting your scraps. And that's going to give you the basis, the raw materials, the nitrogen and the potassium, and to some degree even the phosphorus necessary to start a garden and get that going. I call it chaos gardening. At that stage. You just take all your compost and dump it out in some pile in the back and watch what grows out of it.

Brendan [00:28:57]: Well, you know, there's another person that has, that has that idea of compost gardening (meant to say "chaos gardening"), and that's Gabe Brown of North Dakota, and he throws out tons of seeds out there. I don't know what else and ended up with this … and he doesn't try to control it. That's what we try to do in agriculture so too much is we try to control everything to the nth degree and optimize for one species. He's got this chaos garden. It's just producing so much food of high quality, and it requires no tending because he's got the biodiversity that just maintains a functional system that doesn't require fertilizers and pesticides and management. It's just, they just go out and pick what looks good.

David Wolfe [00:29:35]: I'm so glad you brought that up. This idea of not managing your garden … that's one of the permaculture ideals. Having things close to the house that you will use all the time and stuff that doesn't require management. You want a permanent culture. That's the idea of permaculture. You want a permanent setup that's providing food without you having to work for it. And the way we look at that as we make sure that everything we're planting is doing well naturally. If it's something that, you know, the deer are onto it, and they're just eating it every chance they can get, then that's not what we want to grow. 'Cause we, you know, I live in a forest, there's no, there's no fence. Deer could come in if they want to. We have managed to figure out ways to keep them out by blocking the pathways that they'd like to come in.

David Wolfe [00:30:13]: But if they really do want to come in as they do at the end of the summer, they'll, they'll get in, and so we just, we grow what is there naturally, for example, parsnips, we have wild parsnip is growing in our yard all over the place, wild carrot growing all over the place. We have wild mustards all over the place. I've got mallows and malvas all over the place. It's just coming up wildly naturally. Evening primrose, wild natural St John's Wort. Wow. Natural. This is in Ontario so that we just let that stuff come in and we don't try to put something in there that's not gonna work. For example, like I'm not going to try to grow celery there, it's too cold. We've got lovage instead. Lovage comes in beautiful. Just does great there. It's fantastic. So sticking with, you know, an ideal in spite of evidence is not often a great idea in farming. You know, you've got to just go with what is going to work there.

Brendan [00:31:02]: Right! That's the key to permaculture, and really what we see is when we've got biodiversity, the total yield of a piece of land is much higher, and it's so much more resilient. And so we're really impoverishing ourselves when we try to go with just one thing over a vast area of land. We're just reducing the total food available and the health of the soil and our bodies and all that. You know, in regard to specific types of food, I want to go back to the forest for a second just because so many of the things we love most -chocolate, coffee, vanilla, these great flavors, all these things that carry polyphenols into our body in tasty packages and wonderful fruits and so forth. I'm just curious, what is your, what are your top, most favorite forest foods?

David Wolfe [00:31:48]: Oh, fantastic. OK. Let's talk about tropical farming for a second because we've been talking about Ontario temperate climate farming. When you're in a tropical ecosystem, the locus of action with a high biological activity is at, is up higher. I mean it might even be up two meters, so it goes higher up as the temperature increases and as the humidity increases. So we have yes, action in the soil for sure, but you're going to get various powerful results in tropical ecosystems with compost teas, which is what we, instead of amending the soil so much, what we're trying to do in our clay soils in Hawaii is to open the soil up with sand and calcium and make sure that soil can breathe and of course composted soils for sure so that the roots can get in and start to break up that clay. The locus of action is up high, so the easiest thing to do is just go around, you know, you make your compost tea, you bubble it for 24 hours, and we've got samples of soils in there, and we've got our, we use honey instead of molasses because we're a bee farm.

David Wolfe [00:32:48]: So put honey in there, and we put our favorite little concoctions of, you know, these little mineral things and that little thing from the ocean, and we'll put that all in there, and we'll just bubble it up. And you go around and spray everything. That's the most powerful for that ecosystem. And when you're in that ecosystem you can grow those things that are right in that range. And one of those things is chocolate, which grows right there pretty much at eye level. And then the other one is vanilla, which grows right there, pretty much eye level. And so those are two of my favorites. And, and they're always just right there with you. Every day we grow the chocolate and the vanilla together. Actually, as I learned later down the road after, I think I'd been at it for 13 years, I'm one of the only, I am the only biodynamics certified vanilla grower in the United States.

Brendan [00:33:34]: Interesting. And then all of the tropical ... it's a tropical food, but you're growing ... when you say growing in the United States, do you mean in Hawaii?

David Wolfe [00:33:45]: In Hawaii, yeah! It could be done in South Florida, and people do do it in South Florida. It's harder.

Brendan [00:33:45]: OK.

David Wolfe [00:33:50]: And so, you know, those are, to me, those are like the great flavors. Another one that's in that zone there, Rollinia. Rollinia is in the Annona (*Annonaceae*) family. You know, we may remember the Annona (*Annonaceae*) family from Graviola or Soursop, or you may have heard of Pawpaws in midwestern North America, or you may have heard of Chirimoyas. The Rollinia is like the Queen of them all. And her fruits. Whoa. That is like ...

Brendan [00:33:50]: Ravinia ... Rollinia?

David Wolfe [00:34:17]: Yeah. Rollinia. And this is one of those trees that you just have to keep feeding, keep nourishing it, keep feeding, keep nourishing it. And then one day, boom, it starts coming and they, and they come in heavy and fast with the most amazing fruit ever.

Brendan [00:34:32]: I love what you described about this foliar spray that's ... it's part compost tea and it's part direct nutrition. Again, Graeme Sait, who is doing phenomenal things around the globe with farmers ... one of the things he teaches people is foliar sprays because that goes right into the leaf so you can get a quick response from the plants. And I guess you're saying in tropical areas, because the soil is ... I guess you were saying that the zone of activity is a little higher up. So it's less ... there are less ... I don't know how to describe it, but they're more ... are they more responsive to foliar sprays and less response to soil amendments? Or just like anywhere else it takes longer for treatments of the soil to work their way up into the plant?

David Wolfe [00:35:22]: It's the second; it's the latter. It takes longer for treatments of the soil to work their way through. Foliar spraying is like immediate, and over the years working with some, in my opinion, some of the top permaculture designers out of Australia who have helped me with my farms, we've come to the position that foliar spraying is one of the best ways to get nutrition into a plant. Plants do absorb a lot of nutrition from the atmosphere and from dew and moisture in the atmosphere, and all we're doing, we're just adding a little bit of goodies on top of that to allow them to bring that right in. And we'd like to do that foliar spraying typically in the morning or evening, which is that old Rudolf Steiner style, make sure you get the foliar spray happening when the stomata are open. And that's usually like when the crickets start in the evening, you know, and the insect starting the evening or in the morning. Then they're open, and then the nutrition gets in better.

Brendan [00:36:14]: OK, and I wonder if there's a secondary effect where when the plants are just healthier that they might also be producing more exudates that go down into the soil to feed the soil organisms so that they're making minerals available, and those exudates are working their way through the soil food web, and eventually some fraction of them are becoming part of long-term stable, humate compounds that are capturing carbon long-term in the soil as long as we leave that soil undisturbed. And we keep that—what Christine Jones calls, out of Australia, calls cause the liquid carbon pump—as long as we keep that active and keep all the organisms there, then carbon is being siphoned out of the atmosphere to soil and stored long-term. And of course, all those leaves and twigs and so forth dropping onto the soil, getting digested in the soil, a certain percentage of those are also adding to the long-term soil carbon pool. And so just curious, I don't know if you have any thoughts about that ... does foliar spraying indirectly to help the growth of soil?

David Wolfe [00:37:16]: My observation has been, yes, I think you're onto something there with the way you phrase that. That's been my observation. I would agree with that. Something happens to the overall plant and the growing environment from foliar spraying, and so everything becomes healthier, including the soil underneath the tree, which would make sense because you're going to have some of those materials drip off, that kind of thing. But it is something different than that. When the trees healthier, it changes the soil more radically. I've seen that over the years, every biological experiment you do; it's a genetic variability. Some of those sprouts are going to be, you know, super hardy and they change the soil faster. The hardier ... let's just say hemp plants, for example ... when I dig them out, like the whole thing is full of roots, but the one that just wasn't genetically, didn't have that oomph, came from the same seed stock, just didn't have that oomph, didn't get all the way to the lower levels of the soil and didn't change the soil. So the more powerful that the plant is, the more it will change the soil.

Brendan [00:38:16]: Well, speaking of powerful plants, you described the avocado as a pioneer species, and so tell us about that. What makes it a pioneer species? What does it accomplish?

David Wolfe [00:38:28]: I was fortunate to grow up in southern California, or at least since 1977 when I was seven years old when we came out here. And what's interesting is you could see that this area in southern California is not very amenable to growing tropical trees, like the avocado. But if you can get those avocados into wet feet right where the roots are wet, they'll make it under any desert conditions, as the Mexicans showed us. The Mexicans were really the masters of taking the avocado out of Chiapas and Guatemala and bringing it into climates that weren't really natural for the avocado, but if they could get their feet wet, they're good, and they can handle it. What happens is, is they immediately start that activity of creating mulch, mulch, mulch, mulch, mulch. "One tree, one cloud" as we like to say in permaculture. "One tree one cloud," and over time they can take an area that was a desert and start to pioneer it and convert it back to a rain forest.

David Wolfe [00:39:18]: Because the trees themselves can change the ecosystem. They can change the amount of ambient moisture in the atmosphere, and even change weather, if you've given enough trees and enough time, it's gonna, it's gonna flip it back to its climax system, which is a forested ecosystem. So avocados are helpful in doing that. And what's so unusual about that is for a pioneer species to produce that much fat and oil, very unusual, almost all the fat and oil generating trees like walnuts, almonds and every nut you can think of—macadamia nut—they come at the end of the ecosystem when the established soils, six feet, two meters, full of black humus. Then those nut trees go, "Yeah, now we can get it going." But strangely, you know, you have this avocado that comes in as the pioneer. On the one hand you have avocados, the pioneer. At the end of that ecosystem would be cacao typically, right in those tropical regions where avocados are from. You know, so it starts with avocado as the pioneer species of trees. We call them weed trees because you get avocados going in the tropics, they are a weed! You've got be careful!

David Wolfe [00:40:24]: Avocado is mulch. We feed all our trees, you know, we use the "chop and drop" system in the tropics where we just maintain. We don't chop down the biological diversity that's already there. We just use it as food for the trees that we've planted in there. And then we start with Avocado and we work all the way, all the way to the end, which is cacao.

Brendan [00:40:44]: Nice. God knows it's important to start regenerating forests. One of the other speakers in this event talks about how forests actually are the main source of a particular form of bacteria called hygroscopic bacteria, and they are the chief nucleators of rain events around the world. And that's especially important in the tropics. And so Walter Jehne, that's a talk everybody's got to listen to in this event. And so we basically what it comes down to is a big part of what we're going to need to do to restore balance to our climatic systems and so forth is reforest and revegetate in other ways vast, vast areas of our continents. And that's going to help restore normal rain and water cycles and so forth. There's so many things that forests do it's mind boggling.

David Wolfe [00:41:34]: Well said, and I'm glad you brought that up. So one of the main things that forests do is they bring the salts and mineral layer and water table up and they make it more bioavailable for shrubs, bushes, animals, microorganisms. And essentially that is one of the greatest things about a forest is it's creating shade, and that allows that water table to come up with its mineral materials that come from the deep earth, like salts, because in the middle of a forest in the middle of Germany or in the middle of North America, there's not a whole lot of salt available so that the earth has to bring it up from deeper. That's one of the reasons, by the way, why I use ocean water as a fertilizer on my plants, just to make it easier for them to get access to salts. I have watered my plants was straight ocean water for years.

David Wolfe [00:42:22]: I've never come even close to over salting them, burning the roots, anything like that. So it's straight like three and a half gallons on an established fruit tree of ocean water once a year. No problem. Easy. It could take it probably once a month.

Brendan [00:42:40]: It's interesting, I'm seeing some products pop up that are a ocean water extracts, some of them are desalinated. So you don't create overly, you know, put too much sodium in your soil because that can become a problem. But I just saw something that indicated that, I think it was saying, that ocean water has a fairly high degree of paramagnetic elements. Sodium and magnesium being two of those potentially paramagnetic elements, but so many others. So it might be that that ocean water is helping to enhance paramagnetism in soils.

David Wolfe [00:43:12]: That, that's been my experience. I think there's no question about it. Ocean water, pretty much I've found with like, like in my ecosystem, the trees that are the most troubled are citrus. They're the hardest to keep healthy because the roots can get fungally overloaded, and It's a little too tropical for citrus where I'm at. And what we do to amend the citrus trees just to make sure they don't get into a fungal problem or their immune system stays high, is we pour ocean water on them. Works great! We'll also put ocean water into our compost teas as well.

Brendan [00:43:46]: Beautiful! So David let me ask you a broad question: what is most exciting, fascinating or rewarding about understanding soil and growing food?

David Wolfe [00:43:59: I love the connection with the food that you grow, and we don't even realize what we lost. I guess we had to learn the hard way. We had to go away from farming and growing our own food, go into this mass-produced food, realized that that's not the way to go and then come back. When you do come back, there is an ecstatic feeling. I mean, most people know that feeling because they've grown their own tomatoes and those tomatoes are way better. It's not even comparable to what you buy in a store. So that is, that triggers something; people go, "Whoa, how could this tomato be so much better? You know, the one that I grew?" It's because the plants respond to your energy and your love essentially. And if you have great love for farming and gardening, your plants will, they'll respond. And they will make a meal for you that is satisfying at levels that are hard to imagine coming from the conventional food world. And this is the thing too about wild food. You know, we always go out every day at the end of the day in Ontario, we go out into the forest, and we would go for a swim in a lake and then on the way there, on the way back, we pick wild mushrooms and eat them, and we pick wild mushrooms for tea, so you know, for both purposes. Being that engaged in your forest ecosystem is super important for fulfillment and satisfaction in life. Again, this is something that we lost. We didn't even realize that was important. We had no idea. But when you get back to it you go, "Geez, what was I missing?" And it's, it's just part of being happy.

Brendan [00:45:23]: Yeah. You know, the idea of love and agronomy have never really fully intermingled. But, but Graeme Sait -- again, I learned so much from him at his Nutrition Farming Course -- he mentioned that there's an agronomist, a Canadian agronomist, so this guy's a scientist, and he's one of the top, if not the top one in Canada, and he teaches people certain principles and practices, and one of them is go out and basically communicate with and love your plants. And it sounds totally out there, right? So he tells a story, Graeme does, about how one of the farmers was implementing everything minus one thing, and I guess he had enjoyed some improvements, and then he had a regression in the improvements, and this guy went out walking amongst his fields, and he came back. He was like, just furious or irritated or something and said, "You haven't been loving your plants!" And he's like, "Oh no, I haven't. I didn't think that was really truly important." It's like, it is, you know! There's things going on in our physical and metaphysical reality that we just haven't figured out yet. But eventually we will. But the empirical evidence seems to be there. I mean, this is the kind of thing I've seen other, this is obviously just anecdotal, but there is evidence out there that accumulates around that idea that when you ... this phenomenon of love ... it structures water ... that's really easily documented and has been, and it turns water, it makes water more (meant "less") viscous and more wetting and a better solvent for carrying nutrients and so forth. I mean, just if you look at it just real, just physically like that. But anyway.

David Wolfe [00:47:13]: Yeah! I'm, well I mean I'm way down that rabbit hole the maximum because ... could be because of experience. I know that if you love your plants, they love you back. I also know that they communicate with you so you can have a dream. All of a sudden you're like, "Wait, that plant came to me in my dream, and I've got to water it." Then you go check it, and it's like completely bone dry and "Oh geez, that was really calling to me." I've had those experiences happen. I know other people have too. Cleve Backster wrote a book called *Primary Perception,* and it's about his research on the intelligence of plants and animals. You know plants react to us in real time, and our animals react to us in real time, even if we're not there. So if something happens to us, the plant can feel it. It's actually part of us in some certain way. It's part of our consciousness in a certain way. And so that thing of the ecstatic connection with plant consciousness is also very important part of feeling fulfilled and happy. And what I mean by that is, when you're with your plants, and you're watering your plants, it's really one of the great meditations. I don't know if you come up with something better, meditating in a room in New York City, in a yoga class, it's just not, it doesn't, doesn't do it for me, versus being in the garden. It's just one of those things, you know. It's great to meditate in both cases, but the meditation is always better in the garden.

Brendan [00:48:32]: Yeah. Well, you know, we see so many hints I think of, of the mechanics of how this all works and you know, for people who are super scientific, I mean I have a mystical side big time, but I always am fascinated by how it all plays out. And you start to see the evidence in physics and biology. So you've got quantum entanglement, between your subatomic particles once they, once they've been in communion, let's say, or in contact in some way. They're forever entangled, and the things that happened in one are reflected in the other at infinite distance. So there's a … you know, it really starts to break down our ideas, reductionistic ideas, of how the world works. You know, a bunch of billiard balls hopping around at the atomic level … it goes far deeper than that and beyond what we might think of as matter. Everything is ultimately energy that's a quantum entangled.

David Wolfe [00:49:23]: Well said, well said, and very, very prevalent that that occurs in animals, humans, plants and our direct connection with those. And that's one of the great things that we may not have known about, but when you tune into it, and you're growing the plants yourself and eating them yourself, you're serving other people the food, it's really, it's one of the great benefits of farming, is to have this level of fulfillment and happiness that arises from feeding people and nourishing your plants.

Brendan [00:49:57]: Yeah, So I'm curious, any last tips or good words about how to really farm or garden and enjoy the process?

David Wolfe [00:50:08]: One thing that I've learned in the tropics in a clay soil, I will say this, I use beach sand illegally. I mean, you know, in the sense of like I use more beach sand than any farmer has ever said was OK or any book ever said was appropriate. And I did that based on the Rudolph Steiner biodynamic preparation 501, which is, you know, that you take the silica, you packed it into the horns, you bury it through the summer, and then you pull it out and you take that material and you dump it out of the horns. And then you put it into water and you do it this way for a minute, and then this way for a minute, for an hour, and then you go spray that on your plants. And in the morning, I got the idea from that that there is an anti-fungal element to silica and sand.

David Wolfe [00:50:52]: There's a solar element. I mean, one thing we can say about sand, is that absorbs a lot of the solar energy or what Rudolf Steiner called light ether. And when you get that into a plant like chocolate, like chocolate trees growing in the jungle and all of a sudden they're getting beach sand, beach sand, beach sand, as an amendment. Something really powerful happens because chocolate, if you connect with the energy of it, it's bright. It's like the sun. It's like a … it's gold. It's money. It's like the center of the universe, right? That's kind of the energy of chocolate. And the way we nourish our chocolate trees takes that in mind. And one of the things I got into is putting the silica in there, the sand. And what that does … it's interesting … over time, the soil disperses out, and the sand goes into the soil and becomes diffused into the soil, maybe by the action of earthworms.

David Wolfe [00:51:45]: I've pulled out, you know, like I've shown people like watch this root structure here, pull out the structure out of the, you know, when I planted it in a pot and maybe it had 15 percent, 20 percent beach sand in that pot. When I pull that Cacao out of there to put it in the ground, you know, we sprouted it in that, the aeration in the soil is perfect, it's just perfect. It's like something amazing. So I wanted to bring that one up. And then another one I want to bring up for a more temperate farming, and maybe farming in places like, you know, Mediterranean climates like California, is getting the charcoal in and underneath your beds, in and underneath all new trees that are planted. I planted 50 trees like that this year, and it was the most successful planting yet of my life. I put a bed of charcoal at the bottom of every single thing that I planted this year. And it was, it was powerful what occurred from that.

Brendan [00:52:35]: Awesome. You know, I'm curious David, have you ever had a health challenge that you had to overcome? And if so what happened?

David Wolfe [00:52:46]: Oh Geez. The biggest health challenges that we're always overcoming, you know, like for me, it's always been allergies. Um, but you know, it's always something that like is just, you know, it's a stickler on our side. For some people it's asthma. For me it was allergies and seriously bad allergies where, you know, like my itchy eyes, um, build-up of wax in the ears, swelling in here, sometimes even rashes from being around cats, from being around pollen, from being around ragweed. Um, all that. So over the years, what I've learned is something very interesting I learned from studying plants, and that is the best thing for a sick plant is saltwater. It's the quickest act acting thing, basically in the ratio of ocean water. Ocean water— it's the basic fluid of life. Look into the health of ocean animals versus terrestrial animals. You'll see the ocean-going animals are healthier, much healthier and have vastly less diseases than terrestrial animals. So I got into drinking salt water and what a breakthrough that was. So I know now when I am having an allergy attack, and what it really means is I'm dehydrated. I'm low in water and sea salt. So I mix them together.

Brendan [00:54:06]: Yeah, there's a book out called *The Salt Fix,* and I'm looking forward to reading that. You also mentioned trees, and I thought I should also mention a book out called *The Hidden Life of Trees.* It's been getting a lot of attention including from medical doctors that are mentioning the book. I mean, it's exciting to have as close to let's say the high gods of medicine and science starting to acknowledge that there's more to life than what we have seen so far, and eventually getting revealed in science. We just have to keep our minds open, and it all gets revealed. So thank you so much for those really hot tips. That was awesome. And, and diving deep with me. One more question, I'm just curious … I had the impression when I was in London with you that some things might have changed in your perspective, like, you know, like happen for all of us. We all shift as we mature our perspectives change. I'm just curious if anything has changed in your perspective on anything in particular over the years.

David Wolfe [00:55:16]: Oh, fantastic. Well, I mean, I think all these years of farming because I've been farming all along throughout my whole career. I've been, you know, start with chaos gardens in southern California, and then eventually I got my place in Hawaii and then in Ontario and you know, been there for over a dozen years in both those places. I mean we've got Durians (*Durio zibethinus*) right now that are flowering. That's how long I've been at it. Durians take a long time for 12, 13, 14, 15 years to mature. And so as you grow those things, you start to learn about the food and about diet in general. So certain things that have changed. You have to be very, very careful about, you know, pushing one diet is the right diet for everybody. That's just inappropriate. It's not a one-size-fits-all situation. It's also a situation where, you know, some people can handle more of the junk food than others.

David Wolfe [00:56:05]: And, you know, that's another thing too, is like, "I'm fine and you know everybody should be fine." "Well, no, you're just, you're just have a little bit, you're genetically a little stronger, you've got a stronger metabolism, but one day it'll get you too." So also just being aware of like, hey, you know, not everybody's built the same and not everybody has the same strengths. And so we can work on that. We can build that up through different strategies. And that's what, that's how I've gotten educated in Taoist Tonic-herbalism or Chinese Medicine is to nourish into those treasures. So that, for example, with my allergy problem, that's really, it's really a Jing-related problem when I'm exhausted and wiped out, it all creeps right back in. And so I have to nourish my way, nourish myself in a certain way so that, that stuff doesn't creep in. And it's just … the individuality of diet is something that I address, but I don't like to get too far into it because you're your best guide. You know, you have to try different things and go, that worked for me, that didn't, or that worked, then doesn't work now or that works now and didn't work then, whatever. And what I'd like to get into more is the broader strokes, getting people back gardening again, the importance of understanding the colors and their importance on our food web. For example, black is Jing. Black foods. Black is an incredibly important color for nutrition. Red, that's your Chi, right? Red foods, very important for energy production. But then we've also got to have the great neutralizer in the middle, that magnesium, that's the chlorophyll, that's green. And so those, you know, those more, like the mountains aren't going anywhere anytime soon. The colors aren't going anywhere anytime soon. So we can try to hit those things that are going to be like that, you know, they're pillars that are applicable to everybody. I try to hit those more, and less of the specifics.

Brendan [00:57:53]: That makes a lot of sense because we can get overly reductionistic, and that doesn't help anybody. That's a big problem I think in the health world is people get too focused on, "Oh, this works for these people. It must work for everybody." That's not the case.

David Wolfe [00:57:53]: Right.

Brendan [00:58:09]: You know, I just want to say one thing, I love how you use a metaphor, I think that really integrative, intuitive thinkers are able to use metaphor fluidly. And sometimes it gets misunderstood, but I think that's why we have to nourish our own creative spirit so that we're not too literal-minded and can kind of see the wisdom that comes through metaphors whenever they're used. And they're great for understanding the world of Nature and science and so forth because sometimes it gets really interesting and complex in the world of science, and we need a simpler concept to be able to start to grok how something is working. And so I appreciate that about you. And just the fact that you're a pioneer, like the avocado, in really talking about the outer edges of our understanding and what we can—even before we fully understand it—what we can implement from there to create massive results both in our bodies and in the soil and our gardens and our farms. Biodynamics is on the cutting edge of that and has been for a long time. Rudolf Steiner was onto some things that people still don't understand. We don't yet fully understand what's going on there. Philip Callahan is another person, you know, he's a PhD scientist some people have said should've received a Nobel prize by now for what he's discovered. He was with USDA. There's this book right there. (*Paramagnatism - Rediscovering Nature's Secret Force of Growth*)

David Wolfe [00:59:42]: Yeah ... This is a really good (David holds up the book *Secrets of the Soil*), by the way, which is Peter Tompkins, who did *Secret Life of Plants.* This is the sequel to it. It does a very good analysis of Rudolf Steiner and Philip Callahan in that book. There's Callahan's book. I'm just going to just show a few books that I have at my office. (David holds up *Nature as Teacher* and *The Fertile Earth.*)

Brendan [00:59:58]: That's a great idea.

David Wolfe [00:59:59]: I think it's really good to have books that will help you to farm and learn about gardening. *The Fertile Earth* by Callum Coats on Viktor Schauberger's research. *Nature as Teacher*, also Callum Coats' book of Viktor Schauberger's teachings about fertility and working with Nature.

David Wolfe [01:00:16]: I ... Always have your activated charcoal and charcoal books on hand. (David holds up a book *Activated Charcoal* by David Cooney) I got a ... it's at my house, a biochar very intensely scientific book that really had very powerful impact on me this last summer, you know, where we planted so many trees, and I got the charcoal in there because of that book. I also want to mention this ... this is very important too ... we are so oftentimes thinking that the more recent research is the more valid research, and I would really recommend you go back to reading books in 1800's, reading books, written in 1910. This book right here—it was written in 1904—it's just called *The Soil* ... soil right there, by King. (showing the book to the camera) Very interesting to read these old books on many different subjects, but especially soil.

David Wolfe [01:01:07]: Let's look at this. This is the mycorrhizal fungi, Paul Stamets book, *Mycelium Running-How Mushrooms Can Help Save the World,* to understand that part of the web. Very interesting book here ... *Why Civilizations Self-Destruct* by Elmer Pendell. One of his key theses here is that one the reasons why civilizations self-destruct is they lose the top soil. We lose that rich humus that creates the thinking power. And then of course Rodale's *Healthy Hunzas*. This is about the glacial rock dust of the Hunza people and how powerful that can be as an amendment to soils and as an amendment to trees. And then of course *The Survival of Civilization*, another rock dust book. These are the ones I got into early on, not realizing the power biochar and just the compost, which are absolutely critical. But it's all critical.

Brendan [01:01:58]: Yup. Yup. Awesome. Thank you for that tour, that mini tour of your vastly more expansive library, I'm sure. So thank you for that.

David Wolfe [01:01:58]: No thank you!

Brendan [01:02:08]: Thank you so much for being here as a part of the Eat4Earth community.

David Wolfe [01:02:13]: It's an absolute pleasure to speak to anybody who's interested in living with the Earth better and having more fun in the garden and learn how to plant trees. And one last thing I want to say is you got to also know as you get into this, what your real skills are. For me, I'm a tree planter, so I'm really good at planting trees. I'm not the best garden person. You know, I'm not. I can plant tomatoes. OK, I can plant lettuce.

I love lettuce, but that's not my real forte. I'm a real tree guy. So you need to find out for you what you are, what you do best, and roll with that and go with it.

Brendan [01:02:13]: Nice. Thank you!

David Wolfe [01:02:13]: Great, thanks.

Brendan [01:02:45]: I so enjoyed this conversation with David and his energy, passion and spirit. And I hope you did too.

Alexis Baden Myer Interview
Regenerative Agriculture to Reverse Climate Change

Brendan [00:00:02]: Welcome to the Eat4Earth event. We're exploring how you can heal yourself, your loved ones, and the planet with your food choices. This is Brendan Moorehead, and it's my honor and pleasure to welcome our guest, Alexis Baden-Mayer. Alexis is a lawyer who has worked since 2005 as the Political Director of the Organic Consumers Association, a network of more than 1,000,000 activists committed to creating a healthy, just, democratic and regenerative food system. Alexis is a key organizer of some of the OCA's most popular campaigns, including the Monsanto Makes Us Sick campaign to ban Roundup. Alexis isn't afraid to put her body on the line to call attention to the crisis in our food system. In 2014, the US Health Freedom Congress awarded Alexis the Health Freedom Award for direct actions she's taken that resulted in her arrest, including shutting down the National Organic Standards Board meeting to protest the weakening of organic standards and entering the White House grounds to deliver a petition to first lady Michelle Obama in support of GMO labels, one of Barack Obama's unfulfilled campaign pledges. Alexis's proudest moment as an activist came in 2016 when Bernie Sanders tweeted a C-SPAN video clip of her dumping Monsanto money on the Senate floor to protest the corrupting influence of money in politics. Alexis, thank you so much for being here.

Alexis [00:01:26]: Brendan, thank you for having me.

Brendan [00:01:29]: So, perhaps more than any organization on the planet, the Organic Consumers Association, with its various projects like Regeneration International, is leading the charge to reverse climate change with regenerative agriculture. What are some of the strategies and campaigns that you're most focused on these days?

Alexis [00:01:45]: Well, it's wonderful to see how quickly this concept of regenerating our agricultural system to pull CO_2 that is in excess in the atmosphere and causing climate change, pull that CO_2 into the soil and trap it long-term as carbon. And of course, when you increase soil carbon, you're also increasing the capacity of the soil to retain nutrients and to be more fertile. So this definitely benefits consumers and farmers alike, making farming more sustainable and making food more nutritious at the same time that we're mitigating climate change. And it's been fantastic to see how quickly this concept has caught on. In 2016 at the Paris climate agreement the several organiza—or several countries in the world adopted a pledge and an initiative just around this issue of sequestering carbon in soils. It's called "4 Per 1000", and you can look it up online. It's at www.4p1000.org.

Alexis [00:02:56]: It's a global initiative that's been signed now by scores of countries. And this initiative has countries make the pledge to increase soil carbon by 0.4%, and not adding 0.4% of soil carbon, but just increasing it by that small percentage. If we do that each year for 25 years, we end up matching the same amount of carbon that's going into the atmosphere with carbon being drawn down out of the atmosphere. And at that point we would be carbon-neutral. But if we can get down to zero fossil fuel use, then we begin to be truly regenerative where we're actually pulling the excess carbon out of the atmosphere. Because we're already at 350, or sorry, we're already over 400 parts per million CO_2 in the atmosphere, and that's why we're having the devastating impacts of climate change already. We see increasing and more severe droughts.

Alexis [00:03:59]: We see increasing and more severe floods and storms and forest fires and all of these extreme weather events that are happening around the planet right now. They're caused in part by the global warming problem that's caused by the CO_2 in the atmosphere. So drawing that CO_2 out and down and trapping it in the soil, that is absolutely essential at this point. We need to wean ourselves off of fossil fuels, but that will only begin to correct the problem. We actually need to go from 400 and more parts per million of CO_2 in the atmosphere down below 350, which is what scientists have told us, is the dangerous tipping point. When we passed 350 parts per million, we started to irrevocably disrupt the climate, and we've got to get back down below that level, and this is the only way to do it. But like I said, this is being adopted by nations around the world, and we're even seeing politicians in the United States start discussing this matter.

Alexis [00:05:03]: Now, this was a thrill for me. Just this week, I was at an event on Capitol Hill in Washington D.C. where I work. And Congressman Earl Blumenauer, who is the representative from Portland, Oregon … he has always been active in agricultural policy in the U.S. House of Representatives, and he's always put out model Farm Bills, and he's … you know, we have this bill called the Farm Bill. It's passed once every five years. And it determines agricultural policy. And it's mostly the reason why we have so much junk food in our system. You know, Congress is subsidizing the wrong type of agriculture. So it's been a problem for a long time. And Congressman Blumenauer has always spoken out about it. But this was the first time I heard him give a speech where he said the Farm Bill is actually a climate bill. It has the potential to be an important bill for climate because it has the potential to support the forms of agriculture that can help reverse climate change. So I am really thrilled that even though this project Regeneration International was only started in 2014 at the People's Climate March in New York City, in three short years, we have seen this project really take off. We've seen an international initiative and now we're even seeing U.S. politicians talk about the potential of agriculture to be a solution to climate change.

Brendan [00:06:37]: That's so exciting that legislators are getting on board, and I've seen some other examples as well. And that's a big part of what it's going to take, I think. Now, one of your other campaign's subjects, or subject matter of your other campaigns is glyphosate, and that obviously falls under the purview of this effort to restore soils and rebalance the planet. What does glyphosate have to do with it? And why is it, how is it related?

Alexis [00:07:11]: Well, we became aware of glyphosate because of genetically modified crops. So, you know, Monsanto and other agribusinesses, they like to say that they're feeding the world, and they use technologies to improve yields and make agriculture more resilient to climate change and other forces. But the reality is that genetically modified foods were created to sell the chemicals that these companies produced, so Monsanto's flagship chemical is Roundup, and that's made out of glyphosate, the herbicide glyphosate. And so that's why they genetically engineered crops, so that crops could withstand endless amounts of glyphosate. And they pitched it to the farmers as an opportunity for farmers to have crops that didn't need to be weeded. You could just spray the crops with herbicide all over, and then the crops would live and the weeds would die. And it was designed to be labor-saving in agriculture. So farmers bought into this, and now we've got tons of these crops. Most of the big row crops in the United States, corn, soy, canola, alfalfa, etc., they've all been genetically modified to withstand glyphosate.

Alexis **[00:08:29]:** Now first we learned that, well this isn't good for human beings. Glyphosate was initially designed as an antibiotic. It also chelates nutrients and it chelates things that we need our body to be able to absorb, and so it's got all sorts of health problems. In 2015, the World Health Organization determined that glyphosate was also a probable human carcinogen. It's been linked with non-Hodgkin lymphoma, which is becoming epidemic in farming communities. Farmers and farm workers have had to sue Monsanto because they've gotten non-Hodgkin lymphoma from using the Roundup herbicide. But now we also understand how this impacts farming systems. So the crops that are sprayed with glyphosate, glyphosate is getting into the soil, and it's killing soil microbiology, the soil life that plants need to uptake nutrients and to be resilient. You know, it really kills the soil, just like it kills our gut bacteria. It kills our healthy gut bacteria that we need for good digestion. It kills the soil bacteria that plants need for nutrient absorption, that soil needs in order to retain moisture and be resilient in the face of floods and droughts. It just disrupts that whole system.

Brendan [00:10:00]: So, the biotech industry sold us this idea of genetically modified organisms and crops and of course, this wonderful chemical called glyphosate as a way to feed the world, and they even have arguments for certain GMO foods as increasing the nutrient content of foods, and I believe now they might even be trying to sell the GMOs as a way of creating climate-adaptive crops. I'm not sure about that, but is there any truth, have they fulfilled on any aspect of the promises to feed the world better food and help us create food security, especially in the face of climate change?

Alexis [00:10:47]: I'm afraid not. You know, I wouldn't be opposed to this technology if it were beneficial to farmers, to soil health, to human health, and to our ability to withstand the enormous challenges posed by climate change. But unfortunately, none of these things have come to pass. There are two items that get talked about a lot in the news media. One is golden rice. It's a form of rice, a genetically modified strain of rice that's supposed to have massive amounts of vitamin A. And the idea is that people in the world who are too poor to eat the vegetables that would have vitamin A, they can instead be given the rice that has increased levels of vitamin A and therefore be able to ward off the types of problems that you get when you're malnourished, like having poor eyesight.

Alexis [00:11:44]: So it's kind of a messed up concept to begin with because it's this idea that some people are just too poor to have healthy food. And they should be given a substitute to normal healthy food in the form of a genetically modified version of rice that wouldn't normally have the nutrients that they need. So I don't subscribe to that. I think that everyone on the planet deserves to have healthy real food and that that is an attainable goal. And we know that that's attainable because United Nations has researched this issue in a very broad report similar to the report they've done on climate change. It was a report on agriculture, and it demonstrated that right now the majority of the world's food is being produced by farmers who have less than two hectares of land—tiny little farms. But that's where the majority of the world's nutrition is coming from.

Alexis [00:12:38]: And these farmers would best benefit from the traditions of their communities, the way their grandparents farmed. If they go back to these traditional methods, they can increase food production. They can double food production just by using traditional techniques like composting and modifying your land to hold water better. Using saved seeds that are appropriate to your climate and your microenvironment. So all of these organic techniques are really the key to food production, but increasingly, these small-scale farmers, they're being pushed off of their land onto marginal land as big corporations develop large plantations in the area. So they're getting the worst resources. And they're being sold a bill of goods by the chemical companies who want to sell them genetically modified seeds and want to sell them expensive chemical fertilizers, synthetic pesticides, herbicides. And what we see in countries like India, we see these smallholder farmers with tracts of land around two hectares or less. Tiny little farms.

Alexis [00:13:47]: They're being sold all of these expensive inputs. They don't have irrigation, they don't have good land, which the chemical companies aren't willing to provide them. They are not willing to provide access to land and water, which is the essential thing that a farmer needs. They just want to sell them all these expensive inputs and then the farmers end up going into debt. And in India we've seen hundreds of thousands of farmers commit suicide because of this situation. So this is obviously not the way to feed the world. All of these ideas pushed by the chemical companies are counterproductive. And, even though I don't subscribe to this idea of the golden rice that has the nutrients that you need when you can't get healthy vegetables, they haven't even been able to commercialize that. And they have also talked about creating rice, or, sorry, other crops—in the United States, it's been corn that's drought-resistant. So Monsanto was able to commercialize a drought-resistant corn variety, but by their own data it would be useful only for 10% of U.S. corn growers. And if you think that Monsanto only wants to sell to those 10% of corn growers, we're way off base because Monsanto has a worldwide business model.

Alexis [00:15:13]: If they spend hundreds of millions of dollars developing a new genetically modified crop, they want to sell that strain of corn everywhere, whether it's useful to the farmer or not, and that's what they do. So what they've done cleverly is become a seed company. So they buy up all the varieties of corn. They take the highest-yielding varieties, and then they attach genetically modified traits to these high-yielding varieties. High-yielding is not a genetically modified trait. There is no GMO company in the world who has ever created a high-yielding variety through genetic modification. That's all done through traditional breeding. And then they attach the traits that sell chemicals, primarily, that we've already talked about. So, yes, there is a drought-resistant genetically modified corn variety available in the United States today, but Monsanto is not marketing it to the 10% of farmers who it might actually benefit, if you can predict the weather, which doesn't always turn out to be the case. You know, you'd be in tough luck if you planted the drought-resistant corn the year that you had extra moisture.

Alexis [00:16:20]: And we see these absurd weather patterns where, yes, we do have more severe, more prolonged drought. But then, at a certain point in your growing season you are likely also to get a torrential downpour, because, you know, we have weather patterns where the amount of rain might be semi-constant from year to year, but it's not going to come when it, when expected. And when it comes, it's going to come all at once rather than in patterns that are useful to farming. So we're really playing with fire to imagine that we can solve any of these crises through genetic engineering.

Brendan [00:16:55]: So what I'm hearing is that even some of their creations are actually going to objectively reduce yield, and that maybe, systemically, genetically modified foods, although they introduce certain traits that some people might think are desirable, like resisting a lot of glyphosate applied to the fields, they're actually reducing yield, because the only way to select for yield is through traditional breeding. Is that what you were saying?

Alexis [00:17:28]: That's absolutely right, Brendan, and the Union of Concerned Scientists did a study of all the publicly available data on yields, and they compared the major U.S. crops, and they produced a report that they called Failure to Yield, because, based on USDA public data, GMO crops are not able to be resilient the way traditionally bred crops are. And so GMOs have a slightly lower yield because we're talking about one-size-fits-all marketing. Monsanto spends a lot of money on these GMO crops, and then they want all the farmers to use them. And we would be a lot better off using locally adopted varieties on a region-by-region basis.

Brendan [00:18:17]: So would it be accurate to summarize the situation with GMO crops in this way … that, basically, they've shown that they're not meeting the promise of increased yield. They may in fact be decreasing yield potential, and the quality of the food may be compromised or definitely, I suppose, compromised by the fact that if they're bred to resist a lot of glyphosate, and glyphosate kills soil life, which makes minerals available. And if glyphosate chelates minerals, which makes minerals unavailable, then our food is actually getting demineralized, and our bodies are getting demineralized by eating GMO crops. Would that also be a potentially reasonable attribution there?

Alexis [00:19:05]: That is absolutely right. And we do have data showing that our food is less nutritious than it was generations ago, even one generation ago. So we've had this type of farming for a relatively short time. The GMO crops came out in the late 1990s. Glyphosate, I believe, has been around since the late 1970s, but really wasn't fully—you know, now it's the number one agricultural chemical of all time. But it wasn't used much before the late 1990s when these Roundup-ready crops were developed. So, sadly, we are seeing a new wave of diet-related diseases. In our population today, half of all U.S. adults have one or more preventable, chronic, diet-related diseases. And a lot of people, not just people who work on agriculture issues, but a lot of people are looking at this and realizing that yes, U.S. citizens, we're missing these nutrients that used to be readily available, and our food is less nutritious. And that is one of the causes of the epidemic of diet-related disease.

Brendan [00:20:29]: And then of course if glyphosate is damaging our soils, not only is it affecting the health of our bodies, but the health of the planet if we need soil to draw down carbon to re-stabilize atmospheric climate.

Alexis [00:20:40]: And even perhaps more fundamentally, we need soil to grow food, and all over the United States we are losing soil. And this country is a young country. When it was established by European colonists, they entered a Garden of Eden that was managed by the Native Americans who did agriculture, but they also managed vast hunting grounds. The best example of course is the buffalo. The buffalo were a source of food and building materials for the Native Americans on the Plains. And they managed those buffalo. They culled them, they chased them, and, of course they had their natural migration. We, what became the United States, we had one-quarter of the world's richest farmland, and that was because of the grazing patterns of the buffalo in the Midwest and the prairies, and that's been squandered very, very quickly.

Alexis [00:21:50]: And, we have a situation worldwide, not just in the United States, where we have soil loss, because agricultural practices right now, this hyper-industrialization, and even when we have smallholder farmers being pushed off good farm land, being pushed up into the hills with the poor farmland and continuing to till. Even if you're using relatively organic methods, if you till poor soil too often, that soil is lost. And so we've got a global problem of soil loss. And the United Nations says we have forty growing seasons left. Now, I want to live forty more years.

Brendan [00:21:50]: Forty now? It's forty now?

Alexis [00:21:50]: It's forty! Forty!

Brendan [00:21:50]: Okay.

Alexis [00:22:40]: And, yeah, Howard Buffett, Warren Buffett's son, just wrote a book. I haven't read it yet, but I heard about it, that it has "forty years" in the title. And he's referring to this real, very scary scenario where we are going to lose all of the world's soil, where we just won't have soil that is productive at all, let alone productive at the rates we've come to enjoy.

Alexis [00:23:04]: So we've got to turn this around. We can no longer be dousing our fields with chemicals like glyphosate, with the chemical fertilizers that, as well, contribute so much to soil loss. And we have to change our farming practices and that, you know, changing our farming practices, going to no-till agriculture, that speaks to organic farmers just as much as conventional farmers because this problem with soil loss has been around for millennia, ever since we became an agricultural culture, we have been destroying soil. There's a wonderful book on this subject by David R. Montgomery. It's called *Dirt: The Erosion of Civilizations*. And I read this book recently and it is alarming how, how quickly soils can be worn out through common agricultural practices. So this is a lesson to all of us, whether you farm conventionally or organically.

Brendan [00:23:59]: You raised two really interesting points. One was tilling, obviously, and the fact that even organic farms usually till, and that's a problem. And so, I think you have a term, sort of a modifier for organic farming: regenerative organic farming. And can you just maybe touch on that distinction?

Alexis [00:24:27]: Sure, now we borrowed that term from Rodale, the man who started the Rodale Institute and many publishing houses. Now there, the Rodale name, it's become a family business, and they've been running side-by-side farming trials on their farm in Pennsylvania, the Rodale Institute, demonstrating organic as opposed to conventional. And even if you just farm organically, you are going to preserve your soil and your soil biology a lot better than a conventional farmer even when you use tillage. So organic is always better. But the folks at Rodale also discovered that if they went no-till, they would be even better because then your soil is never bare. It's never exposed to the elements. And then you have much less problems with soil run-off. If you have extreme drought followed by extreme rain, that would normally wipe out the soil off of your field.

Alexis [00:25:32]: But if you can maintain a cover with roots, especially with a root structure, if you just plow it and then they use a tool called the roller-crimper to mat it down so that you can actually feed into the stubble of the last crop. That is the perfect way to really not just maintain but actually regenerate your soils. So even if you're an organic farmer who's tilling, you're probably not going to damage your soil too much if you don't have really bad, extreme weather events. But if you're an organic farmer who does no-till, then you can regenerate your soils and build those soils up. Now that's just the best news ever. Because if we're facing this crisis where most farming methods are causing soils to erode, and we have to suck the carbon out of the atmosphere, we have to do better than just stop the erosion. We have to rebuild the soils.

Alexis [00:26:36]: And most soil scientists who observe Nature would tell you that it takes millennia to build soil. It takes a hundred years perhaps to get like a centimeter going if it's left up to Nature. But the fantastic news is that through organic farming methods that in addition use no-till methods and use soil building methods that have been developed by institutes like Rodale, then we can actually build soil real fast. And you can see this as a home gardener. Another wonderful book that David R. Montgomery wrote that I've read recently is called *The Hidden Half of Nature*, and he talks very poignantly about his wife's struggle with cancer. So it's a book about the benefit of healthy soil for health, and it's also a book about how a backyard gardener can build healthy soil just by composting and then adding that compost to your garden. I'm sure anyone who's listening who is an organic home gardener can attest to the fact that we can build soil real fast. We've got earthworms to help us, and there are composting methods that can take your food scraps and quickly build up—you can make your own soil out of food scraps, out of yard waste, and that is a wonderfully exciting way to contribute to this as a home gardener.

Brendan [00:28:08]: And on the topic of building soil, you also mentioned grazing and how the buffalo existed in the wild and how they were so plentiful, and grazing across broad areas of the country, built some of the best soils, if not the best soils, in the world. And it seems to me, based on everything I'm hearing from other parties in this event is that grazing can be, if it's done right, in a certain way, it can be a real contributor to soil health and to drawing down carbon by building soil quite rapidly. I'm curious if the Organic Consumers Association is it all focused on that subject of including regenerative grazing?

Alexis [00:28:55]: Absolutely. Now I happen to be a vegetarian. And I became a vegetarian in 1990 at age 16 because I heard that the rainforests were being cut down for cattle raising.

Brendan [00:29:07]: Me, too! I tried it for eight years, and now I'm unfortunately a meat-eater again, but I'm trying to cut back. But go ahead.

Alexis [00:29:15]: Well, that's great. I meet very few vegetarians who did it for ecological reasons or for the climate specifically, but that's exciting. But now I understand that there are lots of different ways to raise animals. Certainly, raising animals in factory farms—that's the worst. And nobody who has any sort of diet should ever eat animals from factory farms. So cut that out, number one. But then, how about grazing? Well, there are a lot of good ways to destroy, especially, marginal land by running animals over it. If you just let the animals go wherever they want, they'll go where the best forage is right away, and they will eliminate that forage so that it won't be able to grow back, and that forage will be gone the next growing season. So, if you just put the animals out on the land—cows can do this pretty well, but just think of goats, for instance. You wouldn't let a goat into your garden because they would eat everything, and they would eat it to the point where it would not grow back.

Alexis [00:30:22]: So cows can do this, too. And we've seen that on our really—we have really poorly managed public lands where we allow grazing. And so grazing has really gotten a bad rap from environmentalists just because it's been done the wrong way. And of course, you know, when we're talking about, like, would you rather have a rain forest or pasture land? Well, we decide to keep those forests intact. And so there are a lot of places on the planet where you would never want grazing. But take the prairie. You know, the buffalo, as you said, used to roam there. Now we mostly grow corn there. It would be so much better to return that land to grazing land. That was what it was meant to be. That's what that ecosystem is for. And you can do this in ways that can regenerate the soil and regenerate the ecosystem, even, rather than destroying it, but it has to be done with lots of management.

Alexis [00:31:22]: So there's a scientist, Richard Teague, who's looking at this at Texas A&M University, and he's our go-to regenerative grazing expert. He learned the methods initially, I believe, from Allan Savory. He's from South Africa and Allan Savory is from Zimbabwe. Anyone who's listening who has never heard of Allan Savory, please check out Allan Savory's Ted talk. Just search "Allan Savory TED" and you will find a talk that's been watched by millions of people on this regenerative grazing. And Richard Teague is now demonstrating what he calls "AMP grazing." So, oh shucks, I might blank on the actual …

Brendan [00:31:22]: Adaptive Multi-Paddock. "AMP" is Adaptive Multi-Paddock.

Alexis [00:32:13]: Yes, Adaptive Multi-Paddock. Yes! For a moment I was thinking that the "M" was management because these are management-intensive systems. You have to think about, you have to do the math problem. You have to look at the amount of grazing land that you have. You have to think about the grazing needs of your animals.

Alexis [00:32:31]: And then you have to move them around in such a way that they get the forage that they need without destroying that forage completely and making sure that that land where there's grass growing, that the animals are going to graze, that that land gets plenty of rest before you bring the animals back there again. So, Adaptive Multi-Paddock grazing, AMP, that's what Richard Teague calls it. And so multi-paddock means that you separate your land into lots of little subplots for grazing. And then you move your cattle through those multiple paddocks. And you adapt as your climate situation, you know, if you get more rainfall, you're going to have better pastures. If you're in a drought, your pastures are going to produce less forage for animals. So you have to constantly adapt to changing situations. But the exciting thing about people who use these methods is not only do they manage not to ruin their pasture land, but they improve their pasture land so much that as they go along year after year, they can add more and more animals to the same amount of land.

Alexis [00:33:51]: So not only is this sustainable, we call it regenerative because it is increasing the soil's capacity to produce more forage for more animals. So this is exciting because, you know, I would love to see the population continue to grow. I think that would be a testament to our ability to make things work on this planet. And I'm not in the camp of people who want to see population caps or declines. I think that that would happen naturally if we gave women the right to control our own reproduction. So, I mean, certainly there are techniques that I've, you know, women shouldn't have to have ten babies in their lifetime, but if they get the opportunity to go to school and have a career, they probably won't. But anyway, putting those issues aside, we can produce more food using these regenerative practices and that's what's most exciting about them.

Alexis [00:34:48]: So we don't have to imagine a world of dwindling resources. If we use our resources well, we can actually be better than Nature at regenerating those resources. So, you know, maybe we'll never replicate the prairie and the buffalo, although there are some people in some parts of the world who are trying. And I think that that's a really important project, to see if we can put natural grazing animals back into these environments. So, you know, for instance, the Native Americans at Pine Ridge Reservation, they are grazing buffalo, and they're producing food for the Patagonia brand that's best known for their jackets or climbing equipment. Patagonia has created Patagonia Provisions, and they're selling meat from grazed buffalo. So, you know, I think there are great opportunities, in some circumstances, to return the indigenous animals to the land. But even if we continue with farming, with the same types of animals that people have grown accustomed to eating, we can do it in a regenerative way.

Alexis [00:35:51]: We can restore the soils, restore the ecosystem, and actually produce more food. And even as a vegetarian who probably won't eat much of this food that's produced, I find that exciting. Because the fact is, there's a huge amount of pasture land in this world that many people, especially rural poor people, survive off of. And if you're pushed onto marginal land that isn't great for growing crops anymore, and you have the opportunity to graze animals on that land, to restore that land, and you can use these intensive management techniques, I mean, that's the key to sustainability and to being able to produce enough food to survive. And that's one of the beauties of this natural system that human beings evolved in, where you could eat the milk or meat and eggs of animals that are able to eat plants that you cannot eat. And so it makes food production possible in parts of the world where cropping just isn't an available option anymore.

Brendan [00:37:05]: You mentioned the word ecosystem, which to me is the most exciting sort of revelation that comes out of this regenerative grazing is that not only are they increasing the amount of livestock that can be raised as the land gets more productive, again, if it's been done correctly, but it's recruiting the native species back onto the land. Grass species where the seeds had been dormant for decades under the soil are coming back out of seemingly nowhere and grassland species re-establishing themselves and insects and birds and other wildlife coming back. And some of these areas are now potentially prime hunting grounds for native herbivores like elk and deer. And all of that started with cows being intelligently managed.

Alexis [00:38:05]: Yeah, that's right. I mean, if you're an animal lover, that's something beautiful to behold. There's a great debate happening in the vegetarian community right now about whether to fully embrace lab-grown meat versus vilifying the production of animals that are raised in concert with the living ecosystem that brings back birds and all sorts of creatures that existed in these environments before they were improperly grazed. Like you said, they can be brought back through this proper grazing. So you know, as a vegetarian, I would much rather see meat-eaters eat this regeneratively produced animal food than to give up on the idea of producing food in concert with nature and just go to lab-grown meats, etc. I think that we still have the potential on this planet—it's not completely destroyed yet—we have the potential to restore these natural systems and restore the balance.

Alexis [00:39:18]: And I just heard a marvelous talk by Rattan Lal. He's a preeminent soil scientist at Ohio State University. And he recently published a paper that shows that if we use regenerative food and farming practices, we can return a lot of the land that we're currently using as farmland and pasture land. We can return that land back to Nature, because if we use these regenerative techniques that are so much more productive and can produce so many more animal products, crops from the land, we could actually return a lot of the land back to Nature. And that just blew my mind. And he's not one of the scientists—there are many scientists who do do this, but he doesn't overstate his case. He's always been very conservative when estimating, for instance, the capacity of soil to sequester carbon. So to hear someone like Rattan Lal say we can produce plenty of food for our growing population on less land using regenerative practices and return some of the land back to Nature, I think that is one of the most hopeful things that can be heard at this time.

Brendan [00:40:31]: Absolutely. And of course, Dr. Lal is actually a Nobel laureate (Correction: More accurately, Dr. Lal was actually part of the International Panel on Climate Change when it received the Nobel Prize in 2007). He is no slouch. He is the soil guru on the planet. And like you said, he does not overstate his case. He's conservative. You know this, the topic of eating meat is so emotionally charged and even divisive, and I personally have conflicts about it because my body seems to do better—not just seems, it's very clear that most of the time it does better on meat—and I'm learning how to shift that with my understanding of metabolic types and so forth and various nutrients. But it's encouraging to hear vegetarians looking at the issue as objectively as possible, in terms of, you know, maybe there is a need for livestock on the planet.

Brendan [00:41:42]: At least they are a potentially very helpful tool. The people that are looking at soil regeneration rates, what I keep hearing is that it's not happening any faster than where there's livestock. Livestock are how we regenerate soil very quickly, especially if we combine it with multiple species, crops of various sorts. So it's not just livestock, it's all kinds of things going on, reproducing an agro-ecosystem. And I guess, I'm just curious, what else might you have to say about what some people refer to as an ethical issue with regard to the eating of animals?

Alexis [00:42:22]: Well, you know, I'm not an ethical vegetarian. I became vegetarian with the idea that it would help the environment and help the climate and be a way to feed more people because we seem to waste a lot of land, a lot of our best farmland, growing crops to feed animals in factories. So that's my viewpoint. There are many, many viewpoints, and I do admire ethical vegetarians, and I admire the movement against speciesism, the idea that we're better than the rest of the animals on the planet and so we can use resources the way we want to. I think that, you know, I'm not quite there. I think human beings are special in some ways, but I respect that viewpoint. I respect ethical vegetarianism. But I do want to point out just to show that, if you're a vegetarian and you're interested in veganic farming as opposed to farming with animals, I do agree that it looks like we can restore the most land most quickly if we do integrate animals just because they're a great source of natural compost, and they're good at managing land if managed properly by humans.

Alexis [00:43:50]: You know, that—I won't concede that—but if you want to be a veganic farmer or support that type of agriculture, there are lots of regenerative practices that don't involve animals. And one has been piloted by David C. Johnson who is at New Mexico State University. And one of the nagging things that's been on my mind since I've been an advocate for organic farming is I often hear from conventional farmers—and perhaps maybe not from conventional farmers as much as the input sellers, so this is probably coming from the fertilizer company—but it always nagged at me, cause I thought, well, what if they're right when they say that we actually don't have enough organic matter on the planet to fertilize everything with compost, and we don't have that matter. So you know, one way to make it is to work with animals because they produce copious amounts of organic fertilizer.

Alexis [00:44:58]: But what if that's true, that we would have to cut down trees or something to produce the mulch and compost and fertilizer? Like, what if they're right? That just bothered me for a long time until I learned about what David Johnson is doing at New Mexico State University. He's using an incredibly simple composter. He calls it a bioreactor, and you can put any type of organic material into it, and you can make one of these yourself. There's a YouTube video that he has, so you can go for more information there. But I'll just describe its impact. With any type of materials, say you do have wood chips, you can put those in the Johnson-Su bioreactor. He got help from his wife, Hui-Chun Su, in making this bioreactor, so it's the Johnson-Su bioreactor. So just fill it with any type of organic matter, your food scraps or your lawn waste, and let it sit.

Alexis [00:46:00]: And then, in addition, if you want to make it richer, have worms go through it, and you come up with this extremely rich compost. Now, if I were a home gardener, I would take this by the barrel, or sorry, the wheelbarrowful and heap it onto my garden, because I just, you know, make your own soil that way. But what he did was he took this wonderful compost he made, and he sprinkled it very, very lightly, the lightest dusting possible. And he sprinkled it over the worst land he could find in New Mexico, practically a desert, practically no organic carbon in that soil whatsoever, sprinkled it ever so lightly over the land. And then the other thing he did was he added cover crop seed. So just through these two inputs, just seeds and the tiniest sprinkling of compost, he regenerated the soil life.

Alexis [00:47:01]: So there are lots of crops that make great green manures. And if you're doing this on a home-scale level, the best resource is John Jeavons. And he wrote a book, *Growing More Food Than You Thought Was Possible on Less Land Than You Could Imagine* [*How to Grow More Vegetables and Fruits, Nuts, Berries, Grains, and Other Crops Than You Ever Thought Possible On Less Land Than You Can Imagine*], and so he's famous for this concept of the square foot gardening. You can produce incredible fertility using certain crops, who—the crops are able to pull nitrogen from the atmosphere as well as carbon from the atmosphere and add it to the soil. And then with this light dusting of compost, you inoculate the soil microbiology that way, and David Johnson has documented the most diverse microbiology you can imagine in his soil using just these two inputs. Just the inoculation of compost to stimulate the soil microbiology and then the cover crop. And he's also then sequestering massive amounts of carbon, but maybe more interesting to people who want to survive on the planet, this makes the soil incredibly fertile, incredibly rich in nutrients, and incredibly alive with soil microbiology. So this is amazing 'cause this just blows that idea out of the water that it's just not possible to fertilize land except with massive amounts of organic inputs in the form of compost or animals. If you make your compost right, you can restore land with just those two meager inputs, just the seed of the right types of green manures of cover crops and a light dusting of compost.

Brendan [00:48:50]: David's work is marvellous, and he's gotta be the nicest molecular biologist on the planet. He's a really nice guy. I love watching his presentations, and I hope everybody listening to us now takes a look because he's got quite a lot to teach that's relevant to the everyday person that wants good food and wants a healthy planet, I believe, should learn more about soil, and there's few people better than Rattan Lal, David Johnson, and Elaine Ingham to learn from in terms of our understanding how the way our food is produced is going to make nutrients truly available to us and heal the planet. So, thank you for mentioning him. You know, I'm curious just real quick, because GMO foods are such an issue and because organic is so important, especially regenerative organic … I've been a little bit confused about whether organic can be GMO or not. My understanding is organic cannot be GMO, and yet I think there have been attempts to soften the organic standards to include GMO. And I recently listened to an audio book by a health authority who said that organic foods can be GMO, and I thought he might be incorrect about that, but I just was curious.

Alexis [00:50:21]: Well, it depends how you define GMO. Certainly, the transgenic crops, the GMO 1.0, is firmly excluded from organic. There's a piece of the organic regulations that defines excluded methods, and it defines genetic engineering, but that's genetic engineering in the traditional sense. And increasingly what's happening is, for instance, we've talked about the Roundup-ready crops that Monsanto made. They genetically engineered crops to withstand their herbicide Roundup. Well, there's, I think it's BASF, another one of the GMO and chemical companies. They figured out a way to make a variety of wheat that also was herbicide-tolerant, that tolerated one of the herbicides that they sold, and they were able to do this in a way that didn't involve transgenesis. They used mutations. You can irradiate the cells of crops to produce mutations, and now we have ways to quickly examine the mutations that you've made so you can quickly sift through them using computerization, etc., and you know, actually looking at the DNA, you can check to see if you're getting the traits that you're looking for.

Alexis [00:51:47]: So if you wanted to—you had an herbicide-resistant trait, you could mutate your crop in order to get those traits as well. And that would not be considered genetic engineering. Now mutating your crops to produce an herbicide-tolerant trait, you know, that's what the chemical companies like to do because they sell the herbicides. Now obviously that's not allowed in organic. So we're kind of sitting on the edge of our seats waiting to see if somebody creates a new GMO, a GMO 2.0 that they then do try to use in organic. So far there's not a whole lot of work being done in this area where I think that it's bleeding into organic, but there's a big debate around the CRISPR technologies. It's a type of genetic engineering that's similar to mutation, but is a little bit more technically involved, but they're not taking like—you know, what we normally think of as GMOs, you take the genetic material of a totally different type of being.

Alexis [00:53:03]: Like with the GMO crops that are herbicide-tolerant, they're taking a soil microbe that they've found can resist the herbicide, and they take that and they stick it into the plant. So you're taking life forms that are totally unrelated and mixing them up in the lab. But now the genetic engineering is becoming, I wouldn't say more sophisticated because it's still, it's not sophisticated technology. It's technology that's still pretty haphazard, and you don't really know what sort of unintended consequences are going to arrive. But at least these companies are figuring out that if they want to sell stuff in the European Union and other countries that label GMO foods, where GMOs just aren't used—like, the first wave of GMOs is practically extinct in Europe. They're I believe they only grow one variety of corn, which I believe is the Roundup-ready variety of corn, and everything else that even is allowed in Europe that's GMO just isn't grown anymore because there's been such widespread reaction against it.

Alexis [00:54:17]: Actually I think in Europe it's the BT corn. I forget, but there's only just one little variety of corn that's actually grown that's GMO in Europe. Everything else has just been rejected by the marketplace mostly because of health scares where, you know, for instance, a potato that was going to be commercialized in the U.K., they found that it had severe impact on the lab animals that ate it. So there have been so many health scares around GMOs, and also this idea that you could get all of your varieties of food contaminated. You know, the United States, we're the big—we're the uncontrolled experiment around GMOs. And so we've already lost a rice variety when Bayer contaminated our rice crop in the entire rice-growing region of the southeast. They contaminated it with a pharmaceutical and then they had to give up that variety of rice.

Brendan [00:54:17]: Oh, my God. I didn't know about that.

Alexis [00:55:18]: Yeah, it's crazy. There's a really great GMO contamination database that Greenpeace keeps, and they have a lot of information on the Bayer rice contamination scandal. Recently there was the Syngenta corn contamination scandal where Syngenta started selling a variety of corn to U.S. farmers without getting approval first in China and then China blocked the shipment. And you know, billions of dollars are at stake when you can't sell, like, all the corn in the United States that was grown that year. That's the danger. You know, when you have only six companies controlling all of our major food crops, if they mess up, they mess up royally. So we just have these terrible problems caused by this type of modification, but the companies are getting a little more sophisticated, and they're looking into these technologies that slide under the radar, that don't fall under the current definition of GMO and organic in the United States or GMO as it's defined in Europe when it comes to regulations. So CRISPR is one of those technologies that, you know, in my opinion, should, if you really look at it, it should fall under current definitions of excluded methods for organic or GMOs as they should be regulated in Europe. But the companies are, you know, they can spend a lot of money on lawyers and lobbyists and try to influence the decision makers when it comes to whether or not these new technologies are regulated the same as the first wave of GMOs.

Brendan [00:56:58]: Wow. So, you know, I think that the work of the Organic Consumers Association's gotta be the most important work on the planet and something that everybody should support. And I'm wondering, in terms of the big picture, what worries you the most? What gives you the most hope? And what's it really going to take to create a regenerative food system in places like the United States, where it could be the most challenging, and around the world?

Alexis [00:57:36]: Well, I think what gives me a feeling of security and hope is connecting with local farmers. I'm able to get raw milk here in Virginia, just outside of Washington, D.C. where I live. It's not easy to produce and distribute raw milk. You essentially have to, in Virginia at least, you have to buy a cow, essentially, and do it a little under the radar, almost like you're buying marijuana. It's really ridiculous, the way we've restricted access to healthy whole foods. But now I do have a relationship with a farmer. I have bought my cow, and I am able to get milk from the farm. And having that relationship with a farming family—this is the farm family that I'm involved with—it's a three-generation family and the grandparents and the kids are all running this farm together. They're producing all sorts of value added-products, and I get to see them and hear about their farm every week at the farmers' market. And I do subscription agriculture, CSA, where I'm paying every month to get the things that I need for my family.

Alexis [00:58:55]: And so I feel like making that sort of relationship is the best way to support the farmers in your area and know that they'll be there and also to know that you're getting safe, clean, nutritious food for your family. So that's what it all comes down to. You know, very few of us can produce all of our own food ourselves. So you're going to have to have relationships with farmers. And the more direct those relationships with the farmers in your area can be, the more food-secure you are. The better you know that you have a source of safe, reliable, nutritious food. And that's the ideal. Now, I know not everybody can do this. Not everybody lives in an area that's close to farms. Most of us do. You know, the United States produces eighty percent of the food that we eat.

Alexis [00:59:50]: So aside from things that we need like coffee and bananas, most of us can have relationships with local farmers. There are some great websites where you can find how to hook up with farmers. There's Eat Wild. Eat Wild (http://eatwild.com) is a fantastic source of information on nutrition and has ways to hook up with local farms. Weston A. Price has the Real Milk website (https://www.realmilk.com) where you can buy raw milk direct or enter into relationships with farms so that you can help produce your own raw milk. And there's also Local Harvest (https://www.localharvest.org), which is a massive database of local farms that's easily searchable. You can find out how to buy your thanksgiving turkey. You might need to pre-order that. You should probably do that now if you're listening and thinking about it. There are just countless ways.

Alexis [01:00:47]: And so that's number one, build that relationship. And then in terms of policy, I think I mentioned earlier in the discussion that there's a bill that Congress passes once every five years, and it really determines the type of food that is eaten in this country. And so we all need to be involved with policy. Even if you feel secure in knowing that you've got your farm connections in your area, and you feel like you've got your good source of local food, if you want to maintain that food system, the only way to do it is by getting involved in national policy. Almost all of our food policies are national, unfortunately. There are really strong efforts to create community food systems at the local level and get policy makers at the local level to support that. But unfortunately, our system is primarily dominated by the 90 billion dollars that Congress authorizes every five years.

Alexis [01:01:51]: And the sad impact of that is that Congress supports only a few different types of crops through these programs. And so we're growing a lot of sweeteners, a lot of vegetable fats, and a lot of feed that ends up in factory farms or in your gas tank as ethanol. And with all of our support as a nation, as tax payers, going to these types of crops, that's what most people eat. The average American diet is more than half coming from calories that are subsidized. And that means, you know, all of these big, massive monocultures of industrialized agriculture and then the factory farms that are also run on cheap corn and soy, which is essentially what it comes down to: corn, soy, canola, and I'll say cotton, even though you don't think you eat cotton.

Alexis [01:02:48]: But look at a box of Ritz crackers, and you'll see that you've got partially hydrogenated vegetable oils coming from cotton seeds or corn or soy. So just a few of these crops, along with sugar beets and alfalfa, which is an animal feed, that's the bulk of the American diet. And if we ever want that to change, we have to change this massive subsidies scene. We also have marvelous programs in the Farm Bill, marvelous programs that support regenerative agriculture. There's a program called the Conservation Stewardship Program, and it supports farmers working farms. Not just—you know, the Farm Bill is often talked about—the conservation programs are belittled, saying we pay farmers not to farm. Well there are some programs that help farmers set aside land, but we also have programs for farmers to engage in good stewardship on working lands, and that's the Conservation Stewardship Program. If we funded that as it should be funded and let the farmers access it who want to access it, we could have regenerative agriculture in the next five-year cycle. And because it's got all—it's named a regenerative agriculture practice and the USDA has recognized it. And farmers get support for implementing those practices on their farms, and it is not just for crop farmers, but if you integrate livestock you can be supported for this type of rotational grazing that we talked about.

Alexis [01:04:24]: There are some beautiful programs. But the beautiful programs are receiving a teeny tiny fraction of the taxpayer money, and almost all the money is instead going to subsidize the junk food system. So we need to work on both ends. We need to try to shape the local food system by making connections with local food producers, and at the same time we need to start shifting our tax dollars toward the type of agriculture that we really want to see.

Brendan [01:04:53]: Are there avenues for citizens to have their voice heard about shifting the farm policy so that instead of supporting chemical agriculture, we're supporting regenerative agriculture, through the farm policy, Farm Bill?

Alexis [01:05:13]: Yes, absolutely. Organizations like mine send out countless Farm Bill alerts. I try to make them interesting and teach people about nutrition and climate and environment and keep it fresh so that you're learning something while you're engaging in policy discussions. But yes, hooking up with an organization like Organic Consumers Association, signing up for the newsletter, looking for action alerts and taking action whenever there's an opportunity, that's the work we need to do. And finding out who your legislators are. Not everybody knows who their two senators or their congressperson are, so that's the first step. And then engaging them. And there are so many opportunities. We still live in a democracy and it doesn't always feel like it, but there are many, many opportunities to have your voice heard. You can, if you come, if you happen to be going through Washington D.C., you can walk right into your congressperson's offices, your two senators and your U.S. representatives.

Alexis [01:06:21]: Their offices are open. You can walk right into their offices and talk to a staff member and very often talk to a staff member who actually does the work on these issues. And then of course it's easy to call up from anywhere in the country or to write a letter or to send an email. And I do believe that this type of constituent contact is really paid attention to. I know when I do it, even if I send an email, I'll get a letter in the mail from my senators and representatives, because they do pay attention to constituents' comments. And we can make a difference. I think the problem really with the Farm Bill is it's the most important legislation that you've never heard of. People just don't know anything about it, and then if they do find out about it, they think, "Well, my voice won't count" and so they don't bother getting involved. But I urge everyone who's listening right now, find out who your senators and representatives are and call up the office and say, what is my representative or my senator doing about the Farm Bill now?

Alexis [01:07:37]: Because their staff is thinking about it. You know, there are very few pieces of legislation that every member of Congress is going to have to vote on, and the Farm Bill is one of them. It's going to happen over the next year. The current Farm Bill expires in 2018 and should be completed by the end of next year, and so they know about it. They're working on it. They have staff that they dedicate to this topic. And you don't have to be an expert. You can simply ask about what you know about. If you care about GMOs, if you care about healthy soils, if you care about getting animals out of factory farms and back on the land in a way that is regenerative and not destructive to our environment, just ask about what you know about, and demand that the staff in the congressional offices answer to you.

Alexis [01:08:29]: And most often they'll know something about what you're talking about, and through these conversations you can get the education. And really, you know, I've been at Organic Consumers Association for a dozen years now, but when I started, I didn't know that much. And it was through engaging with staff members in Congress, going to meetings on the Hill, that I learned, step by step, different aspects of farm policy and how the Farm Bill works. But you don't have to be an expert to get engaged. Just go with what you know and start asking the right questions, and pretty soon you'll have a really good understanding of where your legislators stand on these issues. And at that point, you can really start to influence them. And I think that if a lot of people got involved in this discussion, we would have a much, much different Farm Bill.

Brendan [01:09:23]: Alexis, I just really want to thank you and everybody at the Organic Consumers Association for your tireless efforts to defend life on Earth and defend our health from the destructive forces of chemical agriculture and genetically engineered foods. And so on behalf of myself and everyone that wants to eat for Earth, thank you for being here today, and may you be blessed.

Alexis [01:09:54]: Thank you so much, Brendan. It's been an absolute pleasure. I really appreciate the opportunity.

Elaine Ingham Interview
How Healthy Soil Provides Unlimited Mineral Nutrition and the Ultimate Solution to Climate Change

Brendan [00:00:00]: Welcome back to the Eat4Earth event. We're exploring how you can heal yourself, your loved ones, and the planet, with food. This is Brendan Moorehead and it is truly a joy to welcome our guest, the one and only, Dr. Elaine Ingham. Elaine is a PhD soil microbiologist and a world leader in both research and the application of soil health principles to real-world situations. She's best known for the concept of the Soil Food Web that illustrates how soil microbial life provides the foundation for life on land. Elaine is in high demand around the world to work her magic in returning highly-degraded soils and croplands to abundant life and productivity. She's held professorships at multiple universities and served as the Chief Scientist at the Rodale Institute from 2011-2014. Elaine is currently the Director of Research at the Environment Celebration Institute's farm in Northern California, which demonstrates the methods of biological agriculture to grow plants without pesticides or inorganic fertilizers. In addition to her research, speaking, and consulting activities, Elaine has a program that teaches people how to master soil health, and even become a soil consultant. Dr. Ingham, it's so good to see you again. Thank you for joining us.

Elaine [00:01:20]: Thank you, Brendan. It's a joy to be here.

Brendan [00:01:22]: You're the first person that got me excited about soil when you explained the Soil Food Web at the 2015 Permaculture Voices conference. I'll never forget that, or any other of your talks for that matter. Could you give us a crash course overview on how the Soil Food Web works, how it relates to human nutrition and drawing down carbon from the atmosphere to build soils and reverse climate change?

Elaine [00:01:47]: Yes, I certainly can do that. I can't promise it's going to be all that short so you're going to have to hold me to the time. The Soil Food Web is basically pictured here, where we're looking at the Lexicon of Sustainability's poster child. I was the very first picture on their very first year they put together their calendar on sustainability. So that has the basics of the food web. Here's that food web, in maybe a little bit easier form. This is the classic one, from the USDA's *Soil Biology Primer*, that I helped them write. So out of the 8 chapters in the *Soil Biology Primer*, I wrote 6 of them or something like that. So mostly my work, and Andy Moldenke he wrote a chapter on the microarthropods and Clive Edwards on earthworms. This food web chart basically goes through these different kinds of interactions, and of course, everything on this planet starts with the sun, so how do you store sunlight energy? Through the process of photosynthesis where the carbon dioxide in the atmosphere is combined with sunlight energy, and the energy from the sun is put into the bond between one carbon and the next carbon. And that of course is the simplest sugar that exists. If the plant needs 3 carbon sugars or 4 or 6 or 20 or whatever, then it just keeps adding carbons to that chain, but of course, the plant cannot grow on carbon alone. So where is that plant gonna get all of those other nutrients, and that's from the soil. Everything else has to come through the soil, so I always enjoy people who think of the above ground part of the plant as being the most important, when it's in fact your plant only gets 2 nutrients from above ground, energy and carbon, and everything else, all the rest, the nitrogen, phosphorous, sulfur, magnesium, calcium, sodium, potassium, iron, zinc, boron, silica, everything else, has to come through that root system. Basically, the plant's gonna pump that sugar down into the root system, part of those sugars are going to be pumped out into the soil, in order to grow the bacteria that the plant needs to do work for that plant. Some of those sugars are pumped out to feed fungi to do some of the work that the plant requires. So what all is the work that these two groups of decomposer organisms are going to do for that plant? Well, first of all, the plant is telling the species of bacteria and fungi to wake up! The plant needs this work done. And so the bacteria or fungi that utilize those exudates, those sugars coming out of the root system, will wake up and start to make the enzymes to pull the nutrients from the sand, the silt, the clay, the rocks, the pebbles, from the crystalline structure of those materials, those enzymes will pull those nutrients out, and of course those nutrients go directly into the fungi and are now held, or into the bacteria and are now held in a not-leachable form. We aren't going to lose any of those nutrients that are going into either of those decomposer organisms. So those bacteria and fungi happily growing around the root system are serving as a pantry, that's where the plant is going to save all the nutrients that it's going to need. So these organisms accumulate in around that root system are now protecting those roots against diseases, insect pests, and other problem organisms. A root-feeding nematode or a root-feeding microarthropod wandering around in the soil wouldn't even know that these root systems are there, because there is no chemical signature, there's no information coming to those predators and pests to let them know that there's available plant material for them to eat. They are so protected by the layers of bacteria and fungi growing around that root system. So nutrients are being tied up or protecting the root systems, and the above-ground part of the plant will be protected as well, as these organisms are carried up onto the above-ground part of the plant. So protection above ground as well against pests and disease-causing organisms. As the bacteria and the fungi grow, they're going to be making glues, mostly bacteria making glues, that will stick them to the surfaces of the root system. That will stick them to the surfaces of the sand, the silts, the clays, the rocks, the pebbles, organic matter as well, and the bacteria will start gluing together microaggregates, starting to build structure, and pull bits and pieces together so that there's more air space, more space for water, more space for oxygen and roots to be moving deeper down into the soil. The fungi then grow as long strands—they're long threads—and so they're going to be binding themselves, and winding themselves, around the roots, around the microaggregates, around the bits and pieces of sand, silt, clay, rocks, pebbles, organic matter, and holding those materials together in macroaggregates that leave even greater amounts of space. And so all of that structure is built by the bacteria and the fungi to help the plant be able to maintain the aerobic conditions that it requires around that root system. If this area goes anaerobic, oxygen is not going to be available anymore, and plants can't function in anaerobic conditions. As anaerobic bacteria or anaerobic fungi start growing, really toxic chemicals are being produced; the pH of the soil is going to drop to lower and lower and lower levels; and it's going to basically solubilize the root system. So diseases and pests only grow in those anaerobic, reduced oxygen conditions. So having those air passageways, having that structure built by the bacteria and fungi is really important. Now when we look at the ratio of fungi to bacteria. The bacteria are producing mostly nitrates. Aerobic bacteria produce alkaline glues, which pushes the pH of that soil into a more alkaline pH, and therefore the nitrifying bacteria are going to be functioning very rapidly. And so any soluble inorganic forms of nitrogen that appear, those bacteria convert it very rapidly into nitrates, which is fine for plants that require bacterial dominance, but not so good for plants that require fungi to be present. Fungi, when they grow, produce organic acids. They don't produce near as much glue as the bacteria do, and so as conditions become more appropriate for fungi, you will actually see the pH start to drop, and generally you're going to get a pH somewhere between pH 5.5 and 7. Which means nitrogen is NOT going to be converted into nitrate. And so ammonium NH4 is going to be the predominant form of nitrogen. Different kinds of plants prefer different balances of nitrate and ammonium. If you're trying to grow weeds, then you want a strictly bacterial-dominated soil, where almost all of the nitrogen is going to be present as NO3. Perfect for growing weeds. But most of us don't want weeds. We want to be growing plants that we can actually get food from. And so as we start to grow lettuce, we have to have a little bit more NH4 present, so we've gotta have some fungi present so that they will maintain those concentrations of those nutrients that your plant's gonna require. As we're trying to grow most vegetables, we need a little bit more fungal. As we try to grow grasses and row crops, we need a lot more fungal, and equal biomass of fungi and bacteria because our grasses require an equal amount of nitrate and ammonium. As we move on into later succession—perennial plants for example—they need a lot more NH4, which means you've got to be in a fungal-dominated soil to maintain those different kinds of plant species. So not only what is going on in the soil is determined by the food web below ground, but it's also going to have a feedback result on ever-improving the successional stage of your ecosystem. Well, what if you don't want your ecosystem to move along in succession? Well then you're going to have to do something to stabilize the ratio of fungi to bacteria where you want it to be. Now I'm sure you're all probably sitting there going, "Well wait a minute … how are nutrients becoming available to the plant? Because what you're talking about, Dr. Ingham—is that all the nutrients end up inside the bacteria, and they end up inside of the fungi—how do we make those available to your plant?" Because your plant's gonna die if all the nutrients are tied up in your bacteria, in your fungi, in your organic material, in the sand, silt, clay, rocks and pebbles. So how do we get the nutrients out of the biomass of the bacteria and fungi? And that's where the next trophic level comes in. Protozoa eat bacteria. Bacterial-feeding nematodes eat bacteria. Fungal-feeding nematodes eat fungi, and fungal-feeding microarthropods feed on fungi as well. And because the carbon-to-nitrogen ratio or the carbon-to-sulfur, or carbon-to-calcium, or carbon-to-zinc, or any of those ratios, are so much wider in the things that eat bacteria and fungi, that excess of every nutrient is going to be present in the fungal biomass or the bacterial biomass. So whenever any one of these predators eat bacteria or fungi, these organisms are going to release those soluble plant-available nutrients right there in the root zone of your plant. Your plant doesn't have to do any work in order to get those nutrients from the soil, as long as this food web is present and functioning in that soil. So soluble nutrients are made available; the plant takes them up. If the plant doesn't need all of the nutrients that are being supplied by that predator-prey interaction, then the bacteria and fungi who didn't get eaten, are still there and they take up the excess. The pantry is still present, and you're gonna fill in the empty shelves that got eaten by the predators in the system. We do need these higher-level predators because, think about if we didn't have these predators in the system, all of our nutrients would end up in the bacteria and fungi and your plants would die. And so we've gotta make certain that these organisms don't get to be too numerous. It's gotta maintain a balance between the bacteria and their predators and the fungi and their predators. So these predators need to have these predators in order to keep the balance. So we need the predatory nematodes that will eat nematodes and keep their populations down to the proper level to make sure all these nutrients are going to be cycling at the rate the plant requires. We need to have macro-arthropods, the predatory arthropods that eat the micro-arthropods, and keep their numbers in balance and not overeat the fungi or the bacteria. Okay then how do you keep these guys balanced? Then you've got to have the higher-level predators and the higher-level predators. When you think about who's the top of this whole food web, it's human beings. It's our job to make certain that the balances of all of these organisms are present and functioning in the soil so that we can obtain the food that we require, and that food will contain all of the nutrients that we need. And that's one of the problems with the current system where we're putting on just one type of fertilizer, where we're putting just nitrate fertilizer, we're putting phosphate fertilizer, we're putting calcium, lime, into the system. We're only supplying one nutrient. Well, what about all the others? And they're not being supplied in proper ratios. And so your plant's stressed. It's unhealthy. It's subject to disease, and insect and problem organism attack because they're not protected the way they're supposed to. As soon as we start destroying this biology in the soil, we're gonna be in trouble because we're not getting the nutrients we need in our plant materials. We need to re-establish the Soil Food Web and let things work the way they've been working for the last 3.5 billion years, since this nutrient cycling system was put in place by Mother Nature. We are so arrogant to suppose that we know better than Nature, and Nature needs our help to make certain nutrients get into our plants. It's kind of the other way around. We need to work with Nature and not against Nature. Because while we may have won a small battle in the fight against Mother Nature, when you look at who's gonna win the war, yeah, Nature's gonna win the war, not us. We don't know what we're doing and we're causing a great deal of damage. So we need to stop, think about what we're doing and start working with Nature instead of against.

Brendan [00:16:46]: You mentioned the nitrate fertilizers, and I'm curious to know if we're applying nitrate fertilizers, does that mean we're creating our own weed problem?

Elaine [00:16:57]: Exactly. You've got it. It didn't take you long to figure that one out. We're causing the weed problem. We've gotta make certain that food web gets back into the soil, and we stop destroying that nutrient cycling system. Every single inorganic fertilizer is a salt. And when you get to a high salt concentration, the organisms in the soil are gonna die. It's just like you and me. If we gave you salt water to drink, you would be dead in a very short period of time. But it's water! How can you die from drinking water? It's too high a salt concentration. That's what we're doing to the biology in the soil when we put on inorganic fertilizers. Every single one of them is a salt.

Brendan [00:17:46]: You mentioned fungal organisms and the fungal-to-bacteria ratio. And there's a particular type of fungal organism that I've heard about multiple times, mycorrhizal fungi. Could you explain a little bit more about this character in the Soil Food Web story and why we should know, celebrate and protect this wonderful creature?

Elaine [00:18:08]: When we're looking at mycorrhizal fungi, they are a type in this group. One of the really wonderful things about mycorrhizal fungi is that the plant puts out specific exudates to wake up the mycorrhizal fungus that it requires. We need to have the spores of the mycorrhizal fungi within that root system so the exudate being produced by the plant to wake up those mycorrhizal fungi will wake up those spores, and the spore then follows that trail of breadcrumbs if you will, back to the root system, the fungus moves into the spaces between the root cells and moves and grows back to the point where that exudate was being produced and then there's the infection site to allow the fungus to colonize in between the cell wall of the plant and the plasma membrane of the plant. And an exchange is set up. The plant is basically going to put out information, biochemical signals, to say to the mycorrhizal fungus that's colonizing inside its root system, says to that fungus, "Hey, I've been providing you with some pretty good cakes and cookies here, but, you know, that's all over now. You're gonna have to do something for me if you want any more of these delicious cakes and cookies to come your way, there's gonna have to be trade here." And of course, the mycorrhizal fungus says, "Whoa, okay, I need that energy. It's my only source of energy. So, Plant, tell me what you need and I'll go out and get it and we can set up a trade." Bartering system is gonna happen here. So the plant says, "What I need today is a little bit of nitrogen, so find me some nitrogen. Find me some sulfur. Find me some phosphorous. And while you're out there, find me some water. And if you don't, too bad. No more cakes and cookies for you." Mycorrhizal fungus says, "No problem. I already have my hyphae out here into the soil," so going out, when we're talking about an endo-mycorrhizal fungus, going out at least a good 10 inches out into the soil in every direction around that root. Think of all the more soil that that plant can now get nutrients from. So the mycorrhizal fungus goes out, it finds that part of its hyphal network that is already making the enzymes to pull that specific nutrient, so okay over here, here's the nitrogen mine, so we're pulling that in, pumping that nitrogen back. Over in this other place, the fungus is pulling in the phosphate and so that's getting pumped back now. And over here the sulfur. So all of the nutrients that the plant is requesting are brought right back to that spot, the fungus exchanges those nutrients with the plant for the cakes and cookies that the fungus wants. Both organisms grow better. Both organisms are going to survive and reproduce. We will be eating plant material that's much higher in the nutrients that we require as well. So it's quite a win-win-win situation when we're considering those plants that are mycorrhizal. Now, there are plants that are non-mycorrhizal and should never become mycorrhizal. So those really early successional plant species, things like say asparagus, or broccoli, or cauliflower, a lot of the brassicas, the cole and kale crops, should not become mycorrhizal, and it's probably detrimental to them to become mycorrhizal. Typically some mycorrhizal plant is putting out the information to go colonize the root systems of the non-mycorrhizal plants in order to pull nutrients out of them. There's been some work done by Mike and Edie Allen for example showing that a mycorrhizal plant will actually pull nutrients from a non-mycorrhizal plant, and so it supports growth of a mycorrhizal plant. When you think about the fact that most of our weeds are NOT mycorrhizal, this is a great thing. But you're going to have to protect your brassicas, your cole and kale crops from mycorrhizal colonization. And the way they do that, to the best of our knowledge, is around the root systems of the non-mycorrhizal plants, these plants will put out the cakes and cookies to select for microorganisms that are detrimental to the mycorrhizal fungi. So that around the root systems of these non-mycorrhizal plants are the actinobacteria that suppress mycorrhizal colonization. Not all actinobacteria produce these compounds that are detrimental to the mycorrhizal fungi. It's certainly something that seems to be located ... there's this association between the brassicas and the actinobacteria so that they can suppress the growth of mycorrhizal fungi getting into the plant. So presumably those actinobacteria are also serving to help bring nutrients for the brassicas, the cole and kale crops, instead of the mycorrhizal fungi for the later successional plant species.

Brendan [00:23:50]: Okay and I'm curious, what percentage of our crops are mycorrhizal?

Elaine [00:23:56]: It's ... almost everything is mycorrhizal, except for these early successional plants that I was just talking about, these early cole, kale crops, brassicas, things like mustards, things like that. So lettuce for example can be mycorrhizal when it needs to be mycorrhizal, and it can reject mycorrhizal colonization when it doesn't want it. But when you start getting up into the *Solanacea*—like tomatoes, potatoes, peas, beans— they have to be mycorrhizal. They require mycorrhizal colonization. And by the time you get into the row crops, the corns, the barley, the wheat, by the time you're into shrubs or any kind of tree crop, they have to be mycorrhizal. And so there's where with conifers you're going to get into ectomycorrhizal fungi as opposed to endomycorrhizal fungi. Our deciduous trees, deciduous shrubs, perennial herbs, the grasses or row crops are all going to be colonized by endomycorrhizal fungi.

Brendan [00:25:10]: And what happens when we till? Does that harm the fungal organisms?

Elaine [00:25:17]: It harms just about everything. Because when you till you're going to break up that structure, and building that soil structure is a very important part of what this biology does. And when you till you destroy that you've just reduced your ability to hold onto water. You've reduced water holding capacity. You are compacting soil at whatever depth you till. You're going to be pressing down on the soil at that depth and causing compaction, and your roots are not going to be able to grow through that soil very easily at all. Water as it moves through that horizon and reaches that compaction layer imposed by the plow or the tillage equipment that you did, water will stop moving through the soil there and begin to puddle and back up. And that's the part of the soil that will go anaerobic very rapidly, because water does not move through water-logged soil at all. And any organism growing in that area is going to use up oxygen so rapidly that it's going to go anaerobic, and now you have the perfect place for diseases and pests to start to grow. So tillage may fluff the depth of the soil down to the depth of the tillage equipment is going, but below that it's causing compaction. So you've fluffed up above, you've put oxygen in, but you've then reduced the amount of oxygen going into the lower depths of the soil, and you keep doing this over very many years and you're gonna start having massive amounts of disease, you're gonna have insect pests. You can have all sorts of problems. So we need to get this biology back into the soil. The tillage itself of course slices and dices and crushes the fungi, the protozoa, the nematodes, your earthworms, your microarthropods, all those higher-level organisms that we need to have in here in order to make this system work are going to be destroyed by tillage. The only thing that's left are bacteria, and good luck growing anything but weeds if you only have bacteria left in the system.

Brendan [00:27:43]: So it sounds like between nitrogen and tilling and other salt-based fertilizers, we're creating a system that then we grow weeds and under-nourished plants, and then we have to dump more pesticides, herbicides to kill the weeds, pesticides to kill the bugs that are attracted to the smell of anaerobic soils, right? And weakened plants are easy prey, and so they know that. So this wouldn't be the first example of us creating our own problems, would it? (laughs)

Elaine [00:28:19]: No, not at all. (laughs)

Brendan [00:28:20]: And thinking that we know how to manage Nature better than a 3.5-billion-year plan and technology can do.

Elaine [00:28:30]: Yep. It's a little depressing when you start thinking exactly how rapidly we go downhill. Every civilization on this planet that came before us failed because they destroyed their soil. There's a very interesting book by David Montgomery that goes back through all of those examples, what happened in Mesopotamia, what happened to Egypt, what happened to the Romans, every single civilization on our planet has destroyed itself by not understanding the ultimate consequences of the agriculture they were doing. And so their soils fail; they can't grow anything; everybody moves away; and blowing sand covers the ruins of that civilization. We're doing the same thing to ourselves, and we're just doing it faster than any other civilization before us. All of the problems that we're having with water are directly related to our use of toxic chemicals destroying soil structure, destroying our ability to hold the nutrients where they're supposed to be. When we start looking at some of these interactions, I was gonna go through a short little explanation of the ecological monograph, which is probably the original paper that really starts to show what the interactions of these different organisms do in soil. Before, my husband—and that's who is the main author on this article—before the group we started working with, David Coleman at the Natural Source Ecology Lab at Colorado State University, basically the attitude of soil scientists and agronomists was, "Yeah, organisms are just there in the soil. They don't really do all that much important. They're just kind of there. Don't worry about 'em. They just instantly come back after any disturbance." If you understand Nature, of course you're just gonna stand back in shock at that one because Nature doesn't continue supporting something that's not doing the job, not doing something to promote the ecosystem and maintain the sustainability of that ecosystem. So here's a group of people that started to look at what are all these organisms doing in the soil? So basically what happened is, (we) took sterile soil, so we went out collected a real soil, sterilized it to get rid of all the organisms, and then started adding back each of the different components in the food web to really try to discover what it was that they're doing in that soil. So the first set of treatments had just the plant in the system, and of course there were nutrients in the sterile soil, so the plants grew. And I'll show you in a minute how well they grew. The next treatment was plants + bacteria. And then the next was plants + bacteria + fungi. And in all of the remaining treatments here there were protozoa that got into the system. So, plants + bacteria + protozoa + fungi. And then plants + bacteria + bacterial-feeding nematodes + protozoa. And then plants + bacteria + fungi + fungal-feeding nematodes. So increasing the diversity, increasing the complexity of that food web in each one of these different treatment groups. So when you look at growth of the plants, how many milligrams per plant on average, 4 mg ... so you can tell that this is not a very big plant. It was barely surviving. Plant with bacteria: the bacteria alone just didn't really do much to help the plant. Maybe a little bit of nutrient cycling but too much competition between the plant and the bacteria when it's just the plant and the bacteria. The plant + bacteria + bacterial-feeding nematode: look how much more that plant grew, because of the nutrients that were made available to that plant. When you get the plant + the bacteria + the fungi and the protozoa: best growth in here. And then bacteria and fungi with fungal-feeding nematodes, the whole diversity in there. You can see that adding a predator to the system makes all the difference. Because then the plant is getting the nutrients from the sand, the silt, the clay. There are hundreds of thousands of years' worth of nutrients in those mineral components, not plant-available forms. There is no soil on this planet that lacks the nutrients to grow plants. If we kill the biology off then we destroy our plants' ability to get those nutrients. So if you put the bacteria and fungi back into the system, plus a predator, all of a sudden your plants are growing well and taking off. When we're looking at soluble, inorganic forms of nitrogen in the soil, you can see that the ammonium being present, the plants are growing better, and then with the predator in the system, there's a higher concentration of that soluble nitrogen, and that's what the plants are taking up to give that increased plant growth. When we're looking at protein in the plant leaf material, you can see how much higher nutrient concentration is where we have predators as compared to where we don't. So it really gets back to a question sometimes we always argue about with soils people, agronomists, what really is soil. If you go back to Jans Henny [sic - Hans Jenny], the father of soil science, he defined soil as being not only the mineral component, but the organic matter to feed the organisms and the organisms themselves. It's not soil if you don't have the biology. This is a picture of the great plains of the United States. As we started to till and as we started to destroy the biology of the soil, most of our soil blew away. And so this was the original level of the soil in the Great Plains, and after 30-40 years of tilling, look at what we did to that soil. How can you grow anything? Yeah, it's horrifying. These are Dust Bowl days. You've got to get the organisms and the organic matter back into the soil. It's gotta be both, not just one. And so dirt, if you really want to come up with a definition for dirt, it's just the mineral component, the sand, silt, clay, rocks and pebbles. If it's soil, it's got, yes the nutrients in plant not-available forms have to be there, but you also need the organic matter to feed the aerobic organisms that will now allow us to have plants of ever increasing value to us as human beings, to obtain the nutrients that we require.

Brendan [00:36:07]: And you ... oh, go ahead.

Elaine [00:36:11]: Just a couple, just a few more. Because people often don't get it when I say every single soil on this planet contains the nutrients to grow plants. And I like to just quickly show, here's Sparks back in 2003 ... went all over this planet, and collected soils from all over, and then looked at the average concentration of all of these different nutrients. Now I don't have them all on here, but the top important ones. And you can see that on average, let's think about nitrogen, find nitrogen on this list, it's down here. On average in general, on this planet, there's 2000 ppm nitrogen in soil. Most of it is in a plant not-available form. So how do you get the nutrients out of this plant not-available form, and into a plant-available form right around the roots? You have to have the organisms to do that job. Phosphorus. Is there any plant on this planet that wouldn't be able to grow with these concentrations of nutrients? These are way higher than any plant requires. And so we've got hundreds if not thousands of years' worth of nutrients in every teaspoon of our soil. And then if you think about plants can put their roots down 10, 15, 20, 25 … when we're looking at trees, 100, 200 feet down into the soil. There's an infinite amount of nutrients. What we have to get back into the soil is the food web to make it available back to that plant.

Brendan [00:37:59]: I think that point is so, so important. Because you've got people, even very well-meaning people, that are educated about the soil, but they're still stuck on this scarcity idea that we keep harvesting food off the soil, we need to put minerals back. And we certainly need to put something back, if we're mining the soil of something. But the minerals is perhaps not the scarce thing we're mining. What we're mining perhaps is, like you said, the availability. If we're mining the life source of the Soil Food Web in some way, and I don't think mining is the right term … we're just wholesale killing it. The point is the Earth's crust is pretty thick. We're not going to run out of it anytime soon. And plants basically specialize in conjunction with the Soil Food Web at making the Earth's crust into food.

Elaine [00:38:59]: And it always amazes me when somebody says you can't grow plants in pure organic matter. Well just like soil, just like dirt, sand, silt, and clay, you can't grow a plant if all you've got is sand, silt, and clay, or if all you've got is organic matter. But put the organisms back in there, and we grow the best, the highest yields, the best-tasting plant material in pure organic matter with the proper biology. That's what we've messed up on for so long. Human beings just seem to like to kill life. And we don't understand that it's important. Nuke it! You see an insect out there, just nuke it. Never mind that it was a larval stage of a ladybug. Just so sad. We need a lot more education about what actually should be in soil and how it works.

Brendan [00:39:57]: So the cornerstone of your work in restoring life to soil, is compost—many, many ways of creating and using compost, compost teas and so forth, in order to improve the Soil Food Web in a particular location. Using these methods you have generated pretty miraculous results, time and time again. And I recall a case study in which you turned what I believe was a sandy soil into something that looked a behaved like a loam soil in a pretty short period of time, and then blew away some government from USDA representative or something like that. Can you tell us about that?

Elaine [00:40:37]: Yeah, we were working up in North Dakota, South Dakota, and working with a grower that just wasn't really sure. He was still kind of into mineral balancing and that. And so he had invited us to come out and convert his dirt back into soil with him, training him how to do this. And just to establish right from the very beginning, that the soil, the dirt, on this farm was actually pure sand—it was blow sand, that's the only thing you could call it—and so to start everything off correctly, (we) invited the USDA extension service person to come out and do a sample of that soil and then tell us what needed to be added to that soil to make the plants grow. And because it's pure sand, it had a very, in this particular instance, a very high pH, upwards of pH 8. And then it needed calcium, and I was blown away when the USDA person said it needed 3 tons of lime per acre. What would that do to the soil pH up there? But okay we just wanted his recommendation. It needed phosphate. It needed nitrate. It needed just a whole slew of things. It would have cost the grower a small fortune to put all of those nutrients back into the soil. And so just listened to him, but what I really wanted him to say was, "This is pure sand. There's nothing in here but pure sand." And when I finally got that out of him it was like, "Well thank you. We'll see you again at the end of the growing season. We'd like to have you come out here and look at the crops that we grow." "Oh, no, you're not going to be able to grow anything in this soil. This is such poor soil. You couldn't possibly." And when you think about the concentrations of nutrients that were actually present in that material, there was no reason for us to not be able to grow really good crops in that soil. So we started putting out the compost, getting that biology mixed in. We typically do go in and check compaction. So we find out if we need to till that compost in, and absolutely we needed to till the compost in because he had some really deadly compaction layers in that soil. So (we) went in and added 1 ton of good compost to that soil, he soaked his seed in the compost tea, so that we had the organisms on the surface of the seeds. He went in row, and as he put down his furrows, he dripped a little bit of compost extract in front of that seed, and so goes out there and plants his whole field. We come along at first true leaf stage and apply a compost tea to protect the above ground part of the plant. We got the soil into a pretty good place with the organisms that we added in that springtime period, but the above-ground part of that plant was not protected, and so we needed to do that. And of course, when you're applying compost tea to the surface of the plant at first true leaf stage, you're gonna hit the soil too, so we were getting organisms back into that. And then a month later, another application, and a month later, a third application. So really good plant production. I think he got higher than the county yields of, let's see, it was probably corn that we were working with there. He increased his yields if I recall correctly something like 300% as compared to his neighbors.

Brendan [00:44:36]: Wow.

Elaine [00:44:36]: So we then, you harvest the corn. All the residue goes down onto the surface of the soil, and all of those residues start to decompose very rapidly. So just before snow flies, we invited the USDA extension service to come back out and take a look at the soil. And he comes out and he looks at it and says, "Wow, that's great soil. Look at the color." Put his hand in there, look at the structure. And "Okay, so what kind of soil do you think this is?" "Oh, this is a loam. This is just the most beautiful loam I've ever seen." And I went, "No, according to you last spring this was sand. And we haven't added any silt. We haven't added any clay." "Oh no, this is a beautiful loam soil. Look at the texture on this stuff." And he really truly thought that we had dug up all the sand out of that field and replaced it with a beautiful loam soil. When we sent the chemistry test in, and we showed him the only thing in this field was sand when it came to texture. It was again, 100% sand.

Brendan [00:45:56]: In other words, biology trumps everything.

Elaine [00:45:58]: Everything. You've gotta have the minerals there, so it's not like we can forget about that part.

Brendan [00:46:06]: So did all the minerals come from the sand?

Elaine [00:46:09]: I'm sure a lot of the minerals came from that organic matter, came from the compost, came from the teas that we were putting on. I don't care what percentage comes from which. Look at the yields that we've got, and that's really what we'd like to be doing for everybody. So here I have an example of some of the work that we do in landscape. So this is a neighborhood in Boston for example, and you can see where most of the yards are looking pretty peaked. They're really unhappy. You look at the lawn, and all of the grass is dormant. And the only thing that's actually growing are the weeds. All of the shrubs, all of the street trees are looking quite unhappy. It's all being attacked by diseases and pests, except for this yard back here. What's going on here? None of those trees have any insect diseases, whereas right across the street, sometimes the same species are looking really unhappy. Now this shrub is much happier, this is not diseased, how can that grass be this green in the middle of a drought? In Boston in this particular year you could not water your lawn except for I think once a week for x number of hours, and otherwise if you were watering your lawn outside that time you were gonna get a ticket. And so Peter said every night he would get up and he would go to the window and he could see the police car sitting over here.

Brendan [00:47:44]: They didn't believe that they weren't watering.

Elaine [00:47:46]: They did not water their lawn at all. There was not a single drop of irrigation water used, not sprinkled in any way because the root systems on these grasses and on the trees and the shrubs were going down deep into the soil and collecting all the water they needed. They didn't need to be irrigated in any way. No diseases and no pests. And again it was an application of really good compost the fall previous, but it was put on the surface of the soil because we didn't want to till up anything. We didn't want to till up your lawn or your trees or your veggies in the back or your shrubs, so everything went on the surface. In the springtime then 3 applications of the compost tea going onto everything, and that was it. By June we had everything balanced perfectly in this area, in Peter's lawn. So he never got a ticket, but he sure had the police out there. They were so ready, as soon as that irrigation water came on, but it never did.

Brendan [00:48:58]: And part of the reason it was not experiencing a drought on that lawn, would you say maybe the higher organic matter content, whereby I guess one gram of organic matter holds 8 grams of water or something like that?

Elaine [00:49:14]: It holds about its own weight in water basically.

Brendan [00:49:20]: Own weight, okay, maybe I got, yeah. So that lawn, for every 1% in carbon, organic matter, I need to get my terms straight, how much water holding capacity does it have per acre, let's say?

Elaine [00:49:36]: As we put the biology onto the surface, then any plant material that dies and is now decomposed by those organisms turns into organic matter. So you're constantly building the organic matter layers, way down deep into the soil, not just at the surface but all the way down and through. And so we may have put a ton of compost per acre, and when you think about the size of these urban lawns, we were putting on about 10 lbs of compost onto the lawn, and that was it.

Brendan [00:50:11]: Wow.

Elaine [00:50:12]: That doesn't sound like ...

Brendan [00:50:14]: It's the inoculation effect, it's not that you're importing the carbon; it's that you're inoculating the system to become more productive. And then carbon is being fixed from the atmosphere into plant matter, some of it sent, a lot of it sent down into the soil as sugar, that the organisms down there turn into complex carbon structures that persist as humus in the soil.

Elaine [00:50:37]: It's revving up the system. We just have to get the inoculum of the organisms, get them started, make sure that there is a food source to continue feeding them all the time. And this just redoubles and redoubles and redoubles. You don't have to do much work. If you balance the biology in your lawn really carefully you usually don't have to mow that much either. Which is something I've never understood with ChemLawn lawns, where they're out there pouring on the nitrogen fertilizer, so the grass grows faster so you have to mow more, so you have to put on more, it's just such a "more-on" system. Incredible to me. Let's work with Nature and not work so hard. Let her do the work.

Brendan [00:51:25]: Go ahead ... there's another thing you were gonna show?

Elaine [00:51:28]: So this is from Texas. The last example was Boston. Now let's move to Texas, kind of a bit drier. But the principles all hold exactly the same. You just have to understand that food web and how it works. The specific species of organisms in this part of the world are quite different. But they're performing the same functions. The bacteria perform the same functions, fungi the same functions, so that doesn't change. The specific species change. So this is some work on a pipeline. There's a gas pipeline that's now buried in this area that was dug up, and they completely dug up everything. It's a sugar sand, so it blows quite easily as soon as the wind starts blowing. In order to protect the surface and to get the grass growing again, they put on an application of Hydroseed. And you can see where all the Hydroseed has actually blown to. It's all down there, clogging the stream and making a mess. Because all of that nitrate that they put on with the Hydroseed material is now happily destroying the water quality in that stream down there. There's a little bit of the Hydroseed that's accumulated in the fence line, but the grass seed in there isn't growing. It's too piled up with that layer of Hydroseed. A little bit of the grass has started to grow. But this is right after the first rain. And look at what's happened with that first rain. It's already started to erode. You already have a significant amount of this material moving into the stream, once again. And you can see all the streams all the way along as suffering damage from us not understanding what we're doing when we're trying to reestablish systems. You need the biology in here. So the Sustainable Growth Texas group, headed by Betsy Ross, came out here and put on a 2" layer of compost, into which they'd already mixed the grass seeds in the system and had already applied the compost tea, and then just blew that compost onto the surface to a 2" depth. It didn't rain for several days. Finally it did rain and the seeds germinated very rapidly then. Absolutely no loss of the material because the organisms are holding it and sticking it all together. So 6 weeks after this picture was taken — because of course they put the compost on immediately after this picture was taken — so 6 weeks later, that's what it looked like. And of course, as soon …

Brendan [00:54:25]: Is that the slope from the stream?

Elaine [00:54:26]: I would like it if they would learn to take pictures from the same angle. And also they said, "This is where we took the picture." But the first one they took this way, the other one they took this way. So you can see that it's the pipeline, but you can see how well the grass has grown. And of course in Texas, if you've got grass growing, what are you gonna do with it? You're gonna put cattle on it. And that's what all the fencing is for, and that's what all the little pipelines are for. Until they had enough grass they could not have been concerned at all about bringing irrigation water out here. But as soon as you've got cattle going on here, they've got enough pipe to bring water out here for the animals to drink. So very rapidly it becomes a productive area. Now it's not all grass. It's not all big and little blue stem. It's not all the grama grass. There's a few weeds in here. But come in with another little application of the compost tea and get rid of the weeds going in that direction. I've got lots of examples. Do you want me to keep going?

Brendan [00:55:28]: You know what? I'm going to ask you for the South African tomato grower example. I would love to hear that one again because that one is astonishing too.

Elaine [00:55:39]: Yeah, I don't have the data with me for that one. I'm sorry. I do have a couple of other astonishing ones for you. This is some more pasture work. We went out and helped the person, well you can look at all the green pastures, those are the ones that have compost on them. This is his neighbor that has not had compost and they're using toxic chemicals to grow the grass or not grow the grass as the case may be.

Brendan [00:56:11]: Isn't it just a case of left side rain? (joking)

Elaine [00:56:17]: So it is kind of a version of that … because when the rain falls, where does the rain stay? Where does the rain infiltrate and stay in the soil? Well over here where you've got structure. This is purely compacted. You can see where they re-sowed this pasture on this side, and you can see that it's just hard, hard pan. Just the grass can't grow at all over here. So when rain does fall over here it just washes down the hill. But this is in April of 2011, and we had put compost back in October of 2010, which of course in Australia is the beginning of the growing season. So since November, they've actually been able to put their whole herd out and graze on this pasture 5 times.

Brendan [00:57:15]: 5 times, wow.

Elaine [00:57:16]: Five times through this season. That's basically like 1 and a half grazings every month. The person on this side, they put their sick cows out in this pasture once, and that's all it could take. And it's still looking this bad. This pasture was grazed 10 days previous to this picture. And look at how that grass grows. This is what we see.

Brendan [00:57:45]: It's like it could be grazed again almost.

Elaine [00:57:48]: Oh yeah, they could easily put their animals out there. Of course, they didn't have enough animals to go out and graze that much land, so they mowed a lot so that they could have hay for their animals throughout the winter, and of course they increased the size of their herd. So your choice on what you want to do when you have this kind of grass growth. This kind of grass growth has continued ever since. I've never had any of these folks come back to complain to me. We just work with more and more of the dairy farms in the area around Melbourne every year. I have lots and lots of pictures.

Brendan [00:58:26]: This really leads into the next question. Look at those long roots. I believe you have been working on measuring carbon deeper in soil than is normally measured. A lot of times the calculation is 30 cm deep, which is what a little over 10 inches, 11 inches, or is it 12? Anyhow you're looking at measuring far deeper than that so that we can have accurate calculations of the carbon sequestration potential of soil. Will you say something about that?

Elaine [00:59:03]: Yes, because it's like with this grass. This is normal grass that you would use to plant in your yard. It was planted as seed on July 15. We let the plants grow, and this is one of the plants from the plus really good biology. We mowed this to half an inch about 3 days before we took a 10" diameter PVC pipe. Pounded it down into the ground about 5 feet, pulled it up — we had to have some pretty big equipment to pull it back up — took the pvc pipe off, and then washed the surface so you could see the roots. And you can see Hendrikus Schraven, who's the person I did this work with. He's about a 6-and-a-half-foot-tall fellow, and he's holding that grass plant just a bit above his waist. So these roots are going down 4 and a half feet. So again, in 3 and a half months, our root systems are at 4 and a half feet. As time has gone by, the root systems on these grasses have gotten down to 25 feet.

Brendan [01:00:13]: Oh my goodness.

Elaine [01:00:14]: And of course, they're sloughing roots, they're putting off exudates, there's organic matter, there's organisms, so you turn this soil from light tan colored to that rich dark 70% cocoa chocolate color, and you're looking at sequestered carbon. All of it. This is what they mean by terra preta, not bio char. The rich organic material. Some of the work that has been worked on, we're showing that it goes from less than 2% organic matter up to somewhere around 10% organic matter, to 15-17% organic matter through the years, and it's just going to keep going.

Brendan [01:01:04]: What? And this is happening in what period of time?

Elaine [01:01:10]: Since 2002. Since 2002 this location has gone from 2% to 15-17% organic matter. You go back into the journals …

Brendan [01:01:22]: That's a percent a year. That's so far outside of the realm of normal contemplation by soil scientists, and even beyond what a lot of the people that are doing the best. Like Gabe Brown is getting over half a percent a year. Dave Johnson and his research is up to a little bit over half a percent a year. But a whole percent a year … what kind of system is this? I apologize for interrupting you, but I just wanted to clarify because this is mind-blowing, and this kind of thing needs to be documented and replicated, and everybody paying attention.

Elaine [01:02:00]: This is Hendrikus Schraven's compost basically, and he does a very good job of having the right sets of microorganisms in his compost, matching the balances of the bacteria and fungi to the crop that he's growing. So grass needs an equal biomass of fungi to bacteria. You've gotta have more than 10,000 protozoa per gram of soil. And you have to have somewhere around 50-100 beneficial nematodes growing in that soil. Very helpful if you can get earthworms and microarthropods as well. But it's because these root systems are going down deep into that soil and everything's supportive, one of the other, and these are increases in percent organic matter that go all the way down to 25 feet.

Brendan [01:02:56]: So you're measuring that level of organic matter all the way to that depth.

Elaine [01:02:59]: Yeah, we don't always get down that far because that's expensive to go out there with an augur and let it chew its way all the way down that deep. So we haven't done that that often. Or it's when we're digging a big pit we'll take some of this out. So it's a little bit wonky from a scientific point of view, but we are doing these things where very clearly percent organic matter is increasing massively. I look at some of the stuff that Dave Johnson is doing down at New Mexico State where he's showing increases in sequestered carbon, if I'm remembering — I'd have to go to Jimmy Sinton to get him to give me the actual data — but if I'm remembering correctly, they are increasing sequestered carbon by 1-2 tons a year. So right now he's getting 11 tons/acre.

Brendan [01:04:07]: Are we referring to David Johnson? I thought that was per hectare.

Elaine [01:04:09]: Yep, it could be per hectare.

Brendan [01:04:10]: If I recall, what he calls the "transitional" biologically enhanced agricultural management plots (BEAM for short), transitional plots are capturing 10.7 tons of carbon per hectare per year. And the more mature ones are capturing 19.2.

Elaine [01:04:36]: Very good. You remember the numbers better than I do.

Brendan [01:04:39]: Well I looked at it recently, but I'll never forget now because I have a frame of reference to put that in. And the frame of reference is we've got Colin Seis, having reported 9 tons of carbon. It's actually Dr. Christine Jones who reported that Colin Seis over a period of I think 11 years or something was averaging 9 tons per hectare per year with his production of some grain, some sheep, some grass, native grasses and harvesting the grass seeds.

Elaine [01:05:20]: But the work that Christine is doing — she's only gone down 30 centimeters. And remember that ...

Brendan [01:05:27]: So where's the other ... exactly, so many tons more. I hadn't thought of that. All these figures ... the comparisons are meaningless if I don't know what depth they were measuring to. But I'm real curious ...

Elaine [01:05:39]: Ah-huh. It's just again our perception is so influenced by the mythology about soil, where it only goes down as deep as you're tilling. Well, if you've got Mother Nature on your side we're going way deeper than that, and we can sequester so much more carbon.

Brendan [01:06:02]: It's like Back to the Future — "Where we're going there's no roads; where we're going, there's no tillage."

Elaine [01:06:09]: Hey that's a great line. So this is some of the information coming from our farm in California ...

Brendan [01:06:18]: Can I interrupt you for a moment before we go there? Can you say more about how that system was being managed, where you're growing soil to 17% carbon? We're gonna have to give this another context too, which is ... what do the mainstream soil scientists say is possible, something like 0.1% per year or something like that?

Elaine [01:06:38]: That's just silly.

Brendan [01:06:40]: It's like geologic almost inert soils, I don't know. We don't have to go there too much now. But what I want to do is learn quickly … is this being grazed? How is this being managed that these grasses are doing so much?

Elaine [01:06:58]: This is just getting mowed. This particular example from Hendrikus, was just being treated like someone's yard, mowed periodically.

Brendan [01:07:07]: And how often is this special compost or compost tea being applied?

Elaine [01:07:15]: The tea was applied once, and when the seed was planted and mixed into the soil, the compost was put on at the same time. So there's only been two applications of the proper biology in this system.

Brendan [01:07:31]: Are there other examples where a system has taken off like that and maintained this kind of momentum with just such a simple application? The management is kind of like mowing — I mean like grazing but not really — it's just mowing. You don't get all the dung and urine. But you are creating that …

Elaine [01:07:55]: Nutrient cycling is happening. And we're taking any residues of the dead plant material, and it's immediately being converted back into soil. It's just getting the biology into the system and making sure that it's active all the time. There have been a number of different places where we've done similar things. As I've said, our best plant growth is typically in 100% compost. So we do much better under those situations. We don't have to have the mineral component, although to get that organic matter, to get the compost, we had to have once upon a time, had the roots down to the mineral material to collect those minerals, those nutrients. So yeah, just production. Everything we're doing at the farm we are only doing the comparisons of plus biology, no biology, and comparing what the effect is of just adding biology in certain ways. This last year, just this summer, we have added in the conventional system where it will be tilled every year, and we'll be using inorganic fertilizers and pesticides if we need to use them so that we will have that comparison with what we're doing. We make certain that we always have the same amount of nutrients being added to the plus biology as compared to no biology systems. So those are equal. But you can see how much better the corn, for example, is growing where we've added biology as compared to where we have not added biology. Here we're putting the compost, and the applications go only on the surface. And we're watching how long it takes for the biology to rebuild soil structure. So this is where we tilled the soil first. This is the no-biology side. We do have understory plants that we're growing as best we can on this side. Corn in the back, a couple 3 rows, 4 rows, a couple rows of tomatoes, row of okra, a row of cucumber, a row of peppers, and then there were melons down here. So this is August, and you can see that the corn in this portion of this field was just heading out. Most of the plants were looking a little bit peaked. Just not enough nutrient cycling going on. And so if we would look across the center pathway we get to the plus biology side. You can see at this point that's the only difference. I'm going from the no added biology to this dirt, really, to adding all the biology and getting that biology up and going. So we're seeing that all of the corn is headed out. On the plus biology we were getting between 3-5 ears of corn on every stalk. On the no biology side, we only got one ear of corn on every stalk.

Brendan [01:11:30]: So a 5x yield bonus. The bonus part would be the 4.

Elaine [01:11:37]: Plus there are more tillers, and more of the plants survived. So everything was going much better. A lot more peppers. You can see the cucumbers You can't even see the tomatoes because they're so dense in there. And that's very typical of what we see with the added biology. Any plant material that falls to the surface of the soil is very rapidly converted back into soil. So the residues don't stay on that soil surface. This is the okra row, and you can see that even the understory plants aren't growing very well over here. Nutrient cycling is just non-existent. There are only bacteria in this soil, thank you to the people who owned the property before us who absolutely nuked this soil, turning it into dirt. That's really what we should call it. As opposed to here's the okra on the plus biology side, and you can see again the tomatoes and the cucumbers on that side. Just massive amounts of difference. Huge difference in weeds as well. So you can see a number of the different trials that we did, and this is how many minutes it took us to weed the no biology side. Most of the plants were actually weeds, not the crop that we were trying to grow. And then this is the plus biology side. Now just to make it kind of a fair comparison, before we started the weeding trial, we went out and completely removed all weeds from both the no biology and the plus biology sides of the field, and then two weeks later came back in and again weeded, but this time we measured the time it took for us to weed. I don't know anybody who wants to be spending 30 minutes weeding 20 foot rows areas versus 10. Which do you want to be doing? I like the kale, 65 minutes to weed that stupid bed, as opposed to only 5. The weeds don't grow where we get the biology back into the soil. So time and time again we have these kinds of results we're looking at. It's an organic system. They planted the swiss chard, and about the time the swiss chard was one or two leaves coming up, went in and applied compost tea. And this is one week later, the difference between the growth of the chard.

Brendan [01:14:17]: One week.

Elaine [01:14:18]: It just tells you how limited in nutrients this chard actually was in these organic fields. We need to be getting the biology back into the system.

Brendan [01:14:31]: Liberate the nutrients that are already there in the soil just waiting to be liberated by biology. It would be so easy for somebody to forget that and go "Oh yeah compost is bringing in nutrients. Well yeah it is bringing in some nutrients, but that's not the point."

Elaine [01:14:47]: They aren't plant-available nutrients most of them that are in the organic matter in a compost. You've got to have the biology, to again, pull those, decompose that plant material, turn it into bacteria and fungi, and then the bacteria and fungi being eaten by their predators, and *that's* what releases the plant-available nutrients. So one more example and then we should probably just finish your questions.

This is some work in Tasmania that we were doing with an onion grower. And he came to us because he'd been conventional. Well, his father before him had been conventional. He wanted to see what all the fuss about biology actually was. We put together a trial where one of his large paddocks, 150 hectares I believe, he put into the biological approach. In the fall, went out and applied compost, spread it over everything. Come springtime 3 applications of compost tea through the irrigation system. The pictures I'm gonna show you are right before the 3rd application of either compost tea to the field or the 3rd application of herbicide into his field. So he had all his other fields of conventional onions that we could then compare against. So I'm gonna show you first the onion field that was being maintained using all the standard conventional practices. So 2 applications of herbicides, and I don't remember what herbicide was being applied here, but it was a pretty nasty one. I look at this field and I go, "Where are the onions?" Can you find the onions out here? Only when you're looking straight on that row can you see the onions. Otherwise it's like, "Aw man, look at the weeds in there." It's just unbelievable. He's gotta go out there and put on a 3rd application of that herbicide because otherwise he's not gonna be growing onions; he's gonna be growing thistle. That's the kind of weed pressure, and that's in a field that's been treated twice with herbicides. So now let's take a look at the onion field treated with the compost tea. And our onion field is just right over there. See any weeds? And that's what happens when you shift the biology so that the form of nitrogen present in the soil is not something that the weeds can use. There is one weed in this picture, you can find it. It's like Where's Waldo? Can you find it? It's right there, and that's it. Otherwise, and look at the fact that the onions are growing better here. This was planted on the same day as this. Same seed, same everything, but this had the compost and two applications of compost tea before this picture was taken. Just to show you that it's not just the one part of the field that was good, it was the whole entire field that the weeds were just gone. When we take a closeup, this is back in the conventional field, look at all those weeds. Scary. This is one of the little onion seedlings, it's only about 2.5-3 inches tall. The root system is shorter than the above ground part of the plant. And you can already see the attack by the disease-causing fungi. So this poor little seedling is gonna have to be treated with a fungicide if you wanna make a crop. You've gotta be putting out all these toxic chemicals. Or why not, from the very beginning, put out the proper biology? And so this we have to back away and see that we're not nearly as close on the pitchfork. These seedlings are already at about 5-6 inches tall. And the root systems on those plants are a foot and a half down into the ground. Look at the structure already being formed in this field. Lots of oxygen, very easy for the roots to grow down. All the nutrients are coming back into the onions. And so this guy was so happy with this. He made a boatload on this, plus if he played his cards right, he'd be able to convert to organic pretty rapidly.

Brendan [01:19:43]: That's a big deal.

Elaine [01:19:48]: Got lots of examples. Ukraine with . . .

Brendan [01:19:55]: I'm curious if we have anything that we could look at quickly showing different nutrient content in foods grown on ...

Elaine [01:20:04]: I don't have that information. Because I've often gone to nutritionists and asked, "OK, what are the nutrients that we should be looking at in different kinds of crops? So if we were gonna go to grapes, what are the nutrients that should be in a grape? What specifically should we be looking for in grapes?" Because I don't want to do the total nitrogen, the total phosphorous, total magnesium, because every plant has to have the same amount of those nutrients in them in order to grow. So quite often we come up with no real significant difference when we're looking at total nutrients. That's not what you need to know. You wanna know the amount of nitrogen that's in protein. That's what you and I as human beings need to have. And so we need to be asking questions about amino acids and proteins, not total nitrogen. Total phosphorous, your body's not gonna take that up. It's the phosphate that's attached to the organic compounds, and now your biome in your digestive system is going to do the conversions to make that material easily taken up across your digestive system. So if you're just pouring a bunch of inorganic PO_4 into your digestive tract, that's not gonna help you. That's not what human beings eat. We need it in the form of organic compounds. And that's what we're gonna take up. So when we're looking at onions, what precisely are the nutrient forms that human beings get from onions? That's what I want to be measuring.

Brendan [01:21:53]: Don't onions carry a good amount of selenium if it's being made available?

Elaine [01:21:59]: Yep.

Brendan [01:21:59]: I think basically onions and garlic are a good source of selenium. That's what I think we should be looking at is the trace minerals. Because that's one of the most important things that we get from our food is the trace minerals. The trace minerals are in part what enable plants to produce phytonutrients, I believe, and we need those minerals to do our own little enzymatic things and our livers to detoxify all the other herbicides and biocides.

Elaine [01:22:31]: What I want to know is what exactly is the form of selenium that we have to have in our digestive tracts to take up into our bodies. It's not the total selenium. I don't care about that portion of the total selenium pool that might be in a plant that is incapable of being pulled into our bodies as nutrients. So what are the right forms? I'm going to be going to a very interesting conference in Boston the end of November, where talking with Dan Kittredge, he is developing a hand-held UV.

Brendan [01:23:15]: Yes, I've interviewed him also for this event, and we'll be doing other interviews.

Elaine [01:23:26]: And I'm so looking forward to that, if it can actually be measuring something that is actually a useful nutrient for human beings. That's what we need to know.

Brendan [01:23:35]: I can't resist going back to that 17% soil carbon, for one last question on that, then we'll wrap up soon. Is anybody trying to replicate this in an academic research setting? Any of your students, anybody at all? And if not, why not?

Elaine [01:24:00]: We have a lot of disbelievers in the academic world.

Brendan [01:24:03]: That's why I'm asking the question. We need someone, more than one person, to be replicating this and figuring out, you know is there variability in being able to create this effect, and how do we do it and also make sure that there's enough evidence to drown out the doubt.

Elaine [01:24:26]: Yeah, and I'm not aware of anyone that is doing this kind of work, these kinds of tests at university. The people I know are still stuck on total nutrients. Total nitrogen, total phosphorous, total whatever, and that's not the information that we need to know.

Brendan [01:24:48]: Well I'm referring to the carbon part. I mean total carbon is what my focus is on in this example.

Elaine [01:24:53]: The only person I know that is really investigating that is David Johnson at New Mexico State.

Brendan [01:25:02]: Do you have a hypothesis why he's not producing a 1% a year increase? I mean he's doing great … he's still 40-50 times higher than …

Elaine [01:25:13]: Because his biology is still in transition. He hasn't gotten the organisms up to where I would like to see them. So he's starting, he's moving in the right direction. And I think as he's getting a more and more mature food web that's matching the requirements of the plants he's growing. That's where he's seeing these increases. He's still got that variability for that very reason. It's not yet the complex food web that he needs to have to be making boatloads of really good humics and fulvics and complex organic material.

Brendan [01:25:55]: I do think I saw once he said that he sees the potential of an even higher carbon fixation, closer to 30 tons / hectare per year. I could be wrong so I don't want to be quoted on that.

Elaine [01:26:10]: Yeah. You wanna get David on and have him say that.

Brendan [01:26:17]: But that would put it up starting to get close to 1% per year, it'd be like .75% or something.

Elaine [01:26:25]: And I just think we know so little about soil. Think about the ecological monograph; it was published in 1985, and that was the first time when most soil scientists or agronomists, if they cared to listen, discovered that bacteria and fungi and protozoa and nematodes actually do things for plants. And that this is how Mother Nature has been doing nutrient cycling for the last 3.5 billion years. We have only begun to understand this.

Brendan [01:27:06]: It is such a joy to actually see the magic happen. You know something that's really unique about you, Dr. Ingham, is that you've actually created a way for people to learn how to do what you do. I'm referring to the Life in the Soil classes, and the certification to become a soil consultant. I'm wondering if you could just briefly describe the classes, the certification, and what that would enable a student to do.

Elaine [01:27:33]: Basically, we have online courses that you sign up for, we give you a password and you get that password for a year, and so during that year we want you to go through the basic theoretical underpinnings of why the Soil Food Web works. I went over a fair amount of it earlier in this talk. So I think it's like 24 lectures on life in the soil and who and what are bacteria, fungi, protozoa, nematodes, how do they interact, microarthropods, earthworms, in different climates, how do you measure it? How do you go about doing the measurements on the biology? And then the next class is a class on how to make compost. We go through thermal compost and worm compost and a tiny little bit on static compost because I have the attitude that you'd better get really good at making thermal compost before you make static compost. That's the one where most people mess up in a very showy way. As in blowing all the windows for a mile radius in your town or county, and people end up letting you have lawsuits. So really think you need to do the thermal compost.

Brendan [01:28:57]: In other words, going anaerobic and producing hydrogen sulfide ...

Elaine [01:29:02]: And alcohol, and what's the heat of combustion, the temperature that alcohol goes boom spontaneously? Yeah. So thermal compost has ... you gotta know what you're doing ... but static compost is something that sneaks up on people really badly.

Brendan [01:29:22]: Are we talking about David Johnson's style of static composting?

Elaine [01:29:26]: No, he does kind of a merge of the thermal versus static. It's static only as long as you're still taking the temperatures and monitoring that, but you can cool the compost fairly easily with the pipe system that he has. And we've adapted some of that for when you misjudge your high-nitrogen containing material and your compost pile starts heading for 175, 178, and hundred and "Oh no!" It's time to dig a few pipes and punch a few holes in your compost pile, maybe add a little bit of cold water and calm things down. So a class on making compost. A class on making compost extract and compost teas, and of course that comes after the compost because of course you have to make good compost before you can make a good compost tea or extract. And then the next class is the microscope, where we teach you how to use a small shadowing microscope so you can do the measurements on all of these organisms. The quick and dirty way, or the let's be more scientific and quantify everything. A scientist tends to get stuck on the let's quantify everything, and your average grower is gonna do quick and dirty. Let's just get an idea, "Do I have lots of bacteria?" or "Well you know, there's some in here," or "Oops! Nothing." "Lots of fungi," or "Not bad, or "Mmm oops." Same thing for protozoa and nematodes. Quantitative versus more just seat of your pants, and it really depends on what you're trying to do, which version you're going to actually do all the time. Or maybe jump back and forth as you need. So once you do all of the classes, and we require that you pass the quizzes with a cumulative total of 90% or better because it's open book really. If you fail the quizzes you really were not paying attention, so please go back and listen again and again until you get it all figured out. Then after that if you wanna go off onto your own farm and use what you've learned, fine that works. For people who want to go on and do consulting and teaching other people, we ask then that you join the certification program. The certification program is basically that you have to learn how to make really good compost yourself. So we require that you make, sequentially make, 3 compost piles and you start with the standard percentages of high nitrogen green and woody material going into the pile and then you start altering that recipe. By the time you've made your third pile, you should pretty well have a very good understanding of how to make good compost. Usually it only takes people about that long. And once you've made good compost, we're asking that you would make 3 compost teas, 3 compost extracts, again learning one after the other, you learn what you did wrong with #1, then you try what you think needs to be changed in recipe #2, and then you try to get even closer to everything figured out after the third. And so we ask that you have an advisor that carries you through the program. And you compare your counts of the microorganisms with your advisor. So we know that you're getting up to speed on the microscope. And then the final step is to take a piece of land and convert that dirt back into soil. You're going to choose a plant, you're going to do all the measurements that you need to do to start a process out, measuring along the way, ever improving that biology until you can convert that dirt back into soil and end up with really good yields.

Brendan [01:33:53]: Awesome, and this is found at lifeinthesoilclasses.com? (now at https://www.soilfoodweb.com/)

Elaine [01:33:59]: Right or you can go to environmentcelebration.com that also gets you to the classes as well (now at https://www.soilfoodweb.com/). And then of course my website which is soilfoodweb.com the links are also on my website so you can get to them from my website as well.

Brendan [01:34:18]: Great. Well Dr. Ingham, I really appreciate how you bring the topic of soil to life and make it fun and interesting and even exciting. Also thank you for your groundbreaking research, your planet-saving research, your brilliant innovations in composting, and other things, and all-around tireless leadership in restoring sanity in soil, the soil that's so important to every being on the planet.

Elaine [01:34:54]: The faster we can get this information out to everybody, the better it's gonna be. The sooner we can get back to a sane food production system.

Brendan [01:35:08]: On behalf of myself and the Eat4Earth community and the Earth herself, thank you very much for being here today.

Elaine [01:35:17]: Thank you very much for letting me have a forum to talk in. This has been great, thanks!

Brendan [01:35:25]: The biggest takeaway that I want you to have from this presentation by Elaine is that soil is SO renewable if we just know how to revive it. And this is very different from what typical soil scientists tell you. Normally they're coming from a geological perspective, and they see soil progressing on a certain average amount of growth in organic carbon each year. And so they say, you know, it takes a thousand years to build a centimeter of soil, something like that. But Elaine Ingham is a decades-long veteran of soil research; she's one of the co-originators of the whole Soil Food Web concept and the knowledge that these soil organisms are there and doing very important things for the entire ecosystem, for the plants. And the only thing that would hold us back from being able to rebuild soil at a fast rate is thinking that it can't be done and applying chemical fertilizers and all of the rest of it that kills the soil organisms. But what she's able to do and she's done this for hundreds of clients -- I've seen many of her case studies -- he's been able to grow soil very quickly and bring businesses back to life that were just about to have to give up on their soil and got golf courses to detoxify and stop using toxic chemicals. And now they're using compost teas, and now they have fantastic weed-free golf greens that are non-toxic. The one fact I'd love you to remember here and compare this to what you hear out there — because this is supposed to be impossible — one of her students was able to build organic carbon one percent per year for years, and it was only a lawn that was getting mowed. That is very significant. It's quite an achievement to do one fourth that amount, or one fifth. So the issue here is we can rebuild soils and capture carbon at much faster rates than the mainstream realizes. And this is very parallel and analogous to the fact that the mainstream doesn't believe you can heal cancer, doesn't believe you can reverse heart disease and stuff like that. The body is very resilient. Soil is very resilient. We just have to know how Nature works and work with Nature instead of against it. So that's what I wanted you to realize, that this is a presentation you should listen to again if you feel like you want to understand soil better because ultimately it is the most important thing that empowers everything that is important to you. Glad you could be here. That was a very long interview and a very long outro (laughing), so thank you for being here.

Day 2: Our Oceans In Peril and the Food Solution

Shocking News About Our Oceans That We Cannot Afford to Ignore
Reese Halter, PhD
What You Will Discover

- How warming and acidifying oceans are killing the organism that produces almost 2/3 of our
- Why some scientists predict that in 2040 the oceans could be lifeless

Why Oceans Are the #1 Environmental Issue of Our Time, and Healing Our Oceans with Regenerative Agriculture
John Roulac
What You Will Discover

- Why we most move from "sustainable" to "regenerative"
- Why John gives the environmental movement an "F" for communication on the climate change issue
- Why plant-based burgers are a misguided solution to factory-farmed meat and its contribution to climate change

The Real Cause of Climate Change, The True Cure, Plus a 9X Increase of Nutrients in Our Food
Walter Jehne
What You Will Discover

- How carbon dioxide became the focus of climate change models when water is in fact responsible for 95% of climate dynamics
- Why the most important variable in global warming is governed by plant cover yet has more to do with water than carbon dioxide
- The 10 hydrological processes that provide 10 ways to reverse climate change
- How rebuilding the "soil carbon sponge" can draw down 20 Gigatons of carbon per year, safely and profitably, while producing more and better food

Food Solutions to Climate Change from Project Drawdown
Eric Toensmeier
What You Will Discover

- How Project Drawdown determines the potential of various solutions to climate change
- How various forms of planet-friendly agriculture rank as "drawdown" solutions to climate change
- Why these rankings could vastly under-estimate their potential and true rank

Minerals, Microbes, and Reversing Climate Change in a Golden Era for Food
Graeme Sait
What You Will Discover

- Why some fruits and vegetables have almost no nutrition in them
- How to manage minerals, microbes, and plants to grow highly nutrient-rich foods and eliminate pest problems
- How soil organic matter was determined by Australia's scientific research agency to be the #1 determinant of farm profitability
- How increasing organic matter by just 1.6% in global soils could reverse climate change
- Exciting new methods for regenerating dead soils and growing soil organic matter faster than ever

Reese Halter Interview
Shocking News About Our Oceans That We Cannot Afford to Ignore

Brendan [00:00:00]: Welcome to the Eat4Earth event. We're exploring how you can heal yourself, your loved ones and the planet with food. This is Brendan Moorhead and it's vital that we listen closely to what our next guest Dr. Reese Halter has to tell us. Dr. Reese Halter is an eco-stress physiologist specializing in Earth's life-support systems, and he received his PhD from the University of Melbourne Australia in eco-stress tree physiology. Dr. Halter's passion for the environment is life-long, and he's sometimes referred to as Dr. Earth. He's a powerful voice for bees, trees, and seas, nature's wellness plans, and saving Nature now. Dr. Halter is a distinguished conservation biologist, an award-winning broadcaster and prolific writer. His articles appear in publications like Ecowatch, Organic Magazine, Organic Gardener, Huffington Post, and Malibu Times. He is also a go-to expert for the Australian Broadcasting Corporation Dr. Halter has two essential books coming out soon entitled *Save Nature Now* and *Love Nature*. Dr. Halter thank you so much for being with us today.

Dr. Halter [00:01:04]: Yeah, I'm stoked.

Brendan [00:01:07]: Awesome, Dr. Halter, you have your finger on the pulse of the planet, and you're monitoring one of the most urgent symptoms of Earth's dire condition and the forests, the oceans, the bees that deliver essential blessings for our life on this planet are quickly dying. And as they disappear, our own existence is at stake. And this relates directly to how we grow food. It seems to me that the greatest threat of all is what climate change is doing to our oceans. Can you help us understand what is happening to the oceans and what this means for us?

Dr. Halter [00:01:41]: Sure I can. Basically, Brendan, the situation is this. The oceans although they cover over 70% of the face of the earth— they encompass more than 95% of the biosphere or living parts of planet Earth that can host life— and as we have burned fossil fuels since the mid-1700s, approximately 93 percent of all the heat from coal, oil, gas has accumulated in our oceans. That is 300 zettajoules of energy. The oceans are boiling. As a matter of fact, since 1997 the oceans have quadrupled in heat. So what that means for the average person is that the oceans drive our climate and where we are today is we're spoiled in many respects because we depend on regular seasons and seasonal rain that gives us our food, and we are now into what we call climate instability where we can't predict nearly as well as we could have 20 or 30 or 50 years ago the patterns of moisture and more importantly in some areas the incidence of drought and heatwave. The lengths of heat waves are increasing as the temperature increases and that definitely impinges upon crop yield.

Brendan [00:03:29]: And it seems to me that we've got something brewing in the ocean ecosystems itself, themselves that is pretty serious. I believe you've spoken about that before. Can you tell us what's going on with the actual organisms in our oceans?

Dr. Halter [00:03:46]: Well, yeah, I mean as a part of the ocean broiling with heat, they're becoming deoxygenated at a stunning rate. The National Atmospheric Lab in Boulder has made a prediction the year before last that by 2030 large swaths of the Pacific Ocean, including along our west coast and Hawaii, will be missing extreme amounts of oxygen. In other words when the fish or whales or turtles or sea lions come into these regions, they will be suffocated. This is, I mean this is an epic, epic symptom of a warming planet which holds less oxygen in the water. And if that isn't disturbing enough, and it's shocking, frighteningly shocking, as the oceans have digested more carbon dioxide they become acidic. The by-product from the phytoplankton absorbing more CO_2 is a carbonic acid, and that is also a frightening omen because anything made of calcium carbonate— coral reef, shellfish - melt under acidic conditions— and already we've got pteropods, tiny free-swimming little snails along the west coast of America that are showing signs of melting. 54% of them tested by NOAA have begun to melt. The oceans have increased in acidity by 30% over the last half century. It's unprecedented. So we've got less oxygen, and we've got increased acidity, and we've got rising temperatures, and all the critters now pole to pole, equator to pole, they're in such strife that they're migrating as much as five to ten degrees latitude towards either pole in search of cooler waters and in search of food. Everything in the ocean is scurrying for food. It's heart breaking, Brendan.

Brendan [00:06:42]: When you said "melting", are you referring to the exoskeletons dissolving in the water because they're made of calcium carbonate, and then the increased acidity causes them to essentially … I mean they look like they're melting, but they're dissolving.

Dr. Halter [00:07:05]; They're dissolving. I call it "melting", but …

Brendan [00:07:07]: Yeah, might as well …

Dr. Halter [00:07:08]: They're dissolving, their shells now. If you're a lobster, you're any other shellfish, or you're anything along the seashore, the intertidal zone or the coral reefs, you're in terrible trouble. Already we estimate that over 50% of all coral reefs on planet earth, have died or dead, and the coral reefs are home to over a million different kinds of organisms. Up to 30% of all sea life depends upon the coral reefs whether they actually live there year-round or go there to nurse as the cetaceans— the whales, dolphins and porpoises or sharks. They use the coral reefs as nursery grounds and these are glaring symptoms of the climate crisis. And instead of pretending like an addict … addicts, by the way, always pretend that nothing is wrong. When an addict looks … well seriously when an addict looks in a mirror and says "OMG," puts his hand up or her hand up as though they're bobbing in the sea. There are a number of solutions. Our society, parts of our society, are refusing to accept that we are in a crisis. And this is a catastrophe, and it's not getting better. Hello!?

Brendan [00:08:58]: Yeah, and this is hitting us in so many ways. You mentioned that obviously the changes in water cycles are predicted to seriously impact to our food production. I actually think that this, the crisis in the ocean is even more urgent given what's happening with phytoplankton. Do you have any latest data on what's happening with phytoplankton which of course are pretty … I guess there's a base of about 95 percent of the marine food chain. Is that about right?

Dr. Halter [00:09:32]: Yeah, absolutely. The phytoplankton is an extraordinary green plush mat that, that is all … it's ubiquitous. It's in every ocean; it's in every sea. And in the green plush mat we have tiny little critters—

they're called zooplankton— and, by the way, we have most of all of the little eggs, and larvae, most, not all, but most of a vast array of sea life. So it provides what we call a security cover. It also provides the base of the food chain because as the listeners can appreciate when there are small … when there are eggs or fry or larvae of course you're going to get the predators, and it goes all the way to apex predators follow, so at the top of the food chain. What we've seen since the 1950s as the oceans have warmed you see, the cold currents that rise to the surface; they upwell; and they carry particularly iron and nitrogen that are the fertilizer for the phytoplankton. They have in some cases stopped altogether rising, and as a result we are missing in excess of 40 percent of all the phytoplankton in the ocean. Now, the listeners might be thinking, "Aw, you know, that's the ocean. I live in inland. It's no big deal." It's an enormous deal, Brendan, because each of us, the 7.5 billion procreating human race, we rely on the phytoplankton and a blue-green bacteria called *Prochlorococcus* that is amongst the phytoplankton for almost 2 out of every 3 breaths of oxygen. The phytoplankton gives us the air we breathe, and we're missing 40% of the plants and bacteria that give us our air. And as a result my colleagues at Scripps Institute of Oceanography at the University of California San Diego … they have been diligently measuring oxygen content, molecular oxygen content in the oceans and the Pacific Ocean off La Jolla, which is just before San Diego, a stone's throw away from Los Angeles in a way, and in the southern hemisphere on the northwest tip of Tasmania, the island state of Australia, and they have found that since the late 1980s that we are losing at least 19 molecules of oxygen each year. So approximately— per million molecules of oxygen— we've lost more than 600 molecules of oxygen. Now, it's not enough during the day thankfully to disrupt us, but we do know that if you have a sleeping issue, and there are over 70 million Americans who have a sleeping issue, that removing oxygen from our atmosphere is a problem, and it cuts into our sleep pattern. And see, my colleagues at Scripps, 100% ascribe the missing oxygen to burning fossil fuels. Now I would be remiss since we're talking of the oceans not to mention one of the most serious byproducts of burning coal each year is the release of mercury vapor that turns into methyl mercury, a sticky form of mercury, and the oceans have increased in mercury poisoning over the last 40 years by three times. There's well over 80 thousand metric tons of mercury poisoning in the oceans, and it's not just the oceans. We now see mercury turning up in forests, in soils, in creek water, in trees and wildlife. Mercury, for those that are unaware, attacks the central nervous system, it discombobulates it, and it renders humans, insects and wildlife in a shocking condition. It's a debilitating dangerous and eventually life ending poison.

Brendan [00:15:07]: This situation is obviously impacting us in so many ways, and I had heard recently that Scripps came out with a new report. and I don't recall what it was. I think it's different than what you just described. It's new information, not addressing the oxygen part of the situation but something else. Do you know of what I might be referring to?

Dr. Halter [00:15:34]: I mean Scripps is an enormous Institute likely another … I don't follow every press release they issue.

Brendan [00:15:46]: Sure, okay. You know, you mentioned that a lot of forms of life in the ocean are scurrying for food. And I have to imagine one of those is our beloved cetaceans, the whales, dolphins.

Dr. Halter [00:16:06]: Oh, yeah!

Brendan [00:16:07]: And what's happening with them right now?

Dr. Halter [00:16:08]: Well, the whales, dolphins and porpoises are in terrible state. First of all, we've massacred over 5 million whales, and none of their populations have rebounded. We massacred tens of millions of dolphins and porpoises, and they're our brethren! These are extra ordinarily intelligent mammals, and they play a vital role in the ocean because they're the farmers of the sea. So their flocculant fecal plumes— or their feces— is rich in iron and nitrogen. And they alone are attempting to fertilize the ocean and help regrow the missing 40% plus phytoplankton that the fossil fuels have killed. And they are in a shocking state because around planet Earth there's never been more of these seismic surveys for more oil and gas. And let me expand on what a seismic survey is. Seismic surveys release 252 decibels of a blast every 10 seconds, non-stop 24/7 for weeks and sometimes months on end. They're dragged behind these boats up to 40 at a time, and they go back over the water like a lawnmower follows a line and cuts the grass, and they go back and forth and back. This sound deafens all the cetaceans. A deaf whale is a dead whale, and it's not just the cetaceans that are dying from these horrid shocks of sound. It's everything in the phytoplankton. My colleagues at the University of Western Australia earlier this year did a global survey, and what they found is anywhere there are seismic surveys for oil and gas, all the larvae and all of the eggs and anything close by in the remaining phytoplankton is smashed to smithereens. And I guess, you know, at the end of the day, Brendan— and I'm sure most of the listeners can appreciate this— the answer is very elemental. Take the 5.3 trillion dollars globally annually handed to oil, gas fracking and coal as subsidies; take it away. If these industries are so mighty, so great, so benevolent—not, not and not— why do they need subsidized five point three trillion dollars to kill our planet. Why? And the answer is that they don't.

Brendan [00:19:51]: It doesn't make sense, yeah.

Dr. Halter [00:19:52]: It's corruption.

Brendan [00:19:54]: Yup. You mentioned previously in another conversation what's going on with the whales' food supply till you started to touch on it, and it's just heartbreaking. What's happening with the whales as far as, I mean so many of the whales are baleen whales. Their food source ... is the phytoplankton.

Dr. Halter [00:20:17]: Yeah, yeah, and so what we're seeing is a couple of things ...

Brendan [00:20:21]: ... or more broadly the zooplankton. The plant forms and the animal forms in the plankton world.

Dr. Halter [00:20:28]: Yeah, yeah, and another terrible symptom of the climate in crisis, what we're seeing with warming oceans that we've never ... it's unprecedented ... we've never seen this ... the amount of algal bloom. So warm water is growing these algal blooms. In the algal blooms they are rich with demoic acid, a very potent nerve poison and saxitoxin which poison the shellfish. What we're seeing, and what we've seen particularly with the baleen, the filter-feeding whales ... these are whales that take a mouthful the size of a large swimming pool and they expel the water through a gorgeous cartilage that hangs from the upper jaw like a sieve, right, and they expel it, and the sieve catches all of the little creatures, tiny fish. Often they're after krill. There are 80 kinds of krill. They're very small miniature lobsters really, but they're very rich in omega-3 and omega-6 and omega-9 which means they pack an amazing caloric punch for the baleen whales.

What we're seeing, and what we've seen, are these unbelievable mass strandings. We lost … by number, I think it's close to three … it's in excess of 300 Sei Whales two years ago. They're approximately the fourth biggest baleen whale. We lost over 300 of them on a remote shore of Patagonia in Chile. And what happened to those poor creatures (is) they ate a bunch of squat lobsters. The squat lobsters were loaded with demoic acid from an algal bloom, and in Nature as apex predators eat, whatever they're eating has the potential to bio-magnify up the food chain in some cases many millions of times. So if it's a poison it's obviously deadly, and it killed these … I believe there were 331 but too many numbers in my brain, but over 300 Sei Whales. It was the largest mass stranding of big whales we'd ever seen, and man-made global warming irrefutably killed these animals.

Again, these are symptoms of what we're doing, and if we look more specifically at the krill, the southern ocean is the biggest body of water, unencumbered water, on the globe. And my colleagues from Australia each year follow the baleen humpbacks and blues and minkes and the southern ocean right whales. They follow them down to the Antarctic. The way that these creatures have evolved, it's truly a feast and a famine situation. During the summer, they go down to the polar waters in the southern hemisphere. The same is applicable in the northern hemisphere. They go up to the Arctic. But we're talking about the southern hemisphere. They go down to the southern ocean, and they feed sometimes for twenty, twenty-one hours a day, remembering that in the southern ocean during summer, there's almost 24 hours light. In fact, in many parts, it is 24 hours of light, and the animals, the mammals feed, the whales feed, and they pack on megatons, and they store it as blubber. And then they head north to the warm waters, whether it's the Great Barrier Reef, whether on the east coast or the Ningaloo reef on the west coast, and that's where they calve. And the mothers have to have an immense reserve of blubber because the calves being mammals require milk, and the milk is a huge caloric drop. The only way these animals can survive is if they consume megatons of krill.

The krill are another example of an animal that has been shortchanged in a warming world. Their populations have crashed up to 80% in West Antarctica because of both missing sea ice … the krill, although they're very small perhaps quarter maybe even a half an inch long, they can live for up to eight years. It's incredible that a little creature can make it, but in Nature it's getting through the first winter that is the very hardest gig of their lives. In order to do that they require sea ice because the sea ice has both bacteria and phytoplankton, a little bit of algae under there, that's their food source. Missing ice, krill have … when you're in Nature, when you lose your habitat you die. And on top of that we have an insatiable fishery that is wiping out all of the remaining krill. And for those people who believe that eating fish oil is the answer to their illustrious lives, you need to wake up because the krill and the fish oil is full of methyl mercury. And also the krill is whale food. We need the whales to farm the sea, and if you're looking for a magus, please look no further than hemp seed. It's loaded with your omegas. It'll lift you to your next level of wherever you're attempting to get, and you don't have to eat the whale food. So I'm very bullish on leaving the fish oil for the whales, please.

Brendan [00:27:43]: You know, I'll give a little plug for our friend John Roulac and his company Nutivia. He's been a leader in promoting hemp-based foods, and he provides hemp seeds as one of the Nutiva products.

Really good stuff. You know, you mentioned that one of the problems with the food supply for the whales is, is the buildup of these algal toxins in their feed supply because of the blooms that we're generating by heating up the oceans, both through our fossil fuel emissions, and I should mention that there are numerous studies that tag the emissions from our agricultural sources and land use management at a similar level or even higher than the fossil fuels in some cases, depending on how they're looking at it. Anywhere from 30 to 50 percent from how we're oxidizing the soils with too much plowing, all these chemicals, and also burning down forests, cutting down forests, burning sugarcane fields. All of this. So much going up into the atmosphere. Thirty to fifty percent of all of our emissions from land use, including agriculture. And there's something else happening with agriculture you mentioned bioaccumulation. Whatever toxin it is, they tend to be fat-soluble and bio-accumulate in fatty tissues. And of course, the incredibly nutritious forms of sea life are very rich in really, really healthy fatty acids for us, for whales and so forth, and what I want to know is what else is happening, what else is bio-accumulating that's coming from agriculture?

Dr. Halter [00:29:28]: Well, the latest concern that I am aware of, that I've been following say for the last 10 years, banging every pot I own or can borrow a pot to bang, are these wretched neonicotinoids, and we had a heck of a win yesterday. The European Union, and the UK, surprisingly but thankfully, has joined them … they're going to be banning all of these poisons. They're an insecticide, neonicotinoids, they're abbreviated neo-NIC. They're are systemic poisons in many cases, meaning that these chemicals are not sprayed like the traditional crop-dusting model that some may be aware of. Rather, their seeds are dunked in these very powerful poisons, and they are, they attack the central nervous system and they render at … a tick over a dozen parts per billion. The bees lose their minds, and they shake to death. And the poisons move in the plants when they're dunked— many of them, the seeds are dunked— so the plant recognizes that they're poison and it pushes the poisons through their nectar. The bees are attracted to the flower and its nectar because the nectar they take and dehydrate to turn to honey. And the bees also collect plant pollen because that's their only source of protein to feed to the young larvae.

The protein in the bee world just like in the human world builds brains and strong autoimmune systems. And pound-for-pound bees, and a bee neuron, just like a human neuron, or an elephant neuron, or an Orca neuron, pound-for-pound they are identical. The difference in animals is but a degree in the placement and assembling, assemblage in the brain, but the neurons are absolutely dead equal. So the bees are very intelligent, highly intelligent creatures but these neonicotinoids are not just killing the bees. When the flowers dry, after they have pollinated, the flowers desiccate or dry, and they fall onto the ground. The neonicotinoids are then introduced into the soil, and in the soil they kill the soil fauna, and it ripples through the ecosystem where the songbirds and ground birds that feed on all of the billions of different forms of life in the soil, their food. There's no food for them; their populations are down. And by the way, the listeners need to be aware … we're missing a billion and a half birds in North America alone. And it's not just the song birds or the meadow birds. It goes up the food chain to the goshawks and the avian predators. Their numbers are down.

These poisons are hideous. We've been pounding a couple billion pounds of neonicotinoids into the biosphere for the last 15 plus years. And it looks very promising that all of Europe or the European Union nonetheless will back off a hundred percent on these poisons. And that, Brendan, is the biggest win we can really all hope for because these poisons render the soil infertile for up to a decade. And my colleague, Christie Morrissey, at the University of Saskatchewan, has documented 44% of all the fresh waterways in her study in Western Canada are contaminated with these neonics, which can hang around for up to a decade. So we have to be very, very careful. Rachel Carson, bless her, more than 50 years ago reminded us that the technology in chemistry, for chemicals, was far greater than what Nature could contend with fifty-five or sixty years ago. And fast forward to today, it's out of control. So we now know that … by the way, six continents … seventy five percent of all honey sample contains neonicotinoids, and tap water in Iowa has got neonicotinoids in it. We have to be really, really careful with these poisons.

Brendan [00:35:10]: Especially … even if we're totally self-centered, these honey bees, this one pollinator among many, many, many of them that I'm sure are being affected by these poisons … and I think it's 70% of our food supply is pollinated just by the honeybee, or is it by all pollinators?

Dr. Halter [00:35:32]: Well, all the pollinators, the bees are incredible, and by the way, the main reason that the EU has come to this excellent conclusion … there was a long-term study in Germany, and they showed that in Nature reserves all insects were down almost 80 percent because of the accumulation of these neonics in the soils and in the biosphere, everything, and we need the insects.

The insects are food for the birds; the insects are food for some mammals and everything in Nature is time-tested. So, when we look today at a forest or a prairie or a coral reef, it's really important that we understand that that's the end process of 1.1 billion years of evolution; it's time tested and everything in Nature has a very specific role. And when, as you say, when we remove this and remove that, ecosystems unravel. And we need Nature. Nature is our best friend. Nature makes up the life-support systems on our planet, and it's now a matter of working with Nature, not against Nature. And there are thousands of great companies that understand this. There's an enormous burgeoning field of biomimicry which uses Nature to help solve business problems by mimicking. I bring to your attention a book that I wish everyone on planet earth could read, Bill McDonough's, *Cradle-To-Cradle*. Bill talks today eco-effectiveness. Eco-effectiveness solves problems. And in Bill's world— he's an American designer, a very clever man— he understands that pollution is poison, and in Nature there is no waste. And so Bill and all these biomimicrists understand that. And the world that we're moving toward is a world where there's no waste and no poison, because we can't afford that, Brendan, with seven and a half billion procreating people, we got a lot of mouths to feed here.

Brendan [00:38:32]: You know, Bill McDonough, either in that book or in another talk, I heard him say that "design is the first sign of human intention" or something close to that. We've got to ask ourselves, is it really our intention to poison our children, to poison whales, and so forth? And you know, these organophosphate fertilizers, just and mention one type of toxin, are very, very implicated in all of our degenerative diseases. This is fairly new information. We've known it was implicated in cancer. Now we're suddenly seeing it's implicated in heart disease, diabetes, obesity, you name it. They are a big player, and they are so unnecessary.

Dr. Halter [00:39:21]: Alzheimers, dementia.

Brendan [00:39:23]: Because, as you mentioned, if we work with Nature … biomimicry captures the simple fact that Nature's "technologies" are so time-tested, so miraculous, so powerful. We've got all of these, you know, this divine matrix of life ... that it does everything for us if we do it. And we try to replace a little parts of it, and we break the whole machine.

Dr. Halter [00:39:49]: Yeah, we do, and by the way we also had another win yesterday in Europe. Glyphosate, Roundup, it's days are coming to an end there too. And glyphosate ... they just, I mean from autism to cancer and many things in between, it's in the waterways, and sadly it's in our food, and there's no reason for it because here's the thing at the end of the day, Brendan ... the Pharoahs couldn't figure out how to take their riches with them to the afterlife. They sure tried. And we have to understand that we have to be very mindful in how we exist because the Earth's never experienced this kind of a change that humans are driving. We're in the middle of the sixth mass extinction, and it's human-driven. We cannot continue to eradicate everything. My colleague Daniel Pauli at the University of British Columbia told me when I asked him how much death are we looking at in the oceans each year in terms of a number, not the metric tonnage which we think we have an idea of, but again there's so much looting. We're killing at least 10 trillion forms of life in the ocean a year, and my colleagues led by Boris Worm at the University of Dalhousie and on the East Coast (Canada) ...

They've already concluded that unless something very radical occurs, that the ocean sometime in the 2040's, will be lifeless. So we know this. We have the warnings, and we need to get smart. We have the technology. Paul Stamet's group has created the most phenomenal, what I would call, a booster, for plants. That is, they take the extract from certain mushrooms, and they put it, mix it with water, and put it on the fields, and it confers an incredible strength to the plants. And it doesn't kill the insects but the plants have the energy to keep the insects away. The insects will not eat these plants with this extra energy. It's Nature's energy, and it means that we do not need these awful insecticides and herbicides and mitocides, and fungicides. When we work with Nature we can do anything. And we have the technology. Farmers are able to grow Stamet's technology free on their land, and it's a global game-changer.

Brendan [00:43:07]: I hadn't heard of this! I'm glad you mentioned it. And Paul Stamets is brilliant. I mean anybody who's ever, you know, learned anything about his work ... it just continues to amaze and astound. And the mechanism by which, you know, when you make plants strong ... there was a fellow named Phil Callahan, and he found that plants, they emit an infrared light, I guess you could say, (**Halter** Sure they do). And it's like a signal you could say, because either they're strong, and they're emitting a steady strong signal with the infrared light that they're giving off. And if they're sick, they're emitting a sort of a staccato frequency, and it's inconsistent.

Dr. Halter [00:44:04]: And that's what calls the insects in.

Brendan [00:44:06]: Yeah, that's ... and the insects go, "Easy meal" because if they go to a strong plant, that plant is going to have very strong cell walls and going to be really tough on the mandibles of the insect. And their sugar content is going to be higher. Graeme Sait at Nutri-Tech Solutions ... when I took a course from him he mentioned that he did a little backyard research and had ... I guess he put caterpillars I think it was in two different jars gave them leaves from healthy broccoli I think and unhealthy or something like that. And what happened was the— and it might not have been that food source, I don't recall— but the worms that ate the very robust food that had a high sugar content, it turned into ethanol and poisoned them. It fermented in their gut. The ones that ate the weaker plant they survived. So there's a serious risk, for an insect to take on a very healthy food source. And they're … they take out the garbage so of speak, as Graeme says. Just like in the megafauna kingdom where the lions go after the weak and the sick, and even the young. So they don't generally take on the strongest member of a herd because you've probably seen, or you could find on YouTube, examples where lions get gored by a water buffalo, and that lion is now potentially going to die because he's got skin hanging open and bleeding, and it's not like he's got an emergency room to go to.

Dr. Halter [00:45:36]: Right, well everything is … the point is everything is time-tested. And the point is … look, as a human being, we all make mistakes. That's part of being human. If you continue to deliberately make a mistake, like looting our planet for more climate-altering fossil fuels or stealing and killing ancient trees, you're destroying everything for everyone. And our forests are in terrible shape, Brendan. They're dying. All the ancient forests are dying or dead on all continents except Antarctica of course which does not have trees. And this is, it's an epic, epic crisis because the ancient trees give us more than one out of every three breaths of oxygen. The trees are the lungs of the land, and the ancient trees are phenomenal carbon dioxide warehouses. For every one ton of wood the tree has pulled a ton and a half of carbon dioxide out of the atmosphere, and it's given off a ton of oxygen. And the ancient trees grow … we need the ancient trees you see because they do the brunt of their growing in the last half of their lives. So this notion you just grow trees for say 10, 20, 30 years … no. And what we're pushing for is a world moratorium on all logging in ancient forest because we have enough plantation wood, and we also have enough repurposing industry today to use and reuse, become thrifty, with the wood that's already been harvested. And there are industries cropping up on all continents. So that's where we're pushing there because these ancient forests are burning. They're being hit by repeated droughts and heat waves, and we're in an awful shape. So from the ocean to the trees, they're showing us that we have no option other than sustain. And by the way, cane (?) for any entrepreneur is opportunity in disguise. That's what drives the real capital market, not the subsidies … because … we mere mortals on main street are not subsidized so why should Exxon Mobil be subsidized? There's no reason.

Brendan [00:48:34]: And yeah there's so much opportunity just waiting to happen with basically biomimicry-based businesses, and we're seeing that. You know when you mention the forest … Walter Jehne, who is also in this event, makes a really important point about forests and rebalancing the climate dynamics on this planet, and that's an essential conversation people really want to listen to because the forests actually play a huge role in generating normal rainfall events … (**Halter** yeah they do) … that release a lot of the heat from the planet. It's like a heat pump … (**Halter** They're climate stabilizers, Brendan.) Yeah, in more ways than one, and so a big part of what we need to do is reforest the planet, and like you said not just tree plantations that we're cutting down every 20 years for pulp or something. And we get so much of our medicine from forests. I mean we're losing the biodiversity that provides us the most miraculous medicines of all kinds—from many places—but forests having a huge percentage of those extraordinary plants. You're coming out with some books real soon, *Save Nature Now* and *Love Nature*. What can you tell us?

Dr. Halter [00:50:02]: Yeah! *Save Nature Now* is a great book because it empowers us. It's filled with blueprints both of global but more specifically a personal blueprint as the top things that the average listener can easily do. One is switch your diet to become a plant-based diet. It's healthy. It's easy. It's water smart. And it's the single biggest thing that each of us can do to help reduce the carbon footprint. Number two, if you still hold in fossil fuel companies there in your portfolio, divest. Divestment movement has doubled from 2015 to 2016. It's doubled in size, there's over 5.5 trillion dollars that's committed to divesting away from the fossil fuels. And very simply at your home, please plant at least one preferably two food-bearing trees. Use mulch. The woodchips are excellent at reducing the water use. And also they provide important habitat for our friends, the earthworms, these little skilled plowmen (who do) such a terrific job to fertilize our trees and our gardens. We want more earthworms. And of course, as I say, please never use any chemicals of any kind in your yard. A very simple thing that each of us can do in the spring and summer and autumn months, leave a little water bowl for bees. So you take a bowl of water you put a bunch of marbles or stones that a few that poke above the water level so that the bees can perch. Bees need to perch to lap water, they can't consume fresh water on the move, and bees just like people and all other forms of life, they need fresh water, so we can make our little bee bath very easy. And for those that are keen, and I strongly suggest it, do a little bit of above-ground gardening. Get a couple of boxes, and start to grow your own food. It's a terrific way to bring your kids back to Nature. The bounty is ... there's always more than you can eat. And you can share it with your friends or neighbors. And then the kids also see the importance of the bee because the bees are predominantly pollinating most of the foods that you're going to have as bounty from your garden.

Brendan [00:53:33]: Absolutely, and I'd like to add that ... when you mentioned divesting ... I think that we can all look at divesting from the industrial food systems and redirecting our spending too. And I think it will come along. I think the industrial food system will come along as we direct our, just really direct our purchases to producers that are taking care of the soil, and learning much about what that means, what is regenerative agriculture. That's the thing that I want everybody to do in this event is tune into especially every session that has to do with agriculture. It may not be something you normally tune into, but you're going to learn that that's one of the most important things you can understand to make sure your family's getting the very best food, and it's going to make a huge difference in your personal life but for the planet massive, massive difference between spending in ... these two different systems. And I believe industrial agriculture is showing signs of moving over in that direction, but we have to gently force the issue by just redirecting our spending now, and they'll have to come along, or they'll perish.

Dr. Halter [00:54:43]: Yeah, and you know one way, Brendan, for the listeners, for heaven's sake, please support your local farmers market. And when you're at the market ask the vendors ... ”Is this from regenerative agriculture? Is it organic? Is it biodynamic?” And please support the vendors that are doing it right because at the end of the day ... look, you are what you eat, and we really want to be, we really must today be careful because the biosphere is top-heavy with terrible, terrible poisons. And so everything you eat, you put in your body, you want it to be good. Let me, let me leave you with a thought. This is a guy thing, so ladies please take at face value ... but if a guy just got himself, for whatever the reason, but if he just got himself a brand-new half-a-million-dollar Lamborghini, and it was sadly— although Lamborghini has I'm told a new EV— but this is a fossil fuel car. And on this, on the gas tank, it said only use the highest whatever octane ... I don't have a gasoline car so I forget what it is, 91 or whatever ... every guy who had that car I'm sure that would not be putting vegetable oil. They wouldn't put soy sauce. They'll be putting the right fuel in their brand new half a million dollar Lamborghini. So the question, the take-home is this. Each of us are Lamborghinis. Everything you put in your body has to be of the highest quality; otherwise, you're introducing free radicals. And free radicals lead to a boatload of trouble, and nobody wants trouble. In order to have a good life we want more fun. And to have more fun we got to be healthy, right?

Brendan [00:57:03]: Absolutely. The performance that … you know… the high-performance machine that we are really does perform at amazing levels when we do, you know, just the basics to take care of it and then go beyond that as well. And yeah, I like that analogy. But the basics include, it's got to be clean burning. It's got to be clean in general. It's got to be high-octane, and it can't be producing all kinds of really unfavorable byproducts in our metabolism. You know in as far as being what we eat it reminds me of a … that, you know, we are what we eat … it reminds me of something that a Senegalese forestry engineer named Baba Dioum, Dioum I think is how it's pronounced. Baba Dioum. He's been involved in agricultural development and natural resource management, and he presented a paper at the General Assembly of the International Union for the Conservation of Nature and Natural Resources. And he is basically saying that we will conserve only what we love. So we are what we eat, and we will only conserve what we love. He specifically said, "In the end we will only …" excuse me, let me start again. "In the end we will conserve only what we love. We will love only what we understand. And we will understand only what we are taught." So thank you Dr. Halter for, for teaching us more about our precious planet and for being a voice and advocate for Nature and Earth and all beings here. And thank you for connecting with us, with our … you know, reawakening our love of the Earth, and in the power we really do have to make a difference because we do. Agriculture actually gives us more power than we have had in anything else, if we turn it around. How we grow food has more impact than just about anything else we can do.

Dr. Halter [00:59:03]: Yeah it does. And my last words … please protect our planet, it's our only home.

Brendan [00:59:08]: Yeah, Amen.

Dr. Halter [00:59:11]: A woman. (laughs)

Brendan [00:59:13]: (laughs) Thank you.

Brendan [00:59:16]: We covered a lot of shocking ground in that conversation with Reese, but what you're going to learn from some of the next speakers will give you tremendous hope and power to help turn things around, so let the shock of the news we just heard turn your love of the Earth into commitment to action. And the first thing we can do is to simply learn what regenerative agriculture is and the basics of how it works, so that we can vote with our dollars and send our consumer demand signal out into the food system. We can also roll up our sleeves and become part of the regenerative food system as an entrepreneur. Regenerative entrepreneurs usually earn many times more money on less land than conventional farmers, as you'll learn later in this event. Another pathway was just given to us by Elaine Ingham, that of becoming a Life in the Soil consultant. She works with agricultural clients all over the world, helping them grow soil, and in so doing, healing the atmosphere, the oceans, rivers, ecosystems and the whole glorious dance of life all around us. And she teaches her students of course to do the same. And later in the event we'll learn about some pathways to restoring the soil that can save us while feeding our families and building a local community agriculture system.

So stay tuned for more life-empowering and planet-healing information. Thank you for being here, and may you go out and bless the world with your new knowledge, your enthusiasm, and your actions.

John Roulac Interview

Why Oceans are the #1 Issue of Our Time, The False Promise of Meatless Burgers, and Saving Our Oceans with Regenerative Agriculture

Brendan [00:02]: Welcome to the Eat4Earth event. We're exploring how you can heal yourself, your loved ones, and the planet with food. This is Brendan Morehead and I'm excited to welcome a man who was extraordinarily dedicated to human and planetary health, John Roulac. John Roulac is founder of Nutiva, the world's largest organic super foods brand of hemp, hemp, coconut, chia, and red palm superfoods. A leading entrepreneur of the organic food movement, John has made it his life's mission to revolutionize the way the world eats. John is also a philanthropic entrepreneur, having founded five non-profit ecological groups, including GMO Inside, and the Nutiva Foundation, which supports sustainable agriculture and environmental programs. John has been interviewed on over 200 radio programs and been featured in *The Economist* magazine, *LA Times*, *Bloomberg* and the *Associated Press*. He serves as an informed and dynamic keynote speaker on many topics, including the role of regenerative agriculture to sequester carbon in our soils, the link between ocean health and soil health, trends in the organic food industry, creating a purpose-driven company, and the adverse impacts of genetically engineered foods. He is also the also the author of four books on composting and hemp, with 1,000,000 copies sold. John, thanks so much for being here with us today.

John Roulac [01:19]: Good to be here.

Brendan [01:22]: So I would like to start with what I believe is the most important issue any of us could be focused, on and you certainly are. John, you spend a lot of time educating people about the connection between our agriculture and the health of our oceans. Can you tell us what that's about?

John Roulac [01:41]: Many people are becoming more aware that there's a connection between our diet and the way we grow our food and climate change. That's a subject that perhaps a decade ago many, many people just weren't focused on it. And that in fact our diet is the largest contributor, and agriculture, in fact, is the largest contributor to climate change. There was an article recently in *The Guardian*, the UK Guardian, that like three of the largest meat companies in the world produce more greenhouse gas emissions than Germany as a country does. So, how we … how we grow our food has a huge impact … and the connection between our food, our soils and the ocean … is now people … are starting to become apparent. And that's something that I've been working, giving talks, writing articles that the oceans and the soil are all connected.

[02:53]: If we don't have healthy soils, we're not going to have a healthy ocean. If we have healthy soils, we can create a healthy ocean. And the thing to understand is that this mass amount of carbon that's being released from agriculture, from tilling, over-tilling the soil, leaving the soil barren so it blows away … producing lots of pesticides which make huge, huge amounts of greenhouse gas emissions in their manufacture. There's a report that came out how glyphosate, the leading herbicide that Monsanto and other companies manufacture, has such a huge impact. So all that, all that material goes up into the atmosphere. And then at some point it falls into the ocean. The ocean is absorbing about 30 percent of the CO2 and over 90 percent of the heat. So oceans have been, basically been a shock absorber for our degenerative agriculture, degenerative energy policy, which leads to degenerative thinking, degenerative health because we're basically just dumping poisons and destroying Nature.

[04:17]: And so people are now starting to understand there's a linkage that if we can take all that excess carbon, that excess emissions and turn it into a ... turn it from looking at it as quote "bad" ... in the sustainability movement over the last couple of decades ... like sustainability, like, "Oh, stop doing so much bad, just do a little less bad." And we've seen how much that, that's really a failed policy. And they're like, the first wave was just consume resources and pollute. Second wave was, "Oh, let's, let's do things a little less bad" sustainability. And we saw that that wasn't really changing things. And this third wave is regeneration where we can take degraded landscapes and regenerate that by taking that carbon and sequestering it through the plants, through the roots, through the bacteria, the living soil and transform that into healthier soil.

[05:28]: So when it rains, the water goes into the soil. Whereas today when it rains, it's just like a hard pan and just washes away. And so we're missing all that rain. So that's an example of how we can shift what we think carbon is quote "bad" into an asset. And in the process we can help heal the oceans because as the oceans become more acidic, absorbing all of this heat and carbon, then the acidification increases. It's increased by 30 percent since the start of the industrial revolution, you know, in the last 150 years.

Brendan [06:13]: What's happening in the oceans as a result of this increase in acidification, as the oceans absorb so much of the carbon that we've been releasing from burning fossil fuels and oxidizing our agricultural soils?

John Roulac [06:27]: Yeah, well it's a, it's a huge issue because the oceans are the number one provider of oxygen. They're basically our (oxygen) production system, from the plankton. About two out of three of our breaths come from the ocean. And this phytoplankton ... they're these microscopic parts of the food chain in the ocean. It's where ... it's what the whales eat. It's what the sardines eat. It's the basis for life in the oceans. And the plankton is starting to die because of the acidification. And if you accelerate this ... because the plankton need a particular level of ocean health so they can make their bodies and multiply. And when the scientists increase the ocean acidification in experiments to what is the projected ocean acidification by 2040, essentially all the plankton just dissolve.

[07:48]: And already in the Indian Ocean we've lost 30 percent of the plankton, (which) has died from ocean acidification already. So slowly the planet is losing oxygen. And unfortunately, a lot of well-meaning people are repeating Monsanto's and the industrial agriculture's lie of "How are we going to feed 9 billion people by 2050?" That's the mantra. They want everyone to focus on that and how are we going to feed them by 2050? They say more industrial agriculture, more Roundup, more glyphosate, more policies led by Bill Gates going to Africa and saying, "It's illegal now for you to collect your indigenous seeds. We have improved seeds" that old white men from Europe will come and tell you "This is the seeds you can grow and oh by the way, you need to buy chemical fertilizers and oh by the way we have, we can tell you chemical fertilizers and oh by the way, you need pesticides and by the way, you need more farm machinery, and oh by the way, you're gonna need more loans, and oh by the way, you're gonna need an IMF Bank and oh by the way, you know, we have some other things we'll tell you after you implement that." The big lie is that.

[09:05]: 70 percent of the food is grown on less than 30 percent of the land, and it's by small farmers, many of them using regenerative agriculture practices. So industrial agriculture doesn't actually feed the world. What they primarily make is grains (to) feed industrial animals. So that's what they're primarily growing. And oils used in junk food.

[09:37]: So the majority of the food is grown by small farmers, and that's what we're, saying ... we're trying to get rid of. And this whole thing of 9 billion people by 2050 ... the big question is how are we going to create an agriculture, a regenerative agriculture system, that will heal the oceans? Because at our current rate, every fish, every dolphin, every whale will be extinct by ... probably by 2040, 2045. It's coming very rapidly. So there won't be 9 billion people by 2050 according to the scientists who study the oceans. So it's not so much we need this massive more amount of food. It's, we need an agricultural system that restores the soils and is farmed and basically is using Nature as a model.

[10:39]: And the good news is there's lots of people who are doing this, and the people who are focused on this, they're ranchers, they're environmentalists, they're Trump supporters, they're Bernie Sanders supporters, and matter of fact some of the most ardent supporters of soil voted for Trump. And it's just a different world, versus if you go to the coast when you go to the middle of the country. But this regenerative agriculture is a way to bring together people around soil health, around improving income from farmers, healthier food for moms and families and taking care of the planet. So it's a very dynamic movement, this regenerative agriculture. And there's a film that I'm producing, co-producing, called *Kiss the Ground* by the NGO called Kiss the Ground based in LA. And this has been a project I've been working on for the last four years.

[11:45]: Leo Dicaprio's agreed to come on as Executive Producer, which is a big win. It's going to be a 90-minute documentary, and it will be released sometime in the spring of 2018. We're 95 percent done. And it essentially outlines a lot of what I've been talking about on the big screen. It highlights people like Gabe Brown and Ray Archuleta, which are kind of the soil heroes of America today. Gabe was a failing farmer in North Dakota 20 years ago, was going to lose his ranch. He had drought, he had frost, and hail. His crops were going, and someone recommended he go no-till, and he gave up tilling. He has these paddocks, and he grows multi-species grass, grass crops, and then he brings the cows and other animals in. They eat— they're just there for a couple days.

[12:49]: They poop. They piss. They trample the soil. And then they move to the next paddock. And then he can grow crops the next year. He doesn't need to buy any fertilizer. He likes to say he likes to sign the back of the check, not the front of the check. And ironically, I recently wrote an article in *Medium*, the online publishing— I used to write articles for *EcoWatch*, but I switched over to *Medium*. It's a great publication, a blog platform, and it was basically calling out this university of Oxford think tank ... did a study, a so-called

---

study, and said that industrial confined animal feedlot operations or CAFOs ... it's the same as what Gabe Brown is doing in North Dakota where he's producing meat that is grown from solar energy, from the sun and grass that grows on his ranch.

[13:59]: And it's a much better system that avoids all the pesticides, herbicides, chemical fertilizers, all the inhumane treatment of animals, et cetera. So I published this and got some interesting pushback from different people. And uh, you know, I talked about linkages of Monsanto, and how they're linked to universities and Oxford. And then I'm following up with a new article, and it's going to be very controversial. Matter of fact, some people in the food movement are really pissed at me for even attempting this, but it shows why I need to do this because it touches a nerve. And it's essentially the headline I'm working on is "Enviros, Vegans and Monsanto: Strange Bedfellows for Monsanto, Glyphosate, and Soil Destruction". And, and this irony is that the vegan movement has done so much to create great food ...

[14:59]: And when I go out to restaurants, I usually prefer eating vegan. I mostly eat plants, but I do eat some meat. And the vegan movement has been amazing, but they've allowed their focus on not eating animals to basically paint all agriculture that involves animals as bad. And that's a very simplistic view. And so, ironically, they would rather eat a burger like Impossible Burger or Beyond Beef, uh, Beyond Meat, that is sprayed with Monsanto Roundup, grown with chemical fertilizers, creating dead zones in the ocean, huge carbon footprint, putting Roundup in the rain water that can be delivered to grow their veggies. And that's the model for the vegan future that they want. And they want to just say you can do whatever, just don't eat any meat. And they're, they're promoting these kind of false options that are really not healthy. And Silicon Valley and Monsanto are using the vegan community, and the vegans don't even know it.

Brendan [16:15]: Yeah, that's a really interesting irony that you're calling out. And it's something that I've noticed myself and am concerned about because vegans in general have their heart in the right place for wanting to do what's right for the planet and for human welfare, excuse me, well, human *and* animal welfare and reducing suffering. And yet they're somehow maybe not noticing this connection with what these ways of growing food is doing to the planet.

John Roulac [17:01]: They're singular-focused on animal ... and I understand that .... our current animal system is broken. But there's no way that we can feed the amount of people on this planet if we say you can't restore our grasslands using animals. The only way we can restore the grasslands is through the disturbance of hoofed animals. That's the way the planet has evolved over millions of years.

[17:29]: And it's this lack of environmental awareness, and that's the thing. The United States perhaps is the most ecologically illiterate society that's ever seen, ever seen, ever in history, ever in any country. We have such low level of awareness of ecology and systems. And it's a challenge. People really need to ... they need to learn more. Understand the carbon cycle. It's not, it's not like overly complex. There's no more, no less carbon today than there was a thousand years ago. It's merely we've transferred the carbon from the soil and put it up the atmosphere and it's falling into the oceans. We learned that in first grade. Put things where they belong. The carbon belongs in the soil. And the vegans who are more conscious are actually supportive of this concept. People like David Bronner from Dr Bronner's and John Robbins also understands, "Look, if you're gonna eat meat, you should eat pastured meat."

[18:49]: Where you basically are just consuming grasses that the cow has eaten ... And if people want to become vegan, that's their choice. That's a great healthy choice. I was vegetarian for a long time. Great lifestyle option, but I'd like to say if you don't want pesticides in your veggies and your rainwater, you better tell all your meeting and friends they've got to switch to pastured meat. But soon as you say that, they say "Oh, pastured meat leads to more rain-forest destruction." They say that immediately. That's their media go-to because they read that in *Cowspiracy*. *Cowspiracy* is complete brainwashing, not even based on any facts— the premise that you can't do pastured and all this stuff. Yes, they're right that industrial meat is horrible. As I said, the top three meat companies in the world are contributing more than Germany does to climate (change). So we've got to change. They got that right. But this whole thing that regenerative agriculture, pasture grass farming systems is ... they just say it doesn't work. And you know, what's leading to more rain-forest destruction is the soy plantations. So yeah, it's kind of an ironic thing.

Brendan [20:22]: And you know, you mentioned David Bronner with Dr Bronner's, a soap and other products company. He's got an amazing article I think everybody should read. It's called "Regenetarians Unite". I believe that's the title, "Regenetarians Unite". And he makes such important points about how, regardless of our particular choices with food, we need to really look more closely to scratch the surface a bit on all the issues. And he's done that brilliantly in that article. Because, we don't need to agree on everything, but we do need to get one thing right, and that is we've got to rebuild soil. We've got to stop destroying and poisoning the planet and acidifying the oceans. And soil, as Finian Makepeace with Kiss the Ground likes to say, "Soil is the greatest common ground issue of our time." And you pointed out evidence of that and that, uh, well, I don't know if it's direct evidence of it, but in a way it is. You mentioned the ranchers, environmentalists, Trump supporters, Bernie supporters, all in favor of rebuilding the soil. It cuts across all political lines, and we're starting to see some really encouraging bipartisan work in Washington DC to educate everybody, Congressmen and various lawmakers and agencies and so forth about the potential of soil regeneration to solve so many of our problems.

John Roulac [21:59]: Yeah, definitely. I was just with Finian from Kiss the Ground at an event last night for a fundraiser with a lieutenant governor Gavin Newsome, a 2018 gubernatorial candidate running in the November 2018 election and likely to be our next governor of California. And so that was exciting. And I've been working on this event to sit down with him. So I was at the fundraiser and a round table discussion on regenerative agriculture, and Finian was part of that. So was Calla Rose from the Marin Carbon Project and Kevin Bayuk from Lift Economy. And so Gavin was very open to hearing some of these discussions. We showed a trailer of *Kiss the Ground*, which he's actually in because he, he made mandatory composting, the curb side collection, composting, which has been a huge success. People were really upset about it.

[23:10]: He's on the Coastal Commission, and he's also the State Lands Commission. So he has his part of the levers of policy in California. And he was very open to how we can take this excess carbon, return it back to the soils ... we can restore oceans. We'll come back, come back to, to ocean farming if you want. Um, and, uh, see if we can cut some of these regulations ... he's an entrepreneur, you know. I think we've seen the attraction of voters wanting entrepreneurs, and I think Kevin agreeing entrepreneur is maybe the ticket for a 2020 for a United States presidential election. So I think I just shook hands with potentially the next President, as a potential.

[24:08]: So, but at least I think he's going to be governor and you know, California's the sixth largest economy in the world. So that was, that was very positive and Finian from Kiss the Ground did a great job. We all went around, shared, opening up the dialogue, and I talked about the oceans, and he talked about the power of the regenerative approach to healthy soils.

Brendan: [24:34]: On the topic of the oceans, the condition of the oceans right now, do you have any late breaking news or report? What's going on right now?

John Roulac: [24:47]: Yes. Yeah, it's ... people need to wake up. The oceans are the number one environmental issue in the world today. We live on an ocean planet, not a land planet. Over 75 percent of the globe is ocean. And 85 percent of our sardines catch in the Pacific here, Pacific Ocean, it's largely harvested in California, is down 85 percent over the last decade. The cod from Alaska, the Gulf, the Gulf of Alaska, is down 75 percent in the last decade.

[25:26]: And it's attributed to warming and just ocean conditions. There's this ocean blob that's coming back that we saw in 2015. The oceans are getting hotter. The oceans can no longer support our degenerative agriculture or degenerative energy systems. We either deal with this, this is the central issue of our lifetime. It's, it's why people like Finian myself, you know, David Bronner, we are on this, this is our ... this is what ... when we wake up and when we go to sleep, this is what we're working on. And we either deal with this, or we will be another species, along with many other species, that will leave this planet in the coming decades. And, and the sad part is that the environmental groups in my view, get an F for communication. I meet so many people who are college educated, well read, you know— not that a college education means you're smarter or anything— but you know, people who read books. They are open to hearing new information, and they have no idea what I just shared today.

[26:50]: No idea that the ocean is the process of dying. They just think that the oceans may rise three, four or five feet by 2100. For some reason 350.org, The Sierra Club, Greenpeace they're just ... they've been in the battle for so long for the last 20 years, they're so locked into fighting Chevron and Exxon that they've ... they're good people. I see them, I talk to them, and I've written letters specifically outlining a lot of these things. And it's just ... they're just, they're doing what they can. Also their funders want them to talk about how bad coal is. Their funders don't want them to take on Monsanto. You know, the people who give them the money. And it takes money to do these campaigns, so they're slowly starting to shift to talk about soils. But not fast enough.

[27:55]: I mean essentially why, why aren't they Tweeting about this? Why aren't they doing Facebook posts? Why aren't they talking, "The oceans are dying, and what's the cause of it? CARBON." Because when you get with Trump supporters, and you say, "Do you believe the icebergs are melting and climate change, as you know ... And they'll go, "Well, you know, the climate is always changing. You know, I don't know about the icebergs. I've heard it's growing more in the Arctic or the Antarctic." If you just repeat as Paul Hawken from Project Drawdown— it's a great book called *Drawdown*— you just keep repeating the same message they've been hearing that Fox News keeps telling them is a lie. They stopped believing it. It's not going to work. Shouting it more isn't going to change it. But when you talk to some of these more conservative Republican Trump supporters, what have you, and you tell them ... "Do you spend time on the ocean?" or "Do you love the ocean?"

[28:53]: And they say, "Yeah" they love ... they like the ocean. A lot of them maybe have boats, or they go swimming when they do go to the sea if they live in the inland areas. And we tell them what's going on the ocean, they have no idea. When they hear that they go, "Wow, maybe we should be doing something." And it's, it's not a conjecture with the ocean, it's actually measurable. You can actually see, yes it is getting much warmer in the ocean. It is there. It is becoming more acidic. But those basic things are not being communicated. And so that's why I say the environmental groups get an F for communication today.

Brendan [29:32]: You know, and I think some of the education ... I think it's dumbed down. People think that ... the communicators think the public can't handle a little bit of nuance and complexity. And so the message gets dumbed down and over-simplified, and I think that's when people go, "Wait, this doesn't sound quite right". And in some regards, I think people that are skeptical about climate change have a point when there's so much focus on, on the emissions of fossil fuels and the carbon equation. It's a little more complex than that. There's a speaker in this event that everybody must tune into, Walter Jehne. Carbon in our atmosphere is one player. So is water, water vapor. And soils are key, not only in drawing down carbon from the atmosphere, but so that soils primarily with their— according to Walter Jehne, and this is just one perspective, but the UN and the IPC is starting to listen to him— basically soils are not only a place to draw down the carbon that is an excess in our atmosphere and our oceans, but we need to restore the water sponge that healthy carbon-rich soils are, because every increase in carbon, carbon content, organic content of soils has a huge increase on the water-holding capacity and the evapotranspiration that sets up the water cycles that we depend on for regular rainfall and consistent minor events rather than a few erratic extreme events. Like you mentioned, 75 percent of rain from falling in three events. That doesn't work real well for our agriculture.

John Roulac [31:20]: Yeah, we're getting more concentrated rain less often. And again, that's why the ranchers and Trump supporters are like, "Oh, you mean when that water falls on the soil, we can capture that so we can maintain that?" And we're going to have to do that. So, in a sense, the traditional people who've been farming this conventional way, they're realizing they're not going to be able to farm and ranch, what they've been doing, the way their fathers did it. Or grandfathers. They need to change, so when they start having these climactic intense weather events, that their land can deal with it easier and at some point if we put enough carbon into the soil, we can go back to 280 ppm (parts per million), we can go back to a more balanced, natural system, but you know, it all begins if you, as Ray Archuleta says in our film," Kiss the Ground", this 34 year NRCS— it's a part of the USDA soil service— veteran. He said, "Healthy soils equal healthy plants; healthy plants equal healthy animals; healthy animals equal healthy people, and all of that equals a healthy climate."

Brendan [32:46]: Yeah. And you mentioned, when you mentioned NRCS and Ray Archuleta— he's working with Gabe Brown. And Gabe Brown is not an organic farmer, but he's a regenerative farmer. I think the thing to point out in that he is capturing carbon at, according to NRCS point five five percent (0.55%), a little more than half a percent. In other words, a little bit more than half a percent per year in soil. And that's extraordinary. And he's doing that by growing lots of things at the same time, cover crops, and as you mentioned, the holistic planned rotational grazing. It's not your typical grazing. There are forms of grazing, laissez-faire grazing you could say, that have …

John Roulac [33:40]: Destructive, destructive. Yeah, for sure. It's, I mean, you just go along, and they leave the cows … you just see these giant ruts because the cows walking back and forth month after month. And they're developing new technologies and new fencing systems, et cetera that you can do. So very, very innovative. So we, we definitely need to listen to some of these wise farmers and ranchers and start coming back to farming more how Nature intended it. And there's this book also called *Kiss the Ground* that basically goes over a lot of what we've been talking about. And that is just coming out. You can get it on Amazon. And I'm encouraged people to check that book out, you know.

Brendan [34:43]: In terms of the oceans and the acidification of the oceans, what would you say is the single biggest cause of that?

John Roulac [34:49]: Single biggest cause is industrial agriculture (which) is basically carpet-bombing carbon into the ocean.

Brendan [34:49]: Even more so than fossil fuels?

John Roulac [34:59]: More so than the transportation, Exxon and Chevron. Yes. If you asked the Secretary of Agriculture, they used to say it was 9%, then they went up to 13%, but they don't even count like nitrogen-producing synthetic fertilizers. People estimate to anywhere between 35% to 50%. If you combined energy like electricity and petroleum and all that, then maybe that's somewhere between 50% to 70%, and agriculture is 30% to 50%. But the thing is what agriculture can do. It can not only … instead of being a net producer of carbon, it can be a net reducer. We can de-carbonize. So we can grab that carbon from the atmosphere and put it back into the soil. Whereas if we went to green energy, you're still going to produce some (carbon dioxide emissions), but agriculture can really play a play a great role.

[36:15]: So if you had to pick one or the other's solar and wind or regenerative agriculture, you really need to do both. But if you only pick one, regenerative agriculture is going to take the legacy carbon, put it back into the soil. That's our job number one. So we could stop … we could go to 100% solar today, 100% electric batteries, all wind, Elon Musk the dictated energy czar of the world, and if we followed that and didn't address soils, 90% of all species outside of, except maybe some in the soil, will be gone by 2040 or 2050.

Brendan [36:49]: Is that a prediction that ... I'm curious who's making those predictions?

John Roulac [37:00]: I'm making that prediction. If you talk to scientists 10 years ago ... here's the thing to understand about climate science. You talk to scientists 10 years ago, let's say 20 years ago, 20 years ago, they said maybe the oceans might rise three feet by 2100. Maybe we would start to see some changes in weather. Then 10 years ago they were like, "Wow, it's going much faster." Five years ago they go, "I can't believe what's happened." And then their predictions are very, very conservative. And so every two or three years they just said, "What we just told you was completely incorrect, and it's much worse, much faster now."

Brendan [37:46]: Yeah. You know, actually I have heard who some of the predictors are second hand. And so Graeme Sait of Nutri-Tech Solutions, he meets with people at high levels all around the world as he advises various agricultural producers and agricultural agencies in different countries. And he also happened to have been at some IPCC— that's the Intergovernmental Panel on Climate Change— IPCC meetings, where there's people there from big think tanks in Europe as well as the scientists. And, and what he has heard some of them say is, "We don't think there's people here in 2030", and these are people that are looking at the information. They're deeply entrenched in it.

Brendan [38:37]: In order for people to grasp this idea ... there's a fellow, his name is Tom Goreau, and he addresses the fact that ecosystems are highly dependent on thresholds, or they're vulnerable to threshold dynamics. And that's what we're looking at. We're coming up against where if we disrupt climate patterns too much by stalling out the undulating patterns of the jet stream that we've been accustomed to, and you start having no rainfall for long periods and then erratic rainfall falling on a dehydrated soils, massive erosion and things like that, how are we going to manage that? And the human body can only handle so much temperature. There are parts of the world ... there are predicted to be parts of the world where the temperature and humidity will reach points where people can't handle it. And I don't know if we think we're going to live in bubbles or go to Mars, but I think that's delusional, and it's going to be a lot less costly and a lot easier to just do a few things right on this planet than to try to figure out how we're going to get out to Mars and turn even more desolate planet into a ... somehow, turn that into a productive oasis. It doesn't make sense. And we have a paradise here. We just need to turn it around.

John Roulac [40:02]: Yeah, definitely. Unfortunately people are, you know, diverted with their phones and with Facebook and, and you know, with gods, guns, and gays or, you know, bathroom policies. This is where "the great debates" are in instead of some other things that are very important. And that's our challenge. I sometimes am blown away by the way us humans interact and evolve as we move through these years, so sometimes it is a bit frustrating. It's like "Really?? So that's (what) we're going to do?" Such great potential, and I tell all my friends it's important for you to enjoy your life right now because it's likely to be a lot different in the coming decades. And if you have the opportunity to make a difference and leave a legacy ... I was just with someone who was a very successful entrepreneur and, you know, they were looking over their kids, and they said, "John, what can I do? What can I do so this little kid ..." He had a little nickname for his little son who is nine years old … this person is a very successful business person and worked in the finance industry and is a surfer and loves oceans.

[41:37]: And it's like, "What do we do?" A lot of people are having those questions. But at the end of the day, we have to look in the mirror and what are we passionate about and what can we do ourselves? And you can't just expect, well, we're going to elect somebody in 2020 to replace Donald Trump and they're going to fix things, like as if like Hillary Clinton would have really made the changes that we need to turn around … this system. People are delusional about that also. People have to take change. We, we obviously need better leadership, but it's got to start with each one of us. It's got to start with our families. It's got to start with our organizations, our communities, our counties, our cities, our states. Everywhere we go we got to leverage and see what we can do. And at least that's where I'm putting my focus and also having a good time while I'm doing it because if you can't throw some good parties along the way you got the wrong revolution.

Brendan [42:45]: (laughing) Good point. John, I've heard you say that people need to learn to discern the truth. What do you mean by that? And why is that?

John Roulac [42:54]: It's important for people to discern the truth because essentially, you know, this term "fake news", uh, you know, it's just come out in the last couple of years, but the level of brainwashing that exists is at such a high level for so long. We know large multinational corporations that are in the energy business, that are in the commodities, need and want to shift how things operate on a country, political level, across the globe. And that's the way they operate. So example, for Syria … Most people think that we're there in Syria to help the help the Syrian people. What people don't realize is that Syria was … Assad, the current president, was offered a pipeline deal, and there were two routes.

[44:04]: And without getting into all the details, bottom line is he chose the route that the Iranians, Iraqis and the Russians wanted. And he rejected the one that the U.S. and the Saudis wanted. And Turkey. And they basically … we basically … it was the overthrow of Syria. And if you just Google "Robert F Kennedy Jr, Eco Watch pipeline"… So we're funding, we're funding Isis and Al Qaeda through Libya to do this. I mean this is what's going on. And both Republicans and Democrats are in denial of that. And also what's causing the problems in Syria was the lack of rain. So they've, there had been drought conditions, poor quality of the soil. So the farmers were losing their ability to grow crops. Then they go to the cities; they become restless, et cetera. So I'm not saying Assad is this upstanding beacon of democracy. A lot of countries' leaders aren't, but then you look at Libya. Why do we overthrow Libya?

[45:24]: Now, look at all the problems we're seeing from overthrowing Libya. Did we, did we have a plan? Or we just said, "We'll just get rid of him." And they will walk away. And now it's complete chaos. And Hillary Clinton led that campaign to overthrow Gaddafi. Destroyed their school systems, destroyed their whole civil society, and that's America. We are creating destruction and because of our … we have elected these leaders and you know it's sad. That's where people need to discern the truth, just like vegans think that like all cows are bad, and we just need to all go vegan and instead we'll just … and if they have to spray Monsanto everywhere for their vegan burgers, they'll do that and look the other way. It's like, "Hello, wake up." So that's where I'm saying we've got to discern the truth.

Brendan [46:18]: I think we all have to be willing to look at ... to just step back from our most strongly held beliefs and just look at them from a third-party view and just re-evaluate, just to see if we might be missing part of the picture. I don't know. I'm not sure how to explain what I mean so I'll just leave it at that ... and then return back to what moves us and so forth. But I think if we just step out for a second and somehow we might discover something, see a bigger part of the picture, and ultimately we need to think inclusively like everybody needs to be involved in this, not excluding certain people from the process. We have to find the common ground, and soil is that common ground. So anyhow, and there were large ruminant herbivores roaming the planet in similar numbers to what we have now, maybe more, and we had very stable climatic patterns according to the geological records that we have.

John Roulac [47:29]: Exactly. People have a point of view, and we need to learn to look beyond the point of view. But that takes some insight and "know thyself" and be humble enough to look to change. That's important to do. So, it's great to be on your show today, and you have some good knowledge about these issues. It's easier to do a program with someone who's a little more aware of some of these things. So I appreciate your becoming aware and learning about these important issues that are facing the planet and building healthy soils.

Brendan [48:14]: Yeah. And thank you John so much for that. And thank you for your visionary leadership and your long-time tireless efforts to, to help create a liveable world and future for all of us and generations to come. So thank you for being with us here in the community.

John Roulac [48:33]: Yeah, glad to. And I wish everybody has a great day. And let's put our ... put whatever, you know, resources and time you have to creating a regenerative society instead of a degenerative society. Let's regenerate, restore, and make things better.

Brendan [48:56]: Amen.

Brendan's Outro [48:58]: Now that we know what's at stake, it's time to look at the solutions. Walter Jehne is one of the speakers in this event that provides a big picture vision and an actual toolbox for humanity to solve our most urgent crises. My conversation with him might be the most important one of this entire series, and it would be a great one to watch or listen to next.

Walter Jehne Interview

The Real Cause of Climate Change, the True Cure, and a 9X Increase of Nutrients in Our Food

Brendan [00:00:00]: This is Brendan Moorehead and it's my honor and pleasure to welcome our guest Walter Jehne. Walter is an internationally recognised soil microbiologist, climate scientist and innovation strategist with extensive field and research experience at a national level with Australia's Commonwealth Scientific and Industrial Research Organisation and at an international level with the United Nations. He recently presented at an invitation-only UN gathering of scientists and decision makers to discuss including soil in the next report of the Inter-governmental Panel on Climate Change. With his diverse experience in science, government and industry, he is an expert at transforming challenges into opportunities. And Walter has developed a new paradigm that connects Earth's ecological and atmospheric systems to provide powerful solutions for stabilizing climate, cooling the planet and even restoring high nutrient levels to our food supply. Walter, it's an honor and a joy to welcome you to the Eat4Earth event.

Walter [00:01:02]: Yes and vice versa, thank you, Brendan.

Brendan [00:01:06]: First up, you know you have some fascinating things to say about climate change and how we can reverse it by restoring global soils and water cycles, giving us more options and more hope than we might otherwise have. In fact, your model of climate change is a real paradigm shift, that really anyone can buy into. And your model differs in certain ways from the one used by the Inter-governmental Panel on Climate Change. The IPCC rather. How does the IPCC model ... how did it come about, and how does your model differ from that?

Walter [00:01:39]: Right, Brendan. Just a bit of context there ... of course it's not my model at all. It's really ... this is the process, and if you want to call it the model or the blueprint that Nature uses and used to create the global climate and to actually maintain the stability of the climate, particularly the 10,000 years, the Holocene stability that we have been fortunate enough to experience and that has enabled our evolution as a, you know, as a species. So it's not my model, and all we have really done is sort of go back to, well what are the basic, natural processes that regulated climate. How do we understand how they operate? What have we done to them? What are the consequences? And what is it that we can and must do to try and restore them? Okay? So it's not me. It's just simply observation. It also goes back to Climatology 101. Look, it's—and this is really the crux of it—we have had for hundreds of years very, very eminent climatologists looking at these climate processes, dynamics, understanding it and in a very sophisticated understanding. Not that we know everything, clearly we don't. That's science. But they came to a very clear understanding. The punch line is that yes, everybody agrees, climatology agrees, It's actually water, hydrology, that governs 95% of the heat dynamics of the blue planet, has done for about 4 billion years. And this water, this hydrology, governs the climate through a whole sequence of processes. And it's that understanding of those sequences that we were pretty sophisticated, had a good understanding of. But then, basically in the mid 70's—or well, actually Charles Keeling from 1958 when he first confirmed the CO2 rise—but then by the mid 70's this sort of "political" alarm and the political concern and pressure came very much on, "Hey this abnormal, human induced CO2 rise," that Keeling's data had confirmed. And then the question was what the consequence of this CO2 rise, by its small component of the greenhouse effect on the Earth's future climate. And it was really Jimmy Carter in a very positive way, back in the late 70's, who then commissioned Los Alamos and the Scripps Oceanographic Institute in San Diego to say, "Look, please model the actual CO2 component of the greenhouse effect and give me a report to the President, on what are the consequences of this single process." Now, everybody said, "Yes, here's a component of the complex hydrological dynamic that runs the Earth's climate," and it's actually quite tragic because we have so much focused on this one process, that we've in a sense, ever since, I mean amongst some of us, ignored these far more important fundamental drivers of the planet. Now obviously that work was done, that modelling was done. Manabe and Wetherald sort of then reported on it and said, "Yes, it would actually have a minor effect on warming." If anything for the United States it would beneficial because agriculture would be able to extend seasonally into higher productive capacities and really, when that report to the President went to Ronald Reagan in the early 80's it was really sort of taken as fairly benign. But the problem is that that ever since then we've always focused on the CO2 greenhouse effect, rather than the bigger issue of, alright, what governs the Earth's climate and what have we done to those processes? And all I'm doing is actually going back to revisit that knowledge, because in a sense what has been happening—and it was really picked up by Joachim Schellnhuber in 2005 at a big conference in the Hatley Centre—that we are now entering a period of dangerous climate extremes. Accelerating, intensifying, dangerous climate extremes. And it's not the CO2 that's the real problem, it's these dangerous extremes. These extremes are all hydrological. More intense hurricanes, floods, the aridifications, systemic aridification of regions like, you know, California, South West US, droughts, wildfires. And in a sense it's these hydrological extremes that are now already impacting biosystems and their dependent communities. It's these hydrological extremes that really threaten you know, social wellbeing and our future within the next decades. And so I think it is just changing this whole perspective and debate away from yeah, the CO2 greenhouse component and basically really saying well what have we done to the climate in the bigger scale, and what are the consequences? When will this happen, and what can we do about it? Because in a sense, the analogy is we aren't seeing the elephants in the room, because in fact they are far too big to be in the room. The actual driving forces are still outside whereas we have been spending 40 years in modelling, delay and denial, looking at this CO2 component effect of the greenhouse, which quite frankly, governs about 4% of the heat dynamics of the planet and ignoring these processes that govern about 95% of it. And so it's really by only understanding these hydrological processes, this whole Earth heat dynamics, that we have any chance of avoiding and counteracting these dangerous climate extremes that we are going to be facing.

Brendan [00:08:28]: And you have a way of simply … I'm hearing an echo … okay, I'm not sure where that's coming from but it looks like it's stopped. So you have a way of simplifying a very complex heat dynamics, climate regulating system on planet Earth and the three fundamental processes that we can influence and which give us a lot of power to turn things around. Could you describe those three core drivers of heat dynamics and climate regulation.

Walter [00:09:06]: Right, well look basically right from 4 billion years ago it's water that has actually influenced the climate and obviously it's done that through the natural greenhouse effect substantially, because it's actually water vapor that governs 60 - 70% of the natural greenhouse effect. The amount of water vapour molecules in the air. That can be up to 50,000 parts per million. With each water vapour molecule able to absorb significantly more heat in that greenhouse process, than the 400 parts per million of CO_2 that we've got. So in a sense that's the fundamental starting point, the process of why the Earth's temperature and climate, because of the natural greenhouse effect, is 33 degrees centigrade warmer than it would otherwise be. But actually these hydrological processes, apart from that natural greenhouse effect, also govern the actual cooling of the planet. And so there's two other fundamental processes, first is the actual transpiration and evaporation of water from the Earth's surface because every gram of water that is evaporated or transpires, has to turn from liquid into a gas, and in doing so it has to take a lot of latent heat, heat that it needs to do that water to gas conversion and it transfers that heat back up into the upper atmosphere. And when that water condenses in the atmosphere, most of that heat is re-radiated back to space. And so we've got this very powerful latent heat flux, latent heat cooling effect as water is taken from the surface and with that heat, to cool that surface. The third part is of course in the hydrological cycle, now that we've got this water vapour and then water up in the air, how do we actually sort of both coalesce those humid hazes into dense high albedo clouds and then rainfall? Because that is needed to close the water cycle. And again, there is biological processes that drive that. You take water vapour that's in the air ... it will form humid hazes, and those humid hazes coalesce into these clouds, and these clouds can reflect up to 36% of the incident solar radiation coming into the Earth, back out to space and massively cooling the planet. Over 50% of the Earth at any time is covered by these high albedo clouds, and they're having a fundamental regulatory effect on the Earth's climate. Once you've got these clouds, then the next step is how do those cloud droplets again coalesce into bigger rain drops to return back to the Earth to continue that cycle? And again, the formation of those raindrops depends on hygroscopic precipitation nuclei, and again this is where the physics and the science gets detailed. But it's these nuclei that actually then cause the rain, that allow both that hydrological cycle, but all our life on Earth, on land to be sustained. And again, it's the actual types of nuclei, the amount and their processes which then govern that cycle. We can go into the details of that.

Brendan [00:13:02]: Yeah, well I might have been over-simplifying it by describing three, I know you have ten hydrological processes and intervention points we'll get into. In terms of three, it sounds like, here's how I was trying to fit it into three, so you've got, you've described it that water is a very powerful greenhouse gas as a vapour and we've got the—and especially compared to carbon dioxide—and then we've got the ... I have to re-orient myself ... we've got another factor, which is the heat of, or rather the surface temperature of the Earth which is driving how much heat there is to be trapped. That's a fascinating one, I believe, for people to understand. Sort of like the third, if we're going to simplify the three main factors, before we dive into the ten.

Walter [00:14:00]: Okay, Brendan look, if I go back you see, okay, backtracking, right, what I was explaining is here are the three fundamental parts of the water in the Earth heat dynamics and you're right, but the question is specifically okay, what are the three components of the natural greenhouse effect, you know, what drives the greenhouse effect and then how we change that. And if we look at that element of the situation yes, there are three elements okay. And the first is how much heat is absorbed by the Earth's surface okay, because okay, let's go back a bit. We've got the planet, and every day continually it receives about 342 watts of solar energy per square metre average across the Earth's surface, right, 342 watts coming in. To maintain our stable climate, we have to re-radiate, well not we, the Earth has to re-radiate 342 watts going back out, and so it's this balance between incoming heat and outgoing heat for this stability. Because of our interventions we now basically are retaining 3 watts per square metre of extra heat, through this enhanced, abnormal greenhouse effect. That's less than 1 percent of this heat dynamics. So our imperative is, how do we actually cool the planet this extra 1 percent? How do we restore an extra 1 percent of heat leaving this planet? And what we've done is we've disturbed the greenhouse effect, and we've disturbed it through these three principle ways. And the first is, we've totally changed how much heat is absorbed by the planet's surface by clearing forests, by exposing soils, instead of the heat coming in and being reflected, we are basically absorbing it by the soil's surface. By disturbing the hydrological cycle, instead of having that heat being released and going up in these latent heat fluxes, it's heating the soil's surface. And we know that because if we've got a forest the soils under that forest you know, rarely get above 20 degrees centigrade. Whereas when we clear that same forest, have it open, exposed soils, then in summer that soil might go up to 40 degrees, 50 degrees centigrade. Really heating so hot that we can hardly walk on it. Okay, so that's the first thing, it's we fundamentally changed how much heat the Earth's surface absorbs. Just as another factor in this, people don't realise, but we humans have created over 5 billion hectares of man-made desert and wasteland on the land.

[00:17:20]: Okay, so now the point is we've heated the Earth's surface abnormally, massively, but the heat of course just doesn't stay on the Earth, it re-radiates back out into the atmosphere. And this is a critical point, because the amount of re-radiation, infra-red radiation that goes back out into the atmosphere is in fact the key driver of the greenhouse effect. It's how much heat is going up and then how much of that heat is absorbed by gas molecules that can absorb it, water and CO_2, two key greenhouse gases. But it's the amount of heat that's going up that you know governs it. And that's determined by simple physics of black body radiators and the amount of heat is related to the 4th power of the temperature. So if we have two soils which are completely different temperatures, it's the difference in temperatures to the 4th power that regulates that amount of heat that goes up. So effectively, by having bare soils heating, we massively increase the amount of heat being re-radiated that's able to then drive the greenhouse effect. The simple conclusion ...

Brendan [00:18:44]: It's exponential is what you're saying.

Walter [00:18:46]: Well it's, yeah, temperature, times temperature, times temperature, times temperature. It's an exponential, massive thing. And the fact is, you see, by keeping the soil temperature cooler, we can massively decrease how much heat is going up which is driving the greenhouse. So effectively, in simple terms, we can turn down the heat. We can turn down the greenhouse enormously, by simply keeping our surfaces cool, because then there won't be the same amount of heat going up into the air that can be absorbed by these gas molecules, okay.

Brendan [00:19:30]: Yeah that is ... that's like the key, mind-blowing new concept. It's, you know, it's not new to somebody like you but perhaps to those of us out here in the lay public we're used to thinking only in terms of you know, reducing the heat trapping gases, and we're not even thinking about water. And as I understand, the reason the IPCC model of climate change has not really included water, was previously we thought it was too big a factor to influence, is that correct?

Walter [00:20:00]: Right, we haven't included water, or they didn't include water, quite consciously for two key reasons. Water, because of these ten different processes, it's so variable and so dynamic and it changes, different times of the day, it changes in every location, it's effectively impossible to model on a global scale, on an average anyway. Secondly, because they accepted it's such a dominant, powerful factor, that we ... the assumption was that we humans could not have possibly have influenced it, right. But what happened is then that they did the analysis, Manabe and Wetherald did the analysis of the CO_2 component, it only sort of, it showed that now without water vapour included, it was nowhere near accounting for the temperature increases that we're seeing. So the models have in a sense appropriated an element of that water effect and more or less sort of said okay as temperature increases there is more water vapour in the air so we will assume that that's a secondary feedback of the CO_2 warming effect. So they do include some of the water vapour, gas molecule properties but no, they don't include any of this hydrological dynamics in terms of heating and cooling land systems.

Brendan [00:21:31]: And those are the, no go ahead ...

Walter [00:21:34]: No, no, you go Brendan sorry.

Brendan [00:21:36]: So, these are ... and that's where we get into the ten water-related elephants that aren't even in the room right now. And so tell us more about that, I mean we've got apparently ten ways that we can interface with the climate system and with the natural processes that govern it and turn this thing around. Can you tell us more about that?

Walter [00:22:04]: Right, yes Brendan, and in a sense that is exactly right, so Nature works as we said for the last 4 billion years using water to regulate the climate of the blue planet. And there is a sequence of ten sort of processes so they're not totally separate, but if you could imagine here's a water molecule travelling through the Earth's biosphere, the atmosphere, and what have you, and it goes through ten different stages each of which has a profound, you know, cooling or warming effect. And very quickly and we can detail this much more on paper, but the processes are initially these latent heat fluxes right, the actual cooling of the Earth massively as this water gets transpired and evaporated. That water then, so that's one. Two is when you say this water now is in the air, but once it's in the air, if it's there as micro droplets, as haze, micro droplets it will absorb into the solar radiation to warm the atmosphere, and that is in a sense happening at an increased level and we're seeing that as global dimming. And there's again lots of science of global dimming and up to you know, a 15—20% increase in water absorbing incident solar radiation which is causing that dimming. Those humid hazes are again number three, are very, very important in warming the atmosphere because, well, they have a dual warming effect, both in absorbing incident solar radiation, but also absorbing these re-radiated energy, infra-red energy going up by the greenhouse effect. Okay, so basically the water in the atmosphere is a key driver, and so that is why we have to get, we have to accelerate it being removed from the air. And that happens naturally by these haze micro droplets, forming clouds, which are then reflective and cooling and then rain which then returns that water to the soils to restart that cycle. Okay, so we have the sequence of processes. Once you have the rain clearing out the water from the air, you in a sense then allow heat to re-radiate from the Earth at night time, without it getting intercepted by these water vapour and water molecules in the air and these are these night time radiation windows. So when we look at the climate data, we find in fact that 60% of the warming is associated with warmer nights. Nights, you know, not being able to release that heat because it's being trapped in at nights. And that's because there is all this water in the atmosphere. The same thing happens with urban heat islands in cities where you end up with hazes and water in the air and those cities not being able to cool off, compared to the adjacent countryside where it has rained and it can cool. So there are these radiation windows. Another one that follows then, where you've had rain, you've created low pressure zones on that land, because in a sense the rain has taken those water vapour molecules out of the air and created low pressure. And that induces more humid air to flow in, and you end up with these biotic pumps, whereby you get more moisture coming in, more rain, enhancing this whole hydrological cooling cycle. And that's most dominant for example in big regions like the Amazon. So there's this whole sequence of processes, all of which are involved with both cooling and warming and regulating the Earth's climate. And yeah we influence those, each of those in a significant way, because we've disturbed vegetation; we've cleared soils; we've changed the amount of aerosols in the air that make the hazes; we've changed the precipitation nuclei that are critical in forming these dense high albedo clouds and rainfalls; we've blocked off these night time radiation windows; and we have completely disturbed these low pressure, formation of these low pressure cells to let the biotic pumps operate. So, I appreciate it's a bit complex, but there is this sequence of hydrological processes where we've disturbed, and in doing so have induced these dangerous climate extremes and global warming.

Brendan [00:27:18]: And where does soil come into all of this?

Walter [00:27:23]: Well, look soil is fundamental in this sense, because it's the Earth soil carbon sponge that is critical in being able to infiltrate, retain and sustain the availability of water to drive these processes. 420 million years ago we didn't have any life on land, we just had oceans and bare rock and all the water that fell on the land just ran off more or less instantaneously into the oceans. And so we didn't have any of this terrestrial, hydrological cycle. It was only when fungi started forming soils, you know the soil structures so that that soil, that organic matter was able to hold the water, that we created the sponge, with its water, that was able to accelerate these hydrological cycles. It's the formation of soil and then biosystems, terrestrial biosystems, that over the last 100 million years that have enabled the planet to progressively cool, because of these hydrological cycles, in contrast to the actual sun, or the solar intensity increasing progressively. It's a major nuclear reactor that's getting hotter and hotter, but the Earth has been cooling while the sun's been getting hotter because of these hydrological processes. So, look, the soil being the sponge is fundamental in holding the water to drive, enable, all these hydrological cycles. It comes to perhaps the next question of yes, we humans, by oxidizing the carbon out of our soils, by degrading and structurally collapsing those soils, we have completely impaired their capacity to infiltrate and hold water and very much impaired that hydrological cycle. You know, so our soils now hold a fraction of the water that they did pre-industrial humans. You know, whereas we had soils that had up to 10% in carbon, that were very effective, active sponges. We now have soils with often much, much less than 1% carbon, not able to hold water and of course as a consequence, we've got increased floods, increased erosions, increased aridity and all the compounding heat effects.

Brendan [00:30:16]: So what I'm hearing is that, the soil carbon sponge you know holds water, it makes it possible for terrestrial biosystems, in other words forests, grasslands, savannahs and so forth to have a water supply and then the plants transpire that. Let's define transpiration quickly, I'll leave that to you. So transpiration, what is that, we talked about that a couple times how it brings the moisture up in the atmosphere, but how does that work?

Walter [00:30:53]: Well okay, it's very simple, it's basically yes the transfer of water from that reservoir, that in soil reservoir, that sponge … it's basically plant roots taking that water up and releasing it from its leaves, its stomata and its leaves, and in doing so, taking massive quantities of, as we said before, energy, you know, 590 calories per gram of energy for every gram of water that's transpired. So it's that massive flux of energy cooling the surface as that heat and that water's taken up into the upper atmosphere. Without the sponge, without the soil, there wouldn't be the water to sustain that process. It's the longevity of green growth that's critical in that transpiration, and the longevity of green growth is determined by the quality of your sponge, the capacity of your sponge. So that whole heat driver, that first process is all determined by the quality of your soil, its water holding capacity. And that's the starting point of that process.

Brendan [00:32:10]: And then when water gets up into the atmosphere through transpiration carrying all that heat energy, it's either going to be, as I understand, it's going to either turn into humid hazes that keep warming the planet if we have a lot of aerosols and you know dust particles up there from the deserts we've created, from the farms that we're drying out and over-tilling and leaving bare soil and from the particulate matter spewed by our industries and diesel engines and so forth. And so it's either going to turn into water as part of that heat trapping, heat absorbing layer we call hazes, or it can be incorporated into clouds, dense clouds, more natural clouds that have a high reflective capacity to block incoming radiation and then also can be nucleated into rain, and then that creates the heat windows and in that process, actually doesn't it release the heat that the water was carrying in the cloud?

Walter [00:33:16]: Well the … yes, and the heat is released when the water condenses from gas back into liquid, into droplets. But because it's up in the upper atmosphere most of that re-radiates back out to space. Absolutely right, I mean you asked the question about soils … if we have a lot of bare soil, by definition we've got dry, desiccated dry soil, massive amounts of dust, we are now putting 3 billion tonnes of extra dust into the air every year, compared to natural conditions, because of this increased area of desiccated bare soil. We are obviously putting massive quantities of particulates, carbon particulates and pollution into the air, so much so that we've got vast areas of the planet, the whole of the Middle East, the Asian brown haze, where literally the top 3000 or the lower 3000 metres of air is really just a soup a haze of pollutant particles, water molecules and its actually sort of 50,000 parts per million water trapped in that air, and if anything that's from a health point of view is now getting to extreme levels, where that wet heat condition, once it gets above 37 degrees centigrade, is actually terminal for human survival. Humans cannot survive you know, once you get wet heat above 37 degrees, because we lose our whole capacity to cool ourselves through evaporation. And so we are approaching that in large parts of the Middle East and in tropical areas, where if we don't get that haze out of the air humans won't be able to live in those regions anymore.

Brendan [00:35:20]: Wow, wow. And I was just going to say we could visualise—I was just thinking of a way of describing this heat transfer to outer space, from Earth to outer space through transpiration and then rather precipitation of the water and releasing the heat. It's sort of like a geobiotic heat pump, is that accurate enough?

Walter [00:35:52]: No, it's spot on, and it's geobiotic, but it's also sort of, in terms of your heat from the surface, is taken up in these fluxes, taken up into the atmosphere, and then it gets released and then of course that's the whole power that we see in our thunderstorms, you know all the energy in the thunderstorm is all that latent heat energy being released. But from there, that heat very much basically dissipates back out to space, and that's a key part of that 342 watts per square metre of heat, that has to leave the planet continually, to maintain its stable temperature, right. So that and the radiation windows are two of the key means of which to get the heat back out of this planet.

Brendan [00:36:44]: So that's what we need to support, instead of supporting humid hazes. They are going to kill us.

Walter [00:36:48]: Well okay yes, we have to reduce these humid hazes for the simple reason of survival because this wet heat will ... is killing us. I mean literally in the Persian Gulf, communities are now getting to the point where hey, they can't survive. So we have to find a very rapid way of doing that, and the way we do it is yeah, stop the production of these hazes, stop the pollutants, you know the brown haze that sits all over Pakistan, India, all the way to Hong Kong. I mean, it's a massive sort of an Asian brown haze. We've got to get rid of that, and the way you get rid of it is by actually coalescing these hazes into these high albedo cooling clouds and then into rain, and that's what Nature does.

Brendan [00:37:41]: And how do we do that? Yeah, tell us how that works.

Walter [00:37:44]: Okay right. And again, all the physics is all, the atmospheric physics, is all documented by a gentleman Schaefer back in the United States back in the 1940's was you know, leading this. We had a major program in Australia, the CSIRO on this as well, and it's very simple. Water can't fall out of the air as rain unless it is actually formed into raindrops, so they are actually large and heavy enough to fall out under gravity. And to do that, you have to coalesce millions of these haze micro droplets into a larger cloud droplet and then a raindrop which is even bigger to get out of the air, you know, for it to be able to fall out. And the way Nature does this, is through hygroscopic precipitation nuclei. And these are really just simple suckers that actually just suck in millions of these haze droplets into a larger drop, until it's big enough and heavy enough to fall out. There are three types of precipitation nuclei, hygroscopic precipitation nuclei. Ice crystals which form in high latitudes and high altitudes, naturally. Salts, particularly sea salt. And you know that when you're having salt, and it's a humid area its hygroscopic, it's absorbing water. But the most important and the most effective by far and we've done all the work in cloud chamber studies and stuff, are a group of bacterial cells that have got very, very high hygroscopic water suction absorption capacities. And these are being produced by trees from forests, and they actually are driving much of the hydrological cloud forming, rain forming dynamics above those forests. So the whole Amazon, over half its rainfall is driven by these microbial precipitation nuclei produced by those trees, those canopies. And again, a lot of documented evidence of the importance of these microbial, hygroscopic precipitation nuclei in driving cloud formation and rainfall. And again we've disturbed those, we've actually impaired them enormously as we've cleared those forests and have any amount of evidence where we've cleared forests and completely changed the rainfall, because we've removed these precipitation nuclei. So we've got other case studies, exceptional case studies, whereby reforesting areas, by restoring these processes, we have significantly enhanced the natural rainfall of those areas, that can only have happened because of those processes.

Brendan [00:40:53]: Wow, so it really comes down to in, at least for this process, restoring forests. And I think what I'm hearing overall is revegetating the planet so that we have, we are covering soils and not generating so much dust and you know, that creates the humid hazes. But we also need plants for building soil, right, and creating that soil carbon sponge as well.

Walter [00:41:21]: It's one synergistic system, yes we've got to rebuild the sponge, that rebuilds this cooling hydrological cycle, that allows then of course trees to grow. These trees are producing these precipitation nuclei and again the rain in these forests is really a biological symbiotic part of the cycle, right. So rain is actually microbially, biologically driven to a significant degree.

Brendan [00:41:50]: That's a real eye-opener I think, to realise that our system is so biologically driven, even up in the atmosphere.

Walter [00:42:00]: Totally, our rain is a biological determinant, right. Both in terms of the sponge, the transpiration, the cloud formation and its precipitation. And the powerful point is not us, but Nature and we know this, Nature has evolved this over 400 … [inaudible] … and in so doing, has been able, over the last a hundred million years to significantly cool the planet to the point that we were then able to induce the Ice Ages, whereas previously in the Jurassic and Triassic it had been, you know, 4—5 degrees centigrade hotter. And we have basically … the Earth has been able to self-regulate and cool biologically through these hydrological processes.

Brendan [00:42:56]: Would it be accurate for me to say, I've got the echo again… Would it be accurate of me to say that the … I wonder, is there just something that changed on your end that would have created the echo?

Walter [00:43:14]: No, I don't think so, no. No.

Brendan [00:43:19]: So would it be accurate for me to say that the main reason to draw down carbon in the soils and restore vegetation on all landscapes to help build soils and of course grow food and regenerate water cycles … would it be fair to say that one of the main reasons for drawing carbon down into the soils is not just to reduce atmospheric carbon, but to drive this soil sponge, hydrological cycle, that controls even more of the process than carbon dioxide levels?

Walter [00:43:52]: Look excellent and absolutely. And look, that's exactly how Nature created the terrestrial biosphere, through pedogenesis, through …

Brendan [00:44:06]: Which is soil-building.

Walter [00:44:07]: Through the formation of soil building, pedogenesis, which is, by putting organic matter, carbon into those soils to build the structure, to build the sponge, to build its hydrology, to build resilience and productivity, right. So that's how Nature works. We, *Homo hubris*, have come along and sort of said no, we're in the business of oxidizing, burning that carbon out of the biosystem, clearing that biosystem. We've been extremely effective in that destruction. But now, the feedback is, in doing that we have killed that or destroyed a big part of the hydrological cycle. Clearly, the thing that we have to do, and the only thing we can do is what Nature did; we have to put carbon back into those soils, massively, urgently. The beautiful thing— and this is where your colleague, our colleague, Colin sits in—we can do this safely, naturally, profitably. You know we can put 10 tonnes of carbon per hectare, per annum, back into our soils, through more productive grazing, crop management, you know managing our animals and crops more effectively. You've got leading players all over the States, we've got these innovate, regenerative farmers all over the States doing that. David Brand, Gabe Brown, the list goes on and on and on. And so the power, the tool, we've got is to put carbon back into those soils, yes, to rebuild the sponge, to rebuild the hydrology, to rebuild, you know, the cooling and that whole biological system. What we are seeing and what Charles Keeling documented, was in a sense the symptom of our arrogant, ignorant carbon oxidation from our biosystems. You know we have been basically releasing about 10 billion tonnes of carbon net, back into the air every year, you know, basically because of our land mismanagement and of course also use of fossil fuels. And so that's what we have to reverse. But we don't just have to stop emitting … the key issue (is) we've got to put it back into the soils to build the sponge, to build the hydrology. Only that has a chance of now restoring that extra 3 watts per square metre of cooling effect and restabilising the climate of the blue planet.

Brendan [00:47:07]: And you know in terms of how soil affects us very personally with our health, I know that how healthy soil affects how nutrient dense the food is that we grow in it and therefore how healthy we are and I'm curious, what are the nutritional differences that you may have observed or researched between foods grown in healthy living soils, versus foods grown in unhealthy soils? And can you give us an example?

Walter [00:47:40]: Oh yeah, yeah. Look Brendan we are now in a slightly different angle or aspect of this, but it still comes from the sponge, right. As we put carbon back into our soils, we rebuild the structure of those soils. So we rebuild the surface configuration of those soils. Instead of that soil being dense, you know, with a bulk density of 1.8 up to 2, we've got soils that have got a bulk density of 1 gram per cc, which means that basically 60% of that soil is actually made up of voids, of spaces and surfaces. The nutrition of plants is governed not by how many nutrients are in the soil in total, or how much we add as fertiliser—again that's a complete, you know, sad, you know, aberrant—it depends on the availability of those nutrients to the plant, which depends on that surface exposure of those mineral nutrients and the capacity of the plant to solubilize, to access, to uptake and cycle those nutrients in that biosystem. Healthy soils in a sense, are totally, radically different from an industrial collapsed soil because they support the microbial life that is actually driving 98% of the fixation, solubilization, access, uptake and cycling of those nutrients. So 98% of the nutrition of natural plants is driven by these microbial processes. These microbial processes of course need carbon as their substrate, and they need that soil environment to function in. Okay? So it just comes back to a healthy soil will have this healthy soil biology, and so it will have a nine-fold nutritional fertility enhancement, even with the same amount of level of nutrients in that soil. Okay? So it's not the quantity, you know, it's not the amount of nutrients in my soil; it's the life in my soil. It's what Mae West said isn't it? Well, you know I won't go into what Mae West said, but it's the actual life in my soil, not the quantity that matters, right.

Brendan [00:50:28]: That is, I was just going to say that's a really, right there a very Earth-shaking, no pun intended, point right there what you just said. I'm glad that we covered this so thank you, keep going.

Walter [00:50:44]: Yeah, okay, but now it gets a bit more sophisticated. If we go back to 3.8 billion years ago, we had a chemical, toxic, physical world. There was no life. But then 3.8 billion years ago we believe the first bacterial, proto-bacterial cell formed. And it formed because there was a semi-permeable membrane, a lipid sort of membrane film that formed, and that lipid film was able to concentrate essential mineral nutrients across it and exclude toxic minerals, and so the internal cell had a completely different chemical composition to the toxic outside world. And in a sense life evolved through the formation of that first … Okay, we … our connection is unstable now. Hello?

Brendan [00:51:52]: Yeah you got a little choppy but you're coming through still.

Walter [00:51:56]: Okay, okay well I'll continue. Okay, so life evolved through that concentration of essential nutrients and exclusion of toxin into the cytoplasm of that first cell.

Brendan [00:52:13]: So it's not the absolute amount of nutrients in the soil, it's the availability that determines its presence in plants, in our food, in our bodies. And so we'll talk more about that I think at another time because that's a whole other realm, and we need to dive into that because that's fascinating. But so … what can we do now with what we've just discussed in terms of these leverage points that we have, in the hydrological cycles to reregulate the climate and cool the planet? What can we do now?

Walter [00:52:50]: Well Brendan, yeah it's what we can do, but also what we <u>must</u> do. You see because really this is the last chance solution that we've got, but we are extremely fortunate; we are extremely fortunate because there are simple, safe, natural mechanisms that can bring us back to stability. And of course, they are what Nature has used right at the beginning. So if we go back 420 million years ago, how did Nature create the soils, the hydrology, the terrestrial biosystem, our stable climate? What is it … what are the processes?

How do we actually rebuild those, regenerate, accelerate those? And it comes down very simply as in Nature, yes, we've got to put carbon from the air back into our soils. As we've said we can do that, drawing down 10 tonnes of carbon per hectare per annum through regenerative agriculture as our leading innovative farmers all over the world are doing. We've put a big paper to the UN. Yes, we can do 20 billion tonnes of carbon drawdown per annum sustainably, practically, by simply adopting a whole lot of these practical processes. You know, carbon draw down, stopping wildfires, those sorts of things. That is twice, that is twice our current net emissions. So we are going to go negative emissions big time. But it's all about rebuilding that soil carbon sponge, rebuilding the hydrology and from that hydrology, restoring the natural cooling, buffering processes. It is only that cooling, only that hydrological cooling, that can offset the dangerous climate extremes that are now already accelerating, locked in. So the simple action is very much that every square metre of land, every farmer, every community, grass roots community empowerment, of growing green plants, of stopping the oxidation or the burning of that green plant and instead, encouraging its composting, its incorporation, back into stable soil carbon, humates, and glomalin. And very simple, elegant, you know there are long-proven ways of doing that. But it's really just getting the narrative, the information, the imperative across to communities. Yes we can, yes we must. It's that simple. It's that beneficial. Because from that sponge comes our water, comes our food, comes our bioresources, comes our ecosystem services, comes our economies, and comes our social stability. All of them are now at crisis points, you know these planetary boundaries that we are exceeding. All of them can be addressed safely and naturally by rebuilding the Earth's soil carbon sponge. And of course, it's that simple, that simple and that positive, right. And it's that empowering, and it's just a matter of saying, stop talking politics, stop expecting, you know, somebody from upstairs to come down with the solution. The solution is with us, the imperative is with us, it's just rebuilding our soil, rebuilding our hydrology, rebuilding stable, buffered eco systems.

Brendan [00:57:00]: And so what that means for each of us individually I guess, begins with our food choices and supporting regenerative agriculture and making sure that we are buying food that grows soil, instead of food that destroys soil.

Walter [00:57:013]: Wonderful. Yep, absolutely and so that's in a sense, we vote every day when we spend our dollar. Forget about the politics, it's when we spend our dollar and making sure that your food dollar is actually reinforcing and driving these regenerative agricultural practices. Making sure your food dollar is going to food that you know where it is grown, where it has come from, how it has been grown. That it's been grown through these regenerative, carbon-enriching soil processes. As you said we'll talk a lot more about the actual preventative health, nutritional, you know, benefits and dividends that we're going to get if we do that. But let's do that on another day. But the whole thing of using our money that we invest in food, the energy we invest in our communities in re-greening, rebuilding those soils, rebuilding those hydrological, you know, dynamics.

Brendan [00:58:20]: And to do this, to avoid catastrophic climate change and resulting refugee crisis and political and economical chaos, social collapse, God forbid, how much time would you say that we have, to turn things around, and what happens if we don't?

Walter [00:58:37]: Right, so there's an old Chinese proverb that says the best time to plant a tree was 20 years ago. The second best time is now. Right and we are very much in now. We've wasted 50 years since Keeling gave us the information. We've wasted 30 years since we had the UNFCCC committing itself on paper, and we are already seeing these dangerous climate extremes accelerating, be they hurricanes, floods, sea level surges, wildfires, droughts, aridification. And you know, British Columbia was burning, Portugal was burning, Alberta was burning, things are serious. And so the bottom line is, in the next couple of decades, we are going to find that things get very, very tight. And biological systems just don't come down to a soft landing; they collapse. And so we're going to find that yeah, systems are stressed, and then there's a very, very dangerous, rapid collapse and with that comes social instability. And it's that social instability that will be then multiplying, catalytic disruption. You know, so we're going to be the main culprit through that social instability of our risk and crisis. So the more buffering, the more resilience we can put in now at that community level right across the planet is critical. So I would argue yes, we've got ten years perhaps, right. Because we need to build that buffering, that resilience, that secure water, that secure food, you know that secure social stable system. And if we don't, we are going to get that feedback, that blowback from instability. And I mean, you know, I don't want to go into examples, whether you know, it's Syria or now Puerto Rico or whatever. But the point is we are seeing it happening and the challenge, the imperative is what are we doing to void that level of instability? Our, you know, strategic leaders, they get this 100%, they know exactly what it us. Up to know they've been saying hang on, we've got to have security measures to address it. But you can't address it with security measures, you can only address it by rebuilding your soil carbon sponge. Because only that gives you the food, the water, the buffering, the stability, you know, that we rely on.

Brendan [01:01:26]: Well amen to rebuilding the soil carbon sponge. Amen to that.

Walter [01:01:33]: Yeah totally. And the other last thing perhaps on this one —and it's a bit of an ironic thing—is, look we can be very, very confident and relieved that Nature is going to do it, whatever we do, right? I mean Nature is going to rebuild healthy resilient biosystems exactly through the same process she used 420 million years ago and many times since after every Ice Age, after every volcano, after every meteor. That's exactly what she's done, every time, successfully. The only question we have got is, are we going to help her do that, or let her do it after, and without us. Thank you very much.

Brendan [01:02:21]: Yes, ouch. Ouch if she does it without us. So let's avoid the big owie. Walter thank you so much for a real tour de force introduction to an understanding of our planet with staggering implications for each of us and for our world. You're a true renaissance man, you know, in physical science, biological science, agriculture, human nutrition. And on behalf of myself and the Eat4Earth community, I want to thank you for taking on the leadership of bringing this powerful information to the world's stage and to each one of us individually in this conversation.

Walter [01:03:06]: Well thank you Brendan and in all that wrap up, a simple word is don't forget our friendly fungi. Thank you very much.

Brendan [01:03:14]: Amen.

So what Walter just explained to us is that it's actually water that governs 95% of the heat dynamics of the Earth. And he's given us a toolbox for cooling the planet by drawing down carbon from the atmosphere and putting it back into soil and plants and trees around the world. So essentially what Walter is saying is that our current climate models are based on carbon dioxide levels, perhaps for the wrong reasons. We need to get excess carbon dioxide out of the atmosphere into soil, to create the soil carbon sponge that will cool the planet. And also, we need to build forests because that is one of the tools in the toolbox, because of how important forests are for creating rain events, frequent rain events that, instead of you know, infrequent, catastrophic events, frequent gentle rain events, that open up the windows in the atmosphere for heat to escape. And I'll add that we need to get the excess carbon dioxide out of the atmosphere to reduce atmospheric carbon dioxide levels so that the oceans can release their excess carbon dioxide that has turned into the carbonic acid that is acidifying the oceans, dissolving the shells of the phytoplankton and other organisms, but especially the phytoplankton that produce almost two thirds of the oxygen for the planet. So what we're essentially, our goal essentially, is to create a carbon sponge, excuse me, a carbon pump, via the carbon sponge, that pumps carbon dioxide out of the atmosphere, out of the oceans and puts it back in soil and trees and so forth in the biosystems of the planet. And that's where regenerative agriculture comes in, and that is what John Roulac is talking about when he says that we need to create a regenerative agriculture system that heals the oceans because the oceans are arguably our most urgent threat, our most urgent crisis. And regenerative agriculture creates agricultural ecosystems that draw down carbon into the soil and keep it there. And we're going to learn about some specific types of agricultural systems that do that in the presentation from Eric Toensmeier from Project Drawdown and also from specific agricultural innovators that are doing phenomenal things. They're growing carbon, carbon levels in soil, you know, the organic matter in soil, that are beyond what any soil scientists have ever thought was possible. And so stay tuned and enjoy the empowerment and the inspiration.

Eric Toensmeier Interview
Food Solutions to Climate Change from Project Drawdown

Brendan [00:00:00]: Welcome to the Eat4Earth event. We're exploring how you can heal yourself, your loved ones, and the planet with food. This is Brendan Moorehead, and our next guest, Eric Toensmeier, has some of the best news ever! Eric Toensmeier is the award-winning author of *Paradise Lot* and *Perennial Vegetables*, and the coauthor of *Edible Forest Gardens*. He's an appointed lecturer at Yale University, a Senior Biosequestration Fellow with Project Drawdown, and an international trainer. He has studied useful perennial plants and their roles in agroforestry systems for over two decades, and he is the author of *The Carbon Farming Solution: A Global Toolkit of Perennial Crops and Regenerative Agricultural Practices for Climate Change Mitigation and Food Security*—a very, very important book for humanity and our future. Eric, it's awesome to have you with us to share this crucial information that Project Drawdown has put together for us and the whole world, and how food fits into the assessments that have been made by Project Drawdown.

Eric [00:01:06]: Well, thanks very much for giving us the opportunity to be here.

Brendan [00:01:09]: Yeah. I'm really looking forward to this presentation, and you guys have some really great assessments for the various types of agriculture ... you know, best case scenarios, conservative estimates, but I guess you'll explain all of that to us. Like how did you come up with these, what kind of information was used to create these assessments and all of that. So, looking forward to getting into it.

Eric [00:01:33]: Well, Project Drawdown is the brainchild of Paul Hawken. He's one of the great environmental minds of the last number of decades, among other things, and he really kept up with this notion of wanting to pull together an assessment of all of the different climate change solutions that are shovel-ready—that is, are already in motion, are already shown to work, and are already happening out there in the world—and looking at how widely they might be spread, what impact they might have by 2050, and to actually rank them and see which ones were the most effective, because what he found when he was asking lots of experts is nobody really knew how, let's say, changes to the built environment might compare with energy or land use and so on, and how individual solutions within those sectors compared with each other.

[00:02:38]. So Paul arranged ... Paul hired a team of folks from all over the world. I was privileged to be one of the senior researchers there. I worked on the land and food solutions. This team worked on both modeling these solutions and also writing up technical reports on sort of like a narrative of their potential and so on. And basically, what we would do—what I was mostly doing and working with people to do—is to map. Part one is mapping and modeling the solutions. So we worked mostly from data from peer-reviewed scientific papers, but also from some other sources to say for each solution, for these land solutions, how widely are these things practiced now? How many million hectares—and we did it all on metric units, you know, because it's science—how many million hectares are there of such and such a solution of improved rice production, let's say. How quickly are these things growing right now? Can we see that something has been ... like conservation agriculture has been adopted in 79% of prime farmland in the southern cone in Brazil and surrounding agricultural areas and so on. So, how widespread are they now, and how well are they growing? How fast are they growing? We look at their sequestration rates and also their emissions reduction rates.

[00:04:08] In all of these cases, wherever possible, we use meta-analysis where we get as many data points as possible, and sometimes we would do a weighted average or other things. Basically, we try and come up with a number that we feel represents the whole planet, and sometimes there's enough data to actually break it out by region or by climate type. We also looked at some of the financials, although we won't go into that today. What does it cost to establish one of these practices per hectare and so on? And what our model then churns out for us … Ryan Allard and Chad Fishermen and others worked on developing this very sophisticated model where you enter those inputs and others, and it tells you how much growth might there be between 2020 and 2050. What would the impact … how many gigatons of carbon dioxide equivalent would you have as a result, and what would the economic impact of that look like? So, that's kind of our approach on a solution-by-solution basis.

[00:05:10] And we're not looking at the technical potential of these solutions. That is, we're not saying if you took a biochar, and you had all of the biomass in the whole world, and you could make it into biochar, what could you get? We're saying … well actually, that's on to our next solution … we're really looking not at the technical potential. We're looking at the achievable potential in three different scenarios, from what we call optimistically plausible all the way up to optimum. So we're not looking at maximum, if you had all the world's cropland and you put agroforestry on it, what could you get? We're saying, what's the most agroforestry we think you could get based on where we are now and where we're headed currently. And then also the next stage is we integrate these solutions, and in particular for the land solutions, there's only so much grassland, so much forest land, and so much cropland. Within that, we broke it down by climate type, by level of degradation, by slope, by soil type, and so on, all these different ways you can analyze the world's land, because most of these solutions are not applicable everywhere. They're limited by climate or they're limited by slope, like anything that needs a tractor can't be over a certain level of slope or the tractor will roll over, and the tractor operator will die. So there may be limits on, some of them are only applicable to irrigated land and so on. So there are these various divisions, almost none of them can you do everywhere, and when you do one somewhere, you can't do another one in the same place. We're basically having a one-at-a-time approach, and that's basically only because we're not able to get data on what happens when you combine practices. And we'll talk a little bit later about farmers like Gabe Brown, who are combining practices and getting great results. And hopefully, someday there will be enough data that we could say, "Well, what happens if you combine conservation agriculture with agroforestry? What happens if you combine managed grazing with silvopasture?" We just currently aren't able to model that. That's one of the limitations of our approach. Anyway, so we're trying to …

Brendan [00:07:26]: Could I pause you for a moment? I wanted to just … you know, I should've interrupted earlier, but just for people who might not be familiar with the term sequestration, maybe just define that. What is sequestration?

Eric [00:07:39]: Sure. Great. So, I'll pause for a moment and define what sequestration is when we're talking about that. Carbon sequestration is when the … one of the issues, the primary issue causing climate change is an excess of carbon dioxide in the atmosphere. When plants photosynthesize, they break that carbon dioxide … they release the oxygen back into the atmosphere, they take the carbon, and they make various compounds out of it in their tissues—things like sugar and fiber and lignan, like woody parts and stuff. And some of that is released through root exudates into the soil and becomes part of the soil microbiome. Some of that is released back to the atmosphere, but some of it stays there and becomes long-term organic matter. And also as leaves decompose, as roots decompose, over time some of that leaf litter or root matter becomes long-lived carbon in the soil. Plant biomass, roughly speaking, if you dry it out, about a half of it is carbon. And soil organic matter, if you dry it out, roughly 57 or 58 percent of it is carbon. So that's how we're moving excess carbon dioxide from the atmosphere and sequestering or storing it in soils and in perennial biomass. And we're also looking at reducing emissions from agriculture as well. Between agriculture and clearing of land for agriculture, that's about a quarter of all emissions caused by humanity. So we certainly want to reduce emissions from agriculture as well. And we do have solutions that look at that also, though we're not so much talking about those today.

Brendan [00:09:33]: Thank you.

Eric [00:09:34]: Finally, I should add that we're looking at these … We're not just looking at the food production, but we have all these other sectors. We're looking at energy, food demand, which would be like diet and food waste reduction, women and girls, which was some of our most powerful solutions, buildings in cities, land use, which for us is really forestry, ecosystem management, ecosystem protection, and ecosystem restoration, and then transportation and materials. So, we're looking at almost all of civilization, and the Intergovernmental Panel on Climate Change, the IPCC, says we're not going to hit the 1.5- or 2-degree target without transformational approaches to these various sectors, without really overhauling all the sectors of civilization. Drawdown has really taken on that challenge. We're saying, "What are the best solutions in all these sectors? Where can we go with them?" So we'll talk today some about the supply side of agriculture, some of our solutions. Any other thoughts or clarifications before we move onto the next piece?

Brendan [00:10:41]: No, that's great. Thank you so much for that.

Eric [00:10:44]: Absolutely. I get ahead of myself sometimes because I am immersed in this a little bit. So you have to translate for me sometimes, okay?

Brendan [00:10:51]: Okay.

Eric [00:10:52]: But let's look at some of these agricultural solutions. The first one is conservation agriculture, and the way these slides are formatted here is that first we have a definition. We'll show their rank out of the 80 solutions. On the Drawdown model, this was the 16th most powerful. Here's current adoption, that is how widely practiced is this today. Then over here we have sequestration rates. Can you see this little … I'll move that down here. How about that? We have sequestration rates. This is the lowest reported number that we had and the highest, and this is the number that came out of our meta-analysis, so our average, or our weighted average, or whatever it is. In this case, we actually have … for four different climates, we show those numbers. So we had enough data. We had 60 or 70 different data points on sequestration of conservation ag, and we could break it out by climate so we can get more accurate results. We can't always do that. And then finally, here we see this is our three scenarios. Plausible is sort of the … we call it optimistically plausible, where we think we could get, if we assume a favorable policy climate. The Drawdown scenario is the one that helps us achieve our goal by 2050 of getting to the point where the total amount in the atmosphere of CO2, and these other gases, rather than increasing, stops and actually begins to drop down a little bit. And the optimum scenario is sort of our best-case scenario, our fantasy scenario for what we'd like to see, which still isn't the technical potential necessarily of any of these, but is what we think is the very best we could envision. And then for each of those, that's how widely they … the total number of million hectares and how many gigatons of carbon dioxide equivalent over a 30-year period. So, some of that may be way more detailed than people need to know. All of it is on our website. A bunch of it is in the book. We have a lot of the backup technical details on the website, and I'll show that at the end so people who are really interested in numbers can get more.

[00:13:09]. So, let's talk about conservation agriculture. This is a kind of annual cropping. About two-thirds of the world's cropland is growing annual crops, crops that are planted … they live and they die all in one season. Annual agriculture is a major contributor to climate change. Tillage of soil burns up the carbon in soil, burns up organic matter, and emits it as carbon dioxide. It also reduces the quality and productivity and fertility and water-holding capacity and everything else of this soil. So practices that can rebuild soil organic matter we call regenerative practices, broadly, although Drawdown doesn't call it that. We're really aiming to try and restore that degradation, to put the carbon back that was lost when these lands were first plowed up, whether they were in forest or grass or what have you. Conservation ag is one of the approaches to do that. It's sort of … In the U.S. and in many of the industrialized countries, it's very much a highly mechanized practice. In South America, it's highly mechanized. A lot of conservation agriculture in Africa is a very small scale, small holder, maybe like oxen-powered practice. So, it's a diverse set of practices for different scales. Some of it's very chemical intensive, some of it's really not, but it has to have three things to be conservation ag. You have to have cover crops. If you want me to, I can define these things, too, if you like.

Brendan [00:14:40]: Sure, yeah, just a quick definition would be great.

Eric [00:14:42]: You have to have cover crops, which are a crop that you plant not to eat yourself but rather to grow and then burn down or plow under or mulch down. In some way, you're planting that crop to catch nutrients that would otherwise be washed away and to cover the soil so you're not leaving this so bare and vulnerable to erosion. So, that's cover cropping. That's one. Number two is crop rotation, where instead of growing the same crop on the same land year after year after year, you change. This year you grow corn. Next year, you grow soybeans. The year after that, you grow something else. Then you go back to corn again. Or often much more sophisticated systems than that, but by combining different crops, some of them are fixing nitrogen, some of them are not. They're using different kinds of nutrients. They're having different impacts on the soil. That's the way to help to reduce damage and actually increase the health of the soil. And finally, we have reduced tillage. It's really tillage, the plowing of soil that's the great releaser of organic matter in cropland. So when you can reduce tillage or eliminate tillage by not plowing up the soil all the time, you can help to reduce erosion and loss of the carbon in organic matter. Reduced tillage on its own doesn't appear to have almost any impact at all, but when it's combined with a cover cropping and crop rotation in this suite of practices that we collectively call conservation agriculture, we do see some modest rates of carbon sequestration. It is already very widespread and spreading rapidly. The cons of it is that it does often involve a heavy use of herbicide. Instead of ploughing to kill the weeds, you use herbicide to kill the weeds. Personally, I don't think that's an ideal situation at all. Although there are people who do conservation agriculture who use no or almost no herbicide at all. What's nice about this is it does have a very good growth rate. It's growing extremely well. From its beginnings in the early 1970s, it's now at 70 million hectares or more, around the world is very impressive growth.

[00:16:58] And actually, if you look at our adoption and impact bar there, you see as our scenarios go up from plausible to optimum, we actually have less and less land in conservation agriculture. That's because we're taking land out of conservation agriculture. We figured once farmers make that step to conservation agriculture from business as usual—tillage —we're hoping they're going to move to where … we're modeling that they're going to move to a regenerative agriculture. They're going to move from taking one step towards conservation ag to another step to regenerative agriculture. And here's another tricky definition. In the broader world, regenerative agriculture is used to describe any kind of agriculture that leaves the land better than it found it. So, there's a whole suite of practices, and all the things we'll talk about today are considered part of the regenerative agriculture movement. Drawdown, for purposes of this solution and for our book, is defining it much more tightly. We're really looking only at annual cropping systems, not at the kinds of grazing or agroforestry that would also be regenerative.

[00:18:07] And what we're trying to do is there are these two big movements happening. On the one hand, the conventional agriculture is moving in a better direction by moving towards conservation agriculture, by adopting conservation agriculture, by adding the cover cropping and the crop rotation and the reduced tillage, which are all excellent and important. On the other hand, we have lots of organic farms, which are really trying to move in a positive direction as well. They have cover crops and they have crop rotation, they're doing a lot of other cool stuff, but they're not able to reduce tillage very effectively. So, they use tillage to control weeds, and tillage is not great from our perspective. The other farmers are using herbicide to control weeds, which isn't great from our perspective. But they're both in a way moving in the same direction. And I feel like I t… it looks to us like they're starting to merge in a certain way. There are organic farming practices that are not regenerative, where you're really using what you call input substitution, just replacing like chemical input with an organic input that you buy from somewhere else. But we feel like together that these are moving in a new direction. And we're saying if you can have any four of these practices, the three from conservation ag and/or application of compost, use of green manures, which are a subset of cover crops that fix nitrogen typically and are plowed in for fertility … So, basically, instead of buying fertilizer, you might be growing your fertilizer with green manures or applying your fertilizer with compost. And then finally, we have organic practice, the broad world of organic themselves. So, if you're an organic farm that has cover crops and crop rotation and you're applying compost, then we would say you're regenerative. If you are a conservation agriculture farm that also is adding some of your fertility through compost or green manure, we would say that you are regenerative. So we're sort of merging these things together and seeing this as a big coming trend. We think it's maybe the 11th out of the 80 practices. We think it's pretty widely practiced already. It has momentum. It has traction. We see big things for it as an annual cropping practice. But again, the name we use is so … it's important for us to choose names for our solutions that have sex appeal, in a way, but also that can be confusing in some cases. Here, I would want to call this regenerative annual cropping, incorporating elements of conservation agriculture and organic agriculture, but that is really …

Brendan [00:20:44]: That just rolls right off the tongue!

Eric [00:20:47]: That's a paragraph. So, Paul's really good at getting the names short and communicating the essence, but this is my caveat saying we're not actually describing all regenerative agriculture here. We're really talking about annual cropping practices that don't involve livestock and that don't involve perennial elements.

Brendan [00:21:07]: I think I'll jump in real quick and just mention that in probably every other conversation in this event, we're defining regenerative agriculture much more broadly. You know, we're basically throwing in everything that seems to be growing soil. So …

Eric [00:21:24]: And I absolutely agree that that is the definition widely used. That is the definition I use most of the time. For Drawdown, this is the word we chose, the phrase that we chose, to describe this particular practice, but we're not saying that's the only kind of regenerative agriculture, and we're not saying that this solution encompasses all of those other practices. That's an important clarification. Anything else on that?

Brendan [00:21:49]: No, I just … You did it beautifully there. I just wanted to pipe in to give it the context of what we're hearing in the other conversations.

Eric [00:21:56]: Great! We went back and forth on that quite a bit, as you might imagine. Okay. Next one is our last annual cropping practice. This is tree intercropping, and these are agroforestry systems where trees are combined with annual crops. We have three different categories. One is, they're protective, like a windbreak or a buffer along the stream to protect water quality. So sometimes you're protecting the farm crops from harmful weather. Sometimes you're protecting the environment from the farm. That would be protective. Then we have functional systems where the trees are helping the crops in some way, like they might be planted on contour to reduce erosion, or they might be fixing nitrogen to provide fertility and reduce the need for inputs like chemical fertilizers. And then finally, we would have productive systems where the trees themselves are a crop, whether that's timber or fruit or or something else. In reality, a lot of systems merge all of these three different aspects of agroforestry together. The one we have in the photo there is called evergreen agriculture. It's spreading very rapidly in the Sahel region in Africa. And this particular tree, the apple-ring acacia, greatly increases the yields of crops that are grown underneath it. And it largely drops its leaves in the rainy season, when you're growing crops, so it doesn't shade the crops. And then in the dry season, it leafs out when there's no crops growing underneath it anyway. So, that's a really exciting development. In this case, in this image it has been growing with peanuts, and actually, the trees have just started to leaf out because the peanuts are towards the end of their growing season.

[00:23:40] But I love the picture because it shows that this can be done with rows and it's, you know, real farming. We did find this to be a powerful solution widely adopted dating back to … A new study has come out since the book, which shows that 40, 43 percent or 45 percent of the world's cropland has at least 10 percent tree cover on it. So agroforestry is really very, very widespread on cropland much more than we tend to think, and much more than we might see in a place like the U.S., which is not in the lead of countries on these kinds of practices. Sequestration rates are starting to move up. Some regenerative is higher than conservation ag. This is starting to move up as well, although depending on the type of system and where it is, those rates are different. We found that they are highest in the tropics, and we do project a substantial growth and carbon sequestration for this solution … overall impact for this solution. Although I should add here and in a number of other solutions, when you have nitrogen fixing plants like these trees or clovers in pastures or otherwise, or nitrogen fixing cover crops or re-manures, they also emit some nitrous oxide of their own, and we don't incorporate that. All that information basically isn't available yet. Good numbers on that aren't available yet.

[00:25:08] All of these solutions have their drawbacks and their trade-offs. And we need to look squarely at those in order to analyze them as best we can. Then we have managed grazing, and the way Drawdown is defining this is really the way it's defined in the international research community, by the IPCC and the other big players. It's a much a smaller, more constrained definition than some of the other presenters I think you folks will be hearing from today. We're really looking at the management of stocking rates. That is, how many animals are out there on the land, like increasing or decreasing the number of animals, changes in the timing of grazing—that might include things like rotation or resting periods—and also changes in the intensity of grazing. Maybe when the animals come, there are more of them and they graze very intensely for a brief time and you move them on, or maybe you're reducing the intensity of grazing because it was too much and you were wearing things out. So, there's a lot of different practices that fall within that range. And the very sophisticated practices some of today's presenters will be looking at certainly do all of those things, but they do a lot more. We're looking at this very broad definition of managed grazing, and we found that it ranked 19th out of our 80 solutions. That's very, that's a big deal. We're estimating there's 79 million hectares currently in practice, although I think we're going to be reducing that in some of our … as we're drilling down and doing our next iteration of work on these. I think some of that was a little high. Our sequestration rates ranged from … actually, I'm sorry, that's a typo there … from 0.2 actually up to three, was the highest input that we have. But they had averaged out to six, because when you have 50 or 60 different data points and a couple of them are high, most of them are low, and some of them are negative, that's what we came out to. And that's very much in line … or actually, it's above. Typically, you see more like 0.3 when you look at what the international agencies think is going to happen here, what the USDA estimates, what the IPCC estimates were, you know, double or triple what a lot of those folks are estimating even at this 0.6. Certainly, there are examples of people doing higher end, like you said. We do have one in there that's three. I'm sorry. I don't have that typed in properly. So we see very substantial expansion in this practice and very significant impact as well. Moving from 79 million hectares today, in our optimum scenario, up to 626 million hectares. That's a really, really big jump. It's still not all of the world's grassland. There's three-and-a-half billion hectares of grassland in the world. We're using some of that for other things. We're reserving a billion of it for wild grasslands. And we think to go from 79 million to 626 million in 30 years would be a very significant accomplishment for any of these solutions.

Brendan [00:28:20]: And if I could interject again ... for the 626 million hectares, this would primarily, I believe, but I don't know ... how much of that would be already degraded grassland that would probably benefit from this kind of management helping to bring back, you know, better soils and so forth, and all the biodiversity and wildlife that can follow? Just curious.

Eric [00:28:48]: Sure. In this case, I can't specify that, but one would imagine much of it might be ... and, in fact, the places where there's the most potential for carbon sequestration are those where there's less carbon than there used to be. If you're starting with a pristine grassland that never lost its carbon in the first place, there may not be much you can do to increase that. Fortunately (joking), so much of the world's grassland and cropland has been devastated by agriculture, it's not hard to find places where you can improve it substantially.

Brendan [00:29:22]: So, is some of this 626 going to come from pristine grasslands that are already there, or is it just pretty much grasslands that have already been cultivated or been degraded? "Cultivated" is probably the wrong word to use. We use that word in agriculture. We cultivate land, but really what we do is we destroy it with our normal ...

Eric [00:29:45]: We're looking in this case at converting land that is currently in business-as-usual grazing to an improved form of grazing. So we're not converting cropland to grazing, although that is an excellent strategy that it shown to sequester carbon in for sure. We're just going from, let's say, not so great grazing to better grazing. Good question. Good question. Okay. The next solution is also a livestock solution. This is silvopasture, which is the integration of trees and pasture, and that can happen in different ways. The two that we're concerned with are planting trees in pastures—in this photo, these are trees that were planted in a pasture—and also you can allow the managed regeneration of trees growing on their own in pastures by excluding your animals from certain areas so that they don't graze down on the tree seedlings for a certain period of time and so on. There's lots of ways that ranchers and farmers are able to manage their animals to permit the natural emergence of trees and other woody vegetation in their pastures. So there's a lot of ways to do it. The trees might be there for timber. They might be there to provide food for the livestock. In this photo, this is at the University of ... I'm sorry, this is Virginia Tech research farm. Those trees are grafted honey locust trees that will drop pods in the fields for livestock to eat. So, not only does this practice tend to increase pasture productivity, but the trees themselves can actually offer additional food to the livestock. And when you're feeding the foliage of those trees to livestock, typically people use legume trees in the tropics for this, the high tannin levels in those leaves reduce the methane emissions from ruminants by 10 to 20 percent, which is a pretty good bonus impact. The trees might also be there just for shade permanently. And then they can profoundly increase the well-being of animals, and in fact, their weight gain, because they can hang out in the shade and not be in the heat. And as the planet gets warmer, that's more and more of an important consideration. It's also really, like some of those farmers who manage grazing, it's a highly desirable practice from an animal welfare standpoint, which is lovely. So, we estimate this is practiced on 142 million hectares. Some people would say it's much higher. It's very hard to figure out how widely a lot of these things are being practiced, quite frankly. And the sequestration rate we arrived at was 4.8 tons per hectare per year from a range of one to 8.6 from the various data points that we had. So this is really fairly conclusively shown to have very impressive sequestration rates.

[00:32:47] It is limited by climate to some degree. It's basically limited by rainfall. Once you're under, let's say, 500 or maybe 450 millimeters of rainfall a year, it gets increasingly difficult to plant trees. A lot of grasslands are too dry for trees. Those are not good places for silvopasture, but there's lots and lots of grassland that is humid enough for trees to be planted. And there are so many benefits to the environment, to the animals, to productivity. The drawback is the higher establishment costs in managed grazing, and we need robust systems of financing for some of these solutions, including this one, to make it possible for farmers to implement it. We saw 73 to 136 new million hectares for this solution. So, less than doubling. We found that less than doubling the amount of this in the world would make it our highest-ranking agricultural solution, because the sequestration rate is so high and because current adoption is so high. Some people estimate maybe 15 percent of world grazing lands are in silvopasture already, and our numbers are much lower than that. Our guess for current adoption is much lower than that, and very, very serious impact in terms of carbon sequestration under this solution. It's a personal favorite of mine. I'm starting a small silvopasture operation next year myself. Very, very small ... a nut grow, with occasional cow, is really what it is. But globally, this is ... 15 percent of all farmland in Europe is in silvopasture today. It's a very serious world land use, and I think really doesn't get all the ... we're pleased with Drawdown to bring attention to this and a number of other solutions, like refrigerant management and educating girls that don't get their due as solutions. Okay. Moving on, we have ...

Brendan [00:34:48]: I meant to mention real quick. Silvopasture wasn't a term in my vocabulary, or at least at the top of mind, when I interviewed Geoff Bugden, who is a silvopasturist, I guess, in Australia. He does pecans and cattle, a very productive operation.

Eric [00:35:11]: If you imagine often on farms, they'll bring in huge truckloads full of leaves and dump them out on the soil to service mulch or compost. These trees are dropping leaves out in those fields every year. It's a huge addition of organic matter to the pasture. If you put the trees too close together, they shade out the pasture. If you have the wrong kind of tree and the wrong kind of forages in the pasture, that doesn't work, either. It has to be designed properly in order to work. But there are really working models for many, many parts of the world where it is just a marvelous, marvelous practice. Again, I'm biased towards trees, but the numbers are very strong here. Okay, tropical tree staples ... So, about 70 percent of annual cropland—that is, of cropland that is growing annual crops—the great majority of it is growing staple foods, foods that produce carbohydrates and proteins and fats, like soy beans or sunflowers or peanuts or wheat or corn and so on. But there are also trees that produce these products, and trees sequester lots of carbon. We know we want reforestation for that reason. We want afforestation for that reason. We want agroforestry for that reason. Trees do a great job. And it turns out that there are many of them that do very well producing protein, carbohydrates, and fats, but it's really only in the tropics where those perennial staple crops yield as well or better as their annual competition. So, we have chestnuts in the north, but they don't yield as well as corn, whereas breadfruit can go toe to toe with corn or casava or any of the other major staples in the tropics. And in fact, it tends to do better. There are a number of many, many of these tropical staple trees that are already occupying 47 million hectares around the world and growing rapidly. The challenge is much of that growth today is coming from cutting down forests and planting avocados or oil palms or bananas. And if you cut down a forest, there's no kind of farming you could do that can make up for all the carbon you've lost by cutting down the forest. Land use change, you know, forest clearing and even grassland plowing up is a huge contributor. It's about half of all the emissions from agriculture come from land use change, so that's an eighth ...

Brendan [00:37:47]: Holy cow! I didn't know that!

Eric [00:37:50]: An eighth of all human emissions comes from clearing land, and 90 percent of that is for agriculture. So it's a really big deal. So, we're modeling not the cutting down of forests to plant these trees, but the conversion of cropland, the conversion of ...

Brendan [00:38:04]: I think I might have spoken over you. Could you repeat what percentage...?

Eric [00:38:12]: Sure, no problem. Okay. So, of anthropogenic or human emissions total, about a quarter are from agriculture and land use change.

Brendan [00:38:22]: And some estimates are at 50 percent, but we can conservatively rely on ...

Eric [00:38:27]: When you look at the 50 percent figures, that includes a lot of energy use and stuff in the food system, some processing and transport and stuff. The IPCC says that it's about a quarter. So I'm just going along with them. It's still a very impressive figure. So, an eighth of all human-related emissions would be from agricultural production and the other eighth would be from cutting down forests and plowing up grasslands for agriculture. Meanwhile, by the way, we've left over 400 million hectares of degraded land that we've abandoned. We farmed it and ruined it and left it behind. So, another Drawdown solution that we're not addressing today, not profiling today, is the restoration of that abandoned land and bringing it back into production. Why would you cut down a forest when you have perfectly good ruined land that you've left behind? But we do have techniques to restore that land to productivity. And anyway, we're ... so, we look some and draw on some of these larger issues of feeding the world without deforestation by 2050. And I'll just say very briefly that all three of our scenarios were able to meet food demand by, you know, all from 2020 to 2050, without any additional deforestation, because we're producing more by using these practices that increase productivity, but we're also reducing demand by changing diet and reducing food waste. So anyway, these have a very high sequestration rate again. 4.7 was the average that we came out to, which is pretty good. Pretty impressive compared, let's say, to conservation agriculture, which gives you ... I don't remember, we had 0.6 or 0.5 or something for that. So we're forecasting an aggressive growth for this particular practice, these tree staples. I'm happy to eat as many more avocados as they want to grow. I think that's great!

Brendan [00:40:22]: You have no idea what an avocado fiend I am. I eat six a day!

Eric [00:40:29]: It's a pretty marvelous food. It's a pretty marvelous food. It really is. And there are so many others. There's a fruit like that called the safou, or African butter fruit. It's an African analog to the avocado, but it's very high in protein, and it tastes like avocado with olive and lime. That sounds pretty good to me. I'm pretty happy with that. So, okay, moving along anyway, there's lots and lots of those. In the *Carbon Farming Solution* book, I have five or six chapters on perennial staple crops. It's the subject of great interest to me, and I'm really thrilled that Drawdown took it and ran. Our last solution is multistrata agroforestry, our third type of agroforestry here, which is defined as a woody system, tree-based system, that has multiple layers of crops. So, the classic example would be like you can see in the photo here, we have shade trees. These are nitrogen fixing trees, in this case, with coffee underneath. It may be that there are timber trees involved. It may be that there are shade commodities like coffee and cacao. But also people will grow things like coconuts and breadfruits and avocados and bananas in these kinds of systems as well.

[00:41:42]: So there's a diversity of different types of multistrata agroforestry. It's estimated there's about 100 million hectares of this around the world, and it has a very high sequestration rate, seven tons per hectare per year, which is an outstanding rate. Unfortunately, the growth rate is pretty low. It just is not something ... it costs a lot, you know, the establishment costs are high. The sort of learning curve is high. It's limited currently to the humid tropics, although there are people working to bring it to other climates. That's been my life's work, among other things, is bringing it into the cold climates. But even with a very modest impact of ... a very modest growth ... so we started with 100 million hectares, and we went to 118.7. That is enough to make this our 28th most powerful solution. So, small growth with a high sequestration rate can have a really big impact. You don't have to impact all the world's land to do it. And this in particular is useful for a cropland that is really steep, that shouldn't be farming annuals. You shouldn't grow annuals on a steep hill, because you're going to get erosion. You're going to end up with all these problems. That should be in trees. And why shouldn't it be in cacao? I am very happy to have all the chocolate I can get as well. It's right up there with avocado in my book.

[00:43:09]: So, let's compare Drawdown sectors to each other. Here we can see, in each of our scenarios, that the food system—which includes again, not only production but also demand reduction— was actually the most powerful sector, which is a pretty exciting thing as somebody who works in that sector. It's important to know that that's not all from, let's say, carbon sequestration. A lot of that has to do with the emissions reduction. A lot of it ... It's a complex picture, and some of that you could really allocate, let's say, to energy or to transport or something else. But the food system, when you combine production and demand reduction, is a really, really important, a really important sector, really big deal. And here's some breakdown within both the demand and supply solutions. We can see that reduced food waste and a plant-rich diet are by far the most powerful solutions. That's in part because we've avoided land use change—all the forest that would have been cut down that weren't cut down due to the reduction of that demand. We didn't give credit to the productions solutions for their ... that is, if they increase yields—which almost all of these do increase yields— we didn't allocate to them that little tiny bit that would go to them for forests that were not cleared, but reducing demand is huge.

[00:44:43]: Reducing food waste ... right now, 30 to 40 percent of the world's food is wasted, which everybody can agree is offensive and ridiculous. And not only are emissions produced in creating that food, but also typically it goes to a landfill where it turns into methane and becomes a terrible greenhouse gas. So, every part of that is wrong, and I would like to see that wasted food ... well, Drawdown says, "First we're going to feed it to people. We're going to capture it before it goes bad and feed it to people." But another very powerful solution is feeding it to monogastric livestock, to pigs and chickens, that can't get most of their food from pasture. And that's a solution with some real potential as well. So we see the impact, the first column here shows the total amount of carbon dioxide or its equivalent in methane and nitrous oxide that's reduced. And on the right, we see the darker red is their current adoption and the lighter pink, the salmon there, is their projected adoption of those solutions. So, I would say that I don't consider us to be ... that we would all agree this isn't the final word on any of these things, and as more information becomes available, we expect and hope and anticipate that these numbers in projections will change and get more accurate. We hope to be able to make them more regionally specific as well. And of course, what we call coming attractions... or there's a whole number of other solutions coming down the pike for which there either isn't enough data right now or they're just not really in big enough scale yet to be able to be modeled in any way that's helpful.

[00:46:26]: That's not anything against those solutions at all. Like intensive silvopasture or pasture cropping, or the various kinds of seaweed farming and intensive multi-trophic, you know, aquaculture and all kinds of other really amazing things people are out there doing. We're just limited by what kind of data we have. And also, starting with things that are actually already out there being done is not a bad approach. There's a certain realism in that kind of approach. So, here we can see on the left are our top 10 solutions overall with silvopasture as the highest ranked agricultural production solution. Refrigerant management which is number one, which was a surprise to me that the chemicals that we use to provide refrigeration and air conditioning, some of them are two-to-six thousand times more potent than carbon dioxide. It's a huge problem in the food system that needs to be addressed and that people are working on. And then here, we can see our ranking of all of our agricultural solutions overall, including ones we didn't discuss today, like restoring abandoned farmland, various solutions related to reducing methane emissions from rice, reducing emissions from fertilizer. Women smallholders is really just ... women receive globally so much less finance and extension and assistance. Women who farm... that if they were brought to parity in terms of the resources they receive, it would greatly increase yields on their farm by something like 28 percent. And then that enables a certain amount of avoided deforestation. We have some other solutions in there as well. So, for folks who are interested, they can of course get a copy of the book and also visit the website, where we have information on all the solutions. We have summaries for each of the sectors with all kinds of data in there. We have summaries, technical summaries, for each of the solutions that tells more about our math and our process and our assumptions, and also some resources and references for further information for people who want to learn more.

Brendan [00:48:36]: So, that's awesome.

Eric [00:48:37]: There we go!

Brendan [00:48:39]: That is such incredibly inspiring information. And one of the things that really gets me fired up from my perspective, you know, these are very sound scientifically-based projections. You wanted to … I believe, the whole operation Project Drawdown wanted to avoid any kind of overstatement of the potential. And that being the case, we have these outlier data points. Let's say, we've got … I believe number 19 in solutions was managed grazing …

Eric [00:49:25]: Yes.

Brendan [00:49:27]: … and I believe it was 0.6 tons per hectare of carbon sequestered. Is that …?

Eric [00:49:33]: That was what we arrived at. Yes. That's correct.

Brendan [00:49:36]: And what we hear from some people in this event, is some of them are capturing … well, it's all the ones that are saying anything about carbon sequestration from mixed systems, where you're actually stacking, instead of just managed grazing, it's managed grazing, plus cover crops, plus raising some grains and so forth, stacking different enterprises. And that, I guess, is one of the coming attractions, you would say. But these early data points are saying, well, in the last 11 years, we got nine tons per hectare, and some people are saying, well, in this particular four-year, five-year period or whatever, very recent, you know, like it's still going, maybe around 20 tons. And so that is so far out of the range of any of this. Obviously, much more research needs to be done, but one of those data points is validated by the United States Natural Resource Conservation Service. And so …

Eric [00:50:37]: Sure, sure. And there are individual high-data points in all these solutions. So any of these will have some particularly high and often some very low. For grazing, for example, I've seen this is as high as … there was a big study in Africa, where some of them were up to four tons, or losing as much as three tons. So for some of these, there are also examples of loss of carbon from implementing the practice. So, the meta-analysis that we use, one of the advantages of it, is it kind of discounts some of those outliers and brings you to something that's more likely, but that also … one of the reasons for that is it's hard to say that everybody in the world is going to farm as well as the best farmers, that every single farmer is going to farm as well as Gabe Brown. I would love to live in that world, but okay, that might be a little bit of a stretch to some degree. So it's both an advantage and a disadvantage of our methodology, I think, is that some of those high points maybe aren't in there. What we would love to see is some of these … really, there just isn't enough scientifically validated data showing those kinds of very high sequestration rates for, let's say, these very sophisticated kinds of adaptive grazing, these integrated livestock systems like some of these folks are doing, which I think are fabulous. Should at some point those things … should there be enough numbers to plug into a model like Drawdown's and data on how widely they're practiced now and how fast they're growing, then it would be possible to use a model like ours or some other one to really make a projection on the impact of what that would mean. Intensive silvopasture is another one that I'm really bullish on. We could see sequestration rates of up to 10 tons per hectare. The increase of meat production—2 to 10 times more beef per hectare. Enormous! Amazing!

Brendan [00:52:54]: Woah! That takes a lot of pressure off deforestation. I mean, it's not just beef that drives it; I mean, there's beef and soy, various things driving …

Eric [00:53:04]: It could really, really transform beef production. It's is currently limited to the humid tropics. It started in Australia; it's moved to Latin America.

Brendan [00:53:11]: But that's where the biggest problem is, right?

Eric [00:53:13]: Yeah, yeah. Yes. That is where a lot of deforestation is happening. So we … I would love, you know, that's one that I'm a big fan of that has a very high rate and so on. At Drawdown, we call those coming attractions. We say we think these are awesome. We fantasized about doing a whole book of like 100 coming attractions. There's so many of them. They're so cool. We just … We're not yet able to model those things.

Brendan [00:53:38]: You should still write that book. Write it up! Maybe you can't create the model, but just basically, "Here's these outrageous data points. It's exciting as heck! Go for it! Start one of these enterprises yourself." I think that would be a great thing to encourage. You know, a goal—"Here's the most exciting thing you could do with your life!"

ric [00:54:02]: I do think that. I do think that. And some of the things, some of the assumptions that I had when I came into doing this … I started in about 2009 really beginning then looking at the carbon numbers. Some of the things I thought would be really outstanding were not, and some of the things I did not think would be that good turned out to be really great, either on a per hectare basis or just based on adoption. If you have a practice that has a very minimal impact but you do it all over the place, it can have a bigger impact than something with a very powerful per hectare impact that is constrained by being expensive or limited by climate or something like that, or lack of markets for the products from it. So there isn't any one right answer. There isn't any one best practice. There may be one best practice for any individual piece of land that the farmer or rancher can determine. But just because silvopasture is the most powerful doesn't mean it's what everybody should do. It doesn't mean any individual person listening this should do it at all. But it is useful information for us to know that some practices are solidly shown to really work. And I would love to see more people in the U.S. doing silvopasture. The NRCS has it as one of the practices they can pay you to do in many … they'll pay you to do it in many parts of the U.S.

Brendan [00:55:34]: Good!

Eric [00:55:35]: And even in the places where it's not on the approved list, it's on the national list. Even the places where that practice isn't part of the state list, but …. each state takes from the whole huge national list of practices and picks only some they want to do. But in all of them, there's tree planting, and you can use tree-planting funds to plant trees in your pastures and establish a silvopasture. So it also offers a chance to get around saturation. This challenge that … scientists widely agree that at a certain point, you sequester carbon for, let's say, 10 to 50 years, and then you're pretty much full. The soil is full and not going to continue to sequester more after that, or sequestration will be balanced by emissions at that point. So we need to figure out how to hack saturation. One way to do that is to add biochar to soil, which could theoretically continue to increase the amount of carbon above and beyond saturation. With above-ground biomass, we also see this saturation. When a forest gets closed enough … there's a period of rapid growth when a forest is younger … once it's become, you know, mid to older age, it doesn't really grow as fast anymore. And in many forests, it essentially stops growing, although it looks like in tropical forests, it does continue to grow at a slower rate, maybe forever. But with a silvopasture system, let's say, you can grow your timber trees in the field, then you harvest them. If that timber is used as a building material, it's gonna last another 100 years. That carbon that's in that timber is sequestered. And then you can plant a new tree, which is going to start to grow quickly again. And that's one way to get around saturation, and to really make a ruminant production … very, very, very carbon friendly for an indefinite period of time, regardless of emissions of nitrous dioxide and methane and regardless of saturation and soil. So that's one of the reasons I'm really bullish on silvopasture, you might say, to make a very poor pun there.

Brendan [00:57:52]: I actually, unfortunately, didn't catch it, but thank you. That was actually brilliant. Yeah, this is all so very exciting and inspiring. I really hope, you know, Paul and all of you, will write that other book. I just want to thank you for all that you're doing. One quick comment, I noticed we've got all these tree-based or, let's say, tree-inclusive models that are among the highest within the agricultural solutions, according to your assessments. And to me, that also suggests something, a distinction which is between perennial and annual agriculture. Annual agriculture, especially in the degenerative model and the conventional model, being very, very hard on soils versus, you know, we take a step from there and we say, okay, conservation agriculture—still annuals, as you've defined it—but it's better. It's starting to improve things, but then if we go perennial and we go, of course, non-toxic and so forth, we've got far more potential to restore the planet, restore nutritional integrity to our food supply. And I would suspect that in perennial systems, the roots go deeper in general, the plants … So we don't have to just limit ourselves to measuring the top 10 inches of soil for where the carbon's going and say, "Soil's full." Maybe it's growing deeper and deeper into the soil.

Eric [00:59:29]: Yes, absolutely. We want to be going down two meters, ideally, when we're measuring for soil carbon. The general trend is that perennializing is good, and woody plants are good. I don't envision a world ever where there'd be no annual crops. I love tomatoes. I love winter squash. I love bread made from wheat. But how much can we shift in that direction is really the question. Are there lands that are … really, there are prime farmlands that are flat and fertile and not vulnerable to degradation. Those are great places to grow annuals with practices like regenerative agriculture, as we've defined it, or conservation agriculture. But once you get into sloping lands, once you get into the tropics where … there really is no prime land in the tropics, because soils once they're exposed, once they're clear, they just start to degrade really quickly. Sloping lands, various other kinds, certain kinds of soils really aren't suited to annual agriculture unless there's an agroforestry component, or they should be in something perennial or they should be in some kind of a grazing practice. So it's really about trying to match from this pallet of practices, trying to paint on the landscape with the best suitable practices for any given area, that also have to make sense for the level of mechanization, for the markets, for the farmer's individual desires, for other goals, for ecosystem services and other things. It's not a one-size-fits-all kind of an approach. It really has to be from these general principles and generalist practices. It needs to be very decentralized and very regionally adapted, or else it's going to fail, I think. It has to be driven by farmers and based on the needs of farmers and the needs of the land, or we're not going to get where we need to be.

Brendan [01:01:35]: Right. Well, thanks again, Eric. And please send my regards to Paul and thank him for spearheading this. And he's a genius, and he's produced a book that is possibly the most valuable and exciting coffee table book in the world!

Eric [01:01:54]: That was our goal.

Brendan [01:01:55]: Yes. Beautiful pictures, inspiring and empowering information, and I can't wait for volume two. And again, thanks for all you're doing!

Eric [01:02:06]: Absolutely. Well, thanks for having me. Anytime.

Brendan [01:02:09]: How cool that the Project Drawdown team of scholars has quantified the impact of all of these solutions to climate change. It's like a menu or a palate, as Eric put it, to choose what you'll do for the planet and human health around the world. Later in the event, you'll get a chance to meet some of the regenerative entrepreneurs that earn a great living and live exciting lives healing the planet. What they're accomplishing is nothing short of amazing! So, don't miss any of those talks, and thank you for giving this event your precious time and attention. It means a lot, and we're blessed to have you with us.

Graeme Sait Interview
Minerals, Microbes, and Reversing Climate Change in a Golden Era for Food

Brendan [00:00:00]: Welcome to the Eat4Earth event. We're exploring how you can heal yourself, your loved ones, and the planet with food. This is Brendan Moorehead, and I'm very excited to welcome our guest Graeme Sait. Graeme is the CEO and co-founder of Nutri-Tech Solutions in Australia. For over 25 years, Graeme and his company have been world-leaders in discovering a viable alternative to chemical agriculture. Graeme is an internationally sought-after speaker, specializing in soil, plant, animal, and human health and wellness. That emphasis is now expanded into planetary health in recognition of the link between soils and climate. Following his TEDx presentation in 2013, Graeme has continued to create major impact influencing farmers, consultants, doctors, governments, and key decisionmakers worldwide. He is responsible for over 300 published articles and a popular book *Nutrition Rules!* Graeme is a powerful presenter who speaks at conferences and seminars around the globe. His inspiring presentations are often described as life-changing. And I can personally attest to that last point, as (can) folks like Finian Makepeace and Ryland Engelhart who were inspired by Graeme to cofound the Kiss the Ground organization that is doing extraordinary things to advance the cause of restoring global soils to reverse climate change. Graeme, I'm really happy that you could join us today to share your wealth of empowering knowledge and inspiration.

Graeme [00:01:23]: A pleasure.

Brendan [00:01:26]: So, your big focus in humus, which is a topic of your TEDx talk in 2013. What is humus, and why is it so centrally important to human health and the stability of our planet?

Graeme [00:01:38]: Yeah, I had been asked to do a TED talk, and I was actually in LA speaking on the steps of City Hall to a bunch of climate change protesters. I finished my talk and people rushed up and said "what was the word you said"? I assumed immediately they it was this word mycorrhizal—hugely import creature in this whole equation that we'll talk about a little later perhaps. But that wasn't the word. The word was humus. Someone said, "This is chickpea dip, isn't it?" I said, "No, that's hummus. And I realized that here are people giving up their precious time to complain about a lack of action on climate change, and they didn't even know the meaning of the word that was most relevant to the whole issue. So that was the point at which I chose that my TED talk would be based upon explaining the importance of the substance called humus. So, humus is this sweet-smelling, chocolate brown-colored substance that microorganisms make in the soil from organic matter. It's a kind of a stabilized form of organic matter that stepped into the carbon cycle and formed this stable humus. And it serves as the home base, but is also serves several other purposes. It stores moisture incredibly efficiently. It stores minerals. It serves as home base for minerals and moisture, and those two things together are very important for nutrition amongst other things. But it's the humus story simply is that you can't make more carbon molecules. It's the same number of carbon molecules that have been here since the very start of time, and they cycle between three places. The carbon on the planet is either stored in the soil, which is by far the largest storehouse. Or, it's stored in living carbon-based life forms, which is us, and animals, plants, and so forth. Or it can become a gaseous form and store as CO_2 in the atmosphere. And so the same carbon molecules since the start of time cycle between those three places. The big story here is that the largest store house by far, you know, three times what is in the atmosphere, is in the soil as humus, as organic matter. And, the way that we've farmed for the last 10 or 12 decades we've actually mismanaged our soils, and we've lost two thirds of that huge storehouse. We've gone from 5% organic matter down to 1.5% organic matter. And that actually represents almost double all the rest of the carbon we've put out there from coal-fired power stations and industry and motor vehicles and so forth. So, when we look at that story, and we look at our carbon emissions and we talk, and that's all we've done, about reducing carbon emissions; last year was the largest amount of carbon emissions in history, so we're not doing much more than talking. But if we were to cut carbon emissions tomorrow morning, (and) we said, "Yes, the sh_t's hit the fan. We've got to do something. And we cut them 100% tomorrow morning, in 200 years' time we'd drop down to the levels of CO_2 that we had in the atmosphere … basically we'd take us down to 1975 levels. Now, that's still too high, 'cause this thing has been happening for decades—this climate change, this global warming phenomenon. The oceans would continue to heat at those rates and continue to acidify. And you don't find many experts out there who will ever agree that there's 200 years left. So the most extreme version of the only thing we've talked about doing—which is cutting emissions and not doing it—the most extreme version when we cut everything doesn't save the day. We haven't got 200 years, and we can't continue to heat and acidify the oceans and the many other side effects of that story. So, you know, you might say, "Is it all over but the shouting?" It's not, 'cause there is a solution, and that is what my mission around the globe is driving home that there is an answer, and all of us can get involved in that solution. And the solution is simply if you step into the carbon cycle, which is what you're doing when you are working with the soil, and you build organic matter rather than losing it, every little bit of organic matter that you can measure on the soil tests that you build is not new carbon; you've stepped in and sequestered what otherwise would have been in the atmosphere, as direct carbon sequestration. And the figures are all out there. There's the hard science to support the fact that that is the solution. The actual figures are 1.6% organic matter globally, if we could build that, we've reversed climate change. Currently, we just talking how do we keep it at 2 or 3 degrees. Two degrees isn't double our current one degree. This thing feeds on itself. It's exponential. We have no way of knowing what 2 degrees looks like, and we're headed there quite rapidly. This is a way that we can actually reverse that story. We can take 402 parts per million (ppm) of CO_2 in the atmosphere and pull it below 300 within a decade if we embrace this, if we make it almost a military action for everyone to get out there and do it. And that applies to everyone—minding your own patch as a home gardener, even your little spot on the veranda for that matter. You mentioned veranda gardening, but just that role—if you take a calculator and do the sums and say "OK, I've built one percent organic matter for my 1000 square meters …" Now, your contribution—that's the biggest contribution that any human being can make. People need to recognize those figures and understand that they can get involved, and they can make a difference. And we all need to start doing it yesterday. There's an urgency and a serious urgency.

I don't want to get grim, but to give you an idea of the scale of that urgency, certainly in some people's minds, Professor Guy Macpherson from Arizona State University and Professor Emeritus was in New Zealand, my home country, just a couple of months back and was asked in prime time television, "Guy, you know the story. This is your field. Where are we heading with this climate change thing?" Guy looked down the barrel of the camera and said, "I want every last one of you to get out now and do everything on your bucket list because I'm sorry we've left it too late. There's just 10 years left, and there are no human beings left on the planet. Don't leave it for 9 years and 364 days, because the trouble begins way before that. Get out now and do whatever you want to do on your bucket list. Sorry to give you that news, but that's the facts." So, thats what one man, and one quite prestigious and accomplished climate change scientist is telling us. I'm not saying I subscribe to that belief, but I'm telling you there are many people who are that grim, and I meet them almost on a daily basis as I travel the world and speak at conferences and so forth. And the average man on the street sitting back on the couch watching the football is really missing the seriousness of this equation.

Brendan [00:08:05]: I think what's missing also when we hear the most grim prognoses from folks like that is they're missing the soil equation.

Graeme [00:08:17]: Yes, they are.

Brendan [00:08:18]: They don't realize that we do have an option if we choose to exercise it. But we have to get started.

Graeme [00:08:24]: And it was such wonderful news that the French Government at the science level have been the first to recognize that story, and of course their principal initiative from the Paris Climate Change Conference was the 4 in 1000 initiative. And that is not … wasn't really the greatest term, I don't think, because most people say, "What is 4 in 1000?" And they have no conception about what it's about, and it should be instant the recognition of what it means, but it's not. 4 in 1000 means that you aim towards—it's a lofty goal—that you aim and you incentivize your farmers, and everyone else for that matter, to try and build 0.4% organic matter. That's technically 4 in 1000 (4/1000). That's not very clear to the average man.

Brendan [00:08:18]: That's like 4 tenths of a percent—point 4 percent (0.4%).

Graeme [00:08:24]: Yeah, .4%. You can even think .4 in decimals, but .4 is 4 tenths of a percent. The upshot at the science level, is that if we could do that, even if we could get halfway there within about a decade, we've basically reversed climate change. It's actually doable if the whole world was doing it. And there are, I think, 22 countries that have signed on to that French initiative. Unfortunately, Australia is not one and nor is America and not going to be for quite some years to come by the look at your current President. But yes, not a good story on that front. But, yeah, that's basically the story … so that has been my mission, and I'm frantically trying to—at governmental level in many countries—drive home the fact that we've got to act, and we've got to act pretty soon. But it's doable. That's the good news.

Brendan [00:09:57]: Yeah, 4 tenths of one percent … I have encountered various people who are doing that, and usually it seems to be a combination of livestock and crops, something like pasture cropping like Colin Seis does in your lovely country, and also people in the US doing the same thing.

Graeme [00:10:18]: Yes, well the figures for the US figures are that you guys are putting out about 8 billion, slightly more, but about 8 billion of the 36.2 billion tons comes from 5 percent of the world's population of putting out almost 20 percent of the CO2. But if you were to step in—and this is not the grazing lands 'cause grazing is actually a more effective way of building humus than intensive cultivation—but if you were to take the cultivated lands in the US and build 1 percent, that pulls back 4.5 of your 8 billion, and that's more than what's needed to save the day. So this is a very doable thing, but we've just got to recognize that and begin doing it very, very soon.

Brendan [00:10:56]: Did you say, you said, one percent of something? I didn't quite catch that.

Graeme [00:11:00]: I said, basically you guys are pouring out 8 billion. That's 20 percent of the world's total. If you just built one percent organic matter in just your cultivated lands ...

Brendan [00:11:11]: Got ya. On our 400+ million acres.

Graeme [00:11:16]: Yeah, if you built 1 percent on that, that pulls back 4.5 billion of your 8 billion, and that's more than what's needed to save that day. That equation is more than what saves the world. So it's absolutely doable because you can do it even better on—there is much, much more land that's involved in grazing land—so really, really doable. But we just got to start doing it! You know, there's this short timeframe, and we are sitting around apathetic or in total denial. And someone says there aren't many people in denial, but your President is one of them.

Brendan [00:11:48]: I think it is important to make a quick distinction about the type of grazing we are talking about. We're talking about grazing—there's Holistic Management; there's rotational; there's cell grazing, different names for the same thing, but mimicking ...

Graeme [00:12:04]: Yes, I call it intelligent grazing. It's just the recognition that you can do the thing much, much smarter. And you can have all different strategies, but the very simple part of the equation is that you retain 4 inches—and we talk in millimeters and centimeters—but we'll call it inches. Four inches is the benchmark. No matter how you do it, you try not to graze below 4 inches. You leave some solar panel, as you know, you well and surely know.

If we look at the most fertile area ever in the history of mankind, it was the Great Plains. And if we look at what drove that fertility, we discover that it was buffalo coming in these huge herds with that sort of mob grazing effect, the predator effect, keeping them together, eating everything. They weren't choosy because another head was next to theirs at the time. So there's massive amounts of urine and dung and a huge soil fertility-building exercise associated with that mob-grazing model. But interestingly, if we say, OK, the definition of the word science is adherence to natural laws and principles, so what can we learn from the most productive areas in history. What we see the animals did, the herds did, was at four inches they moved on. They sort of knew, and so you can say "why did they do that?" Well, it's so basic. The leaf is the solar panel that photosynthesizes and pumps half of the sugars it makes it down into the roots, and 60% of that half is pumped out into the soil to feed the soil life, and some of that becomes humus. So that's a hugely, hugely important strategy or model to understand, and if you graze … the roots are actually based on how much solar panel is supporting them because the above-ground are supporting below ground. So if you've got four inches, you've usually got somewhere around about four inches of roots below. If you graze back to three inches the roots prune themselves, because three inches can only sustain three inches of root. You go back to two inches, one inch, or half an inch, you've got half an inch of roots. And so you've lost your entire humus-building model. Your whole soil fertility model is gone when there's no leaf supporting the biology and the humus-building apparatus beneath those leaves. And so, it's so simple. Leave it at four inches and graze and develop models. And there are many of them, but the central, driving thing is 4 inches. You've got to leave four inches. However, you do that doesn't matter. You try to leave 4 inches as Nature did in the most productive soils ever.

Brendan [00:14:27]: Right, and unfortunately that's not how most people are grazing. They just kind of let the cows do what they want, and our domesticated cows have even lost that intelligence gene to not, you know, graze down to the roots.

Graeme [00:14:42]: They're not given a choice because they're in a confined area you know and that's the way they've managed …

Brendan [00:14:48]: Right, it's true that they're not getting moved on. But it's also, I think, true that when they're given free rein over an area, and they stay there too long, and they pick and choose, and they chew the good stuff down to the stubble and leave the more thorny stuff.

Graeme [00:15:00]: But see, they're not marked, they're not in the herd like they used to be. The herd that had predators that kept them in a herd, so you stayed close because you had wolves eating you on either side. So, you're sort of bunched in, and that effect we've got to create that because obviously we don't have the predators there, so we've got to create that with confined areas and bring them in for short times and so forth. You can do it. You don't necessarily have to have enclosed paddocks as we call them, or fields, or whatever you call them. You can do that with just a long electric course, electric course wire. And the animals will mob up beside that wire as you gradually move it around the field on large fields, and you can get that mob grazing effect at the edge of the line. And you can do it many ways, but the bottom line is just that simple thing is you're trying to leave the solar panel, and you're trying to achieve large numbers of animals in one area for a short time that creates all that dung, and all of that urine, and all of that soil fertility effect. The animals become your principal fertility tool in that model. And that's how Nature did it. We're just learning from what we were supposed to do. We're supposed to learn from this perfect blueprint, not think that we could do better than that. And that's been our downfall, and that's got us on our knees staring down the abyss at the moment—the concept that we thought we could do better than perfect. It's an arrogance beyond conception that only Homo sapiens would be capable of.

Brendan [00:16:21]: When it comes to the human nutrition, you know, human nutrition, human food, and you're teaching farmers how to grow food for humanity in a way that builds humus and maybe sometimes livestock are involved, maybe sometimes they're not, but you mentioned that humus is so important in the soil that it's even more important than the ratio of minerals, which you also teach is quite important. The ratio of minerals because that affects soil structure, but humus apparently even trumps that if I recall correctly from the course. Can you explain a little about that?

Graeme [00:17:00]: Yes. Well, what we work with, and what we call Nutrition Farming is this understanding that it's all about balance. Balance is a critical word whether you're talking about the balance between calcium and magnesium or the balance between fungi and bacteria, whether it's biological, whether it's mineral, balance drives everything. Even in our bodies there's huge balancing mechanisms. Simple things like estrogen versus progesterone and many, many people, for example, are progesterone deficient, and all of the problems associated with excess estrogen, which include our largest killer, prostate cancer, and our second largest woman killer, which is breast cancer, can actually be countered by balancing out that ratio between estrogen and progesterone, and taking a natural progesterone cream, so the balance works whether it's the soil, the plant, or the animal. And then the soil, we look at key ratios, and we talk about the most important ratio being the calcium to magnesium ratio, but we go through six key ratios. And then there are other ratios even on leaf testing. But in the soil, the ratios are really important because they govern the two most important things that you manage when you're looking after a soil. When you're looking after a soil, you're managing something called gas exchange. How freely does the most important of all nutrients, oxygen, of the most important of all elements, oxygen, is more important than any other mineral in the soil. It drives everything, including us. We'd live for maybe two minutes depending on how long we can hold our breath. That's the same deal as a hugely, hugely important thing—how freely does oxygen move into that soil? The roots use it for everything. The organisms that surround those roots use it for everything, and then they breathe out. And of course, they breathe CO2, and the CO2 diffuses from the soil, the plant leaf is waiting with thousands of tiny little mouths called stomata under the leaf, to capture that CO2, combine it with water and sunlight, and so begins the most important process on the planet, by far there is nothing even slightly close to the process of photosynthesis. So, photosynthesis builds the glucose-building blocks of all carbon chemistry, of all life, us included. That's where we come from. It all started and all begins with the process of photosynthesis and the building of the glucose-building block for all carbon life. So, a hugely, hugely important process and interestingly at the nexus of the single most important process on the planet—and there is nothing that comes close—is the most important principle, because the plant creates this building block that it uses for everything, pumps half of it down to the roots, and then gives away—you know this is the unusual thing—it literally gives away 30% of its total production of its most important substance. So, what we're seeing here as I said, is learning from Nature is the most important principle: give and you shall receive. And that's a universal principle that applies to our lives as much as it does to this most important process. I mean people work in jobs they don't like; they retire; and they finally donate their time and become volunteers or whatever and then feel the sense of peace and harmony they've never experienced. And that's part of that law—you can't actually receive what you don't give. And when you do give, that's when you receive. And so there, as I said, there's Nature as a teacher at the most important process on the planet is the most important principle. So, the plant gives away 30% of its most important substance and in return, when it feeds up that army of soil life around the roots, the soil life reciprocates. It actually gives more than it gets, and of course, fixes nitrogen, and delivers minerals, and protects from disease, and makes humus, and all of these things, the wonderful things that soil life grants us, all begins with the plant feeding and looking after that workforce.

And so your role, back to the farmer's role, is how do I manage gas exchange. How freely does the oxygen move in, get utilized by the roots and the organisms around the roots, and then move out to drive this process of photosynthesis? And the better you manage gas exchange, and that's gonna apply to you home garden, that same story. You want to have a friable soil that allows the oxygen and then the CO2 out. And the better you do that, the better you do. And of course, that applies to everything, including building humus because the organisms all need oxygen, and they do better, and they build more humus and so forth. So that ratio, the most important ratio, that determines how well the soil can breathe, is called the calcium to magnesium ratio. Calcium is a huge ion with two positive charges that grabs all the little particles of clay and with its positive, because clay is negative charged, and pushes apart the clay and opens up the soil, and that's called flocculation. And magnesium conversely tightens the soil, because it's much smaller, and it pulls together the clay and lessens the soil's capacity to breathe. So you might say, "I'll just do some lime, and I'll fix the calcium," but there's a second role that you're involved in as a grower. As a vegetable grower, as a farmer, or a gardener, and that second role involves the management of the green pigment in the leaf called chlorophyll because that's the sugar factory. That's where the whole process of making photosynthesis takes place. So the better, the more green that is, the less pale colors and blotches and so forth in the leaf, the better you've managed chlorophyll. And the better you manage chlorophyll, the more sugar factories, the more production of that glucose-building blocks, the more humus, the higher the quality of the plant, the less disease pressure because the plants can fire everything with all of that glucose. So the whole process is down to your management of gas exchange and chlorophyll, and that's why you can't forget magnesium and the calcium to magnesium ratio because the centerpiece of chlorophyll, the most important single mineral, just like iron is for our blood, magnesium is for the blood of the plant, the green pigment, the green blood called chlorophyll. Magnesium is the centerpiece of the chlorophyll molecule, so we can't forget magnesium. We just need to get the ratio right, and that varies between the light soil and heavy soil. For example, there's an ideal calcium to magnesium ratio for every soil, and you know, certainly, in agriculture it's very easy to look at a soil test and determine what that is and aim towards having a soil that can breathe perfectly. And that involves the perfect calcium to magnesium ratio. So, that's just an example of one of those ratios. I won't go through all of them, but all of them have their own importance.

Brendan [00:23:08]: Yeah, I know it takes a whole two days to do that.

Graeme [00:23:09]: Yes. There's the phosphorus to sulfur ratio, and the iron to manganese ratio, and the phosphorus to zinc ratio, and the magnesium to potassium ratio, and so forth. All of which have got their own their own logic and reason for working, but the interesting thing and this is what your question finally coming back to the answer for your question is that basically those ratios become less significant the more organic matter you've got. Because organic matter is the home base for the organisms that do all of the things that you want to happen in your soil, and the more you've got, the more of that that happens, and all of the inhibitory effects of poor mineral ratios become less significant. You've got so many microbes doing all those things anyway, you can get away with having a soil a little bit more out of balance. Humus, organic matter, is the great forgiver in the soil, so the higher the organic mix, so really it overrides everything because you've just got so much soil life performing all of those roles that the importance of that balance become slightly less. So humus is the most important substance.

The National Bank, our largest bank in Australia, said "Well, OK, we've got so many farmers wanting to get bigger or get out, and wanting to borrow money to buy their neighbor's farms, and so we go through the set of criteria and we tick the boxes and say 'yes you qualify' and then a huge number, an unacceptable number, of those loans are falling over. So we need to review what determines profitability when you're farming in agriculture. Is it your size of your tractor or the amount of NPK you used, or your management skills, or your marketing skills? What is it that determines?" So, they spent three years on 800 farms with our central scientific body, the CSIRO, looking at that and to the surprise of everyone, what absolutely head and shoulders above number two, what determines your profitability was the amount of organic matter in your soil. It was the moneymaker in the farming enterprise, and you know that makes it really exciting to realize that we've already got 22 countries that are incentivizing farmers via the 4 in 1000 initiative to build organic matter. And they're building the very thing that's going to make them more profitable, so you're getting paid to become more profitable. That heralds the dawn of the golden era of agriculture, in my opinion. It's an exciting time to be involved in farming.

Brendan [00:25:23]: And so is it … when we say organic matter, carbon in the soil, and humus, we're essentially, not precisely, but essentially talking about roughly the same thing?

Graeme [00:25:32]: We are except there are two types of organic matter, and that's quite important and not widely understood. There is what's called active humus and organic matter, and active humus is like taking your lawn clippings and throwing them in a corner and four months later you've got a pile of compost. And that's been made specifically by bacteria in the soil, or bacteria in this case, in your lawn clippings. And they've created a compost, and you take that compost and put it on your garden and you'll see the soil change three shades darker because you can put on huge amounts—it's just the home garden. You couldn't afford to do that in farming. Um, but six months later you come back to get your tomatoes and put something else in, for example, and those three shades darker have gone back to the original color. That's called active humus. That's bacteria. You know we've got several creatures in the soil. Bacteria is the most dominant and one of the smallest. But they've made this humus that is not very stable. It oxidizes and returns as part of the carbon cycle, and that's what's happened in your garden. That's not what you'll get paid carbon credits for, and that's a huge part of the story.

Now we start talking biology rather than minerals, is this recognition that fungi, beneficial fungi in the soil, are lacking in almost every soil you look at. They're easy enough to bring back, and we can actually brew them up, we can feed them up, we can very easily bring them back into our soils. But perhaps not continue to kill them off so much with some of the herbicides, and the miticides, and the fungicides. But, still you could really inoculate them here and keep them there and feed them and so forth, but they're hugely important because they take some of the bacterial humus, and they take humus they make themselves, and they wrap it up with some clay and create this clay humus crumb that totally stabilizes and changes the nature of that humus. So now, it stays in the soil for 35 years. One of the greatest breakthroughs in composting science, you put a little bit of clay-based soil into the compost and now the humus that you've created in that compost will stay in the soil for 35 years. And, of course stay out of the atmosphere for that time. So, you know, a hugely important strategy is this recognition here we've got to bring back the fungi in the home garden, on every farm on the planet. We've got to bring back fungi into the equation. There's, you know, a very famous fungi that I mentioned earlier called mycorrhizal fungi that burrows into the plant root and expands out and gives us 10 times the original plant surface area and provides so many benefits. But one of its huge claims to fame was only discovered in 1996 by a woman called Sara Wright. And, basically what she discovered was that the most dominant strain of those organisms, called the glomala strain, produces a sticky, carbon-based substance called glomalin that we now know—and she didn't really know at the time how important that finding was — but it turns out to be the triggering mechanism for about 30% of all the organic matter in the soil, in which, you know 30% of the organic matter in the soil is actually about what's in the atmosphere with you know being just as a crude comparison. Uh, and that creature that makes it is not in our soils anymore. Nine out of 10 soils don't have it. Ninety percent of mycorrhizal fungi had been killed off with modern agriculture. So we need to bring them back into the equation. We can inoculate them; we can feed them up; we can even … compost stimulates mycorrhizal fungi, whatever you've got left. So we need desperately to understand their role. And then the second creatures in the realm of beneficial fungi are these creatures that are called saprophytic or cellulose-digesting fungi who are also decimated in our soil, not quite as badly as mycorrhizal, but pretty bad. But they can be so easily brewed up for a couple of dollars an acre, literally, or fed up with things like humic acid or cover crops, and so forth, to get that fungal component working again and then sort of create the stable humus that pulls the carbon out of the atmosphere and stores them in the soil for 35 years, and that can save the day and really will save the day if we can just recognize the importance of it.

Brendan [00:29:30]: And in terms of our nutrition, if I understand correctly, so that the fungal organism … having more of these particular types of fungal organisms in the soil will help build stable humus, and humus has some kind of ion exchange that holds the nutrients in the soil for the plants. Explain that because that's where the connection is to human nutrition as I understand it, right?

Graeme [00:29:59]: Good question, yeah, So there are two storage systems in the soil to store the minerals that are the basis of everything. Minerals determine every aspect of our nutrition you know in the soil, in the plant nutrition. If we look at research showing copper deficiency, if your soil is copper deficient, for example, the plant, our food will be deficient in carotenes and vitamin C, because copper is a building block for those two phytonutrients that make food part of the story that makes food medicinal. You know the founder of modern medicine, and it's a bit of a cliché, but he said it, you know. Hippocrates said, "Let your food be your medicine and let your medicine be your food." And what we're discovering now with the science over the last decade is just how profound that statement was—this recognition that we can take all the supplements in the world but there is no comparison to the nutrition found in our food. Food contains, you know … it might be something high in selenium, for example, like Brazil nuts. Well, there are cofactors that determine the uptake of selenium, perhaps the most important of which is vitamin E. Well, you never find selenium by itself in any food as there's always going to be vitamin E present there. And that's just one of multiple cofactors that determine food that's supposed to be our medicine. And the medicinal quality of that food is all about the soil that you grow it in. And so you know we are what we eat, and what we eat comes from a soil is a shadow of what it used to be. And if we can change that story, and humus and mineral balance are the two parts of that equation, we change that story. And of course, soil microorganisms ... it's a three-part equation—it's minerals, microbes, and humus, and their interrelationship determines directly our health. And there's a huge parallel between what's happening to the external stomach of the plant. So, the plant produces this glucose-building block and then pumps out a third of it, or 30% of it, out into the soil to look after its external stomach. So, we've got a similar, we've got a tube that runs between our mouth and anus that contains 10 times more cells than our total community of cells that is who we are. So many of us picture ... have described us as, you know, as a community of interrelated ten trillion cells.

And then we have a whole separate thing, of course, called our soul. But physically we are this community of cells all of whom can communicate at thousands of times a second and allow us to be this wonderfully functional, multicellular creature. But, um, there's actually more of something else within us and on our skin and that's called our microbiome. And there's actually 10 times more. There's 100 trillion, instead of 10 trillion, a 100 trillion of these organisms, so you could say we're a sack of microbes walking around because we literally are.

And the recognition of the importance of that has just exploded in recent years. In 2000, there were 239 published papers on the microbiome, the organisms that live within and on us, and this last year 2,720. And there's a huge explosion and interest in recognition of the importance of these organisms. But when you look at those organisms and their role, which is every aspect of our health including mental health, is directly linked to these organisms. I mean the studies that they actually ... that have been conducted in Australia here on something called fecal transplants are actually mind-boggling. I feel they're almost Nobel Prize-winning thing, these studies, where we're seeing, for example, people with what used to be called manic depression and then that now called bipolar, which is considered to be sort of you know, pretty difficult disease, as they call it, to counter ... they're taking people with bipolar killing off all of their gut organisms completely with a series of antibiotics, reintroducing healthy, you know, bulletproof gut organs—they actually pay people to poo, basically. And then from that poo of people who are super resilient, they brew up these organisms, and that fecal transplant involves putting them into someone else that's had all of their life killed. And you've literally transplanted a healthy person's gut system, microbiome, into someone else. And it's unbelievable. I mean, bipolar disappears. Long-term chronic inflammatory diseases disappear almost instantly. It is like, it is one of the greatest breakthroughs. Even this work in Australia here on animals ... they take a bunch of chickens that are struggling, and in comparable conditions, then there's one chicken that's doing incredibly well, they take, however many, say 20 other chickens, kill off all their organisms, introduce the poo from the healthy bird, and suddenly you've got a flock of super healthy animals. It changes everything.

Brendan [00:34:34]: That's extraordinary.

Graeme [00:34:35]: I mean, you can see the whole world's gonna … this is like absolutely world-changing, game-changing stuff, in terms of where we're heading on multiple levels with these findings. And it's actually Australian scientists that have been pioneering some of this stuff, so that's quite exciting from that perspective. But, so we now know basically every aspect of their health is … and we look at what these organisms, our internal stomach, you know this life within, the sort of things that they do for us, and then we look at the external stomach of the plant that it feeds to maintain these huge number of organisms around the roots, and it turns out to be almost identical. The same substances that produce the same supportive immune enhancing substances, and the delivery of minerals is as dependent on microbes in our gut as it is in the soil, and so forth. It's a really fascinating equation.

And it turns out that we've slaughtered and compromised our internal organisms with multiple things, including the consumption of processed food. You know that's just such a basic thing when you see what you know, what's in most people's trolleys in the supermarket lanes. You know the cornflakes, for example, you know food lasts for a week or maybe two weeks unless we preserve it or salt it or dry it or whatever. But now we can take food that lasts for two years on a supermarket shelf, and what changed? Well, we included something called "food grade stabilizers". It's a nice innocuous term, but what food grade stabilizers are, of course, are biocides. They're materials like sodium benzoate and so forth, that kill single-celled organisms, so that you have no spoilage organisms and now you've got extended shelf-life from the food. But why would you think when your child is eating that tablespoon of cornflakes that last two and a half years on the shelf, why would you think that that 2.5 percent stabilizer that kills microbes is going to stop working when it gets down into your stomach? And of course, it doesn't. It's one of the biggest single players for what's called dysbiosis and the killing off of some good guys and some of that diversity, all-important diversity in our gut, is related to the amount of … you can actually pick someone's health based directly on how much processed food they're consuming because they're impacting their gut so seriously with that whole story. So, you know, we look at what's called probiotics in humans and what good guys can you reintroduce. We look at the longest living people on the planet eating lacto-fermented foods, sauerkraut, kimchi. The Koreans are right on the longest living Asians. They eat kimchi twice a day and that's repopulating the entire system, you know, because even if you're not killing it off with stabilizers or antibiotics, you're still pooing out a little bit each day. So the longest living people into the 100's are Georgians, always consumed lacto-fermented food and no difference now with the Koreans and so forth. And it's a hugely beneficial thing for us to reintroduce those organisms, but there's the same story in the soil that we can make compost teas. We can feed up, you know, like in our guts, we call it prebiotics.

On my farm I've gotten wildly enthusiastic about a plant called yacons. And yacons are a root vegetable, and I've got huge numbers of them not fully grown, then it'll be the largest growing in this region of that particular, because I started researching that and discovered that the most powerful prebiotics … prebiotics of foods that stimulate the gut organisms and fire up whatever you've got to counter the damage you've done to them. And so this is a really important thing. They're estimating that the prebiotic industry is going to be worth, and you know, two or three billion in the next decade as people recognize the potential.

But the two most important prebiotics are called inulin and fructo-oligosaccharides, which often is just called FOS. Well, it turns out that this root vegetable—they're so easily grown that any home gardener can grow it—called yacon, is so sweet and it's delicious. They call it Peruvian apple. It's crunchy. It's just a really, really nice vegetable you can eat raw or you can juice it, and the syrup is perfect for diabetes because it tastes sweet, but it doesn't have any negative effect for diabetics. But basically, the entire sweetness comes from inulin and fructose. It's literally a prebiotic food. More so than any other food. So it becomes incredibly medicinal for all of us to just, you know, that's so easy to grow. They grow a couple of meters high, and you can get ten kilos per plant, and then you can … that lasts, that root vegetable actually gets sweeter when you store them. Anyway, I've got hundreds and thousands of them that I'm planting here at the moment. It's one of the multiple 50 enterprises on the farm is going to be producing a living prebiotic called yacon. Sorry that was a long answer.

Brendan [00:39:14]: I didn't, you know, I didn't know all of that about yacon. I've heard of yacon syrup. I've heard of it as a prebiotic sweetener. And now I want to grow yacon, so thank you for mentioning that because that sounds awesome.

Graeme [00:39:29]: And, you mentioned what can you do on a veranda. What you do you just get one of those plastic sort of rubbish bag-type planters that you can buy for a dollar, fill it with compost and soil, and plant your yacons in there, and you'll have that whole thing filled with these tubers that are so delicious, and it grows with nice flowers. So, it's quite a … it's a member of the sunflower family, and it has all these beautiful flowers, so it's a nice thing to have anywhere. But what a wonderful benefit.

Brendan [00:39:55]: So when we're talking about soil quality, building humus and, you know, all the nutrients getting into the plants because the microbes are doing their job because they're being fed by the exudates of, you know, some of the glucose that the plant produces through photosynthesis, and then we're not killing those organisms and destroying them with all the chemicals, all the plowing and so forth, and so if these minerals are getting to the plants, the plants are able to produce, you know, their phytonutrients. And then we consume food that supports us. But, that's not what's happening overall with most of the food supply yet. And that's when you know we've got so much degeneration in the human species as a result of this. But you know, I came across a video from the 50s with William Albrecht, great soil researcher, and he was making a point that he was showing tomatoes next to your two tomatoes next to each other, two stalks of celery, two bunches of celery next to each other, he says you can't necessarily tell the difference in nutrient quality just by looking at it. But you, Graeme, have a have a couple of tips I believe, for you know, how can we assess foods' nutrient quality even if we don't have, you know, some kind of a high technology tool to analyze it. How do we know?

Graeme [00:41:19]: Well we do, we do actually have a high technology tool, and it's just called your taste buds. I mean because you know like that celery that looks identical will be hugely different in flavor or because you can pump things up with nitrogen, and because we pay very little with this horrific model that we've developed for food production where farmers have literally become serfs to the supermarkets who demand that they get bigger and bigger, and more and more efficient, and yet when they do that, they still fall over, and they still commit suicide. And you know the strawberry industry for example in Florida has gone from hundreds down to dozens, and we still have suicides every year and failed businesses every year. It doesn't matter how big they got; they still play them off against cheap Mexican imports, and that model that farmers have been price takers rather than price makers has to change if we want agriculture to be successful. We've got to have a model where we recognize the value of food and where farmers have some say. And they're guys doing all the work. They're making the smallest part of the margin. They've literally being drawn and quartered with the current food production and food marketing model, and that has to change. And that's what's great about things like farmer's markets and why we all need to support things like that. We need to look after the most important profession on the planet which, is farmers. There's nothing that comes close to the importance of food production, and those people have got one of the hardest and worst jobs. It's not in the sense …. because I'm doing it myself, I absolutely love it … but they're not treated well, and the whole model is essentially fatally flawed, and it needs to change. And so that's one of the many things that I'm driving.

Now, the other kind of mission currently for me, for me, is almost as important as this recognition of the need and the link between the soil and the climate change issue, is this world's most widely used chemical glyphosate. Your country is horrific. I actually, I've got to be honest, apart from the wonderful people that come from your place, I hate being there and eating your food. And I don't know how the hell you guys can put up with it and can accept it because you've had this pollution through your food chain, with your major food crops now of course being genetically modified across the board. And we're talking about things like soy, which is in every loaf of bread that you eat and many, many other foods. And we're talking about corn where the sugar from corn, for example, the syrup is in every soft drink and every sweetener, and its corn is fed to the entire food chain. And both of those crops, because they're Roundup Ready, and we're talking about Roundup, we're talking about glyphosate the world's most widely used chemical, is sprayed onto those crops three times during the crop cycle on average. And so you've got you know really, really ridiculous levels of residue of this material. And we were told that it was harmless. You know, everyone was told years prior, "You know its biodegradable. There's no issues." It wasn't true. It was absolute bullsh_t, and we need to wake up really quickly to this. And many people are calling it the new DDT. This makes DDT look like a kindergarten party, and it's totally polluted our planet. We've got to stop it, and we're going to get in and do it quite soon.

But in your country, you've gone so far down that path that there's breast milk levels of 250 parts per million of this. I need to explain to you why it is so serious. And most farmers across the globe, and I say, "You explain to me how glyphosate works." They have no understanding at all of how the chemical they use more commonly than any other, it's whole mode of action. Here's why it's such an issue. Glyphosate works on the principle of several things. It was developed originally as a chelating agent to clean manganese from boilers that would have deposited on the inside of boilers, and then it was discovered that could also kill plants. So it remains a very powerful chelating agent which can lock onto minerals and reduce their availability. So that has a big impact when minerals are tied up in the soil and so one of the most powerful is manganese, a mineral called manganese, is really important for plant protection amongst many things including photosynthesis. Manganese plays a major role on the whole starting process of photosynthesis, but then it also kills off manganese reducing organisms. Organisms that make manganese available in the soil.

But a central mode of action—these are just side issues—is that it shuts down a pathway, a biochemical pathway, called the shikimate pathway. That's how it actually works. The chemical doesn't kill the plant. You actually shut down a plant's immune system and any opportunistic organisms always present in the soil comes in when the plant has no immune capacity and immediately kills the plant. And that's what kills the plant with glyphosate. If you take your soil—this is the case for anyone—put it in a microwave, which hopefully you don't do with your food, and nuke everything in that soil, and so it's completely dead soil, look put chlorine or whatever, but kill everything in it, and then plant a plant into it and spray glyphosate on it. You can never kill it. You can't kill the plant because there's no organism, you killed everything good and bad. There's no opportunistic pathogens that can kill it because that's how it dies. You knock out its immune system.

Now, the way that the multinationals got away with introducing this, they said mammals don't have a shikimate pathway. Too bad that we've given a form of AIDS because we've really compromised the immune system of every other living creature, which is all soil life, plants themselves, birds, fish, I mean everything in Nature other than mammals, has this really important shikimate pathway that you shut down and you've literally compromised the immunity. It's like giving the whole world a form of AIDS. The fatal flaw with, you know, three sprays on your major food crops—in fact, you know our bread contains your imported soy, and it's a disgusting thing that every child's gone off to school with three sprays of glyphosate on their sandwich. And there needs to be a recognition of that. The fatal flaw in saying, "It's not a problem with humans because we don't have a shikimate pathway" is that we do have 10 times more of another creature than there is of us that does have a shikimate pathway. And we nuke our immune system. 85% of it is in the gut learning from these gut organisms—that's how we develop immune competency. And now we've compromised the immune systems of the very organisms our immune systems … look are you going to get? Well you've got the fastest growing group of diseases, autoimmune diseases. You've got direct and absolutely incontrovertible links to the plague of autism. I mean where are we heading with autism, for example. Currently within 13 years, one in two people in your country is going to be born with autism. I mean, you know, I don't want to be horrible to kids with autism, but I'm just saying literally you're going to have one half the world that can't communicate with the other half. I mean, we can try and prove that, but it's going to be a fairly miserable kind of scenario if we don't put a stop to it. And there is a huge link between autism and glyphosate. There's a huge link between one in four of us now succumbing to Alzheimer's—massive link to glyphosate. It is mind-boggling when you get into it.

I spent time on stage recently with the hero of mine, professor Don Huber, who's been a major whistleblower and an incredibly accomplished scientist who's been driving this understanding that we've made a huge mistake. We've got to pull it back. We've got to stop this thing, and we got to do it really soon for a variety of reasons. So it's a huge issue, and as I said, and in your country its everywhere. And the levels, when you measure blood levels, are frightening. And you know that gut organisms are all impacted and everything. Our whole capacity to fight the fight and be resilient is compromised with this terrible chemical, and it really has to go. So I tell farmers everywhere, and they say "Oh, we can't grow no-till without glyphosate." You're going to have to learn, because it's got to go. That's the reality.

Brendan [00:49:00]: Every time every time you speak I hear about somebody amazing that you've been meeting with or speaking with and I recall a story from one of our last conversations about how you were with

James Cameron the filmmaker with, you know, the Avatar films and so many blockbusters and I'm just curious, you know what happened to that conversation if you could recount that? And also, I'm curious, have you met with him again?

Graeme [00:49:25]: You know, well, it was actually, it was involved with Suzy, his wife, who is running this very wonderful school called the MUSE School based upon, you know, a different model of education where you choose someone's passion, and they learn on the basis of that passion, and that opens the doorway to an enthusiasm for learning generally. And it's a wonderful model. I've been into the school a couple of times when I've been over. You know, it's a model that should be everywhere. But because of that, I was invited to their New Year's Eve party in New Zealand. James is over. He's got a 3,000 acre farm. There's actually some prime grazing land that he's purchased, and he's making of course Avatar 2 3 & 4 in New Zealand at Weta, at Peter Jackson's studio. So yeah, I went up to the party. Was a great party, and it was all organic food and so forth, and some of the little local farmers were there and they were all saying, "What the hell is this stuff, you know, where's the meat?" because they're vegans. But my argument ... so we had a discussion with James at the end, and then we went outside, and there was sort of a bit of a raging argument. But the thing, the whole argument was based on the fact that while I've got nothing against veganism, although it needs to be intelligent veganism, because most people that we test, and we do a lot of testing in our course because we give you sort of a bit of a report card for heavy metals and trace minerals and so forth and other nutrients. And you know most vegans are B12 deficient and are missing a couple of amino acids and iron and zinc, which is more ... better uptaken in animal forms and so forth. So there's a couple of issues, but if you take care of that, and you're aware of that, then veganism is a great thing, and that's very healthy and so forth. But, if we recognize that animals may be the most important link with this, what we've just talked about, the way we graze, intelligent grazing, and that we can build humus more rapidly.

Look at the work of Dr. Christine Jones, a wonderful researcher, in Australia here who's been looking at that model of cell grazing and pasture cropping and so forth and how efficient that is for building humus. And it really is the best way to build humus because the soil is undisturbed. So fungi, who like to be undisturbed, can thrive, and if you stimulate them up with that mob grazing model and so forth, you can seriously build some humus into that equation. So animals, what I'm saying is animals may well save the day. They may well be the key because most of the world is grazed; it's not intensively farmed. So, if we just were to incentivize the electric fences and the watercourses and so forth that would allow wherever it was appropriate to adopt that model, we can save the day really, really quickly. And of course if we're not eating animals, why would they exist? You know sure you're going to have a few sheep for wool, but I mean the model, most of the animals that do most of the grazing, are going to be there if we're not eating them. There's got to be a reason for their existence. I agree totally with the vegans from the perspective of our mismanagement and our horrific story of confinement animals and this one we're talking about free-range chickens, and we're talking about free-range pigs, and of course free-range beef, and so forth. And it's important and all of the kind of principles of looking after, nurturing, and respecting those animals who wouldn't exist if we didn't ... if we weren't eating them. You've got to recognize they wouldn't even be there, but if we can give their lives, you know, that they can be treated humanely and have a decent life while they're alive, at least there's a little more justification.

But the important thing is they may well be the key to saving the day. So veganism has actually it has got a negative in that context because you say he's taking three thousand acres and growing soy or something new, you know. And that model, in that context is a little flawed, and that was my argument with James and it was a good argument. He's intelligent, and we had a good argument. He said come and see me when you're here next time, which I've not been back, but I will at some point. So yeah, it was just an interesting debate because we do need animals in my opinion.

Brendan [00:53:17]: And I think on that regard, I want to make a quick point about free-range, because in the United States, the term 'free-range' on a package of chicken eggs or you know chicken parts or something is absolutely meaningless. I want to make that point real quick for our listeners. And so we have to, what we really need to, and there will be other people, and there's other people in this event talking about the labeling issues. But we've got to get really specific. We need to start asking questions. We as consumers need to start asking specific questions. Is this animal spending their life roaming naturally all the time? Maybe sheltered from the elements inside of a house, but with ample space. Not crammed together with supposed access to a 10 by 10 area through a door that's open five minutes a day, and there's no way that any of those chickens are making it out there, and that's called free-range in the United States. It's disgusting.

Graeme [00:54:15]: Yeah, well I mean it's not it's not simple because, I mean, I see all these things, obviously I'm in fields all day. And you know if you set up the current model where you've got a barn with a whole area that they can free-range, but the barn contains all their food and the warm conditions, and what happens is the animals just go back in the barn. And you can have it open 24/7. You can have it go for the go out there but they've got all this food. They've got all the things. It's just like us sitting on the couch and eating fast food, you know. There's a whole model that's kind of flawed. You have to change everything. You've got to have some decent nutrition in the pasture so they've got a reason to go outside. And you can't just have them walking around on dirt and say that's free range because the whole model is, you know, that whole concept as I said is flawed. So, there's quite major changes.

Will be interesting to hear your other speakers speak on that issue because it's a major issue. But it's multi-dimensional, and it really needs to be looked at right back to the whole way that we feed them and what we feed them and the pasture, you know, you can put 40 different herbs into a pasture, deep-rooted, herbal medicines, high-protein herbs that really can change the whole nature of that chicken. I mean the chickens we're growing here, the eggs that we're grown here, they set up on the plate you know twice the height and three times the orange color of a normal egg, and they're so delicious you know. They are genuinely out on a decent pasture sort of thing. And they eat less grain as a result. You know and because that I've got some nutrition in their pasture, so you've got to take care of both things at once essentially.

Brendan [00:55:46]: You know I'm curious, Graeme, since you're on the cutting edge of everything soil, farming, food, and health, and climate, planet, you know, and you told me not 2 years ago about some technology that it was going to help us grow soils faster and so forth. I'm just curious what's got you excited these days. What's on the cutting edge?

Graeme [00:56:10]: There's probably three things that well, I'm always excited about something. but you know, people bring things to me because I'm in suddenly, you know, 33 countries in the last 12 months. And there's a technology from South Africa called Pure Care that involves basically the delivery of a whole lot of different oxygen species that you actually use a UV tube to ozonate water, but only tiny, tiny amounts of ozone. And then you, under pressure, combine it with hydrogen peroxide so you've got $H2O2$ and $O3$, create something called peroxone which is a whole bunch of different forms of oxygen. And then you deliver that via irrigation at six parts per million, which is exactly the level of oxygen, that's only one form of oxygen, that you brew microbes in. So that's kind of like your brewed up your soil. And the changes with—when I talk about how important oxygen is—the changes are just mind-boggling. I've not seen anything comparable. I mean soil structure changes completely. Earthworms come back. The humus-building capacity of the soils returned within two to three months. It's only obviously relevant to irrigated soils, but there are a lot of them out there, and all of them could be transformed with this technology. It is the most exciting thing I've seen. I mean I say there's no such thing as a magic bullet, but this is as close as what I've ever seen because it transforms dead soils, you know soils that have been growing GM crops and have been poisoned with all sorts of crap. Even those soils are recoverable in a short time. It's the sort of thing that someone like Elon Musk should get behind and finance on a global thing and get it out there rather than spending his money dreaming about going to a godforsaken red hole and ...

We've got this glorious jewel that we've mis-managed and we understand so little about, so many parts of it, when we look at the Nature story, and we look at soil life and some organisms we barely know what their roles are. You know ... say nematodes, and we think, "Oh that's the bad guys that are chewing into our roots. Well that's 20,000 ... that's a small percentage of this 80% of nematodes are the good guys that perform a whole range of roles, but we don't even know those roles or understand them. We've named 20,000 forms of nematodes, but we know from DNA analysis, which identifies completely different life forms, that there are over a million. So 990,000 God or whoever you think put them there, are all with a role in an interrelationship, and we don't even know what that is. And yet we're so 'I'm gonna go and try and build a plastic bubble on some red God-forsaken hole that's going to cost trillions of dollars. I mean where is the logic behind when you're living in this perfection that we've messed up that we can reclaim, why wouldn't you put your money into reclaiming it? And I just get angry and frustrated because you know Richard Branson ... they're all doing this similar thing with ... they're great; I really admire, particularly Elon Musk. I think you know this is wonderful return to the entrepreneurialism where you're doing something of value, but then he's sort of blowing it in my opinion with this ridiculous dream of spending trillions on some other place as if there's no hope for this one. And this is perfection. This is the most beautiful place, and we can so easily bring it back to that. Anyway, yeah, that's just my opinion.

Brendan [00:59:25]: Amen! So, what you know one of the themes of this event of course is voting for regenerating the Earth with our food choices, with our dollars, with our Australian dollars, American dollars, with you know every currency on the planet, and everybody who's listening, please vote with your dollars at the supermarket and ask questions and learn how things are actually being grown. Don't necessarily, you know, just go by every single label. Find out what it really means. And you mentioned, you know, take responsibility for any plot of land you can and grow soil, or grow humus, grow delicious life-regenerating foods. What else? Is there anything else that people should be considering?

Graeme [01:00:17]: Well, um, I mentioned you know the three things. And, so I've mentioned one of them which was that Pure Care technology. I'm also, you know, really excited with just what I've seen recently with the use of … we talked about microbes, soil microbes, then we talk always about the aerobic guys, you know, how we can grow up compost teas, and we can really bring back that all-important biodiversity. See the simple rule is … okay, so science is adherence to natural laws and principles. So I'll say, "What's the most important principle in Nature?" Well there were no doubts about it. The most important principle by far is diversity, biodiversity. And that's just what Nature thrives on. So we find with the model of cocktail cover crops for example, a huge in my opinion, massive breakthrough, this recognition that if you can have five families of plants—and I mean home gardeners could do this for that matter —but five families of plants, and you can have more than one of each of them, but only when you get those five families together you get this messaging between the roots and this outpouring of these substances called phenolic compounds, which is why we drink green tea because those antioxidants impact our cells very beneficially. Well, it turns out that these trillions of multicellular organisms and single-celled organisms in the soil also respond to those antioxidants that get, in this case, poured from the plant roots only when you've got five families together. If you've got four, it doesn't work. So there's a major finding from a Brazilian agronomist whose really important finding, so the five families just so you know, cereals, grasses, brassicas, legumes, so you could get a blend made of those four. But the missing link usually it's called, I think, you guys say chenopods, but we say chenopods. So chenopods are a small family, they own just everything from the beet family, like silver beet and beetroot and sugar beet. Spinach is a chenopod. Amaranth and quinoa, that's pretty much the group. But you only need one percent, so you know it might just be sugar beet in your country because you get the seed easily. Only 1% of your total blends, but you've got to have it there. You know, you might have five or six percent of brassica, so that just sort of like the seasoning, and then most of it might be legumes or grasses or cereals and you cover crop. But at least what the cover crop opportunity gives you that … it's totally anti-science, our current model of monoculture—that never happens in Nature. You never have one thing and nothing else. Plants love each other. The more the merrier is the central principle of Nature. And so at least within that monoculture model that we've developed—it's easier to harvest and all the rest of it—we can bring in some biodiversity because what's above-ground determines what's below ground. Every plant feeds different groups of organisms, and the more variety—it turns out this having the five families, but maybe two or three of each, the more the merrier—gives you this tremendous response. You saw it begin building humus again. The organisms are fired up, and it's almost like—the results from what I've seen—seem almost like three or four cover crops happen in a single short four-month cycles, like you quadruple the impact of cover cropping, which feeds the soil, and changes the soil structure, and so forth and stimulates soil life. Well that just goes into hyperdrive with a simple inclusion. And so someone should be putting out a blend for their home gardens. Buy a little pack. You can spend a moment where there's nothing on there. Nature abhors a vacuum, and it was the bare ground of Nature so we're learning from Nature, and you put out these five species, and you grow this soil-changing scenario. So I'm really impressed with that scenario, but as I mentioned, when we talk about soil organisms, and soil life generally, we talk about beneficial aerobic organisms.

But there's also another group of organisms. So, the guy called Professor Higa identified from Japan—he called his product EM—but this is a group of anaerobic organisms, actually many of which are similar to what's in our gut. So, there's probiotic yeasts, and there's many, many strains of *Lactobacillus,* just like on our skin and in our gut, exist in the soil. And it turns out that they perform almost as important roles as the aerobic guys. So, for example, we have a new product which is kind of an extension of EM called BAM (beneficial anaerobic microbes). And I'm seeing things, particularly in my home trials where I've been trialing it, and I mean it's just wonderful. You can make a compost in a quarter of the time, and there's no turning, and there's no loss of carbon as you turn it. You know, normally you take a ton of organic matter, and you get 670 kilos on average of end compost. That's the conversion rate. And a lot of that as you turned it has gone up as CO_2 and so forth. And you've had to add extra moisture, and you've had to have that carbon footprint turning it all the time, and so forth. But with these anaerobes, with this BAM concept, you can make your pile up, but then you got to cover it, and turn it into a completely anaerobic, like a silage pit. And a home gardener can do this with a simple cheap tough tarpaulin plastic tarp, but you just put some blocks and seal it off so that it's just, and then … you make your pile … two months later you come back, lift that plastic tarp, and you've got this beautiful black compost that's so protective against all sorts of diseases, to create a disease-suppressive soil. It doesn't involve chemicals and so forth. It works better than conventional composts in a shorter time. Conversion rate is 910 kilos, so it's 25 percent more actual composting carbon. Instead of sending some back to the atmosphere you capture everything. It really is … and farmers don't have to do any work. You just set up a pile, and you've you know it takes you a couple of hours to set a decent-sized pile up. If you've got a machine or something to do it on a larger scale, have a large tarp to cover it, and then two months later you come back, lift it, and there's this beautiful compost. And that excites me because the hardest thing about making compost—and compost is the most important single thing to changing the day; there are many, many things, but compost is right up there at the most important. You know there's a division of the of the U.S. AG department involved in soil health. They did some trial with putting a ton per acre of compost on multiple sites in two states. Now a ton per acre over three years, three tons per acre. Just so you know it takes about 20 tons of compost per acre to lift organic matter one percent, so to take two percent organic matter on a soil test to three percent takes 20 tons of compost. They put, from memory, well it was three tons, a ton an acre per year for three years, and then they did the average soil test to see what increase they should have got an increase. They should have got an increase—well, we're talking in my terms, but 0.15 percent is what three tons equates to. The increase was 1.38%. I mean it was like seven or eight or nine times more, so then what that's telling you is compost, the role of compost, is that you will reclaim in your soil's capacity to build humus. You've brought back all the organisms that you killed that can take some of that glucose that's pumped down and some crop residues and the roots as they died off and converting them to humus. Most cells have lost that capacity because we killed off all the organisms that do that. Compost brings them back, brings back that biodiversity, reclaims that potential to build humus and can save the day. So, we've got to all start looking at composting, and here's a way to compost anaerobically that's faster, quicker, or more efficient, and more likely for farms to take it up, so that excites me.

Brendan [01:07:28]: So basically, really good, intelligently created compost is like a catalyst for the liquid carbon pathway that sucks carbon out of the atmosphere through plants' photosynthetic process, which they then exude a large portion of into the soil to organisms, and if there's enough biodiversity there with the fungal species too, then we get stable humates, humus, that lasts a long time and doesn't go back into the atmosphere.

Graeme [01:08:00]: Yeah, and that catalyst is about the organisms, the biodiversity. A teaspoon of compost has five billion organisms in it and many … might be 30,000 different types, and your soil has nothing like that. So you're bringing all that biodiversity and all that workforce back into your soil to be able to start building humus in that soil, and that's what we need to do. So compost is just like … every council needs to be composting. Every home garden that can compost do it. And with this anaerobic, well, anyone can do that. You know you can have a little pile in the back, chuck a little plastic over it, come back and there's your compost. You can be a lazy bastard, as we say, over here if you want to be because it's easy, you know, and that makes more people do it, and that's what we need.

Brendan [01:08:40]: Graeme, I absolutely love your excitement and your extraordinary dedication to just keep pumping out that message, keep traveling, keep educating, innovating, setting an example for everybody, and so …

Graeme [01:08:56]: Well, it's not some kind of … it's important to understand that it's not some kind of heroic sacrifice on my behalf. It's the best spot in the world, you know. You live life when you're doing this job, traveling the world … you know, I'm sure there are assholes, and there are pricks, as we say, out there, but the farmers that have recognized the need to change, they're the brightest, they're the most intelligent, they're the most love-filled … I mean you just … this honestly … you live life … doing this job is like living life through rose-colored glasses. You only meet all these wonderful people, so it's just an incredible life. I mean I couldn't ask for anything more. I'm so grateful to even be able to do it, and of course now I'm farming myself seriously, and that's just so much fun it's ridiculous. It's like the best fun you ever had. Compare that to smoking a joint or something—there's no comparison. You're going, "I bet there is!"

Brendan [01:09:49]: (laughing) Well, that's kind of what I meant by the example. I mean, you're showing the whole world that this is fun; this is exciting; it's the most inspiring purposeful work that we can possibly have. And we need to also start appreciating the people that have been bringing our food to us unfortunately often through a system that abuses them and doesn't value them—the farmers.

Graeme [01:10:14]: Well, in that context, you've got a President talking about, you know, devaluing Mexicans and throwing them out and putting up a wall. For God's sake, California produces 89% of the fruit and vegetables, and everyone producing it's Mexicans! You should be lauding those wonderful people because none of you will go out and do it. You should be appreciative of what they're doing, not throwing them out. Anyway, that's just ... I get angry.

Brendan [01:10:39]: Yeah, that's for another conversation for sure.

Graeme [01:10:42]: They actually like the soil, and they're a farming community, so that's hugely important. You should be absolutely embracing those people, because they're growing your food. That's the reality. That's so important, and they've been abused and misrepresented, and so forth. But anyway, I won't go there.

Brendan [01:10:58]: Well, on behalf of myself and everybody in the Eat4Earth community, I just want to thank you for being here today.

Graeme [01:11:05]: A pleasure, great to see you again.

Brendan [01:11:08]: Wasn't that amazing? Graeme can fire up your passion to save the world like nobody else. I really want to retake his Nutrition Farming course. and if you ever get a chance to do that, you must, even if you'll be gardening rather than farming. You can check out the Nutri-Tech Solutions website for the schedule of upcoming courses around the world including the US, Canada, Australia, New Zealand, UK, and I believe other places. And if you get interested in becoming a regenerative entrepreneur, or if you just really want to understand better how to identify what regenerative food is and how it's produced, some of the other speakers in this event will give you ideas, as they share about their business models. And it's pretty amazing actually if you compare to what we normally consider as farming. This is another world, so stay tuned and enjoy yourself.

Day 3: Conquering the Plague of Cancer

GMOs, Allergies, Cancer, and the Great Threat to Our Economy
Robyn O'Brien
What You Will Discover

- The far-reaching danger of GMO foods
- How Robyn found the strength to stand up to Big Food
- What a group of oncologists say about the cost of cancer treatments

Cancer Myths, Nutritional Deficiencies, and 7 Steps to Conquer Cancer
Véronique Desaulniers
What You Will Discover

- The role of heavy metals in causing cancer
- The food with 50x the anti-cancer nutrients of broccoli
- The superfood that helps fights cancer in 5-tablespoon doses

Minerals, Metals, & Different Diets for Different Cancers
Manuela Boyle, MD
What You Will Discover

- Why 90% of cancers are not related to inherited genes
- Two very common mineral deficiencies connected to cancer
- Why some cancer treatment diets can include meat while others should not

Pancreatic Enzymes as Cancer Surveillance & Metabolic Individuality for Custom Anti-Cancer Diets
Linda Isaacs, MD
What You Will Discover

- Why pancreatic enzymes may be the body's way of avoiding cancer
- Why some people beat cancer with meat-centered diets while others beat cancer with vegetarian diets
- The powerful detoxification strategy that disappeared from *The Merck Manual* after the 1970s

Extraordinary Stories of Healing with Juicing, Souping, and Anti-Cancer Nutrients
Cherie Calbom
What You Will Discover

- Wild stories of healing cancer with juicing

- The plant food that is exploding onto the anti-cancer research scene
- When to use souping and when to use juicing

The Definition of a Carcinogen, Starving a Cancer, Emotions and Cancer Risk
Ty Bollinger
What You Will Discover

- A surprising reason certain people did not get cancer from Chernoble's radiation
- A dietary strategy that starves a cancer of its preferred fuel
- How emotions affect your immune system

Robyn O'Brien Interview

GMOs, Allergies, Cancer, Our Children, and the Great Threat to Our Economy

Brendan Moorehead [00:00:00]: Welcome to the Eat4Earth event. We're exploring how you can heal yourself, your loved ones, and the planet with food. This is Brendan Moorehead, and our next guest triggered an allergic reaction in the food industry when she asked, "Are we allergic to food or what's been done to it?" A former financial and food industry analyst, Robyn O'Brien has been called food's Erin Brockovich by Bloomberg and the *New York Times*. From a conservative Texas family, Robyn earned an MBA on a full scholarship, graduating as the top woman in her class before going to work as a financial analyst that covered the food industry. And while working as an equity analyst, problems with our food supply hit very close to home and led her to discover serious problems with the health of the American food system, as documented in her first book, *The Unhealthy Truth: How Our Food Is Making Us Sick And What We Can Do About It*. Her work has been featured on CNN, CNBC, Bloomberg, the Today Show, Good Morning America, Fox News, in the *Washington Post*, and countless media outlets, and she wrote a very popular column for *Prevention* called "Inspired Bites" while serving as the executive director of Allergy Kids Foundation and doing strategic advisory work for companies making trend-setting changes in the food industry. Her focus is on restoring the health of American families in order to address the burden that disease is placing on our economy. All of her initiatives and work address the needs of the one in three American children that now has allergies, autism, ADHD, and asthma, and the growing number of American children with cancer. Robyn has received broad acclaim, including being named by *Shape* magazine as a woman to shape the world, by *Forbes Woman* as one of the 20 inspiring women to follow on Twitter, and by the Discovery Channel as one of its 15 top visionaries. Her work is recognized and supported by renowned individuals such as Dr. Oz, Robert Kennedy, Jr., Ted Turner, Bonnie Raitt, and Prince Charles. So Robyn, thank you so much for being here with us.

Robyn O'Brien [00:02:07]: Oh, Brendan, thanks so much for putting this all together. It's great.

Brendan [00:02:10]: Yeah, so I guess in a nutshell, what happened to turn you from a conservative Wall Street analyst into a dedicated food activist confronting some of the very same companies that you probably trusted and even admired previously when you covered them?

Robyn [00:02:27]: Well, as you mentioned, I grew up in a conservative Texas family, and I went to business school on a scholarship. I was recruited by Exxon and Enron. There was no environmental awareness. We just ... we weren't exposed to it in any way growing up in Houston. And I knew that I didn't want to go into oil and gas. I had a tendency to get bored easily, and to me the equity world just seemed fascinating. The ability to meet with different management teams every single day to cover different industries, to learn different business models, to see different CEO styles and types. You really were just kind of at the feet of these titans of industry, and it was a fascinating job. And I truly loved it, and still to this day I miss it. I'm still close with the guys that I worked with. I loved finance. Everything that I had pursued in business school sort of led me to that path, and it was such an incredible job to have at a very incredible time. As the only woman on the team, when the guys said, "You can cover the food industry, and retail," I thought, like, *I'm not the right person for this*. I don't know how to cook. And I really, you know, had always given up Diet Cokes for Lent. I wasn't at all dialed into anything food aware, and I just covered the industry as an analyst. And so it was very black and white, simply learning these business models. I wasn't trying to out think anything. I simply was trying to better understand how they were driving profitability, how they were getting at their margins. And at that point in time, a lot of these companies, what they were doing was they were swapping out real ingredients and swapping in these artificial ingredients.

And we saw what that did for profitability. We saw what that did for margins. But at the time, I never thought to ask what it actually does to us. You know, what's the impact of swapping out a bunch of ingredients that have been in our food system for hundreds and thousands of years and replacing them with a bunch of artificial ingredients that had been created in a lab as recently as the 1970s, '80s, and in some cases extremely recently. And it wasn't until we decided to start a family—and at that point we relocated to Colorado—and I was saying goodbye to the guys on the desk, fully intending to go back to it. I had all of those contacts live and stayed very close to all of the guys that I worked with, all of the resources that we had out of New York. And it wasn't until our fourth child was born when all of a sudden, she had this acute allergic reaction one morning over breakfast. And I'm thinking, *What is happening to this child?* And I was so unfamiliar with what a food allergy looked like, that I didn't even recognize it as that. And her face was swollen shut, so we took her to the emergency room. It was a Saturday morning, and the doctor says, "This looks like an allergic reaction." I'm thinking, you know, *since when*? Because I'm sure as you can relate and absolutely anybody over the age of 40 can, we didn't know anybody growing up that had these food allergies. You know, we all went to school with a PB&J or a carton of milk, and these things weren't considered loaded weapons on a lunchroom table. We all grew up eating kind of the same candies and snacks, and we didn't have to worry about two kids in every classroom now having a food allergy, which is what the statistics are today.

And so the analytical—there were two things happening that day, and I remember it so vividly—the analytical part of my brain is trying to process the data and thinking, *What has happened? What is going on? Why all of these kids?* They don't just fall out of the sky. Epidemics don't just happen. What is triggering an epidemic like this where we now have two kids in every classroom? So that part of my brain was going off. At the same time, my heart was feeling absolutely suffocated because I thought, "How as a mother can I protect the health and life of my child if she is allergic to food?" And again, that felt very radical because as a mother, you know food is meant to sustain these kids. And all of a sudden food groups—like dairy or soy or wheat or fish or shellfish or eggs that you thought of as standard food groups—suddenly, those are the top eight allergens, and you're thinking, *What's my kid going to eat if she can't eat these foods?* And then, here I was a mom of a house full of children under the age of six, and none of them at that point really knew how to read. And so I thought, they can't read the sides of these labels. I mean, they could read a basic little kid book, but they cannot read the sides of these labels. And so it was just this gripping terror of how do you protect the health of your children? How was I feeling so incredibly flat footed at this point, and what did I not know? And I kept coming back to that because I thought, here I cover the food industry, but we had never talked about the number of kids with food allergies.

What did I not know? And so at that point I just went into this massive research dive and this data dive to try to figure out what was happening to the health of American children. And so when you go into some of these government agency sites and portals and things, and you're trying to extract how many kids have food allergies, you don't just get food allergies. You also get the number of kids with asthma; you get the number of kids that have type 1 diabetes, the number of kids that have type 2 diabetes; you get the number of kids with pediatric cancer. And so as I started trying to find more information on food allergies, which is actually very difficult to find ... The CDC does not actually count the number of deaths from food allergic reactions.

Brendan [00:07:48]: Oh, wow!

Robyn [00:07:49]: They will count the number of deaths from asthma, and in some cases a food allergy death is marked as an asthma death because the airway shut down—and so it's the inability to breathe that, ultimately, is what is marked as the cause of death, even though it may have been triggered by, you know, a sandwich in a mall or a peanut butter cookie. And so I was sort of ... you're running blind because you're thinking, *The CDC is not counting these deaths*. The data at that point, was sort of this foam data, you know, and it felt very ... it didn't feel solid. And so as I kept trying to find more information, I started to sort of reach out to different mothers, reach out to different groups. And in some cases, some of them, like this woman that had run *Allergic Child* in Colorado Springs, they were phenomenal. I mean, they were just allies from the very beginning and said, "What can we do to help? What can we do to help?" And then there were other organizations where I was asking questions about "Why the epidemic? Why is this happening to our kids?" And those organizations didn't like the questions.

And so this is, like, the first couple of months into all of this, and I'm thinking, at this point a lot of parents are sort of marginalized. A lot of mothers are dismissed thinking they're being alarmist or attention seeking. I'm trying to kind of cobble this data together and pull it from all these different resources. And it was so big. And yet at the same time as a mother of four, we were seeing what was happening in the preschool, and the preschool director was like, "Open this cabinet, and look how many of these auto injectors that are in here. And it wasn't like this 10 years ago, Robyn." So we were seeing the data in real time. They would say this is anecdotal data, but we were seeing it happening in real time, and yet these agencies ... still to this day, the CDC does not count the number of deaths from food allergic reaction. So, it had its gray space, and as an analyst, I thought, *that just doesn't work; that doesn't help us protect the health of our kids*. And so I started pulling together information, and as I was trying to learn about food allergies, there were some sites we sort of had to pay for this membership. And I thought, *that is crazy*. If my child had been diagnosed with anything else, the information would be free, and I felt very strongly that the information should be free to parents.

So I started this little site *Allergy Kids*, and at that point in time, I was really just trying to raise awareness, join this kind of tribe of moms that I saw, help create an understanding—a better understanding—and help show the data, because I thought the numbers could tell their own story. But as I continued to do that, and I made these little carrying cases and stickers with this little symbol. The media loved it. And so they reached out, and it was all local news here in Colorado and in some other stations and things, and they all reached out and they're just like, "*This is so great.* You know, you took action, and you did something." So I started appearing in the press, and there was a non-profit in DC that just flipped out, and basically, they sent this email suggesting that everything had to flow through them. And I thought, that does not feel right, you know, as an advocate, as somebody working to protect children. There are so many mothers and so many dads, grandparents, and caregivers who are fighting for these kids, and we're foot soldiers. So why wouldn't you want to embrace these parents as the foot soldiers that they are? So I started asking around, and it turned out that other people had experienced the same sort of shut out from this nonprofit. And so, you know, it just didn't sit right, and they were really aggressive, trying to kind of keep me quiet, and so I pulled their financial statements because that's what I knew how to do.

Brendan [00:11:26]: (laughs)

Robyn [00:11:26]: I just thought, I don't understand why they are trying to silence these moms. And so I pulled their financial statements, and that's when I realized that they were funded by Kraft. And at the time, back in 2006— this was early, early 2006, probably February-ish, March— I learned that they were funded by a company up until that point I had not heard of called Monsanto. And so their medical board was working on allergenicity issues with Monsanto. So as an analyst, I'm thinking, *who is Monsanto?* I grew up in Texas. We didn't talk about this company. And so I punched in their ticker symbol—and it's MON, you know—and it pops out. At that point it was over $70,000,000,000 in market cap. It's this massive chemical company. And I'm thinking, *What in the world does this have to do with food allergies?* And so we start kind of doing this dive into Monsanto, and I set up a system—an analytical system that I used to employ when I was an analyst on the desk—and it was to capture headlines and capture data so that every morning when I'd sit down at my desk between like 6:00 and 6:30, I kind of have the current headlines and stories and news and anything that was relevant.

So I did the same thing on food allergies, on children's health, and on this company, Monsanto, because I was trying to sort of come up to speed on what they're all about. And in October of that year, this headline comes through, and at that point the EPA had issued a very small grant to a university in Michigan, and it was, like, $440,000, which is not a lot for a grant that is supposed to cover something as huge as this. And the title of the article that was talking about it was, "Do genetically engineered foods cause food allergies?" So at that point, again, the Texan in me is thinking, *I don't even know what a genetically engineered food is. What is it?*

So I'm doing this deep dive—what is Monsanto, what are genetically engineered foods?—and all of a sudden, I'm thinking if these foods … if you go to the USDA and you pull this data, and you're realizing that these foods were introduced in 1996—they had never been in our food system before—and then in 2006, 10 years later, the EPA is issuing a grant saying, "Do genetically engineered foods cause food allergies?" I'm thinking, *Why in the world are we only studying this now 10 years after these things have been put into our food supply?* And then on top of that, they had never been labeled, so parents, nobody—none of us—had any clue that the stuff had gone into our food supply. So at that point I pick up the phone, and I call this researcher in Michigan, and I just start asking questions. I said, "I'm new to this. I'm new to the food allergy space because of my child. I'm an analyst. I'm kind of trying to learn as much as I can about this company, Monsanto and GMOs and genetically engineered foods. And can you explain to me why you're doing this study if these things have been in our food supply for 10 years?"

And I'll never forget what he said. He said, "We don't have the animal testing models to know whether or not this is definitively going to cause an allergic reaction or not." He said, "You know, we're not going to knowingly put an allergen into a product." There had been a bunch of studies ... the Brazil nut, you know, all these things that had come before. He said, "We're not going to knowingly do that." He said, "But the problem is that in the process of genetic engineering, in that insertion process, the concern is that maybe something has been created in that process that doesn't even have a name yet that could trigger an allergic reaction."

And so I'm thinking, so in this blast of genetic engineering where you're inserting a different trait into a plant, like a soybean or corn, it's that blast that then creates these kinds of unintended units or proteins or whatever this guy was going to study. And I'm thinking, *you mean we've done this, and we don't know if that process is kicking off or producing these unintended consequences?* And on top of that we've been eating this for 10 years, and on top of that these things aren't labeled.

And so I stepped back from that, and I remember kind of stepping back and thinking, *What is the rest of the world doing?* My mom is from New Zealand, and so we grew up with this kind of wide-angle lens of what's happening around the world. And I thought, I wonder what is New Zealand doing? New Zealand doesn't allow genetically engineered crops to be grown in the country, and they're not allowed to be grown at all. And France is a similar country. They don't allow it to be grown. And then over 60 countries around the world that have allowed it into the food supply say that they have to be labeled, so the consumers can make an informed choice.

And so that was that was an incredibly difficult time because I'm sitting on this information. At that point, you know, most people were just like, "Robyn, you have gone way too far down this rabbit hole. This is ... are you sure you want to be talking about this?"

I didn't want to be talking about it. I remember looking out in the backyard one day at these four little, tiny little kids—I mean, they were like under the size of my knee running around—and thinking, *if I don't talk about this, who will, and how do we talk about it?* And so what has been fascinating to me the whole way through is that as I was getting ready to launch *Allergy Kids* and the site—and that was Mother's Day of 2006—I wasn't yet up to this level of awareness. But right before we launched, I was contacted by a Dad whose daughter had died from an allergic reaction after eating a sandwich at a mall. She'd eaten at the sandwich shop dozens and dozens and dozens of times—and it's always the same sandwich—and then this one time she went into an acute allergic reaction, and she died. And her death was marked as an asthma death because it was her inability to breathe, and she was 13. And I remember thinking, *no matter how terrified I am, like that is the biggest terror any parent could face, and I have to keep going.* And as that story unfolded, as they tried to pursue justice for their daughter, I realized how much we were up against as families. And as I continued to tell the story, you know my work was kind of starting to get covered by the press: CNBC News covered it, *New York Times* covered it, and it started to make some headlines. And in some cases it was very much kind of, this can't be true, this is crazy, shoot the messenger. And as I learned, as I studied more about the tobacco industry and different industries, when you're bringing an issue like this to light, "shoot the messenger" is a pretty popular tactic, and it's pretty easy to pick apart almost anybody. And I remember standing and facing that and thinking, *what do I do?* At this point, what do I do? And I couldn't unlearn the information. I couldn't *not* do anything.

I remember being at the gym one day and a six-time Ironman that I used to swim with, he swam beside me. He's like, "Are you ok?" And I'm like, "No, I'm not OK, not OK. I don't know what to do." And at that point it was incredibly stripping, and I felt this enormous responsibility. The isolation was profound. My own parents were struggling with it. You know, a lot of people just really weren't ready to hear this information yet, back in 2006. And I remember sitting there talking to this friend—he'd won six Ironmans in Hawaii—and he said, "You need to know my best friend." And I said, "Who's your best friend?" And he said, "His name is John Reganold, and he is a professor at Washington State. And he studied all of this, and he actually introduced the first organic agriculture major in the country." I thought, *OK, I'll talk to him.*

So I get on the phone with this guy, and he was absolutely phenomenal because at that point, I was pulling data as much as was available, but I'm not a scientist. And so I thought, I'm always going to have to be in close contact with some of these scientists to really have a better understanding of what they are doing in practice, and then also as resources to be able to reach out to them. And at that point, he was already studying and doing research on the impact of pesticides on butterflies, and you think where we are today and the conversations that we have today. Well, this guy was talking about it, you know, back in 2005, 2006. And he was the first scientist where I realized there are a lot of people that are worried about this stuff and a lot of people that don't know what to do.

And so as I began reaching out to different pediatric researchers because I was trying to get a better understanding of what was happening in their practices, there was another pediatric researcher who had been studying food allergies. He called them the four A's: allergies, autism, ADHD, and asthma. And he'd written a book and in his work he cites one in three children now have these conditions. And he had also reached out to that food allergy non-profit in DC and received the same sort of shut out. And all of a sudden, we're sitting there thinking, *maybe this is a bigger story to tell.* And as I began to tell the story, Robert Kennedy invited me on his radio show. A lot of people who hadn't wanted to hear it were suddenly like, *why, wait, what?* Robert Kennedy had you on his show? How's that possible? What'd you do to do that? And I got a lot of that, and for me, it was just so critical that the information get out, and I think as terrified as I was about the food allergy piece, because that was so personal to me, it was really when I got to unearthing information about cancer ...

And that was a couple years later in 2008. The President's Cancer Panel released a report, and the panel had formed under George Bush, and then the report was released under Obama. And to me that was *so* important that it was a bi-partisan effort because the way I looked at it, you know, cancer and food allergies and autism, they don't care if we're Republican or Democrat or Independent. They do not care. They will take apart our families no matter what. And as I was reading this report, it said one in two men and one in three women are expected to get cancer in their lifetime, and that cancer is the leading cause of death by disease in American children under the age of 15. And you can't unlearn something like that. And I remember it was like at page 113 or towards that area where they have a specific section saying pesticide exposure ... we need to be reducing children's exposure to pesticides, and I'm thinking, *we have genetically engineered our food*. We introduced these new crops in 1996 to withstand increasing doses of this pesticide, and we didn't get told that this was happening. And that felt so incredibly un-American to me: that freedom to know how our food is grown, to know that other countries either are not accepting it or are labeling it so that consumers can make an informed choice.

I then spent time in Iowa and Kansas and Wyoming with farmers to try to understand what they were seeing. Because, again, I know what I'm good at analytically. I also knew where I needed to build out better understanding. And so the farm was one of those places. And I'm actually named after a farmer who battled breast cancer and also battled cancer in one of her own children. And so as I was meeting with these farmers, you know, it was, I knew from my own godmother who I'm named after that she didn't want to hear it. You know, she did not want to hear about glyphosate. She did not want to hear about it, and she's a single mom. Her husband had died. She needed it to manage her farm. So I had such an acute sensitivity for how difficult and how personal these decisions can be. And as I was meeting with these farmers, they said, "We don't have MBAs, Robyn." You know, they're brilliant in what they know, but in terms of running that business model and being able to purchase fertilizer when prices are down or manage costs, they're really kind of at the whim of the system. And one of the farmers in Kansas, he said, "We call them the fertilizer mafia because we never know what they're going to do with the price of fertilizer—if they're going to jack it up, if it's going to come down." And so trying to financially manage that as a farmer for some of these farmers is really difficult. So this particular guy went back to business school to get an MBA, and then he financed a holding tank so that he could make better manage his costs on his farm. So I'm thinking, you know, it's impacting the farmers.

At that point I had farmers who worked for Syngenta, and another farmer put me in touch with them. And I remember going into that meeting, and I just remember thinking, *What in the world, like, what am I doing here?* They were all grandfathers, and it was fascinating to hear them talk about the patents that had been put on these crops, who was benefiting, how these multinationals were benefiting, how they were struggling financially as farmers, how their children didn't want to step into it and take over the farm. And I thought ... *we're all on the same side of this issue where a system has been put in place that is doing a tremendous disservice to a lot of us.* So then how do you build out? And for me with a finance background, I still to this day come to this place where we've got to help farmers finance that conversion. We've got to help finance the conversion of the food system and these farms. As you know, for a farmer to go from conventional GMO soy or something like that to organic, it's a three-year process to basically allow that conversion to take place.

And so much of that is the soil gets contaminated with Roundup and these pesticides and herbicides that are applied, and so this process has to take place so that the soil then is in a place that it's allowable to grow these organic crops. So what happens is you've got this three-year period to a farmer who's not rolling in cash in the first place ...

Brendan [00:25:50]: Right.

Robyn [00:25:51]: ... who's got to figure out a way ... "What do I do in that three-year period? I can't *not* sell anything because nobody wants these kind of middle crops." And so it's been fascinating in the last couple of years to really see how the food industry is starting to respond. I gave a TED Talk in 2011, and at that point I was able to tell my story completely, 100% in my words as me as a messenger. And when you're working through a book, there was so much that ... there was so much detail that had to be in that book, and there were 60 pages of end notes. And yet, for a TED Talk, you know, it's just 18 minutes on a stage, and the vulnerability I felt in that was massive. I didn't want to do it. The week before I thought, *how do I back out of this? I don't want to do this.* The vulnerability of just standing on that stage and having to tell the story. And it was fascinating to see the response from that talk. And I think probably what was the most interesting was—there are plenty of families who responded and plenty that responded relating to the food allergy work—but it was a multinational food company that contacted me, a CEO, and he said, "You can say things I can't say." And I thought, *this is crazy.* And I talked to my friends, and I said, "He wants me to come out, fly out there and do this kind of hands-on meeting with his team." And they were like, "That's crazy; they're never going to change." And I thought, *how do you, how do you change anything if you're not willing to sit at the table and have the conversation?*

So I flew out to some management meeting, and it was fascinating. It was me, and they had somebody in from the top levels of McDonald's, and I just remember thinking this is crazy, you know, like, this is such a long shot.

And yet this CEO literally was at my shoulder the whole time. And at one point I just turned to him, and I just said, "You obviously understand this." You know, he had something personal with one of his boys. And I said, "You obviously understand this. What are you afraid of?" And he just didn't hesitate and looked me straight in the eye, and he said, "My board of directors." And so at that point I thought, *we've got to educate Wall Street, too.* So much of my work had been consumer-facing, especially the food allergies piece and connecting with those mothers, and I've taken incredible heat for it as you can imagine. I mean, the trolling and everything else that happens, it's incredible.

But what I have really come to is we have to educate the capital because now we've created this incredible awareness and this incredible demand, and 8 out of 10 households are buying organic. You see companies like Nestle buying companies like Garden of Life. You see General Mills buying Annie's. You see Hormel buying Applegate. These big companies get it. Like they get that that's the engine and that's the revenue growth, and they've got to buy in. And they don't have it in their DNA, so they're acquiring it to try to kind of uptake this DNA and figure it out, you know, how they can better play in the system. But to me, if they don't figure out how to convert that farmland, this growth will stop because less than one percent of our farmland in the U.S. is organic. And so what that means is, even if you're the CEO of one of these organic food companies, much less one of these multinationals, even if you want to convert a product line—let's say, you know that General Mills wanted to convert half their portfolio to organic—that supply chain does not exist in the United States to do it. So they're bringing in all these inputs and things from China and Australia and Romania and Uruguay, and they're trying to source organic from all these different countries around the world because we don't have the supply chain here. And to me, that's the most incredible opportunity confronting our food system today is for these companies to really commit to growing organic in the United States. I mean, if it's less than one percent of our farmland, but 8 out of 10 households want it, you start to convert that farmland and all of a sudden those farmers who weren't in a position to be financially secure because they're kind of looped into this operating system that companies like Monsanto have created, it gives them the ownership back. And I think, as someone who is named for a farmer, that's just incredibly important to me.

And I think those opportunities are in front of us. And as you and I have talked about, we're starting to see these really unlikely allies in this work. It was probably three or four years ago where I wrote an article for Maria Rodale, and I basically said, the Grocery Manufacturers Association is a relic. They've completely missed this. I didn't understand why any of their members would continue to pay fees because the consumer was clearly shifting at that point. And they still were not embracing it, and then on top of that, they were financing these campaigns to shut us up. And as so somebody who had worked on all these different labeling campaigns from California to Washington to Colorado and literally spent so much time on TV and all these places really advocating and being pitched against by these Monsanto's spokespeople, I thought, the Grocery Manufacturers Association is completely trying to shut up their own consumer, which is the death of a business.

And so at that point I said, they're a relic, and why these member companies are staying in here, I do not know. And, you know, really kind of targeted, like watch the Grocery Manufacturers Association because it's ... something's about to shift. And sure enough, here we are a couple years later, and Nestle has left, Tyson, Unilever's leaving by the end of the year, Theme Foods, Campbell's, and it's just disintegrating in real time before our eyes, which five or 10 years ago, nobody *ever* could have anticipated. And yet in that ... I think it's going to be interesting. In a meeting yesterday, I was saying it's, there's going to be this period of "now what?" because they sort of could huddle under that umbrella for a long time, but I look at it and I think these companies need to be banding together to secure a better supply chain for their future, for our future, for our farmer's future, and our country's future. Because to me food security is national security. It starts with these farms. And so if we're just growing all this GMO corn and GMO soy that nobody wants—like now in the U.S., nobody wants it, and it was never anything anybody else wanted either—we're realizing that the GMO corn that's been grown for ethanol, that that's creating all these unintended side effects, too. So you've just kind of got to bite the bullet on this one and start to convert these farms. And to me, it's not like it's going to take a decade. It's three years, so it's very doable and very fixable.

Brendan [00:32:48]: Aren't there some companies that are actually starting to actually fund farms to turnaround?

Robyn [00:32:55]: Yeah. And so it was Kashi. Again, so unlikely because Kashi was an example I gave about one of these companies that had been acquired, and I use it as a verb, and Annie's was being acquired by General Mills. I said the last thing you want to have happen is to get "Kashi-ed" where you have a strong brand that then got acquired by Kellogg's, survived for about four years, and then just disintegrated, and the quality of the ingredients started to slip, and all of a sudden they lost that core consumer base. And so when Annie's was acquired by General Mills, John Foraker was fierce and saying, "No, we're going to preserve the integrity of this brand." And it's still, as you watch these acquisitions over time, you really have to stay on these bigger companies not to water down those ingredients and kind of let stuff start to slide, because it doesn't happen in the first year or two. It's always by like year four where you really start to see the erosion of the ingredients and other things. And so when Kashi came to me, they said, "We've been watching you talking about how less than one percent of the farmland is organic, and we have a program."

I thought, *this is crazy! This is awesome*. And the woman who was in charge of this thing has been with Kashi since the early 2000s. She's got young children, and she had this vision for basically helping their farmers convert to organic because the challenge they saw internally was ... Kashi said that we didn't have enough almonds to meet the demand for organic almonds. And so what they had wanted was to be able to put organic almonds in all their products. Well, the U.S. doesn't make enough organic almonds for just Kashi to fill their products with organic almonds, so they thought, how can we help our almond farmers convert their farms? And so they launched this third party—they don't own it—certified transitional program, and it's certified with Quality Assurance International (QAI)—it's another system well-known in the food industry—and every time you purchase one of these boxes that carries this "T" for "Certified Transitional," part of those proceeds are going to support these farmers who are converting their farms. And the numbers that they have already put up are impressive. And my sincere hope is that others in the food industry get past the politics of what they've come through with the Grocery Manufacturers Association and just say, this is a good idea. Because what they're doing is they're tapping the consumer for her capital, too. And so we always say, "Oh, vote with your dollar, vote with your dollar." Well, that's a pretty powerful vote to help a farmer convert from conventional to organic. And where I may not want every product in my grocery cart to look like that, I would definitely say, "I'll take one out of every five that can look like this, or maybe one out of every 10," and that way you know you're helping to convert these farmers. So, I think what's important with that one is they don't, they don't own it, and they don't want to own it; it's third party. It's not Kellogg; it's not Kashi. I'm, they're just hoping that others will, will participate in the program. So they've got an example. You know, Patagonia is doing stuff. Nature's Path is doing stuff.

The Farm Bill is the big legislative piece that could address it in a really meaningful way when it comes to capital. But as you can imagine, we've gotten to 95 percent, 92 percent genetically engineered corn and soy because those chemical companies are so powerful with their lobbyists in DC. So to create noise around that Farm Bill really is the next step. And it's been building over the last decade or two for sure. It truly should be named the "Food Bill" because it's how those assets are allocated across our food system that affects all of us from people that are on food stamps and payment plans to the farmers that are growing the stuff to what's happening in school lunch programs. There are so many places where our government touches our food system. And ... if you had an opportunity to check a box when you were voting, do you want your tax dollars to be used to grow genetically engineered crops and all the pesticides used on top of those, or do you want your tax dollars to build out an organic food system that makes that more affordable and more accessible to more Americans? If we actually got that choice with our tax dollars, we'd be having a different conversation.

Brendan [00:37:31]: Yeah. You know, I'm curious—just to go back to sort of the food allergy issue—what I wonder is, what's at the core of that? Is it that these novel proteins are being created? I mean, I heard that in the average genetic engineering process, it's 5% novel proteins are created that no organism on the planet has ever seen before, something like that. And ... is it *that*, or something else, maybe the fact that ... and also on that point, is that getting also into our ... obviously we've got corn and soy in so many products, and those are the chief main bioengineered products, but then also because that's used as feed for animals in the industrial animal agriculture system. Is that getting into our milk and meat ... and their fat or something because of bioaccumulation? I'm just curious, what does the evidence suggest that is actually causing allergies?

Robyn [00:38:38]: So, you raise a lot of really good points. And I think what can be so intuitive to a mother who is feeding a child, nursing a child—as you know, whatever I was eating when I was nursing the kids went straight through, and the kids would respond to it—and so you think about it in terms of the way we feed our animals, the way you feed a cow and then take the milk from a cow. What we do know is that 80% of the antibiotics that we consume—that the U.S. uses and consumes—80% of them are consumed by livestock. And it was Michael Pollan who in his books really kind of started to look at this genetically engineered corn-fed diet. What's it doing to the health of the animals?

And there have been plenty of books and plenty of films that have come out sort of touching on that. Again, you know as I started with, the data is, is very ... it's shallow, and it's sort of that "don't ask, don't tell" policy. And when you speak with these farmers who have shifted from one feeding system to another—you know, from something like genetically engineered soy to organic—you do hear stories about the health of the livestock. The scientists who tend to be funded by the companies like Monsanto will say, "Oh, those are just anecdotal; it's just anecdotal evidence." But we've seen multiple accounts of parents who have switched a child's diet, have taken, in some cases the sort of trigger foods out—whether that's dairy or soy or eggs— they'll remove the trigger food, and things that you're not even realizing were part of that—the kind of conditions that can be associated with food allergies—go away. So for example, an acute food allergic reaction is what we hear about or read about in the news where somebody kisses their boyfriend, and they die because the boyfriend ate a peanut butter and jelly. With these sorts of sensitivities, or these other symptoms that can be associated with food allergies, are things like chronic eczema, chronic ear infections, chronic mucus, and it's speaking to this kind of inflammation that can happen. And as I was working with different scientists and researchers in the beginning, it was that chronic inflammation that truly concerned me because I thought, if a child is in this kind of low-grade inflammation all the time, and you're trying to just kind of quell it with anti-histamines or whatever—without actually getting that offending trigger out—what happens to a body that lives in that chronic inflammation all the time?

And so as we were coming through it, I thought, *how can I reduce my kids' exposure to some of these inflammatory triggers?* And for me, the first thing was, the things that have come into our food system in the last 20 years, let's get them out. And so we just started at home with trying to remove some of these novel ingredients, and whether it was things like high fructose corn syrup or things like artificial colors, the more that I did research on that and the more that I saw the artificial colors, for example ... There was a study called the South Hampton study that I learned about in 2007, and it was a double-blind study. So the parents of the kids didn't know, the researchers didn't know, and these kids were fed different products that had either the artificial colors and artificial ingredients in them or not. And the evidence was so conclusive, so overwhelmingly conclusive when the children consume these artificial colors. Hyperactivity was off the charts—the behavior was just out of control—versus the kids that were consuming the natural ingredients that had always been in the food system. And so as a mother, I was thinking, I have four kids, and if I can just try this at home—you know, reduce the kids' exposure to artificial colors, reduce their exposure to artificial growth hormones—that's something I can try at home.

And that was where I was so grateful for the organic industry because I didn't know what organic was. I hadn't eaten it. Even after we'd moved from Texas to Colorado, I still wasn't at all aware of what organic was. And so to come into the knowledge that by law it's the production of these foods without artificial ingredients, without artificial colors, without artificial dyes, artificial growth hormone, without genetically engineered ingredients, without things like these pesticides, these synthetic pesticides, I thought, they're producing food without all these chemical additives at the same time that these other companies have just embraced it like crazy to drive profitability. And, and I mean, I get that. I was an analyst. So we started to shift back and now, thankfully the medical community. You have people like Dr. Mark Hyman who talk about it. You have people like Dr. Frank Lipman, Dr. [unintelligible] and Kenneth Bach, and they really do speak as MDs—as fully certified MDs—to these conditions. And I'm so grateful for them because it's very easy to marginalize or dismiss a mother. It's very easy to marginalize and dismiss somebody who is just talking about the finances of it. The scientists, a lot of them have to get funding from different corporations, but it sees doctors who are willing to say, "You know what, this is what we have to do," and more of them are starting to come forward, thankfully. And I think the more that this information can get into the hands of mothers at an earlier stage, into the hands of parents, caregivers, the more that we can make this pivot and start to exercise more precaution and prevention in the earlier years to hopefully start to stem some of these conditions. Healthcare costs in the U.S., I mean, we spend more on healthcare than any other country on the planet. It's almost 20 cents of every dollar that's spent on healthcare and disease management, and we know because it's like, yeah, you go down the street and you ask your neighbors what they're dealing with, and the numbers are off the charts. So you know, whether it's the skyrocketing prices of EpiPens® or the skyrocketing prices of insulin medication, it's impacting all of us. And the pharmaceutical industry has done tremendously well. Which I also think is why we're seeing this enormous awakening happening right now around food because people are realizing there is actually a lot that I can do. And it may feel like a really out-of-control situation, but there's a lot I can do.

Brendan [00:45:25]: I'm curious, what do you see happening over the next few decades with the costs to our economy of having this ... we've got the trajectory we're on right now, so we've got a situation we're going to arrive at. How bad is that if we don't turn this ship around, and what can people do—just regular folks do—to help turn that ship around?

Robyn [00:45:50]: You know, again, I would turn back to the doctors, and it was in the *New England Journal of Medicine* a few years ago, where some oncology doctors wrote in and said, you know, if we don't address the skyrocketing costs of cancer medication, it will bankrupt the economy. And that sounds so dramatic, but you know, again, these are oncologists writing in ...

Brendan [00:46:10]: So just one disease, cancer, is predicted to bankrupt the economy by cancer doctors themselves.

Robyn [00:46:17]: By cancer doctors themselves. And then at the same time, you have doctors that treat diabetes saying the same thing, and it *will* cripple the economy. I think we're starting to see a little bit of it right now with the healthcare debate. The problem is it gets enormously political, and as someone who has worked in the food industry for 20 years under multiple administrations, this is not a Red or a Blue thing. Both sides of the aisle have failed to do what needs to be done here, which is really clean up the food system. We could have a system where prevention is actually discussed in healthcare instead of just the system that we currently have, which is sadly where sickness sells. So I will be very grateful when the day comes when our healthcare debate includes food. You know, we go through presidential debate after presidential debate year after year after year, and food never comes up when these candidates on both sides of the aisle are talking about healthcare. And to me, the greatest form of healthcare that we have is what we choose to put on the ends of forks.

Brendan [00:47:26]: Yep. And that's why I'm doing this. It's my passion, my obsession to transform food, turn it back into the medicine it was always meant to be, and have our food system be an expression of our love for this beautiful planet and the children that deserve to inherit a safe, healthy place that supports their full potential. And so I really want to thank *you* for being such a leader in this part of the picture and obviously it's not just GMOs ... you've got your finger on the pulse of many things. I'm glad you brought up what Kashi is doing with transitional organic foods and brands so that we can, we can help support our farmers in that transition. Is there anything else that occurs to you that I, as a consumer, can do to help support this transition so that I have ever-increasing choices of healthy food that I understand and that supports my body and the planet?

Robyn [00:48:35]: Well, you know, I think the most important thing is to not be afraid to say something. The work that I've done has connected me with mothers around the world. When we were bringing the cost of

EpiPen® to light, it was mothers in the UK that were phenomenal, and they have been. They were amazing back in 2007 when we were first starting to address the issue of artificial colors that were being put into American foods that weren't being used in foods in other countries. And I think it's that realization that this really is a global issue, and what we choose to produce here impacts families and farmers around the world, and to really not underestimate the power of one person. Because the first talk I gave, six people came, and one was my pediatrician that I invited, and another was a friend who is a nutritionist. And you can't be afraid to start small. You vote with your shopping cart every single day. So choose organic wherever you can. Get to know those farmers. A lot of people will say, "Oh, you know, only farmers markets," But you know, that's not a reality for a lot of people, and you have to be mindful of the fact that there're all social-economic levels that are impacted by this, and all social-economic levels are really craving better food. And so that opportunity that's in front of all of us to help shift the system, and it's not going to happen overnight. With less than one percent of our farmland is organic, the opportunity there is huge. It's not going to happen overnight, but the opportunity to get it to 10% of U.S. farmland, to 20% of U.S. farmland—it's right in front of us. And so to me, that's what's so exciting. The fact that you have companies that are starting to engage and respond in a way that five years ago, there's no way we would have even considered that. To me, you know, that's a really exciting opportunity.

Brendan [00:50:27]: Yeah. And I believe that we're all truly called to follow your example and speak up and just, you know, just have it be part of our conversation and have it be something that we commit to with our pocketbook at every opportunity that we can. And together, we can have a collective impact, and we already are. I mean, everybody who's already buying organic, buying regenerative, buying biodynamic ... this is what's driving it. So, let's just keep doing it, doing more of it. And thank you so much for bringing us an update from the research trenches. And thanks for all that you do and being here also in the Eat4Earth community with us.

Robyn [00:51:10]: Awesome! Thanks, Brendan.

Brendan [00:51:11]: Thank you!

In this conversation with Robyn, she helped us realize that cancer isn't just a threat to our health; it's on track to cripple our economy, which makes it an urgent national security issue. The Farm Bill subsidizes the soil-destroying chemical and GMO-based agriculture that is substantially driving the cancer crisis and the climate crisis. That's why Robyn is essentially saying that the Farm Bill is actually a Healthcare Bill [Correction: Food Bill], and Alexis Baden Meyer describes the Farm Bill as a Climate Bill. So, let's make some noise around it this year because every Farm Bill deeply affects our lives for many, many years, and we don't have much time left to avoid catastrophic consequences that have been building from years of misguided Farm Bills.

Next up, we have four cancer specialists who are going to help protect you from—or help you protect yourself from—the dreaded plague of cancer. Because even eating organic and having a healthy lifestyle isn't always enough to avoid it, as Veronique Desaulniers discovered when she was faced with breast cancer.

Véronique Desaulniers Interview
Cancer Myths, Nutritional Deficiencies, and 7 Steps to Conquer Cancer

Brendan [00:00:00]: Welcome to the Eat4Earth event. We're exploring how you can heal yourself, your loved ones, and the planet, with food. This is Brendan Moorehead, and we're speaking with Dr. Véronique Desaulniers. Dr. V as she is known to her clients and students, decided to "retire" after 30 years of active practice and devote her time sharing her personal non-toxic healing journey with breast cancer. Her years of experience and research have culminated as The Seven Essentials, a step-by-step coaching program that has served women in 35 countries around the globe. Dr. V is a number one best-selling author and has a number one best-selling book on Amazon, *Heal Breast Cancer Naturally*, in seven different categories. Dr. V, thank you so much for being here with us today.

Dr. V [00:00:48]: Thank you so much for having me, Brendan. I'm excited.

Brendan [00:00:51]: Me too. Dr. V, you are a bioenergetic chiropractor by profession. Tell us a bit about your background and the type of practice you had.

Dr. V [00:01:02]: Well it all started way back when, when I was 16 years old, and I sat in a lecture that my local chiropractor gave, and it was one of those light bulb moments where I knew I wanted to bring wellness to the world because it was such a positive, vibrant message that he was talking about. So fast forward a few years, I graduated as a chiropractor. And after I'd been in practice for about three years, my father was diagnosed with pancreatic cancer. And basically, traditional doctors gave him no hope and gave him six weeks to live, which he bought into that, and unfortunately within six weeks he passed away. But that was a real turning point for me because I realized that there was something that could have been done for my father. I went to the library, I mean back then, 1983, no internet, so I went to the library, called a few cancer clinics, and realized that there was something that could be done with reversing disease and cancer. So took that fire in my soul, and brought that to my practice, and started applying all kinds of different principles using homeopathy, bioenergetic testing, lots of nutrition, exercise, all these things, and educating our patients into what it would take to reverse disease. And we saw amazing results, cancer reversing, autoimmune diseases, children with allergies, and really sick people that were getting well because they were applying the laws of Nature, the laws of the universe, and they were taking responsibility for their health. So that was an amazing journey to be able to work with thousands of people over those thirty years.

Brendan [00:02:44]: Wow, and your journey with breast cancer, you as a breast cancer survivor, was not a traditional one. Tell us a bit about your journey and why you chose a much less traditional route.

Dr. V [00:02:58]: Well, I saw in my practice people who use traditional methods, and unfortunately most of the time it did not turn out very well, and I just knew that the body, my body, had an amazing ability to heal if I put the proper pieces of the puzzle together, and I saw that with my patients as well. So I've been in practice for about 25 years, I'm getting ready for work, I jump in the shower and felt a lump on my left breast, and bam, that was a life-changing moment. It was definitely, my life was never the same again, both professionally and personally. And so I realized that there was something that I was missing, I mean I was doing everything right, or so I thought. I ate organic before organic was in style, I had home births, breastfed all my children, I exercised, I was under chiropractic care, I was doing all these amazing things, but yet, here I was faced with breast cancer. How is that possible? And so there was a lot of soul-searching, a lot of deep dives down the rabbit hole to see what pieces of the puzzle I was missing. And I found myself feeling very frustrated, and confused, and overwhelmed, and had those 3 a.m. sweats where I was wondering, *am I going to be okay? Am I going to see my children grow up*, and that led me to kind of have an aha moment, and if I felt like that after being in practice for 25 years, how much more so would the average person who didn't have all this professional experience. So that led me to create what I call The Seven Essentials System. It's a very simple step-by-step guide that takes the confusion out of the healing journey and brings clarity and confidence because it's a very simple guide to follow.

Brendan [00:04:48]: That's really good news because cancer strikes me as a very complex disease, and in fact, I believe that the confusion, and fear, and complexity starts with certain myths. Can you tell us anything about myths that surround breast cancer specifically?

Dr. V [00:05:06]: Yes. When it comes to breast cancer, first of all, a myth that's really promoted heavily by traditional medicine is that our hormones, women's hormones, cause cancer. Well if that were the case, then every twenty year old on the planet would have cancer. So it's not our hormones, but it's all the chemical estrogens, the xenoestrogens the xenoprogesterones that we're exposed to from the environment, from pesticides, herbicides, the things that we put on our skins, metals like aluminum are classified as metalloestrogens that stimulate and mimic estrogen. Mercury and amalgam fillings … mercury is classified as a metalloestrogen. So we have all these chemical estrogens and hormones that are stimulating this production in our body. So the key is, number one, remove yourself, remove your body from all those things, and be very conscious about what you bring into your environment and what you put on your body and in your body. And then secondly, understand if you have the ability to break down those aggressive estrogens. There's a process called methylation, and if you're not a good methylator, you're not going to break those estrogens down, and they're going to recirculate, and yes it can increase your risk of cancer. That's a big one for me because I see women that are in fear of their hormones, and we need our hormones to function properly, for brain health, bone health, cardio-vascular health, our immune system needs it, so suppressing our hormones with toxic drugs is not the key to getting well.

Brendan [00:06:49]: If I'm not mistaken, I believe diet, as in food choices, has recently replaced smoking as the number one lifestyle influence on cancer. It's either that or something very similar. I have to look up to be exactly sure, but it's predicted that one in two men, and one in three women alive today, will experience cancer. You touched on endocrine disruptors as a specific trigger for cancer. Is there anything else that you have learned is related to food, other toxins, nutrient deficiencies, things like that?

Dr. V [00:07:28]: Absolutely. Look at the standard American diet, the acronym is SAD, which it really is a sad diet. It's processed, it's overcooked, it's full of chemicals and toxins, GMOs, it's literally making people sick. And so essential number one of the Seven Essentials System is to look at food as your medicine because the body has an amazing ability to heal, and what you put in it with food is either going to turn off your cancer protective genes, or turn on your cancer promoting genes. So it's very important to look at food, the deficiencies that we have, even in organic foods, because as you know with the work that you're doing, our soil is extremely deficient of nutrients.

Brendan [00:08:19]: Say a little bit about the Seven Essentials, because I know that part of your mission is to inspire women to be proactive and then making informed decisions, and obviously that all starts with food. Tell us a little bit more about the other seven essentials.

Dr. V [00:08:33]: So number two is reducing your toxic exposure, and that could be everything from environmentally, to looking at what's in your home, looking at electro-pollution which is a huge toxin that affects billions of people on the planet, as well as our agriculture and our plants and our animals. Number three is balancing your energy, which means balancing your hormones, your sleep, your exercise. Four is healing your emotional wounds, because we know that there's a huge component in how you think about your body. and how you think about your future, and how it affects your immune system. Number five is biological dentistry, which means, get rid of those amalgams in your mouth and talk to a biological dentist about the problems with root canals and how they can suppress your immune system. Number six has to do with repairing your body with therapeutic plants and herbs, specific supplements, specific nutrients that turn on the protective genes, turn on the immune system, detoxify the body. And lastly, seven is practicing real, early detection, not what the Pink-movement professes but really specific tools that will find and detect cancer when it's the size of a pin head vs. when it's a size of a golf ball and it's a lump or a bump, and by then it's progressed quite a bit.

Brendan [00:10:01]: I'm going to circle back to food, because that is the topic of this event. I firmly believe that cancer is more complex than nutrients and toxins, that the emotional part is very key as well, and you mentioned electro-pollution. So, I'm not simplifying at all the realm of the causation, but I wanted to ask you, because there's the question of processed food vs. fresh food intake, and in particular, lots of fruits and vegetables, but over the last hundred years the nutrient content of our food supply, our whole foods, real foods, has declined to a point where sometimes oranges don't even have vitamin C, tomatoes don't even have lycopene, which of course is a protector against cancers, especially in the prostate for men. A comparison was made between the average iron content of a bowl of spinach in 1953 with a bowl of spinach from 1997 and at that time it would've taken forty-three 1997 bowls of spinach to be equivalent to one bowl from 1953. I can imagine what the comparison would be right now, but obviously minerals like zinc and selenium are important to the body's detoxification process. You mentioned that as an important one of your seven essentials, and plants also need these minerals to actually make the phytonutrients and antioxidants and vitamins and so forth that also confer cancer protection and healing benefits. So, I'm curious, do you think that in addition to the inadequate intake of fresh foods and vegetables that we're also fighting an uphill battle with the depleted nutrient levels even in our whole foods.

Dr. V [00:11:59]: Absolutely, one of the things that we highly recommend for women who are in a healing journey or who are being proactive with prevention, make sure that you have basic trace minerals in your supplementation and through real food. For example selenium, you want to make sure that you get plenty of selenium because selenium is key when it comes to your immune system. Eat some organic Brazil nuts because those are chock-full of selenium. Zinc is responsible for over three hundred enzymatic processes in the immune system. So again, zinc, very, very important. Magnesium, low magnesium levels, it's actually a pro-carcinogen, so if you have low magnesium levels, it can instigate an issue with cancer. And we know now with the study of nutrigenomics, which is the study of the phytonutrients in the food and epigenetics and how the nutrients in the food affect our genes, we know how powerful it is to have the proper nutrients to turn on those cancer protective genes and turn off those cancer-causing genes.

Brendan [00:13:11]: It's extremely powerful when we look at the research, plants are amazing; nutrients are amazing. And on the toxins side, I wonder if you could say any more about any particular toxins, classes of toxins, especially the ones we get in our food, I know it's also very important to consider the ones we're getting from sources we can't control necessarily. But there are some we can control, our health and beauty aids, and the food we put in our mouth. What might you be able to share about toxins in our food that it would be best to avoid?

Dr. V [00:13:44]: Well, obviously, staying away from GMO foods. We know Jeffrey Smith and his research on responsible technology and how toxic GMO foods are. It's Franken-food, it's a foreign food, our body does not know what to do with it, and so it creates problems with the digestive system, the immune system, causes tumors, I mean there's a whole list. Removing yourself from GMO and eating foods that are non-GMO verified, that's a big step. Moving towards organic, or freshly grown in your own yard, or you know the farm to table movement. Support your local farmers that are doing organic foods because that's where you're going to get the best nutrients available.

Brendan [00:14:35]: It's interesting, on the topic of organic, there have been some publications that say organic is no better as far as nutrient content, and then there are others from Rodale Institute that say well sure it is, here is the data. I actually think it comes down to how regeneratively those organic farmers are farming. And that's covered in different parts of this event, as far as how the soil is actually being treated, but that's for another conversation. But yes, in general, organic foods in my experience have so much more flavor, and to me that is the indicator, and again we're going to talk about that in other parts of the event. But that's the first indicator of the nutrient value of foods—how does it taste? Does it taste more like broccoli than other sources of broccoli? And you also mentioned GMOs—by the way, let me let you respond to that. What would you say about that in regard to the tongue and taste?

Dr. V [00:15:33]: Oh I mean there's no comparison. You mentioned tomatoes have no lycopene, commercially grown tomatoes have no lycopene. I mean just the way they feel, just the way they cut and slice, and taste— it's like eating rubber, versus you pick a fresh tomato off of a plant, or you get it from an organic farmer—it's juicy. It's soft. It's red instead of pale orange. And it's fabulous. I mean that's just an example of the difference in taste from organic to not.

Brendan [00:16:07]: I truly relish my organic foods, and I wanted to also respond … you mentioned GMOs, and I was really intrigued to learn recently that one of the reasons GMOs can affect us—you mentioned gut health—is that they bring in lectins, certain plant proteins that are plant defense proteins, and they put them in GMOs to fight off the pest and make the plants more resilient to pests. Well guess what, those things also affect us. And of course, we've got Bt-corn that's producing a toxin, and it's inside the corn, it's genetically engineered into the corn, and those genes are sometimes called "jumping genes" because they might be able to get into our own bacterial genome, and then we've got a Bt-toxin production factory in our guts. And I'm just curious if there's anything else to say about GMOs.

Dr. V [00:17:05]: What can we say? It's toxic, it's poison. There's just so much evidence out there, and of course, we look at the big "M" company that's promoting all the GMO seeds and the glyphosate pollution that's affecting so many of us. Even if we try to eat as clean as possible, we're still affected directly or indirectly by pesticides like glyphosate. It's a planetary problem.

Brendan [00:17:37]: And that's the thing with these GMOs and glyphosate, and more specifically Roundup, because glyphosate is applied as a Roundup with these carrier molecules that basically, the intention behind them is to carry them into cells and cross membranes and so forth. So these things go straight into our cells and even our mitochondria in a way that glyphosate alone wouldn't do on its own necessarily as effectively, but it's a thousand times more effective in Roundup, which is how it's applied. And the glyphosate creates a change in our intestinal lining that opens up the tight junctions, and that's why we're having such a breakdown of intestinal health, in part. That's just one of the many things, and Dr. Bush talks about that in this event as well. I think we are seeing yet another example of how disease begins in the gut as naturopaths and chiropractors have known for decades. Modern medical research is finally discovering why, so hopefully it's going to catch up eventually.

Dr. V [00:18:49]: We're getting there.

Brendan [00:18:50]: Right now, people like you have the methods that were discovered to work a long time ago before it was known exactly why they work and all of that. So let me ask you, in terms of eating, are there any particular dietary or eating guidelines that you use with people for prevention and for intensive intervention with cancer and so forth, and of course remaining a survivor and avoiding recurrence.

Dr. V [00:19:16]: So I'm a conqueror, not just a survivor.

Brendan [00:19:18]: Yes, that's right.

Dr. V [00:19:20]: Survivor means you've just barely survived, so that's why I'm labeled the breast cancer conqueror, that's our mission.

Brendan [00:19:28]: Unfortunately, I have to eliminate my indoctrination into the language of the machine, this survivor language.

Dr. V [00:19:35]: That's right, that's okay. Let's see, what was your question again?

Brendan [00:19:42]: Any particular dietary guidelines for using food.

Dr. V [00:19:48]: Well, when it comes to food, one of the questions we always get is what's the best "anti-cancer diet", what's "the one". Well, I can tell you from my experience in this industry for 40 years, I've tried them all, I mean all of them. The most recent one that I experimented with was the ketogenic diet. That led me down a path to really help me understand a little bit more about cancer and the mitochondria, and we know that cancer is really a metabolic disease because of high insulin resistance, inflammation, not enough oxygenation, and we also know that it's a mitochondrial disease because when the mitochondria don't get enough oxygen and when they don't get the proper nutrients, when they get things like the glyphosates, they mutate, and there we have a pathway for cancer. But to really understand the balance that there has to be, obviously, we encourage lots of cruciferous vegetables, lots of leafy greens, if you're on a healing journey, minimizing your fruits. Lemons and limes and Granny Smith apples are acceptable. Minimize your protein. If you chose to eat protein, make sure that it's a clean source, grass-fed beef and wild-caught fish, but only two to three ounces, minimal amount. The key is to keep your blood sugar at a minimal, to increase your ketones with lots of healthy fats, coconut oil and avocado oil, and sprouted nuts, all the things that bring us ... the olive oil ... you know, the good fats. And making sure that you get plenty of oxygenation. When you combine all of those three together then you stand a better chance to reverse and to create vibrant health and to get well and stay well. Some people have gotten well by juicing twenty-five pounds of carrots every day, and some people have gotten well by doing ketogenic. You have to really individualize it and look at your gut health, look at your genomic make up, what weaknesses do you need to support. You have to look at your blood type, and the type of cancer you have, your journey, where you are. It's not a quick fix, a quick answer for the dietary habits.

Brendan [00:22:14]: And I'm curious, in the world of consumables I'll say, beyond food. Actually, I think herbs should be considered food. I was going to call it a supplement, but really herbs are our food, and I'm just curious if you have anything to say about particular herbs and the wonderful plant kingdom out there beyond what we normally think of as food.

Dr. V [00:22:34]: Well, one of my favorite foods are broccoli sprouts, part of the cruciferous vegetable family, but the sprout has twenty to fifty times more of the phytonutrient called sulforaphane which literally turns on over two hundred protective genes and turns off the inflammatory genes and helps to detoxify the aggressive estrogens and chemicals in your body. Things like spirulina. You can take, according to research, five teaspoons of spirulina as a "therapeutic" dose to kill off cancer cells. Bloodroot is a plant that has a phytonutrient in it that literally kills cancer cells only. It will not affect your healthy cells. Medicinal mushrooms. I mean there's so many medicinal mushrooms out there like chaga and turkey tail and maitake. There's so many of them that are so beneficial for us. There's a list of them. We can talk for a whole hour on the medicinal aspect of foods and minerals and herbs and supplements.

Brendan [00:23:48]: I'll say just briefly, medicinal mushrooms have been magical for me. It was a big part of my recovery from chronic fatigue immune deficiency syndrome. My natural killer cells were really not performing very well, and I started with some maitake D fraction. That was powerful for me, and then I started using some products from a company that had some combinations of reishi and so forth, and that was powerful, and it made a world of difference for me.

Dr. V [00:24:24]: Absolutely, I mean the studies are there. I did want to point out to your audience that what we're talking about, and what I'm talking about specifically, is not just something I pulled out of my hat, but everything that I teach and everything that's been in my book and on my website is based on science and based on studies. We always do a lot of research. Pubmed is a great resource where we can read about all the studies, and I tell naysayers or people that are a little skeptical, just go to Pubmed https://www.ncbi.nlm.nih.gov/pubmed and put it in the search bar, "cancer and medicinal mushrooms", or "cancer and bloodroot", "cancer and vitamin C", "cancer and selenium", and you'll see that the proof is there.

Brendan [00:25:10]: And you mentioned detoxification, and I see a strong connection between nutrition and detoxification because we can't necessarily detoxify if we don't have the nutrition. For example, you mentioned sulforaphane from broccoli and broccoli sprouts, which upregulates phase one and phase two enzymes in the liver, and I'm just curious if you could say more about your particular approach to detoxification.

Dr. V [00:25:40]: There's so many things that you can do, obviously for me it starts with food, and then there are specific pathways that you want to make sure that you clean up. You want to clean up the colon; you want to clean up the liver. You can do that through liver flushes or specific herbs and supplements. Fasting is extremely beneficial for detoxification. Coffee enemas are great because they stimulate the liver and the gallbladder to help release a lot of those toxins. Sweating, infrared, far infrared saunas, near infrared saunas, extremely beneficial. Moving your body, rebounding, lymphatic drainage. There's so many great things out there to help detoxify your body.

Brendan [00:26:27]: I can personally attest to the importance of liver detoxification. I used to be a habitual overeater for emotional reasons. I was stuffing. I didn't realize it. I was always filling the void with food. I didn't become obese. I just don't have that metabolism. I have some kind of other fierce metabolism that does something with no matter how many calories I eat. But what happened was, my liver got very congested, and I was pretty surprised when pretty much decades almost into my healing journey, somebody said you've got to do repeated liver, gallbladder flushes, and I did those, one a month for thirteen-fourteen months, and I still do them, and I still, I'm still not done. I'm just mentioning that because some people might think that it's a three-day process or a week process. You hear of the three day, the seven-day cleanse out there, and there's a certain amount you could accomplish with that. But for me, given how far down I was, and how much had occurred in a relatively short period of time in my early adulthood, there's some stuff to do. But it can be done, and it's very liberating.

Dr. V [00:27:45]: It is, it's a process, and it's a journey. And I tell our clients all the time, "It's a marathon. It's not a sprint. It's taken decades to get you to where you are today, so it's going to take time to turn things around." You mentioned the liver flushes, I don't know if you're familiar with Hulda Clark or not. She was a naturopath back in the days. She's no longer alive, but she was a firm proponent of the liver-gallbladder flushes. And her opinion was that unless you pass two thousand stones, your liver is still congested, so that's kind of a bench mark for us who are doing the liver flushes, because if you pass four or five at a time you've got a ways to go.

Brendan [00:28:33]: I lost count a long time ago. Unfortunately, I didn't start counting. I don't know where I'm at on that continuum. What I have noticed is the things that made the biggest difference came from the plant kingdom. They were gold-thread I think, gold-thread something, I have to look it up again, it was a particular product that contained gold-thread something, I think it was grass or something, Gold Coin Grass, excuse me, Gold Coin Grass, that's what it was, and it was breaking up liver stones very effectively. And then also just some regular food. When I have beets and dandelions and so dandelion greens, I don't necessarily see stones come out as the result of that, but I know that, I can tell my liver, because it's increasing bile production. It's what beets in part can do, along with artichokes and so forth. Any time you're increasing bile production, your liver is able to excrete more toxins. It all seems to come from the plant kingdom aside from a few other things that help loosen stones like malic acid which you might want to take as a supplement instead of having so many apples that you've got your fructose content over the moon. That might not be a good idea.

Dr. V [00:29:51]: That creates other problems.

Brendan [00:29:55]: So, I want to have you say more about the other parts of your program, the emotional side, anything you feel is really important for women to understand in regard to conquering breast cancer.

Dr. V [00:30:12]: Well you mentioned you were a good stuffer, which ... that's interesting because I use the same phrase as well. I was a really good stuffer. I grew up in a very dysfunctional, alcoholic family, sexually abused between the age of three to five by a convicted a pedophile back in the 50s, which was unheard of, that he would've been convicted back then. But, as I came to realize all these things, I realized that I was living the life of a wounded child in an adult body, and many decisions I made were not always the best, but once I realized that and I was able to learn to forgive myself, to forgive others, learn to self-nurture, and to self-love. It's so key because your thoughts, every single thought that you think is going to create a protein messenger, and everything that you think is communicated to your cells, chemically as well as energetically. And once I realized that, it was a big shift for me in choosing happiness and choosing joy and choosing to let go, and it was such a big turning point in my life to be able to choose those things and not live in that grey, gloomy path that I had. So sharing that with women and helping them to realize, you know, as women we're trained to be care givers, we're always taking care of everybody else, but if you're on a healing journey, you must take the time to bring down your stress level; you must take the time to meditate; you must take the time to journal and to really heal those wounds that have kept you captive because you have breast cancer for a reason. It just didn't happen to you because less than 5% of cancers are genetic anyway. Everything that you've done in your life so far has brought you to this point. The good news is, you can change all those things and start living a happier, transformational life.

Brendan [00:32:25]: You are reminding me of the work of Candace Pert with molecules and emotions. She's a phenomenal scientist and worked at the National Institutes of Health and then also Bruce Lipton with his biology of belief.

Dr. V [00:32:42]: Yes, absolutely.

Brendan [00:32:44]: Absolutely documented. What you just said is totally founded scientifically. There are physical things that happen in our body in response to our emotions.

Dr. V [00:32:55]: To the point of, it affects our DNA and our genetic expression. It's so powerful. Dr. Dean Ornish, a medical doctor who's done a lot of research with prostate cancer for example, and simply by teaching men to manage their stress, and to meditate, and to make dietary changes, the difference was amazing in the genetic expression, turning on four hundred and some positive genes and turning off hundreds of cancer-promoting genes. Just simple lifestyle changes like that can have such a huge impact on our health.

Brendan [00:33:36]: You were just at a major cancer-related event called The Truth About Cancer: A Live Symposium, I'm just curious, did you learn anything new there, anything exciting, eye-opening, mind-blowing?

Dr. V [00:33:56]: [laughs] Where's my notebook? It was, what can I say, we're always learning new things. Off the top of my head I can't think of them, but I know there were some because I took a lot of notes. I would have to say that just the overall energy of this community that understands that we can't poison our way to health with traditional medicine, and if we take responsibility for our health—you know there was always an underlying theme, which was nutrition, which was detoxification, which was emotions, dental, you know all these things that I talk about all the time—but to see a community that is so supportive of that and to hear story after story after story of people with brain cancer, prostate cancer, breast cancer, stomach cancer, I mean, you name it, reversing diseases, these are live people and so it's just, you know, sometimes we get stuck behind our computer, we're doing our research and our work, but to have that connection with real live people was so amazing for me, it just really touched my heart.

Brendan [00:35:05]: It must've been a beautiful experience, and there were people there like Thomas Seyfried who has really brought the mitochondrial and metabolic model of cancer to the fore, and so that's somebody that's really shifting how we understand cancer.

Dr. V [00:35:23]: He's a genius. I have so much admiration and respect for him. And you know that he's taking a lot of hard hits and a lot of hard blows. He's a warrior. He's a pioneer. But it's common sense. It just makes sense what he's discovered, and again it's not the end-all-cure-all. Is the ketogenic diet the only way to eat? No. You have to find balance, and that's one thing that I really stress with my community. Test to make sure that what you're doing is working for you. If it's not working, go to plan B. Don't be so stuck on the type of diet or a type of regime. If you're not getting the results that you want to get, then shift and try something different.

Brendan [00:36:06]: That is such wise advice. My personal journey had a lot to do with discovering metabolic individuality, my own. And after years of trying to fit myself into this approach, and that approach, and the other one, and when I came across systems for understanding metabolic individuality, that's when I got real control of my energy, my detoxification processes, and just general wellbeing. So I'm really glad to hear that you have that innate understanding, that there is individuality, we've got to just look and see, well how am I responding to this?

Dr. V [00:36:45]: Exactly.

Brendan [00:36:46]: And the ketogenic diet has its place, and overall I think humans are designed to cycle between different eating regimes because that's what we faced in the past.

Dr. V [00:36:59]: Exactly. We didn't have a grocery store that was open 24/7 that we can get strawberries or bananas in the middle of winter. There was the feast and famine aspect of life a few hundred years ago and for thousands and thousands of years. And so it just makes sense that we put our body through that metabolic challenge and create that autophagy where our body can break down and recycle those unhealthy cells, and to me it just makes so much sense.

Brendan [00:37:33]: And it's so much fun that the way we get to heal is through food, which of course is pleasurable. It's one of the main gifts of being human is being able to eat food, delicious food. As I mentioned earlier, our food, even our real food, fresh fruits and vegetables, even organic, is not the same as it was a hundred years ago. A hundred years ago basically all of our food was effectively organic, yet there were flaws in our agricultural system, our plowing and tilling and so forth, and other people will speak to that in this event, that affected ultimately the sustainability of our methods and the nutrient quality of our food, but in a hundred years, we've lost so much. I'm curious if we were able to put that back, if we were to put back the high nutrient-density, I mean it's literally more than ten times the nutrient density that we have now on average, at this point, if you go all the way back a hundred years. And I'm just curious, what do you imagine the impact would be on cancer rates, cancer conquering if we had a food system that produced toxin-free super food, super nutritious, there wouldn't be a distinction between super foods and regular foods. They would all be super foods.

Dr. V [00:38:50]: It would equip us to be able to handle all the other junk that's out there, the electro- pollution and the other toxins that our body may be exposed to. It would help us to stay centered in spite of certain stressors in our life. We would sleep better. We would feel better. We would detox better. So it would obviously have a huge impact. And we know, as you mentioned, food is just so much fun—the color, the flavor, the experiment, the experience that goes with it. It's part of our being, part of our culture, and if we could experience that on a much higher level, then it would definitely have an impact on our health long term.

Brendan [00:39:39]: Dr. V, one more question for you. In regard to breast cancer, is there anything else you would want to say to women about breast cancer right now?

Dr. V [00:39:51]: I would have to say that when you're initially diagnosed, there's the shock and the fear. And the coercion of traditional medicine is to put you on that conveyer belt—let's get you started and let's cut, burn, and poison. But to really step back and to recognize you have the time. For the most part, breast cancer is not a life-threatening disease. You don't need to end up in the ER room and have surgery right away. So you have time to look at your options. You have time to get a second opinion. You have time to do your research. And it's so important to look inside and do what you feel is best for you. If doing chemotherapy and having surgery is best for you, and then you balance it out with proper nutrition, then that's awesome. But if you believe that those things are going to poison you, and they're not beneficial, then don't do them. You have the time to make those decisions for yourself. This is your body. This is your life and you get to choose and decide.

Brendan [00:41:01]: Dr. V, breast cancer has been such a frightening disease, and it doesn't have to be, and I'm hearing you say it doesn't have to be so frightening at all apparently. And you're empowering people, and you're demystifying this disease. And the way you're addressing it is so holistic. It's just a tremendous service to women all over the world in 35 countries and growing. And I just want to thank you for your leadership in the treatment and prevention of breast cancer and other forms of cancer.

Dr. V [00:41:32]: Thank you so much for having me on your show, it's been a pleasure.

Manuela Boyle, PhD, NMD Interview
Minerals, Metals, and Different Diets for Treating Different Cancers

Brendan [00:00:00]: Welcome to the Eat4Earth event. We're exploring how you can heal yourself, your loved ones, and the planet, with food. This is Brendan Moorehead, and it's my pleasure to be speaking with our guest, Dr. Manuela Boyle. Dr. Boyle is an integrative oncologist and a PhD scholar who treats cancer. She is regularly invited as a guest speaker at key conferences around the world and is the published author of several peer-reviewed papers. She's also a peer reviewer of the prestigious Breast Cancer: Basic and Clinical Research Journal -- Libertas Academica. She has recently been accepted as an external expert by the European Center for Disease Prevention and Control in Stockholm, Sweden, in an honorary position aimed to provide independent scientific opinions, expert advice, data and information, and to maintain scientific excellence at all times through the best expertise available. Dr. Manuela, thank you so much for being here with us today.

Dr. Manuela [00:00:58]: Thank you for having me, and Hi from Brisbane, Australia, yes, all the way from here.

Brendan [00:01:06]: A beautiful part of the world, I can attest. I was there in November and December … not the whole months—I wish I was—but for three weeks, staying in November and December of 2015.

Dr. Manuela [00:01:18]: Wonderful, great. Thank you again for having me, it's a real pleasure. I'm an admirer of your work and really honored to be here and be your guest today.

Brendan [00:01:28]: Likewise. So, Dr. Manuela, it's predicted that one in two men, and one in three women alive today will experience cancer. Do we know the key factors causing this pandemic of cancer?

Dr. Manuela [00:01:43]: Well, sure, we do. There are several theories of cancers, why somebody has cancer, why somebody does not have cancer. The genetics theory whereby if somebody in your family has cancer, basically pretty much you're predestined to have cancer yourself—it is a theory that still is part of it, part of the broader picture. It's all so linear, however. There are families whereby cancer maybe has occurred in grandparents or parents but then not in the newer generation. So the genetic is not so much a linear progression of disease. In fact only 5 to 10% of all cancers seem to be related to genetic inheritance of susceptibility to cancer. In fact 90% or so of all cases are in fact due to epigenetic changes. So what's epigenetics? Epigenetics is all about changes that have been a chromatin of our DNA deeper in our cells. But what makes those changes then? Well, you have to look outside, away from the genetic factor, and you have to look at environmental factors, factors that have such an impact onto our body to be able to change the folding of the DNA inside the smallest part of our body which is the cell. Then the question would be: "Well, can we prevent epigenetic changes and things that are external factors?" And the answer is yes we can. And so the theory of cancer in the last ten years have been really related to or being referred to as, like I said, environmental factors, food, for example, stressors, bowel infections—yes, they've come through, and they also have been related to the onset of cancers. But basically it's about all changes coming from an outside source into our system. And overtime those changes can create such an impact as then to create the onset of cancer. So research in the last perhaps ten years or so has been very much concentrating on the stem, the epigenetic source of cancer, and to do something about it basically. So genetics is yes, surely it can create a predisposition and susceptibility for somebody to have an onset of cancer, but really by large it's about external factors and the external environment.

Brendan [00:04:28]: I'm curious since a big focus in this event is the connection between personal health and the quality of the foods that we eat. I'm wondering how big of a factor is diet, and are there any particular dietary patterns that you've noticed or have seen in the literature, among people that are getting cancer that may be coming into your office, and how do those patterns generate cancer?

Dr. Manuela [00:04:54]: Yes, food has a significant impact on the heightened risk of cancer. All of us have to eat. All of us have a lifestyle. And all of us have some kind of a stress in our lives. If you look at those, it's really very basic factors in people's lives that you could say, "Okay, we're talking about epigenetic changes; maybe we have to look into those three drivers," so food and diet, absolutely. The change of food, then again really, the food industry has a lot to answer—a lot of problem here—has yes, a great impact. In specific colon and colorectal cancer, plenty of literature points to the fact that certain types of dietary patterns can, in fact, and have been shown to contribute to the onset of the disease. So much so that studies from a public health view point were conducted in a particular population like the American people and the Australians, British, who all pretty much follow a similar diet called the western diet. It's also called the SAD diet that stands for the Standard American Diet or even the standard Australian diet. They're very similar. And in that population the numbers of patients, even the younger population, really, with the onset of colorectal cancer is really very high. The comparison was drawn with the eastern countries—I'm talking about Japan, China or South East Asian countries—whereby their type of diet is really completely different. One of my interests has been also to very much explore the population of India and Sri Lanka whereby their type of diet is based on spices; it's based on raw vegetables, based on a quite large amount of turmeric and a few others, what we know as healthy foods. Sri Lanka for example has the lowest amount in the world of colorectal cancer, whilst for example in the United States, well there you go, we have a high amount of colorectal cancers, so what's that all about?

Let's have a look at the food that we eat, food that really doesn't have fiber, food that does have a lot of additives, overcooked food, fast food. It's not food though, fast food. I mean I don't even call it food because it doesn't have any nutritional element in there. So these kinds of pseudo-foods are the ones that create an imbalance in the gut, the microbiome. The gut has a number of wonderful gut flora, wonderful little live bacteria which actually help us, keep us on track, and actually fight back against the carcinogenic elements. So if you don't look after your gut's flora, because the food is so bad, you can't expect that your immune system and the gut flora itself will help you get rid of carcinogens, or other types of so-called foods, and there you go ... now we're having irritable bowels which then can descend upon the colon disease and ulcerative colitis. and then sooner than later, now you're one step away from colon cancer. So, when we look at food, yes there's a lot that the food can and should answer. The pandemic of diabetes type 2—it shows even then how the gut's dysfunction can create a chronic, reversible, but still chronic disease. With cancer, we look at it the same way. So, what can we do with that? Well, we have to learn how to say no to certain foods, so-called foods, and think about really our health in a way that is preventive. Once the colon cancer, or any other cancer, are set, well, it's a lot more complex then to resolve the situation. We do have great successes but it's a lot of work, and a lot of sacrifice, and a lot of disease and illness. And it's a lot of issues that affect somebody with colon cancer. So let's look early around your life and think, "Okay, well you know what, we can say 'no' to certain things and say yes to others". But even within food that we think it's okay food—well, what about, is all food created equal? Well, we have foods to eat in supermarkets and other types of outlets which are not exactly the same as foods that you have from farmers markets. Foods that are sprayed on with anti-bugs, and those overly clean food, the non-organic foods. Well, are those actually foods? I don't know. That's a big question mark. So what I suggest to my patients who are ready and that we train, and we are quite successful, so that we get them back into an optimal life, is to absolutely don't even go into supermarkets anymore. Try to find a farmers market. Ask a farmer. Go to those organic farmers markets. The farmers know. They know what's in season. They know how the fruits or vegetables are grown, which conditions the fruits and vegetables have been exposed to. And whatever goodness that you find in there is what you actually have. So, when we think about preventive medicine, it's about loving yourself. It's about recognizing your own self. It's about respecting and giving yourself the goodness that's out there. Try to find that goodness, and keep yourself in health. So love yourself enough to make good choices. it pays off long term.

Brendan [00:11:15]: I think what I hear you saying is that nutrients matter. That's one of the things I can hear you saying because you mentioned fast food doesn't even have nutrients. Well, we know it has protein, fat, and carbohydrates, but I'm not sure how many other nutrients are in there. And then you mentioned supermarkets where this food has travelled a long time since it was harvested, and in that period of time a lot of nutrients start to break down. And then if it's irradiated, which pretty much all non-organic produce is irradiated, so that may cause further damage to the nutrient molecules, plus it sterilizes the food, which as you mentioned, it's not so good to get totally sterilized food necessarily. We evolved with "dirty" food, and we need that to replenish our microbiome perhaps, especially—and I probably if I should insert a caveat—if that food is grown on healthy soil because if it's grown on soil that's questionable and it's been nuked with agrichemicals maybe it's not going to be as beneficial with the microorganisms. So what that leads me to ask is ... you know, we've had a striking decline in the minerals in our food supply. And that's starting with the soil. There are also other factors, but it starts in the soil, and depending on what minerals we look at and what time frame we look at, it's pretty frightening. There's declines up to 50 to a 100%, not a 100% excuse me, 90% over the last hundred years, if you look a hundred years back. A lot of the comparisons only look forty years, and that's not enough to see the whole decline in certain minerals. It's pretty astonishing.

Dr. Manuela [00:13:13]: You're absolutely correct. An important fact is also the speed on which food is grown. Now there is a movement in Europe. I'm Italian; I originally coming Milan in Italy. And in Italy some years ago there was this Slow Food Movement. I'm not sure if you're aware of it, whereby what is grown has to actually have a natural growing process. So whatever it takes for an apple to become a ripe apple. It takes a little while, nature takes some time to do so. So speeding this up has actually shown to deprive, to take away, the nutrients that are fundamentally and vitally a fundamental part of this apple. Now if we speed this up, we're not going to get the nutrients that come from it. It's interesting. What I suggest to my patients and others is, "Well, look, if you don't have a chance to go to a farmers market then you really are pretty much stuck by going to the local supermarket". Ask yourself the question, "Alright, why does the vast array of food, for example, are they all in season?" because you cannot have winter foods and summer foods in the same time. Some of them would've had to be frozen, would have had to be been there for a while, and you know they're not going to be okay for you because likely they don't have what's needed in there. So just to be a little bit smart about what is there that you can actually use. Number one. Number two is—you're absolutely right—there are farms in Australia, and certainly in Europe ... they're called biodynamic. What does it mean, "biodynamic"? It means that of course, a lot of attention is given to the quality of the soil. The soil has to have all the nutrients, all that richness to be able to grow our vegetable or our plant or our herb. And it has to be done in a way that is not chemically laden because it's not just enough to be organic anymore, it's also about the soil, just like you said. So the soil which if it's left in the original condition does have minerals and it does have a good amount of nutrients to feed and make this plant of fruit or veggie grow in a right environment.

There are, unfortunately, however in general, yes, we know that even the soil is deprived for example in Australia which is relatively I suppose a healthy country from the outside I guess, but we do have a significant deficiency in magnesium, significant deficiency in selenium, significant deficiency in other minerals which are basic minerals in the soil. So much so that of course some of the foods have to be either fortified or, certainly if you do some kind of tests in preventive medicine for patients or individuals (who) really don't have those minerals, and then you have to say, "Okay maybe it is the soil." But the soil originally, it does have those minerals. It's the way in which the soil has been treated or mistreated, and basically we don't have those minerals anymore, so it becomes a significant problem. Additionally, of course, it is ... look for the [unintelligible] it is driven by food industry, no doubt, and for the food industry the mantra is really to produce more, faster, and to such an incredible rate, so much so that certain types of very important steps are avoided and you go into super-drive, trying to get food out there. I guess in a way because the consumer has this idea that yes, you can have anything that you want, and yes you can have all the fruits, all the veggies, all the meats and everything else is so available. Well, it's not natural to do it that way. It's definitely unnatural. So, the cattle industry for example. Australia is just like the United States—it's a cattle country. You've got a lot of cows, a lot of meat, but even then, what are these cows fed on and need, to support and produce so much milk and to get so much meat, such a big turnaround. Well, they have to be fed on something and often times you have hormones there injected so that they can produce more milk, it can be more [unintelligible].

What about salmon? Salmon in Australia or around Australia and New Zealand used to be a wonderful food. It's not sustainable anymore. So the salmon is farmed. How is it farmed? Well, because of the demand you have from a little salmon into a huge big salmon in the speed of light. I went unfortunately to see—I say unfortunately because it was kind of shocking—to go and see the salmon in farming. Over there it grows because salmons are fed hormones, they're fed growth food that makes them grow very, very quickly. You have additives, all kinds of things in order to have a big salmon, and that can go straight onto the fish market and onto the super markets. And there you are. But then again, how do we get, how do we eat anything … do we get anything that has actually been put onto these animals as come onto us, and the answer is yes. So when we go back to cancer, and there is this high number of hormonally-driven cancers which are prostate cancer for men, breast cancer for women, uterine cancer and ovarian cancer also for women. The problem with the hormonally-driven cancers is because you have a high amount of hormones. Where do these hormones come from? Well, the majority of them come from xenoestrogens or xenobiotics, and those ones again come from foods that have been manipulated with hormones and grown in an unnatural way. This is not just a theory, this is a fact. It has been proven in a number of studies, it's proven every day with functional testing, with pathology testing that we do on our patients in our clinic and many other clinics around the world.

Brendan [00:20:16]: So we've got over-processed foods; we've got hormone-contaminated foods; and we have nutrient-depleted foods. And it occurs to me to mention that two minerals, one of which you mentioned, selenium, and zinc, which are pretty important for detoxification processes for our immune system … and so we're being assaulted with chemicals, but our foods are not supplying us those minerals, and a big reason is that the soil organisms are being killed by the fertilizers and by the pesticides, and how we grow, and we over-till the land and so forth. And then the plants don't have the minerals to produce the phytonutrients that make plant food be the medicine it was always meant to be, and still is if those compounds are in the food, and sometimes they are and sometimes they aren't. There's tomatoes on the market without lycopene basically.

Dr. Manuela [00:21:15]: Basically, yes.

Brendan [00:21:19]: I'm just wondering if this depletion of the minerals and the phytonutrients is another factor in the genesis of cancer, is that our detoxification and our immune system are not functioning to par.

Dr. Manuela [00:21:38]: Absolutely. Of course that you absolutely cannot live, I suppose, in a bubble. I mean I suppose it would be nice, but we cannot live in a bubble. So the body is so wonderful that we have an organ called the liver, and we have an immune system, so we're all born with this wonderful ability to detoxify from toxins coming from the outside. The point is that, when there are too many toxins, when it is too much, when the liver is overloaded, the liver is not going to work anymore very well. The liver goes into a phase two detoxification whereby it's actually built there to deal with the excess estrogen that we get, or the hormones that we get from our food, dealing with xenobiotics, or make-believe estrogens, deals with toxins coming from all type of food and other elements. The liver is there as our detoxification organ. However, it gets overloaded, and it doesn't … the overloading of the liver, people sometimes they think, "But I don't drink alcohol so my liver should be fine." Well it's not so simple. It's not anymore just drinking alcohol, but certainly alcohol contributes to an overloaded liver. But it's about everything else that our body rejects because clearly we know that certain types of toxins, certain types of pollutants don't belong, so our body goes into a very natural way of trying to detoxify, getting rid of those toxins. But if the liver doesn't function, then we are pretty much in a situation where those toxins then become part of us and then start making those really huge negative impacts onto the cellular level. You just mentioned earlier about the chromatin, really, really deep inside the cells.

But what does the liver need, for example, to detoxify? Well, it needs things like selenium for example, and so now we are in a situation where we don't have selenium naturally because our soil doesn't have it anymore. We then have a liver that is overloaded, and we don't have now our ability to detoxify, so now you go full circle, and there you go. And then what you do? Well, at this point you have to get supplements. You don't go to food anymore because we know selenium is not there, so you have to look somewhere else. And then you have to go into nutraceuticals to be able to actually compensate.

The liver is really essential to, like I said, to modulate and to detoxify, conjugate, and secrete this type of toxins. At the same time of course, the other factor is about the ability of our immune system to actually also help in a way, the liver, in a sense, in keeping up and making sure that we can really keep this inflammation down and for the body to be able to deal with pollutants and other type of hormones and xenobiotics and all of those. Now the immune system is this very sensitive part of ourselves; it's actually our body guard, a little guardian angel. You can call it whatever you like, but truly do love your immune system. If you abuse them, well, make friends out of them. For instance, they are there to keep up the balance in the microbiome, and that is their very main function. The second function is to fight back if we do have pre-cancer cells. How do you know, I mean, you don't feel that you have precancerous cells until they are full blown cancer tissues. But it's a process that starts earlier on with precancerous cells. So if you don't feel your pre-cancer cells; you go along with your life as normal I guess. The liver, the immune system is there fighting for you, and if you don't look after them, like I said, they're not going to do well with that fight. And then there is the occasion actually where the immune system gives up and says, "Okay, can't do this" and the precancerous cells become cancerous and there you are, and then you've got a problem. And the immune system typically is suppressed, and we don't know why it's not working out, why it's not helping us, and, well, like I said, you have to go back a few steps.

The immune system is … how can we keep a good immune system in function? Well, the food for example is one of them—good food I'm talking about. The other one is considered the pre and probiotics which we can also have from food, if food was functional. If it was assimilated as it's supposed to be, it would give us exactly what we need to keep our immune system up and alert. However, this often doesn't happen because once again we don't have enough fiber, prebiotics, we don't have enough fiber from our diet as a choice, even if we choose fiber, well, we need to make sure that we get the right vegetables in the same way as we discussed earlier on. When we get the right choices though, fiber is fantastic, it's essential, it's important. And it is there to feed and help the gut microbiome as well as help the immune system. So we've got everything in Nature, and it's actually cheap. That's nothing very complicated about that.

Brendan [00:27:23]: In terms of our liver health, it occurs to me to mention that glyphosate, the main ingredient in the herbicide RoundUp, is toxic to weeds and most forms of life, in part because it chelates minerals, so it binds to minerals like zinc, iron, manganese, boron and so forth. So it not only kills the weeds, it kills a lot of other things including beneficial soil organisms that would normally make the minerals available in soil to plants. That's a big part of the soil organisms' role, different bacteria and fungal organisms and a lot more than that actually. So when these nutrients like zinc are not sufficiently available in soil to plants, plants instead take up toxic minerals like cadmium that have similar physio-chemical properties to the nutritional minerals like in this case zinc. So, ultimately, the scarcity of beneficial soil organisms can actually cause toxic metals to accumulate in our food and in our bodies.
You've researched the impact of toxic metals on health. Can you tell us a little bit about what you found?

Dr. Manuela [00:28:31]: Yes, absolutely, that's right. There are a number of toxic metals, and like you said, cadmium is another one of them. It's interesting how we often come across to a certain high amount of arsenic. And you feel like, "Arsenic, where did that come from?" Well, arsenic for example comes from, unfortunately, another [unintelligible] but there are ways where rice grows in fields which are highly polluted because of [unintelligible] and others whereby arsenic is present and so populations that use quite a lot of rice in their daily food, they have unfortunately a very high amount of arsenic. It's derived, it's being cultivated in a way that unfortunately the food industry is trying to do. So that has to be taken into consideration. Of course cadmium is another one of them. Nickel is another one of them. There are lead and mercury for example, so we have these toxic metals that are part of the way in which the food grows because of things like Roundup and other types of spraying, and other ways in which the industry works in terms of getting rid of bugs and getting rid of other types of little creatures. But unfortunately, that impact goes inside … it goes into the soil, and because it goes into the soil basically it goes into the produce. And if that happens, then we also unfortunately inherit that. It's really important … it's very interesting to actually do some research into the heavy metal load that every patient, as a preventive as well as for patients who are in treatment … what type of heavy metal load does this patient have. So we do that and often come across amazing things, sometimes off the chart.

Let's not forget that these heavy metals not only are behind and contributing to the onset of cancer, but they do contribute to a lot of other chronic diseases, for example Alzheimer's. We know the mercury crosses the blood/brain barrier, and it gets inside the brain, and it creates such a problem that then you go into onset dementia. What about Parkinson's disease? That's another one. But as far as cancer goes, yes, definitely. Our body is not meant to really deal with heavy metals. The body goes into some type of little panic mode. That's not [unintelligible] heightening the lymphatic system .. puts them onto the liver … the liver doesn't know what to do with that because it's too much, too difficult to deal with. It's overwhelmed by it. And so they live with us, something that doesn't belong to us lives with us. Something that's highly toxic then lives with us, and then you feel like, "Surprise, patient has got cancer." Well, you know, the thing is not a surprise at all.

Other things of course that also become quite toxic is also, let's not forget, apart from heavy metals is the way in which food is cooked. Because let's say in the ideal world, an individual gets fish which is non-farmed, it is from the sea, from the ocean, it's relatively [unintelligible] and heavy metal-free to a degree, but then instead of cooking it, or baking it, or cooking it in a healthy type of way, this type of food like fish is chargrilled. It's put on to a barbeque, it's grilled, and it becomes black or really overly burnt on the outside. That is also very toxic for the individual. It can create in fact a lot of difficulty, a lot of problems in the gut that eventually will lead up to have irritable bowel disease, and then colon disease, and then can go into colorectal cancer. In Australia in particular, it's a country with overall good weather, in general, the practice of barbecuing or having barbecued meat or fish is so wide spread, and unfortunately we don't realize that you don't have to eat the dark, black part of the piece of meat or the piece of fish because that is toxic to you, so cut it off. Get rid of it. Or don't even cook that way. Cook it differently. There are some strategies that can be put in place in order to avoid not only carcinogenics [sic] from food and food sources, but also the way in which the way is cooked. Toxic metals are difficult. Once toxic metals are found in tissues of a patient, the chelation, the detoxification from these toxic metals takes a while, and it has to be done well. It has to be done in a manner that makes sense. You cannot move out of the system toxic metals all of a sudden, for example, all at once. There would be significant issues related to the ability of the patient even to sustain such a detoxification. The detoxification needs to be done slowly. Potentially the toxic metals have been there for a very long time, so you cannot really overwhelm the individual and just do a quick detoxification, particularly if it is from a heavy metal. So it takes a while. Typically post chemotherapy, which is another big amount of toxicity put upon the system, it takes at least two years to detoxify patients from heavy amount of copper for example.

Brendan [00:35:04]: Wow.

Dr. Manuela [00:35:05]: Two years of an everyday slow but steady detoxification. This is just an example but yeah.

Brendan [00:35:13]: So I guess it's important for people to realize, "Hey, don't just abuse yourself while you're young because you're not going to just fix it over a weekend. You're going to be spending some time on it". And I've heard from doctors that specialize in detoxification, like Dr. Joseph Pizzorno who's also in this event, is that there's evidence that the effects of this toxicity often don't show up until middle age, so somehow you defeat the symptoms for a while, and then suddenly bam, you're feeling it. I recently just heard the term "gerontogens", as in gerontology, so these toxins are actually pro-aging influences, and it's kind of unfortunate that we have so many sources of toxins, and ultimately, they're making us sicker and shortening our lives, and technology can only do so much. We've got to go back to diet. And I imagine when somebody's in an act of detoxification with you, you have nutritional protocols. In fact, I understand you have individualized nutritional protocols, and I'm just curious because there's so many research-validated diets in the literature. Can you tell us what you do, and how is it individualized for each person?

Dr. Manuela [00:36:34]: Right, okay, so there are of course some protocols for detoxification. I guess number one is to find out what type of heavy metals the patient has to be detoxified from. So there is some, of course [unintelligible] investigations about the type of toxins that are part of the individual and then the way in which the toxins, how they behave. And so for each toxin, there's a certain amount of time given in terms of chelation and detoxification. Before any detoxification can go through all these degrees there's an understanding of liver function, gut function, bowel function, and so making sure that they execute in a way that they are ready for that. So that's a very long, but very successful method to do so. On the other hand in regards to diet, in regards to nutritional protocols for cancer patients in particular, of course they do different ... unfortunately, there's no one size fits for all in terms of diet that would be easy and would be fairly linear and straightforward. There are several different diets depending on the type of cancer, which is interesting. If you do a search in the literature you'll find at least a dozen validated cancer diets. So what's good about them? Are they all good? Are they all bad? Which one is what? Well, really the attention has to come from the type of cancer, not so much from the type of diet. Cancers really work quite differently in the way of, well, first of all, you have [unintelligible] cancers, then amongst them you have those cancers that are hormonally-driven and others perhaps that are not. So already you can see there are some differences. In general, obviously, we're all looking at plant- based diets as long as those plants are grown in a right way, really on a plant-based diet. Why plant-based? Because plants have minerals, like we discussed before, which is so important to balance out and really fight against cancer. And secondly is because what's really very important is to keep the insulin very stable. So cancers, no matter which cancer, all love very much high cycle growth factors like insulin, like sugar, high glutenated, all of that. They need that because they need to live on it. They need to have other daughter cells to take over the host. In general, a plant- based diet is one that would apply to all cancers. Then you go a little bit deeper, and you look at the individual. Number one, you look at how aggressive the cancer is, how far gone the cancer is. Are we talking about an isolated tumor, or we're talking about metastatic cancers. We have to look at those other variables.

So, for example, let's have a look at gastro-intestinal cancer or pancreatic cancer which is a very fast aggressive cancer that actually comes from prolonged gastro-intestinal dysfunction. When you look at the pancreatic cancer, pancreatitis is sometimes before pancreatic cancer's onset. Then you have to look at this cancer, that is aggressive, that is impairing the release of pancreatic enzymes, so you really know that this is a cancer that has to be stopped just about above everything. So plant-based, green juicing, making sure that the patient is sustained with a certain but very, very low amounts of protein because (of) the inability to digest these proteins, and second because it's really ... even when you look at protein, you couldn't help but to understand that aggressive cancers also feed on protein, so it's not just sugar anymore. But there are proteins like gluten, for example. Gluten is a fuel for cancer. So you have to look at all aspects of these cancer cells, and say "Alright, you are aggressive, fine, I'm going to starve you". And patients are not going to die because they're not going to eat. Nobody is going to die because you are reducing the amount of food. As long as liquids and as long as certain types of low caloric intake is kept in place, a patient can manage, can handle. Of course we do other things with pancreatic cancer, including the pancreatic enzyme therapy, which is very important. This is the type of, I guess possibly the most difficult cancer to deal with, because it's so aggressive. So we starve that. The patient is sustained, We check the weight of course every step of the way. We use botanicals and nutrients to compensate for the type of really reduced caloric food, and we've had very good results with that.

Let's talk about colon cancer, as we mentioned before. Colon cancer patients, they basically say goodbye to meat for a long time. They say goodbye to meat, processed food. They say goodbye to a lot of different types of meats, rich foods. They still have to have some proteins, but certainly not red meat. Why? Because when we eat red meat, we chew it, we digest it, and it goes to the large intestine. Well, from then onwards it takes about eight hours to really be excreted, so it's a long path that we have in the large intestine, and at this point, it becomes putrefactive, perhaps there is a decrease in the gut flora, in the larger intestine. The meat at that point, the putrefactive meat is pro-inflammatory, perhaps we don't have enough fiber. There you go. You have something that you really don't want to have there because you really have a problem. So no meat, but once again, plant-based food, a lot of fiber, and a lot of fruits and vegetables, they are quite fine. So it's more like a vegetarian diet.

Let's talk about now blood cancers. Blood cancers are different, patients are typically highly anemic. The problem there is blood and iron-based food. With them we emphasize iron-based food, let's say spinach, chickpeas. Sometimes they have to take iron tablets, but they can have one meal of organic grass-fed lamb. It's okay for them. It's not a big deal, but for colon cancer you never get to that point.

What about hormonal cancers. Well, (with) hormonal cancers we know that the hormones are the problem. They're hormonal cancers. Well, what makes hormones? What are they made of? They're made of cholesterol, so would you want to give patients with hormonal cancer (a) high amount of fat, even goose fat. Well, no maybe not so. You probably want to have a look at something else like lycopene for example. We talked about tomatoes and lycopene, very important, well studied, particularly with prostate cancer. I remember for example I went in Germany only a few months ago, and it was very interesting that they took out the Budwig diet for example. The Budwig diet is a cancer diet that is based on large amounts of fat, meat, a lot of butter, a lot of oil. Is it good? It may be good for brain cancer patients, sure. But not for hormonal cancer patients.

Why brain cancer patients? Well because for brain cancer patient a ketogenic, potentially high fat diet is perfectly fine because that type of tumors live on and thrive on sugar and glycolysis, so we take away sugar. Well, how's the brain going to work? Well it's going to work on high protein and high fat. It can work that way. Brain tumors we know don't feed on those proteins as well as fats. So every cancer is different, apart of course, on top of that if the patient had gone through chemo therapy and/or radiation therapy of course their ability to digest and to absorb is also quite compromised. It's not just the type of diet but also the amount of the ability to absorb that's also very important. I'm glad to say that I have a great nutritionist who works with me in Australia, as well as in other clinics overseas where I consult, and they are great. They really are smart. They do individualize each and every diet for each patient based on the type of cancer, based on ongoing issues such as with the digestive system, and really patients truly thrive. Nothing like … forgetting the type of diets, what we call the hospital foods. No, I mean, they're not okay. And I have been able to actually observe these not just in Australia, but I consult also in Dubai, in Milan. I do some consulting in London and at times in Sri Lanka, and my goodness, hospital diet is the most consistent diet that you find, the most international diet that you find anywhere in the World. Same thing. You know it's not really great. Really.

Brendan [00:47:09]: Yes, well it's kind of a version of I guess the standard American diet exported to every hospital in the World. But since plants seem to feature in all or most of the anti-cancer diets and cancer prevention diets, I envision a future in which soils are super healthy, plants are therefore brimming with nutrients, and food is toxin-free and fresh and delivers more than enough nutrition to keep our livers working, our immune systems, everything functioning. And cancer and other chronic illnesses become as rare as they once were.

Dr. Manuela [00:47:51]: Absolutely. Look, one of my mentors—I'm very lucky I've got a number of mentors who are just amazing people. They're authors of books, and they are speakers. They are great, great contributors to overall health and population health. One of them told me when I was a younger girl, "Think about this, put it this way, junk food is like junk mind", so it is true. Look, the two are very well connected. We know all over the world that there are crazy things happening, right? There are people who are in mental health, or certainly affected by mental health, and they can just give rise to all sorts of tragic events in the world. Sure, we can think of poverty as one of the factors we can about (affecting) some crazy things going on. Think about the nutrients or nutrition. Would that have any connection? The answer is yes. So mental health or functional mental health also has got a lot to do with nutrition. For example, we know that microbiome has a lot to do with the mental health. Depression, anxiety, free-floating anxiety, many depressors, even post-traumatic stress disorders can be helped to be resolved if we have a good nutrition. So the gut has got a lot to say in all kinds of things, in cancer which is my specialty, but also in other aspects, and we see it in diabetes type two. We see it in medicine more often in degenerative disorder but really also in the mental health. This has to be really a very, very significant impact in a number of diseases and wellness.

When my patients go through cancer, they come out of cancer, (and) they go into what I call rehabilitation and very much so maintenance program. Do you know, none of them, I've never come across one, and I've had hundreds of patients really, none of them have ever said to me, "Well, you know what, I want to go back to the same diet I used to be on before cancer". That never happened. In fact they're very happy. They feel great. They've recuperated really well. They're back into wellness, and they like to stay in wellness. So they say, "Oh doc, can I still stay on the same diet?" "Of course you can." They don't need to have my permission because they know by then that they feel so much better than before, and they vow they are absolutely intending not to go back to the same kind of lifestyle and [unintelligible] that they had before. And so they continue on really well, and they embrace exercise. They do things they've never done before, even when they were supposedly healthy before the onset of cancer. So they have like a second chance, and they embrace the second chance and become strong advocates for proper food, for plant-based food, for food that has to be grown in certain ways. I have so many of my former patients—of course they're not patients anymore; now they're fine—who are speaking to their own communities and making and raising awareness about that. So they're great. They're all doing really good. Yes, people are rethinking about this, and they're taking their life in their own hands a little bit more than before, which is very good. It empowers (them) now they know what to do.

Brendan [00:51:45]: Well, Dr. Manuela, by including nutrition as part of your cancer treatment program, I'd say you're part of the movement to return food to its rightful place as everyday medicine, and that is a very noble path. So, thank you for your leadership in that and for your contribution here to help build the movement for a regenerative food system. And all of us in the Eat4Earth community thank you for being here with us today.

Dr. Manuela [00:52:14]: Thank you Brendan. People like you that make this happen … we are sometimes isolated voices, but we need somebody like you to really further give the bits and pieces of information, and hopefully even if whoever is listening to you takes even ten percent of what I said and runs with that I'll be a really happy person because look, when cancer is there, well, it's a different world. It's a world, unfortunately, of fear; it's a world of sacrifice; it's a world of sadness; it's a world of heavy work; it's just so bad to be there. Do something beforehand, absolutely. And if food is the way, and it is the way, well, embrace it. So thank you for making this really a valuable tool. Well done.

Brendan [00:53:11]: To me it's fascinating that different types of cancers require different types of cancer-healing diets. We're also going to hear from Dr. Linda Isaacs about how different people, with different types of metabolisms, require different diets to help them heal their cancer. She's also going to talk about pancreatic enzymes as part of the body's surveillance system for preventing and beating cancer.

Linda Isaacs, MD Interview
Pancreatic Enzymes as Cancer Surveillance & Metabolic Individuality for Anti-Cancer Diets

Brendan [00:00:00]: Welcome to the Eat4Earth event. We're exploring how you can heal yourself, your loved ones, and the planet, with food. This is Brendan Moorehead, and I've been looking forward to this conversation with out next guest, Dr. Linda Isaacs. Linda L. Isaacs MD is a graduate of Vanderbilt University School of Medicine and is certified by the American Board of Internal Medicine. She offers individual nutritional protocols for patients with cancer and other degenerative diseases, as well as protocols for those who wish to maintain their health. She worked with her colleague Dr. Nicholas Gonzalez for more than twenty years, and during that time they published articles together about the remarkable results they saw in various types of diseases. Dr. Isaacs, thank you so much for being with us today.

Dr. Isaacs [00:00:43]: Well, it's a real pleasure to be here.

Brendan [00:00:46]: Dr. Isaacs, so often we hear nutritional authorities recommending a very specific diet for all people, or for specific diseases, but I believe you do something quite different. If I'm not mistaken, you treat people in part by looking at their metabolic individuality and giving them individualized nutritional protocols. Could you give us some background on the basis for your approach to individualized nutrition?

Dr. Isaacs [00:01:14]: The work that I do, and the work that Dr. Gonzalez and I did together, was based on the work of another practitioner named Dr. William Donald Kelley. Over the course of his career he treated a lot of different types of people with individualized diets. What he found was that some people did well on a more vegetarian diet, some people did well on a diet that was fairly heavy in animal protein, and there are people that did well with diets in between those two spectrums. We're finding that to be true in our practice as well. The idea behind it is that diet can affect our autonomic physiology. That's the branch of the nervous system that controls a lot of functions that we don't have to consciously think about, like our digestion, our blood pressure, our heart rate. But the diet that we eat can affect that physiology, and that can affect our health. Actually there's a book out by Dr. Gonzalez called *Nutrition and the Autonomic Nervous System* that goes into quite a lot of detail about this. There are also rather lengthy recordings that he did, or that I've done, available elsewhere. But that in a nutshell is the reasoning behind why we use different diets for different people.

Brendan [00:02:36]: Is this Dr. Kelley the same one that wrote *The Nutrition Solution*?

Dr. Isaacs [00:02:41]: No, that's somebody else. William Donald Kelley was an orthodontist who practiced orthodonture in the 1950s and 1960s, but then his professional career changed when he himself developed what was almost certainly pancreatic cancer. He devised a method of treating himself that involved nutrition, a lot of pancreatic enzymes, detoxification, and he succeeded. And after people saw him change from looking like he was on the verge of death to back to his usual self, people started to come to him looking for help with their cancer. And so his orthodontic practice changed into an alternative cancer treatment program.

Brendan [00:03:25]: What is the foundational science or observation that he made around the autonomic nervous system and how different nutritional regimes affect it?

Dr. Isaacs [00:03:40]: What he found on a purely practical level first was that he himself had healed from his own illness with a more vegetarian type of diet, but then he thought that everybody should do that. But then what he found was that there were some patients that he would put on that kind of a diet, and they would feel absolutely terrible. Eventually he started trying, in desperation, tried something completely different which was meat, and found that they then flourished. He found that a lot of the supplements that made him feel better made them feel worse, and vice versa. From there, looking back at some of the other nutritional literature, he looked at the work of somebody named Francis Pottenger. There's a group called The Price-Pottenger Nutrition Foundation that is dedicated to preserving the works of Drs. Price and Pottenger. This Dr. Pottenger had done a lot of work with the autonomic nervous system, looking at the effects of diet and things like basic minerals, like calcium and magnesium and potassium, and what he had found was that different people have different metabolisms, different balances of those two halves of the autonomic nervous system and that he could affect that with those minerals and with diet. So Dr. Kelley after kind of serendipitously observing these things for himself also found the work of Dr. Pottenger, which backed up what he was saying.

Brendan [00:05:08]: It's interesting, my own experience with understanding my metabolic individuality has been absolutely instrumental in coping with, surviving, and coming a long way of recovery from a full-blown chronic fatigue syndrome. And this was a big part of it, just understanding my metabolic leanings, and being able to address those with food choices, supplement choices. My understanding from what I've read, I've read several different sort of popular books, layperson books like *The Metabolic Typing Diet*, and the other Dr. Kelley's book *The Nutrition Solution*. My understanding has been that on one side of the spectrum there's like a protein-type you could say, and then on the other side more of a carbohydrate-type, and that there may be two types within each of those. And I'm curious, so from my understanding is, let's say the protein-type has one that's more parasympathetic nervous system-dominant or what they sometimes call fast oxidizer, and then on the other side the say carbohydrate-type, they've got more of a sympathetic nervous system dominance, or maybe it's both, slower oxidation rate in cellular respiration. I'm just curious if that's the same kind of thing that you're looking at and how the respiration rate might relate to the two branches of the autonomic nervous system.

Dr. Isaacs [00:06:38]: I'm afraid that much of what you're talking about is something that was added on to Dr. Kelley's work by another practitioner, and I'm not really as familiar with its use. Based on my own clinical experience it sounds like it may be getting excessively complicated, but unnecessarily so. But I really can't comment on that I'm afraid.

Brendan [00:07:01]: Okay. So this individualized nutrition affects the body in ways that are applicable to all or most conditions, or is it especially pertinent to conditions like cancer?

Dr. Isaacs [00:07:14]: Well I think it's applicable to a wide variety of different types of illnesses. I know that my practical experience is that it's relevant for most people, regardless of what kind of problem they have and that even in very informal settings, in other words, not patient-related so to speak, but just talking to people that I meet that want to know what I do and then get very interested, that I wind up giving them something to think about and something that I've heard has helped their health, even if they're not formally a patient. In other words, if you have somebody who you know that they're feeling very tired and very spacey and it turns out that they've placed themselves on a vegetarian diet a couple of years earlier, well what that can do is push the system to be very, very alkaline, and I know in some circles alkaline is supposed to be good, but there's a happy medium for just about everything when it comes to human health. So someone on a vegetarian diet who's very, very alkaline as a result, can wind up having trouble focusing, having trouble concentrating enough to get basic functions of life done. Those people, if they eat a cheeseburger, they can actually wind up feeling considerably better. This kind of work can apply to a lot of different situations. It's not just about cancer.

Brendan [00:08:39]: I definitely relate to that example. That has been one of my key issues, sort of brain-fog, spaciness and so forth. When I try to eat more vegetarian, often times that creeps in rather quickly, and the only way to restore balance is to go for some animal products, and usually more on the red meat side of things. Or I have found that certain minerals help shift me, and that I can shift how much that influences me by increasing, for example—I'm not asking you to endorse this or anything—but in my own personal experience and based on some practitioner manuals I found from a particular metabolic typing chiropractor I guess. If I raise my calcium to magnesium ratio for example, or my zinc to copper, or my molybdenum to sulfur, those are some of the ratios that I have found very powerful in shifting me away from the meat monster mode, as I call it sometimes, more towards a little bit more vegetarian, lighter proteins, and so forth. I'm just curious if that is similar to kinds of things that you see.

Dr. Isaacs [00:09:55]: Yeah, that's a good example of the kinds of things that I'm talking about. There's some people who by nature have a very overactive sympathetic system, and those people for the bulk of their life will do well with relatively little animal protein. There's some people who genetically are just carnivores. They do best with a lot of meat in their diet, and that's going to be how they'll function for the course of their life. There's some people whose metabolism is more balanced. Their autonomic physiology, the two parts of it work fairly well in tandem. For those people, they need to eat a variety, or different types of foods. And the biggest hazard for them is reading a book that sounds very convincing that says that everybody should be eating in one of those two extremes. For a balanced person that will just shift them in the other direction so to speak, and they wind up getting sick because they ate an extreme diet. What they need is balance, a variety of different types of foods. And in many ways I think that a take-home point, so to speak, for a lay audience would be that for the most part people are attracted to what's good for them. There are exceptions. One of them is sugar. We all love it. Nobody should eat it. But having said that, most people will gravitate towards the diet that's good for them as long as they're not reading too many things that persuade them that nobody should be eating in a particular way. Your typical person with an overactive sympathetic system doesn't want to eat a steak every night. They don't feel well if they eat that way. The people that do well with the steak, if they eat a vegetarian diet, they're miserable; they're starving. If people would listen to what their body is telling them, for the most part, will come out in the right place.

Brendan [00:11:54]: That strikes me as a really important point to reemphasize. We've got so much information out there in the health realm and people seem to find that whatever worked for them and maybe for the cohort of patients that seem to be attracted to them, suddenly they have all the evidence that they feel they need to decide that this is the optimal diet for all humans, and apparently it's just not that way. Some people yes, they're going to thrive on a more animal product heavy diet, and some are not going to do well, and some have to go in the middle and have a ton of variety as you're saying across those different angles. I actually call this, I have a term for it, with regard to say dietary ideology for a lack of a better word I call it an idea virus. So, these idea viruses get out there, and everybody catches it and they latch onto it, and we also just call that a health fad or something. But now we've got so many that have been out there for a while, just fighting with each other it seems. And we don't need to fight, we just need to respect maybe metabolic individuality.

Dr. Isaacs [00:13:06]: Right.

Brendan [00:13:08]: And I'll make one little point here on the topic of beef, you know this big, big controversy, and a big topic of this event which is -- not all beef and not all red meat, not all animal products are created the same. It matters so much how they're produced. They can either be horrific influences on our planet and our health, or they can be very nourishing, for both our bodies and the Earth. So other speakers and I are addressing that in this event.

Dr. Isaacs [00:13:38]: That's really important, I'm glad to hear that.

Brendan [00:13:43]: Yeah. So I'm wondering, are you free to share any case histories that illustrate, and again, not for people to say, "Oh, well that sounds like me", you know, you've got to realize you need professional guidance sometimes to be able to figure it out. Then again trial and error is not too harmful when it comes to food. That's what people are doing anyway, they're doing trial and error. Can you give some illustrative case histories?

Dr. Isaacs [00:14:10]: Well sure, the case histories that I'm going to talk about are actually some that were included in an article that Dr. Gonzalez and I wrote in ... I think it was published in 2007. These are both patients with cancer. One was on a more vegetarian type of diet, the other was on a more carnivorous type of diet. So, the first one is a woman who in November of 2000, she went to her doctor because she wasn't feeling well, and she'd lost a little weight. And her doctor, very astutely did a CAT scan which showed a three-centimeter tumor in her pancreas. It took a little time to get the biopsy done but eventually in early February of 2001, a needle biopsy was done and showed that it was pancreatic cancer, and the tissue was actually reviewed again at the Mayo Clinic, just to confirm the diagnosis. There are more than one type of pancreatic cancer, but it was confirmed that she had the aggressive kind where life span is usually measured in months. So she started with me on a protocol that we offered in April of 2001, and as of last month she's still alive and doing just fine. So she is now seventeen years out or something, that typically kills. You know, seventeen months would be remarkable actually. So she's seventeen years out almost with this very negative diagnosis. So she's done very, very well. Her diet was one that was high in vegetables basically, very little animal protein. A lot of magnesium and potassium, very little calcium. That's the type of protocol that she was on.

Another patient of mine is a gentleman who in 1995 developed some swelling in his abdomen and his feet, and a CAT scan was done which showed multiple masses in his abdominal cavity that were putting pressure on various things causing the swelling further down in his body. He had a biopsy, and he had a type of lymphoma. Lymphomas are cancers of the lymph nodes and in his case it was one called follicular lymphoma which is one of the less aggressive ones but it still can certainly cause plenty of problems, and it was certainly doing that for him, he had the swelling in his legs. So he was offered chemotherapy, but it isn't terribly effective at least at that time, what they had available then, for the type of problem that he had. So instead he came to see me, went on his protocol, and the swelling in his lower abdomen and in his legs resolved. We're not big fans on doing a lot of scans here just because there's radiation exposure involved, but he has had several CAT scans since that time that have showed complete resolution of the lymph nodes that were in his abdomen. The last time I spoke with him was about a year ago, and at that time he was doing great. I had given him a call just to check in on him, and he was actually out back—he was building a house, wasn't doing all of the work himself, but he was doing quite a bit of it, so he was in the middle of working on a retaining wall when I spoke to him, which is pretty good for somebody who's pushing 60. He is doing just fine. He was put on a more carnivorous diet with a lot of red meat, very little things like greens. No alkalinizing foods because his body tends to be too alkaline in the first place, so that's an example of two patients and the different ends of the metabolic spectrum.

Brendan [00:17:57]: You know, this issue of alkalinity vs. acidity, I know a lot of us had heard the work of Dr. Otto Von Warburg. Is it Von Warburg or Warburg?

Dr. Isaacs [00:18:11]: It's just Warburg.

Brendan [00:18:17]: I'm just curious if you have any thoughts on that because that was the idea that perhaps the more alkalinity the better, related to cellular metabolism, but was that maybe more of a downstream effect or just a way of looking at part of the picture, or is it not something you'd really comment on?

Dr. Isaacs [00:18:36]: Well, I don't think getting more alkaline in and of itself is going to take care of anybody's cancer. I think that your typical alkalinizing diet is usually very much a plant-based diet, and what we believe is that the surveillance mechanism against cancer is actually pancreatic enzymes. A very alkalinizing diet because it's very low in animal protein, is going to free up some of the body's own enzymes to go to work against the cancer, and so while there are a few people out there who have done well with an alkalinizing diet and that's all they did, I think that the mechanism is actually not what they think it is. I think it has more to do with enzymes being freed up to work on the cancer as opposed to just getting more alkaline. I don't think it's as simple as buying a box of baking soda basically, I think there's a little more to all of these things.

Brendan [00:19:35]: Can you say more about pancreatic enzymes as a surveillance mechanism, I think that's how you described it.

Dr. Isaacs [00:19:45]: Sure, well, Dr. Kelley, our predecessor in this work, who had what was almost certainly pancreatic cancer, and I say it that way because he never had a biopsy. This was early 1960s, so they would've had to take him to the operating room to definitively prove what he had. But he had lost about 50 pounds and had a visible tumor in his abdomen, so they said, "You probably have pancreatic cancer. You need to go home and get your affairs in order". He put himself on a vegetarian diet, an alkalinizing diet, and in fact stabilized, but he still was having enormous trouble with digestion, a lot of gas, just poor digestion. He started on pancreatic enzymes to try to deal with that, the theory being that if you had pancreatic cancer, it probably wasn't making pancreatic enzymes. But then what he found was that the character of the tumor changed as he started to take quite a lot of pancreatic enzymes. He then went to the medical literature to see if anybody else had ever expressed an idea that pancreatic enzymes might work against cancer, and what he found was the work of a man called Dr. John Beard.

Dr. Beard was an embryologist by training, which means he studied the very early stages of development of the embryo, when things are just a few cells. What Dr. Beard had noticed was that there's a tissue in early development called the trophoblast. It's the earliest stages of the placenta which is a connection between the mother and the baby that allows the baby to get the nutrients that it needs and to get rid of waste. The early stage of the placenta is called the trophoblast, and what Beard observed was that the trophoblast in its behavior and in its appearance is a lot like cancer. The trophoblast's job as the embryo enters the uterus is to latch on to create a connection between the embryo and the mother. The trophoblast invades, it creates a blood supply and it fools the immune system into thinking that there's nothing to react to here, even though the mother's system is very different from the baby's, genetically speaking. The mother only contributes half of the genetic material. But there's one big difference between the trophoblast and a cancer. The trophoblast knows when to quit. At a certain point it stops invading, matures, turns into the placenta. And that will then peel neatly off after the baby is delivered, leaving the uterus intact for another pregnancy. But cancer just keeps going. The trophoblast knows when to quit. Beard's theory was that if you could figure out what the signal was that told the trophoblast to stop invading, that he might find an answer to cancer. He looked at a lot of different things happening in both the mother's body and the baby's body, and what he found in a number of different species, including humans, is that at the time that the trophoblast changed its character, the baby started making pancreatic enzymes. Now pancreatic enzymes in regular physiology are thought to only digest food, and they have no other role. Babies aren't going to see a meal for another seven months, so the question would be -- why is the baby making pancreatic enzymes so early. Nature tends to be fairly conservative; things don't happen until they're needed. But if the role of the enzymes is to control the behavior of the trophoblast, then it makes a lot of sense that enzymes would be made that early. This is the theoretical basis behind the use of enzymes. Some practitioners at Beard's time used them and had some good results, and there's been a scattering of people over the years that have used them since then with some very positive results. In terms of basic science support on a more modern level, there are experimenters who have agreed that the trophoblast and cancer look and act a lot alike and use the same mechanisms to get their job done. There's receptors on the surface of the trophoblast cells and also on cancer cells that will be like the catcher's net for enzymes that the pancreas makes. So there's definite suggestions that it's quite possible that orthodox science will make its way back around what Beard was saying a hundred years ago, at some point in the near future.

Brendan [00:24:26]: Am I understanding that pancreatic enzymes communicate or do something so that cancer—we actually don't know what they do exactly—but that tell cancer cells "don't be a cancer cell", "don't be like a trophoblast that doesn't know the boundary between itself and the baby", and the baby of course enforces that, perhaps, if that's the mechanism, with pancreatic enzymes. Is there anything else specific that we might know about how pancreatic enzymes might rein in or stop cancer cells?

Dr. Isaacs [00:25:02]: Well not for sure. My own feeling about that is that I have a significant number of patients who've done extremely well. That's why I do what I do. I think that modern medicine is very focused, it almost seems as if you have to know exactly how something works on a cellular level before you're allowed to use it, or to believe that it might work. An example that I use sometimes, the time that I went through medical school and did my residency, nobody knew how nitroglycerin worked to open up the blood vessels around the heart, but we gave it to people who were having chest pain because we knew that it worked. We didn't know how it worked. The nitric oxide pathways as they're called, weren't found until the 1990s. So I think that the real reason why I use pancreatic enzymes in treating patients, is not because I read an article about exactly what they're doing on a molecular level, it's because I've treated patients, and I've seen them get better.

Brendan [00:26:08]: So in other words we're talking about empiricism, clinical results as opposed to just knowing the mechanism. You're just saying, "We're getting results. They're consistent enough. We're going to keep doing it". And there's no evidence of any harm.

Dr. Isaacs [00:26:24]: Exactly. That's right, and I personally think that that makes sense. What I'd say is there's a lot of drugs out there, and there'd be an elaborate mechanism described for them, and they'll create them— "translational medicine", that's the term, you figure something out at the bench; you create a drug; it's going to do exactly what you think it's going to do, except that it doesn't. Just as an example, I saw a patient today as a matter of fact who's been on medication that's used for chronic myelocytic leukemia, and it's supposed to be very specifically targeted to a very specific problem or area, but it also creates terrible vascular disease that can be crippling, can be very, very serious. Nobody had any idea that it was going to do that, but that's what happened. So between using a drug whose side effects will not be determined for a few years vs. using something that I've seen work in patients, and that is really pretty nontoxic as well, I'm going to keep doing what I'm doing.

Brendan [00:27:36]: This is similar I suppose to this idea of using things that work, are safe, and we just don't know how they work perhaps. In naturopathic medicine for a long time physicians knew that detoxification was important, they didn't know all the mechanisms and more recently we've been discovering what the mechanisms are and just how important toxicity is in the generation of disease processes. So I'm curious, do you use detoxification in your protocols and treatments?

Dr. Isaacs [00:28:18]: Yes, we do, and again that was a big part of what Dr. Kelley was doing all those years, and the positive results that Dr. Gonzalez found in his practice, so we continue to use those things. The main thing that we use on a day-to-day basis is a procedure called the coffee enema. That is something that mainstream doctors typically find absolutely ridiculous. All I can say is they probably never tried it because most people feel tremendously better when they do them. They actually have a very long history in the medical literature, and they were in nursing text books right up through the 1950s. In one text book called *The Merck Manual* they were present from the time they started printing it up through the 1970s. I found some literature from the eighteen hundreds where doctors talked about their use in poisonings or in severe infection. I actually found one article describing a lecture by one of the Mayo brothers that started the Mayo Clinic, and in that lecture he was saying that coffee enemas were absolutely critical for post-operative care. There were a lot of competent observers that thought that they were valuable. My own feeling is that orthodox medicine kind of discarded them as pharmaceuticals came in, but I actually think that they are tremendously valuable and that regardless what their mechanism of action might or might not be, we find that first of all patients feel much, much better if they do them, and secondly the patients that decide that don't want to do them or don't have to do them, don't do as well. So I think they're critically important.

Brendan [00:30:00]: My understanding of how they work is that they are a cholinergic influence, in other words they stimulate bile flow in the liver and perhaps other processes, so it's basically stimulating the liver to kick out toxins at an accelerated rate. Is that your understanding?

Dr. Isaacs [00:30:22]: It's quite possible that that's correct. There are some articles from the 20's and 30's where actually enemas of various kinds were used pretty widely in regular medicine, and there are some articles from that era suggesting that that is indeed what happens. The thing is that nobody's really investigated this in the modern era where we've got techniques like ultrasound for example, to actually see what's going on. There's a theoretical aspect to that, we don't really know for sure. But again, I personally am quite comfortable going ahead and using something if I feel clinically it works without necessarily needing to do extensive studies to find out exactly how.

Brendan [00:31:07]: I should add perhaps that proponents of coffee enemas suggest that there's a vastly different influence between drinking coffee and using a coffee enema and that the hepatic portal artery or vein in the colon area is absorbing the undigested coffee right into the circulation; it goes straight to the liver instead of to other cells first. Would that be what you think is happening?

Dr. Isaacs [00:31:44]: I'm not too sure about that one. All I can tell you is that patients who have been coffee drinkers and then done coffee enemas can tell you that the way they feel afterwards is very, very different. In terms of the direction of flow of whatever is absorbed across the intestinal wall and getting into the blood stream, all of that from the stomach down to the colon is going to go straight to the liver. To me, in a way, I tend to shy away from creating a lot of theories about how something works if I'm not absolutely sure that it's correct. My own philosophy or theory is that perhaps the stomach works on, if you think about it, the stomach's job is digestion, and it may be modifying the coffee in some way when you drink it than when you do it as an enema it doesn't happen.

Brendan [00:32:38]: That makes sense given that in the stomach things are exposed to such a low Ph, so much acidity is going to transform a lot of things.

Dr. Isaacs [00:32:46]: Exactly.

Brendan [00:32:47]: Why do you suppose that toxicity is becoming an ever-increasing issue for our health. Why are we accumulating so many toxins, any thoughts on that?

Dr. Isaacs [00:33:00]: I think since the 1950s we've really had an explosion of different types of chemicals that are used every day. If you think about it, we're surrounded by it. Even if you go to your health food store and you purchase your grass-fed meat, and it's neatly packaged up in plastic that's adherent to every aspect of that meat. There are chemicals everywhere. I try my best to minimize my use of plastic containers and cartons and etc, and yet I find that my trash can is full of it at the end of the week. All of that, the production process means that chemicals wind up in the air, and the water, in the food we eat, in the ocean. We have surrounded ourselves with a lot of chemicals, and while any one of those might've been tested on some animal or a cell culture model and found to be safe at some very high concentration, we're dealing with a lot of low-volume exposure all day every day. And I think that can't help but have an effect on our health.

Brendan [00:34:13]: It's funny you should mention the plastic because—it's funny and not funny—the not funny part is that it's got phthalates which are very key toxin that we need to be aware of and it makes plastic softer. It's in those plastic wraps, and there was a book that was actually I suppose written in jest, I don't know the title, but basically it was saying that the healthiest diet is one with no plastic, no wraps around it. I haven't read it myself, I'm saying this second-hand, but it turns out that that actually is an influence. Foods wrapped in plastic are delivering phthalates into your food, and that's something to be aware of and avoid whenever possible. Aside from nutrition and detoxification, are there any other important elements of treatments that you use that you might call attention to?

Dr. Isaacs [00:35:13]: The three components of what I do are: diet, supplements, which I suppose both of those two could be put together as nutrition, and then detoxification. I certainly think that emotional and spiritual aspects can play a role as well, although I don't get into prescriptions on that one. I think there's many different ways for people to deal with emotional and spiritual issues, but I do find that the vast majority of our patients will tell us that the way they look at life and the way they deal with things has changed as a result of all of this. I think it's important for patients to find some joy in life and to not harbor about negative emotions like anger of lack of forgiveness, that kind of thing. Again I don't tend to be prescriptive there, but I do think it's very, very important.

Brendan [00:36:09]: These people that are getting so much benefit, how long was it that you said that the person that had pancreatic cancer, how many years or months out are they from a death sentence?

Dr. Isaacs [00:36:21]: She has made it sixteen and a half years from the time that she was given her diagnosis.

Brendan [00:36:29]: Just extraordinary. I'm curious, I mean, are these people getting well entirely on this type of treatment, there's nothing else that they're doing that you're aware of?

Dr. Isaacs [00:36:38]: Not that I'm aware of, no.

Brendan [00:36:40]: Wow.

Dr. Isaacs [00:36:41]: Certainly not standard therapy. I think she may have done a little additional alternative type stuff, but nothing of any duration. And actually what she did, she had it well after she should've been gone so to speak. In the early stages all she did was this protocol.

Brendan [00:37:02]: So in other words metabolically individualized diet and supplementation, plus detoxification and psycho-spiritual healing perhaps, or that might happen, I don't know, it's something...

Dr. Isaacs [00:37:21]: In her case actually, she's a very devout Christian and a wonderful person. She's somebody that definitely walks her talk, but she was that way when she first came in. I don't know what she would say in terms of any spiritual or emotional changes, but she seemed like she had that pretty much together, from my point of view. What she needed was to adjust her diet and take a lot of supplements, and with that she's done well. Our general philosophy is that cancer can potentially be like diabetes. If a diabetic doesn't eat properly they're going to get into trouble, but if they do what they need to do, it can be managed, it can be controlled. From our point of view, this is not a protocol that one does for three months, or six months, or two years, or whatever. A common question that I get is "When can I quit?" Apparently Dr. Kelley's answer to that was, "Whenever you stop wanting to feel better". In other words, if you stop doing what you need to do to take care of yourself things are going to go back to where they were. So this is a marathon, not a sprint.

Brendan [00:38:37]: Are there any particular patterns that you've seen in terms of what might be generating cancers for people?

Dr. Isaacs [00:38:47]: I think in general cancer is an illness of uncontrolled cell growth, and so what can stimulate that, I guess the question would be. There are some people that are creating more cancer cells than their body can handle. We're all creating cancer cells all the time, but our surveillance mechanisms get rid of them. From my point of view one of the big surveillance mechanisms is pancreatic enzymes, and so if you're eating a diet that requires more digestive enzymes than your body can make, then you may get cancer. People whose sympathetic nervous system, the fight or flight system, is overactive, their sympathetic system is basically telling their digestive tract "Not now". If you think about it, if you're about to get eaten by a lion, digesting your lunch can wait. You need to put your energy into running as fast as you can. So when the sympathetic system is overactive it shuts down the digestion which includes the pancreas, and you can wind up not having enough pancreatic enzymes in circulation to deal with cancer cells. Then there are things that can make you grow more cancer cells than you would have otherwise, things like smoking or radiation exposure, all the chemicals that we're exposed to. All of those things can go into making more cancer cells than our system can get rid of.

Brendan [00:40:17]: That's interesting, I had never ever thought of that as far as metabolic individuality influencing potentially cancer risk via mechanism, just too much fight or flight activity in the nervous system suppressing digestion in general. So I'm curious, in regard to your approaches to cancer, are there some people for whom this would be more appropriate and some people for whom it would be less appropriate, or is it not possible to really say?

Dr. Isaacs [00:40:52]: Well, what I would say in terms of cancer treatment is that there are some cancers where standard treatment can be very, very effective and under circumstances I would recommend that somebody do it. For instance, surgery for localized breast cancer or colon cancer. From my point of view, I think people should do that, and so that's what I would recommend, what I do recommend when somebody in that circumstance comes to see me. There are other conditions like some types of lymphoma for example that again standard treatment could be very, very effective. Beyond that though, it starts getting more about the approach of the patient, and so again if somebody is physically unable to swallow a lot of supplements, that can happen with the esophageal cancer for example, then this is not going to be a program for them. You've got to be able to swallow a lot of supplements to do this. That kind of characteristic of the patient would be what I would be assessing at that point.

Brendan [00:42:00]: Dr. Isaacs, you've got a very unique approach to treating cancer and I really appreciate how personalized it is. I'm kind of on a crusade in part too to help people understand that there is something that we might call a metabolic diversity and that the world of health and the planet itself would be much better off if we are honoring that in ourselves and also adjusting our food systems, how we grow food, so that whatever we're raising, whether it's animal products or plant-based products, that it's done in a way that is in harmony with Nature using Nature's natural pest control methods, its natural self-fertilizing mineral availability enhancing mechanisms. It's all there in this amazing technology called soil and biodiversity. And we are smart enough to harness that system, and that's what this event is about, is reintegrating that back into the human experience, and when it comes to cancer it's so important to have somebody like you who has this perception, this awareness and these nuances to share and help people heal and also help people realize that, "Gosh, a diet with animal products could be the best thing" for that person, and especially or as long as it's coming from animals raised in a way that puts good nutrients into the meat and gives the animals a good life and grows soil instead of all the opposite that comes from factory-farmed animals. The world is very fortunate to have a physician like you and we here at the Eat4Earth event and this community, are very fortunate to have had you here with us today, so thank you for sharing your experience and your expertise.

Dr. Isaacs [00:44:07]: Well thank you for having me, I'm really glad to hear the work that you're doing, and I hope that all of this can help the world change to be a better place.

Brendan [00:44:18]: It's so great to hear a doctor talking about metabolic individuality. Not many people know about that, much less talk about it, but I believe it's at the heart of why some people can thrive on a vegan or vegetarian diet while others seem to thrive only on diets with animal products. It also helps to explain why some people thrive on red meat while others only on light animal products like fish and poultry. Next, we're going to hear from a mostly vegan eater that had cancer and beat it with a vegan diet and lots of juicing, Cherie Calbom, also known as the Juice Lady. She's going to talk about some of the cancer-preventing and cancer-fighting nutrients in plants.

Cherie Calbom, MS Interview

Extraordinary Stories of Healing with Juicing, Souping, and the Anti-Cancer Nutrients in Plants

Brendan [00:00:00]: Welcome to the Eat4Earth event. We're exploring how you can heal yourself, your loved ones, and the Earth, with food. This is Brendan Moorehead and I'm very happy to welcome our guest, Cherie Calbom. Cherie is a leading authority on nutrition, juicing, souping, and detoxification. Known as the Juice Lady, George Foreman's nutritionist, TV chef, and celebrity nutritionist, she's helped pioneer the fresh juice movement around the world. Now she's pioneering the hot new trend called "souping". A graduate of Bastyr University with a Master of Science degree in Whole Foods Nutrition, Cherie is the author of thirty-four books, including her latest *Souping is the New Juicing*, featuring the wildly successful watercress soup diet which offers immediate weight loss along with unique health benefits and anti-aging effects. She has sold over three million books around the world, with many of her books in translated editions. Cherie has lectured worldwide on nutrition, juicing, detoxing, and fasting. Her blogs and books on health and nutrition have helped millions of people live healthier lives. She's appeared on CNN, Fox News, WCBS New York, along with numerous infomercials including the infomercial that introduced the George Foreman Grill. Her articles have appeared in New York Daily News, Newsmax, Miami Herald, LA Times, Essence, Vogue, First for Women, and Women's World.

Cherie thank you so much for being here with us today.

Cherie [00:01:33]: Thank you. Thank you for inviting me.

Brendan [00:01:36]: Cherie, you have a most extraordinary story of trauma, poor health, and miraculous healing. Can you tell us something about the events that led up to your interest in juicing?

Cherie [00:01:47]: In my late twenties I got really sick. I had chronic fatigue syndrome and fibromyalgia, and I couldn't work any longer. I had to quit my job and move back home with my father and step- mother. Life seemed pretty abysmal. I was sleeping twelve hours a day and getting up tired and shuffling through the day and back in bed again, and never feeling well. I felt like I had the flu all the time, and very, very fatigued, and I ached all over. And I was very discouraged because no one knew how to help me, and so I decided I was going to have to help myself, and I went to a variety of health food stores and doctors. At the health food stores I learned about juicing, and that's when I decided I better do something myself, like start juicing, and change my diet. I was eating all wrong, and I noticed that everyone was telling me "no junk food", and I love fast food, I like to go to a little fast food restaurant and go home with my little bag of whatever junk, and that was my dinner. My breakfast was sort of whatever I could grab. My lunch I went out to eat at a restaurant from work. That was kind of my lifestyle, and it appeared to be all wrong. And so I got my first juicer. I went on a five day vegetable juice fast. On day number five my body expelled a tumor the size of a golf ball with blue blood vessels attached.

Brendan [00:03:28]: Oh my God.

Cherie [00:03:29]: Totally got my attention. Having no science background, no information to go on, I was absolutely flabbergasted. I didn't have it tested, I just got rid of it because it was shocking to me. But I thought "Wow, having gotten rid of that, I should be well tomorrow. Maybe that was what had made me sick". Oh, no. My body was detoxing, and I had days where I felt a little better and days where I felt worse. But I decided that this was the only path that had gotten any kind of results, so I going to stick with it, no matter how bad I felt. Nobody told me about detoxing and that I could have some detox reactions, but I just plowed through it. That's probably why I've written so much about juicing, and detoxing, because I want people to have a lot of information. But one day, having stuck with my diet of juicing and eating vegan, all of that three months of summer—I just ate a pure diet and vegan foods—and I woke up one day, one morning, felt like somebody gave me a new body in the middle of the night. I felt absolutely fabulous. It wasn't just that one day that my body healed, it had been healing all along, but it was a realization that day of the good wellbeing, the feeling of wellbeing that just kind of bubbled up, and I knew I discovered something pretty powerful. But I called it a cure, and it's a big misnomer. Having called it a cure, I thought it was cured, and I could go back to my old way of living, which was not what you teach, living from the Earth. My symptoms started coming back and scared the daylights out of me. I thought "Oh no, I've tasted health, good health, I don't ever want to lose it. I guess this is a lifestyle, I guess I can't ever go back," which was right. I had to have a healthy lifestyle. Once I really embraced that, then I was able to enjoy vibrant health.

Brendan [00:05:41]: What have you seen happen for other people who juice-fast?

Cherie [00:05:46]: I have stories that could paper my room, my office.

Brendan [00:05:52]: You've been at this for a while, you've been the Juice Lady since 1992 I think.

Cherie [00:05:58]: Yes, even a couple of years ...

Brendan [00:06:00]: That's about when I first got my Juiceman juicer, in '92ish, something like that. I first learned about juicing at the exact time you were starting to become the authority. For some reason I only heard about the Juiceman and not the Juice Lady.

Cherie [00:06:15]: Well, I was working with the Juiceman, that's how I got my title. I was working for the same company and telling my story for many of the Juiceman lecture series. Since that time, I've encountered so many people whose lives have changed. I'll tell you a few dramatic stories. I have ones that aren't so dramatic, maybe I'll just mention that first like pain leaving, that's one of the first things that people acknowledge, "Oh, my pain is gone", arthritis types of pains, and carpal tunnel and headaches, and all sorts of elbow, knee, and back, and neck, and shoulder, and plantar fasciitis disappearing within days. But I have some dramatic stories to tell. One was of a woman that was sent home to die. She had cancer, and the treatments they gave her didn't work, and they said there's nothing more we can do for you. She found my book on juicing and decided to do a three-week juice fast. And she had tumors throughout her body. She said one day, a little over three weeks into the program, all of a sudden she felt this pain in her body and the only way she could describe it was a ripping or sort of tearing, and awful, excruciating pain. And she was so mad at me, she said "That Cherie Calbom, that diet, look at what it's doing to me". And all of a sudden her tumor fell out on the floor, a great, big tumor.

Brendan [00:07:53]: Fell out of where?

Cherie [00:07:58]: I don't know, I didn't want to ask. But from that moment on, she progressed toward healing, and she said four years later she looked ten years younger than she had four years before that. And she was running up steps that she said, downtown, she couldn't even hardly walk up. Her whole life changed, she was cancer free, and she was living a vibrantly healthy life.

Another lady came to me, they had sent her home to die too, she had seen both a naturopath and an allopath, and they didn't know what was wrong with her. She'd gained fifty pounds of water weight, everything they tried for her wasn't working, and she couldn't walk hardly. She couldn't even walk down her driveway, she said, to get her mail. She couldn't clean her house. She couldn't do anything. And she truly did feel like she was dying. And they said they thought she was too. Both of the doctors said there's nothing more they could do for her. I was her last-ditch hope. She said "What should I do?" and I did a diet assessment, and her diet was fairly good. So I said, here's what you do, you add a green juice before every meal, that's going to give you powerful nutrition, and your system sounds like it's so shut down that you're not digesting your food well, and it sounds like it's just going through your body without you gleaning many of the nutrients. But the juices are broken down so well that you can. So she did that, and thirty days later called me back, and she'd lost most of that fifty pounds of water weight. She was walking a mile a day. She said, "I just chopped a cord of wood and stacked it all. My whole life is changed, thank you. You gave me my life back". I said "Wow."

Brendan [00:09:56]: I received a lot of those stories on your website, there's so many.

Cherie [00:10:00]: Yes, many, many, exciting, life-changing, life-giving stories. That's what juice is, it gives you life. It is the goodness from the Earth, broken down, predigested I call it, so that your body can take those nutrients right into your cells. It's like an infusion of nutrients going right into the cell, and that's what's changing people's lives. That's why I'm so passionate about juicing, and especially juicing those dark leafy greens that we don't eat enough of.

Brendan [00:10:34]: And juicing, in part, the way it works I believe, is through detox, detoxification. How does juicing help us detox?

Cherie [00:10:45]: Juicing has so many of those phytonutrients, those wonderful little nutrients that bind up free radicals, bind up toxins, carry them out of the body so they don't damage your cells. That is so extremely important that we detox, because we live in such a toxic world. There are toxins in our air, our soil, and our water, and we are bombarded daily with these things. It's in our food, and pesticides and preservatives, and then de-natured food where our nutrients are destroyed. And so, between all of that, we're not getting the nutrients, and we're getting the toxins. I, along with many health professionals, say that any kind of illness, disease, it has two factors: toxins and malnutrition. Not getting enough nutrients that we need. When we start detoxing, getting rid of the toxins, when we start feeding our body pure nutrition, our body begins to heal. It does what it's supposed to do. That's why I believe juicing is extremely important for every single person, it's not just, "Oh if I'm sick" or "I don't feel very well today, I'll go juice". No, it's a lifestyle. I juice every day. I had a big glass of juice this morning, and I made one for my husband, and I've got some extra sitting there, so I can have some more in a little bit. Juicing is powerful to detox and to feed your body super nutrition.

Brendan [00:12:21]: I noticed that you recently did a talk on juicing as a complement to a ketogenic diet. Could you say something about that?

Cherie [00:12:30]: Yes, for cancer, the ketogenic diet is being prescribed by so many doctors right now, and in the holistic field. Not so much the allopathic yet. They're not prescribing anything. "Go eat whatever you want". But in the naturopathic and holistic field, yes, ketogenic is ... there are a lot of studies on the ketogenic diet, which is very high in fat, 80% fat, about 15% protein, and about 5% carbohydrates. I like to change that up because 5% carbohydrates includes their vegetables, and that's too low. We need many more vegetables, and I talked at the Truth about Cancer symposium on this, and showed some of the vegetables, and some of the phytonutrients that actually cut off angiogenesis, and I'm glad we're talking about this because I talked a moment earlier about those blue blood vessels that were attached to that tumor my body expelled. My body expelled it from my colon, so I assume that's where it had been attached. But what cuts that blood supply off and what starts that blood supply first of all. Our body gets stimulated with chemicals, cancer-causing chemicals within the body, stimulates those, they call them tubules, or blood vessels, to go out to the tumors, or to the cancer cells, and feed them. Because they're rogue kinds of cells, they don't have the normal metabolism of the healthy cells. This feeds them, and what cuts off that blood supply are many of the phytochemicals in vegetables, and some fruit as well. Things like celery, and carrots, and watercress and kale are all fabulous, and there are a ton of these phytonutrients like luteolin and apigenin and isothiocyanates. I mean big long words that you have to go take some biochemistry to say, but they are powerhouses, and you can't ignore those. We can't cut those out of our diet, so I modified the ketogenic if somebody wants to that route, which does allow some meat or animal product that would be of course organic and free range, but I upped the carbohydrates. In fact, I don't put a limit on vegetables and vegetable juicing. I advise people to drink at least two quarts of vegetable juice when they have cancer. That goes way back to early studies of the early nineteen hundreds in Europe, where they were doing that. I had thought, where did somebody get this magic two quart thing, but I've had great success working with people with two quarts a day. They're getting better, they're getting well. But I wonder, where did that come from? - Well it came way back in Europe to 1905 when they started working with people with juicing, I didn't even know they had juicers then.

Brendan [00:15:44]: I didn't either.

Cherie [00:15:45]: But I found that, and I presented that to my group—I have a group going, What to Eat and Juice When You Have Cancer—and I presented that old, old research that nobody talks about anymore because we've gone to the cancer drugs, but they were using that with great success way back then. That's why I recommend that if you're going ketogenic, which, I'm all for getting the good fats, like the avocados, and the coconut oil, and the extra virgin olive oil that's organic. Those are excellent. But 80% of that would be a lot of fat, so I cut down on the fat, the protein can stay at about 15% if that's what people choose, if they choose animal protein, but way upped the vegetables. And the way to get them—we couldn't even possibly chew up two quarts worth of juice of the vegetables to make that juice, and who's going to sit down and chew on a kale leaf, or a chard leaf? You probably aren't. How many salads can we eat with those things in it. Juicing is your answer, and besides, so many people that are ill have digestive systems that just aren't processing the food well to get all those wonderful nutrients. So that's why juicing is just very powerful.

Brendan [00:17:07]: You know, I think with juicing sometimes it is often let's say prescribed with a lot of fruits, so I suspect, and that's obviously high sugar, I suspect that if you're trying to complement a ketogenic diet, you would stick with low-carb vegetables, and those are the ones that have the highest nutrient-to-calorie ratio. Kale as the king of nutrient density. Things like that.

Cherie [00:17:37]: Yes.

Brendan [00:17:38]: Is that correct? Would you probably steer that community away from using fruits in their juicing?

Cherie [00:17:46]: I do, and that's one thing that even holistic doctors are saying you can't juice because it's too much sugar.

Brendan [00:17:55]: They get separated from the fiber which slows the sugar down.

Cherie [00:18:00]: That's why, they're thinking about a fruit juice, just like you said, or high sugar vegetables. I am all for getting the sugary fruits out of your diet completely. In fact, in the ketogenic, the only fruits that are recommended would be the berries, and lemon and lime, and unsweetened cranberries would be the fruit. Of that you can choose the lemon and lime and the unsweetened cranberries and even the berries, I recommend that you just eat whole and not juice, or put them in a smoothie, blend them up, but keep the fiber with even the berries. Get the green juices, you are right, and I love all the greens. There is so much new research on watercress. Watercress was something we never even talked about. It was a little garnish on the restaurant plate, and nobody even ate it, they pushed it off to the side. Now watercress is coming, zooming into center stage for cancer research, and they've found amazing results with healing cancer. Watercress got a perfect 100 score when they compared it to all the vegetables of all, you know full complement of nutrients. So here is this little, tiny, leafy watercress—it's a cruciferous vegetable—and I'm telling people, "Juice it. Blend it. Make raw soups with it. Put it in salads. Get a lot of watercress." Get a lot of kale, a lot of chard, celery. Celery, that little celery stick on the hors d'oeuvres plate that people just pass by, or maybe they have one. Celery is a little power house, it is a little work horse in fighting cancer and fighting disease. And carrots, even though carrot is your higher sugar vegetable, there are a lot of studies on carrot juice healing cancer, so I like to dilute it in a variety of ways, either with a lot of greens like, cucumber gives you a lot of water, it's a great thing to use with carrot to dilute that sugar and then add some other greens, of course, in there.

And some ginger ... ginger is a wonderful spice, spicy root to add in. It's anti-inflammatory. If any kind of condition going on in your body, or you just want to prevent heart disease or prevent cancer. I juice ginger every day. It's great if you're starting to catch something like a cold or the flu. Juice up extra ginger. I juice up a lot of things like that. With carrot too, they found in studies that it has more cancer- fighting properties that are utilized when it's combined with fat. So you can add coconut milk, organic coconut milk with your carrot juice. Put in some ginger, a wonderful spice, it absolutely is delicious. I love to add a dash of cinnamon. Cinnamon we haven't thought of except something that goes in pumpkin pie. Cinnamon has wonderful, powerful, healing properties. It lowers blood sugar which is extremely important if you have diabetes. So many things, everything practically we could touch from nature, from the Earth, has something amazing in it for our bodies.

Brendan [00:21:25]: Ginger is phenomenal. I recently learned that it's antiviral, that it helps protect and heal your kidneys. In regard to cinnamon, isn't there a particular type of cinnamon that we should focus on if we're going to be taking...

Cherie [00:21:41]: Yes, I'll keep it simple. It's the more expensive one.

Brendan [00:21:47]: Ceylon cinnamon. You don't save on cinnamon, right?

Cherie [00:21:50]: Yes, and If you go to your health food store, it will be the more expensive one. People always ask me, "Oh, I forget, what is it?" So I always say "Go by price".

Brendan [00:22:02]: Also I want to add though it's C-E-Y-L-O-N.

Cherie [00:22:05]: Yes.

Brendan [00:22:06]: How it's spelled. Is there a difference between juicing and blending, and what are your recommendations for each?

Cherie [00:22:13]: There is a big difference, and that is the primary question I get asked by everybody. What is the difference, they buy a Vitamix or a Ninja for example, those are the two most popular blenders, but they were told that they were getting juicers. The people who sold that to them said, "Oh, no, this is a juicer". Those are blenders because it keeps everything in one container. If you've got it all in one container, all mushed up, that's a blender. If you've got pulp separated from juice, that's a juicer. That's an easy way to distinguish the two. Both are good. There's nothing bad with either one, both are excellent, but they do different things. It got broken down to me very well by one doctor who said the blended, fiber rich, is for your colon, and of course other things, but separate it there, and the juice is cellular. It's like an infusion right into those cells. It's broken down so you're just getting like a direct hit of nutrients into your cells. So do both. I often do both, and today I will do both. I make a big batch of juice, I drink that first thing in the morning, because what do we need when we get up in the morning? We need energy, and that juice is so energizing, it gets down to your cells, it revives those little cells. You've been fasting all night. That's why it's called breakfast, breaking the fast of the night before. You want to put something that's easily digested, easily absorbed into your body, to break that fast. That's how you break a long fast. If you did three, five, or ten day juice fast, you would want to break it with something that is easy on your system and easy to digest, like maybe a smoothie. The juice is even easier to digest, that's why I love the juice first thing in the morning, and then you can have a smoothie after that if you want. What I do, is to pour some juice in my Vitamix, I add an avocado, I add some leafy greens to that, because those blend up very easily, beautifully, and then I add some supplements. Maybe a drop or two of iodines, liquid minerals, I jazz it up a with a little more nutrition, and that's my green smoothie. And then you can put some ground raw nuts on top, or chopped raw nuts. I love that as a little extra protein and some fat. There's so many things that we can do. But I always say, do both. Don't just do one. If you want those green smoothies, at least get some juice in also, each day.

Brendan [00:24:53]: Right. So you're getting the nutrient infusion and you're getting the fiber.

Cherie [00:24:58]: Yes, doing both.

Brendan [00:25:00]: And having more fun. I mean anytime you could put chopped nuts on anything it's a home run.

Cherie [00:25:07]: I'm with you, I love a little crunch.

Brendan [00:25:12]: So what is this souping thing about, this trend?

Cherie [00:25:16]: There's a trend called "souping", and I call it a catch-all name. People didn't know what to call those blended concoctions that they were told was juice —It really isn't juice—to raw soups, to gently warm soups, to the all-day old fashion simmer-away soups. That's what souping is. It's a catch-all name for all of that. And it certainly is a trend because people now with all their Ninjas and their Vitamixes are blending a lot of stuff, and that I call souping, and right up to simmered chicken soup for the soul, chicken soup for the body, old fashioned simmered soups, your lentil and your split pea, and on and on it goes, soups. They're souping.

Brendan [00:26:11]: I was speaking with Dr. Zach Bush about transitioning into a plant-based diet. So what he was saying is that, for some people with a destroyed digestive tract it's important to begin with actually cooked plant fibers as opposed to raw. So in addition to the juicing, perhaps before adding blended raw vegetables, it would make sense to add the soups where the vegetable fibers have been cooked and would be easier on the digestive tract until the microorganisms have developed sufficiently that they're digesting the fibers for you.

Cherie [00:26:53]: Yes, I so agree with that. There are people with such compromised digestive systems, and they aren't doing well with all the raw food. Raw food is powerful, and it's a powerful healer, but you're right, many people have to heal enough to transition to that point where they can take all of that raw fiber. I have a lot of beautiful juices—not juices, soups—for somebody in that category, it's better to have puréed soups. I have a lot of puréed, different, vegan soups. And you can take almost anything and purée it, blend it up, any soup. That's much more digestible. In that category too, if you've got compromised digestion, and you're going plant-based, of course, you don't want the dairy, but people like the creamy soups, so I've got a whole bunch of ideas for people on how to make creamy soups without the cream. From butternut squash to yummy carrot, or spicy carrot soup with the ginger in it, to different types of vegetable soups and watercress soup. I use things like soaked nuts. In my watercress soup I have almond butter. You can have brown rice or quinoa in there that will add a thickness when you blend it, so there's a variety of ways to make your soup creamy without adding any dairy to it.

Brendan [00:28:31]: I would imagine that some really good quality Thai coconut milk or something like that would be amazing.

Cherie [00:28:38]: Oh, yummy. I love coconut milk in anything. So yes, you can make, and it looks like and tastes like you've put dairy in there, like you've got milk, but you don't. And it's so much better for you.

Brendan [00:28:55]: Let me ask you ... why is eating, juicing, blending, souping with organic ingredients so important? I've heard you mention that.

Cherie [00:29:10]: Yes, I'm so adamant about getting organic as much as you possibly can into your diet because it's been proven—they don't want to talk in the news, you won't hear about it in the news—but it's been proven that all of these pesticides do cause diseases, and cancer is right up there at the top of the problems that we face with eating pesticide-sprayed food. People often say to me, "I can't afford organic." A couple of things I want to say about that. First of all, our health is so important. Invest in your health because there's the back end. We don't think about it, but it's running to the drug store for all those medications over the counter even that adds up to often times a lot more money than we would spend on organic produce. Then, what is your health worth? Invest in yourself. I love that one commercial, it's a credit-card commercial, and they say that the price of this is bla-bla-bla and the price of that is bla-bla-bla, and they get to the end and then they've got something spectacular, and they say "priceless". That's you. That's your body. That's your health. It's priceless. And so we want to invest in that; we don't want to one day get some horror diagnosis. For now we've lost everything we've saved for. Many people lose their homes. They lose all their life savings in that effort to get rid of that disease. No, no, we don't want to end up there. We don't want those pesticides. But here's a good rule of thumb, if you say, "I just cannot afford that organic lemon," because those seem to not have come down in price—many things have. There's the dirty dozen and the clean fifteen. Go to ewg.org, and you can get a downloadable app to put right onto your phone so you can look at it when you shop. That's a very practical thing to do. You always want to avoid the dirty dozen. They are the worst sprayed, worst offenders. Apples are always on the list, and strawberries, all the berries are on there, all those thin skinned fruits, the little leafy greens. Just all of those things, absorbing that pesticide right into the structure of that fruit or vegetable, it's in the matrix, it's in the water of that. You cannot wash it off, you can wash maybe a little bit off of the outside, but it's in the water, in the juice of your produce. The clean fifteen on the other hand is way down toward the bottom, and there's very little pesticides sprayed that they found on those. Avocados are on there, and onions always seem to be on that list. Lemons and limes are not too far from the clean fifteen. So I say if you absolutely can't afford organic, take off the peel, and that may be okay for you. But as much as you can afford it, and find it, get organic.

Brendan [00:32:24]: And I'd say that since celery and cucumber are so central to juicing, it'd be important to get those organic, I'm pretty sure those are on the dirty dozen.

Cherie [00:32:36]: Or close to it if they're not. I always look at what's close to it. I go down to twenty or twenty-five, not just the top twelve because they'll list it in the order of the pesticide residue amounts. So there are different types of pesticides that they find on that particular type of produce. But I always get organic cucumbers and organic celery. What is so exciting to me, is that, it's more and more readily available, the organic. And the price is not outlandish like it used to be. I can find organic cucumbers and organic celery almost everywhere I go these days. My local regular supermarket, to Trader Joe's, to once in a while even one of the big box stores will have organic celery or organic cucumbers. Not always. And of course our health food stores, and things like Natural Grocers. Many towns now have a Natural Grocer in them, Whole Foods. It's definitely worth it to scout it out, wherever you are. And here's what I always say, vote with your dollar, because the grocery store wants to sell. They're there to make money, and they want to provide to you what you want. So always ask for the organic, and they'll start ordering it for you. And the more people that buy it, the more the price will come down, nd the more it will be available. We have been, as Americans, voting with our dollar, because I'm seeing more and more organic everywhere I go and the prices being more reasonable, and occasionally I have even seen organic for less money than the conventional.

Brendan [00:34:20]: Really? That's interesting.

Cherie [0:34:22]: Not often. I like to compare.

Brendan [00:34:27]: Another thing about organic food that I don't think gets discussed very often is the fact that—well, some people will dispute this—I mean there's mixed research on whether organic food has higher nutrient levels, and that's largely, I believe, due to the fact that many organic growers are not necessarily doing the fully organic thing and building soil. That was originally part of the definition of organic, you're building the organic matter of the soil, and when you're doing that, by definition, you're doing that by enhancing the microbial life in the soil, and it's the microbes in the soil, beneficial microbes that make the minerals and so forth available to the plants. Helps minerals to create phytonutrients, and that's the medicine in the food. And my experience, pretty much across the board, almost all the time, is that organic produce tastes better to me. Sometimes I do side-by-side comparisons for the heck of it, and especially, well, just certain foods that I do, where the pesticide content is not going to be as bad because it's maybe close to the clean fifteen or it's on the clean fifteen. But I also want to make sure that I'm getting good nutrient content. And the only way that we have right now to gage that is taste and smell, and a few other things as well, but that's for another conversation.

So I think that's one thing to consider as well. If we're trying to heal ourselves, if we're trying to be our best and reach our full potential on a day-to-day basis, we've got to have the nutrients coming in, and so that's another reason organics come in. I'm imagining, and I want all of us to imagine, a food system that entirely eliminates farm toxins, restores high nutrient levels to food, all food, and heals the planet, and it does that by rebuilding soils, and that's what some of the other speakers in this event are talking about, and it's often referred to as regenerative agriculture, and it's very exciting when you start to learn just enough about how soil works to go, "Wow, this is really Nature's magic right here." And this is the true, big time, all-around solution to so many issues, starting with our own health but also all the way through the planetary system, the water cycles, the carbon-cycles, and re-establishing balance in our atmosphere and in our water supplies and so forth. And soon there's going to be labels specifying whether foods were grown in ways that regenerate life or degenerate it. And so that will be amazing and will give us a chance to transform our health, the food system, and the planet every time that we buy food.

Cherie [00:37:27]: Yes, I would love to see that. It should be a new label. "Look for this."

Brendan [00:37:34]: There's some of them coming out, and I don't have the names for them yet, other than one. One is called Land to Market, and that's specifically for, at least I believe, it's specifically and exclusively related to animal products that are grown in ways, basically raised pastured, because as you know animal agriculture is one of the worst influences on the planet when it's industrialized the way we have industrialized it. But there is a way to raise those animals that actually helps restore the planet. This brings up initially a question for you, personally. What is your long term health maintenance? Are you a vegan now or was the vegan juicing diet and so forth a temporary healing diet, but are probably largely plant-based still? I'm just curious if you're vegan or not.

Cherie [00:38:31]: I'm not a strict vegan, but I have a lot of days that are vegan. I have a large plant- based diet. My husband and I have gone on, we call it our salad kick. We're having main course salads for lunch and dinner, and then the juice and smoothie for breakfast. And it's been very energizing, and I feel enlivened, I guess I would say. And I'm noticing the change in my skin getting all those vegetables constantly. So both my husband and I have found that we do well if we get a little bit of pasture-raised, organic fed, animal protein here and there, so we're doing that. That's my lifestyle these days, and it's the best one that I have found, to eat that way. So occasionally we have an egg that's pastured and organic grown. I have a friend who has lots of chickens on her place, and hers were the best because they're just fresh. So that's my lifestyle, and I would encourage that kind of lifestyle for everybody really, unless you're ill, and you've got to do something different, more aggressive in your diet.

Brendan [00:39:57]: I find the same thing, that I thrive with just some pasture-raised animal products, and I've been able to reduce the amount that I've been eating over time, that's been going down, and down, and down. I've been doing that via some methods, nutritional methods, metabolic modulation as I sometimes call it, that I talk about at other points during this event. I won't get into it right here, but it's been a life saver for me and I think it will help other people thrive on less animal protein, because most of us that are meat eaters, we eat way too much, but there's a way to change that, and thrive on less, and truly want less. I actually want less, far less. It's astonishing.

Cherie [00:40:52]: Same here.

Brendan [00:40:53]: Yeah, okay. You know the nutrients in our food and the toxins that we're exposed to and the detoxification are even more important than we usually consider, and that's because our own personal nutrition strongly affects our unborn children, if we're going to have any. And when I learned a little bit about your story I saw that you believe that your health issues started before you were born. I'm curious, I don't know that part of the story as far as what you believe might've happened. Could you say more about that?

Cherie [00:41:28]: Yes, I'm glad you asked. My mother had cancer when I was very young and she died when I was six years old. They say that cancer has been growing in a body for quite a few years probably before the diagnosis comes. She was diagnosed when I was four years old, so I believe that she had cancer before I was born even. I believe that that greatly affected me in some ways. With a weaker immune system, I've always had to work hard at staying healthy. Now that I've learned to treat my body in the way it needs, I don't feel like I'm working hard at it. I feel like I've hit a stride, and it's doing what it's supposed to do. But my mother, I looked at her diet based on what relatives could tell me, like my grandmother and my aunts, and her diet was terrible. Her diet was the same as my diet, only she didn't have all the junk food options back then, but she loved sweets. I did too. She did not like vegetables, didn't eat vegetables, and liked to exist on baked goods.

My grandmother was a wonderful baker, made homemade bread and cinnamon rolls, and cookies, and all sorts of wonderful desserts, and my mother loved that and did not eat right at all. And I was following directly in her footsteps, so that leads me to, is it genes, or is it lifestyle? I don't know. That's a big tossup. We would have quite an argument going probably depending on who we had on with us. But for me, I say it was my lifestyle because all through these years doctors have told me, "Well you're probably going to get cancer like your mother did" and I keep saying, "No, I'm not going to get cancer like my mother did, because I'm doing something very different with my lifestyle than she did".

Brendan [00:43:47]: Yeah lifestyle trumps genes, hands down. That's what we're discovering with epigenetics. Our genes express themselves according to the environment we put them in, and it turns out that we actually inherit two things from our mothers, so your intuition that you got possibly something happening across a generation from your mother. Well, basically we inherit all of our mitochondria from our mothers because the mitochondria in the sperm cell are in the tail which falls off when the sperm and the egg join at conception. So all of our mitochondria come from our mother, and mitochondria can be in good health or not in good health, and they can degenerate and also regenerate. It's possible that you might've received some weakened mitochondria in that egg.

Cherie [00:44:49]: I'm sure.

Brendan [00:44:52]: So your children can start with an inheritance of weak mitochondria. That's what I have picked up somewhere. I can't cite a study. It might've been from a book, from a credible source recently. They all start to merge together. Fortunately, mitochondria can be repaired if the damaging influences are removed and healing influences are produced, and I believe one of the sources would be the bio-photons from ... could you say more about bio-photons that we get from fruits and vegetables, and do we only get them from raw or do we also get them from cooked?

Cherie [00:45:35]: We only get bio-photons from raw. There is a lot of research now on photons, it's been going on for several decades. It started in Germany. and they have looked at and photographed actually, raw vegetables, raw fruit, and seen beautiful light rays of energy. It's called Kirlian photography. I don't know if they used that particular photography with the bio-photon research, but that's what it is. There are those light rays of energy emanating from the plant that indicates that you've got the photons there. The plant absorbs the photons from the sun, and that is the energy that's going into that plant. And when you cook it, you destroy it. So all cooked foods do not have bio-photons, and maybe with lightly steaming you might have a tiny bit left, but when you really cook it you've got none left at all. And they've photographed the raw vs. the cooked, and the cooked is like dead. It has no life coming from it, and the raw has light. Those photons are so important for your mitochondria. In the research they've looked at that, and the photons, the bio-photons, feed the mitochondria. So I really believe that my mitochondria has regenerated because of all the raw that I do, all of the juicing, and the salads, and the smoothies, and the raw foods recipes that I make. It's been life-giving. Why do we need that? So many people are dragging around tired telling me, "I'm so fatigued, and so exhausted".

Well, bio-photons feed your mitochondria. Your mitochondria makes ATP or energy fuel. If you're not making much energy fuel, of course you'll be tired, absolutely. You'll be fatigued and dragging around. When you start getting this raw food, raw juices, live foods into your diet, and wow, your little cells come alive. And I liken it to seeing a plant ... you've got a beautiful plant in back of you ... what if it was all wilted and kind of limp, and lying on its side, and then you pour some water on it, beautiful, life-giving water. And then the next morning you see it's back up. It's got, I call it the hands raised to the sun. It's come to life. Your cells are like that. What's going to bring your cells to life? It's the raw foods. And of course, you start with the juices because they're so well broken down that it's going to get right into your cells, and you're going to get those wonderful, energizing, mitochondria-healing nutrients, bio-photons.

Brendan [00:48:22]: I think that there's another inheritance that we get from our mothers, I'm not a hundred percent sure in this, but we get telomeres either mostly through our mothers, or entirely. [**Correction:** Each of the chromosomes we inherit from our parents have telomeres. Telomere length is likely influenced by both the mother and father.] And telomeres of the of the end caps are in our DNA chromosomes that protect genes each time our cells divide, and there's a strong connection between the length of the telomeres and how long we live, as well as how healthy we live. And telomere length is heavily influenced by toxins and nutrition and damaged by toxins, basically. Damaged by toxins, fortified by nutrition. So by applying abundant nutrition with juicing and souping, that may lengthen telomeres, I say may, but it does, I'm sure, and at least slow the shortening of telomeres and thereby increase lifespan and health span, so pretty exciting stuff. And that might be an additional explanation as to why you experienced possibly some influence from your mother's lifestyle in your own. So, we all need to learn more about this, and the research is going to be pretty amazing I think over the next few years about this. So that we can kind of see, you know what, it's not just our own health, you've got to take responsibility if you're going to have children, for their health, with what we eat today.

Cherie [00:49:48]: Absolutely, and I tell every mom who wants to have a baby, wants to get pregnant—this is a thing you do. You start this before. And you start it as soon as you possibly can, detoxing, and feeding at the cellular level because this is going to be your answer for having a healthy baby. It starts with your healthy cells.

Brandan [00:50:14]: Cherie, are there any other recommendations, and even if it summarizes what you have already said, what are your top three recommendations for achieving optimal health and even miraculous healing?

Cherie [00:50:27]: I haven't talked yet about acidosis and the acidity of many people's bodies. Juicing, and of course our souping, and our green smoothies, are made with a produce that is alkaline, and helps to bring balance to the body. But most of the American diet is around acid-forming foods I call it. They're not acid in your mouth, or in a test tube, but they're acidic in the final breakdown in your body, and they measure that by the minerals left in the final ash of metabolism. If you're eating a diet, and here's the acidic foods, and it shocks people: meat, dairy, grains, sweets. Any kind of sugars. Coffee is very acidic, black tea, and soda pop, junk food, fast food. All of that is going to be extremely acidic. Sports drinks and energy bars with all the sweeteners in them. All of this is acidic. I've named the American diet, breakfast, lunch and dinner. I would say, "What's killing us?" I have a slide when I do a lot of presentations, "Do you know what's really killing Americans? Breakfast, lunch, and dinner" because we're eating this stuff three times a day at least. So what we need to do is bring an alkaline balance to our bodies. Why do we want to do that? For so many reasons. To prevent disease. Cancer cells thrive in an acidic environment—they do not like an alkaline-balanced environment—they thrive there. An acidic environment is very bad for our muscles. My husband has discovered this with back pain and all the acidity in his diet because he loved a lot of meat. That's why we've gone way away from that and into salads because that's your healing hope. If you've got back pain, if those muscles are like shoe leather, tight as a drum, if you've got pain throughout your body, you've probably got too much acid, and you need to alkalize your body, bring alkaline balance. That's one thing that I talk about a lot. Get those alkaline rich foods, and they aren't very many. It's vegetables, fruits, sprouts, seeds and nuts primarily, maybe some of the beans but, primarily it's your produce that's going to bring alkaline balance. And get more raw in your diet. Most people do not have enough raw food, and if you can't eat raw food, of course juice is your answer because if you've got a very compromised digestive tract, which many people do today, having grown up on all of the gluten and the sweets, and the preserved foods, and it's just been very damaging to the digestive tract. Bring healing back and bring the nutrients in through juicing. Get high nutrient-dense produce as much as possible, just like you mentioned. If you know local growers that do compost, and you can meet them at farmers markets in the summer and find out who they are. That's where you want to go. In my town it's Saturday morning, and that's where you want to go to get your produce, at least in the summer. Get as much nutrient density as possible and eat a variety of colors. Isn't that what so many people are saying now. Look for all the different colors. We get stuck in a rut, right? We think, "Oh, these are my favorites, and I'm just going to have these all the time", but we need a variety and so get as many different-colored, beautiful, brightly-colored vegetables into your diet. Try some new things. If there are things you say, "I don't like that at all" well, tuck a little bit of that into a nice juice blend.

And how do you make a nice juice blend? I didn't cover this either. Since I don't use apple—some people do say they have to have some apple to make it taste good—it's just a little too much sugar for me, but carrot apple makes a great base which you can tuck anything just about in, and it's going to taste good. But if you can't have apple ... which I don't seem to do well on any kind of fruit juice, except lemon, I do carrot-lemon base and to that I add cucumber, and celery, and dark leafy greens. I've got some chard, some great big giant chard leaves right now. They look like fans. I add some chard. I get fresh turmeric. That's a wonderful way to get that anti-inflammatory spice into your diet. Or if you can't find fresh, you can stir some into your juice. I juice big chunks of ginger root every day. Ginger is an excellent anti-inflammatory. So get those anti-inflammatories into your diet as well. This is what's going to prevent disease, keep you healthy, keep you strong, help you sleep well at night, help you wake up in the morning feeling good. I'm all about feeling good and having that energy to make it through the day. Those are my top three.

Brendan [00:55:49]: Awesome, thank you. Every day we have the opportunity to build health for ourselves, and I'm saying for the Earth as well, with the new regenerative agriculture. It's been around for a long time, but I say new because we're going to actually see more and more of it. We're going to have the opportunity to ask for it, to see labels, and I encourage everybody to learn about soils, so we learn what questions to ask. It's a really fascinating conversation, really, when you start to geek out just a little bit on soil. Thank you so much Cherie, you're a courageous and dedicated soul. Courageous for continuing to put one foot in front of the other until finally healing on all levels. I know personally how hard that is, I'm still in process. And dedicated to bringing healing through clean, whole foods, to the entire planet. Thank you for your travels and all your books and articles, and your global leadership and contributions. Thank you from me, and the Eat4Earth community for being here today.

Cherie [00:57:00]: Well, thank you, thank you so much. I send it back to you, thank you for what you're doing and making us so aware of our soil, our wonderful soil that is so important and has lost so much through the years or agriculture, commercial agriculture. So, bravo to you and the Eat4Earth community. Thank you for inviting me on your program today.

Brendan [00:57:24]: Cherie just gave us some very important and inspiring information. Plants are so powerful, and I love that she brought up souping because for certain vegetables and certain people, souping is a delightful way to get a lot of vegetable into your body, especially the ones that are more suited to souping than juicing. And of course you can add spices more readily to soups which brings in that whole world of plant nutrients and medicine. Today Cherie and Véronique mentioned mitochondria in conjunction with cancer. Tomorrow we're going to be hearing from speakers that will show you how to support your mitochondria with a ketogenic, fat-burning diet.

Ty Bollinger Interview

Definition of a Carcinogen, Starving a Cancer, Emotions and Cancer Risk

Brendan [00:00]: Welcome back to the Eat4Earth event. We're exploring how you can heal your body, your loved ones, and the Earth with food. And today I'm speaking to somebody that many of you probably know well. Ty Bollinger. Ty is a health freedom advocate, cancer researcher, documentary filmmaker, radio show host, author, former competitive bodybuilder, and all-around great dad and father. After losing several family members to cancer, he refused to accept the notion that chemotherapy, radiation, and surgery were the only effective treatments available for cancer patients. So he began a quest to learn all he possibly could about alternative cancer therapy and treatments, and the medical industry itself, and what he discovered was shocking. And I can tell you from what I've learned from *The Truth about Cancer*, I was shocked. I learned a lot. So we're going to dive into some of that, and it's great to have you here with us today, Ty.

Ty [00:59]: Yeah, thank you Brian, I appreciate it. Looking forward to the conversation today.

Brendan [01:02]: Awesome. So, you know, with all the research that you've done, and all the cancer survivors that you've talked to, and the cancer experts, what are some of the lessons and discoveries and, you know, let's say, even unexpected things that you've come across in your search?

Ty [01:23]: You know, there's probably a couple of things that stick out to me. Number one, you know, we got into this, my wife Charlene and I, back in 1996 when my father was diagnosed with cancer and died in 25 days. I'm 50 years old as I stand before you today. My Dad was 52 when this happened to him. Way too young, right? He was dead in 25 days. We began to research cancer and nutrition and "alternative" treatments, and we began to learn there's a lot of effective treatments out there that we didn't know about and that doctors don't even know about. So, I think one of the main things that stuck out to me, and it shocked me over the years, is just how natural cancer treatments, how to be healthy ... this knowledge that should be available to everybody ... it's been suppressed. People just don't know. They don't know how to treat cancer. They don't know how to be healthy. So, that's one thing that stuck out to me.

Another thing that's really stuck out to me over the years is just the importance of nutrition. As basic as it seems, as mundane as it seems, it's like, "Yeah, well, duh! Of course nutrition matters." It's shocking to me, Brendan, how many medical doctors will tell you that nutrition does not matter. It blows my mind.
You have somebody that's sick ... let's just take this scenario: you have a cancer patient that's sick, their immune system has been compromised, and they go in for chemotherapy which further sickens them, further destroys their immune system, and they ask the doctor, "What should I do as far as my diet's concerned? Should I change my diet at all?" And the oncologists will tell them, "It does not matter what you eat. It will not affect your body. It won't affect your cancer. It won't affect your health". That is insane! And it just blows me away that this is protocol nowadays. Dozens, hundreds, maybe thousands of cancer patients over the last fifteen years that I've spoken to or emailed, have told me the same story. Literally, probably in the upper

hundreds. "I went in to get a CAT scan or a PET scan or an MRI. I was diagnosed with cancer, I treated the cancer, and I asked the doctor, "What should I do differently in my diet?" And they said, "Doesn't matter." Wow! I just can't imagine. I mean, can you imagine if you went in to take your car in to the mechanic's, and it wasn't running well ... which is really what's happening to our bodies when we get sick. They're not running properly ... and the mechanic would tell you that it doesn't really matter what you put in the fuel tank, that you can put alcohol or Kool-Aid or, you know, just oil. You can put oil in the gas tank. It won't really matter. It won't really affect your engine. It won't affect the way that your car runs. You would fire that mechanic in a heartbeat and go find somebody that knew what they were talking about, right?

Brendan [04:13]: Right.

Ty [04:14]: Isn't that what oncologists are telling you? "The fuel for your body doesn't matter. It won't affect the way it runs." That is asinine. That is the most absurd thing I've ever heard. And that's some of the lack of education, the disinformation that we fight against, to educate people that food matters. Nutrition matters. The way that you regain your health is you provide your body with the fuel that it needs so that it runs properly.

Brendan [04:35]: Right. Now, let's unpack that. Let's, like, dive in a little bit. There's a number of different anticancer diets and different ideas about what's the best way to prevent cancer with diet. What have you seen? Like, what are the main commonalities that have come up?

Ty [04:54]: The best preventative diets are diets that are as close to Nature as possible. As close to pesticide-free as possible. Stay away from genetically-modified ingredients. So, you might say, "Okay, that's pretty easy." Well, is it, really? If you're eating the modern diet that's packaged, canned, processed foods that never deteriorate. They never rot. They have a shelf life of twenty, thirty, fifty, a hundred years. Is that really a healthy diet? And the reality is ... it's not. We're not eating close to Nature. I did an interview with Dr. Mercola for *The Global Quest*, the documentary that we released a couple of years ago, and he said the key to health is three words: Eat real food. So, if we would eat real food then our bodies would be able to assimilate it and be healthy from it. The problem is we're not eating real food anymore. Corn, soy, canola, and a whole host of other fruits and vegetables have been genetically modified. We know that GMO corn causes cancer. The *Séralini* study proved that. Monsanto says it doesn't. They're lying. We've read through the studies. It does cause cancer. Pesticides like glyphosate, herbicides ... they cause cancer. World Health Organization admits that they cause cancer, but we still spray it on our crops. We still spray it in our yards, okay? So, that's not natural. That's not what we had a hundred years ago. We weren't exposed to these toxins a hundred years ago.

A hundred years ago, the rates of cancer were one-in-eighty, now they're one-in-two men and one-in-three women. Why have the rates gone up so much? Because their diets have changed. A hundred years ago you couldn't go into the grocery store and buy canned, boxed, packaged stuff that lasts forever. You had to pick it, eat it close to Nature, and whether you're eating vegetables or fruits or roots or meats, eggs, whatever it is ... they grew it. If it was an animal, they slaughtered it, they cooked it there on their property, and ate it. My grandparents are a prime example. My granddaddy was a rancher in west Texas. He had cattle. He had hogs. He grew his own garden. My grandma made their own bread every day. He cooked, you know, they ate fresh eggs and bacon every morning from their pigs. They ate fresh vegetables and potatoes that they grew on their farm and they both lived into their eighties. They lived a long life. Why? Well, because they ate real food. I don't advocate any particular diet. I think that that tends to divide those of us that are into trying to be more healthy.

Brendan [07:31]: Amen to that, by the way. One of my soapboxes is—can we please stop arguing about the best, most healthiest diet? Maybe there's bio-individuality.

Ty [07:43]: Exactly, Brendan! And I agree completely. Certain diets work for some people, and they don't work for others. Some people are going Keto, some people are going vegan, some people are going vegetarian, some people are going Paleo ... I don't care what you go! Just eat as close to Nature as you possibly can. Stay away from GMOs, stay away from pesticides, and eat as close to Nature as you can, you know? The natural state of food, whether it's roots, vegetables, herbs, seeds, grains, spices, meats, animals, eggs ... whatever it is, is as close to Nature as possible, and you're going to be a lot healthier than if you're going to a fast food restaurant three times a day or going through the packaged isles of your grocery store and eating a bunch of processed crap. You're just going to be healthier. So I agree, let's all band together. Let's all get along because we're all fighting the same enemy, and that enemy is really a lack of education about how to be healthy. And that enemy, that lack of education, is being perpetuated by Big Agra, Big Food, the pharmaceutical industry ... that don't want you to know that your food matters.

Brendan [08:48]: You know, one thing that I've learned from reading, or actually listening, to *The Truth About Cancer* audio book ... one of the things that really stood out for me that has kind of been coming to the forefront ... and this is really obvious, like, this should be really obvious ... we are creatures that live on oxygen, right? And then there's the whole other half of the world that we need badly, which lives on carbon dioxide, and we trade back and forth. So, there's the plant world and the animal world. I didn't realize ... this sounds so simple ... but I didn't realize what you revealed there is that Otto Warburg defines a carcinogen as "a chemical that inhibits the availability of oxygen to the body".

Ty [09:30]: Yep. It's fascinating.

Brendan [09:31]: Yeah! And, so, when you look at it, that's what a carcinogen is. It's all these chemicals that are just interfering with oxygen metabolism in various ways. They're deranging different enzymes, hormones, whatever it is. And I recently listened to Catherine Shanahan's audio book version of *Deep Nutrition*. She makes a really good case for how processed vegetable seed oils are also a big part of this whole disease epidemic, cancer and all the diseases, and I think there's a connection. I'm curious if you've heard anybody talk about any kind of connection between the way that processed vegetable seed oils might interfere with oxygen metabolism. They certainly interfere with various things.

Ty [10:18]: I'm not familiar with the way that the processed seed oils are, but I know that the hydrogenated oils ... the trans fats that we're all familiar with ... they do inhibit ... they damage the cell wall and inhibit oxygen absorption. That's one of the things that Dr. Johanna Budwig, who is the founder of the Budwig Diet ... she realized that. She found a way to get around it through better oxygen deliveries through flax oil and cottage cheese, which allowed the oxygen to be delivered to the cells.

Brendan [10:46]: Oh, is that what that does.

Ty [10:50]: One of the things that you mentioned, though, with Dr. Otto Warburg ... He was a Nobel Prize winner in 1931 or 1932, I believe, and he did a lot of work on the mitochondria, and he did a lot of work on oxygen and, you're right, one of the things that you realize is that cancer cells do not do well when there's oxygen available. They only exist, *typically* they exist—not *only,* there are exceptions—but they *typically* exist in environments that are anaerobic, which means there's a lack of oxygen. As a matter of fact, the primary way that all cancer cells produce energy is through fermentation, and fermentation only occurs when there's a lack of oxygen. And, so then, the cells resort to fermenting sugar in order to produce energy. It's a very inefficient burn. It's a very inefficient way to produce energy but that's the way cancer cells produce energy. Through fermentation. And that only happens when there's a lack of oxygen.
So, we have certain types of treatments, like hyperbaric oxygen chambers, that deliver oxygen to the cells, and they've been very effective at reversing cancer. That's why it's so important that if you are sick with cancer or if you want to prevent cancer, make sure you exercise, and you get enough oxygen in your body as best you can. You don't want to be stagnant. That's another reason why it's so important that if you have cancer, that you want to move. You want this up and down motion, like jumping up and down on a rebounder is so good for you because it pumps the lymphatic system which removes toxic debris from your body. All these things are interconnected, Brendan, as you can see. Oxygen in the cells, movement, detoxification, healthy food, healthy soil ... They're all interrelated.

Brendan [12:30]: You know, one of the other things that came up, too, in your book, that really surprised me, and it ties in with all of this—actually, let me ask this a different way. Let me see if it comes out. What else was surprising to you or just sort of mind-blowing? Anything in particular?

Ty [12:47]: You mean along my cancer research journey?

Brendan [12:50]: Yeah, what else jumped out?

Ty [12:52]: One of the things that really blew me away was the fact that, you know, if you talk about there being a suppression of cancer treatments, if you talk about there being this "conspiracy," right? To suppress health and certain professions like chiropractic ... You know, I've heard about a conspiracy to suppress chiropractic. I always thought that was kind of nutty.

Brendan [13:14]: Yeah, every time I hear of "conspiracy" or "suppression", I'm like, really? I mean, is it really just that? And then like, "Yeah, it was!"

Ty [13:21]: Yeah. That's what blew me away because I'd always been ... I'd grown up a child of the seventies, watching TV, believing everything that we were told on television. You know, the government wouldn't lie to us. And then we'd find ... I began to do research ... found out that there's a report that's in the appendix to the Congressional Record of 1953 called, "The Fitzgerald Report". Benedict Fitzgerald was an investigator for the Interstate Commerce Committee, and he was tasked with determining if there was a suppression of cancer treatments, natural cancer treatments, in the United States at that time. His determination was that there was a "conspiracy of vast proportions to suppress natural cancer treatments" at that time. This isn't the ... this is a Senate investigatory committee. It's in the Congressional Record of 1953. You can read it. They determined there was a conspiracy!

We fast forward to 1987. Judge Susan Getzendanner was the judge at a court case, *Wilk vs. AMA*. Chester Wilk was a chiropractor. He sued the AMA. He sued them with the accusation that they were suppressing chiropractic treatments. That they were actively lying about chiropractic in order to make chiropractors look like quacks. Judge Getzendanner, in 1987, ruled that there was a "conspiracy by the AMA to suppress chiropractic." So, we're talking about a Superior Court judge. We're talking about the United States Senate. They've both used the term "conspiracy" to describe what's going on today with healthcare, with cancer treatment, with chiropractic. So, it's not a conspiracy theory anymore, Brendan. It's a conspiracy fact. There actually is ... there are conspiracies to suppress these treatments. And why would there be conspiracies? Because there's much more money to be made in treating than in healing or curing.

Brendan [15:18]: And it can be so, so, so simple, actually. And so this is where my soapbox comes in, which is we just have to simplify our food system and get it back to Nature in the sense of using ecological principles. It doesn't mean we go back to Nature as far as, like, we abandon all of our technology. It's nothing like that. In fact, we can combine the two, as long as we're not meddling too much where we're combining, we're trying to turn genetics into a technology. That's where I think we get into a serious danger zone, as we know.

But, one of the other things that really jumped out at me from the book was the fact that there was a population in the Chernobyl area that did not get cancer. Three million people got cancer and then there's, like, three thousand that were kind of untouched and it was something ... it was the water! They were getting highly hydrated by drinking Caucasus mountain water that has special properties. And in another place in the book you mentioned that when we're dehydrated, detoxification shuts down. I think one of the big challenges that we're facing is that we're assaulted with so much toxicity. We have stress in our lives. All of these things stress the kidneys, require the kidneys to work harder, require more water, so we, literally... I think humans have to drink more water than *ever* in history to keep apace with that. I'm just curious what you have might have to say about all that.

Ty [16:51]: Yeah, that's a great topic, Brendan. You were talking about the interview that I did with Dr. Igor Smirnov. Dr. Smirnov was actually on the Russian scientific team that investigated Chernobyl. He's a Russian, he's from Moscow, and he was there when it happened. And he was tasked with determining why there were certain populations of people that were exposed to the same radiation from Chernobyl, but they didn't get cancer. And they found that the difference was they were drinking this water that was from the Caucasus mountains. It was exposed to certain frequencies, certain natural vibrations, I guess you would think of it. It's actually called the Schumann resonance. It's the natural frequency of the Earth that they were exposed to that changed the structure of the water, and it caused the people that drank the water ... it caused their bodies to protect themselves against the radiation exposure. It, basically, made their bodies unaware that they were being exposed to the radiation because of the frequency of this water. We could kind of equate it to ... if you take a dog whistle, and you blow it as loud as you can right here in this room with me, I wouldn't hear it. It would not affect my hearing. It would never hurt me. But, if our German shepherd was next to me and you blew the dog whistle for a period of time ... I've read, upwards of 24 hours ... if you did it straight, you would literally drive the dog mad. And the dog would hear it. It would affect the dog, and it could give the dog disease because the dog hears the sound. It's the same principle with radiation. The water actually made the people to where they didn't know there was radiation. Their cells ... the radiation was invisible to their cells, and it didn't hurt them. So that's really the principle. So, I do agree with you. A lot of times sickness results from dehydration. So we need to ... if you don't have access to this Caucasus mountain water, it's okay. Drink more water. Drink more clean water, drink more filtered water, whatever kind of water you want to drink. I refuse to get into the great water debate over which water you should be drinking. I think you should drink clean water.

Brendan [18:54]: It's kinda like the great diet debate, right?

Ty [18:57]: Yeah, it's like, drink more clean water. Drink the cleanest water that you have. And, you know, I hear people say, "Well, if you can't get alkaline water with a Ph of 8.9, you shouldn't be drinking it." I'm like, "Are you insane?" Of course, drink whatever water you can get. Just stay away from the sodas. Stay away from the sugary pop drinks. Stay away from all the stuff that has loaded chemicals and drink as clean a water as you can, and you'll be better off. There was a medical doctor in Iran that was thrown in jail. His name was Batmanghelidj. They called him "Dr. Batman" and he treated thousands of prisoners that were ...

Brendan [19:28]: He was thrown in jail? I didn't know that. I'm sorry for interrupting! You're talking about the author of *Your Body's Many Cries for Water*?

Ty [19:36]: Dr. Batman, yeah. Batmanghelidj. Yeah. So, he wrote the book, *Your Body's Many Cries for Water*. He was, literally, thrown in prison in Iran, and he treated, literally, hundreds of cases of sickness. Maybe thousands of cases. I'd have to go back and read the book. I've got the book here, but it's been a long time since I read it. But he treated hundreds of prisoners that were chronically ill, and he got them better by doing only one thing. He got them to drink more water. And his theory was that you're not really sick, you're dehydrated. And because you're dehydrated, your body can't detoxify. And if you'll just drink more water, your chronic illness will go away. And he literally turned around chronic illness in hundreds of patients in prison. And it wasn't even with clean water. It was with dirty water that was all they had access to in prison. But he still got them better by drinking dirty water because they were hydrating their bodies. Our bodies are 80 to 90 percent water. If you're not drinking enough water, your body's not gonna function properly. So, that was his mantra, "You're not sick. You're just thirsty. You're dehydrated."

Brendan [20:37]: Yeah, that book blew me away. He talks about how when people get dehydrated, their capillaries kind of shut down to conserve the fluid mass in the most important organs ... the brain, the liver, and so forth. So, the muscle tissues and the various peripheral parts of the body get less hydration. And the mechanism used by the body to do that, according to him is histamine.

Ty [21:02]: Histamine, yeah.

Brendan [21:03]: So, dehydration is actually inflammatory according to him. So, when you hydrate, you actually ... oh, and another thing he says is you should go for walks. Drink a lot, and then walk because you've got to get your heart pumping ... push the fluid ... push your body's fluids back into those capillaries. Push them back open so you hydrate your tissues. Otherwise, the water may just keep kind of circulating through your major organs, and so forth, but not re-hydrate the ones that have been a little shut down in your dehydration.

Ty [21:31]: Yeah. Also ... and I don't know that this was Dr. Batman's position ... but this is actually another reason that you should walk and have the motion is because walking, moving up and down ... my favorite exercise is jumping on a mini trampoline. That stimulates the lymphatic flow. So, you don't have to do anything to get your blood to pump. Your heart does that. And if it didn't, you'd die.

Your lymphatic fluid is just as important as your blood, but there's no pump to your lymphatic system. The lymph carries nutrients to the cells. It also detoxifies. It helps to detoxify the cells, and it carries the toxins away. If you're not moving, if you're not going up and down, if you're not walking, if you're just stagnant, the lymph doesn't pump. It doesn't flow. And that's another reason so many people are sick, is they're not moving. Because the lymphatic system is very important in overall health. But, if you're not making an effort to pump that lymph on your own, it doesn't get pumped. Unlike the heart, which pumps the blood, you've got to do some movement each day to pump the lymph.

Brendan [22:34]: Yeah. I want to go back to food for a second, too, since that's my big soapbox. I've been hearing, here and there, that a lot of plant-based diets are involved with healing cancer because they're ... actually this ties into hydration, I think. A big part of the reason I've heard other people postulate this is, if you're juicing 25 pounds of fruits and vegetables a day, you're getting hydrating water. I mean, the phytonutrients are super important, of course, but there's something to that water, as well as coming in with those. So that could be a big part of that picture. But, what I've also heard is that diets like the Gerson diet are actually observed to be less effective than they were, let's say, in the seventies and the sixties and so forth, and some people have postulated that that's because the nutrient content is way down. So, you're getting all this great real food but the nutrient content is down and that that's related to soil health. And I'm just curious, did you have any experts talk at all about soil health?

Ty [23:40]: You know, peripherally, I probably did. I don't remember any Earth-shattering conversations I had about soil health, but you're absolutely right, though. It's not postulation or theory now. It's clear; it's fact that the foods aren't as nutritious as they used to be. And the reason is that the soil has been depleted ... the micronutrients, the microbes in the soil, all the things that contribute to healthy soil ... the soil has been depleted by, you know, farming the way that the modern farmers farm. I mean, you know, you do the same crop year after year. You don't rotate, you don't give rest to the soil ... it's just over and over and over. The soil's depleted. It's totally different than the way that we used to farm. We'd rotate crops. We'd give certain lands time to recuperate and replenish, and you'd go farm other parts. And it's a rotation system, and the crops were rotated. Even the animals on the land were rotated. The cows went from pasture to pasture.

The chickens would follow them. You'd have different types of microbes in the dung from the cows, then the chicken. And, so, you're totally replenishing the nutrients in the soil year after year. After you rotate the crops, you rotate the animals. That doesn't happen anymore. And, so, as a result, you can have all these healthy fruits and vegetables that you're eating. But the nutrient profile is not as good because they were grown in soil that was depleted.

Brendan [25:00]: Yeah. And I've been hearing from the folks at Kiss the Ground ... Kiss the Ground is an organization that's trying to get our attention back on soil through regenerative agriculture ... and they're in touch with a fair number of organic farmers. Even organic farmers are saying, "My produce is smaller." This and that ... So, there's something that's been missing across the board, organic and conventional agriculture. Obviously, conventional has the disadvantage for the soil of all these chemicals that kill soil organisms and so forth, but also in organic, they're doing too much tilling. So, that's where organic can go more regenerative is stop tilling. They actually till more, meaning plowing, because they're not able to use the herbicides. So, then, they control weeds more with tilling. But the way to control weeds, and I won't get too far into this is, is simply to have healthier, more robust biodiversity in the soil and the plants above. Stop monocropping. It's when we monocrop that we have those problems.

So, along those lines, as far as soil health, one of the things that comes up in that ... I mean, when I talk to various doctors and so forth, especially Dr. Bush ... He's amazing! Dr. Zach Bush. He's going as far as saying things like the microbes in our soil may actually be ultimately responsible for the phytonutrients in our vegetables. And they're certainly responsible—we've known this for decades—they're responsible for the minerals being able to get liberated from the parent materials in the soil—the sand, silt, and clay—into the vegetables themselves. Otherwise, vegetables are just passive recipients of whatever minerals are in the ... what's called the transpiration stream, this moisture that's being sucked up from the soil through the plant into the atmosphere. But the microbes are needed in healthy populations and balances to actually make specific minerals available to the plants. So, if we want to have a phytonutrient-rich diet and a mineral-rich diet from plants or animals or whatever, we've got to have healthy soil.

And, something that caught my attention in the 2016 *The Truth about Cancer* live symposium was that you guys had a product that was a mineral supplement product. And I was just curious what got your attention on minerals? Was that something that came up for a little while in your interviews or, I don't know, I was just curious.

Ty [27:28]: Yeah, I'm thinking it's maybe the Multi-Vita-Maxx product. I can't remember specifically, but it's a multivitamin mineral product that has fulvic acid, and humic acid delivery system which ... again, the key to health is to absorb nutrients, not to ingest nutrients, but to absorb them. So, if we ingest them into our body and our body doesn't assimilate them and we just excrete them out, that doesn't do us a lot of good. The key is absorption. And so that's why a lot of the products that we've created ... I'm part owner in a supplement company called Organixx [Note: Ty is no longer associated with Organixx] ... but, the products that we create, they all are fermented, sprouted and they're in a fulvic acid and humic acid base, which helps the bio availability. In other words, it helps your body to absorb the nutrients. So, you're probably thinking of the

Multi-Vita-Maxx, which is a mineral vitamin in a fulvic and humic base, and that just helps your body to deliver to your body those nutrients.

If you look at the store shelves of the big box stores, you buy just an ABC multivitamin, you know, whatever it's called. They're useless. They're not food-based. They're not whole food. They're chemical synthetics of what a vitamin or mineral could be. We look at vitamins and minerals and then we can create those in a lab. They're chemicals. They're not real whole food. All of the products that you should be taking as your supplement should be whole-food based, not chemical-based. And so that's why you might as well just take the bottle, if you buy it, and dump it down the toilet because you're not going to get any delivery. It's not going to help you. Not that there's not some good use from the inexpensive products on the shelves. There certainly are some cheap products that you can use, and you can get a little bit of effect from. But most, as a general rule, they're not effective, and your body does not absorb them. And you really don't want your body to absorb 'em because it's chemicals.

Brendan [29:23]: Well, also, they lack the cofactors, many of the times, because there's little trace minerals and so forth that are needed to ... you know, it's a whole symphony, basically.

Ty [29:36]: It is! That's exactly right. It's a symphony. In order to get nutrition, it's like a symphony. And what we tried and ... unfortunately, we've been told it's not a symphony, that all you need to do is to go get the saxophone player to play in a couple of notes for you and then ... then it'll sound good. Okay? That's a rude, crude example. But, that's not the symphony, right? It's the sax plus the bass, plus the drums, plus the clarinet. That's what makes the symphony. So, you've got to have the cofactors. You've got to have the enzymes, the probiotics, the vitamins, the minerals. All these things work together for health. And what we've tried to do is isolate one thing and think that that's going to get us healthy, when the reality is you need the whole. And that's why it's so important to eat a whole-food based diet, to take whole-food based supplements. Because, if ... do you remember back ... I graduated college in the early nineties. In '91 I got out of Baylor ... Do you remember Ephedrine? It's like the over-the-counter speed?

Brendan [30:36]: Yeah! I always pronounced it e-PHE-drine. Yeah, that was big. The Ma Huang herb which was ...

Ty [30:42]: Ma Huang, yeah! So, that was taken off the market. The FDA made that illegal to sell over the counter because there were several heart attacks that people had because they're taken too much ephedrine. Well, that's the prime example of us taking what God has made ... these natural foods, roots, herbs, whatever ... and trying to improve it. Or, maybe just trying to patent it so we can sell it and make a lot of money. I'm not gonna try to tell you what the motivation was. But ephedrine was an extract of the ephedra plant. You've heard of Ma Huang, which you just mentioned. There is no toxicity level if you eat the whole plant or the whole herb, if you take the whole herb. It's got that one active constituent in it, ephedrine, which causes the natural speed effect, which people want. The truckers were taking it so they could stay awake and drive long hours, and it was like, you know, over-the-counter speed. But it made your heart race, and it could cause a heart attack. But, if you took the whole plant, there was never an instance of anybody overdosing or dying from it. Why? Because that was one active of dozens, if not hundreds, of actives in the plant, and some of the active ingredients actually counter-effected that speed to where it didn't hurt your heart. But, when you took the one thing out, then it could cause a heart attack. That's just one example of how we try to improve on the things that God's made out in Nature, but we never actually improve on them. It just makes them less effective or dangerous.

Brendan [32:12]: Yeah, completely. I mean, I think that reductionism is, like, one of the key diseases of the human mind, and we've got to recognize that. Where we keep going, "Well what is *it*? What is the *thing*?" and looking for that one key, active ingredient. And that's when we start creating problems. And we did ... we've done that everywhere. If you look at agriculture, I mean, because that's my soapbox (laugh), we basically said, "Okay, the soils are getting depleted," and, this is years and years ago, hundreds of years ago. The soils were getting depleted back then ... so they were looking at what's essential. What are the rate-limiting nutrients? So, they came up with ... you know, there was research done that said, "Okay, well, that's phosphorus, potassium and nitrogen ...

Ty [33:02]: N-P-K.

Brendan [33:03]: Yeah, N-P-K: nitrogen, potassium, phosphorus. And, so, that's what we've reduced our whole agricultural fertilizer system to. Chemical N-P-K. And we're suffering the results. And the other speakers and I go into the depth of what that actually does to our bodies. So, that's ...

Ty [33:23]: You know, Brendan, I believe we've also done that when it comes to cancer. And here's how: we have reduced cancer to a tumor. And, so, if you're diagnosed with cancer, the doctor says, "We've got to do whatever we can to shrink that tumor, whether it be with poisoning with chemotherapy or we radiate it, we burn it with radiation therapy, or we cut it out with surgery." That's what I call the "Big Three" treatments. That is the reductionist theory of cancer. "You've got a tumor, let's shrink it or get it out because the tumor is the problem." The reason that modern cancer treatments aren't working is because the tumor is not the problem. The tumor's a symptom that something's gone wrong in your body. Would anybody think that that I were a wise truck driver if my truck ... the check engine light in my truck started going off, and I just smashed it with a hammer, and I thought I was better? The truck was better?

Brendan [34:19]: I'd think you're hopped up on pseudo-ephedrine.

Ty [34:22]: You'd think I've been taking too much ephedrine, right? Because that's a warning light. That's a symptom, right? It shows that there's something wrong in my truck, and I need to go in to the mechanic and figure out where the real problem is that's causing the light to go off. And then if you fix that problem, the light goes off. I don't need to smash it with a hammer. But with modern cancer treatments, that's what we do. And I'm not making light of the fact that sometimes the tumor can be a real problem, especially if it's a brain tumor. You know, we had an event in Orlando last year, and there was a man that had a brain tumor so big that his eyes were bulging out of his head because it was pressing up behind his eyes. Now, that man's cancer free now, just so you know. And he was given a month to live, at that point, and he's cancer free. One of the doctors that I know, Dr. Daniel Nuzum has treated him, and his cancer is gone. And it's amazing stuff! But that's a situation where the tumor can be a real problem, and there are times when we just need to cut the tumor out. I'm not saying that surgery does not have its place. But after the tumor's cut out, we still need to try to get to the root cause of why the tumor grew because the tumor is a symptom that there's an imbalance in the body. But modern oncology looks at the tumor as the cancer, and if we cut it out or we shrink it, you're cancer free. Well, that's why there's so many people, so many hundreds of people ... it's so sad ... that I've been contacted by over the years that said, "I went through chemo radiation. Those tumor markers were down. The doctor said I'm cancer free and now it's back, but it's all over my body, and now they've given me two weeks to live." Well, why does that story keep repeating over and over? It keeps repeating because we're treating the wrong thing. The tumor's a symptom something's wrong in the body, and we need to fix the underlying imbalance in the body.

Brendan [36:15]: What are some of those other imbalances? We've sort of touched on oxygen and things that are affecting our ability to use oxygen, whether we have enough nutrients, whether we're toxic, and toxins there are carcinogens ... they're interfering with oxygen usage ... but, what else? What else is there to look at?

Ty [36:31]: I think with cancer, we look at two ... cancer is primarily a disease of a compromised immune system that results in deficiency coupled with toxicity. So, just remember, *deficiency* and *toxicity*. Almost everybody that's got cancer is deficient in good nutrition. Nutrition causes your body to run properly, and if you don't have good nutrition, your immune system is compromised. And your immune system is your army that's fighting off the bad guys, the cancer cells, so to speak. If your immune system's compromised, you don't have the soldiers out there to fight. And, so, because of the fact that you're nutritionally deficient, your immune system can be compromised. But it can also be compromised by the toxicity that we're always exposed to, right? The environmental toxicity. You mentioned it earlier. We're bombarded with toxicity in our food, water, air, and invisible toxicity now in the radiation that we're exposed to that we were never exposed to before, all of which can compromise our immune system, which makes us toxic. And as a result of that ... if we're not detoxifying, if we're not drinking enough water, if we're not moving, if we're not stimulating our lymphatic system ... then we become toxic, and those are the things that lead to cancer. Those are the underlying imbalances in almost everyone's body that has cancer. They're toxic, they're nutritionally deficient, and they they've been exposed to these environmental toxins that we don't even see oftentimes that have compromised their immune system ... that have let cancer get a foothold.

Because the reality is, Brendan, we've all got cancer. Everybody that's watching this summit has cancer. Now, we may not have been diagnosed with cancer but we've got cancer cells. But if our body's working properly, if our immune system is functioning properly, then our immune soldiers are able to see those cells. They tag them. They kill them. And we don't get cancer. But if the immune system is compromised, that cancer can get a foothold in our body, and that's when it can become life-threatening. So, it sounds simple. But we've got to hydrate. We've got to take in good nutrition so that our body runs properly ... so our immune system runs properly. We've got to do the best we can to detoxify from this toxic exposure that we're bombarded with on a daily basis. And if we do those two things, we've got a pretty good chance of living a healthy life and living a life with cancer. I think one of the problems, Brendan, is that we look at cancer as this exterior force that we've got to have this battle against. And the problem is ... you know, President Nixon declared this war on cancer in 1971. There's casualties in every war, you know, and, unfortunately, a lot of times we become the casualty to the treatments in this war on cancer because we're fighting it like it's some external force that's got to be destroyed. When the reality is, if we feed our body good nutrition and we detoxify our body, sometimes ... that "check engine" light, right? That tumor, it just goes away because the imbalance has been corrected. Just like, if you've got some sensor on your tires that's incorrectly functioning, it's going to cause that "check engine" light to go off or your "check tire" light to go off. If you fix that sensor, the light goes off on its own. So, if we fix the underlying imbalance, sometimes the tumor just goes away.

Brendan [39:53]: You know, one of the things that ... another thing that popped up, that kind of relates to this because ... you know, I think how our body gets rid of the cancer cells ... obviously, we've got to have a good immune system function. And another part of the picture is what you brought out towards the end of the book ... autophagy. So, our body ... and I don't know if this is considered part of the immune system necessarily or not, but ... our body can go through a process of looking for the defective cells and then we, literally, digest our own cells, and we turn them over into raw materials again to build a healthy cell again. And, so, it's called autophagy, self-eating basically. That brings up the issue of ketogenic diets and then, of course, because cancer thrives on sugar, should we be eating sugar and so forth. So I kind of want to throw in these controversial topics and see what you think as far as the role of ketogenic eating preventatively, therapeutically, and then, also, how much sugar, even from natural sources, is safe or desirable. Some people are healing people on these massive fruit diets, and then others are saying, well, you know, really slow down on the fruit. We should be cautious about that and be more ketogenic most of the time. So, I'm just curious what your perspective is on all that.

Ty [41:10]: Yeah, that's a great question. And, yeah, I remember, at the end of the book, we did deal with autophagy which is basically self-eating. We've got immune cells, like our macrophages, which are phagocytes, part of our immune system that actually devour. They're white blood cells that go and they'll eat ... It means "cell eating." Macrophages does that. They'll go eat other cells that need to be taken care of, like cancer cells. When our immune system's compromised, the macrophages don't work very well. A lot of times, one of the problems is that cancer cells have a coating of protein around them that make them invisible to the macrophages and they're not able ... they don't know that there's a problem with that cell, so they don't go digest the cell. You talked about the ketogenic diet. I think that's a good topic to go into here real briefly because, as we mentioned earlier, cancer cells produce energy via fermentation, right? They ferment glucose, which is sugar. Now, if you remove the glucose, they don't have a source of energy, right? So, it seems logical to me that if you want to get rid of the cancer, there's not a better way to do it than to starve it, because then if you starve something and there's no fuel, it goes away. One of the problems is when cancer cells have fuel, they tend to live forever. That self-terminating, which is called ... what's the gene?

Brendan [42:31]: Apoptosis?

Ty [42:32]: Yeah, it's apoptosis but it's the gene, the p56 ... I can't remember the gene. I'm going to Google it real quick, and I'm gonna tell you because I just drew a blank here, but ... apoptosis and it's a p-*what* gene? P53. I said p56. So p53 gene is a gene that causes cells to commit apoptosis, which is self-destruct. For some reason, in cancer cells that's been turned off or been damaged. And so one of the things about cancer cells is that because of the fact that the p53 gene has caused them to no longer commit apoptosis, they will continue living as long as they've got fuel. So, doesn't it make sense that we would get rid of the fuel? And the fuel is sugar. Ketogenic diet works because we removed the fuel. When you're eating a ketogenic diet, you're eating a high concentration of fat, medium protein, very, very low-carbohydrate diet. As a result of that, your body goes into what's called "ketosis" where it produces energy through ketone bodies, which are basically fat cells. It's fat. It eats fat instead of producing energy through carbohydrates. Cancer cells don't use fat very well for energy. It's very difficult for them to produce energy with fat. So, if we can get our body into a state of ketosis, the cancer cells ... the <u>normal</u> cells in our body, especially the brain, work very, very well with ketone bodies. That's why a lot of times when people start eating a ketogenic diet, they'll say that their mental fog went away, and they had mental clarity and that they did much better with remembering things. And it helped their mood, helped alleviate their depression and all kinds of things with the ketogenic diet. That's why. Because our normal cells, our brain cells, work very well with ketones to produce energy, but the cancer cells don't. So, one of the things that ... and this was a diet that resulted from some of Dr. Otto Warburg's theories back in the early 1930's, the one that won the Nobel Prize that we talked about earlier. He talked about the mitochondria producing energy, and the way that cancer cells produce energy with fermentation. The bottom line of the ketogenic diet is that if you remove the source of energy for the cancer cells, they go away. They die. They self-destruct. And that's what you told me about earlier ... the apoptosis that I totally forgot, which is a term that I've used about a million times. So, maybe I need to get back on a ketogenic diet! (laugh) But, one of the things that resulted from Dr. Otto Warburg's work is the fact that we can cause those cancer cells to commit apoptosis, and the way that we do it is we remove that fuel by a ketogenic diet.

Brendan [45:08]: Yeah, yeah. Awesome! Now, we've covered some of the physical causes. Would you say there are any nonphysical causes and remedies for cancer?

Ty [45:18]: Yeah, that's a great question, too, there, Brendan. Did you see the documentary that I produced about half year ago called *The Truth about Pet Cancer*?

Brendan [45:27]: I did not see much of that at all, yeah.

Ty [45:30]: So, this is a study that one of the veterinarians told me about, but it wasn't done on dogs. It was done on people. So this applies to your question. What effect do emotions have on cancer? Well, we've talked about the immune system, we've talked about the white blood cells, we've talked about the way that your immune cells will digest bacteria and pathogens, and that's what they're there for. This was an experiment that was performed several years ago. But they took a group of people and they put them down in a movie theater, and they had them watch this slapstick comedy, like *The Three Stooges* or something just totally silly where you're just rolling laughing because it's so funny, you know? Maybe it wasn't *The Three Stooges* because my wife thinks that's just insanely stupid, and she doesn't think it's funny. Most men like the three stooges for some reason. Most women don't. I'm not trying to be sexist, that's just reality. So, I doubt it was *The Three Stooges*. But they expose these men and women to something that was just so funny, they were rolling laughing. And then they drew the blood of these people as they were laughing or after they had finished laughing. They put the blood in a petri dish, and they examined the activity of the immune system in the blood. And they found out that their immune system was, like, hyperactive at that point, attacking bacteria and pathogens and invaders in the blood. They took the same group of people, and they made them watch the ending to an extremely tear-jerking movie with a horrible ending where everyone in the audience was crying.

Then they drew their blood, and they put it in the petri dish and they found out that the immune system was not functioning. It was dead. They had watched death, and their immune system was dead. It wasn't working.

What does that tell us? It tells us that our emotions have a huge impact on the ability of our immune system to function. So, when we think of fear, anger, stress, resentment, sadness ... those are emotions that are going to happen. But we don't need to live in those states of emotion because we know that that detrimentally affects our immune system. On the flip side of the coin, when you're laughing, when you're happy, when you're living in joy, you're living in a peaceful state, you're forgiving people ... people are going to wrong you. The only person you're hurting when you're bitter towards them is you! You're not hurting them. Most people ... They did a study that, like, 75 to 80 percent of people that people will hold a grudge against, didn't even know they were mad at them. They didn't even know they had done anything. But people held a grudge against them, and it was only hurting them. So, my suggestion is if you're bitter towards someone, if you're holding a grudge, just let it go because you're not hurting them, you're just hurting you. And, so, live in states of joy. There was a survey that was done on kids and ... there was a study that was done, it wasn't a survey, but it was a study that was done, and they monitored adults and children through their everyday life over a period of a couple months, and they found out that the average adult laughs less than 40 times a day. The average child laughs 400 times a day.

Brendan [48:27]: Really? Holy cow!

Ty [48:29]: Yeah, so, what does that tell you? It tells you their immune systems are working. Their immune systems are out there fighting the bacteria and the pathogens. That's why, as you get older, it's one of the reasons that, as we get older, we tend to get sick. We're not laughing as much, and our immune system is not functioning at that high capacity that it needs to. And that's not the only reason. I'm not saying that we're sick because we're not laughing, but that's one of many different factors.

Brendan [48:53]: That's really sound advice right there. Like, just ... just watch cat videos. Do it.

Ty [49:00]: You know what? I love to watch *The Three Stooges*. I love to watch the old Pink Panther movies with Peter Sellers and inspector Clouseau. I like to watch movies. Like, *What About Bob, Napoleon Dynamite,* just stupid movies. I just think they're funny.

Brendan [49:14]: *Idiocracy.* I love that one. Hilarious!

Ty [49:16]: Oh, *Idiocracy*? Hilarious! Those movies are great! Watch 'em. You know, have you ever watched a movie late at night that's, like, a scary, nail-biter, that's got a horrible ending and you have bad dreams at night? I mean, I have. That's why, at the end of the night, I won't watch anything like that. But what you've effectively done is you've shut down your immune system, and you shut it down through the night, too, because you're still thinking about those things. Watch something funny before you go to bed. Wake up in the morning, and just list two or three things that you're thankful for. Just live in that state of gratitude. Thankfulness. Because we all have things that we can be thankful for.

You know, we're living here in the United States. We've got a lot to be thankful for. A lot of things that we take for granted, people in other lands ... they don't even have. They don't have access to the food, to the water, to the nice style of life that we have here. Let's just get up and be grateful. There's always going to be ... you know, one of the peeves that I have, and I'm not trying to go political here, but one of the peeves that I have with everybody in government, whether it's Republican or Democrat ... they're all the same ... they create this class warfare between everybody where you should only stick with your kind of people and just disagree with *them*. Whether it has to do with the racial or with class warfare or whatever. We're all people. Let's not be bitter, let's not be wishing that we had this or that. We live in the United States. We should all get along. We should be thankful for each other. We should be friends with everyone, and we should just try to be thankful for what we've been given, because we live in an awesome country and, if we can remember that, I think we can drastically improve our health.

Brendan [50:55]: And if we all start growing our own food, I hear that's a great way that people with opposing viewpoints actually start to come together—for the share of food. I can't recall who I heard say that but I was, like, blown away. These people, they were in a courtroom and they were fighting with each other, and then they got outside and somehow they ended up talking about growing food. And then, suddenly, they're, like, trading tips and stuff. So, this person has a theory that growing your own food actually connects you with other people that are also growing their own food. Then we can stop worrying about Republican versus Democrat and all that.

Ty [51:26]: Yeah, I agree! And that does bring a lot of people together, growing your own food. There's a lot of ... you know, when we were talking about health freedom ... you know, I'm in this fight for health freedom, and that's all we do. We fight for people to have the right to choose how they want to be healthy, to eat the food they want, to take vaccines or not take vaccines if they want, to take chemo or not take chemo if they want. We're all about personal choice. I've found that I'm teamed up with a lot of people that I disagree with on a whole bunch of things, but we're on the same team in this issue. And I think if we focus on what we have in common, instead of the things that separate us, we can be a lot happier.

Brendan [52:03]: Amen! Well Ty it's been awesome to have you here, and I just so appreciate how long you've been fighting this good fight as, you know, a crusader for *The Truth about Cancer* and helping people escape the death sentence of a cancer diagnosis. So, you know, hats off to you and keep going ... keep trucking!

Ty [52:26]: Thank you Brendan, I really appreciate it.

Brendan [52:27]: Trucking without pseudoephedrine! No pseudoephedrine on those truck rides of yours!

Ty [52:33]: Definitely not, man. Brendan, I appreciate all that you're doing, man. It's been a blast talking to you today. I hope the summit goes over great, and keep up the great work, man. We're all on the same team, brother.

Brendan [52:42]: I'm so grateful for Ty's work in bringing out the truth about cancer. Ty, his wife, Charlene, and their whole team have introduced millions of people to many of the world's top cancer therapies and doctors, some of whom you're seeing in the Eat4Earth event. I wouldn't have known about these extraordinary doctors and their life-saving treatments without *The Truth about Cancer* docu-series. Thank you so much for your presence and your participation in the Eat4Earth event.

Day 4 – Ketogenic Eating and Lifestyle Strategies

Fat for Fuel: Live Long and Healthy with Mitochondrial Metabolic Therapy
Joseph Mercola, DO
What You Will Discover

- Which type of food is most damaging to your body (not what you think)
- How to empower your mitochondria to produce more energy and reduce disease risk
- The detox supplement you've never heard of that removes radioactive isotopes like cesium 137 (from Fukushima)

End Food Cravings and Skyrocket Your Energy and Performance with the Keto Reset and Metabolic Flexibility
Mark Sisson
What You Will Discover

- The difference between metabolic flexibility and ketogenic metabolism
- Why you should transition gradually in several steps to metabolic flexibility
- The only things you need to measure to develop ketogenic adaptation

The Emotional Journey of 6 Months to Fat and 60 Days to Fit
Drew Manning
What You Will Discover

- Which is more important to health and fitness … food quality or exercise
- Why a calorie isn't just a calorie
- How much protein Drew eats to support his 6'2" 193-pound muscular body
- The #1 factor for success in changing your diet and transforming your body

The Ripple Effect: Lifestyle, Success, and High Performance
Greg D. Wells, PhD
What You Will Discover

- What Greg has learned from studying sick children and elite athletes
- Which is most important starting point for optimal health … food quality, exercise, or sleep?
- How lifestyle influences hormones, appetite, cravings, etc

You Can Be Stronger, Healthier, and Happier … and Together We are Unstoppable
Erin Elizabeth
What You Will Discover

- Fake news, fake fact-checkers, and Google's censorship of health information
- The unsettling trend in holistic medicine that she has been monitoring
- How Erin got through her health challenges and ultimately triumphed

Joseph Mercola, DO Interview

Fat for Fuel: Live Long and Healthy with Metabolic Mitochondrial Therapy

Brendan [00: 00]: Dr. Mercola is a true visionary who champions freedom of thought and of choice on all matters related to health. He has empowered millions of people around the world to take control of their health and has led the charge to implement much-needed changes to our current health care system and our food system. He has been a board-certified family physician for over three decades. In 1997, he founded his website Mercola.com which has become one of the most visited natural health websites in the world and made him one of the leading health educators of our time. A four-time New York Times best-selling author, Dr. Mercola's latest book *Fat For Fuel* has recently been the number one sold nonfiction book in the U.S. Dr. Mercola welcome to the Eat4Earth event.

Dr. Mercola [00: 43]: Well, thank you for having me … appreciate being here, Brendan.

Brendan [00: 46]: You've recent written this fantastic book, *Fat For Fuel*, about a particular type of ketogenic diet that you call "mitochondrial metabolic therapy", and I'm going to ask you about that in a moment, but first let me just address the general audience. Many of our listeners have probably at least heard of the concept of a low-carbohydrate, high-fat ketogenic diet, usually as a means of achieving weight loss and improved energy, and what's exciting to me about this topic is that as I've started to experience this way of eating for myself in order to have more stable energy, it occurred to me that this is actually a powerful way to "eat for Earth" because it not only helps us thrive while consuming … I mean it helps us thrive while also allowing us to consume fewer of foods that are damaging to the health of our planet and our bodies, namely excessive carbohydrates and protein from conventionally grown GMO-based, pesticide-laced corn, wheat, soy, and factory farmed animals. So speaking as somebody who until recently needed to eat almost, or at least felt I needed to eat, almost a pound of meat a day to feel energetic, I'm just kind of amazed at how much my appetite for protein has plummeted since starting to eat this way, so I'm excited to spread the word about this. Dr. Mercola, what are your thoughts about the potential planetary impacts of ketogenic diets? And what are the differences between mitochondria metabolic therapy and other ketogenic diets?

Dr. Mercola [02: 17]: Well, one of the primary ones is the one you referenced earlier, and that there's a really strong focus on decreasing the amount of protein which of course has secondary benefits from a sustainability perspective. And in fact the pound of meat that you're eating a day … there is no not a micro doubt in my mind that it was killing you prematurely. That is far too excessive protein, and you might wonder why or you might be a bodybuilder and say, "I need that pound of meat." Well, if you choose to make that decision, then it's important to understand the consequences of making that decision, and that is that you're going to activate one of the probably the most important metabolic signaling pathway in your body which is mTOR. Most physicians have never heard of this. It was discovered about 15 years ago, but it's a really very primitive pathway. It's been highly conserved throughout the animal kingdom, and it's in many different species. And it's short for "mechanistic target of rapamycin", rapamycin being an anti-cancer drug, very potent effective anti-cancer drug. So that may give you a clue when you eat a lot of meat you're going to activate this pathway very similar to activating insulin. And so if rapamycin is an anti-cancer drug and suppresses it, then it works for cancer. Well, wouldn't it make sense that one of the best ways to prevent cancer is to keep that pathway inhibited most of the time, not all of the time. So that's the key, and there's another book that was recently published which I really admire the author, Steven Gundry, who wrote *The Plant Paradox.* It's all about lectin-based … and it's interesting that we reached, coming from two different perspectives, we reached almost identical conclusions. I wish I would have read his book before I wrote mine because I would have integrated the lectin issue into it. So I think it's important also, but I couldn't agree more with his conclusion, which is that we … ideally, I would say avoiding animal protein is a wise strategy long term, but we probably should have some, and the best animal protein would be small fish because it's high in DHA, resolvins, and protectins and also devoid of many important things, and Gundry's really fond of—I thought it was brilliant—it's not so much what you eat, it's what you don't eat that makes you healthy. So if you're not eating a pound of meat, and you're eating like two to four ounces of meat on days that you're working out, great, because you … most of us only need 30 to 50 grams of protein a day, and you get a pound of meat you were probably getting well over 200 grams I would imagine because that wasn't your only source of protein. So that's just absolutely excessive, going to increase your risk for cancer, heart disease and kidney disease, and if you already have kidney disease it's one of the worst things you can do. So obviously when you reduce animal protein … most conventionally raised animal protein of course is a significant environmental burden … when you're eating small amounts … so ideally you would engage in the practice of eating small fish regularly because it's probably the best source of DHA, which is the most important fatty acid you can eat. DHA is so important. That is really the only fat that you eat that isn't burned for energy. It's actually integrated into your cell membranes and used for a variety of metabolic purposes. Specifically, it's integrated into the mitochondrial cell membrane. So really important to get it, and you can get it from supplements, and if you are unable to eat fish for whatever reason then that's certainly useful to do, but I think the better approach … because you know one of the other basic strategies is to eat real food, which means avoiding the processed foods, avoiding the industrialized farming raised foods, the ones certainly genetically engineered and sprayed with herbicides like glyphosate. So all of those … everyone who's watching this probably understands that already, but you know there's some important principles in the *Fat for Fuel* book that go into great detail about how to support your mitochondria, your mitochondria being these organelles integrated in nearly every one of our cells—not all our cells—our skin cells and our red blood cells don't have them—they get their energy from other mechanisms. But most every cell in your body has a few hundred to a few thousand, and they produce ATP, the energy currency of the body. And if you don't have a supply of ATP, you will be dead in literally seconds. You don't have water you're dead in hours, but probably … or days for sure. Some could go through a few weeks, a few months for some people, but if you don't have ATP you're dead in seconds, so you need it. It runs your entire body. So the key becomes how do you improve the quality of your mitochondria so that they're able to produce energy efficiently. And one of the best ways you can do it is to re-teach your body how to burn fat fuel. Pretty much everyone who's born healthy has that ability, but we lose it when we eat continuous large amounts of refined carbohydrates and processed foods and damaged fats, damaged fats probably even being … you know damaged fats, which are responsible for the epidemic of heart disease in the early part of the 20th century, are probably more pernicious than excess carbs, and then probably following that would be excess protein, and finally carbohydrates. So people look at this as a low-carb diet, but the reality is it's a real food diet, removing all the damaged fat and limiting your protein to adequate amounts and then the carbs come secondary here. I mean you could cheat in the carbs and have a lot less consequence than on the others. Because if you have damaged vegetable fat—it's industrially processed—you are just looking for metabolic trouble. There's just no way … because it's integrated all in your cell membranes. It's responsible for almost every metabolic function your body has, and if you put the wrong building blocks in there you will have trouble that's just inevitable. There's no way around it, and then the excess protein as I mentioned earlier will stimulate the mTOR pathway, which also has its own complications, and then finally the carbs will increase insulin and leptin resistance leading to further metabolic damage.

Brendan [08: 35]: You mentioned that your favorite source of DHA is small fish, and I think you mentioned in the book that you don't favor so much algae oil. I'm just curious what the reason for that might be.

Dr. Mercola [08: 51]: I don't favor algae. Well, algae is not a fish.

Brendan [08: 54]: Right, no I mean DHA from algae oil.

Dr. Mercola [08: 57]: Oh yeah, because algae … because essentially it's a processed food. When you eat DHA from fish it's a real whole food. And when I open my can of sardines, and I have a can of sardines probably four to five times a week … the other two days I have probably some … well, when I have it in supply … it's really these five bird meatballs that are literally two ounces. I get them from Will Harris's farm, White Pastured Oaks Farm (White Oak Pastures) in southern Georgia, made from … it's probably one of the best regenerative agriculture farms in the United States so I get, you know, that's good. So that, but the other days of the week … and you know, when you open up these cans of sardines, these are whole fish. I mean the heads are taken off, and the guts are gone, but it's a whole fish so you're getting not only the DHA, you're getting the EPA and probably half a dozen rather really important essential fats. And when you get DHA from algae, yeah, it's probably better than nothing, but it's unbalanced, and you can cause metabolic disturbances if you just get an isolated source like that. So I think the ideal, the way we were designed, is not to take that algae extract. I mean, where did you get that in Nature? You don't, but it's probably better than nothing if you're a vegan. And I actually recently interviewed Dr. Kate Shanahan who wrote the book *Deep Nutrition*. I don't know if you've heard of her. Really a good deep thinker, and she changed my position on this too because most of the studies that were done are pretty clear when you review the literature, that there's compelling evidence to suggest that we don't make a lot of DHA from the plant-based omega-3's, the ALA. Because the studies show … you know, it's like 1 or 5%, but then she challenged me, and I think that there's probably some validity to this in the concept that most of these studies were done on an unhealthy populations. They're eating bad fats, they have high processed food you know, so they're not the ideal situation and not a physiological optimum for sure. So in that population which is anyone who's following the recommendations in the book you would be in their group pretty soon but that your physiology is probably a little bit different, and you may be able to make more DHA from the ALA and the plant-based sources. So we don't know actually, and I haven't seen any studies done on it, but I think it's an interesting concept, and I think there's probably some validity to it, so rather than the 1 or 5% of DHA conversion it might be as high as 10 or 25%. It may be significant, and maybe you don't need it. I don't know, but I would rather err on the side of caution and have the fish. Because I think there's such compelling evidence, and if you look at the blue zones of literature and all these long age populations where they have high percentages of centenarians or super centenarians, that fish is a small ... well, fish was a big part of their diet. The studies of course show people that are over 100 years old, so most of the damage from the fish was when they were probably in their mid-aged to being elderly. So when they were eating fish, even it was large fish, they were relatively healthy because that we didn't have a chance to contaminate the world, the oceans of the world by then. But now it's a different story, so you have to pay careful attention. If you're young this is a serious issue because large sea fish are contaminated with mercury, PCBs, dioxin, PBDEs which is the flame retardants. You know these are all toxins that get bio-accumulated in these large fish, and it's something if you do eat them yes you'll get the DHA, you'll get the beneficial fats and the resolvins and protectins, but you'll also get this load of other toxins that you're going to have to spend a lot of time getting out of your body, and that's probably one of the topics of my next book is how to optimally detox because there's ... it's not a simple strategy ... it's really a whole complex set of interventions that are required to get this stuff out of your body.

Brendan [12: 57]: And unfortunately you're talking about sushi, many people's favorite food right.

Dr. Mercola [13: 02]: Well no, sushi, no, sushi is it is a term that literally just means raw fish, so it depends on the type of fish. If you have raw tuna, absolutely. But if you have ... I guess you could put anchovies in there or sardines you know. I don't know if they have them. I don't frequent sushi restaurants. But as long as it's a small fish, the smaller the fish the better. Ideally like 2 or 3 inches or even smaller, like anchovies are. I think some of the sardines I see are like maybe 4 inches, but you know the smaller the better, the less long they had to be alive and bio-accumulate the toxins that are in the waterway.

Brendan [13: 40]: Got it. On the topic of fat ... you talk about saturated fat, which has had such a controversial history, and I wonder if you could elaborate a little bit on that issue from the book.

Dr. Mercola [13: 56]: Well, the conventional physician for the longest time ... saturated fat has been vilified, and that's largely related to studies that were also done that were flawed for a wide variety of reasons, the two primary ones being that there was no effort in most of these studies to isolate the pernicious fats and much of the damage was done to trans fats. And in others of these studies ... the devil's in the details ... so if you could pull up the study, go into the methods section you'll find ... what were they feeding these animals that they thought was a saturated fat diet? Well, they were giving them food that was traditionally thought to be saturated fat, but actually it was from animals that were given guess what?? All these rancid, industrially processed vegetable oils! So they actually never analyzed the fat that they were given, they just assumed it was okay, but it was it was industrially processed animals. So the fat that they were giving them was actually essentially damaged vegetable oil fat, not really saturated fat. So there's two primary flaws in this, but even considering that, when you look at the epidemiological reviews, there's been a large number of studies and a meta-analysis that show pretty clearly that there is no risk from the saturated fat. Now Gundry is in his latest book *The Plant Paradox* actually refines it a little bit more, and there are things called lipopolysaccharides or LPS or what he calls "little pieces of shit", which is an appropriate term. Essentially many people have damaged microbiomes and these bacteria, these LPS molecules can migrate out and cause lots of problems, and what they do is they punch holes in your in your gut wall, which is a very thin lining, and so he recommends avoiding saturated fat in the initial first few weeks, and I think I'm going to modify my program to recommend that too. Even though it's a healthy fat, if you're not healthy it can be a problem. So you know, rarely is there ever a simple answer to things. Typically the correct answer is always "it depends", you know, and it depends on many variables that you have to go into great details. So you know, I'm always amused when they when you go to medical school one of the things that's actually drilled into you is you've got to talk to the patient. You just can't ... you've got to do an extensive thorough, comprehensive history. They just can't tell you they have this problem, and then they expect you to treat it because it depends on all the other variables that are connected to it, and it's almost always the case. So you need a really ... the most important part of a treatment program is really look at the history done by a skilled clinician.

Brendan [16: 47]: Right. You know a lot of ketogenic diets promote specific percentages of carbohydrates, proteins and fats. But in your book you seem to point out that different people will have different needs for protein, different tolerances for carbohydrate, and you provide some ranges of those, and I wonder if you can expand on that.

Dr. Mercola [17: 12]: Sure. Typically, the most important thing to measure ... and one of my mentors in this is Ron Rosedale who has been studying this a lot longer than I have. He's a physician who taught me about the importance of insulin physiology about 23 years ago now. And I believe it's true ... is that the most important nutrient to measure is protein as we talk to referenced early and the reasons why. So it's really critical if you get that thing right, and the way you get a right is to actually measure it, and the way you measure it is, if you don't have it already, is go to Amazon, buy a $10 or $15 electronic kitchen digital scale that you can weigh your meat. Now you don't have to weigh all of your food, like if you're eating sardines, and it has a can, and it will tell you precisely what's in there. But most food that you buy in larger quantities you're going to have to actually weigh that out because you're not going to have a full serving size. So you weigh what you're going to eat, and then you need to look it up in a nutrient database, and there's a number of them online. My Fitness Pal is a popular one, but I recommend Cronometer (Cronometer.com). It's free. Just weigh it, put it in, and they'll tell you exactly what it is. So how much do you need? As I said earlier 30 to 50 grams for most people, but more precisely if you want to measure it, it's about one gram per kilogram of lean body mass. And you calculate ... you have to figure out how much percent body fat you have. If it's 20 percent, like many people, then you're 80% lean, so 80% of your total weight in kilograms which is divided by 2.2, and then you have that many grams of protein. Now a gram of protein is not a gram of meat, so your pound of meat is not 454 grams of protein. Actually, that would be yeah that's a pound ... it's 454 grams, kilogram is 2.2 pounds but so 454 grams. So no I don't actually eat much meat, so I don't remember what the conversion is for, you know, an ounce of meat versus how many grams protein, but you just look it up because it's different for different cuts of meat. So you look it up in this database, and it'll tell you precisely, and you measure out you know 66 grams of meat, or like when I'll have shrimp I get shrimp from Alaska and not from Indonesia, and I'll have like maybe 70 grams. I know precisely how much ... that's 18 grams of protein for me, which is ... you know, I rarely go over 20 so I try to keep my total protein intake below 60 for sure, and sometimes it's closer to 50 unless I'm doing strength training days which is what I actually did today. Twice a week of the strength training which is good to do because it helps prevent sarcopenia. But anyway getting back to your carbohydrate question ... so that's how you measure your protein which I think it's the most important. And then carbohydrates is also the same. You've got to measure them, and you usually calculate. The recommendation is based on net carbohydrates, and that carbohydrate being defined as a total carbohydrate minus the fiber. So if you had like, you know, eight ounces of kale, which would be 240 grams that's not 240 grams of total net carbs it's probably closer to 15 or 20 because most of it is fiber that you're not going to be able to digest and break down to glucose, but your gut bacteria will break it down and the short chain fatty-acids which will nourish your gut microbiome and secondarily nourish you. So you want to keep your net carbohydrates down to about 20 to 50 grams. 50 is kind of on the high end, and if you're really are treating terminal cancer or that you have a serious illness, then closer to 20 might be more reasonable. But even better, if you're like 70% of the population United States—probably not that percentage for other people who are watching this—you're overweight. 70% of people in the US are overweight. So if you're in that population then you may want to consider a fast, which is zero carbohydrates, and it's zero protein. Probably could integrate some fat because fat doesn't stimulate insulin or mTOR. It kind of a goes for a free ride. So an example of that would be like butter and coffee that didn't have cream or sugar of course, or MCT oil. MCT oil is a shorter chain version of mostly coconut oil, but it can be derived from palm oil, and it typically has 8 and 10 carbon chains in there, fats, and the MCT oil from caprylic acid or c8 is even better, and it converts ketones which converts to energy real quickly. And it's a really useful tool that people can use in the transition phase. Because ultimately these recommendations are not done forever. They're done until your body develops the ability to burn fat as its primary fuel. And how do you know that? You measure ketones, and when you're generating ketones then you've made the transition, and that means that you are metabolically flexible again, and you can burn fat or sugar depending on what you're doing. Now you can always lose that flexibility by going off a program, but when you have that then it's important not to stay in ketosis for long-term. Many people don't understand and embrace it, and I certainly didn't. I had to learn the hard way even though it was known by some, but certainly not by me, or people I was reading. So that's when you do cyclical ketosis, so then you have higher carb like 100, 150 grams of net carbs and higher proteins, especially on the days that you are training. You do that once or twice a week, and then you go down to the lower levels on the other days, and you cycle back and forth, and your body loves it. It loves this cycling because rarely you know it's so unusual where you're going to have health benefits by eating the same thing all the time. You need to integrate variety and not only variety in the foods, but in the variety in the concentrations and the ratios of your foods. And it's all based and customized on how you are feeling and how your body is metabolically responding to this. So that's why we don't give any magic formulas, but really give guidelines where people do and test themselves. You can test your blood sugar is another way to do that. When I was doing this program I wore a 24 hour continuous glucose monitor. It did measure my blood sugar every five minutes. So I got to know my data pretty well, and

I think there is great value in measuring your blood sugar. It gives you that immediate feedback. The equipment is cheap as can be, it's seven bucks to pick up a meter on Amazon and less than a quarter to measure one blood test, so it doesn't cost you a lot for $10 you get a lot of blood tests for that $10. So most people can afford that, you don't have to go to the doctor. You do it with the means at your own home, so you do a fasting blood sugar test before you go to bed. You've got a lot of good data that will show you how your body is responding because literally one in three people in this country have diabetes or prediabetes, and there's a significant percentage of them no doubt in my mind, of the people that are watching this, that do fall into the category diabetes or prediabetes. And that is a core … it's a fundamental metabolic aberration that is, not a prerequisite, but it's a significantly contributing risk factor for almost all chronic degenerative diseases, including Alzheimer's and heart disease and cancer. So if you've got diabetes going on you're just looking for trouble. It's not just diabetes, absolutely not. And you know it's one of the risk factors … and blindness, you know, age-related macular degeneration is another complication of that and diabetic retinopathy. So these are all complications from a dysfunction of your metabolism that ultimately leads to disruption in the way your mitochondria works.

Brendan [25: 00]: So we're talking about food as medicine in the context of ratios of carbohydrates, proteins and fats, which can be pretty easily calculated using tools like the one you mentioned in your book, Chronometer, but I wonder how accurately can we calculate our food-based intake of micronutrients like vitamins and minerals given the fact that the USDA has been reporting declining levels of micronutrients in our food supply for decades. So when those tables were created I don't think macronutrient ratios in foods have changed but the micronutrient ratios perhaps have. I wonder what your thoughts on that are?

Dr. Mercola [25: 37]: There's no question, and you know that part of the arrogance that we have as a professional, a profession, is to think that we know it all and can measure these things precisely and figure things out. but you're right. Much of this data is very dated, and it's based on analysis and assays from plants that were grown many decades ago, and the topsoil had a complete different nutrient density, our ability to provide nutrient density into the plants. So that is a concern there's no question that's why ideally you want to grow your own food. I grow a significant amount of my own food, and I'm passionate about that. And we can talk about how I do that, but you know, so that's one way to get it. But I think there are certain minerals that most people need. Not only because of the soil depletion in minerals but also because of the toxic exposures we have. So what are those minerals? Iodine really important, selenium useful for making glutathione, detoxing, also your thyroid, which also selenium and iodine work for, magnesium which most people are deficient in, and then zinc, another big one most people need, and probably sulfur, and there's a lot of ways you can get sulfur. You can probably, one of the best ways is soaking in magnesium sulfate epsom salts. This way you can get magnesium and sulfur, or you can take something like MSM so those are five important minerals I think most people should be on. A lot of people you know 10-15 years ago the big focus was on calcium, and I think calcium is important to get, especially if you're excluding dairy which usually is a primary source of calcium. So if you're excluding dairy I would do it, and would you like to know my source of calcium?

Brendan [27: 22]: Sure.

Dr. Mercola [27: 23]: It's not one we sell on our site. (laughs)

Brendan [27: 26]: It's not what?

Dr. Mercola [27: 27]: It's not one we sell on our site.

Brendan [27: 28]: Okay!

Dr. Mercola [27: 29]: It's one … I basically save the egg shells from the pastured eggs that I eat, and I don't I actually saved the whites, and I give the whites to my personal trainer, but I have the yolks. So I consume the yolks, about two a day most days of the week, and I discard the whites. And then I save the shells, let them dry, and then I use a coffee grinder to pulverize the shells. And I take about a teaspoon of that, and that's my calcium source. There's not only that calcium but some of the other micro minerals, especially if you have, you know, non-CAFO bird eggs that you're consuming. So you can assume that these birds are eating some insects and have access to true pasture that hasn't been … where the topsoil hasn't been decimated. So that's a pretty interesting way to get some of your other micro nutrients. Not only calcium, but there's some other nutrients in there like silicon, and I probably … I think there's another important one too that I think that most people would benefit from because we're toxic to aluminum, but also thallium which is now in the gasoline that's replaced lead, and tin, and then cesium, cesium 137 from Fukushima, the radioactive isotope. So all these can be actually detoxed out of your body with a form of silica called orthosilicic acid commonly implemented as Biosil. That's a really good use. It's sold as a support for collagen and hair and nails. It really does do that, but more importantly it's in a powerful and effective detoxer of these toxins that we tend to accumulate over time.

Brendan [29: 19]: Wow I've never heard that.

Dr. Mercola [29: 22]: Yeah, I got to tell you something you've never heard, right?

Brendan [29: 25]: You've told me plenty. (laughing)That calcium in an eggshell isn't that calcium carbonate, and if so I'm just curious would it be more available to the body if you took it with a shot of apple cider vinegar or something like that? I'm just thinking out loud here.

Dr. Mercola [29: 42]: I don't know the form I don't think it's calcium carbonate. I'm pretty sure it's not. It's I just don't know the form, but it might be calcium carbonate, I don't know. But I like apple cider vinegar. I go through about a pint, almost a pint a week actually. It's a very useful ketogenic supplement because basically it's acetic acid which is a nourishing fuel for the microbiome, so it'll help improve your beneficial bacteria and suppress pathogenic bacteria. So I think it's great. We actually sell a form of apple cider vinegar, but if you want to get it you want to get the real thing. One that has a "mother" in it that's organic. You don't want to buy the cheap stuff because it's not going to be as beneficial. I love apple cider vinegar.

Brendan [30: 33]: I wonder if you could say more about the issue of how we're growing food, and you actually mentioned in your book because obviously how would grow food affects soil quality, affects mineral availability, affects our health, and you mentioned in your book another factor that's rampant in our food supply that is affecting our mineral assimilation, that's glyphosate commonly known as Roundup when combined with certain carriers. What can you tell us about that?

Dr. Mercola [31: 02]: You know I think most of your audience knows the dangers of that so I don't have to expand on the problems with glyphosate, but it does … it's … it was basically patented as an antibiotic and as a mineral chelator, specifically zinc and manganese, so it definitely causes problems there, and it also decimates your microbiome in your gut and really destroys or impairs many of the tight junctions in your endothelial lining of your intestinal tract. So you obviously don't want to have any herbicides, especially glyphosate, pretty pernicious. Probably it's on its way it's out, and it's already marked as poison in California, which is a big step in the right direction. So but ultimately, I think it's really important that most people grow some of their food, and even if you live in a college dorm you can do that alright. Let me show you actually this is ready to harvest so it actually works out pretty good for the timing of this. These are my sunflower seed sprouts.

Brendan [31: 58]: Wow. Oh my God, that's a bumper crop. Is that a day supply? A week's supply? A month's supply?

Dr. Mercola [32: 06]: This is like 3 or 4 days, and this one it's coming up to close behind so you can see it's a lot smaller.

Brendan [32: 18]: Are you putting something special in there to grow them so vibrantly?

Dr. Mercola [32: 22]: Yeah there's some little tricks of that maybe we talked about this because anyone can do this, even if you're a college student in a dormitory you can do this. Literally it took like two square feet, and who doesn't have two square feet in their house? I guess some people may not, but virtually no one watching this. So you know because that's a big issue for many people. They rent a house or they're in an apartment, and they don't have the space, and you know there's a lot of reasons why they wouldn't be able to do that, but anyone can grow sunflower seed sprouts, and it's really one of the most nutrient-dense foods that you can grow, at least vegetables. Thirty times more nutrient dense than most vegetables that you grow. Now it doesn't have a lot of polyphenols in it like some of the other vegetables do, which can be very useful for other reasons you know like rosemary or garlic or broccoli, you know, so these are useful for other reasons. So you need ideally you should have two or three dozen different types of vegetables or plant-based materials that you're eating every day. But you grow these … the reason these that look so well is for a number of reasons. You soak them overnight. Organic sunflower seeds … you have to have a good source because if you have bad seeds to start with it's never going to work no matter what you're doing. So organic sunflower seeds from a reputable company. Soak them for eight hours. I use a … I'm actually starting my third batch, so I have a little sprouting cup that pulls up, and then I don't know if you can see that. So it just drips and then then you could hold it. and then it'll drain. It's in the soaking phase now about another hour or two, and then I'll take it out of there and then just let it drain for like a day, and rinse it out every eight hours or so. And then it's ready to plant. And the key that most people don't understand is that when you plant them it's crucial to put some type of cover over it, like I've customized a ceramic tile cut to fit that shape of the container. And then you put that in and squash it down. And then you put ... I put two five or 10 pound rocks on top of it. You weight it, and it needs that weight because that's the exercise for the plants. If it doesn't have that weight they won't be healthy. They'll be just small and tiny. So it stays on for almost two or three days until it literally pushes up, and in fact there's so much power that comes up through those plants that you could literally stand on that plate and it will push you up. Yeah, there's a lot of force there. So you don't have to worry about damaging the plants. We all ... see, we all need stress, stress is an important part. you know lots of us want to avoid it, but stress is crucial. Well, it doesn't have to be hormetic stress, that's one type of stress, but there's a lot of other stresses, just like not eating food is a stress, and exercise is a stress, and it's certainly not a hormetic stress. So in fact I look at exercise, and fasting as really similar. They're both stresses to the body. And the magic of that stress ... this doesn't occur because if you were just actually to exercise all the time aggressively, like five hours a day for continuously every day for, you know, after a short time you'd be in such a deep hole that you'd be bed-bound and very damaged, right? Because the magic of exercise occurs not in the exercise but in the recovery from the exercise. Similarly, the magic of fasting occurs not so much in the fasting but afterwards. It's when you refeed because you stressed your body; now it's ready to take advantage of the nutrition. But you need that cycling back and forth, that stress off and on. That's why you don't exercise every day typically, and you don't fast every day or you don't feast every day, you know, you cycle in and out. It's the same thing. You exercise and recover. You feast and famine and recover. So it's an important principle just philosophically to understand and once you do, you can factor it into a lot of other strategies in your lifestyle choices. It really has application for just about everything.

Brendan [36: 37]: Yeah. Now a lot of people seem to have challenges getting into ketosis and transitioning and there's probably a lot of different variables, but I am curious about, since you mentioned in the book, that if manganese is deficient or unavailable because of glyphosate, that mitochondria are not working properly, and I'm also wondering that with this evolving theory, the mitochondrial theory or rather the metabolic theory of cancer, and since I've always thought that pesticides were one of the major causes of cancer correctly or incorrectly, and of course other environmental toxins, I'm wondering ... do pesticides and possibly the deficiency of minerals in our food supply together generate mitochondrial dysfunction that's generating cancer and other conditions.

Dr. Mercola [37: 28]: Yeah, the ultimate mechanism is not genetic damage as a primary cause. It's the secondary result of the mitochondrial dysfunction that generates the genetic damage. So anything that disrupts mitochondrial function is going to increase your risk of those. And toxins, mineral deficiencies, can do that. Manganese is important, but it's relatively unusual to require manganese deficiency because it's needed in such low amounts. I'm not even sure of how you ... I mean sure I know there's assays for it, but it's not a common one, and we don't typically prescribe manganese although some people I'm sure benefit from it. So if you have a healthy diet for that has a wide variety of plant sources, especially seeds and nuts organically grown and hopefully in soils that are not nutrient-depleted, you're going to get enough manganese to compensate, but especially if you're avoiding glyphosate but speaking of glyphosate, on our site we have a test that you can order it's not inexpensive. It's a $100. But it's done up from a lab in Davenport, Iowa. The People's Lab, and they will tell you how much glyphosate is in your urine, how much have you been eating. Yeah, it's pretty good. So I did mine a few weeks ago, and guess what it came back out? Zero! It can validate if you've done it properly or not, so you don't have to guess anymore. You can see if you're eating clean, or you know that little processed food you've been sneaking in now and then is really making a difference, so it's easy to check now.

Brendan [38: 54]: Awesome now I'm going to look at that myself but more for other people than myself. I studiously avoid conventionally grown foods.

Dr. Mercola [39: 02]: Yeah, well, you know, and the key thing is processed food, so a conventionally grown vegetable isn't necessarily a danger. Some are worse than others, but once it's processed that's when the escalation and the exponential damage occurs. That's where the damage is. You really want to focus on real foods, ideally organic, but if you're eating real food you're most of the way there that's the key thing.

Brendan [39: 33]: Okay, you know Dr. Mercola more than more than possibly any other health educator I'm aware of, you've advocated not only for sanity in the nutritional world, but also you've helped support better food policy, labeling for foods, GMOs in foods. You've conducted interviews with producers that are growing food in ways that regenerates soil, that don't require pesticides, herbicides and so forth, fertilizers that kill the soil. And I believe you're a founding member of Regeneration International. Is that correct?

Dr. Mercola [40: 17]: Yeah, and we've also catalyzed the American Grass-fed Association, which is the best way to find true, authentic grass-fed and grown in the US and processed in the US because most of the grass-fed meats are coming from Australia, and that's just crazy. Like we can't grow it here? The problem is we don't have the processing plants, so there's some infrastructures that need to be resolved. But we we're finally able to get that passed like within the last year, so it's great, and we're very excited about that seeing the transition. You know I mean there's some effort and work in it, but it's really, you know, you just see the problem and you just address it, which is one of our strategies are. So we're happy to be involved in that process.

Brendan [41: 03]: Great. Well I really appreciate your time today Dr. Mercola and all of your support, your pioneering courage really. You're very clear spoken and outspoken and just kind of tell it like it is, and you've been doing that for decades, so I thank you for that.

Dr. Mercola [41: 21]: You're welcome! If anyone wants to learn more obviously the website Mercola.com, but also the book *Fat For Fuel*, which is literally … I mean it's the first book I've ever written— I've written like a dozen now—that was actually the number one non-fiction book sold in the US, which is … so there's been a great demand for this I think, the timing was good. But I'm excited because of the information it has that can really change people's lives, that can save people's lives, so they don't have to suffer needlessly and die prematurely like so many people are because the catalyst for the book was 1600 people die every day in the United States from cancer, the vast majority of which do not have to die from cancer. And it's just it's just an abomination that this scenario exists. And *Fat For Fuel* discusses not only diet but a lot of other mitochondrial biohacks you can do that we did not discuss like cold thermogenesis, intermittent fasting, and the importance of photobiology, photobiomodulation, and detoxification. So all these are being discussed in the book that can further enhance cyclical keto-genesis.

Brendan [42: 29]: Yeah, I'd say you did a phenomenal job at both contextualizing ketosis or ketogenic diets and presenting clear simple guidelines for anybody to kind of customize it for where they are and what they want to accomplish.

Dr. Mercola [42: 45]: Thank you!

Brendan [42: 46]: So thanks again for being here and for your collaboration and helping us all eat healthy and eat for earth.

Dr. Mercola [42: 53]: Absolutely.

Brendan [42: 54]: Dr. Mercola's book *Fat For Fuel* was my introduction to ketogenic eating patterns and as a result I've been able to cut my consumption of animal proteins by about two thirds, and I'm far less dependent on regular mealtimes. When I do intermittent fasting it's not hard for me to go 18 hours or more overnight without eating. It's really made a difference for me. Dr. Mercola and I spoke for another half-hour after that interview and he shared some really interesting facts in the conversation.

Mark Sisson Interview

End Food Cravings and Skyrocket Your Energy: The Ketogenic Reset and Metabolic Flexibility

Brendan [00:00:01]: Welcome to the Eat4Earth event. This is Brendan Moorehead, and together we're exploring how you can heal yourself, your loved ones, and the planet, with food. Our next guest, Mark Sisson, is one of the early pioneers of the paleo, primal, ancestral health movement, and an ex endurance athlete. We're going to be discussing how to gain the amazing benefits of a ketogenic metabolism without the struggle often associated with the transition to a fat-burning metabolism. Mark is the *New York Times* best-selling author of *The Keto Reset Diet*, best-selling author of *Primal Blueprint* and *Primal Endurance*, and blogger at top-rated health and fitness website, Marksdailyapple.com. He's the founder of several companies: Primal Blueprint, devoted to designing state-of-the-art supplements that address the challenges of living in our modern world; Primal Kitchen, delivering uncompromisingly delicious—I can attest to that—nutrient-dense foods that are always dairy, gluten, grain, soy free and full of beneficial fats and high quality protein; Primal Kitchen Restaurants, a franchise of primal, paleo aligned restaurants that offer healthy, clean and organic, fast, casual dining options; and Primal Health Coach, an unparalleled and fully rounded health, coaching and business education program. Mark shares over three decades of research and experiential learning that unlocks the keys to building metabolic flexibility and becoming a fat-burning beast and basically taming hunger and cravings forever, which excites me because I've lived with that for a long time. So, Mark, it's awesome to have you with us today.

Mark [00:01:37]: Thanks for having me, Brendan, great to be here.

Brendan [00:01:41]: So, ketogenic metabolism is just plain awesome, and so let's do our best to take people from zero to sixty and kind of give people a quick summary of the pros and cons of ketogenic fat burning metabolism vs. sugar burning metabolism, to start off with, and then dive into it a bit.

Mark [00:01:58]: Sure, so, the operative word here that we want to strive for is "metabolic flexibility". What that means is the ability for our bodies to get energy from whatever substrate is possible or available in the moment. So it means burning fat when there's fat on your plate, it means burning fat when there's no fat on your plate, but there's fat on your body. It means burning glucose if you've just eaten carbohydrates. It means burning ketones if your liver is starting to make ketones. It creates this wide array of opportunities to derive energy. In the absence of metabolic flexibility, when we're not good at burning fat, we're not good at burning ketones. We rely too much on carbohydrates to convert into glucose, what we know as blood sugar, and as a result we go from meal to meal throughout our entire lives, every three or four hours, refueling, trying to get this carbohydrate, this glucose, into the system. A ketogenic eating strategy is one that reconfigures your original factory setting at birth, which was to be really good at burning fat, and re-teaches your body. You learn once again how to become good at burning fat, how to become good at making ketones, and you develop this metabolic flexibility. That's probably the best possible explanation I can give for it.

Brendan [00:03:24]: Okay, and how about issues like affecting athletic performance, disease risk, things like that. Is it possible to say anything about that?

Mark [00:03:35]: Of course. Having achieved this metabolic flexibility, and having unburdened yourself from having to eat every three or four hours to get energy from the one source that you know how to get—and that is the sugar-based metabolism—a number of things fall into place. First of all, there's a decrease in inflammation, and that's pretty much a standard testimonial that we get throughout the realm of people who enter this fat-burning phase. There's typically an increase in athletic performance, especially if you're any kind of an endurance athlete. If you have been doing 10Ks or bike races, or anything that takes some amount of time to complete, the fact that you've become good at burning fat, means that you can get more energy, race at a higher level, using fat as fuel, as opposed to having to take in the energy gels and all of the stuff that goes along with that. I noticed an improvement in my sleep when I engage in a ketogenic eating strategy, and we'll talk about what that means a little bit. My body composition which was pretty good before I went keto, became better, training more toward what I would call my ideal body composition as I burned off more body fat, as I retained lean muscle.

Probably the single biggest element of a fat-burning, keto-adapted lifestyle, is this freedom, as you acknowledged earlier on, from hunger, cravings, and appetite. The ability to wake up in the morning and have all the energy I need without having to eat, the ability to go long periods of time without losing my focus, my mental concentration, because I'm thinking, "Oh my gosh, it's noon, I better eat, or else I'll get 'hangry' in the afternoon, or I'll have energy issues, or I'll want to take a nap". When those go away, you really do realize that your productivity increases, your energy in general increases, and as a result your mood improves; you're not so moody as a result of low blood sugar, things like that. So, really, this metabolic flexibility opens this whole amazing world of possibilities all of which are better than it was before. It's not to say that everyone who's not keto's life sucks. It's just that, and I was the best example in this, I thought everything was awesome in my life, I was low-carb paleo for fifteen years, had good energy, never got sick, had good body composition, felt like everything was pretty much dialed in, didn't feel like anything was broken, but I'm just one who chases performance all the time, so I'm always looking for what's the next thing. And because I'd written about keto for a long time, and I spent days in a keto state where I was taking in less than 50g of carbs a day, but I never really did a deep dive in it. So about a year and a half ago, I did a deep dive, two months keto, and just because I noticed from myself an increase in all of these basic metrics that I was looking at, even though everything was great before, it got better. So I thought to myself, well, jeez, if it gets better for me, and I was already in pretty decent shape, imagine what possibilities await people who are stuck, plateaued, who've had frustrating experiences with whatever type of eating strategy they tried, and it hadn't worked, who have medical conditions that are not responding to the drugs, if you will. And that's really what got me most excited about writing this book *The Keto Reset Diet*, all of these possibilities. So you might ask "Well, then, who is keto good for?" and I'd say "It's good for everyone". If you have the willingness to try it, it certainly is the sort of thing that anyone can try and just experiment and see what the results are for you and choose from there.

Brendan [00:07:42]: As somebody who, you know, you're seeking performance, other people might be more seeking just living a great life, and so is there any contradiction there? I understand you would be somebody who loves food and loves living well. Did you have to compromise at all going ketogenic?

Mark [00:08:00]: That's a great question. That is a very important caveat. I love food. There was a degree of added mindfulness that I needed to take on in order to stay keto every day for sixty days. It was basically being aware that while I was already low-carb, I was already in that 100 to 120g a day total carb arena, and basically eating everything I wanted to eat, I mean, the idea there is, I sound like I wanted to eat Cinnabon and pizzas and liters of Coke, but of all the foods that I gathered for myself that I felt were good for me, healthy, fit the paleo, primal bulk, I did not sacrifice any of those because I was trying to adhere to some rigid standard. So when I went keto I did have to go "Okay, I'm at a 110g of carbs a day, eating whatever I want in that big list of food. Can I find 50 or 60 grams of carbs a day not to eat from there. So that was the only real, if you want to use the term "sacrifice". But one of the things that happens when you go keto is within a couple of days into this cycle, you start to realize that some of those things just aren't, you know, I was giving up. I wasn't having sweet potato once in a while. I wasn't having potato salad. I wasn't having a couple of pieces of bread that I might have—some grain-free gluten-free bread. Really simple fixes. I was eating lots of vegetables, big salads, lots of vegetables, a little bit of fruit, mostly berries. So it was a very easy transition for me from where I came from, and that's one of the strategies that we use in *The Keto Reset Diet* book. You don't jump all in from a standard American diet of 350 to 400g of carbs a day to 30grams of carbs a day. You can, but it's awfully painful. It's a real tough transition that way. But we stairstep you down, and so we take you into that, first of all, just eliminating all the stuff that we know you shouldn't be eating, and you know you shouldn't be eating too: the sugary drinks, the pies, the cakes, the candies, the cookies, all of the processed foods. And we boil it down to lots of vegetables, meat, fish, fowl, eggs, nuts, seeds, little bit of fruit. It's all stuff that we know we should be eating. Even in that realm, you can still get to where you're in a 100 to 150g of carbs a day, but that's so removed from what most Americans who depend on the governments pyramid for their guidance, six to eleven servings of grains a day and all this other stuff. It's so removed from that. That first phase really does signal to your body, "There's not going to be a lot of sugar. We're not going to have an opportunity to just depend all the time on making glucose and using that for fuel, but I have to start learning how to burn fat more efficiently." But we're not going to get crazy about it; we're going to ease into it so that you develop this metabolic machinery that enables you to burn fat efficiently, and then you could apply that to your workouts, and you can apply that to your moving around throughout the day. And then once you've gotten to that level, and we allocate three weeks in the book, a twenty-one day kind of reset. Once you get to that point, now we can go into the keto phase of this and really start to get the benefits and do so having proven that we're already pretty good at burning fat, and we're not going to off the rails because we've elected to remove another 50g of carbs. Does that make sense?

Brendan [00:11:56]: Totally, and there's something very unique about that system. I'm not an experienced keto dabbler. I'm a newbie, but there were a couple of tips I picked up from my first run. So I'm on my second listen through your audio book, and I'm realizing "Oh I should've actually read this too so I would make sure that it landed" because I started to rush it, and I'm like "I've been dabbling in this for a while", and so I started to break through with the help of your tips, but I didn't follow your system precisely enough, and I fell back. And so what I, I want to get into that, because this is something that could happen to anybody so easily, your system totally addresses all of these things—it's awesome. Because when people try to go at it too fast, as you said, it's painful, it's easy to fail out. There's a lot of people, a friend of mine that I just talked to yesterday is convinced it just doesn't work, and it's unhealthy, and all this stuff. But I asked him one question, and I'm like "Okay, you already messed it up". One thing, he was having too much protein. It's really worth doing this. I mean, aside from performance, feeling better, thinking clearly, having freedom from cravings, I mean, the improvements in the immune system function and everything else, reduction of disease risk, what I've seen described with references all over the place. It's really worth it. It's actually used to treat cancer and so forth, with very, very promising results.

Mark [00:13:26]: So, Brendan, one thing I want to make clear is when I say painful, I don't want people to think it's painful-painful, it's just one of those things where it's uncomfortable if your brain has been used to getting glucose all the time, and whenever you were hungry you reached for the bagel or the coffee, or whatever sugary snack it was to top off your blood glucose. A brain that is used to that, that is then deprived intentionally of lots of sugar, and is sort of forced to start to build metabolic machinery to burn ketones, that brain gets a little woozy, gets a little hangry, it gets a little cranky. So it doesn't really hurt, it's not painful-painful. Maybe I ought to rephrase that.

Brendan [00:14:18]: Well I use expressive language sometimes myself, figuratively. But for me actually, I will use, I'll own the word painful because I have had such a struggle with brain-fog for a long time after having my microbiome decimated and so forth. I've probably mentioned this numerous times in this event. For me, I have to be able to make it work, otherwise I just abandon stuff. So I've been struggling, and as I started to break through, it was like the clouds parted, like "Oh my God, this is amazing". I added two pull ups to my pull-up capacity like overnight, as I started to feel that things were shifting. And then I botched it. I'll explain that in a minute, but I was just going to mention that what seemed to help, one of the things that helped me shift, was exercising in the morning, gently, at aerobic or below threshold, and then fasting a bit, and then breaking the fast with fat. Another thing that I don't know if you've ever heard of this or looked into this but, when I started to feel the shift happening it was just after starting to take some CBD oil for the first time in my life, and I looked it up very quickly. I just thought "Oh it looks like there's actually a connection between cannabinoids in our system and ketogenic metabolism". Do you know anything about that, is it possible?

Mark [00:15:54]: I haven't seen good research on that yet, and I'm interested in it, and I've tried the CBD oil, and I think that the problem right now is that everybody's making really outrageous claims for CBD oil for everything. There may be some benefits to it. I mean I've tried it, and haven't really gotten that much noticeable change. I suspect that we have cannabinoid receptors throughout our bodies, so that CBD oil that would then attach to those receptors might have some signaling effects that would be beneficial. But I haven't really seen a lot of good research which isn't to say that ... I mean, as we go through this interview, you're going to realize that we're in a whole new realm with this keto way of eating that there's not a lot of great research. There's a crap load of anecdotal stuff that's amazing. So I suspect that the research will eventually bear a lot of this out. Clearly there's research that looks at athletes over six weeks and sees amazing results in those people. There's some great research in the medical field with kids with neurological issues that respond extremely well to a ketogenic diet because the brain loves ketones. It would rather burn ketones than glucose in most cases. But for the general population, and looking at all of these things that we sort of check off the box, there still are not a tremendous number of broad studies. They might look at fifteen people and see some great results, but I can't wait until we look at a study that looks at twenty thousand type 2 diabetics who underwent a keto eating strategy, and I will predict we will see basically cures from type 2 diabetes from that. You asked earlier who might benefit best from that, I would say as a population, type 2 diabetics would absolutely, under supervision of a physician, would absolutely see pretty amazing results because this is really about getting off of that blood sugar, that glucose dependency. It's about reacquiring the ability to dispose of glucose through insulin and through other means, insulin sensitivity. That's what I can't wait to see, these larger studies that I think will be eye-popping.

Brendan [00:18:23]: Yeah, and getting into ketosis for the first time or getting back into it if you've fallen out of it, I wanted to touch upon that. You've raised the issue of certain lifestyle factors also have to be in place. Not just the macronutrient ratios and so forth. What I did that knocked me out was, I was feeling so good, and I was working obsessively on something, I stayed up until three, and I'm not good at sleeping in so I woke up four hours later, I felt great. I don't know how many hours later I went and exercised. I was very fasted, under-rested, feeling great, exercised extra intensely.

Mark [00:19:10]: Classic.

Brendan [00:19:11]: Not too long later, I started to feel really hungry, but I had a meeting with a friend, and all I had to grab was a few teaspoons of coconut flakes, and it wasn't enough. And after that for days, and that's where I'm at now, I'm struggling, I'm back in the blood sugar thing. So I never fully broke through, I just started experiencing something, I thought "Oh, I'm here". So it's been fun and interesting.
I wonder if you could talk about the pitfalls and the various lifestyle factors that have to be in place for this to work. Because you can do everything right dietarily, and it wouldn't work for you.

Mark [00:19:52]: Sure. So a couple of things, first of all, we are trying to develop metabolic flexibility. Let's go back to that original premise. What it means is with metabolic flexibility, on those days that there's no food available, you're really adept at taking that fat out of your body fat stores and burning it as energy. Taking some of it, sending it to the liver, making ketones, sending that to the brain, using the ketones instead of glucose for energy for the brain. So this metabolic flexibility is what really gives you that ability to go through the day without having to think about "What am I going to eat?" and "When's the next meal?" But it takes a while to develop that metabolic flexibility. You could be in ketosis and you could be making ketones and have your urine strips be purple and be three, four, five millimolar on your blood ketone analysis, but still not have developed yet the metabolic flexibility which would allow you to then, in the presence of a lot of, let's just say you had a day where you had a 170g of carbs, to get out of ketosis but not even notice the difference, not feel like "Oh one day I was in ketosis, the other I wasn't". If you're metabolically flexible you're able to get energy from all these different substrates. And that takes a while, so that's why we recommend six weeks of being in keto to really develop that kind of metabolic flexibility. Otherwise, if you get out in the first couple of days or the first couple of weeks, you haven't built the metabolic flexibility yet, so now you're sort of suffering from having gone off the rails a little bit, or gone off the program.

In your case, and let's talk about that, one of the things, one of the responses that the body has initially to a low blood sugar, when the brain is still sort of craving glucose, the brain sends signals to the adrenals, the adrenals secrete cortisol, cortisol is an emergency, flight or fight hormone and the effect of cortisol, one of the many effects of cortisol is it encourages gluconeogenesis, it encourages your body to make sugar because this is a flight or fight sort of effect. At the same time it encourages your body to store fat and not want to take fat out of that storage. So now you have this dual mechanism—you're making sugar, which is raising the blood sugar; you're not able to access the fat that you otherwise so readily were able to take out of your fat store and use for energy. Now you go to the gym, and you really can't do much of a workout, you don't have much glycogen in your muscles and the gluconeogenesis part of that is struggling to keep up and can't really produce glucose at that high a rate, to do a hard workout. So when we don't get a lot of sleep, and sleep is one of the most important aspects of this, and the most overlooked elements of this. When we don't get a lot of sleep, cortisol goes up, when we're under stress, working hard, we've got projects going, cortisol goes up and so our ability to manage that aspect of this process is critical because, as you say, you can get all of the macros right, you can get all the fat, protein, carbohydrates numbers dialed in and go "Dude, I'm doing what you said. How come I'm not getting the results?" It's because there are really critical other aspects of this that need to be addressed, otherwise you'll get into that no man's land of being low carb but still sending signals to your body to require sugar. And it's taking this evasive action. So that's probably what was going on with you. And that's why we spend a lot of time, as you know in the book, addressing these other lifestyle factors. And by the way, these aren't unique to the keto lifestyle, everybody needs to get their sleep dialed in, everybody wants to lower the amount of cortisol they produce as a response technique, it's a stress response. It's just that now it really starts to show up in your experiment of one.

Brendan [00:24:12]: We also need to be moving. It's a really good point you make in your book. We need to be moving consistently because just being … well, define the active couch potato syndrome, because I'm one of those people, Gosh, darn it.

Mark [00:24:32]: I've seen a lot more research on this. It's pretty cool. Something that came out a couple of months ago which looked at energy expenditure over broad populations. They looked at hunter-gatherer societies, and they looked at urban societies. And they realized that the body has this fairly narrowly defined window of energy it's willing to expend in a day, and if you're an athlete like I was, and I would be out just busting my butt running twenty miles a day, riding a hundred miles on my bike, or whatever, that's a lot of energy that's being expended, and so the body has this compensation mechanism that then wants me to go home and watch TV and sit on the couch. So the active couch potato syndrome kind of refers to people who just go to the gym and do all the work at the gym and then don't do much the rest of the day. They might still take the elevator to their tenth floor office job, or they might still park their car right in front of their work, or they might whatever. They don't benefit from the movement that we talk about as being so critical to not just the keto strategy but to life in general.

So the active couch potato would be all of these people who think that they're doing the right thing by going to the gym and putting in a workout but then that's where they've used all their energy for the day, and there's none left to go about the day. What we suggest is you dissipate the energy throughout the day. Find ways to move throughout the day easily. And when you move more easily at a low level of output, guaranteed, you're only burning fat. So that's improving your fat metabolism doing that. And then for the most part, fine, if you're going to do a workout, do a short hard work out, or do a longer slower workout, but just make sure that you're moving throughout the day, rather than just putting it all into this one forty-five minute concentrated period, and then saying "Okay, I did all the movement for the day. I'm done. Check that off the list".

Brendan [00:26:46]: What's shocking to me is the research that's coming out indicating that if you're sedentary for long periods during the day, there are things that happen to the body that are not necessarily fixed by just getting into the gym for 45 minutes every day or every other day. That's the thing that I have to address, and I'm not active enough either, but rather than a couch potato, I'm more of a not active enough desk jockey, and even if I don't get in the gym a lot, I need to be getting up and walking around every hour.

Mark [00:27:20]: Are you sitting now, or are you standing?

Brendan [00:27:21]: Yeah, I'm sitting.

Mark [00:27:22]: I have a stand up desk. I'm standing right now.

Brendan [00:27:27]: Fantastic.

Mark [00:27:28]: Here, I don't know if I could show you this but, this is my … can you see this setup here?

Brendan [00:27:33]: Yeah, yeah.

Mark [00:27:35]: So I've got a leaning post, and I'm leaning right now, but I'll just stand up right now. But I mean, I stand, and I can sit, and whatever all day long. But if I'm going to be talking to you I've got a leaning post. It keeps my hip flexors wide open, so I'm not seated like boom-boom [gesturing to indicate a 90 degree angle between torso and legs]. I'm more like about like that, or even more like that [gesturing to indicate about a 135 degree angle between torso and legs] as I'm leaning on it. And then I have a pebbled mat that I stand on so I get the tactile sensation of being on rocks while I'm working at my desk and doing whatever I'm doing, creating. So these are little hacks, I guess you call them, that you could put into life. I mean I take frequent breaks. If I take a phone call I'll walk around the house or outside. I work out at my house, but I'll walk around the yard and pace while I'm on a phone call. Those are the ways that I can find to move throughout the day.

Brendan [00:28:34]: I've got to check that out. I had not even heard of a leaning post, but I totally get the biomechanical advantages there as well as physiological-metabolic ones from moving a little bit all the time and not being stuck.

Mark [00:28:50]: What's interesting is that even the people who are big on stand-up desks, would say, you still need to move, standing isn't the cure. I don't know if you know who Katie Bowman is, but she's a bio-mechanist, and she's big on this fact that even if you have a stand-up desk, you still have to change positions, you've got to change the height of the desk up and down, you can change the tilt of the desk so your arms are in different planes of motion or ranges of motion throughout the day. It's kind of a fun challenge to figure out ways in which to move and still get your work done and not piss your boss off.

Brendan [00:29:26]: I'm already pissed off at my boss which is me [laughs]. One of the things that appeals to me about the ketogenic diet is that it is inherently a low to moderate protein diet. So I believe it has the potential to contribute to a reduction in the consumption and therefore the cultivation of grains and grain fed animals which are two of the worst contributors to ecological destruction on the planet, especially in our conventional chemical industrial system. Actually, both types of products can be in a regenerative system so it's not just an "especially", but in those models. And what I find and probably other people do as well, is one health book to another, one food philosophy to another, the protein requirements vary all over the map from the less than half a gram per kilogram of body weight to even more than two in some rare instances.

Mark [00:30:33]: Yeah, bodybuilders.

Brendan [00:30:34]: How do you come up with yours, and what research is that based on?

Mark [00:30:40]: We sort of took a weighted average of all of the systems out there, and then we also looked at the recent science, because again, this whole concept shifts a little bit when you are keto. When you're not keto, when you're a sugar burner, the protein requirements are probably a little bit higher because you're a sugar burner. The fact that you only know how to burn sugar—I say only, but you're not very good at burning fat; you're not very good at burning ketones—so if you're a sugar burner, and you haven't built up the metabolic machinery to burn fat, when you run out of glucose, like you skip a meal, again, that whole mechanism, the brain says "Whoa, there's no blood sugar; there's no glucose, I don't know how to function without this fuel", cortisol gets secreted. Cortisol then goes and literally one of its effects is to strip amino acids from muscle tissue, sends those amino acids to the liver to become glucose, to be made into glucose, so it may be that a sugar burner has higher protein requirements simply because they waste protein. They burn it. They combust it, and that's probably the absolute last fuel you want to reach for even if you're metabolically flexible. The order of events would be, if I'm metabolically flexible I want to burn the fat off my plate first; I want to burn the fat off my butt second; I want to burn the ketones that I'm creating through my liver; I want to burn the glucose that's in the food I'm eating right now; I want to burn the glycogen that's in the muscles; the last thing I want to go to is protein as a last resort fight or flight mechanism to create glucose.

In those cases, a lot of these original metrics for determining protein requirements probably, knowingly or not, account for loss in the combustion of amino acids as a fuel source, when it probably shouldn't be. So when you are keto-adapted, when you're fat adapted, one of the major benefits of this is, the body starts to look at protein, and says "Well, we're not going to burn it; we're so good at burning fat; we're so good at burning ketones, so we're not going to burn protein; we're not going to take in so much in excess that we have to deaminate it and pee it out" because that's what happens to a lot of people taking excessive protein. They either turn it into sugar, or it's too much for the body to handle or more than the body wants, shall we say, and so the body has a process to deaminate the amino acids and then pee them out. In the case of a ketogenic eater, and one who's developed this metabolic flexibility, one of the effects of being keto is an upregulation of these genes that preserve protein, that preserve amino acids, that keep the amino acids within the body, and we have lots of storage capacity for amino acids in the body, it's sort of an amino acid pool or amino acid "sink" that we refer to. So it may be that your daily protein requirements when you're keto are 50, 60g a day if you're a man, 45g if you're a woman. And what I've learned from myself is that in no case, when you are well metabolically adapted, do you really ever need more than say a 100, 110g of protein in a day. And that winds out being for most people 0.7g per pound of lean body mass, something like that. And that's a high end. Guys like Ron Rosedale, Dr. Ron Rosedale, which say even that's too much because you're so good at recycling protein when you are keto that maybe it's 45, 50, 60g a day. I don't go that low, but I'm really intrigued by the research that would suggest that the efficiency … I talk about metabolic flexibility, and then I also talk about metabolic efficiency, the ability not only to burn different substrates to extract energy but to do so with great efficiency so that you need fewer calories to get you throughout the day. And that addresses your point that you made earlier on about, feeding the world. I've found that since I improved my metabolic flexibility I need 30% fewer calories now than I did five years ago when I read all the Harris Benedict equations about "Well, I'm a guy who needs 2600-2700 calories a day." No, I only need 2100 calories a day, 2000 calories some days. The other thing which is pretty cool about keto and metabolic flexibility is you not only unburden yourself from having to eat every meal, you unburden yourself of having to think about macros every day because now we talk about not just a day at a time but, as long as I've got all my protein requirements for the weekend, it didn't matter that I had 120 on one day and 40 on another, and 70 on another, because it all evens out because the body has this new-found capacity to manage protein throughput in a way that … it's a skill that you never developed when you were just a sugar burner.

Brendan [00:36:18]: But that same flexibility with the protein, doesn't necessarily apply to the carbs, correct? In other words, there's got to be a daily limit on carbs, is that correct?

Mark [00:36:32]: Yes, when you're building the metabolic machinery, when you're keto, you want to limit the carbs every day. Having done that—and this is the most important thing about The Keto Reset—I called it "keto reset" because you're resetting your metabolism, and if you do it appropriately and you spend enough time keto, in most of the research, guys like Dom D'Agostino who's like the number one, I would say the go-to guy in the ketogenic world, would say, six weeks is that sweet spot where you get 95% of the benefits you're going to get. From six weeks on, you can choose to stay there forever. I know people that have been keto for ten years. But going back to one of our original premises, I love to eat different types of food, so I'm not in keto all the time. I'm in what I call "the keto zone" which means I did the work. I did the reset. I built a metabolic flexibility. I spent two months keto, and I'll do that every year with great precision. Having done that, somedays I'm at 30g of carbs, totally a keto day. Some days I'm at 140g of carbs, totally a not keto day. But what's important is I don't notice the difference in how I feel, I don't notice any difference in how I feel. You'll see people who have been keto for a long time or some amount of time, and say "Well, jeez, if I have 80g of carbs in one day, I'm kicked out of keto, and it takes me three days of feeling like crap to get back in". That's not metabolic flexibility, that's a damaged metabolism. The metabolic flexibility goes back to our ancestors, if you look at evolution, you look at how elegant this system is. We're wired to overeat because food was so scarce, whenever we came across food, we're kind of wired to overeat, and then we're also genetically wired to store excess calories as fat. How cool is that? You can carry a gas tank around with you, in the context of evolution. And then when there's no food available for a day, or two days, or three days, draw upon that gas tank for energy and not have it affect you negatively, not have you pissing and moaning, and whiney and hangry, and "Oh my gosh, the world is coming to an end, and if I don't eat lunch, I don't know what's going to happen". No, this was how we're designed, we're designed to have this metabolic efficiency to be able to store it very well and to be able to take it out of storage and burn it very well and with that in mind we would understand then that our ancestors wouldn't be focusing on macros all the time, like "Oh my God, I ate too many carbs today. I'm going to feel like crap".

Brendan [00:39:19]: Could you imagine the survival odds in the Ice Age world?

Mark [00:39:24]: No! So the intention is to develop this sort of metabolic flexibility and efficiency so that given the fact that you're not eating crap, okay, we've got to assume you're not eating cakes and pies, and candies and cookies, sweetened beverages and all that stuff, you know, a lot. This metabolic flexibility just allows us to say, "you know what, I'm going to have a sweet potato with dessert"—not dessert, well, maybe "For dessert tonight I'm going to have a bowl of berries and a little bit of whipped cream on it" you know, some amount of flexibility there to not be so rigidly keto. So that's why I call it "the keto zone" because some days, at the end of the day, I go "wow, I was like totally keto today. I had 20g of carbs all day. I only had one meal"—a piece of steak and some broccolini or something. Other days I go "Wow, jeez." I had somebody sent me a paleo treat as a sample. I tried that. It was good. But because I've built this flexibility, I don't notice the difference from one day to the next, and that's the definition of metabolic flexibility.

Brendan [00:40:35]: Got it. I'm curious, we're speaking about this, and we haven't mentioned it but, obviously you are one of the fathers of the Paleo-Primal-Ancestral movement so clearly your research and experience has led you to believe that humans require animal protein and animal fat as part of their diet. There are other people who obviously prefer to use an entirely plant-based diet, and I'm curious, do you know anybody using keto for a plant-based diet, maybe somebody who's actually a researcher and an educator, and what's been the result there?

Mark [00:41:18]: I don't know any researchers or educators doing a totally plant-based keto program because first of all if it's totally plant-based … and I have a lot of people who claim to be vegetarians and then I find out they're eating eggs, egg protein.

Brendan [00:41:32]: Well that would be a lacto-ovo vegetarian, it wouldn't be a vegan obviously.

Mark [00:41:35]: Correct, not a vegan. I think that being a vegan, I can give you an example of somebody who might do well on this, and that would be somebody who's morbidly obese, who has a lot of body fat to cut into, who would take advantage of some of the plant-based protein supplements that are out there now and then who would eat mostly plant-based throughout the day. I could envision a vegan opportunity there to completely go keto without using animal protein. You could use MCT oil because that comes from coconut, you could use coconut oil, you can use avocado oil, so clearly you can get your healthy fats. Historically the problem with vegans has been that they've also avoided fat. Even a lot of the plant fats. If you're vegan, and you want to go keto, you have to embrace the concept of having significant amounts of healthy fats in your diet. That would be the shift. But I feel pretty confident that I could work with somebody who's got a lot of weight to lose, who wants to be plant-based, who wants to be vegan in this pursuit and then start to take advantage of some of the plant-based proteins that are out there and use those to be sure that that person is getting an adequate amount of protein along with the fat, and then I could make it work.

Brendan [00:43:05]: But if they're not extremely overweight, are you suggesting that maybe a vegan approach wouldn't be as good for them?

Mark [00:43:13]: Well it's just, it's difficult because if you're not significantly overweight, or if you're at a good weight now, and you're trying to be a plant-based keto eater, the only way that you could get into ketosis is by forcing your body to make ketones because the body says there's not enough carbohydrates. So if your diet is largely carbohydrate, because plants have a lot of carbs in them, you either are eating a lot of grains to get the carbs, or you're eating a lot of vegetables. And if you eat a lot of vegetables which I'm a 100% in favor of, you can't get, I don't know how many pounds of vegetables you'd have to eat in a day to get enough carbs to keep you going. So you'd have to take your intake way down so your carbs are still under say 80g of carbs a day, and that would limit the amount of plants you can take in. And then obviously you'd have to up your fat intake through the oils, and probably supplement with some protein powder to make it work, so it could work but you probably have to enter ketosis more from the low-cal side of things, than just the low-carb side of things.

Brendan [00:44:32]: I guess as long as you have adequate fat, as long as you have...

Mark [00:44:35]: Right, unless you have adequate fat. But then again, for most vegans, the reason they're vegan, well there's two, one is animal concern, but the other is that they're eschewing fats of most types.

Brendan [00:44:49]: I don't think you can make that generalization any longer. It might've been the case.

Mark [00:44:52]: Well if you're the type of guy like McDougall ...

Brendan [00:44:54]: Yes, certainly McDougall and the starch, but I would say not all ...

Mark [00:45:00]: Yeah, I know, I agree.

Brendan [00:45:01]: ... [not all] vegans are starchivore-based.

Mark [00:45:03]: Well, I'd love to see more research, and even more anecdotal stuff on vegans who are attempting to go keto. For sure. It's just a lot easier if you avail yourself of animal protein.

Brendan [00:45:15]: Right. I lost my train of thought there, what was I going to say.

Mark [00:45:23]: In terms of the animal protein thing, if we sort of have a grey area of eggs and milk, you know, dairy products and cheese and stuff like that, that allows a lot of people who are lacto-ovo vegetarian. I mean there are even a people who say I'm a vegetarian but I eat fish, not really a vegetarian but ...

Brendan [00:45:48]: So I've heard Nora Gedgaudas say "If you look at my plate, at first glance you're not going to realize that I eat meat, you're going to think I might be a vegetarian, because there's so many vegetables."

Mark [00:45:58]: Same here. Totally, same here.

Brendan [00:46:59]: Same with you, same with me.

Mark [00:46:00]: Oh I have a big, big, big bowl of salad every day. That's my main meal. By volume it's like 95% vegetables but I have 25, 30g of protein on top of it. I douse it with the Primal Kitchen salad dressing, so I have some healthy fat on there. That's my major meal of the day. I can take the meat off that salad, and it would be a great keto vegetarian meal as well. At the end of the day I have some form of protein, maybe some fish, maybe some chicken and a triple serving of grilled vegetables. I've made this comment many times: I think I eat more vegetables than most vegetarians.

Brendan [00:46:45]: Right, because they're typically eating so many grains and beans. Now, for people that struggle metabolically in various ways, myself being one of them, I've created a lifelong obsession now with food quality, with nutrient density in food, with how our food system either restores nutrient density to our food supply or continues to erode it. What I'm wondering is, do you think that people that struggle more making the transition might have an issue with mineral deficiency and/or an accumulation of chemicals either from our food or from the environment that are metabolic inhibitors?

Mark [00:47:27]: Could be both, could be one or the other. We're all metabolically the same in terms of how we process things, how we make muscle, how we burn fat, how our immune system works. It's just the degree to which these things happen that vary from individual to individual, and in some cases many of us are more sensitive to environmental toxins. Some of us have decades of metabolic damage that is not going to be undone or fixed in six weeks of keto eating. Clearly the produce grown today does not reflect the produce grown in the 40s when the RDAs, and when they were analyzing the mineral content of so many of the vegetables and fruits and things that we're depending on. So I sort of grieve for our lands today and all the damage that's been done, and how every generation of a new crop has less and less nutrition in it. So I would agree with you that the mineral issue with people who are embarking on a keto eating strategy, you should pay attention to minerals. A lot of people would say "I'll take up just a bouillon cube that's got some sodium and chloride and magnesium or potassium or whatever," and take a mineral supplement as part of a strategy to keep you on track, because if you're just depending on those vegetables for your minerals it may be that they're probably not providing what you think they're providing.

Brendan [00:49:12]: Right. Last question real quick, what do you think of exogenous ketone supplements?

Mark [00:49:18]: It's a mixed bag because if you're metabolically efficient, and you've built the metabolic ability to burn ketones, you've done the work, then ketone supplements can be very beneficial in certain circumstances. I use them on occasion before I go to the gym and do a heavy leg day, or before I play Ultimate Frisbee on Sunday because I'm going to be sprinting for two hours with twenty-somethings. And sometimes, by the way, I've used them ... like I take a ketone supplement maybe a half hour before I give a talk, if it's at three thirty in the afternoon or four o'clock in the afternoon, and I haven't eaten that day. So I use them as performance-enhancing drugs, but to think that you could take ketone supplements to get you into ketosis and speed up your process, I'm not buying that because I think that this works because your body gets signals that it has to increase the number of mitochondria, that it has to increase the efficiency of the mitochondria, that it has to learn to become better at burning fat, that it has to build the enzymes to take that out of the storage, and it has to do all this work to create this system, this metabolic machinery that you can then use to burn off your stored body fat and preserve your muscle tissue. So just taking a ketone supplement to raise ketones, doesn't do anything. It's like, people who get into ketosis initially ... by the way, let's talk about ketosis and what it means. Ketosis means an excess of ketones in the blood stream. Ketosis doesn't mean you're burning fat. It doesn't mean you're burning ketones. It just means you have extra ketones in your blood, because you either took ketone supplements to raise them or your liver started making more ketones because you were low on glucose, and you're a sugar burner, you know, and then sent a signal to your brain, "We've got to make ketones, because there's no glucose". You don't "win the game" by having high blood ketones. In fact people that have been in ketosis for five, ten years, who are consuming 20 to 30 or 40g of carbs a day, every day, religiously, they might show 0.5 millimolar or 0.4 millimolar in terms of ketones, which would by definition "not be in ketosis" but they're clearly keto, and the reason is, they've become so efficient in their use of ketones, that the liver says, "I don't need to waste this energy in the urine, I can just make enough ketones that the brain is happy, and that's all I need to make. I don't need to pump massive amounts of ketones into the blood stream." That's an ironic kind of place where you arrive at when you realize that those who have been keto for a long time show the least amount of, not the least, but they show minimal amounts of ketones in their blood stream just because they've become so good at measuring how much ketones they need. The body becomes so good at titering the amount of ketones. It doesn't waste it. And the body doesn't want to waste any energy. That's why different people tend to get fatter, and fatter, and fatter over time. The body says, "I don't want to waste energy." Otherwise, you have to force it to waste it.

Brendan [00:52:30]: That's a really good point to complete on. It's not about necessarily the readings in this case on a meter. It's about the result of your body having adapted to hormetic stressors, essentially that's what it is, and we need those hormetic stressors, and this carbohydrate restriction is just more of them, at least that's my interpretation. Would you say that's accurate?

Mark [00:52:54]: I wouldn't refer to it as hormetic stressor because to me a hormetic stressor is the forty-seven degree pool that I jump in every night before I go to bed.

Brendan [00:53:03]: This is more like just factory blueprint, like "stop abusing your metabolism".

Mark [00:53:06]: This is making food choices that signal your body. You trick your body into thinking there's not going to be glucose or carbohydrate for a while, and we need to make alternate plans. It's not a stressful event. I don't even like to use the word "stressor" for the body. You're just guiding the body to an alternative metabolic pathway that it is fully designed to do, under the right circumstances. It's just that in our modern time we never give it the right circumstance. We always have carbohydrates available, every minute of every day there's carbs available, and that's kind of how we guide ourselves down that path. Well, if we get ourselves off that path and start judiciously restricting carbs the body goes "Hey, I know how to do this, I've been doing this for two and a half million years, so you just got to give me the right signal." So what we're doing is we're figuring out what the signals are to create this metabolic flexibility.

Brendan [00:54:09]: Mark, it's been so awesome to receive the benefits of your hard-won experience, your dedicated research because, and in this case in particular, ketogenic metabolism is a game-changer. You're a game-changer, your book is a game-changer, it's a great handbook and resource, *The Keto Reset Diet*. So thanks for creating that and the great products you're creating, and thank you for being here with us in the Eat4Earth community.

Mark [00:54:34]: It's my pleasure.

Drew Manning Interview
The Emotional Journey of 6 Months to Fat and 30 Days to Fit

Brendan [00:00:00]: Welcome to the Eat4Earth event. We're exploring how you can heal yourself, your loved ones, and the planet, with food. This is Brendan Moorehead, and I'm excited to welcome our guest Drew Manning. Drew is the host of the hit A&E TV show *Fit2Fat2Fit*, a *New York Times* best-selling author of the book *Fit2Fat2Fit*, an NASM-certified fitness trainer and creator of the Fit2Fat2Fit brand. He has appeared on *The Dr. Oz Show*, *The Tonight Show*, and *Good Morning America*. Drew is best known for having gone to extreme measures to help people overcome weight issues, improve their health, and create the body of their dreams. And not only that, he has inspired many other fitness trainers to take their dedication and effectiveness to the next level by following his Fit2Fat2Fit example. Drew, it's great to have you here with us today.

Drew [00:00:47]: Thanks for having me, Brendan. It's my pleasure, man.

Brendan [00:00:50]: I was moved by listening to your *Fit2Fat2Fit* book on audio book. First I was moved by the fact that your commitment to helping people is so strong that you would risk your own health and everything it depends on in order to better understand the challenges faced by your clients. I was also impressed by the humility and compassion that you bring into helping people shift to healthy eating in order to lose weight and gain a healthy and fit body. Drew, why did you decide to go from super fit and healthy, to gaining sixty pounds on purpose and then losing all that weight and regaining your health and fitness?

Drew [00:01:26]: That's a great question, and honestly it was because I grew up my entire life in shape and that's all I knew. I played football and wrestling from a very young age, and so for me when I became a trainer it was hard for me to connect with my clients who were mostly overweight, and I couldn't understand why it was so hard for them just to do what I was telling them to do. I would give them their meal plans, their workouts, and say "Okay, there you go. Do it." And they would be like "Oh, I messed up. I had soda, even though you told me not to order it" and, you know "I had a hard day at work. I didn't go to the gym that day." And I would get frustrated like, "Why don't you just do it. It's not that hard. You just eat healthy, and you exercise, and boom, you'll see the results. I don't understand why it's so hard." And they'd tell me, " You know, Drew, you don't understand because for you it's easy, and it's always been easy. And for me it's really hard". And I kind of took that to heart, and so I was thinking of ideas, of ways I could better relate to my clients. And for whatever reason, the idea of getting fat on purpose—I know this sounds ridiculous and crazy—but it came to my brain, and I felt like, "Okay, this is my calling. I need to do this". It was so weird, but I really felt like it was something I needed to do. And that's the reason why I decided to do it, it was to gain a better understanding of what it was like to be overweight for the first time in my life. Because I never knew anything differently, I used to see it as something that was so easy until my clients were telling me otherwise, and I decided to step out of my comfort zone and try something kind of extreme, kind of crazy, to gain a better understanding.

Brendan [00:02:49]: I would assume that the hard part would be getting back into fitness, but was it also hard to break the healthy habits and gain the weight?

Drew [00:03:05]: Yes, for me it was really hard because I was more obsessed back then with my physique and working out, and eating healthy. And to let go of that was really hard mentally. I remember there were days when I was so jealous seeing people running on the side of the road, and people going to the gym, and I'm like, "Oh man, that used to be me". Because here's the thing—when you grow up your entire life in shape, part of your identity is based around what your body looks like, and so once my six-pack was gone, my muscles were gone, I kind of freaked out because I didn't know who I was anymore, I didn't know what my purpose was. I wanted to go to complete strangers and tell them, "Hey, I'm not really overweight, this is just an experiment. Here's my before picture, go to this website, this is what I used to look like", because that was who I was. And once I lost that it really caused me to reflect on "Okay, there's more to me than my body." But it really played a role in my self-esteem, my lack of self-confidence, as I got bigger. That was the hardest part of the journey, it wasn't just physically gaining the weight, but mentally and emotionally being overweight, in public, in front of my wife at the time, I would cover up in front of her, I wouldn't want her to see me naked, I didn't want to see myself naked. Those kinds of things I wasn't prepared for, and that was a lot of the surprise was on the mental-emotional side.

Brendan [00:04:20]: That sounds like the beginning of where you started to really get insight into where your clients are coming from that haven't had the decades of just being nothing but fit like you had.

Drew [00:04:32]: Yeah, and that's where I needed to connect with my clients. It was on the mental-emotional side. Because before all I could connect with them on was the physical side, changing up their macros, their calories, their meal plans, their workouts, but I didn't understand how to connect with them on that mental-emotional level because for me. I used to see it as something so easy that you just will power your way through, and you just do it. And then as I was getting bigger I started to realize, "Oh, this is so much more a mental and emotional transformation; it's so much more mental and emotional than I ever imagined." And that's where I was really humbled, and that's where I started thinking, "Okay, this is what my clients have been telling me".

Brendan [00:05:10]: When you began your journey back from fat to fit, for the first month you chose to only change your diet and not add exercise workouts. Why did you do that, and what did you notice and learn from just changing your eating habits?

Drew [00:05:23]: I wanted to show people the power of nutrition because so many of us think, "Oh if I just work out harder and longer, I'll get a six pack." Like "If I do a thousand crunches a day I'll have a six pack."

That's kind of the mentality of a lot of people here in America unfortunately. So I wanted to show people, "Hey, if you really want to see results, it's more so in your nutrition than it is with exercise," and there's new scientific studies backing that up, showing exercise really doesn't do a whole lot for your body composition. It's so much more in the nutrition. And so I decided to skip exercise for thirty days. I went from 5000 calories of foods, like Cinnamon Toast Crunch, and Mountain Dew, and white bread, and Spaghetti Os, and macaroni and cheese—all of these delicious processed American foods—to 2000 calories of real whole food for thirty days. That's the only change I made, and I dropped nineteen pounds in the first thirty days which was expected, but then all my blood work went back to normal levels. So I had non-alcoholic fatty liver disease. It developed within six months, which is crazy. I didn't drink any alcohol during my journey, but a lot of soda. A lot of people think, "Oh I don't drink alcohol," but they drink a lot of soda, and they don't think it does a lot of damage, but it does. And then my blood pressure was 167/113 at its highest. My testosterone dropped to the low two hundreds. All of that stuff within those 30 days of just changing my nutrition, went back to normal levels. My testosterone more than doubled, my blood pressure was normal, my HDL, LDL, triglycerides, fasting glucose levels, were all in the green after those thirty days of just changing my nutrition.

Brendan [00:07:02]: Did you notice your taste buds change when you went from the healthy diet to the unhealthy diet and then back?

Drew [00:07:10]: Yeah, that's a really good question I get asked that a lot. I really do believe your taste buds do change and adapt. Here's the thing—the highly palatable food that we have here in America tastes really good. Cinnamon Toast Crunch, Twinkies, Mountain Dew, Doritos, Pringles, all of these foods taste really good. I had it straight for six months, and I understand how it creates an addiction for some people when you eat these foods every single day. Now the interesting thing, one of the biggest lessons I learned was on the journey back to fit. So I transitioned from eating those foods to cold turkey now eating broccoli and spinach and kale and mushrooms and chicken and turkey and all these healthy foods, and I remember the foods did not taste nearly as good. On top of that the withdrawal symptoms were way more powerful than I thought. It was like I was going through a detox where my body wanted the high from those processed foods again, but I was giving it these healthy foods. And I thought ,"Okay, I'm going to feel good again" but no, I felt like crap for two weeks. I had headaches, I was moody, I was grumpy, and here I am an advocate of eating healthy, but finally it clicked for me, this is what my clients go through when I try to put them on a meal plan of eating healthy whole food because their bodies have been adapted to eating this way so long, and the food doesn't taste nearly as good. It's not as highly palatable. Any kid in the world is going to choose marshmallows over broccoli, for the most part. Same thing with adults. We've been trained to eat that way for so long, and now you're saying, "Okay I'm going to eat healthy" and it takes a while to adjust your taste buds, I believe, to adjust at some point, but you've just got to be patient with yourself.

Brendan [00:08:46]: So how long did it take for you to start to relish broccoli and spinach and so forth?

Drew [00:08:53]: After about two weeks the cravings became manageable, and the food did become tastier I would say, because I did start to eliminate those foods out of my body and just was constantly eating those foods. So I would say a good two to four weeks is when I started to notice some changes in my cravings. I started feeling better again, higher energy. But for each person it's going to be different. Some people might still think broccoli tastes horrible. To each their own, but if that's all you have available, then you're going to eat it, right? You're not going to starve if you have something as healthy as broccoli to eat, but anyways, I would say two to four weeks.

Brendan [00:09:32]: What I've noticed, I mean, I've been a healthy eater for a long time, but I go in and out of, let's say vegetable-intensive periods punctuated by some periods where I have some ice-cream, and it's feeding the bacteria in my gut that love ice cream. And the science is now showing us that that's actually one of the big drivers -- whether we're feeding the black wolf or the white wolf in our intestines. That's the one that tells us which food it wants, and tells us which salad bar or which drive-through to go to. I've found that I totally crave, the more salad I eat, the more I crave it.

Drew [00:10:16]: Yeah, basically gut bacteria and how that drives some of our cravings, right? I've read some new science about that and how that actually drives cravings. And so that bacteria wants it, and it'll get it, and that's what causes us to want that food sometimes. So it is scary, but it is possible if you can stay consistent. If you choose ice cream over broccoli 90% of the time, it's going to be hard to initially wean off of that. But it's really interesting how addictive it can become for some people.

Brendan [00:10:46]: In your book you make some distinctions between dieting, eating, and lifestyle. What's the difference between those and between eating as a lifestyle and eating for weight loss?

Drew [00:10:57]: Yeah, so for me, the diet mentality that we are obsessed with here in America is "What's the quickest way to lose the most amount of weight with the least amount of effort?" That right there is the diet mentality that so many Americans are obsessed with. That's why we always watch these TV shows where it's like "What's the new diet?" and they read the magazines like, "Lose ten pounds in ten days". That's the diet mentality that we're obsessed with here in America that we see all the time. People can do these short term things where they sacrifice their wellbeing and their happiness, to starve themselves or whatever, to lose a lot of weight. But it's not sustainable for 90% of people because they're depriving themselves of calories and nutrients and all kinds of things, and they focus all of their value on just weight loss alone. For me, lifestyle is something that's sustainable over time. It's nothing extreme. To make a lifestyle change, in my opinion, the difference is knowing how to overcome your mental and emotional challenges. Diet you can do short term for thirty days and just hunker down and just sacrifice and do it and lose the weight. But then you're like, "Okay, that has an end date". A lifestyle, there is no finish line, there is no end date. It's something you continuously do, that you make a priority every single day in your life. That's the difference between a lifestyle and a diet in my opinion.

Brendan [00:12:18]: Does this require a lot of, I mean, the lifestyle that you embrace and teach, does it require, it sounds like it's not requiring a lot of deprivation but maybe some discipline.

Drew [00:12:29]: Yeah, any kind of lifestyle change, whether is a health lifestyle, or financial lifestyle, or a religious lifestyle, where you're trying to live a certain way, any kind of lifestyle change is going to require some type of discipline. There's no easy way to get through life. There's no easy path in life. Whether it's a health, or financial way or religious, you have to sacrifice something and you've got to be disciplined. But if it's a priority and you have a strong enough "why", then I feel like you're going to make it a priority in your life. If you have a "why" of why you want to be healthy, that's more than just "I want to look good." If it's more like "I want to be healthy for my kids and teach them good examples, and be around for grandkids" and things like that, those kinds of "whys" that are bigger, that stick with people, that help them make it a priority and make it into a lifestyle change.

Brendan [00:13:21]: And having a torso like Drew Manning doesn't hurt either.

Drew [00:13:25]: Of course not. But what I want to do is help people realize it's not about the looks. Healthy looks different on everybody. We think healthy is what we see on Instagram models, or in the magazines, "Oh, that's what I need to look like to be healthy", but I can tell you straight up that there's a lot of people with six packs that are skinny, that are dying on the inside. Just because you're losing weight, just because you're skinny, doesn't mean you are healthy. Focus on the healthy habits and the process, and let the results fall where they may. And yes weight loss and looks can be a byproduct of living that healthy lifestyle over time, but don't equate physical looks with health all the time.

Brendan [00:14:05]: In regard to different approaches to eating, there's quite a few different trends, we've got intermittent fasting, and of course there's relationships between them but, intermittent fasting, ketogenic diets, and the old calorie counting, you know, calories in minus calories out, there's calorie restriction, which has been a part of all the historical diets you were kind of alluding to, and then other dietary strategies, avoiding lectins and so forth. I'm just curious what your take is on these and how they fit together in your approach.

Drew [00:14:41]: For my personal journey, it has been interesting, I kind of was more of the bodybuilder type of diet years ago when I got into the fitness industry—you know, six small meals a day, Tupperware container, bringing it with me everywhere I go, counting your macros and calories and things like that. And then I got sick of that. And yes, it works. I looked great. And so I maybe transitioned into the ketogenic diet about three years ago, and here's the interesting thing—my physique didn't really change. My performance in the gym was about the same. But I went from eating six meals a day to two meals a day. My brain felt so much sharper, my digestion was a lot better, and I didn't have any lags in energy throughout the day, my improvement in cognitive function and mental clarity was like night and day from where it was before. That's why I fell in love with the ketogenic diet, for me it was because it felt like it was more so nutrition for my brain, and I didn't have to be a slave to food as much. But I really do think that different things work for different people.

My advice to people is you can read all you want about keto, and paleo, and vegan and whatever it is. Become your own self-experimentation, find what's optimal for you, and the only way to do that is to do your research and then give each protocol a try for at least sixty days. Don't try it out for a couple of days and say, "Well it didn't work for me, I didn't lose weight." Do at least sixty days of a certain protocol, maybe take some data down, some markers, before, like a baseline, and then see how things change. So get your body fat tested, get your blood work done, do some measurements, and then measure it again in sixty days and see if you're moving in the right direction. And if you are, then maybe it's a good thing for you at that time in your life. And then from there move forward. But I have to always be open to upgrading and tweaking things as I move along, because I think what works for you one day, won't always work for you twenty years later. You've got to be open to new things that are changing as our bodies change. For me right now the ketogenic diet with intermitted fasting and some periods of extended fasting which I've started doing recently, have been a game-changer. I just finished a three day fast, two days ago, and I feel fantastic. Last year I did the seven day fast, and it was a great experience, but it was a little bit long for me being as lean as I am, so I brought it down to three days, and I felt fantastic.

Brendan [00:17:06]: I think those are some really wise comments that bear repeating, not repeating, but emphasizing, where you said that certain things may work for you now, they may not work for you later depending on what's going on with your body. The impression I get from a lot of health educators or let's say diet educators like, "This is the way to go. You do this." There's so many approaches that work for different people at different times. Our metabolism goes through phases, we go in and out of detox phases, out of anabolic phases, we're re-building, you know, there's a lot of things. I can go into my whole spiel on metabolic typing, but what you had to say about ketogenic eating I feel is very relevant to the Eat4Earth event because you're talking about, in contrast to let's say the Atkins approach to the ketogenic diet, which is very heavy on protein, yours is lighter on protein, potentially very light on protein which can make it a more planet-friendly diet. What can you tell us about the role of protein, and particularly animal protein I suppose, in your approach to ketogenic eating?

Drew [00:18:21]: That's a great question. Here's the thing, the body building mentality that I kind of adapted when I first got into the fitness industry was you know, one gram of protein per pound of body weight. If you're two hundred pounds, you're trying to get in 200g of protein and you're chugging protein shakes and eating as much tuna, steak, chicken breast as you can. That's a lot to get in. When I went from that to a ketogenic diet, I cut that in half, even maybe more than a half some days, where I'm getting an 80 to 100g of protein and that's it. And I'm not losing my muscle mass because we've been taught you need protein to put on muscle. Right now my calories are about 70% fat, 25% protein, 5% carbs, so it's not nearly as much protein as I normally had back in the day. For me, I don't need to be taking supplements, protein shakes, whey protein, I don't take any of that anymore. All of it comes from mostly eggs, sea food, or fattier cuts of animal protein, but not in large quantities. I'm eating one to two times per day, and that's pretty much it, and I can't get in a 100g of protein in one meal, it's sometimes hard to get 50g of protein in one meal. It's so much easier to digest, my digestion is so much better. I don't have to meal prep all the time, and wasting food because if I meal plan too much, and there's too much and I don't get to it, I have to throw it away. Whereas now I'm only preparing one to two meals per day, and I'm good to go. My physique, my body composition is about the same; my brain performs so much better; my digestion is better. So it's really different than what we've been taught, especially people in the fitness industry, they still are slow to come to this conclusion, thinking, "Oh it's not going to work," but until they try it. So we're slowly getting there.

Brendan [00:20:09]: When it comes to sourcing animal protein, for people who are eating animal protein, is there anything in particular you look for, sourcing quality and let's say planet friendliness?

Drew [00:20:21]: Yeah, I'm a big believer and this wasn't just until recently, maybe a couple of years ago. I wanted to become more mainstream, and I've had doctors come on my podcast and educate me and others on the importance of the quality of the meat. Because we say you are what you eat, and one of my buddies, Sean Stephensen, that has that really popular podcast from *The Model Health Show*, he says "You are what you eat ate", or what that cow ate. Things that were put inside that cow, you're eating parts of that, and that affects us at the cellular level. Once I realized that then for me, I've always tried to buy healthier meats, not just the factory-farmed cheaper meat, but knowing the importance of grass-fed beef and free-range chicken and no hormones and no antibiotics. Now you see companies jumping on board with this and finally labeling those kinds of things. When in reality it shouldn't be that way. If you put antibiotics and hormones you should have to put that on the label, that you added this to it. Instead of the other way around when we have to let people know, "There's none of this, none of this, no, no, no" like you see all these labels now with these lists of things that aren't in them, which is how it should be naturally. So I definitely invest in that and being a dad to two daughters I will invest more money, because I know it's more expensive, for now, to get that high quality meat, but for me it's important for my girls to have that quality of meat as well.

Brendan [00:21:45]: I don't know if you're familiar with the book *The Plant Paradox* by doctor by Dr. Steven Gundry?

Drew [00:21:50]: I haven't read it, but I've heard of it.

Brendan [00:21:52]: He talks about how if we're eating factory-farmed animal products, those animals are raised on corn and soy, carrying corn and soy lectins that we haven't evolved with, our gut microbiome hasn't evolved with. And then we've got all the genetic modifications, genetically-modified corn and soy, bringing a protein from the snow plant in the case of Bt corn (**Correction:** Bt corn carries genes from a bacterium called *Bacillus thuringiensis* that produces the Bt toxin), which affects everybody, and now we're getting this into our body if we're eating chicken and beef and pork that were fed corn and soy, which all of it was, if it's not sourced from a strictly naturally. I shouldn't use the word "naturally" because that's a word that doesn't mean anything in food labeling. But if it's truly pastured and not fed these grains. He's (Dr. Gundry, author of *The Plant Paradox*) actually got clients that had to drop all chicken, beef, and pork from commercial sources to heal from certain diseases because after they dropped everything else, they were still getting problematic plant lectins and tag-along toxins through their meat sources, even if they were organic. Organic chicken was carrying corn and soy lectins that their body and their gut flora were not able to handle. Their gut flora was nuked by antibiotics or whatever and couldn't digested it, or those foods just hadn't been around so much in our diets for thousands of years that we could adapt. But some people do seem to tolerate, or not tolerate these things, better or worse than others. That's something to consider, that's sort of a hidden danger and health hazard sort of simmering away in the background is even organic but grain-fed animal products.

Drew [00:23:42]: Yeah, because that's not naturally what they would eat in Nature. That's a cheaper source of food for them. I'm a big believer in that, and the problem is a couple of things. One is education, letting people know the importance of that because I feel like all the studies done on meat have always been done on factory-farmed meat, low-quality meat, and that's where a lot of the problems we see with digestion in the country. The other problem is how much more expensive you're paying for grass-fed, pasture-raised meats that are available. You're going to have to pay a premium price. And so it's hard for your average person to be like, "Okay, I'm only going to eat this," and they're paying not almost double, but you know, sometimes it's more expensive. The more demand there is for it, it's going to drive those prices down, but how do you feed a whole nation where some people live in New York City where there's not a lot of farms around, or LA, so I don't know what the solution is. I'm just saying I see some of the problems, but we've got to fix it because this is what a lot of the illnesses and diseases of today are caused by, so it's a big, big problem.

Brendan [00:24:46]: Fortunately there actually is room on this continent to grow a lot more grass-fed beef, if it's done in a way that's called Holistic Management. For people who want to check that out, it's going to be featured, other speakers are talking about that in this event. But basically they're coming out with a certification that will make it easier to identify animals that have been raised naturally on grass, and I shouldn't use the world naturally—it means nothing—but raised in a way that actually grows soils, restores biodiversity and potentially mitigates climate change. And that's one of the big messages too in this event, if we're going to eat animal products, we've got to do it differently, and it can have a benefit for the planet instead of being extremely destructive like factory-farmed animals are, as well as being healthier for us. So when it comes to the price difference, sure it costs more right now, and that may change, but if we're eating a low-protein ketogenic diet, or lower protein anyhow, then maybe it's going to be a wash, maybe it's going to be net benefit, plus we've got all the beneficial fatty acids instead of the detrimental ones, we've got a higher omega-3 to omega-6 ratio in pastured animal products vs. inflammatory high omega-6 to omega-3 ratio in the commercial animal products. It's really a big reason like you pointed out, probably behind why animal products show up as carcinogens in the studies. We've got to look at how these animals are being raised.

Drew [00:26:29]: Exactly, but it's exciting times, we'll see where it will go from here.

Brendan [00:26:37]: So, just to kind of bring this around even more to food, when it comes to real food like spinach for example, do you notice differences for weight loss, health and fitness between spinach grown conventionally with pesticides, without taking care of the soil vs. spinach grown in other ways that are more holistic?

Drew [00:27:02]: That's a great question and there's a lot of controversy around this. For example in the whole world of "if fits your macros" right, there's a battle between the quality food vs. just, "You can look good, and get a six pack with lower quality food as long as you fit in a certain macro-nutrient range," which I've seen before. So pure weight loss and pure body composition can be manipulated with no care of the quality of the food, and I've seen that. The problem with that, when people see that they think, "Okay, well I'm just going to buy the cheaper stuff if I can look that way," because people think that's what healthy is, to look that way, when in reality healthy is on the inside, not so much on the outside with a six pack. You can look that way with lower quality foods. What you aren't taking into account is autoimmune diseases, digestion issues that a lot of people have, inflammation, so as younger kids sometimes in the fitness industry, you're a little bit stronger, and you seem more invincible, but it's setting you up for long-term disaster later on down the road. But people don't feel that right away. If they have Cinnamon Toast Crunch and Pop-Tarts and donuts and soda, and if it's fitting into their macros, and they have a six pack, and they don't feel like they're going to die, they feel like, "What's the big deal?" It's not like it instantly hits you. The damage creeps up over time, and so it's hard to tell people that have a six pack and they're ripped to say, "Hey man, you're killing yourself by eating these junk foods," and they're like "Oh, I'm good". You have to convince them like, "Hey, you gotta stop buying that." Maybe at some point the people they look up to will start to come around and preach kind of what this message is of quality over quantity. A calorie isn't just a calorie. It's more about your medical health first rather than looks. Does that make sense?

Brendan [00:28:55]: That's a great way of summarizing it. So from a practical standpoint, if somebody's beginning their journey from fat to fit so to speak, what's the number one key to making that transition?

Drew [00:29:07]: Honestly, it's more so on the mental-emotional side. That's what I preach now, and I help people on their mental and emotional challenges because I don't think it's the lack of knowledge. With YouTube and Google and how much information is available for free out there, it's not a lack of knowledge, it's a lack of application and application falls on the mental-emotional side because we've become lazy as a society because our society is set up to make it harder to eat healthy. You have to go out of your way almost to eat healthy, to get the healthy food. Whereas the unhealthy food is so convenient, and it's an uphill battle. I think the battle is won on the mental-emotional side.

So two things that are key for helping people transition into a healthier lifestyle. One is to be accountable to somebody, or an online group, to provide you with some type of accountability to motivate you in those times when you want to give in and not live a healthy lifestyle. And then also that leads you to have a support system. So a support system is your friends, a gym partner, your spouse, your loved ones, an online community of people that have the same goal in mind with you, that will help you, give you love and encouragement and let you know you're worth it to be healthy, but also a kick in the butt every once in a while because sometimes we need that. We need the balance of those two things. I feel like accountability and a support system, and with social media it's so easy now. You can start a blog; you can start a vlog on YouTube; you can post your meals on Instagram; you can join private Facebook groups where people are all helping each other out towards a likeminded goal; or you can go to a Cross-Fit gym or a Zumba class where you know the people there that are doing the workouts with you. The power of community is available out there. And I feel that accountability and a support system are essential no matter what lifestyle you choose to live, no matter what diet you do, no matter what workout program you do. You've got to have those two things: accountability and a support system to help you make it a lifestyle change rather than, "Okay, I'm just going to do this for 30 days."

Brendan [00:31:10]: That makes a lot of sense, and in fact your book is I think an important part for anybody that wants to take that approach because you've got some practical advice on being prepared, just logistically and also just kind of relating to it emotionally because you have a family and your family had certain responses to what you went through. So I think if people are going through a similar journey they're going to really see themselves in your journey because you really put yourself right in that situation, right into those shoes. And that is awesome, just amazing. No wonder you have a TV show about it, because it just spawns reality, it's like, "This is what's real." You mentioned social media, you're super active on social media, very helpful to your followers there, I can see. Is that the best way for people to connect with you and one of the various resources that you provide to help people with their journey?

Drew [00:32:07]: Yeah, social media. First of all is all Fit2fat2fit, Facebook, Twitter, Instagram, YouTube. And my website is Fit2fat2fit. So is my book. The TV show you can find on A&E, season 1. Season 2 comes out in 2018. But the things that I do now to connect to my followers is honestly setting up these private Facebook groups where it is a paid membership. But you can access this group, and you get access to me and my coaches, but also to the community. And these are complete strangers from all over the world that are in this Facebook group together, and they're posting their struggles, their successes, their weigh-ins, their failures, their meals every day. If one person needs help, they have a question, there's a dozen or more people to help them with their questions. And then when that person sees someone else needs help, they'll jump in to help that person. So it's really powerful to see these complete strangers that never met, come together with one common goal, helping each other out. There's probably millions of Facebook groups out there that you could join and be a part of to receive that support, but that's what I do. I run it. I kind of manage it, and I jump in on Facebook lives, answering their questions and connecting everybody. It's amazing the world we live in. With the technology we have nowadays, people from all across the world can join together on a weight loss journey with people they've never met and have a connection with someone like, "Wow, I love your story. Thank you for posting this. This helped me today in this." And it's just really cool to see. That's available all through my website fit2fat2fit.com, and I try to entertain people on social media as much as I can.

Brendan [00:33:50]: Well you're a true innovator, you really are, and an amazing leader in this world. And I want to thank you on behalf of myself, and the Eat4Earth community, for bringing all of this together today.

Drew [00:34:06]: Yeah, and I just want to say thank you, Brendan, I appreciate what you guys do and the movement that you guys are a part of in bettering our world, so I appreciate you and thank you for having me on.

Greg D. Wells, PhD Interview
The Ripple Effect: Eat, Sleep, Move, and Think Better

Brendan [00:00:00]: Welcome to the Eat4Earth event. This is Brendan Moorehead, and together we're exploring how you can heal yourself, your loved ones, and the planet, with food. I'm actually quite awed by our next guest, Dr. Greg D. Wells. As a scientist, broadcaster, author, coach, and athlete, Dr. Wells has dedicated his career to understanding human performance and how the body responds to extreme conditions. Dr. Wells is an Assistant Professor of Kinesiology at the University of Toronto, where he studies elite sport performance. He also serves as an Associate Scientist of Physiology and Experimental Medicine at The Hospital for Sick Children where he leads the exercise medicine research program. There he and his team explore how to use exercise to prevent, diagnose, and treat chronic illnesses in children. Throughout his career Dr. Wells has coached, trained, and inspired dozens of elite athletes to win medals at world championships, The Commonwealth Games, and The Olympics. He has studied athletic performance in some of the most extreme conditions on the planet, like the Andes mountains and the Sahara Desert. Dr. Wells' latest book, *The Ripple Effect*, is a fascinating look at the power of simple changes to transform your health and performance, drawing on his world-class scientific and athletic expertise. Dr. Wells is also the author of *Superbodies: Peak Performance Secrets from the World's Best Athletes*, which explores how genetics and DNA, the brain, muscles, lungs, heart, and blood, work together in extreme conditions. Dr. Wells has also spoken at top events like TEDx, and The Titan Summit, alongside Sir. Richard Branson, Robert Sharma, Steve Wozniac. Dr. Wells is also a frequent contributor to *The Globe and Mail* and has been an expert source to other top media outlets like ABC News, 20/20, The Discovery Channel, TSN, CBC, and CTV. Dr. Wells, it's really awesome to have you here.

Dr. Wells [00:01:52]: Yeah, amazing to be here, thank you so much for the opportunity. We're going to have fun.

Brendan [00:01:56]: Yeah, so Dr. Wells, you've studied elite athletes, you work with sick children, so you've got two extremes on a spectrum here, and you've identified ways essentially to help anyone from elite athletes to mere mortals like the rest of us, to perform better in life by accessing what you call the holy trinity of healthy living: eating better, moving better, sleeping better. I'm curious, which one of these would you say is most foundational as the place to start the ripple effect?

Dr. Wells [00:02:25]: Yeah, it's really interesting, we always sort of parse them out like "I'm on a diet" or "I'm going to start going to the gym" but I think it's really important, believe it or not, to do more than one, because they have ripple effects on each other. So, for example, if you get a great night's sleep, you control the hormones leptin and ghrelin that control and regulate your appetite and satiety, how full you feel. So if you get a good night's sleep, suddenly you're eating better. If you eat better, you recover better from a physiologic perspective, and your workouts get better. If you start exercising more you improve slow wave sleep, and your sleep gets better, so it's this positive circle. So as much as people always want to say, "What's the one thing?" I actually think we need to do a different approach because what we're doing isn't working. We have 58% of Canadians, 68% of Americans who have overweight or obesity. We have one in five North Americans—the statistics are similar in Australia, and the UK, and Europe, and it's becoming similar to India—but we have one in five people who struggle with mental illness. We have 85% of our population that doesn't get enough physical activity, so we actually need to adopt what I would believe is just a holistic lifestyle. It's healthy because ultimately that opens up our possibility to perform at a world class level. We'll do better at music, drama, sports, business, teaching. Whatever it happens to be that you care about the most, that will benefit from taking this type of an approach to life. But if you held a gun to my head and said, "What's the one thing that you're going to do better?" I would say "Always start with sleep" because if you sleep well, everything else becomes easier. But I really want everyone to start thinking about "How many different pieces of the puzzle can I add to my life to enhance the way that I'm living, and open up my potential?"

Brendan [00:04:13]: So, is it sleep for everybody, in other words, beginning with a sick child all the way through elite athletes. Is sleep always the starting place in your opinion?

Dr. Wells [00:04:23]: Well, I do exercise medicine, and I'm an exercise physiologist so usually my role has something to do with exercise, but when I begin to look at the research, and when I studied this "ripple effect" concept, beginning at about 2012—t's literally taken me about five years to pull it all together—the research is just so clear that we need to sleep well. If you sleep well, your brain recovers and regenerates. You can check out Jeff Iliff's TED talk on some of the new research on how the brain washes itself when you sleep. Some amazing data that just got published literally about six weeks ago that actually images that. You can see the penetration of fluids into the brain when you sleep. So we know that the brain washes itself out at night while we sleep, and that sets the stage for better learning—we learn when we sleep; we don't learn during the day—better creativity. We're creative and we problem solve during REM sleep, which happens in the second half of sleep. So all of these factors are just so incredibly important, and we're now beginning to make all of the scientific connections to really explain what's going on. And the imaging techniques that are available now enable us to look inside the body and see the changes that are happening when we do things really well and also when we don't do things as well and we get really sick. So that's a factor when we're doing sports. Most sports teams are now hiring sleep coaches. The Seattle Seahawks have been quoted as saying—their coach has been quoted as saying—that "Sleep is our weapon." And certainly we're beginning to look at sleep as a more important factor when it comes to chronic disease management—Alzheimer's, cardiovascular disease, cancer. There's now been some cool data that shows that melatonin, the hormone that's released when we sleep, has a direct impact on cancer cells, so it is a huge factor when we talk about elite sports and also in the medical world as well.

Brendan [00:06:21]: And since food is the subject of this event, I'm curious, what's the interplay between sleep and food consumption, assimilation, metabolism, and vice versa?

Dr. Wells [00:06:33]: Right, so there's really interesting work that's been done on how sleep regulates the hormones that control our appetite and also our satiety, how full we feel. So if you get a great night's sleep, you're not going to be as hungry. Your decision making around food is going to be better, and you'll feel more full.

Brendan [00:06:51]: Boy have I noticed that one.

Dr. Wells [00:06:53]: Totally.

Brendan [00:06:55]: If I don't get sleep I'm so ravenous the next day. I guess my ghrelin is through the roof, right?

Dr. Wells [00:07:01]: Yeah, totally, and you can't control that. That's just a physiologic reaction. You're hungry. Your blood sugar is low. You have to go kill something so you can eat it. It's an evolutionary response that we have. It's hardwired into our DNA. And so that's normal, whether it's going out hunting on the savanna of Africa or you're driving by Starbucks, and you need a scone. It's the same response.
When it comes to eating better, sleep is I believe absolutely foundational. Also, there's really cool data that shows that what we eat influences what happens when we sleep. If you eat foods that are a little bit higher in carbohydrates, you can increase tryptophan in the brain which helps us to sleep a little bit better. I'm not a huge fan of adding carbs late at night mainly because of—the vast majority of North Americans need to improve their body composition—but if you're in a healthy place when it comes to body-comp, and you want to have a little snack that triggers your ability to sleep better, that's an option for you. We also know that adding some proteins late at night increases growth hormone release. Growth hormone is the fountain of youth hormone that repairs all of the different tissues inside of our body. There's also data that shows that high fat consumption late at night disrupts sleep because it's so hard to digest. So what we eat in the afternoon and the evening has a very clear impact on the quality of our sleep. So what I say to people is, use yourself as a laboratory, don't just react but actually respond, take some notes, think about what you're doing and how you're sleeping and then reverse engineer a great sleep and find out what works for you.

Brendan [00:08:37]: Tryptophan is a really interesting one, and I just heard recently that it's a particularly delicate amino acid. I'd be curious to know it you agree with this or not. I haven't run down any research on this, but I heard that it's particularly susceptible to damage by toxins in our environment and in our food.

Dr. Wells [00:09:03]: I haven't heard any of that data, so I have to look it up, check it out. It sounds interesting.

Brendan [00:09:08]: I just heard that last night, so ... The other thing about tryptophan, I guess, is if we get enough light during the day we're going to be converting it into serotonin, and then we're going to have enough serotonin, so that when the lights go down, assuming they do, assuming we're not staring at blue screens and we put on our blue blockers at night and dim the screens, then it's going to convert more readily to melatonin and help bring on sleep. That's one of the tryptophan pathways we've got to protect.

Dr. Wells [00:09:39]: Yeah, interesting. I'm a big fan of the digital sunset—taking your phones and your devices and turning them off at least an hour before you want to be falling asleep, hopefully even earlier than that. For sure obviously activating the night shift feature if you've got iOS and the iFlex feature on an Android or whatever it is that you are using. I've done that for my iPhone, my iPad, my computer screen, and we've also installed dimmer switches throughout our house so that in the evening we can replicate the sun going down, and dim everything. So we're having dinner, and the lights go down a little bit. The lights upstairs as we take the kids up towards bed go down, and we want to replicate that.

I love reading fiction books before sleep because that seems to make a huge difference in the quality of my sleep, not checking industry reports or scanning Facebook or social media or whatever else it happens to be. So protecting those last couple of hours before you go to sleep, makes a huge difference in the quality of your sleep, and your ability to recover and regenerate.

Brendan [00:10:40]: Yeah. Well I'm curious, in terms of food, what is the most important factor in your opinion, is it the amount of nutrients we're getting per calorie, the meal timing, macro-nutrient ratios?

Dr. Wells [00:10:56]: I think it's health equals nutrients over calories. I think there's a number of different strategies that you can use around meal timing. I think that there's loads of different strategies you can use around macro-nutrient ratios, but the one that I believe—and the research has shown over, and over, and over, consistently to improve outcomes—is health equals nutrients over calories. The more nutrients that you can get into your system per calorie in general the healthier you're going to be. Very clear research on the amount of vegetables that you eat improving your health. There's clear research on links between plant-based nutrition and cardiovascular disease, plant-based nutrition and cancer, healthy nutrition, high nutrient nutrition on depression. There's been even some cool research for example on the compounds in green tea and mental health. So all of these polyphenols, all of these flavonoids that are in the plants that we can eat, have tremendous and wide-ranging health benefits. And most of those polyphenols and flavonoids we haven't even identified yet, so we're just getting started going down that road. I've seen different strategies used effectively in macro-nutrient ratios, so it depends on what you're looking for. We know that the extremely low carbohydrates, higher protein, higher fat strategy is very good for epilepsy and cancer for example, so it really depends on what you're trying to accomplish when it comes to that. And then I also think that there's been some interesting research recently on food timing and meal timing with the advent of intermittent fasting. Although I'm not really a fan of any sort of quote unquote "diet" strategy, I think there's healthy eating, and I think there's less healthy eating. But the data on intermittent fasting is very, very interesting. So I've been exploring that mainly because it appears to have a positive effect on the ability to tolerate chemotherapy, on brain function and neurogenesis, apoptosis, and a number of different physiologic factors.

So I'm exploring that at the moment. It seems to be pretty interesting. That's an area that I foresee evolving quite a bit in the coming years.

Brendan [00:13:07]: You know, of course in this event we're talking a lot about nutrients per calories, as far as nutrient density, not only in types of food, as you mentioned plant foods being potentially the highest nutrients per calorie, but also the quality of those vegetables as it pertains to the soil quality. So soil health is what's governing how much of all the different trace minerals are getting into the plants, and so they can make those compounds, and so that are in our bodies we have enough minerals as the cofactors that work with all of this. I think there's massive potential, like literally, manifold orders of magnitude potential to increase—at least one order of magnitude—to increase the medicinal power of our food supply.

Dr. Wells [00:14:00]: I couldn't agree with you more.

Brendan [00:14:02 I think it's something we can all get behind and just become a little bit aware of how important it is, and then advocate for it through the food chain, through our purchase decisions.

Dr. Wells [00:14:13]: Absolutely, voting with your pocket book is a really effective strategy of creating societal change and corporate change. I love what Brazil did recently. They basically threw away their food guide because it wasn't working, similar with the US, similar with Canada. Our food guides are a disaster. They threw away that and recommended that people eat real food that they recognize as food, that they make it themselves, and that they eat with family and friends. It's incredibly simple. We don't need to overcomplicate it. The solutions are right in front of us. It's blatantly clear. And if we can start to not worry so much, focus on time, the quality of time that you spend with family and friends when you're eating, and take the time to make your own food. I'm incredibly busy. I've got two labs. I've got a business that I run. I'm a public speaker. I write books, flying all over the world. Judith my wife's a chiropractor and acupuncture massage therapist. We're super busy. We have two little kids, but we decided three years ago to invest in taking the time to make our own food. And all of us—every single person of our family—our health is sky-rocketing. Our mental health is improving, physical health, mental health. And so it really does come down to making that commitment to prepare those foods yourself, get access to the right types of foods, vote with your pocket book, and it's possible to eat a very healthy diet on a budget. I've heard so often, "Oh it's too expensive, I can't do that. it costs too much," to which I reply, "It's eminently possible to eat healthy on a budget. Beans, legumes, lentils— there's all sorts of options for getting loads of nutrients into your system in a cost-effective way as long as you're willing to take the time to make it yourself and to invest in that as a family".

Brendan [00:16:02]: Yeah. Nora Gedgaudas hired somebody to do a little research on that, a little analysis, put out an e-book called *The Primal Tightwad*. So it shows that you can eat the highest quality diet including animal products, which we tend to think of as the most expensive, and it will cost less than the standard American diet. If you look at the numbers—and Diana Rogers did a similar analysis, I think, and I think there's an article on her blog, basically it's showing the dollars—it was either per calorie or per nutrient or something, or maybe both—and you're paying a lot more when you get processed food, and you're getting so little for it. It may be the cheapest per calorie but not the cheapest per nutrient. Like you said, what's most important is nutrients per calorie, so ultimately it is so much cheaper and affordable in every way.

Dr. Wells [00:17:06]: Yeah, if I could just push that out to people, share that information. Let's blow up that misconception and share that type of real ... because it's a real world strategy. "What do I eat? How do I afford this? How do I do ... what's in my shopping list?" We've got to get that information out to people so they can make the right decision at the right time for their family. So those are brilliant references.

Brendan [00:17:25]: And it can really have an impact. Just recently I was watching the *Prosperity* film ... You know what, it looks like you're muted.

Dr. Wells [00:17:35]: Yeah, I just muted myself so I could ... I'm doing that deliberately so I don't get feedback.

Brendan [00:17:42]: Right, got it. If you have a mic, you could plug that in real quick. So somebody in the *Prosperity* film that Pedram Shojai created said that some study or analysis indicated that if the world stopped buying chewing gum, that whole industry would vanish in four weeks. So it's like "Hello?" We sustain everything. We're entirely responsible for everything that we perhaps would like to see change and transform. So we can do it, absolutely.

Dr. Wells [00:18:22]: Yeah absolutely, and we're seeing that happening quite a bit. The amazing new information that's been coming out, and people's access to websites like *Pubmed* where they can get the latest scientific information—not opinions, not a blog post—but actual real scientific articles available to everyone. Pubmed.com. You could go in there, and you could search the links between vitamin D and cancer, or various different, literally whatever you want to explore—vegetables and cardiovascular disease—it's all there— plant-based diets or Mediterranean diet and cancer. There's some amazing information there, actual real research studies. And I think that that's critical because we live right now in an era where people are confusing emotions for facts, and where we really need to make sure that we're paying attention to what actual research says, what actual science says. But also of course a big note of who's paying for that research. That's the one sort of variable that you have to consider, to look at those acknowledgments, look who funded the study, and that can give you a second level of insight, but there's amazing research that's available to everybody, and we can access that. We can read it. We can make some great decisions and inform ourselves based upon the best practices, not on whatever industry interest is pushing out advertising that may influence our decisions, that may not be the healthiest for us individually and for our families.

Brendan [00:19:45]: The way I see the food and health crisis is we've got a nutrients per calorie crisis that's originating both in the soil and in processing of foods—how we deliver nutrient vacant, calorie dense foods, so those two things. Then we've got all these tag-along toxins, farm chemicals and so forth, and I'm curious, from your perspective, is it more of an impact to have the low nutrients per calorie or the high toxins per calorie, or is it kind of like hard to choose which is the worst.

Dr. Wells [00:20:29]: That's an interesting question. I don't know if I've seen any research that evaluated those two things, one against the other. My focus right now personally is on the H = N/C nutrients over calories, I think that that's foundational because we use those, and we have to have them. Without those, problems emerge very quickly. The body has an incredible capacity to manage toxins and to eliminate them through our kidneys, through our liver, we filter everything all the time, we're very good at that, so I personally worry a lot more about the H = N/C than I do about the toxin side of things. Having said that, we eat largely organic because I believe there's pretty clear data that shows that organic foods have a lower pesticide load than non-organic foods. There's clearly no difference in terms of proteins, carbohydrates and fats—the macro-nutrients—but there's a clear difference in micro-nutrients, vitamins and minerals and also especially in pesticide loads, which I just simply don't want in my system. So that's a decision that we've made as a family, that does cost more, no question, but we've made an investment in that. We got rid of cable, and we eat organic. So that's sort of like a decision that you've got to make, and that's how we're approaching it in my family.

I actually had a communications person from a large pharmaceutical organization that's involved in food start trolling me on Twitter and battling me on that specific issue saying a whole bunch of stuff which I won't repeat, but it forced me to go into the research. And she was quoting nothing, and I went through and quoted almost twenty research papers, had a little Twitter spat on a Friday evening, which was great because it forced me down into the research to prove what I was saying. And one of the studies that I came across was an amazing study by Stanford University—a very large scale study that's often quoted in the pro-GMO the anti-organic food lobby—but it was interesting once you dive into the data in that study because it does clearly show, no difference, carbohydrates, fats, proteins are roughly the same. There _are_ differences in micro-nutrients which is one of the important things, and it does show a decreased level of pesticides in the foods, as do many other studies. So it's quite interesting when you get to break all of that down and explore it in a little bit more detail. There's also the whole GMO argument which I'm not an expert in—I'm an exercise physiologist, not a specialist in that area—but I think that is sort of a population level experiment that's run right now. I don't think that we know, yes or no on either side, where the data really proves with regards to health and wellbeing, but we'll find out hopefully over the next few years, as studies are done, hopefully more independent studies are done.

It's an exploding area. It's very, very confusing, but back to the original question—toxins vs. nutrients. We focus on nutrients first and foremost and then minimize toxins as much as possible. We consider these the essentials, and these to be, you know, do the best that you possibly can given what you're able to do over here. That's how we're approaching it, and it seems to be working really well for my family. I've had all of my blood work done recently, and it looks fantastic. So it appears to be doing what we're hoping that it does when it comes to actually breaking down the physiology of it.

Brendan [00:23:47]: Awesome. Now, I'm curious, since one of the themes in this event is to explore the different food philosophies, so we've got plant-based, we've got omnivorous, we've got ketogenic and so forth, and I'm just curious, as far as optimal human performance, what are your thoughts on plant- based, omnivorous, ketogenic, or is there just too much bio-chemical individuality and metabolic individuality to say, "Oh, this is the most optimal for everybody"?

Dr. Wells [00:24:19]: I think that saying that all humans should eat exactly the same thing is probably not correct. We all need to find out what works best for us. There is very clear research that certain styles of eating are very good for certain groups of people. For example, the ketogenic diet has been shown to be very effective for people with epilepsy. It's very effective for people with certain types of cancer. So for example if I have cancer, if I have epilepsy, I'll go all in on the ketogenic diet. I think the research is extremely clear that the more plants that you eat the healthier you are going to be, especially when it comes to cancer and cardiovascular disease. Plant-based nutrition or vegetarian—it's usually researched as vegetarian or vegan— has many health benefits. I'm beginning to see a lot of athletes adopt that strategy, especially in the ultra-endurance world that sort of began there, but it's now in the NFL. It's now in bodybuilding and some other places as well. I don't worry about the dogma associated with vegan or vegetarian. If you want to go down that road, fantastic. I just say plant-based, aim from 90%, you're going to get most of those benefits, and it gives you that freedom not to stress yourself out. The other style of eating that's been shown to be pretty much universally beneficial for human health is the Mediterranean diet. It's very clear that that has positive effects on cardio-vascular disease, cancer, mental health, so that's another strategy that you could adopt if you wanted to go down that road.

There's one that I think has been researched at the University of Toronto by Dr. David Jenkins and his team, which is the blood-type diet and that's been pretty much universally shown in the research there's absolutely no validity whatsoever. There's zero evidence that that actually works by blood type. However, all four diets that they recommend are infinitely better than the standard American diet. So if you adopt any of the four, you're going to end up better off. So it's really important to dig down and make sure that you're not just following a blog, but dive into the research. Find out what works for you. Think about your own personal situation, what you're trying to accomplish, and get some help. There's some experts out there. Consult with them, a really good naturopathic doctor. Consult with a really good progressive dietitian. There are people out there that you can look to, to look at your diet, break it down and take a look at what you need to do to get healthier. So it's my thirty thousand foot overview of those different styles of eating, but the main message is, think about what works for you. Test it out. If you seem to be physiologically better, if you're improving your body composition, if you're improving your energy, if you're improving your mental health, then that's something that's probably going to help and work for you. And then titrate it from there.

Brendan [00:27:01]: One thing I'll mention about the Mediterranean diet that I thought was an interesting commentary by Dr. Steven Gundry who wrote *The Plant Paradox*, a fascinating book. He contends that the Mediterranean diet has been perhaps a little bit misconstrued as high carb, in the sense like, "Oh, eat lots of pasta" and that he feels, if I'm correctly recalling and quoting the book—I recommend people read it—that basically what makes that an amazing diet for people is it's high in polyphenols. They eat a lot of great vegetables and so forth, and olives that are amazing. They're eating a lot of whole olives, I believe, as well as a lot of good quality olive oil. And that's another topic because you can find olive oils that are not good and that are cut with soy oil, and you don't want that. So relatively high fat content of the diet of high quality, which makes polyphenols available. It's really hard to assimilate polyphenols without fat. That's what helps bring them into the body. Also, a moderate quantity of small fish. A lot of Omega-3, super high quality, easily assimilable fish protein, usually anchovies I think, in that certain region that he was looking at, Grecian isles I believe.

Dr. Wells [00:28:31]: And another great way to go after that is to check out all the work that's been done by the Blue Zones people, Dan Buettner's Blue Zones work, which is really interesting. I've sort of broken that down and looked at it, and I think that's another very important, clear way of making some decisions around what you're eating. So exactly, I love all the stuff that you said about the Mediterranean diet. I agree with that. If you look at it it's not a lot of pasta. It's lots of plants. There's some meat involved. There's some fish involved. There's a little bit of grains, and it's a variety of different things all which contribute together to improve health in that population. So yeah, I love what you're saying. Sorry to interrupt.

Brendan [00:29:11]: Yeah, not at all. And another point he makes, I'm glad you interrupted me because I wouldn't have remembered to say this. He makes the point that in the plant foods that they eat, especially these New World foods that are fairly new to much of the human population like tomatoes, cucumbers— things like that, actually I'm not sure about cucumbers, but squash and so forth, eggplant—they come from the New World, the plant lectins, which are proteins that bond to sugar molecules and are actually plant defense systems. They can derail our physiology if they get into our body, and he contends that the longer the human microbiome has been exposed to certain plant lectins and passed down through the birth canal of mothers to their children and so forth—of course we share our microbiomes in other ways ... I think just human intimacy with other people will actually ... you will get some of their microbiome—and so it's not just in the birth process, but that's a key inoculator. So what he's saying is, these new plant lectins ... well, the Italians noticed that what they had to do with tomatoes to make them more assimilable was they had to take the seeds out and peel them, to minimize the reactions that they would have. And then they of course cooked it because that helped to make the lycopene more available. So that's how tomatoes are largely consumed over there. They do the same I think with some of the other New World plants. They deseed them and skin them, peel them. Obviously there's some nutrients lost in the peel, but they're also eliminating a lot of the plant lectins so he feels that's a really important component of what made the Mediterranean diet helpful, is they had their own intelligence through whatever intuitive discovery that they needed to do certain things to process those foods, to make them kind to their digestive tract and their whole body.

Dr. Wells [00:31:18]: Interesting. I've heard that discussion around lectins, and I haven't had a chance to dive into the research on that yet, but that's certainly on my to-do list for 2018. But it looks like an interesting area.

Brendan [00:31:33]: Yeah, I think it's real cutting edge, and I think that the decimation of our micro-biome by antibiotics has made us more susceptible to things that we used to handle quite well. There are various plant lectins that we've been consuming for a very long time but we're killing the microbiome with antibiotics and other things like triclosan in our hand washes and so many things, the glyphosate residues in our food, decimating our microbiome. But I'm curious to know, back to you and your specialties, with children, what kind of illnesses are you seeing that are maybe growing in recent years that are a subject of your work with children?

Dr. Wells [00:32:28]: So, to tell you a little bit about what we do. We've built up the Exercise Medicine Research Program at the Hospital For Sick Children, and that began working with children with cystic fibrosis which is a genetic lung disease that gradually destroys lung tissues over long period of time. We've made some tremendous gains in that area. There's some fantastic new drugs that appear to be lifesaving with this population. My role there is to explore how exercise interfaces with that disease to improve outcomes, which it does. We sort of hope that exercise can keep people alive long enough to make it to the cure, which is going to come from some gene therapy and some pharmaceutical therapies, and that's really exciting work. Another area that we've spent a fair bit of time in, is in helping children with leukemia, blood cancer, and how we can use exercise, nutrition, sleep to improve outcomes once they've made it through the treatment phase. 80% of kids now survive childhood cancers which is amazing, however in the years following the cancer many of them are at a higher risk of having secondary disease like type-2 diabetes and metabolic syndrome and cardio-vascular disease because of some of the challenges associated with radiation and chemo. So we're really interested in trying to help those children using exercise post therapy. And that's become something we've also tried to do in cardiology, we've started doing in inflammatory conditions, and it's just taken off.

When I started there I was all alone by myself, and then over the last ten years it's grown, and grown, and grown. And now at our last conference which was a couple of weeks ago there were 90 people there from within just the hospital where I work in the local area. The whole idea of exercise as medicine, lifestyle as medicine, has really exploded. I'm happy about it now. It used to be something that was not considered at all. There's now a new course that's gone into the Medical School at the University of Toronto where I'm at, that actually teaches physicians exercise, which never existed before. My goal is that hopefully we have not only exercise, but we have courses on sleep, courses on food, the medicinal power of foods so we wake up the entire system. I'm very holistic in my approach. I want kinesiologists, physiotherapists, medical doctors, naturopaths, nutritionists, dietitians, chiropractors, all to be working together and respect each other's areas of expertise so we can provide really powerful information for patients and for the general population that's based on evidence and based upon science. That's the real trend that we've seen, this awakening to the power of exercise, the power of sleep, the power of food to actually have an influence on our health and wellbeing and in many cases also includes outcomes in diseases. I prefer using lifestyle medicine to prevent disease from ever happening. Obviously once you have a disease you need to go at it with every tool that is available to humanity to try to get through that, and also help get back into lifestyle medicine, to help people recover from those diseases once they've gone through that battle and come out the other side.

Brendan [00:35:35]: Since you mentioned that, as we know, inflammation is at the core of so many illnesses and of course with children, I think that it's possible that the decimation of the human microbiome in our guts, with children getting too many antibiotics when they're young or maybe being born by C sections and not having good ... getting a hit of antibiotics. Not to harp too much on the same thing, but I just realized I didn't actually make the connection a few minutes ago, and I thought this might be a way to tie it all together, but basically it seems that inflammation is so often beginning in the gut because of several factors like losing the healthy microbiome and becoming more susceptible to plant lectins because the organisms that used to help break them down for us—we coevolved with certain plant lectins in our diet and with certain microbes that were helping us digest them—now that that situation has changed, the microbiome has lost a lot of its diversity in many of us. And also we've started to modify the plant lectins, at least through the soy and corn with genetic engineering and a few other plant crops. We've actually changed the lectins, so they're novel entirely to the whole food chain, the microbiome as well. That could be—and this is partly what is suggested in *The Plant Paradox*—this could be a big part of the influence on inflammatory syndromes in our bodies. That may be something to look into for children. I believe that there's a combination of fecal transplantation into children—it's already been shown that with autism it's amazingly effective to massively reduce the symptoms. In some cases, I think they're calling it full reversal, but I can't say for sure. I haven't really looked into it in great depth. But that could help these children reduce the inflammation that's driving so many things aside from autism. What were the specific conditions you see most with children?

Dr. Wells [00:37:56]: To follow up on that, I really have not seen or have not looked at any of the research on lectins and inflammations, so I have to fully acknowledge I know nothing about that.

Brendan [00:38:07]: Sorry to throw you such a curveball.

Dr. Wells [00:38:10]: No, that's why I love interviews, I love these conversations because every question that I don't know the answer to triggers an investigation. If I knew all the answers that would not be very much fun, so I'm fully respective of that and honored and privileged and appreciative of that.
Into the inflammation issue, there is I think some fairly consistent agreement that inflammation is one of the common pathways amongst many different conditions. We know that it's related to cardio-vascular disease. We know it's related to stroke. We know it's related to cancer. We know it's related to mental health, especially depression. And so we're very interested in trying to lower inflammation in our athletes, and our patients.

One of the simplest ways to lower inflammation in our body that most people aren't aware of is stress. Stress increases inflammation inside the body. Inflammation is a great pathway. We need it, it needs to happen, it's good for us because that's how our bodies repair, that's how we regenerate. If you go do a workout and your muscles are sore, that's the inflammatory process working to heal your body to make it stronger. If you cut yourself, inflammation happens, it heals you, that's phenomenal. The problem exists when our inflammatory levels are kept high consistently for a long period of time, and that's where we need to build in periods of recovery, regeneration. That's why meditation is so effective, why taking a break and actually using your vacation days, America, and Canada and everyone - we need to like take some time to get away, and recover and regenerate. Lower that stress. It's the easiest way to lower whole body inflammation. Another great way to do it is cardio-vascular exercise which appears to lower inflammation as well. There's the initial inflammatory response during the exercise itself but then overall there's a lowering of the whole body's inflammation.

So there's a number of different healthy ways that we know are universal human truths that improve those physiological markers. We've actually done some research on the use of omega-3 to reduce inflammation which is another reason to up that in your diet. One of my grad students did that work. Another one of my grad students did some really interesting work on cold immersions and cold tubs which also improves inflammatory outcomes as long as the water is not too cold, and as long as you don't stay in there too long. Obviously that's used by a lot of athletes. You see them in cold tubs after exercise. Another great way to lower your inflammatory markers—a study that we just finished this week that we're submitting for publication—is all in and around massage therapy, which decreases your inflammatory markers inside your body as well. Another great way to speed our recovery, not to play you out of the nutrition area with sort of getting into inflammation …

Brendan [00:40:47]: No, it all works together.

Dr. Wells [00:40:49]: Totally, it's a very holistic approach, and those are some of the things that we've been investigating in my lab recently and all because inflammation appears to be critical for improving human performance if you increase inflammation and then decrease it so the body can recover. And then also considering inflammation as a common pathway among many different chronic illnesses that people are faced with these days.

Brendan [00:41:12]: Yeah. I'm curious, what about sleeping quality and the influence on inflammation.

Dr. Wells [00:41:17]: Sleep is directly related to inflammation, and that's one of the main reasons why sleep is related to cardio-vascular disease. We know that sleep is related to cancer. We know that if you get more sleep you have a lower risk of recurrence of breast cancer. We know that if you have better sleep you have a lower risk of depression and that the amount of your sleep is an independent risk factor for depression. You can treat depression with sleep. So there's all of these different, and they're all related to all of these different pathways, the common factor being in many cases inflammation in addition to melatonin and some other issues. But if you want to live a long life, we know how much sleep you need. There's very clear research that shows around seven and a half hours is the amount of sleep that you need to have the lowest risk of all-cause mortality, and it's like cancer, heart disease, getting hit by a bus, all wrapped up in one. And also, if you get less than six hours a night, your risk of all-cause mortality starts to increase. So bare minimum six, ideally seven and a half, seven to eight is a good strategy. The younger you are, the more that you need, and it's because it's related to all of those different chronic illnesses.

Brendan [00:42:18]: Of course, seven and a half hours corresponds to a multiple of about five times the typical ninety-minute sleep cycle where you go through a full cycle. Do I have that correct?

Dr. Wells [00:42:29]: Yeah, absolutely, and that's exactly what I tell people. I say work backwards from the time you want to wake up in the morning and make sure you get four or five cycles of ninety minutes. So either six hours or 90 minutes, and it's actually really cool, if you look at the new operating systems on many of the different phones, one of the things I've noticed is that in the clock app, the middle button is a bedtime alarm, and so I now no longer use a wake-up alarm; I use a bedtime alarm. And it can calculate the amount of hours that I've got there, and I know what time I'm waking up. And I'm free and clear. So I'm like 9:30 to 5:00. I got my seven and a half minutes (probably meant to say "hours" not "minutes"), and I'm up at 4:45 usually, and I got my seven and a half hours, and I can crush my days and feeling better. So use those tools that are available to you to make sure you figure out when you need to go to bed which is far more important than what time you need to wake up.

Brendan [00:43:18]: Got it, yeah, good point. I'm curious, in working with elite athletes in extreme environments pursuing the next record of some kind, is there anything you've learned … I mean these guys and gals have to be so precise and focused about everything they do, I'm just curious, if you've learned anything from them that applies to an average person in their life, if they're trying to crush it with a sales presentation that's coming up, or anything, everything's on the line kind of moment, at least they could make it that way, they could hold that opportunity in that way and then focus on it like a corporate athlete so to speak, borrowing the term from, I think, The Energy Project.

Dr. Wells [00:44:05]: Yeah, I've got the book (*The Power of Full Engagement: Managing Energy, Not Time, Is the Key to High Performance and Personal Renewal*). It's here somewhere. I've got that book. Actually, it's right in that thing over there. So if you wanted to look at, I've worked with a couple Olympians, I've been to three Olympic games as a commentator, and the one thing that I would say determines whether or not an athlete is going to be successful at an Olympic games, once you've done the training, you're at the Olympics, is whether or not you're able to stay focused because there's so many distractions. There's media. There's your parents. There's the crowd. There's your competitors. There's a million different things that can draw your attention away from what you're supposed to be thinking about. Attention is the word that I love your audience to sort of contemplate. And controlling your attention is really key, whether it's in music … Imagine someone playing music and being distracted and how their performance would go. It would be terrible. Someone giving a speech to the public gets distracted. We have to control our attention, and we live in an era of non-stop, constant distraction. We have our devices. We have social media. We have text messaging. We have e-mail alerts. And what I ask for people to do is to really contemplate a time, and set up a time during the day, when you can do your best work in a completely undistracted environment. I love to do ninety minutes, first thing in the morning. I learned this from Robin Sharma, author of *The Monk Who Sold His Ferrari*, the ninety ninety-one formula, ninety minutes for ninety days on your number one most important task in your life and everything will change.

I love spending time with my children when I'm at home in the city. I put my kids to bed. It's simple. It takes me about an hour, but I do it every single time, completely undistracted. No phones in and around the dinner table. When you want to check your e-mail, check your e-mail. When you want to do social, do social. That's totally cool. Send text, send text. It's just what we have a break between what we're doing and what's going on. So say you're at the dinner table having dinner with your family, but you're checking social. You're not actually at dinner with your family. That's when problems begin to occur. If you're playing baseball, and you're a hitter, and you're in the batter's box, and you're trying to detect what pitch is coming next but your mind is elsewhere on your finances, on your family, you'd have almost no chance of being successful.

Our ability to control our attention is a game-changing principle for people moving forward. I believe the best way to train that in yourself is mindfulness and meditation. So I love my Headspace app. Calm.com just won app of the year. This is a next big wave of health, I think. It's going to be meditation much like yoga has been over the last little while, last twenty years. And so we really need to focus on focus, and to pay attention to our attention. I just made that up. That's kind of cool. I should write that down. But that's the game-changer. That's what I've seen at the Olympics, and to be honest with you I also see it in the hospital. People who are able to focus on positive progress have a different likely outcome than people who are focused on the problems and the negativity. That's very easy in our world. The easiest way to capture someone's attention is fear. And we see that being used far too often right now. You have people jumping and worried and anxious and scared in order to get their attention, and that works for almost every single human because of our evolutionary history. But what we need to do is control that attention deliberately to consciously pay attention to the things that we want to pay attention to—reading that book, spending time with your children at the park, having a great meal with your spouse, delivering a world-class presentation, coming up with a new solution. That's a way of completely changing your life. It's the simplest, fastest, most powerful way to change your performance during the day to get a completely different outcome of your life.

Brendan [00:47:48]: Yeah, multi-tasking has recently been—first of all I confess I have been the worst multitasker and I'm working on improving that, transforming that—but research on it is shocking. You actually reduce your intelligence by multitasking. Then of course you're damaging all of your relationships, your performance, your job potential, your income potential, your athletic potential. And on the flip side, like you said, the research on meditation is amazing. What happens when you improve your ability to focus—your intelligence increases, your effectiveness increases, physiological markers improve. It's kind of like the "OMG" effect, I mean "What is going on, oh my God", transforming so many things. So I have to turn the trinity into a quadrinity or something and add …

Dr. Wells [00:48:46]: The "think" component? Well I actually did, the title of my book is *The Ripple Effect: Eat, Sleep, Move and Think Better*. At the last minute I did add in "think" because of that exact issue that you brought up. Meditation and mindfulness are just so incredibly powerful. Focus is so critical. Humans are incapable of multitasking. We actually cannot do it. We just task switch quickly. So I recommend people think about single tasking. You want to up your game … you want to take it to the next level … you want to improve your performance … improve your health … find ways of single-tasking. And even … just test it out. The next time you walk into a meeting with someone, really look at them, really pay attention to them when they are talking to you. Go all in on what they're saying to you and try to understand. Don't have your phone on the table, not even turned over. Put it completely away. It's so easy to differentiate yourself in that way now because people are constantly sitting off to the side checking this (holding up his mobile phone). And I'm not opposed to this (pointing to his mobile phone). This is probably the greatest invention in human history. It's transforming the world in a good way, but I think that the way we are using it is problematic. And you can quickly differentiate yourself and take your game to the next level by doing things just a little bit differently. Work on controlling your attention and giving people your attention, which is this incredible gift that you can give that ups their game, ups your game, and completely changes the psychological environment that you're in when you're doing time with your family, when you're in a meeting, all sorts of different things, in sports, playing music, all of it. So it's powerful.

Brendan [00:50:17]: That is so true. The most impactful moments I've had with another human being were in proportion to how present they were and how present I was.

Dr. Wells [00:50:27]: And think about that with your kids in this world, or think about that with your spouse or with people who are working for you, or when you're on stage, or when you're in an audience. It's a total game-changer in today's environment, and it feels good when you do it. It's good for you, it's good for them, it's relaxing, it improves your mental health. Again not to say you can't be on social media. You should be on social media. Fire it up. You can have a positive influence if you positively comment. So there's lots of benefits to it. We just need to control it a little bit better, and if you do that, awesome things can happen.

Brendan [00:50:58]: Awesome. One last thing, is there anything else in the realm of where your attention is on these days, and has been for a long time, that you've discovered, like if I want to be as healthy as I can, and I want to feel great as long as I can, in other words improve my health span and life span while having a super high performing life, is there anything else I need to keep in mind?

Dr. Wells [00:51:22]: One of the things I was speaking about a lot probably in the last week … I attended an amazing event on the weekend it's called The Titan Summit which was incredible, and I learned some really interesting things there. And I had four speaking engagements this week. I've been pulling information out of that and speaking to people. There were workshops this week, so sort of deep dives into what we've been talking about so far today. But one of the things that I've been saying that really shocked people was how much time you need to spend planning. Just literally disconnect from the world, all the devices off. Get out of your normal situation, book a hotel room, take your family away and spend three to four days thinking about, let's just say right now it's the middle of December. 2018 is coming up. What's 2018 going to look like for you. What are you going to do? What habits are you going to install? And then on a quarterly basis take a day, a full day. Break down what you're doing, deconstruct it, plan the next quarter for your health, and then do that quarterly every single week. Take an hour; plan your week. Every morning take ten minutes; plan your day. That way you have control over what you're doing, and you're spending your energy on accomplishing your priorities. I want people to shift away from time management, and I want them to start doing priority management. We get derailed by the demands on our time, and we don't spend enough time on what's of high priority to us. So I put my kids to bed at night. I try to have dinner with my wife as often as I can. Now we're about to go away for a three-week holiday over the December vacations. Planning is everything. Schedule the time. Go away. Create a different environment. Think differently, and set your life up the way that you want it because I truly believe that lifestyle determines your success. Success does not determine your lifestyle. And so if you control your lifestyle you're going to control the success that you have in your life.

Brendan [00:53:17]: Thank you for that. That's a great, great note to end on. And again one of the other things that I'm working on is becoming a better planner. (laughing) Thank you so much for helping us access more of our potential at a time when, I think now more than ever, human beings are called to perform at a higher level in service to the world. And I'm touched by your big heart for children and the fact that you dedicate a huge part of your life to helping children with exercise and the other aspects of the holy quadrinity. So I want to thank you on behalf of the parents of the world and thank you for what you're accomplishing. It's uniquely valuable and important. And thank you so much for being here in the Eat4Earth community with us.

Dr. Wells [00:54:07]: Yeah, my pleasure and thank you for what you're doing for the future of our planet. So it's important work, and thanks for getting the message out there and for doing what you're doing because we need help. So I really appreciate this opportunity.

Erin Elizabeth Interview
You Can Be Stronger, Healthier, and Happier ... and Together We Are Unstoppable

Brendan [00:00:00]: Welcome to the Eat4Earth event. We're exploring how you can heal yourself, your loved ones, and the Earth, with food. This is Brendan Moorehead, and I'm so pleased to welcome our next special guest, Erin Elizabeth. Erin Elizabeth is a longtime activist with a passion for the healing arts, working in that arena for a quarter century now. She's spoken to thousands of doctors since 2015, and courageously seeks out truth no matter what it is, or where it is to be found. She has starred in various documentaries such as *The Truth about Cancer*, *The Truth about Vaccines*, and *That Vitamin Movie*. Her website, Healthnutnews.com is just a little over three years old but has already cracked the top twenty natural health sites worldwide. Erin I really want to thank you for being here with us today.

Erin [00:00:47]: Thank you Brendan, it's an honor to be here. Thanks for having me.

Brendan [00:00:50]: My pleasure. So, Erin, like so many of us that end up health nuts, often by necessity, you've been through a lot, and you've come out the other side healthy, fit and as beautiful as ever. And I'm probably blushing. What was it that inspired you to start your website Healthnutnews.com?

Erin [00:01:12]: Well, I think initially I figured it would be more of a lighthearted site than it might have become over the last three plus years that I've had it. Initially I really wanted to do a lot of things in the kitchen, that was the plan because I'd run health retreats for a number of years here on the coast, and had speakers and chefs from around the world, known in the health community. But then I realized right away that, no surprise, I'd worked for a non-profit a number of years and was more of an activist, and I think that it became bringing people breaking news but also being an activist and letting people know about important matters going on that needed attention. So I think it became a little more serious, although I think that letting people know what I eat or new recipes or healthy organic food, that's important as well. But it just took a little bit of a different direction than I initially planned.

Brendan [00:02:10]: Recently you gave a talk entitled "The Future of Florida, Fake News, and Food". What was that about?

Erin [00:02:18]: Yeah I spoke at The Truth About Cancer in Dallas, which would've been some time back, and then not that long ago I spoke about The Truth About Cancer Orlando, and so I know a lot of people were speaking on the issues of cancer. And the year before I suppose my speech had touched upon that more, but this year I just felt those were really important issues, some of the things going on here in Florida, as well as people knowing about fake news. And I know that may encompass a lot when I say "fake news", but unfortunately sites are being silenced, for a lack of better word, like my site or Dr. Mercola's or other health sites because Facebook has brought on Snopes, which they've announced Snopes as the fact checkers. And Snopes meanwhile is embroiled in a huge court battle allegedly—it doesn't matter—they defrauded the company for illegal activities. But also then they begged for money online and raised in just days over a half million dollars. I think they raised near a million dollars now. They asked for half a million on a Gofundme account because they said they may be shutting down, so they were asking folks for money. But what was most interesting is that mainstream pushed that narrative so hard. I do a lot of videos now in my presentations, which I didn't initially, and in the videos I showed that Snopes— their own video—was shocking to many of the audience where they show the mainstream saying "Snopes", "snopes.com", "snopes.com" all of these different people saying "Snopes.com, they're really in need of money, we've got to help keep them alive." And why mainstream is doing that is because they know that they can't really survive without sites like Snopes. So even though Snopes is ... I mean, I hadn't been around but a few months when they tried to debunk an article I did about a missing doctor, and they put the wrong location. I think I put the location, and they said "No, actually, he was in this state" or whatever. I don't think they got the state right, and unfortunately—thanks Snopes—he's still missing almost three years later. So, it's sad that they have anointed themselves a kind of God of what's true and false, and I don't think that people understand that 98% of the United States thinks that Snopes is gospel pretty much. They go to Snopes. That's where they go find out. They've been around over twenty years. So unfortunately besides Snopes, Facebook has also admitted that they're disabling functions of pages. I've got two main pages about three quarters of a million, and if you count in followers and likes, it's well over a million. But they have disabled any of my abilities to boost a post. Maybe I'll have an article kind of going viral, or I want to boost something, so they're taking that away, and they said that that's because they do not like my business model. Well, I don't have a business model. I don't sell anything. So I found out that this was a canned letter they were writing many people, and it says, "This decision is final." And it was done most frequently to the health sites or, not just health but some of the sites that really are going out on a limb, more investigative journalists just bringing the truth. And sure they might do it to a few hoax sites, but the crazy part is you'll see these hoax sites every day that still do hoaxes: "So and so died", a celebrity that didn't die. And you can see these crazy sponsored ads selling whatever some kind of package, and flipping homes and all that, but if you're doing something that's really helping then yeah, they're immediately going to take away the functions. I'm on a thirty day [untelligible] presently. I'm on them several times a year on my personal page. But I think that the fake news is not just with mainstream as far as that they are Pharma-controlled, by pharmaceutical ads and big agriculture but also the social media.

One more thought on this one, when the massacre happened in Las Vegas ... I won't go into that ... I just was out in Las Vegas lecturing and stayed at The Mandalay Bay, which was not easy, but I wanted to kind of investigate what was going on, but within hours or at least a day or so after, back when the Las Vegas tragedy happened, and tragedy struck, the largest mass shooting in modern history, Yahoo said, "Well, we weren't going to roll it out for a while, but we're going to roll it out now." "Well, we don't allow conspiracy video." And really this is our news now. I mean, YouTube is the number two site in the world, so Google being number one, they own each other. One owns the other; Google owns YouTube. So they said, "We're going to roll this out now, early, because of this horrific tragedy, all of these people dead, where we're not going to allow these conspiracy sites, we're going to kind of stifle them." They come up first a lot of times on the search and the YouTube search engine. Yes, because people want to see what really happened in Las Vegas. The timeline changed. They didn't know where the alleged lone shooter was. And so that happened, and then Google changed their algorithms, which they announced, and I think between all three, the top three sites in the world, which really are our news if we're not watching mainstream television, which so many people are cutting the cable, as we have, but that is our news. They're definitely stifling, silencing, strangling the truth tellers, which they're calling conspiracy theorists, so we're kind of used to that. Whereas before, when you would google an article I wrote, it would come up number one. Now it will show Snopes with their fake diatribe that they've written—that's already been debunked—trying to debunk me. And I think most sites, as you know, in the health, the people you've interviewed, we're doing our best to bring the truth, whereas Snopes just wants to spend a lot of time—and I think they're very biased—to just debunk others. And that's pretty sad. And then you have to defend yourself, which is kind of silly. The good news is that I think we are headed towards more of a grassroots roots route, where news, the real word, would be spread through the internet, but the problem is you have some of the top sites trying to stop that from the truth getting out.

Brendan [00:09:03]: Yeah, this is a real problem, and I recently read an article where somebody was trying to debunk a particular health-educator's information about glyphosate, and when you look at their arguments, it's typically … well, I wouldn't say that I've studied it enough, but I kind of have this sense of that a certain way they approach trying to debunk something. They'll pick up on one little nuance that they'll … it's almost like they intentionally misinterpret it, like, "Okay, we can spin that as if they're saying this", and they attack even though that's not what the person is actually saying. In this case about how glyphosate … I have to go back to the article, I hope I saved it because I actually wanted to start a file of these bogus debunking articles and sort of deconstruct them and look for the way they're doing it and then kind of do an analysis and an exposé and like, "Okay, here's how the trolls 'think'", quotes around the word "think". Here's how they create the appearance of debunking something when it's total nonsense. Or it's a trivial point they make; they might make a point that, OK maybe there's some angle there that there's some truth to it, but it's just irrelevant or not substantive. And you know, Ronnie Cummins with The Organic Consumers Association mentioned to me that his traffic, Dr. Mercola's traffic, just a couple of months ago just fell in half, and that's a problem when the Organic Consumers Association is doing so much to defend human health, the health of the planet, they're doing some of the most important work on the planet.

Erin [00:10:55]: Oh definitely, yeah, and it's sad to see that non-profits like that who Dr. Mercola and I supported for so long and just believe in, and others as well. They're trying to even … I mean they are great non-profit grassroots organizations, Ronnie Cummins is great. And then they're literally stifling them. I mean that's insane. Because they're getting the truth out. That's why.

Brendan [00:11:23]: Is there anything else to touch upon maybe from that talk that you had? I'm just curious about the juxtaposition of Florida, fake news, and food. Florida makes me think about climate-change; food makes me think about agriculture; and fake news, go ahead…

Erin [00:11:52]: So as far as Florida, I talked about a number of things, the event was taking place in Florida with several thousand people for The Truth about Cancer. Some of the folks were coming in from around the world. I think we had 27 countries represented at this last one that I'd spoken at. I wanted them to be aware of some of the issues happening in Florida, so one of the things I touched on—and people were shocked at this—that our governor Rick Scott has—I can't take credit for it because it was Florida Bulldog which is a non-profit watch-dog group with a fitting name, out at Fort Lauderdale that broke the news—that his wife owns millions in stock in mosquito spray. So when you see these editorials that USA Today, I mean they just have no ethics whatsoever, and they publish this by the governor of Florida, and he's saying "For the sake of our babies, we have an epidemic with Zika." He says, you know, "You don't understand, we must spray because otherwise we're going to have microcephaly in babies, shrunken heads for your children, so they're not born ..." And already I think at that point, or around that point, this was a while back, The World Health Organization had announced that it wasn't an epidemic. Zika wasn't an epidemic, and the studies show, which now since he did that article, CNN did an article that said—I mean it's funny because it takes CNN for people to believe it—but even CNN did an article stating that the spray, which would be Naled, the name brand being Dibrom which is morbid spelled backwards, which is kind of morbid to me.

Brendan [00:13:34]: Goodness.

Erin [00:13:35]: And it's been around for so long, but they weren't doing it, I don't think they are doing it aerially as much, at the rate they're doing it now, which is insane, especially after the hurricanes, and it's banned of course in all of the European Union, and so is malathion, another one, but they said that it can cause ... and it's been shown to be linked or can cause developmental delays. And then also even Huffington Post did one a year or two back, saying that they're going to spray Puerto Rico, which now I think after the hurricane, poor Puerto Rico had to finally give in after Maria devastated them. But prior to that they were trying to spray Puerto Rico, and the governor there said "Heck, no." And the Mayor of San Juan ... they sent the planes back and said "We're not going to allow you to spray this" because as Huffington Post showed that the published studies, science shows, that not only does it cause developmental delays but birth defects. So straight up birth defects in long term studies. So those are published studies, but it doesn't seem to matter, I guess. People are like, "Yeah, but we can't get a mosquito bite, because of Zika" when it's not Zika; it's the spray. So sorry, they want you to believe it's the other way around. They want you to think "It's not the spray; it's the Zika". But that's kind of frightening.

I'm trying to think of some of the other issues we talked about. I would imagine climate change, and I know people have different feelings on this. I think definitely I know that's a controversial topic whether water is rising. I mean I can see that that's happening here, and for the first time ever, because we had a house we were selling, an old little house that we lived in, I had around twelve years, and I've owned this house, and for the first time ever—it's three four houses off the intercostal—but it reached all the way almost to our door, our front yard. And that's never happened, we've heard it from people whose ... just sometimes with some of these houses, their parents' or their grandparents', it's been handed down ... and in this case I just bought it ... but some of the people had been there for generations because it is a historic district ... I'm near the center of town, and they've never seen that, ever. I mean we have records kept as well. That's never happened in the history where that kind of flooding happened during Irma. So we definitely have bigger, stronger, more frequent hurricanes, or just with weather in general, with the water level rising. So yeah, it's definitely an issue that I think people don't always want to talk about.

We have a gas pipeline coming through the state, and we're solar here, so we have fifty solar panels. And I think that that used to be ... I still don't talk about it much because as soon as you say that, there seems to be this stigma, and it's "oh, you're smug", maybe because the TV show, or South Park or whatever. We have an electric car that'll run on solar, and then it's just a two-bedroom house, but we don't have an electric bill. If you tell people that, it's surprising how angry people will get that you're using sunshine here at the beach to power your home. "Oh, people can't afford that" or "Isn't that nice. You use sunshine. " Would it be better if I were using fossil fuels? I'm sorry.

We just had a leak yesterday of 210.000 gallons with the Dakota pipeline, with the Key Stone pipeline in the Dakotas on the border of North and South Dakota. But when I posted about that I had people first say it was fake news. I mean this literally went like that old saying by I think it was Gandhi … I don't remember actually who said it, but it might've been Mahatma Gandhi. They first said, "It's fake news. This would be on the news." So then I said, "Here it is. CNN", "CNN is fake news" "Okay, here it is on Fox" "Well, it's probably just sabotage." But I'm not sure why. It's some strange thing in this country that people may enjoy paying … we pay billions as *New York Times* has said, not that I particularly like them, but the figures are there in black and white. We pay billions upon billions a year, not one, two, three—more than that—billions per year to Big Oil, you know these tycoon billionaires of Big Oil. And I'm not sure what the resistance is from people to switch to sustainable clean energy that is not going to hurt anyone … people aren't going to die in explosions. And again people would like to just kind of be able to write off that Naled or Malathion are safe to spray from planes. Here they literally use helicopters so it's even scarier. They somehow, not everyone—there are a lot supporters, my readers who most get it—but still even a few of my own readers are real resistant about alternative power, and they don't know how it works. Sometimes maybe people don't like things that they don't know about, so I do my best to educate them.

Today Tesla came out with their … my dad's an engineer, and if I get it wrong … it's not a sixteen wheeler … I should know … but it's a large truck … it's a semi … and Tesla just came out with their first fully electric or solar—you could easily power it with solar as opposed to electric—semi. And Walmart already ordered … I don't know if it was … first it was ten, then I saw fifteen, and it looked like the number was going up from there, but Walmart did announce that they're going to start using those trucks for transportation.

Brendan [00:19:26]: Well that's awesome, and I'm excited to hear that. It's really cool to have a company like Tesla to kind of lead the charge. I think our country worships the entrepreneurs, especially the sort of moonshot entrepreneur that has huge visions, makes big things happen, and I believe Elon Musk is helping to hopefully overcome any skepticism or bias or, I don't know what it is. You're identifying defensiveness around the issue of solar like, "Oh, are you too good for petroleum?" I'm not sure what the idea is when people are having an issue with that, but there was a movie called *Carbon Nation* by Peter Byck. You saw that?

Erin [00:20:24]: I didn't see it, I have to make a note and remember to see it. No I didn't. I always love to hear about movies.

Brendan [00:20:30]: So what he discovered in interviewing people on both sides of the political spectrum, is that as long as climate change wasn't used in the conversation, or wasn't the issue, if it was about simply intelligent, responsible, independent energy policy people were on board. He found people that were conservative, Republicans, Libertarians, whatever, over more to the right, and of course people on the left. They were all about having a renewable energy economy. It's just that in certain conversations "climate change" would suddenly throw it off course. So it doesn't need to be part of the conversation. The same thing is true here in terms of regenerative agriculture and restoring our soils, it doesn't even have to be about climate change. We have to restore soils. We've got sixty harvests left. I think everybody likes to eat, and obviously everybody likes nutritious food, and so what we're showing is that we can grow as much food—I say "we"—I mean these food system innovators—some of them are in this event—we can grow as much food with higher nutrient density, with less of these chemicals that affect us all, and that's regenerative agriculture. It doesn't have to be about drawing down the carbon from the atmosphere and what that may do for the future of our planet.

Erin [00:22:05]: I talked a little bit probably in regard to food. I think we talked about growing our own, and sometimes I understand that people ... I was talking about hydroponic ... I did an article about hydroponic ... we do a lot of articles on the site on hydroponic growing ... and people are like, "Well, don't use PVC", and I understand their concerns. So there isn't anything that's perfect, and some people said they prefer growing in their own soil. And then people are saying, "Yeah, but whatever spray that is happening," say if it were Naled, "then that's affecting the soil." But yeah, I do think that there's hope, and you want to look forward to the future with hope. And I think that is great, that we can do more sustainable growing methods. And that is the other thing, misconception maybe. I think people are waking up ... I definitely see that, but I think even five-ten years ago people knew what GMO was, or genetically modified food, or genetically engineered food that we'd be eating that they thought that was the sustainable way, but now they realized the price that you pay, and also it's not sustainable. And I think people are opening their eyes to that, but yeah that's great. I imagine that with some of the guests you've had interviews thus far that they're on it—and I know Joe is too— so it's nice to see that people are awakening.

Brendan [00:23:31]: So you've been talking to a lot of doctors lately, for a few years, what are you speaking to them about? Are you speaking to them in groups, speaking to the individually? What's that all about?

Erin [00:23:45]: I ... and I don't know if ... you could always just say, since we didn't discuss it, if you want to skip this ... but it depends. I'm speaking at Cal Jam coming up for the third time in I think early March, so third year in a row, which will be exciting. I've spoken at Florida Chiropractic Association. Usually both of those will have three thousand plus. Same at Parker University. I spoke there about a year ago, and that was about 3400 chiropractors for that event. So some are chiropractors, and they're doctors too, or doctors of chiropractic. And then other ones will be MDs and DOs. I just spoke out in Las Vegas not that long ago to a group of doctors, and not always, but definitely part of the reason they flew me out to Las Vegas to do this event—I spoke for a hundred minutes on that one without stopping, which is what they wanted; they wanted a hundred minute key note—and it was mainly about holistic doctor deaths. Did you know that?

Brendan [00:24:55]: Yeah, I'm aware of this, I haven't been following blow by blow, but I have seen certainly your Unintentional series about what's happening. And of course somebody's going to paint it as a conspiracy theory, but it's uncanny.

Erin [00:25:16]: Well yeah, it is uncanny. And back in November I was lecturing at a medical conference, and they had kind of one side for doctors and the other side for the public. I was the MC. Somehow I ended up MC-ing the event, which was great because I got to introduce all my heroes at this event. And then I was a lecturer as well. And I only touched upon the holistic doctors briefly during that because I don't know if the general public had heard about it, but then they had. This one was a general public audience, and then we had doctors who [unintelligible] ceremonies that night. And it really—I don't want to say validated for me because it's not really a validation for me—but I was curious what some of the holistic doctors who had died, (what their) family members were feeling. And I've met some of them before, and I know a number of them. And we were friends or colleagues of the holistic doctors, who in the Unintended series who died. So sometimes you're writing about your own friends you've just talked to, or they've been at your home, or you've been at their home. And it's a little macabre, but they had awards that night for Nick Gonzales for instance, and they seated me next to … this is like the third event where I've been sat next to his widow Marybeth Gonzalez who's amazing. He was an MD in Manhattan—just to touch on this briefly—who was putting patients under remission. And at his funeral the church was really just jam-packed in New York with patients who had been like late stage pancreatic cancer and now were on remission still twenty years later. So they basically cured them of cancer as many would say. They still don't know the cause of death. They thought it was heart attack, but the autopsy showed he was healthy. He was relatively young and healthy, so it came as a shock to people. But she was the first one to accept an award on his behalf, and then—I haven't had the site that long so—and Joe, Dr. Mercola, got an award. There are a lot of mostly doctors who had passed, and then the family members. I got "Truth in Journalism" (an award), and that was really great, but of course I dedicated it to the doctors even though they were just talking about the site overall, but I didn't want it to be about me, and I figured I said with well over seventy who have died that I think it warrants an investigation. But what was shocking to see—it wasn't shocking but it was surprising—people were very supportive, and they did a standing ovation. And I hope that that was really for the doctors because we've had these fallen heroes who we've lost. And I don't know if they're connected or not. I get … especially with some of the latest who have died … and it's been pretty shocking deaths … and of course, I mean, it's either alleged suicide, murder, or murder, suicide in all these different families that are dying. And so they get angry and say, "How dare you say Pharma did this. You don't know", and I actually never say that. That's what people don't understand. These are not usual readers of the site, maybe a friend had shared it with them or something, but what they don't understand is that I'm just presenting all the doctors who've died. Obviously, the overwhelming majority are holistic, and if they've died in a shocking manner, whether it would be—I know it's a little gruesome here but you know—whether it would be a sudden death, kind of like Nick Gonzales, or an alleged suicide or established murder, or a death where they can't figure out how they died when they were found dead. It's been difficult but I just saw the pattern, starting in the beginning with Dr. Bradstreet and felt that I had to report on it. And I never ever thought with the name of the site, first of all that I picked, that I'd be writing about that. And I never thought really—as I say it aloud it sounds so strange—that I'd be lecturing to doctors about this, but I always want to let them know, Brendan, that I don't want to instill fear because some of them do get afraid. And especially, I don't know if it's more at the beginning or more now, but they would write, and strangers, some of them total strangers, or ones that maybe Joe, Dr. Mercola knows, but I hadn't met yet, now I've met, and they were fearful and some of them were thinking of not practicing. And so the whole message was that if anything, you want to make your voice louder, and to speak out, and let people know that you're not afraid, and you won't be silenced and to really turn up the volume. So hopefully somehow through this strange … I mean it's very sad and tragic … but these strange deaths … it had been somewhat cathartic or to try to help those doctors. So they know "Look, I know I'm writing about the series. Don't shoot the messenger here, but I also want you to know do not be afraid. Keep doing what you're doing. Speak out louder than ever." And we don't know if these are connected or not, but I don't want people to be fearful or go into hiding, because if it is connected, that's exactly what they would want, whoever they would be. I mean just to say hypothetically.

Brendan [00:30:36]: In terms of speaking out, you did mention an example ... I don't think you mentioned the whole story on the spraying in Florida ... but you're speaking out a lot and all of us need to speak out, and in particular, I'm going to sort of move back to the topic of food, and food and agriculture.

Erin [00:31:04]: I know yes, we did go off here.

Brendan [00:31:06]: Well no, I asked you those questions, and I wanted to go there. So I wanted to know if you could sort of tell me, I mean, we have examples, a lot of times with all these things happening, people can feel like, "Oh my God, there's these colossal forces influencing everything, our food, our agriculture, and our environment." And people feel sometimes powerless, like, "What can we do?"
And the reality is we actually can do a lot. Consumers have tremendous power. We're the ones that buy everything. We're the ones that keep every business in business, and we can actually ... if we speak up especially unison together one big voice, it has power. The first time I really noticed that in the food world was in the 90s when the FDA wanted to try to regulate supplements as drugs and the public voice and opposition was so strong that we won and supplements in this country are still considered food. We can't make drug claims but hey, no need to. So I'm curious to know aside from this example in Florida where they were going to spray, and I guess there was another organization that rallied people to protest,` and then that spraying was cancelled.

Erin [00:32:33]: Yeah, it was cancelled in just a couple of counties north of us here in Florida, which was great.

Brendan [00:32:39]: And that was going to be against the Zika, the idea was Zika. That's what that was.

Erin [00:32:45]: What happened was it started, and I don't even know if I did an article on it, but I had seen that the county, and gosh are there so many people that I've worked on campaigns, of course for ... and also it's sometimes by the city, of course for our county ... they go by county ... and so there was the head of mosquito control, some call it "vector control". I promoted someone who I thought has spoken out against Naled —at least that he doesn't want to use that, it would be more comfortable with BTI or something less harmful or no spraying at all—to get elected for Collier county. And now the name is escaping me, but they're just I think two counties north—it's just outside Jacksonville, Orange Park would be in there—but basically they were going to do aerial spraying, and they posted, just letting people know about, a notice, and so what I did on my one page, maybe I did it on both, but to over half a million people I said ... and I don't usually do this ... I mean I know that trolls will send people to my page all the time because they don't like what I'm talking about ... but this is going to literally affect our health because just up the road they're going to be— and my family is there as well, which was another reason why it was near and dear to my heart—that they're going to be spraying. So I said "Guys, look." I didn't say "Hey, go there any say something", but they did, and the reaction was so strong. Also, oh gosh, I think Hope Springs, and I just can't think the name of the county, but all of these different counties, Jacksonville basically, just west of Jacksonville and Jacksonville's one of the biggest cities—which people don't realize—in the US. And so between that and then just their locals being so outraged and waking up to it, they did cancel. And then I did an update because they said, "We've cancelled the aerial spraying." Now, what they still do (is) some residual spraying by trucks. I think I had heard that they were trying, but if they're aerial some say it's eight times stronger when they're dropping it on you from a plane. And I had shared a video that a friend who's an organic chef because food is so important, and people do worry about our food. And she has an organic garden in her yard, and she's a local chef and prepares food for different people. And she was just outside with her grandchild, on a little time off helping babysit, and a black helicopter came over and sprayed. Now, it was BTI. It wasn't Naled. But she got it on video. It literally showed there was no warning. It was 8:30 a.m. on I think a Monday or Friday. It was either the beginning or the end of the week, and she was just literally out in her backyard, and you can imagine a helicopter going over. And they got the nozzles open the spray is coming down on you and your one year old baby.

Brendan [00:35:39]: It's ridiculous.

Erin [00:35:41]: And so she was concerned about her garden after that, and even if it were BTI, and you never know what they're spraying, they actually did call recently to warn me that they were going to be spraying, and I thought it was a friend pranking me except I could see the number on my cellphone. He said "We're going to be spraying", and I said "What are you going to be spraying, you have to tell me." And he said "Just some Kontrol", [laughs] "We're going to be spraying some Kontrol" and I thought this is somebody. And I actually called back and already the director's not thrilled with me because he allowed me to record him for an interview which you can hear where I'm telling him I'm recording him, and then he didn't like it because I think there was a huge backlash when the video went viral on YouTube and on the internet. But with this particular, they have to call me. Even if I'm a journalist, I'm a resident, and "Call Joe or me." So they called, and I said "It's Kontrol, and it starts with a 'K'." And yeah, I mean it sounds innocuous, but it really is scary, maybe not as bad as Malathion and Naled, both of which—especially Malathion, which they spray as well—are banned in the European Union, all those countries. It's banned I think in all of Europe, and they've been shown to—this isn't like BBC, this is in international news—that those pesticides, the birth defects aside, and everything else what they're doing to our children, is that they are ... I think they said wildlife literally is decreasing by I don't know, one study was saying like 90%.

Brendan [00:37:21]: Oh my God.

Erin [00:37:22]: Yeah, it's just killing, it's just like us, we're life, we're beings on this planet. So are they. Bears. I think in the particular article that I saw there was a picture of a poor bear out there trying to make it, but whether it's people, bears, I mean it's absolutely ridiculous, and of course, our planet. But they did try to, Osceola county, one of the spokespeople at another county, huge county which encompasses kind of part of Orlando, they had written me, and they didn't like my picture and they said "You can't use the picture." And I said "No, no, no, I bought it, I own that picture. I can use it." And they said "It's misleading. It has five planes spraying, and that was like after Andrew" the picture I used. We had to do a lot of spraying after hurricane Andrew, which was actually a strong hurricane but relatively small, just went across and just devastated South Florida in '92. But yes, it was horrible in the areas it hit. Homestead Florida, etc. were absolutely devastated by spin-off tornadoes etc. which I've been through before. But it wasn't that big of an area, but of course they brought five planes out after people have been through hurricanes, tornadoes, lost their homes. Now they're being sprayed, and he didn't like the picture. And he said—and I can say this because I have the e-mail—he said "Well, the *Orlando Sentinel*," or someone like that, "they would just do this and fix it." And I'm like "Oh, really, they would just do what you say because you work for the county. Well, I don't. I've got news for you." And they haven't bothered me ever since. But it was amazing that they said it would scare people, and I said "That's not my intention." It's to educate people and tell them to not be scared but be prepared.

Also another thing was ... there's a great guy down there ... I think he's running for some smaller political office in Miami, Michael de Felipe, but someone had introduced us, and I interviewed him about a protest they were having down there in Miami. So that gets more attention, and CBS evening news did a national news coverage on that where they had people there with, I mean with half the size of this room, with banners so big they could barely carry them. Some of them had the governor Rick Scott on there like him in an airplane and crazy stuff. And also they had a great billboards, large signs that were well done—they looked like they were done by artists—that were giving the scientific facts about what they're spraying. So that got national—it was CBS evening news—so they're down there covering that, and they were interviewed. And he had just set it up the night before. We did an interview. I think that there was a third person in on the interview. We just did it through our phones on Facebook live. It went viral to hundreds of thousands, and thankfully they had more people than they knew what to do with there, and I mean, the more people that protest the better. But yeah, I think that what it comes down to is not only are people concerned about their families, or their animals, or the planet, but also their food because it does affect the food. And I think that's probably why I see more people wanting to, I mean, yes, I think ideally and inevitably we want to stop the spraying, but also we want to have ways to ... I understand why people are doing ... whether it's hydroponic growing or doing green houses, growing in the ground ... at least it's a little better growing in the ground in a green house. I don't know if it protects that much because the land could get saturated outside, but they are taking precautions because they are upset because of what's being done. And it's not just Florida, it was New York and Texas especially after Harvey. Southern California. I lived in Southern California eight years, Brendan, and I don't think I ever saw ... I had animals back then, and I always had a door just cracked because I was on the second story of an apartment, and they could go out in the big balcony and come back in and hang out, lie in the sun, get their vitamin D, and there was never a mosquito, I'd never seen a mosquito in Southern California, but yet, they're also doing aerial spraying there as well, so...

Brendan [00:41:36]: Plus it's not as moist, I think. There's so much standing water sometimes in Florida that maybe mosquitoes become an issue, I don't know. I mean, do you actually not see many mosquitoes in Florida either?

Erin [00:41:47]: Not as bad as people would think. Orange County—well, they sprayed in Orange County California, where I used to live in that area—but Orange County Florida, which is Orlando, for years, and I have to look this up ... there was so much going on with hurricanes, I didn't get to look not too long ago, and we have been rebuilding since then .. but Orange County didn't spray for years, and the reason was they said that Naled or any of these ... they're definitely neuro-toxins, they're deadly, they're poison ... but they say, "Oh but it's in a small concentration." They said they're not affective for the *aedes aegypti* mosquito, which is the thing that everybody was worried about, which was Zika. And also they said that the people had spoken out, and they weren't too keen on it, the Orlando people. There are some pretty hip folks there, and they're in the city;

they're city-dwellers, and they don't want that, especially Orange County is really Orlando. The people are smart, they've done their research, they're educated, they don't want it.

Now I had heard that they were trying to spray since then, but they had ceased all aerial spraying of at least Naled. They may do more of what they call these organic pesticides which are controversial, but at least they weren't doing that. And that went on for years. But I've been told by scientists that they're not particularly effective against the *aedes aegypti* mosquito. You'd be better as the head for vectors mosquito control, at least I think he says, for Collier County, explains that you go out and … gosh he has that special word … but when people see the mosquitoes, a lot of times it's standing water, like you said, so there's a name for them, and I've just slipped my mind. In a "container", they call it "container". So container mosquitoes. You empty the containers. I mean it's great collecting rain water for the barrels, but have it so they can't get in there and breed, or empty your containers if it's just something you have lying around, or open all these containers. And that they can do that and people can make a huge difference as opposed to spraying poison down from planes upon us. And that would be much safer for our food, especially if you're growing your own or crops in the area.

Brendan [00:44:05]: Totally. There's so many alternatives to pesticides, and this reminds me of the organization Parents for a Safer Environment. They're doing some phenomenal things because they're showing people that people can go and influence their local cities and counties and so forth, that are spraying, unfortunately, like 2,4-D everywhere. This is part of Agent Orange, and it is being applied in public spaces, in parks and so forth, like crazy. And it doesn't have to be. And there's actually a process by which mothers and fathers and any community-oriented people can engage the local authorities in a process of implementing Integrated Pest Management, IPM. And there's actually, I think in all cases, at least in most cases, there's policies at the state level that counties would follow in most states, where they have to at first try Integrated Pest Management before they use these more toxic compounds. And people can get on board with that and shift this risk profile because it's huge. There's a lot of pesticides people are getting from their parks and so forth, their pets are getting through their feet. 2,4-D doesn't stick well to whatever it's sprayed to, so it's easy for it to suddenly get up into somebody's body that's walking on it. It's also kind of floating up in the air depending on how recently it was applied and so forth. So, Parents for a Safer Environment are doing great things in that regard. That's another way that people are having a real impact just by speaking up, learning what the process is. I'm curious if you have any other examples especially in the world of food and agriculture, let's say, where people have spoken up and made a difference. I'm thinking you know, there's the Dolphin Safe Tuna campaign from back in the 90s. Anything else that comes to mind when I mention that?

Erin [00:46:18]: I'll be quick because I met the man who did that Earth Island Institute and my biological mother who I found some years ago, no surprise, the apple didn't fall far from the tree, but she's a journalist and a scientist PhD, so I was able to have dinner in San Francisco because of Earth Island Institute, who because of that, the man especially the people who filmed on that boat with the fishermen and showed the dolphins being caught. I do think that I've seen definite cases where people have spoken up and had changes and as far as food. I think somebody like Ronnie Cummins doing, so I don't want to sound biased and say Joe or Dr. Mercola of course, but I mean he's obviously made a difference. And I think another good one, Pam, I remember her name Pam Larry. Even though it didn't pass … she's Pam Larry, and she's really just an amazing woman. She did Prop 37 out in California. She began it. She's a grandmother who started the proposition, and it didn't pass only because the big agriculture was sending out advertisements, literally like villifying. My friends would show them to me, because I lived there for so long, in Southern Cal. They'd show me, "Hey, look I got this flyer, and it said 'Dr. Mercola is a quack, and do not listen to him on this'." Or other people. But she started that, and her initiative became a proposition that people were voting on, to label genetically modified foods. And I think that that's so important. But I think she would be one where, I mean it was so close, it was so very close, and I think people were just misinformed. But that's another thing where I'm always encouraging doctors that I speak with or just readers on my pages or my newsletter, which I don't send out enough, to all these people, letting them know that they can have a voice even if it's just, whether someone wants to start something local in their community. And when I was at the event with some of the holistic doctors' families and a lot of doctors who are still alive and well and their families, we were talking more about how they need to have more grassroots efforts to connect people within a state, or even a county, so people can get together because there's power in numbers. So that's so important.

But even it can take one voice like someone like Pam Larry, a grandmother who's just such an awesome human being, that would start something like Prop 37 and came so close. And if nothing else I think it raised real awareness, and despite the fact that Prop 37 didn't pass, and I think if it had in California it would've hopefully had a wave then all the way through to the East Coast and where you live eventually, that it did raise awareness about genetically modified foods and let people know that ... there's a misconception I think that people say, "Oh no, it's going to hurt the farmer." Well, of course there are factory farms or there are farmers, and they feel forced to use genetically modified foods. And I've talked to many of them, and I grew up in the Midwest. We're both from Chicago, but I actually grew up, was adopted and grew up in Indiana, in the heart of that, with farmers, the heartland literally. But some of them, they don't want to. But they just feel like that's just kind of forced upon them, and I think that can change since it's only been since the 90's with the tomato being the first, that breed of tomato, being the first genetically engineered food. That can change. I think that people can, Brendan, they can speak out and encourage other people to do the same and form groups. I guess I've been doing that since high school. And kids too, I don't think they realize how much power they have. Children can make a difference because they are our future of this planet, and if they speak up ... we have a boy here—and this is a good example in Florida and still it's an epidemic I think—but he spoke up about the food that they throw away with the grocery stores. I mean thousands of tons literally tons, and tons of food, literally that are thrown away, and that if would be instead ... they'd have a system where that food was given to the poor. But still they will grind it up so that the homeless aren't able to eat it, in some areas, and I think that it's still ... whereas France and the whole country of France doesn't allow them to just throw away, you can't just throw it away, "Oops, it's going to expire, we're just going to throw ten thousand pounds of vegetables in the garbage." And they can have an alternative where people can, they can salvage before it goes bad, and people can have it who are less fortunate.

Brendan [00:51:30]: Yeah food waste is a huge part of this issue, I mean we're talking about the impact of agriculture on the planet, I guess about a third of the food just goes completely to waste. Maybe it's more like 40%, I've seen that, maybe a few different numbers on that. I think Dr. Mercola is a hero for how much support he threw behind Prop 37 in California. Big kudos to your partner. I worked on that campaign a little bit, just for signature gathering. I was in Los Angeles, living there at the time.

Erin [00:52:09]: And people are probably pretty passionate about it.

Brendan [00:52:11]: Big time. 80% of the country wants genetically modified organisms labeled. It's not a question, and it is a right to know what we're eating. And there's so many things that don't even have to be on the labels at all, and that's one of them. There's many more—some of which will pop up here and there in this event. They're really important to know about—that affect our ability to digest food really, to assimilate it, to absorb it, for the micro-organisms to survive in our guts so that they can do their part of the job. It's serious. We need to know what's in our food. And the best way to speak, or let's say the easiest way—there's no best way—there's many ways to exercise our voice, but the most profound one is just choosing what we buy. We are voting every time we pull out our wallet, and so the question is how much do we know about what we're buying, and that's where sometimes we have to get into activism because we're eating things that we don't know we're eating, and we deserve to know.

Erin [00:53:18]: Oh yeah, definitely, and that's another thing where people, again, where they have the power, or even just an individual, like you said where you can vote with your wallet, because you're right, you do every time you use it. And I think more people are doing that, and we've seen it change so much even at more conventional grocery stores where even in Florida because we're a little bit behind—I lived in California a long time—we're a little bit behind here as opposed to California or even maybe Colorado. But I think it's catching up because now I see whole organic sections of food and even with dairy. I mean, that's another controversial issue, but now they have a2 milk because people are realizing you don't want to drink a1, or they're having grass-fed and not factory farmed. And I think that's a start. I know there are some people that don't want dairy or have dairy alternatives that are actually healthy, so that's great too.

And another thing, of course, besides the conventional supermarket and besides growing our food, of course, we do our best to support farmers' markets, which I know ... I had a sticker on my car, and it dates me but back in the late 80s saying "Support local organic farmers. " And I mean I was a teenager, but I think then I would have people ask me "What's organic?" But I think that now of course it's changed, and people are changing. And they can also support local farmers, and they can save money. I mean some of the farmers' markets are expensive, but sometimes you can find one that's not certified organic, but they aren't using any pesticides or anything. And we have one like that here. It's expensive to certify a farm, or maybe they're doing biodynamic farming, which I know Joe talks about. And so you can do that yourself, or if it's obviously on a small level, maybe just on your property. But you can then—farmers who can grow much more food than we can at home—we can support them as well, so that's important. "And I know people say it, but really if we go to those farmers' markets, I think people are resistant to that a little bit too. But when they go, they're like, "Wow" and it's amazing what they can find.

Brendan [00:55:29]: Yeah, absolutely, I love farmers' markets. Do you have any final thoughts or recommendations for how people can really take back control of their health, the food system, and the environment around them?

Erin [00:55:48]: I would say it can be difficult, and it can be a little overwhelming to do your own research. I mean each person is different, and you're going to have to take things with a grain of salt. You may not agree with everything I say, or maybe not agree with everything with anyone out there you're going to listen to or read would say, but to do your research and to know. I think another thing is, it's really important, having been through many health struggles, and I was over 50% body fat; I was obese—I give away a free book of how I overcame the weight loss and the Lyme and all that, Lyme disease—but to know that there's light at the end of the tunnel. If you're making changes and wanting to implement healthier eating habits or foods into your diet, incorporate that into your diet, it may seem like a bit of a struggle at first. You're just like, "Ah, it's not making a difference." Maybe the weight's not coming off, or you're still having auto-immune challenges, or if you're overcoming cancer, which some of those doctors like Nick Gonzalez were healing through food. He was not using any kind of drugs, or anything really extraordinary except doing it through very specific healthy organic diets. And that people know that they can make amazing changes. And at first it might be difficult, but they know that there's light at the end of the tunnel, and that they can come out the other side and be stronger and healthier and happier. So that would be my advice.

Brendan [00:57:31]: Beautiful, thank you. And in terms of, speaking of Dr. Nick Gonzalez, I believe he is the Nick Gonzalez that was working with Dr. Linda Isaacs, and does he do pancreatic enzymes?

Erin [00:57:46]: Yeah, I do think he does. I should know that. I know there's so many. We're talking about Nick in particular tonight ...

Brendan [00:57:55]: Yeah there's so many. The reason I bring him up is Dr. Linda Isaacs is also in this event, so ...

Erin [00:58:01]: Oh okay, yeah, I think it might've been pancreatic enzymes, and I know I've heard of her and respect her very much. That does ring a bell. So I think that's probably the case with the pancreatic enzymes. So yeah, I mean obviously there are some supplementations, but really I think listening to his lectures, and knowing him before he passed away, or died suddenly of unknown reasons, but yeah I realized how crucial diet can be, not just for you know "You could change your diet," lose weight and all that, but really just changing your body, your mind, everything. It's so important, and we just had a, just closing that holistic health coach that was in the news here. I did an article today about that. She was fined, and she was threatened with jail time for giving diet tips, which is crazy because unless you're a dietitian in the state, even if you're a certified health coach or whatever, you can't do that. But I think that now they have several attorneys, and there's a couple of different non-profit organizations standing behind her, with attorneys, saying [unintelligible].

Brendan [00:59:07]: Good.

Erin [00:59:09]: Yeah, so I think we're going to see that as well, because people don't always know maybe the healthiest foods to eat, and now I think the word is getting out, and people are learning and realizing that our old food pyramid may not be so healthy after all, and that's the old standard. Just keep doing your research and know it's going to get better. And especially with the internet, the power of the internet, we're grassroots, and that we can grow, and there's nothing that can stop us.

Brendan [00:59:41]: Awesome, that's a great note to end on. There's nothing that can stop us. Truly we can be unstoppable. We just have to commit and join arms and get loud and have fun doing it.

Erin [00:59:55]: Exactly. The journey is a big part of it.

Brendan [00:59:59]: Well Erin you are, you are truly an unwavering champion of truth. I really appreciate that about you, and I think, you know, for truth, health, and medical freedom really. So I believe I speak for others as well, everybody here at the Eat4Earth event in thanking you for your leadership as a journalist, as an advocate. I believe you've also been a health coach and probably don't have as much time for that lately but...

Erin [01:00:29]: I miss doing that kind of things.

Brendan [01:00:32]: So thank you so much for spending this time with us today.

Erin [01:00:35]: Thank you, thank you, it's been an honor. Thanks for having me, I really appreciate it.

Day 5 – Detoxify and Re-Mineralize Your Body

Food, Water, Toxins, Your Brain, and Your Success
Alex Charfen
What You Will Discover

- 2 new artificial sweeteners that don't have to be disclosed on food labels
- What you need to know about "toxicity threshold" and "operational drag"
- What achievement-oriented people need to know about food to create momentum and reach their potential

The Toxin Solution: Essential Keys to Safe and Complete Detoxification
Joseph Pizzorno, ND
What You Will Discover

- Why you must detoxify these organs in this order
- A stunning new research finding about the primary cause of heart disease cancer, diabetes, and most other diseases (not what we've been told)
- The "health food" that carries arsenic into your body, even from organic sources
- The very common heavy metal revealed to be a primary cause of osteoporosis (and which results from farming practices we must change)

Minerals, Heavy Metals, and Advanced Detox Strategies and Technology
Wendy Myers, FDN-P, NC
What You Will Discover

- The #1 way heavy metals are getting into your body (not what you think)
- 2 toxin binders you should consider using
- The detox strategy shown to reduce all-cause mortality by 40%
- The new detox technology that makes detoxification faster and easier than ever

Minerals, Spiritual Attainment, and a Technology to Measure the Nutrients in Your Food and Power the Grassroots Movement for a Regenerative Food System
Dan Kittredge
What You Will Discover

- A handheld tool that will enable you to measure the nutrient density of food before you buy it
- The surprising conversation Dan had with Whole Foods about his technology
- Dan's fascinating experience in the Himalayas developing high-level spiritual practices
- A stunning revelation about the untapped genetic potential of food crops

Minerals That Heal & How to Increase Food's Mineral Content 10X
Robert Van Risseghem
What You'll Learn

- Why turmeric from India has high levels of phytonutrients like curcumin
- The potentially cancer-fighting mineral you've never heard of that is deficient in American soils
- The essential mineral that correlates strongly with low incidence of cancer and AIDS around the world
- Crucial roles of the mineral molybdenum in the body that you've never heard of
- A simple step to increase the minerals in food by 10x

Newly Discovered Ways GMOs Can Harm You
Jeffrey M. Smith
What You Will Discover

- The vegetable that is supposedly safe to eat non-orrganic but is actually getting sprayed with RoundUp / glyphosate
- The new GMO technology that may be the most dangerous yet
- How to share information about GMOs with other people without making them defensive

Why Lymphatic Drainage Should Be Your First Step In Detoxification
Kelly Kennedy
What You Will Discover

- How to avoid ever having a "Herxheimer" reaction again during detoxification
- The seven factors that thicken lymphatic fluid and block lymphatic drainage
- The five most common indications that your lymphatic system is stagnant
- The big mistake most people make when trying to stimulate lymphatic drainage, and the correct way to unblock your lymphatic drainage pathways
- The all-in-one device that accelerates healing via lymphatic drainage and improving parasympathetic nervous system tone for accelerated healing

Alex Charfen Interview
Food, Water, Toxins, Your Brain, and Your Success in Life

Brendan [00:00:00]: Welcome back to the Eat4Earth event. We're exploring how you can heal yourself, your loved ones, and the planet, with food. This is Brendan Moorehead and I'm excited to have our next guest, Alex Charfen. Alex Charfen has studied greatness for decades, in particular in regard to the entrepreneurial personality type. His entrepreneurial career began at age eight and has spanned multiple industries including tech, real-estate, and entrepreneurial consulting. Alex believes that the most important work he will ever do is helping other entrepreneurial personality types prosper and understand themselves so they can make the difference that they're intended to make. His book *The Entrepreneurial Personality Type* published in 2016 has become the handbook for entrepreneurs around the world looking for answers. He's spoken on the biggest stages, appeared on TV, and in print for major media outlets such as NSN DC, CNBC, Fox News, *The Wall Street Journal*, *USA Today*, *Investor's Business Daily*, and MX Open Forum to provide his unique views and insights. His next book *Momentum* will publish in early 2018. Alex, I think this is going to be a really fun and eye-opening conversation, and I really thank you for being here today.

Alex [00:01:12]: Thank you Brendan, I'm excited to be here, I love this topic.

Brendan [00:01:16]: Yeah, you and I apparently are both equally obsessed. So, Alex, as a life-long student of greatness, you pay a lot of attention to physical and lifestyle influences on performance, things like diet, exercise, movement, sleep, water. So if somebody is focused on achievement and performance in work, business, entrepreneurship, relationships, life in general, how important are lifestyle factors in the scheme of things, and in particular the food we eat?

Alex [00:01:47]: Brendan, you know, I'm not going to say that you can't be successful if you don't eat healthy because there are definitely people out there who have achieved financial success without paying attention to self-care, or nutrition, breathing, hydration and movement, but I don't think they're happy. I think that true success comes from earning what you think you're worth and making an impact on the world and making your contribution, and helping people with whatever it is that you do. But I think it also comes from feeling good, feeling vital, feeling energized and being excited about being alive every day. I work with some of the most successful people in the world and the coaching that I give them is all about how to grow in scale a business, it's how to put the right systems into their companies, it's how to have the right communication structure. But then we back away and I take a holistic view of the individual and say, "Are you eating right?", "Are you breathing right", "Are you drinking enough water?", "Are you moving enough?", because when we start focusing on ourselves as a holistic organ and we look at that in addition to trying to grow the business, suddenly the business grows faster. I've said this for years Brendan and people laugh at it and snicker until they try it. Hydration will make you more money. Eating healthy will make you more successful. Moving, breathing and getting more into your body, connecting mind and body will make whatever you're doing in the world exponentially stronger. And I think so many of us run by that, and I did at one point. I ended up almost

300 pounds, running a $250,000,000 a year company, with fourteen offices throughout the US and Latin America, a massive staff, and my doctor told me I was his most likely candidate for a heart attack.

Brendan [00:03:37]: Wow.

Alex [00:03:38]: And when I heard that in my early thirties, thirty to thirty-one years old, when I heard that and I woke up, I realized, "Hey, this is not going to work. I can't just keep trying to push this thing called 'success', without actually taking care of myself". And when I started taking care of myself, my entire world transformed.

Brendan [00:03:56]: I think that for at least some period of time, most achievement-oriented folks have relied on processed foods for convenience and just expedience, getting through the day, and obviously you've looked at this, what are the short-term and long-term influences on performance of relying on processed foods?

Alex [00:04:19]: Oh gosh, this is such a hot button for me, Brendan. I tell my clients the only processed food that's safe to eat is the one that you process yourself because today more than any other time in human history, we cannot trust the food supply. When it comes to anything that's processed anymore, we are part of this massive human experiment where the amount of hyper-processing and chemical-additives, chemical-preservatives, colors, dyes, artificial sweeteners, added sugar. What we're eating today when we eat processed foods, aren't really foods, what we're eating is calorie-laden, rich products that have high flavors, but it's hard to call it an actual food supply. Can you live on it? Sure, but the problem is we are getting more and more overfed and undernourished because when you look at most processed foods they have very little, and I mean most—I'm not saying some—*most*, the vast majority of processed foods, have very little bioavailable nutritional quality. But they do have calories, and what's ended up happening is this focus on trying to get enough calories, or trying to get enough macros, you look at most processed foods, and they will meet those requirements. But the fact is, we're no longer getting the enzymes, the phytonutrients, the real building blocks of human, being vital, being alive and rebuilding your body. When you look at the population, it shows. In the United States over 60% of the population is overweight; 30% of the population is functionally obese; 13% of the population is morbidly obese. These are numbers that don't make sense. In the 1950s, less than 10% of the population was overweight—not obese—overweight. We completely reversed this dynamic by creating this food supply that is literally toxic every time you sit down to eat.

Brendan [00:06:17]: It's interesting because I just learned that these toxins, both the ones intentionally put in our food supply and the ones that end up there as residues from our farming practices are actually now being called "obesogens" because they actually generate weight gain because they mess with our hormone systems and so forth.

Alex [00:06:36]: Oh, Brendan, it's so much more than that. If you look at artificial colors, artificial sugars, artificial flavors and chemical preservatives, most of them are excitotoxins; they're nervous agents; they're neurotoxins. Let's just take the case of artificial sweeteners which I think are the most egregious product that has ever been introduced into the market. If you look at just crap products like Aspartame and Splenda, the newest abomination of food, Neotame, and Advantame. Aspartame is one of the worst products ever introduced in the history of the food market and 75% of the complaints that come into the FDA are about Aspartame-related products. The FDA in 2006 published a paper that there are 92 known reactions to Aspartame and these are the things like brain-fog, hair falling out, mania, hyperactivity, feeling completely ungrounded, crazy stuff that the FDA has published papers on, but we don't pull the product off the market. Now, food manufacturers are reacting by removing this neurotoxin called Aspartame from products, but here's the problem—they're replacing it with even more neurotoxic products. And I think—you might already know this—but if you're watching, here's why I say you can't trust processed foods: the FDA and the food manufacturers have this revolving door where they just switch people who make the rules with people who break the rules. It's absolutely true. Here's the latest: 75% of the complaints coming into the FDA are about Aspartame. Well, there's two new products: Neotame, which if you know anything about Greek and Latin roots, they're saying "new tame"; and Advantame, "better than the old tame". Isn't it crazy? Those two products ... Aspartame is about three hundred times stronger than sugar. Neotame and Advantame are twelve and twenty thousand times stronger than sugar. So, check this out: they just got it approved by the FDA in the past two years that Advantame and Neotame can be added in any food product without being on the label ...

Brendan [00:08:42]: It's unbelievable.

Alex [00:08:43]: ... because they use so little. So now you can buy a product that says 100% natural, organic, and legally it can have Advantame or Neotame in it. And so we don't even know when we're getting an artificial sweetener. Here's what you know with a 100% certainty: there will be no complaints to the FDA about Advantame and Neotame. It will be the cleanest sweeteners ever introduced into the market. Just watch ... ten years from now, they're going to be saying that they're the safest sweeteners ever because there's no complaints. There's no complaints because nobody knows they're eating them, and that's the level of manipulation we're subject to today.

Brendan [00:09:17]: Wow. So, let me see if I've got this right, you said that these can be added without being mentioned on the label?

Alex [00:09:27]: Without being on the label, and here's the justification: it's twenty thousand times stronger than sugar; you use such a little amount that it doesn't need to be on the label because it's trace amount. So let's be really clear about these products, what does an artificial sweetener do? It hits your tongue, and it causes a nervous reaction that tells your brain you just ate something sweet. Well throughout history, when we ate something sweet that meant that our body was about to get a rush of nutrients. We were going to get carbohydrates; we were going to get phytonutrients; we were going to get micro-nutrients, and a ton of vitamins, enzymes and more that comes out of the foods. Like an apple, we get a sweet taste; you get the entourage effect of everything in the apple, and everything you need to have that be bioavailable is right there. Well you take something like Aspartame, or Neotame, or Advantame, you put it on the tongue, and the body gets this sweet response that's a neurotoxin. Artificial sweeteners, most of them have been made by accident in a lab when somebody was trying to do something else, and they got some on their mouth or on their fingers and realized it was sweet. In one case they were making a pesticide. So a lot of the pesticides with all of the chemicals in it that kills bugs, you water it down, water it down, water it down, and the only nervous system reaction you get in the short term is a sweet taste, but you know based on the research that's been done, that if we use artificial sweeteners it actually triggers our body to eat more. It tells our body, "Hey, you should've gotten nutrition." Now you need to go find more.

Brendan [00:11:00]: And that's why it's totally irrelevant what the particular quantity is of this sweetener in the food, because it's what it's doing to our insulin response.

Alex [00:11:12]: No doubt. And it's what it's doing to our entire physiological response to tasting sweet, because as soon as sweet hits the tongue, the stomach starts producing more acids, the saliva in the mouth changes because the body doesn't know the difference between a neurotoxin and an apple. The body treats them in exactly the same way. The body doesn't, "Oh this is a calorie-free sweet product, so we don't need to do everything that we do". So, you run into people who are drinking a lot of Diet Coke or sodas, or they're using artificial sweeteners. The most egregious is when I meet someone who's like diabetic, and they've been told by their doctor that they should only use artificial sweeteners. If you look at the math there, these absolute neurotoxins affect every other system in our body, and most people who use them put on weight. It's not some, it's most; it's 80 to 90% of people who use artificial sweeteners actually have their weight go up. And here diabetics are being told, "This is what's going to help you". It's like catching somebody who's having trouble swimming and handing them a boat anchor.

Brendan [00:12:17]: And avoiding the word "artificial" on packaging and so forth, I mean there's so many foods that are labeled "natural" that really shouldn't qualify as such. I wonder if you have any examples of that.

Alex [00:12:30]: Sure, I mean just pick up any product these days, not any, but the vast majority of products that say "natural flavors". Here's what a natural flavor can be today, you can start with a grape derivative, like grape sugars, or grape concentrate, and bombard it with chemicals to the point where it doesn't even slightly resemble what an original grape flavor would've tasted like or what a grape concentrate would've tasted like. You end up with this chemical franken-food, that's allowed to be called a "natural" flavor because there was a natural product in the beginning of the processing. Here's one of the most frustrating for me ... there is a good sweetener on the market ... stevia is a good calorie-free sweetener. In Latin America it's been used forever. You throw some stevia leaves in your tea, and it makes it taste sweet. They use it in deserts. They use it in all kinds of stuff in Latin America. Well in the United States, because the lobbies from these food manufacturers were so huge, they weren't allowed to sell this natural product that has been used forever in other parts of the world. So for years the government banned it. Then they finally approved it. Why? Because Pepsi and Coke wanted to start using stevia, and then there were other manufacturers that wanted to start making the product. Well now, you can see, you can go to a shelf and see a product called Truvia which says stevia, and what it really is is that natural product that's been bombarded by chemicals, and by the time you are eating it you're no better off than if you're eating Aspartame. Well, you might be better off than Aspartame but not much. Aspartame is poison. Truvia is chemicals, and at the end of the day, here's the challenge with our food supply and these "natural products": there may be some testing on some of the chemical components of the foods that you eat if you're eating processed foods, but what's never been tested is the joint effect of all the chemical components in a processed food. Last Easter I was up at a local supermarket here called HEB, and I walked in and there was this whole table of Easter desserts that were on sale. And I picked one of them up, and there was over forty different chemicals in a cake. The ingredients were this big, and they were 8-point type. You read it and it's overwhelming. There were four or five different types of dyes. There were two different sweeteners. There were preservatives, thickeners and emulsifiers. And you start looking at all of that mixed together and it's really hard to say that you're eating food.

Brendan [00:15:13]: It's horrifying, unfortunately. I mean if you do live in Texas, and you're going to the HEB, there's a huge produce section in the HDB stores as I recall—I was in San Antonio last summer—and so there's a lot of real food there, too. Just stay away from the middle of the store.

Alex [00:15:31]: Well here's the challenging thing—and you might be noticing this—but I watch supermarkets closely because I coach my clients to shop on the outside of the supermarket, and you'll be okay. Stay away from the middle with all the boxes, bags and cans, and shop on the outside of the supermarket and everything will be better. Well, here's the problem: if you go to the outside of the supermarket now we start to see processed food sneaking into the produce area, sneaking into the fruits and vegetables, sneaking into the deli and the meat counters. And when you look at it today, in my opinion, the move is as fast as we can towards processing our entire food supply. And I think as somebody who wants to perform at a higher level, who wants to do better, who wants to actually survive longer, you have to fight every day to keep those products out of your system because you're part of this human experiment that nobody really knows how it's going to end up.

Brendan [00:16:31]: What are some of the other ways that … I mean, are there some other ways that our food supply has been made more toxic?

Alex [00:16:39]: Oh, sure, Brendan, one of the biggest challenges that we have—and every once in a while I get into a big fight with somebody online about this–is that we have completely changed the definition of what it means to farm foods. So, you go back 50 years—and here's what I meant "to farm" foods—you had land that you respected; you rotated crops; you made sure that there was the right amount of nutrients, the right amount of time for a field to replenish; you tilled the soil, and you put the crop back into the soil; you made sure that you had really good nutrient-dense earth that would grow foods. Well, today we don't do that so much anymore. We take really bad soil, and we put hybrid genetically modified seeds into the soil. And then we bombard them with basically—let's be honest, there is a little bit more—but the fact is, it's essentially three different nutrients: it's nitrogen, phosphorus and potassium. And we have this NPK, which we know, here's what it does: it creates foods with very high yield and terrible nutrient value. And what happens to our bodies whether we want to admit this as human beings or not … what's happening is our food supply is getting so corrupted that we have high-yield, low-nutritional value. So if you eat wheat from one of these fields, or corn, or soy, or rice, here's the problem—your body takes on this physical product that has very low nutrient value, and here's what that means to our bodies—throughout all of evolution, low nutrient value, high yield meant spoiled, toxic, bad, so our body fights against it. We actually start with … our immune system starts fighting against the foods that we have, and what you would expect to see in the population if we're eating really bad foods that our body is treating as toxic is you'd expect to see an epidemic of adrenal fatigue, hormone issues, auto-immune diseases, challenges with the digestive system, challenges with being present and aware, and depression, and frustration, and anxiety, and Attention Deficit Disorder, and all of these things that we're seeing blow up at double digit rates. You can say it's technology. You can say it's television. But let's be really honest here. We are chemically affected, and there's a hormonal consequence for everything we put in our mouths or on our bodies. And the more depleted those foods are, the more depleted those things are, and the more chemical input we have that our body isn't used to processing, the more it has an effect on every single one of us. And when you look at the population at large, it's pretty easy to see exactly what that effect is.

Brendan [00:19:19]: So what are some of the effects on performance and ultimately success of having hormones disrupted, having mitochondria that aren't getting the nutrients they need and the good phytonutrients which are like tuners, fine tune ups for mitochondria, and so forth and not having the zinc and selenium to detoxify these things in our livers? And these things are adding up. How is this influenced in performance?

Alex [00:19:45]: Brendan, you can see it every day, all you have to do is go out and walk in any public place, and you know. I've been overweight; I was 300 pounds at one point. And I'll say two different things. One, fat people aren't lazy. Fat people are working way harder than everybody else. I know. I was there, and it took a tremendous amount of effort to do anything when I was 300 pounds. Today I feel like I have it easy. And the fact is, no one ever said, "Man, I want to go gain a bunch of weight so I can do more." And the problem is that when you're taking on toxic foods, one of two things is happening: you're either gaining weight that's visible, or you're gaining fat internally that isn't visible. We have a lot of people who look healthy but are struggling internally because they're thin, and they have fat on the inside. It's called "TOFI". I had a dietitian tell me this recently. There's actually a term for it: "thin on the outside, fat on the inside" where people have metabolisms that are taking processed foods and are actually creating fat around the internal organs inside their bodies. And so when you look at performing or creating at the highest level or contributing at the highest level, any operational drag you feel, any pressure and noise that you feel in your body is going to reduce the amount that you can do.

The challenge today is that in so many ways, we don't just excuse processed foods, we've created like a movement around processed foods. Let me explain what I mean by that. When I go out and I say to people like, "Hey, you shouldn't eat that," people start looking at it in a way like, "I have a right to eat this." So it's literally become like "I have a right to poison myself." But people don't understand just how challenging it is. And this is how endemic it is, processed foods have become a part of some people's family traditions. I have a brother in law that on Thanksgiving expects to have this broccoli Velveeta corn flakes or something casserole, and if it's not made with all the processed stuff, it doesn't remind him of his childhood. Well, holy crap, so what we're saying now is if I don't have a big bowl of frozen conventional vegetables topped in like a Franken-cheese food, I don't feel like I had Thanksgiving. Think about what that's doing to us and the future generations. It's like we're driving ourselves further down the path of being overfed and undernourished.

Brendan [00:22:09]: I can't help but wonder if part of the reason that children are slipping into obesity and so many other health challenges very early, is that they're inheriting shortened telomeres because that's one thing that gets passed from parent to child. You get telomeres ... in case we need to explain that, those are like the endcaps on the chromosomes of our DNA and as they shorten, we start to see accelerated aging and sub-optimal performance of our systems. And as long as we keep them long we can stay healthy, provided all the other pieces are in place. And basically, nutrients tend to help lengthen telomeres, and toxins tend to help shorten them. And those actually get passed, the length of our telomeres in our parents' body, tend to be passed—I guess as an average length or something, maybe chromosome by chromosome—to the children as demonstrated by Elizabeth Blackburn, the author of *The Telomere Effect.*

Alex [00:23:16]: Then there's more to it. That's one part, the toxicity, the challenges that affect the telomeres in the body. But if we look at the other side of it, when we look at gut bacteria, science is now finally realizing ... "science" because today so much of it is bought and paid for, and it's just complete garbage. We don't do hypothesis anymore; we do prove whatever outcome you want. The challenge today is, when you look at gut fauna, science is realizing we have a brain in our heads, and we have a brain in our gut. And the brain in our gut affects the brain in our heads. And there's an exchange of information that happens here. The healthier your gut bacteria are—the healthier the fauna in your digestive system are—the healthier you are as a human being. What we now know is artificial sugars—anything that creates toxicity in your body—artificial sugars, artificial colors, sweeteners, artificial unnatural flavors, chemical additives and preservatives, and processed foods in general, dramatically affect gut bacteria. They reduce gut bacteria. They reduce healthy bacteria. And so if you are a parent who has a child ... if the mother has a child and has unhealthy gut bacteria, so does that child because it's almost a duplication of what's going on in the mother's system. And then if the child's lucky enough that the mom breast feeds, they're still getting a depleted replenishment of their gut bacteria because the mother's has been so affected. So epigenetically we are affecting multiple generations with the processed foods we're eating today.

Brendan [00:24:47]: It's remarkable how much the microbiome affects things like mood, mental clarity, energy levels, athletic performance, anything you want to name.

Alex [00:25:02]: I mean yeah, the ability to take on nutrients, digestion, the ability to be aware and present, how often you do or do not experience brain fog. We're now realizing, medical science is realizing that's driven from the gut.

Brendan [00:25:16]: I'm somebody who has lived that for a long time. My whole health journey involved having my microbiome nuked, and I still haven't been able to correct it. And I experience brain-fog all the time because I haven't fixed that yet. I've got to get a fecal transplant probably, which means flying to another country because I don't have *Clostridium difficile* which is what I would need to get a prescription here in this country.

Alex [00:25:41]: In this country we don't like to use anything that doesn't have a pharmaceutical tied to it.

Brendan [00:25:47]: Or that needs prescription.

Alex [00:25:50]: Like if they can't give you a prescription, they're probably going to ban it in the United States.

Brendan [00:25:57]: There's many ways that we've been alluding ... many ways that our physical health affects mental performance. I'm curious if there's any particular mechanisms you think it's important for people to understand, the relationships between how this system or that system functions in the body and how that reflects in our day-to-day performance?

Alex [00:26:19]: I think the most important thing is this: there's this entire population in the world who thinks they're okay because they're asymptomatic, and again, asymptomatic is almost impossible, if you're eating a lot of processed foods. It's affecting you in some way, but it's not affecting you in a way that you care about yet. And here's my belief: as you take on processed foods, as you use prescription drugs, as you take on toxic chemicals that are in so much of our health care products and our shampoo and deodorant, and everything else, our body's absorbing those things. We've found that artificial colors and dyes, don't leave the system. They get stuck in the lymph nodes. We've found that a lot of artificial chemicals get stuck in subcutaneous fat, or they actually get stuck in your cell tissue. And when we look at that toxicity that we're taking on over time, I think the biggest challenge we have is this: somebody takes on toxicity, takes on toxicity, takes on toxicity and they feel fine, they're asymptomatic. Then they hit this toxicity threshold when literally from one day to the next brain-fog, hair falling out, challenges with hormones, challenges with the endocrine system, challenges with digestive, blood sugar, and it's like overnight people start falling apart. And I wouldn't say this if there wasn't so much evidence in the world.

When we look at even psychiatric disorders, which most, let's be honest, most psychiatric disorders are made up by the APA. But you do have a classification of symptoms that they look at, and when we look at children, tell me why is it that for boys under the age of 18 we're in double digit growth of Attention Deficit Disorder. Are we really saying that there's that many kids that are defective, that are broken? There's got to be something that we're doing wrong. Part of it is that they're in way too high of a strict and restrictive environment at school. But the other part of it is, we're sending little children out into the world with the worst nutrition of any other class of person. All you have to do is go to any restaurant in the United States and look at the adults' menu and look at the kids' menu, and you know, kids get screwed. The kids' menu's always the worst food in the entire place. Even if you're in a healthier place, the kids' menu's terrible. And when I look at how we are conditioning people to eat today, kids can go out to eat over and over again and never eat anything fresh, never anything that was live. They're literally eating everything out of a fry basket, and if we expect to have any type of performance, it's like putting sugar in a gas tank. You can't run the car.

Brendan [00:29:01]: That's so true, and with children in particular, they respond very quickly one way or the other to toxins. Well, they probably have more resistance …

Alex [00:29:13]: They have more of a capacity to …

Brendan [00:29:16]: Yeah, to handle it. But what's fascinating is that once good food is restored, they can come back into normal behavior, better performance, better attendance at school and so forth, less fighting and bullying. There have been several studies on this where they took schools that had serious problems with that, and they put whole foods into the cafeterias instead of the egregious junk that you see in these places, and within a matter of months those measures of behavior, and performance and attendance and so forth were totally turned around. It was extraordinary.

Alex [00:29:55]: It changes everything. I have this theory, Brendan, that I've shared with a lot of different organizations, and it's funny that the people who I work with—I work with a lot of physicians, with a lot of scientists, with a lot of medical doctors who have done their own research—and they come to me because my organization has done an exhaustive amount of research around how does the body really work. You look at the average doctor today, and if you look at medical schools and how much they learn about breathing, hydration, nutrition, and movement, which are arguably the four pillars of health, in the average medical school curriculum, there's none. No learning at all on breathing, hydration, nutrition, and movement. Zero. They learn chemical processes, they learn physiology, they learn a ton about prescription drugs, mostly because the curriculums are created by those companies, but they don't learn about how to actually keep people healthy. The theory that I have is, look, our bodies are made to survive, not to thrive. They're made to survive. So if we don't have all the resources we need, your body will do anything it can to survive. So if we don't take on the right amount of water, and nutrients, and movement, and oxygen, here's what happens: your body goes into this survival mode where it says, "Hey, resources aren't present, conserve all of the resources we can so that we can survive." And in survival mode, the body will literally slow the metabolism, you'll have that low-energy crash feeling, you'll stop purging and eliminating as much because it actually stops or slows your digestion. You have foggy, racy, unclear memory issues. In survival mode your body will conserve resources, so it will hold onto water, you get bloating, muscle pain, joint pain, it will slow calorie burn, it will only burn sugar, it will slow everything down, it will use the easiest nutrients first, sugars before fat, and then it will store everything else. And then the biggest thing that bodies do in survival mode is they store nutrients. It will store fat, grow fat cells, multiply fat cells, and hold on to fat to survive. All we have to do to reverse that is give our body abundant resources, abundant food, breathing, hydration. Or hydration, nutrition, movement and oxygen, and what happens is we go into a thrive mode where your body says resources are abundant, let's use all the resources and your body thrives, and here's what a thriving body looks like: you have a natural thirst instinct that compels you to drink water all day, your body weight will naturally regulate, your hunger comes and goes naturally based on activity and how many calories you're consuming, and your body will want functional movement and breathing. The challenge for most people is they're operating their bodies in survival mode, and then they want to go work and work out and get in shape and exercise. And I hear this from people all the time, "Alex, I want to work out so bad. I just don't have the energy." "I want to get in shape so bad. Just every time I walk into a gym I can barely move. By the end of the day I can't see straight." Those people are operating a 100% of the time in survival mode. You are literally pushing a boulder uphill every day with your life.

Brendan [00:33:09]: I think we really have to move beyond sort of the RDA mentality with nutrition because it's very survival-oriented: "Hey, you shouldn't have any deficiency syndrome as long as you get this much vitamin C, vitamin A, magnesium, calcium."

Alex [00:33:26]: And let's be honest, the recommended daily amount allowance is such a joke. Have you ever looked into how those were established? Because I did. I'm like, "What does RDA actually mean?".

Brendan [00:33:36]: Yeah tell us about that.

Alex [00:33:37]: Okay, so it's just like the American Psychology Association. First, I'm not a big committee guy. I think that when you have a committee, you're usually going to hear crap. And here's how those recommended daily amounts are established for each vitamin class. There's a committee for vitamin C; there's a committee for vitamin D; there's a committee for vitamin E; and they get together and they look at all of this research and then they decide what the recommended daily allowance is. Have you ever noticed how the RDA is not weight-dependent. It's just for everybody. It's the most non-scientific science in the history of man. Everybody should have these vitamins lined up every day, and then everything's going to be okay. I call complete and total BS. If you've got a vitamin D deficiency, go outside, because what you're taking in a pill is an isolate of a vitamin that you're expecting to put in your mouth and without any entourage effect, any enzymes, any carriers that's going to help that be absorbed into your body, we're fooling ourselves into thinking we're curing a vitamin D deficiency. What we're normally doing is just increasing the toxicity that our liver and kidneys have to deal with because when in human history has the body ever had to deal with a mega dose of vitamin D or and isolate of any kind? And today every time I go on Facebook, and I see somebody swallowing a big hand full of pills and being proud of themselves because they're getting healthy, I feel bad for them because they don't really understand what they're doing. I've worked with clients where we've sat down, and we've looked at their supplement load, and they're getting twenty or thirty times as much vitamin B as they need; they're getting fifteen or twenty times as much vitamin C as they need; they're getting a hyper dose of vitamin A. You bombard your body with isolates every day, and your body is going to start working around those isolates. There's a reason why when you take that big handful of supplements, you pee neon orange. It's not natural.

Brendan [00:35:33]: Let me ask you this, what are some of your top tips, let's say your top three tips for improving performance and, go crazy but maybe with a focus on the food world.

Alex [00:35:45]: So, number one is the most important nootropic. The most important supplement and the most important bio-hack for anyone who wants to perform is water. We don't talk about it because it's free, and there's no water lobby, and there's no government agency around water except for the one that puts all the fluoride and crap in it, but there's nobody out there saying, "Hey, drink more water" because nobody's getting paid for it. But it doesn't matter what you do in your life, you can have a perfect diet, be on all the right supplements, workout and do everything that you should do, but if you're not drinking water, your body is not going to optimize because every system in the body requires water. 100% of systems in the body are either supported by water or water is a catalyst. And here's the biggest one: toxicity in the body. There's one path for the removal of toxicity, water. And we don't think about that. When you don't drink water, here's the math: when you're fully hydrated your body will detoxify; when you're dehydrated your body absorbs and keeps toxins, period. And so, for me, number one, I get all of my clients to do our water program. If anyone wants to try it, you can go to getthirstynow.com, and we have this ten-day natural thirst program where within ten days, everybody who's taken it so far, except for a couple of people, get to the place where they're drinking more water than they ever thought they could in their lives. Actually, I have a couple of people who like went ten days and still didn't feel like they were drinking as much as other people. But, Brendan, we've had thousands of people take this program, and the results we get are insane. We've had people get off of insulin, lose a hundred pounds, stop taking prescription antidepressants and accelerants, stop taking stimulants, all from drinking water. So, number one, you can't beat it.

Brendan [00:37:35]: I totally agree, that's been one of my life lines, maintaining my hydration while everything else was jacked in my microbiome.

Alex [00:37:45]: If you look at research from a hundred and fifty years ago to six thousand years ago, water was a cure-all for everything, and there was so many different studies, so much different research, so much anecdotal evidence throughout history that if you drink water things will get better. Well, about a hundred and fifty years ago we started experimenting with these things called medications and tonics and different drugs that we could put into the market, and water became a by-product of the medical industry. We don't even think about it anymore, but for me that's number one. Number two, if you want to get the biggest bio-hack there is, is get outside in the morning and walk. Just go for a twenty-minute walk in the morning. I coach not only some of the most successful people in the world, but also some of the most intense and driven and in-shape entrepreneurs, like half of my clients look like bodybuilders. They look like fitness models, and there's a reason. They really care about how they look. But I take people who are marathon runners, body builders, intense cross fit people, and we get them to go outside and walk for twenty minutes in the morning. And if you look at the scientific evidence around walking, the studies that have been made around walking, here's what I believe it does: it knocks us out of an adrenal cycle and into a dopamine and serotonin cycle because our bodies recognize fight or flight. Fight or flight is a physiological syndrome and a cognitive syndrome, and both work in concert to create fight or flight. When we get somebody outside to walk each morning after four or five days they start realizing they're more present, they're more aware. It's really funny, I have a friend of mine who's also a client, who is a marathon runner, and I had to talk to him about walking, and he's like, "Alex, I do thirty miles a week, or when I'm training for a marathon I might do sixty miles a week. What is walking going to do for me?" And I explain to him, "You get out of fight or flight, it's going to make you more aware; it's going to create dopamine and serotonin." Well here's what's interesting. He started doing the walks. He started realizing that if he walked in the morning, his training runs were infinitely better. He started realizing he felt less depleted, and he even got out and walked in the morning that he ran the London marathon, and he had a personal record.

Brendan [00:40:00]: No way, that's awesome.

Alex [00:40:03]: Absolutely, and if you look at it, Brendan, I believe there's an evolutionary reason for getting up and walking and what that does for us. You get up in the morning; you go on that walk; it resets the body; it calms the upper body; it makes us relax. One of the big suggestions that I have for everyone is do it barefoot, or buy some Vibram Fivefingers or buy minimalist shoes so you really feel the ground. Walk in the grass, walk in Nature, even if you just have to walk next to the street in the grass and look like a weird person that's not using the sidewalk, don't let it bother you because if you get out there for twenty minutes, give me seven days of walking for twenty minutes in the morning, and you won't recognize your mornings.

Brendan [00:40:47]: There's so many things walking does. You mentioned water and walking so far, and that reminds me of the book, *Your Body's Many Cries for Water,* where the doctor that wrote that, one of his key strategies in his program for hydrating people is that you've got to walk after you drink the water so that it can push its way into the tissues. You've got to raise the heart rate and the circulation because water-dehydrated capillaries are constricted to keep the bulk of the food in your core and in your brain where you need it most, and so the muscles and maybe certain other organs that aren't being used as intensively, those capillaries are constricted a bit. So when you go out and walk after you drink water, or while you drink water, it helps to push open those capillaries and then you're actually really rehydrating otherwise that doesn't happen.

Alex [00:41:39]: There's no question. Each morning me and most of my clients go through this morning routine that we developed, it's a scientifically supported morning routine where everything here is meant to get our bodies physiologically, cognitively and chemically awakened and ready for the day.

One of the first things that you do is hyper-hydrate which means you drink 16 ounces or more of water, and then one of the next things you do is you get outside, and you walk for twenty minutes. That combination of hyper-hydrating and going out and walking … you literally get breathing, nutrition and hydration and movement all at the same time just by doing that, and it's a complete game-changer.

You asked for three tips, I've got the third one. The third one is when it comes to nutrition, if you haven't done an elimination diet yet, do it. There's only one way to know which foods you should be eating. You can't test for it. You can't get blood-tested. You can't get allergy tested. No doctor can tell you. The fact that people say they have a diet that works for everybody just shows that they don't understand nutrition. Because there's no such thing as a diet that will work for every person out there. The fact is that we all have different sensitivities, reactions, allergies and issues in our bodies that make certain foods untenable for us. And if you're willing to commit the time to do an elimination diet, we have one that we call the "Low Risk High Reward Elimination Diet". I'm biased. I think it's by far the best one on the market. But when you're willing to do an elimination diet, what happens is you go through a period where you eliminate the toxins and the allergens and the reagents in your body that are causing reactions and then you start testing foods.

And Brendan, the first time I did an elimination diet prior to the elimination diet I was eating wheat all the time. I was eating pasta. I was eating wheat. I was eating whole wheat. I thought I was healthy. I did the elimination diet. The first food I tested was wheat, and prior to the diet I would've told you I didn't have a lot of symptoms. On day thirty-one when I tested wheat first thing in the morning, I was curled up in a ball in pain, and it was because I had gotten rid of all the toxicity in the body. I had lowered that toxicity threshold. I ate the wheat, and the body said, "Hey, don't do that again." And I have this emotional … you know, when I go to a party, or when I'm out somewhere, and they serve pastries or cake or anything like that that has wheat in it, people are shocked at the fact that I don't even have an inclination to move towards it. I run away from it because I have that experience of eating a piece of bread and being curled up on my kitchen floor and thinking this is what it has been doing to me. I didn't know that I had the symptoms before because I was reacting to everything all the time. But that happened for me with wheat. That happened for me with soy. And to a lesser effect it happened with corn. But I don't even consider eating those foods anymore because I have a clear memory of just how horrible they made me feel. So for anyone who's watching and wants to really optimize and have a defendable customized diet that you can explain to anyone, go download the elimination diet and it will be a game changer for you.

Brendan [00:44:45]: Yeah I think it's a really good point where you mentioned that you didn't notice the symptoms before, and that was probably because the body habituates. The symptoms get more and more muted over time. It's like a neurological habituation. If you keep tapping your hand you'll kind of stop feeling it. It will get kind of numb. So you have to get reset, re-sensitized, to know what's actually happening.

Alex [00:45:07]: There's no question. In fact, just yesterday I had one of my high-end clients who's in our top Mastermind, a physician, and I had him and his wife in town, and he was talking about how now that he is drinking water, he's gone through our program, how he's drinking sometimes ten liters, fifteen liters a day when he's active.

Brendan [00:45:30]: Wow. That's a lot, that's even more than I drink, and I drink an obscene amount of water, but that's got me beat.

Alex [00:45:37]: Well, Brendan, I have clients who get up to three, four, five hundred ounces of water in a day which a lot of physicians will tell you will hurt you, but here's how I instruct everybody to do it: follow your natural thirst. If your body tells you you're thirsty, drink. And here's what I see with people who start the hydration program. They start and the water consumption spikes. Once you start taking on the water, your body tells you you're thirsty all the time, and then it slowly comes down to like maybe two to four hundred ounces a day. Here's my theory for that: you start drinking water, and your body finally says, "Okay, hey, let's get as much of this as we can and detoxify". Well yesterday Adam was talking about how four weeks in he had a day where his urine was just dark, like dark yellow, dark brown all day. So four weeks in on being completely and totally hydrated, drinking tons of water, he has this day where the body finally decides to purge toxins, finally decides to let go of stuff, And now he was saying that if he goes an hour without water, he instantly recognizes brain-fog, instantly recognizes a mind-body connection issue, instantly starts feeling a little bit lethargic, a little tired—his eyes are hard to keep open. Well my contention is you're feeling that all the time. Now you know the difference.

Brendan [00:46:56]: Right. It's so important that achievement-oriented people hear things like this and that all of these things you shared today, and that you continue to share on your website and so forth, all of these things that sabotage health span, life span, performance and ultimately interfere with them fulfilling their dreams, creating their legacy.

Alex [00:47:21]: Just happiness, like overall just being happy in the world.

Brendan [00:47:25]: Yeah, I'm just trying to speak to the achievement-minded people because they don't even care if they're happy, some of them. They just want to achieve. But hey, you know what, happiness is the killer app, I hear.

Alex [00:47:37]: Yeah, exactly. And I think that when I say happy for an achievement-oriented person, here's what I think happiness is ... here's what I know happiness is for someone like me and for my clients: happiness is being able to say, "Here's what I want to do," being able to assemble the plan to get there, and then making it happen over and over again. The challenge with that is that if you're an achievement-oriented person, you are different than the rest of the world. You get up every morning; you go into the future; you create a new reality; you come back to the present; and then you demand it becomes real. And in order to go through that process you must be fully present. You want all the faculties that you could possibly muster. You want to be completely and totally engaged and aware of what's going on because then that process works. And I don't believe that achievement-oriented people can be happy or satisfied or any of those things unless they're making that happen. I look at it as a momentum. We are in momentum when we're making thing happen, when we're achieving, when we're doing what we want to do in the world, and anything that doesn't give you momentum is taking it away. It's binary. It's on or off. And if you're achievement-oriented, you know how much momentum means to you. You know how much it means to you to be moving forward, to be making things happen. So, anything that is holding you up, you have the responsibility to yourself, and to every other person who's trying to do things in the world, to get rid of it. And then you'll reach your full potential.

Brendan [00:49:07]: You know the concept of momentum is so, so profound, and of course that's the topic of your next book. I can't wait for that book. Alex, thank you for being here today with the Eat4Earth community. It's been a lot of fun.

Alex [00:49:21]: I appreciate it, Brendan. As you can tell this is a topic not only that I've researched extensively, and I'll be honest, obsessed over, but it's also a topic that I'm really passionate about because in my career as a consultant, when I was younger in my twenties, I worked with some really amazing people, and I helped some of those people build ten figure businesses or nine figure then ten figure businesses. I helped some of those people take small companies and make massive organizations. I helped some of those people become better executives better C level contributors in companies, and some of those people died, and at a very young age. I had a friend who at 54 years old was entering his prime, just about to kick off a huge new venture and stood up from his couch and had a heart attack. I had a friend who went on vacation, got away from work for a week and died on a beach, lying on a folding chair or lying on a beach chair. And, Brendan, to me those memories will never leave me. Dave Schmeiser, the 54-year-old, was a good friend of mine ... he was a mentor. He was a client. He was just a great guy. And I realized young that if we don't take care of ourselves and start eating right, it can be lights-out. And the fact is achievement-oriented people, we don't pay enough attention to ourselves. We pay far too much attention to what we're trying to do, and one of the things that I tell all of my clients is self-care is a path to success. Self-care includes taking care of yourself, getting the right nutrients, the right amount of oxygen, the right amount of movement, and the right amount of water. And if more achievement-oriented people like me would do that, we would see a lot more contribution in the world. And let's be honest, we live in a world that needs to change. And if you don't think you can change it, I believe you are wrong. Every one of you has a capability.

Brendan [00:51:23]: Thank you for that. Thank you for leaving us with that message and this call to action. A lot of people aspire to be entrepreneurs and look up to entrepreneurs. I think entrepreneurs are major culture creators, so I salute you for being an entrepreneur that is shifting entrepreneurial cultures so that people will stop looking at it as acceptable to eat devitalized processed food, to make it to some promised land that they might now really enjoy if they ever make it there.

Alex [00:51:59]: Yeah, there's no question Brendan. I really appreciate you having me and letting me share this message. I don't think we talk about it enough, and for anyone who wants more information, I have a podcast where I share a lot of this. You can go to momentumpodcast.com you can check it out. And Brendan, I applaud you for doing this summit, for putting this information together, for giving the speakers together because this is one of the most important topics we can talk about today, and nobody's talking about it.

Brendan [00:52:31]: Well, that's what we're here to do. So thank you. And as soon as we get done chatting I'm going to go drink some water.

Alex [00:52:37]: [laughs] Same here, Brendan. Thanks, brother.

Joseph Pizzorno, ND Interview
The Toxin Solution: Essential Keys to Safe and Complete Detoxification

Brendan [00:02]: Welcome to the Eat4Earth event. We're exploring how you can heal yourself, your loved ones, and the planet with food. This is Brendan Moorehead, and I am honored to welcome our distinguished guest, Dr Joseph Pizzorno. Dr. Pizzorno is a world-leading authority on science-based natural medicine, the term he coined when founding Bastyr University in 1978. A naturopathic physician, educator, researcher, and expert spokesman, he is the editor-in-chief of *PubMed*-indexed *Integrative Medicine, a Clinician's Journal*. Treasurer of the Board of the Institute of Functional Medicine, member of American Herbal Pharmacopoeia, and a member of the science boards of the Heck Foundation, Gateway for Cancer Research, and Bioclinic Naturals. He is licensed in Washington state and the recipient of numerous awards and honors, such as the Linus Pauling award, the American Holistic Medical Association's Holistic Medicine Pioneer, and the American Association of Naturopathic Physicians' Naturopathic Physician of the Year. He has been an intellectual and academic leader in medicine for four decades, was appointed by Presidents Clinton and Bush to two prestigious commissions advising the government on how to integrate natural medicine into the health care system, and he is the author or co-author of five textbooks and seven consumer books. Dr. Pizzorno, it is such an honor to have such a dedicated and decorated physician with us today. Thanks for being here.

Dr. Pizzorno [01:35]: Thanks for the kind introduction and invitation. I'm delighted to talk with you today.

Brendan [01:39]: Dr. Pizzorno, in your recent book, *The Toxin Solution*, you say that the major source of toxins is the food that we eat. Some food-born toxins are added in the manufacturer of processed food, of course, and some are due to our agricultural methods. For a long time, it was assumed that agricultural chemical residues in food were harmless, so what research has been revealing that this is far from accurate and that we are in fact already experiencing serious consequences of toxins from many sources, including our food and agricultural methods?

Dr. Pizzorno [02:15]: I think this is the key question, and the research is actually very clear right now. Let me do a little historic comment on this. The very first class that was taught at the then called John Bastyr College of Naturopathic Medicine way back in September 1978 was the "Health Effects of Environmental Pollutants". I taught that class, and it was a very frustrating class to teach, because of course when you teach a class, you want to have a textbook, and the textbooks at that time on toxicity and toxicology were only about industrial exposure, and they adamantly stated that although these chemicals and metals are a problem for people working in industry, the general population, the consumers were not affected by them at all. I knew that was wrong forty years ago, because I was seeing patients showing signs of toxicity, and it appeared to be coming from the foods they were eating. At that point I couldn't prove it. I could just see it clinically. Since then, particularly in the last fifteen years, there's been a huge amount of research published showing that the toxins in the foods are becoming major causes of disease. And in many ways it's a double whammy. So when we eat our food, we expect the food to be very rich in nutrients, vitamins and minerals, and things like this. But if you look at the trace mineral content of food over the last hundred years, it has dropped between fifty and eighty-five percent, according to a trace mineral, for example, copper which is eighty-five percent lower than one hundred years ago. Now, the reason that is significant is that the way our bodies work, we are basically enzyme machines, and enzyme machines are made of protein, made by our DNA, and then a co-factor, typically a vitamin or mineral, and those co-factors are actually critical for the enzyme to function properly. The way most toxins work is by displacing the vitamin or mineral in the enzyme system, and so the enzyme system doesn't work anymore. So we have a situation where not only are we eating food that no longer has the trace minerals you need for the enzymes to work, but we're actually eating foods that have toxins in them that are poisoning the enzymes that are struggling to function because not enough trace minerals are available. So then we started looking at the research showing when we look at people with the highest toxic load, compared to people with the lowest toxic load, we see dramatic results. So for example, looking at diabetes, and diabetes has the most research, which is not surprising I guess, because if you look at the incidence of diabetes over the last fifty years, it's increased by a factor of ten. I remember after I started practicing back 1975—it is kind of macabre to say this, but I was excited, when I finally saw a diabetic patient after six months of being in practice, and I was booked every day, so it was, "Great, fine, now I've got a diabetic patient." And now diabetes makes up a significant portion of everybody's practice every day. What happened? It turns out that the research is showing that the diabetes epidemic is primarily due to the environmental toxins, primarily coming from food.

Brendan [05:32]: That is earth-shaking in a way, because we have assumed that diabetes is primarily due to overdosing on carbohydrates and sugars and so forth, and now we're seeing that it's more complex than that. Certainly that's a factor, a big one, but with chemicals actually …

Dr. Pizzorno [05:51]: Let me give you a fascinating piece of research. Everybody knows that obesity is one of the biggest risk factors for diabetes. And it's clear, when people are obese they get more diabetes. And most people are saying the reason for this diabetes epidemic is because people are obese. I want to be very clear on my following statements. I'm not saying obesity is good for you. What I'm going to tell you is, if you look at obese people, and then differentiate them according to their toxic load, and you look at people who are obese in the bottom ten percent of toxic load, they have no increased risk for diabetes. What did I just say? Everybody knows that being obese causes diabetes. But if you're obese and don't have a high levels of toxins, you don't get diabetes. So there's something else going on here.

Brendan [06:42]: That's amazing. And I believe you've coined the terms obesogens and diabetogens, or at least they're out there in the …

Dr. Pizzorno [06:50]: I didn't coin them. These are the terms coined by the researchers. In other words, researchers are looking at diabetes and saying, "Wow, the more toxins people have, the more diabetes and the more obesity they have." So they coined the term "obesogens" and "diabetogens".

Brendan [07:04]: Got it. So are there other conditions that are clearly linked to these agricultural toxins as well as toxins from other sources?

Dr. Pizzorno [07:12]: Absolutely. How about ADHD in children? ADHD did not exist fifty years ago, and we know, for example, that the organophosphate pesticides, which kills insects by poisoning the neurological system, that these things cause ADHD in children. We know, for example, what about another condition ... how about IQ in children. The higher the child's level of organochlorine pesticides, the lower their IQ. How about arsenic in rice? If you grow rice in water that is contaminated with arsenic, the rice will absorb it very efficiently. When we look at arsenic, the CDC, the Centers for Disease Control, considers arsenic the worst of the environmental toxins that we're being exposed to. And as I started looking at the research on arsenic and a multiplicity of diseases, arsenic came up again and again and again—things like cancer, things like gout, dementia ... all over the board, arsenic is a huge problem, and we're contaminating our food with it.

Brendan [08:18]: There was an interesting piece of research in which the researcher was checking a correlation between many factors in childhood obesity, and the number one factor was eating chicken, and it was determined, I believe, that that was due to the high arsenic load in chicken, commercial chicken, that are eating all of these commercial grains that have been raised with rock phosphate fertilizers that carry a lot of cadmium. And of course they actually give chickens arsenic for various reasons in the commercial methods of raising chickens. Now cadmium. I mentioned cadmium. I believe that you also have spoken or written a bit about chemical fertilizers and how they bring cadmium into the food chain.

Dr. Pizzorno [09:19]: Yes. So in a study in Seattle, which is where I'm from, and the researchers were looking at osteoporosis in women, and they were noticing more osteoporosis in women and finding that the women with osteoporosis, there was an unusually high level of cadmium in these women. Now, in the past it was easy to differentiate who had high cadmium and who didn't because basically smokers have twice as much cadmium in the body as non-smokers. But they're finding cadmium toxicity in non-smokers, and they're seeing a lot of osteoporosis. They then tracked down cadmium to eating conventionally grown soybeans, particularly in the form of tofu, because conventional soybeans were being grown with high phosphate fertilizers, and high phosphate fertilizers, many of them are contaminated with cadmium. And for some reason the beans family of foods likes to absorb cadmium from the soil, particularly if that soil is deficient in zinc. And think of those trace minerals that are much lower now than it used to be.

So what's happening here is cadmium is probably the most toxic of the metals that we are exposed to in the environment. And because it's so toxic, our kidneys are very, very good at clearing out the cadmium. The half-life of cadmium in the blood is one to two days. We have to get rid of it as fast as possible, because it is so toxic. The problem is that it is gotten rid of by the kidneys, and once it gets into the kidneys, the kidneys are almost unable to get rid of the cadmium. The half-life of cadmium in kidneys is sixteen years. Once it gets into the kidneys, it then causes constant damage to the kidneys, particular the mitochondria, but other areas as well. When you damage the kidneys, you can't convert vitamin D to its most active form called 1-25 hydroxy vitamin D, and that's what's necessary to get calcium into the bones. So you put cadmium in the kidneys. You poison the kidneys. Then the kidneys cannot produce vitamin D, and then you have osteoporosis.

Brendan [11:23]: Wow, I didn't know that's the mechanism. That's fascinating. So a major theme of the Eat4Earth event is obviously the connection between soil health, nutrient levels in food, and the influences of nutrient levels and toxin levels on health and disease. And aside from the influences of food-borne toxins on disease, how important would you say that it is to make sure we have high nutrient levels in soils, high availability of nutrients in soils and therefore in our food, how important is that to the toxin levels in our bodies and our ability to detoxify from the toxins that we get from all sources?

Dr. Pizzorno [12:06]: Very, very important and it's a very good point. So health begins with the food that we eat. The average person eats seventy-five tons of food in their lifetime, so we eat a lot of food. And that food is supposed to be rich in nutrients. So the nutrients are there not only to make our enzymes work, but those nutrients play a critical role in our detoxification enzymes as well as our antioxidant enzymes. And it turns out that if we're eating foods that are low in nutrients and high in contamination, many of these contaminants not only poison the enzyme system for proper functioning, they poison the enzyme systems for detoxification. And they poison the antioxidant enzymes that we use to try to protect ourselves from the damage of these toxins. So I look at patients—I no longer do primary care; I'm really focusing my time on writing, research, lecturing, etc—but I still see some patients, some kind of concierge patients. My regular patients now is that they come to me with this some kind of disease, this that or the other that I can help them with. I say to them, "Ok, well that's your disease. You know, I'm not really interested in what disease you've been labelled with. I'm interested in how your body is working, and I know your body's not going to work properly if you don't have enough nutrition and if you have a lot of toxins." So now with these patients, I say, "First off let's assess your nutritional status; let's assess your toxic status; get the nutrients up; get the toxins down; and then let's see what's left." And for the vast majority of them, that's all I have to do! It doesn't matter what the disease is named. Get nutrients in; get toxins out.

Brendan [13:43]: Wow, that does simplify things a bit! So is there any evidence that eating organic foods helps reduce the body's toxin load and disease risk?

Dr. Pizzorno [13:57]: It is dramatic and unequivocal. Again, I'll quote a study from Seattle, not that research is only done in Seattle, but since I lived there I pay more attention to what comes from Seattle. So one group of researchers from public health did a study looking at children who were eating conventionally grown foods versus children eating organically grown foods. So what they did is they stood in front of Puget Consumers Co-op, a local health food chain in the Seattle area, and if the children were eating at least 75 percent of the foods organically grown, then they put them in the study. And then they stood in front of a conventional grocery store, and they asked the same question of the children—were the they eating at least seventy-five percent of their foods conventionally grown? If they said "yes" they then put them in the study. What they found was that the children eating conventionally grown foods had nine to ten times higher levels of organophosphate pesticides and organochlorine pesticides in their bodies, compared to children eating organically grown foods. And so you start looking at these children, and you see dramatic increases in all the diseases and lower IQ. The good news is that we put a child on organically grown food, within about three days their blood levels will come down to pretty similar to kids who always eat organically grown foods, but unfortunately their fat stores, and their brain, and their bones, and everywhere else in the body is still saturated with this stuff, and it takes months to years to get rid of it. But it is very clear that as you detoxify, people can get their toxins out, their disease level decreases.

Brendan [15:33]: Well, that's exciting. So what I hear you saying is that we need to get the chemicals out of our diets, need to make sure the vegetables and fruits that we buy, or meats, or whatever we eat, actually has high nutrient levels, as they are supposed to have. Right now the standard way to do that is buy organic, and soon we'll have food labels that will also specify whether these foods are grown in ways that actively build healthy soil, because sometimes organic, as it has been carried out, doesn't necessarily remain true to the roots of the organic methods. And so there's a new labels coming out, I believe it will be called "regenerative organic" that will make sure that those producers are actually actively building soil, and when that happens the minerals become available to the plants, and we get much higher nutrition.

Dr. Pizzorno [16:33]: I've not heard about that new labelling coming, but it sounds fantastic.

Brendan [16:37]: Very new. I may be speaking about it a little bit early, but it's coming, and there are some other labels as well in the works. One is called Land to Market, and that applies, I believe, primarily if not exclusively, to animals raised with methods that grow healthy soils and restore natural grassland ecosystems, as opposed to … it's just more intelligent management, that actually is more productive for the producer. But it's a bit counter-intuitive, so people don't necessarily stumble across it by trial and error. It took some thinking to develop and a lot of practice, and now it's implemented on tens of millions of acres worldwide and producing phenomenal results.

Dr. Pizzorno [17:29]: I'm happy to hear that. So I think I'm so concerned about the food supply that I'm growing more and more my own food, and this past spring I put in about three hundred square feet of raised gardens to grow my own vegetables. So I've been really working on it to practice what I preach. And as part of the preparation for this, I read a book on biodynamic farming, and I was fascinated to read the book because as I was reading it through they would say here's how you create the soil as healthy as possible, with organisms, et cetera, and then now if you're seeing this particular problem with your plants, you need to put in this particular nutrient. If they're being attacked by particular pests, you need to put in this particular other nutrient, so give them this nutrient. And then also, you know, try to collect rain water to water your plants rather than city water because city water is contaminated with so many chemicals. Now, as I was reading this book, I was thinking, "Wow, these guys are thinking about plants the same way I think about patients." Get nutrients in; get toxins out. It just makes so much sense.

Brendan [18:40]: You know, you raise an important point. I've entirely overlooked the biodynamic label that's out there. That's a certification, you know, you don't see it. I don't know if I've ever actually seen it on packages and so forth. I'm not even sure where I would get biodynamically-produced food locally, but they absolutely are currently perhaps the best standard for building soil health and nutrient density into our foods. Now, when it comes to selecting foods, which are the most important ones to avoid purchasing conventional and to either purchase organic or to grow in our own yards?

Dr. Pizzorno [19:26]: That's where the Environmental Working Group is so helpful. They publish a list of which foods are the most contaminated and which are the least contaminated. I might do some of the food priorities a little differently than theirs because I have more clinical perspective, but nonetheless it is a great place to start. So, for example, number one on the list almost every year is apples. And so that's one of the foods you should eat organically, always, or not eat them. One of the challenges I have is that I travel and lecture literally all over the world on environmental toxins. So I'm travelling, and what do you eat, OK? [laughs] So every day you just have to make the decisions which foods are least contaminated and which ones are most contaminated. So if I want some kind of fruit juice on the airplane, I get orange juice rather than apple juice. Not that orange juice is not contaminated, but apple juice is one of the worst contaminated. So you just try to make choices. And so the Environmental Working Group has something called the Clean Fifteen and then the Dirty Dozen. And those serve as a great place to start (www.ewg.org).

Brendan [20:32]: Yeah, I use that myself. However, I do make the point when buying food to always choose the very best that I can afford, and not choose … for example, avocados are very expensive organic. At least they can be a lot more expensive. The difference is actually not that big, now that I think about it, but that's one that I buy conventional a lot of the time. But when I'm feeling flush financially, I try to buy organic entirely, or it is going to become biodynamic and regenerative organic and so forth, because I am voting for the planet, not just my own health. It is not just my own health, beyond my own body's load of pesticides, and again, you mentioned certain crops don't carry that much, and it may be that is because those crops don't require that much. But my standard, my ultimate standard, is no toxins applied to our ecosystems, our agroecosystems, and also that we are actively building soil to draw down carbon from the atmosphere and restore water cycles and so forth. So really that's my ultimate standard for what I choose to purchase.

Dr. Pizzorno [21:59]: Excellent. 100% agreement. We only buy organically grown foods. If it's not available organic, we don't buy it. Pure and simple. Well, that's not quite true. I would say we're probably at about a ninety percent ratio now organic to non-organic. And as you say, it is not just our health. It's also our planet's health. And it's also not just our health, it is our children's health as well. So, again, when I lecture on this area, I have a lecture I just presented for the first time last June on environmental toxins and neurodegeneration. And there is a lot of very strong research showing increased neurodegeneration with toxic load, but also with children having lower IQ with more toxic load. So after I show the studies. Like there's been three studies now on organophosphate pesticides, showing that the kids born to mothers with the top ten percent of organophosphate pesticide load, compared to kids with the bottom ten percent or organophosphate load, these children have a seven point drop in IQ. And it's proven now with three studies. And one of the studies followed these children for seven years, and they don't get their IQ back. You get permanent damage to the brain to have a fetus developing in a mother that's toxic. So I look at the audience and ask people, "OK, everybody who's been told by their family and friends that they're stupid for wasting their money on organically grown foods please raise your hand." Of course in the audience, over half of them raised their hands. Now I look at them and I say to them, "Not only are you smarter, but your children are smarter. Think about it."

Brendan [23:31]: It is really important that you are raising the intergenerational issue, because that damage is permanent, as you point out. And there are other inheritances that children get from us, the health of their mitochondria, the health of their telomeres, all of which determine how much energy they're going to have, how much health they're going to have, how long they're going to live. But like you mentioned, IQ and mutagenesis, that can be final. Also, there is the fact that some people are more susceptible to these toxins. Can you say something about that, not just agricultural, but any toxins? What is it with individual susceptibility?

Dr. Pizzorno [24:20]: That's a very, very good question, and it comes down to the fact that because of genetics, we have a huge variation in how well people detoxify those kinds of toxins. If you look at some of the key enzymes in the liver, one of which is called cytochrome P450 2D6, which is called 2D6 for short, and you look at its activity—and the way you look at its activity is by giving a person a drug or toxin and see how fast it is detoxified—there is a one thousand fold variation between people with the fastest version of this enzyme versus people with the slowest version of this enzyme. This means that people with the slowest version of the enzyme, when they're exposed to toxins, they can't get rid of them, and they cause more damage. That's why, if you look back at the cigarette advertising in the fifties and sixties, it had this old geezer, a hundred and five years old, smoking. I remember one advertisement in particular. He was about a hundred and two years old, "I have been smoking since I was five years old, and I didn't get lung cancer." Well, you had the right enzymes. You broke those toxins down. But how about his spouse—I don't know if it's true or not—who died forty years earlier because she got lung cancer from breathing his cigarette smoke. We have huge variations in how well we detoxify, and it's not just genetic. It is also nutritional as well because these enzymes require trace minerals and vitamins to work properly, and if you're on a diet eating food depleted in nutrients and high in toxins, your enzymes cannot get rid of them. So yes, big, big differences.

Brendan [25:57]: I wonder if you could give us a five minute crash course in phase one and phase two liver detoxification and how they work together.

Dr. Pizzorno [26:05]: As we evolved as a species, we were exposed to toxins, and you can determine how much we were exposed to those toxins by the half-life of the toxin in the body. So if the half-life is really short, less than a day, that's pretty clear evidence that that we were exposed to similar chemicals or metals as we evolved as a species. Whereas something like cadmium, with a half-life of sixteen years, means we have not been exposed to those things, so we don't know how to get rid of them. The primary way the body gets rid of chemicals is in the liver, through a two-step process called phase one and phase two. So phase one are what are called the cytochrome P450s. These either directly detoxify a toxin. For example, cytochrome P450 1A2 detoxifies caffeine. There is an eight-fold variation in how it works. So for someone like me, for example, that enzyme works very poorly. I can have a cup of coffee morning, but if I have a cup of coffee in the afternoon, I can't sleep at night because I can't get rid of the caffeine. So a number of chemicals get broken down quickly that way, but the majority of the chemicals, particularly the most toxic ones, are actually changed by phase one into a more active form called an "activated intermediate", which then goes right to the phase two enzymes. They are then bound to another molecule. It is called conjugation, and the typical molecule they are bound to is glutathione. They are then bound to this other molecule that either neutralizes them directly or makes them water-soluble, so that they can be excreted through the kidneys. So when everything's working properly, or phase one is working fine, we can directly get rid of the toxin or make it activated, so then phase two gets rid of it very quickly. So when phase one and phase two are working well, we're going to be much more resistant to toxicity. When phase one is not working very well, we are much more susceptible to toxicity. If phase one is working well, but if phase two is not working well, we actually get a much more toxic reaction that's actually probably the worst of all situations because you have the phase one producing all these activated intermediates, which are much more toxic, a good example being cigarette smoke. The carcinogens in cigarette smoke are made much worse by phase one, because phase one is getting set up so phase two can get rid of them, but if phase two is not working properly, they're actually worse. And it turns out that there are many things we can do to both improve phase one activity or to impair phase one activity. So I mentioned the glutathione conjugation with phase two. That's a really, really important phase two in the system. The problem with conjugation with glutathione is that we can deplete glutathione, depending on our toxic load. So, for example, if you're a heavy drinker of alcohol, you deplete your glutathione, so all of the active intermediates that are supposedly conjugated by phase two and eliminated, now the body cannot do it quite as well. You get much more toxicity, and this is not a rare situation. For example, I'll ask our listeners, "Do you take acetaminophen?" With acetaminophen, the key mechanism for detoxification is phase one activation followed by phase two glutathione conjugation. If you take acetaminophen and are drinking alcohol at the same time, you make the acetaminophen far more toxic. And what it does is it burns out people's kidneys, and it burns out their livers. So you have to be careful. I'm not saying don't drink alcohol, OK. but I'm saying don't drink alcohol if you are also being exposed to chemical toxins. Over-the-counter drugs and prescription drugs are considered by the body in many situations—or I should say most situations—they are chemical toxins. The body has to detoxify them. And if you're not detoxifying properly, they are much, much more damaging to your body.

Brendan [29:58]: You mentioned the phase one enzyme that is involved with detoxifying caffeine. I must have that same slow enzyme because I'm definitely a cheap coffee date.

[**Dr. Pizzorno:** That's funny!

Brendan [30:06]: I've recently learned that an unhealthy dysbiotic microbiome, in other words, unhealthy species of bacteria overpopulating our gut, usually starting with hitting it with antibiotics and not repopulating it with good bacteria, can interfere with the excretion of toxins that we've conjugated in phase two, and specifically bacteria like *Klebsiella*, *Clostridium*, and *E. coli* produce enzymes that de-conjugate these things we are trying to excrete from the body. So how significant a factor do you think this is, and how can we avoid the issue?

Dr. Pizzorno [30:57]: A great, great example. An old-time naturopathic adage is that disease begins in the gut.

Brendan [31:07]: Now we know why.

Dr. Pizzorno [31:09]: And now we know why. These old-timers observed that a hundred years ago, but only now do we understand what is going on. So once the liver conjugates these toxins, they are either dumped through the bile into the gut, or they are excreted in the urine by the kidneys. Now when they are dumped into the gut, if we have the wrong kind of bacteria in the gut, they break down those conjugated chemicals, and the chemicals are then reabsorbed back into the body by a process known as enterohepatic recirculation. So one of the things I do with my patients, when I am trying to detoxify them, the first step is actually to detoxify the gut. Actually, the first step is to stop putting toxins into your body. So stop that. That's what I talk about in the book. I say that we will go through an eight week program. In the first two weeks is … you need to become aware of where the toxins are coming from because there is no point of detoxifying if you keep putting toxins in your gut. The second two weeks is detoxifying the gut. *And* you have to get the right bacteria in your gut and make sure there is enough fiber, because what the liver is expecting is when it dumps those conjugated toxins through the bile into the gut, it's expecting there to be fiber in the gut to bind to those toxins and get them out through the stool. Well, our body developed these systems back when we were consuming between one hundred and one hundred fifty grams of fiber every day. Now the average person consumes fifteen to twenty grams of fiber a day, so fiber is not there to get rid of the toxins to bind them and get them out through the stools, but not only that, because of all of the antibiotics that we have been taking, we now have bacteria in the gut that are more effective at de-conjugating these bound toxins, and so it is now it's easier for them to be reabsorbed into the body. So when we're looking at toxicity, you have to stop the toxins coming into the body. You have to clean up the gut. You've got to clean up the liver, and you have to clean up the kidneys. And only after you have got all these things working properly, do I put the person on a detoxification program.

Brendan [33:06]: So when it comes to the gut, it sounds like we need to take about ten times as much fiber as the average person is currently taking in. That's one thing, and I'm going to go back a second because I mentioned that typically a dysbiotic microbiome begins with antibiotic use, but I shouldn't leave out the fact that there are many forms of antibiotics that aren't included in our food intentionally, such as artificial sweeteners that damage the microbiome in our gut, and herbicides and other pesticides. The glyphosate in the Roundup herbicide is very devastating to our microbiome. And it's in everything conventional, and it is even getting into the rainwater and therefore maybe getting in small quantities into organic foods. So there are many things affecting our microbiome, and just the fact that a person might not have been subjected to pharmaceutical antibiotics does not necessarily mean they don't have something to check into as far as their microbiome health.

Dr. Pizzorno [34:11]: Yep, very well said, and another source I suspect most people aren't aware of is - how many people are taking proton pump inhibitors? So somebody has heartburn, or GERD—that's what the technical term for it is—and they go to the drug store, and they buy one of these over-the-counter antacid compounds that are blocking acid secretion in the stomach. Well that sounds fine because you have less symptoms when you regurgitate your food. The problem is that we need that acid not only to break down our food to get the nutrients out of it, but the acid in the stomach protects us from naturally-occurring bacteria in the foods. So a person eating foods of commerce, which can be contaminated, and they're taking proton pump inhibitors, they can't kill bacteria, like for example *Clostridia*, and research has shown that the more proton pump inhibitors a person consumes, the higher the levels of *Clostridium* bacteria in the gut, and the Clostridia, as you mentioned earlier, are some of the worst kinds of bacteria to have in a person's gut.

Brendan [35:10]: So you started to mention your general strategy for detoxifying effectively and safely. And you go into a lot more detail in your book, which is fantastic. I guess I'll leave it at that, because people need to get your book. I've listened to it on audio book three or four times. What are your top three recommendations for minimizing toxins and maximizing detoxification capacity?

Dr. Pizzorno [36:03]: That is a very, very good question. So of course, if you're going to avoid toxins, here is the primary way of doing it: number one, eat organically grown foods. Number two, do not buy organically grown foods that are stored in plastic or cans because those packaging materials could get into the body. Once I get organically grown foods back home, I do not cook them on Teflon-type type, non-stick coatings because some that is going to get into the food. So you basically have to decrease your toxic food exposure as much as possible. The second area is you have look at your water supply. Amazingly, ten percent of the public water supplies in the US have arsenic levels known to increase disease in humans, and only half of the public water supplies have even been even tested for arsenic, so you've got to make sure your supply is not contaminated. If you live anywhere in a city, or within one hundred yards of a major highway, you need to have air filters in your house, because there's a lot of particulate matter in that area that is very, very damaging to the body. We don't let anybody come into our house wearing their shoes. We have them take off their shoes when they come into the house. And finally health and beauty aids. Make sure you are using health and beauty aids that are low in phthalates, and make sure your lipstick does not have lead in it, and just these kinds of obvious things. So number one, you just have to avoid the toxins, and then number two is that you want to help your body detoxify. And there's two primary methods that are easiest for people to do and are the least likely to have adverse effects. Number one is increase fiber. I believe everybody should get at least fifty grams of fiber every day. Now, don't all of a sudden take fifty grams of fiber because it can take your body awhile to adapt to a particular bacteria in the gut. But the good thing about the fiber is that if we take the right kind of fiber, it actually promotes the growth of healthy bacteria in the gut. And then a dietary supplement that I recommend that everybody who lives in civilization should consider is NAC, also known as N-acetyl cysteine, and N-acetyl cysteine is quite an interesting nutrient in that it increases glutathione production in the body. And glutathione is our most important intramitochondrial, intracellular antioxidant, protecting us from the damaging effects of these chemical toxins and metal toxins as well.

Brendan [38:34]: So what I'm hearing is how important it is to minimize toxins and also to make sure we're getting the right nutrients to be able to detoxify. A lot of those come from our food. In fact, all of them should, really. I guess it doesn't hurt at all to have the benefits of modern technology and being able to produce concentrated forms of things like N-acetyl cysteine. And I've taken that myself. Essentially every day we have the opportunity to build health for ourselves and for the Earth by learning how our foods are grown and asking for what we really want in our food and what we don't want in it. So Dr. Pizzorno, with scientific detoxification being so central to human health and potential, I just want to say we are all very blessed to have somebody like you that has dedicated so many years to this. Thank you for your work to understand and demystify safe and effective detoxification, despite skepticism and outright opposition from conventional medicine over the years, for creating an institution, Bastyr University, that has magnified the reach of natural medicine exponentially over the years, and for being a true pioneer and resource to us all, and all of us here at the Eat4 Earth community. Thank you for being here with us today and sharing your hard won wisdom.

Dr. Pizzorno [40:05]: Well, thank you for your kind compliment. I appreciate it. And, I just want to leave with your audience that only twenty percent of disease is due to genetics. Eighty percent is due to choices we make. So if you make healthy choices, you're healthy. If you make unhealthy choices, unless you got really, really lucky at genetic roulette, if you make unhealthy choices you get disease. And it is just as simple as that.

Brendan [40:29]: Dr Pizzorno and I recorded an entire second interview that covers detoxification in even greater depth, including genetic differences among individuals, called single nucleotide polymorphisms, or SNPs for short. This is included in the "Day 9" interviews.

Wendy Myers Interview
Minerals, Heavy Metals, and Advanced Detox Strategies and Technology

Brendan [00:00:00]: Welcome to the Eat4Earth event. We're exploring how you can heal yourself, your loved ones, and the planet, with food. This is Brendan Moorehead, and it's time to learn some secrets of detoxification and rejuvenation with our expert guest, Wendy Myers. Wendy Myers is founder of Myersdetox.com. She's a detox guru, functional diagnostic nutritionist, and NES bio-energetic practitioner in Los Angeles, California. She is the number one best-selling author of *Limitless Energy: How to Detox Toxic Metals to End Exhaustion and Chronic Fatigue*. She has the Detox for Energy course coming soon. This is a revolutionary metal detox program to regain energy and brain function. Passionate about the importance of detox to live a long disease-free life, she is a sought after speaker appearing on countless summits and podcasts. Go to detoxforenergy.com/free to download her free check-list: The Top Ten Tips to Detox like a Pro. Wendy, thank you so much for being with us here today and on such short notice.

Wendy [00:01:06]: Thank you so much for having me.

Brendan [00:01:08]: Wendy, most of us could use a little more energy, and some of us could use a lot more of it. I was one of those people for a long time. In fact, it is frequently reported that fatigue is the common complaint that people bring to their health-care providers. What do you believe are the most common and important factors causing people to experience fatigue?

Wendy [00:01:33]: Well, there's a lot of reasons people have fatigue, and it's been the number one complaint of all of my clients. I've had thousands of clients that I've worked one on one with. I don't work with clients any more, but when I was, everyone's tired. Even people that have energy want more energy. What I have found over the years in my research is that there's a family of toxic metals like arsenic, aluminum, tin, thallium and cesium that poison enzymes that transfer nutrients into our mitochondria. And our mitochondria are our body's powerhouses. And if they don't have the right nutrients that they need, they're not going to be able to make the energy, or not be able to produce the amount of energy that our body needs,. And then if you don't have enough energy, you won't have enough energy to sleep. It actually takes energy to sleep. It's a very energy-intensive process. You're not just lying there. You're fighting infections, and you're regenerating tissue, and you're detoxing metals. Your liver is detoxing at night. Your immune system is fighting things. So it's very energy- intensive. And that's why a lot of people find, they go to sleep, and they're trying to sleep more, and they just don't wake up refreshed. They just aren't producing enough energy. And then there's other factors as well of course that reduce people's energies like EMF, electromagnetic fields. These are also things that reduce energy production in the body. And then there's infections that can impede energy production. But a big factor a lot of people aren't really thinking about are these toxic metals that cause fatigue.

Brendan [00:03:15]: Why are people so toxic?

Wendy [00:03:18]: Yeah well, it's one of those things where everyone is exposed to toxins like metals and chemicals in our air, food, and water. It's completely unavoidable, everyone has metals and chemicals in their body. I know there's a lot of people listening that may be eating really well, and they are trying to sleep, and they're exercising and they're taking supplements, and they're generally taking really good care of themselves. But for me, I was doing that—I was doing everything perfectly—and I still didn't feel good. I still was having trouble losing weight. I was not sleeping well, and I didn't have the energy levels that I wanted. And I was having a lot of different issues and eventually in my own healing journey discovered that metals and chemicals were preventing me from meeting my health goals, preventing me from the energy levels that I wanted. I was having troubles with my hormones and various other health issues. Through detoxification I was able to solve them, so that really set me on a path, on a mission, to want to help other people and bring some awareness to where they're getting toxins and how they can detox them out of their body.

So, first let's start with the food. There's lots of different metals in our food, and it doesn't matter whether it's meat or vegetables, or what not. All foods have some sort of metals. Even supplements will have metals in them, especially herbs that are grown in China or India. So plants unfortunately can be watered with waste, like waste water treatment plants. They'll take sediments from that and use that as fertilizer and that can have really high cadmium levels. That's approved to use, the sewage sludge, and those can have high levels of cadmium like I just said. Then there's water … water is a big source of toxins, the water that we're showering in. Even if you're drinking filtered water, you could be showering in water that's full of fluoride and chlorine, medications, birth control, and not including …. metals, like in my water. I have uranium, and I have antimony. And a lot of people have arsenic and uranium in their water. Your skin absorbs all of these metals, and the skin is a wonderful vehicle to absorb nutrients, including metals and chemicals in water. That's a very common source people might not be aware of. And then there's air. Air is actually the number one place people get toxins and breathe in metals and what not. We breathe in aluminum and mercury and cadmium and other problems because of coal burning that we are using for our energy sources. Thallium is also another metal that we're breathing in. Just burning all these hundred-million-year old petroleum resources that are full of thallium, and thallium is a huge factor in chronic fatigue. These things are just … you need to be aware of them, and you don't need to get too worked up about it or depressed or "Oh my God, it's hopeless". It's just a fact of modern life, and you just need to have a sensible detoxification regimen to add to what you're already doing for your health.

Brendan [00:06:48]: So your focus is toxic metals and the fatigue that they tend to cause. How do you test for that, and how do you treat it?

Wendy [00:06:59]: So when I work with clients, we have a program where we use hair metals analysis to test clients, and we also use urine metals analysis, and stool metals analysis. Different metals come out in different ways in the body. My first love though is hair metals analysis. It's where I like to start with clients. You don't even have to test to start detoxing. It can be nice to do some tests to figure out what exact metals you have but by no means are you required to do that.

Brendan [00:07:34]: How about treatment? I think you have a somewhat unique approach to detoxification treatment.

Wendy [00:07:42]: So I have a course that's coming out in January. That course will help give people the basics. I think it's going to be called "The Detox for Energy Course". But that will give people the basics on how to detox. Some very simple things you can do are binders. You know binders are something you need to do to absorb metals and chemicals in your body. PectaSol-C is a fantastic one. It's a modified citrus pectin, and that has a number of benefits in your body. Then there's also something called Biosil which is also really cool. Biosil is a silicate, a special type of silica, and that's going to bind onto arsenic, aluminum, tin, thallium, and cesium, and grab onto those metals, mobilize them, and then the PectaSol-C will bind to those metals and remove them from the body. So Biosil is a very, very effective chelator. Chelators will grab on to the metals and remove them from the body. There's a myriad number of supplements you can take to detox. I outline a lot of them in my book *Limitless Energy*, and essentially that's kind of the very basics.

Typically when people do testing, they'll find out exactly what metals they have, and there's different supplements that work best depending on what metals you have. So typically when we work with someone, we'll give them a customized supplement protocol for the metals that they have in their body.

But everyone needs certain basics, and doing the PectaSol-C and Biosil is a great way. I've also have been working more bio-energetically with clients. I think that bio-energetics as a way to detox is probably the most compelling and easiest and cheapest way, a most effective way to detox the body. And I've been definitely moving my research more in that vein to detox people.

Brendan [00:09:33]: So what is the bio-energetic approach? How does that work?

Wendy [00:09:36]: I'm doing a heavy metal summit in January, Theheavymetalssumit.com, and I've interviewed a number of people about how to detox bioenergetically. There's different approaches there as well. Essentially, the concept is you have your physical body, but you also have an energetic field. The main way your body communicates is energetically, and essentially when you correct your body's energetic functioning, you neutralize any toxic chemicals, and you neutralize any heavy metals in your body. It's kind of hard to believe, but the metals, the frequency at which they resonate, just doesn't happen anymore in your body. They just disappear. I know that sounds really hard to believe, but I have doctors that I've interviewed on my Heavy Metals Summit that have been doing this for fifteen years, and they do testing to corroborate that. They do testing before helping someone and working with them bio-energetically, and they do testing afterwards, and the metals are completely gone. There are some exceptions like mercury. It can be very difficult, but it can still be addressed bio-energetically, but it's just a little bit more difficult to work with. And then there's also mold. Mold mycotoxins could be a little bit more challenging to work with bio-energetically. But it's really incredibly effective, and it's something that I've just been learning about this over the past year, about how to detox bio-energetically. And it's really, really exciting. I think it's just going to really change the face of detoxification because I've worked with thousands of clients, and there are some people that are so sick they can't take a ton of supplements. Or they can't afford to take a ton of supplements. Or they are just so sensitive they react, and the detox just really hasn't worked for them. Bio-energetics is the way to go. It's the wave of the future. Even Dr. Oz says the wave of the future of medicine is energy medicine, and so that's really where I've focused more of my research and messaging with people to kind of just steer them to a better way to address their health and their toxins.

Brendan [00:11:55]: I'm curious, are some people more vulnerable to accumulating heavy metals and other toxins?

Wendy [00:12:05]: Absolutely. When someone is mineral deficient, they're going to be more prone to accumulate and not release heavy metals. So we all get the same exposures typically. We're all exposed to a lot of different metals and chemicals. But there's some people that are having a very mineral- deficient diet, or they either like, they eat of processed foods and carbohydrates. They have a lot of stress. Those are also going to reduce minerals even further. And for instance, if you're deficient in zinc, if you don't eat any red meat, you eat a processed carb diet and what not, you won't have enough zinc, and your body would be forced to accumulate cadmium to repair your arteries, to repair your ligaments and your tissues, and your skin and things like that because it just doesn't have zinc to do the job. So very, very important as a basis for detoxification to mineralize your body. And you know, our food today is deficient. Even if you're eating organic food, the soils just don't contain the minerals that are required to support our health, the levels that we need. So I always start with clients mineralizing their body and taking magnesium malate, taking zinc. I really like Oceans Alive Marine Phytoplankton to get all the trace minerals and all kinds of other minerals, and that's the foundation of any health protocol and detox protocol also.

Brendan [00:13:35]: So in other words, a heavy metal like cadmium is like a toxic mimic of zinc. It performs some of the functions I guess, or can be used because of some similarity at the atomic level, but it has a toxic influence as well, heavily so.

Wendy [00:13:49]: Absolutely, yeah. Zinc and cadmium occupy the same binding sites in the body, so they can be used interchangeably to do the same job. But obviously cadmium is the inferior building material.

Brendan [00:14:02]: In my own experience I have learned that mineral ratios are very, very important for maintaining proper energy function and so forth. I'm just curious if that relates to this at all, how do mineral ratios play into the mix?

Wendy [00:14:18]: Yeah, I mean, when you're using hair metal analysis to kind of evaluate and use it as a guide for supplementation, you're looking at mineral ratios. And definitely a goal of trying to balance some of those minerals is giving them a sort of combination of minerals and supplements aimed towards not only increasing the individual levels of minerals but to balance the ratios of minerals, to balance sodium to potassium or calcium to magnesium. And that's just a delicate balancing out that can be guided by hair mineral analysis. But yeah the body functions better when you have adequate stores and the minerals are balanced to each other.

Brendan [00:14:55]: So I'm curious, is there like a target ratio that is ideal for people and then people come to you and their ratios are just all over the map, and then you're trying to move them toward the ideal ratio that increases function to its optimum, or how does it work?

Wendy [00:15:11]: It probably would be beyond the scope of our talk today, but it can begin very, very complicated, but yeah, everyone comes in, they all have a completely different hair test, but we're all kind of guiding them to the general ideal levels of mineral ratios and mineral levels.

Brendan [00:15:30]: Okay, so as I understood, I think, in the past you had a big focus on using minerals, like as a person mineral sufficient it helps them move the toxic metals out. Is that correct, and is that still a focus of yours or are you shifting so much toward perhaps a faster and less expensive approach which is the bio-energetic?

Wendy [00:15:51]: Yeah, well, you know, even if you're using bio-energetics, you still have to tend to your physical body, so you still have to take minerals in and supplements and nutrients and things like that. But yeah, definitely, everyone needs to take magnesium every single day. I really like magnesium malate. Everyone needs to be taking a multi-mineral or a marine phytoplankton to get the minerals that their body needs so that it can function. Minerals are the spark plugs of the body and they push out metals, they displace metals. But I'm just more a fan, just over the course of working with so many people, and just my own personal results working bio-energetically, that you have to work on both planes. Bio-energetically is definitely the way to go, but you also have to work physically—you have to take binders, and you can still take chelators, and you want to take minerals as well.

Brendan [00:16:42]: How about saunas and things like that, are there any other particular approaches you think are important and that you typically advise?

Wendy [00:16:49]: 100%, I love infrared saunas. Saunas are a great way to sweat out metals and chemicals and different toxins, and they're really, really healthy for you. There was just a finished study that came out that was done over twenty years, and the people in this study they were doing a sauna four to five times a week had a 40% reduction of mortality of all causes, including heart disease. I mean that's pretty incredible, pretty incredible result. And part of that is because of the health benefits, the immune system benefits that are imparted by regular sauna use, but also because of the detoxification effects as well.

Brendan [00:17:30]: You mentioned food earlier, about how cadmium for example can get into our food supply from sewage sludge and also gets there via forms of rock phosphate fertilizers that carry cadmium into the soil—and that type of fertilizers is not used in organic agriculture from what I understand—but I'm just curious if you've seen differences in people that are already eating organic vs. not eating organic, or in different parts of the country where they're accumulating more metals and also what kind of dietary changes you advise to move in the right direction?

Wendy [00:18:07]: Well everyone is different, and depending on where someone lives, what type of diet they're eating, the water that they're drinking, the water that they're showering in, their air quality, everyone has a different profile. It's definitely good if you're eating organic, that's much better, but even organic foods still have toxins landing on them. There's still typically toxic water that they are being watered with. The soils are still mineral deficient. The soils still can have metals in them. If you took a conventional farm, and then an organic farmer bought it, and now he's using organic farming, there could still be metals and toxins in the soil from previous pesticide use. There's a lot of banned pesticides that had lead and arsenic and other metals in them. They're no longer in use, but they're still present in the soils. And so eating organic doesn't absolve you. Organic does not mean free of metals. Organic foods are not tested for metals. and a lot of the organic food from China that's sold at Whole Foods is grown in incredibly toxic soil, air, and water. So unfortunately eating organic does not mean non-toxic. It just means no pesticides. And that's definitely a part of the problem, and I think organic foods have more nutrients in them which helps to protect you from accumulating as many toxins, but it's a small part of the solution, but definitely part of the solution.

As far as diet is concerned, I generally tell people to not worry too much about what they're eating as far as toxins are concerned. I mean certainly I'm not a person that says avoid fish even though we know it contains mercury and cadmium and other metals because again there's so many health benefits to fish. And there's research that shows that you have more health benefits of eating fish than you do by avoiding them, even for pregnant women. There's a study that showed that children of pregnant women who avoided fish had I think five point lower IQ. I mean really this changes the course of a child's life. The Omega-3 fats are more important to a developing fetus than are the potential mercury exposure that they may be getting from that fish in the diet. So the recommendations are completely wrong pertaining to fish consumption, especially for pregnant women. And so it's one of those things where you don't avoid fish. I certainly don't myself. You just need to have a sensible detox plan, and also you want to avoid simple carbohydrates and sugar because that places a tremendous burden on the liver. And when your liver is dealing with that 911 emergency, which is your high blood sugar, it can't detox. It's not detoxing you. So you have to think about … your liver only has so much work that it can do in a day, so you want to not give it, throw jobs at it, that are unnecessary, that prevent it from doing other more important jobs like breaking down metals and chemicals and taking out the trash. There's some common sense things, typically avoiding supplements and herbs from India and China. It can go a long way to reducing metal exposure. And drinking clean filtered water, and if you can do a whole house filter so you're not showering and bathing in toxic water.

Brendan [00:21:54]: You know, on the topic of fish, that's a big one I think for a lot of people. It is for me, and I'm wondering, the data that you looked at, did they distinguish between large fish and small fish, because small fish like herring, mackerel, sardines … they have a ton of the essential fatty acids, the omega-3s, and they are bio-accumulating less mercury, so I'm thinking those would be better than the larger fish which are usually the ones most often recommended to avoid, and I'm curious if that study made a distinction between the different sizes of fish these people were eating.

Wendy [00:22:30]: Yes, exactly. It makes sense to avoid tuna, but not all tunas are bad. Skipjack tuna that's going to be far, far lower in mercury content because they're much smaller, they live less time than say an Ahi tuna that you eat in sushi. And I typically avoid ahi tuna and whatnot. But typically the canned tuna, the Skipjack are perfectly fine to eat. The study did make mention of that, that the canned tuna is typically ok, but it's the larger migratory Ahi tunas that are to be avoided.

Brendan [00:23:08]: And I think eating lower in the food chain is obviously going to have a lower impact on the planet. I don't know if I can say obviously. but they're faster-reproducing, and of course there's tuna species like the Blue Fin and they're basically endangered.

Wendy [00:23:21]: Yeah, absolutely.

Brendan [00:23:23]: So we shouldn't at all be supporting that fishery. A lot of people would argue we shouldn't support any fisheries because the oceans are really under a lot of stress from overharvesting, so it brings up the question of vegetarian-sourced omega-3 fatty acids, which typically are in the short chain that then the liver has to assemble into the long chain eicosapentaenoic and docosahexaenoic acid. So I'm curious what your take is on that because traditionally people say we can only convert those vegetarian sources at about five percent. I sometimes wonder if people with a healthy liver could do a lot better than that. There are certainly vegans, a few of them that seem to be surviving for a long time on a vegan diet. Others succumb to problems in ten to twelve years. I mean it could take a while.

Wendy [00:24:17]: I think it's one of those things. I think everyone is different. For me, I tried a vegan-vegetarian diet. It's not for me. I just can't do it. It's not healthy for me. I suffer pretty severe health issues doing that, but everyone is different. If you think of the whole bell curve. There are some people that do fine on the vegan diet. I think the majority of the people do not. There's some people that do great on an all-meat diet, but the majority of people are not going to. So I think it's just more about listening to your body, what your body is craving. Your body will always tell you what you need to be eating, and I think people are very good at reading a book and then following that, letting their mind override their body's innate intelligence. So I'm just kind of like the, "I see food, I eat it" kind of thing, and I just listen to my body. If my body's craving broccoli, I eat broccoli. I mean not unhealthy cravings, not sugar and things like that. I'm talking about healthy cravings. You want to listen to your body, and I think as it pertains to needs. And I think people really get into trouble when they try to follow like a doctrine or a diet, and then they're not listening to their body. They will get in trouble, and people can suffer some pretty severe health issues as a result.

Brendan [00:25:31]: I totally agree. After many years of doing that to myself I came up with, I sort of had this idea that " diets" are like idea viruses, and they take hold, and then they control you and make you sick if it's not the right idea.

Wendy [00:25:47]: Exactly, that's a very good way to put! [laughing] Very good way.

Brendan [00:25:52]: And on the other hand the tongue is an extraordinarily sensitive bio-sensor, you could say, so it knows what is a fit, and I use that every day and every meal. I actually had to do that because my mind became so dominant. I'm so analytical, I had to become more of a sensory being when it came to eating food. And from one day to the next, one meal to the next, fish can taste like the most amazing thing or the most revolting thing.

Wendy [00:26:17]: Yes.

Brendan [00:26:18]: It totally depends on where my body's at.

Wendy [00:26:20]: Yeah, if you're eating something and it just tastes like the best thing you've ever tasted, your body wants that, it needs that. And there's other times when I'm sushi, sushi, sushi, like I have to have it, and other times I'm just not thinking about it at all. Your body will tell you what you need. Yesterday I was craving red meat. I went and I had some lamb. So I just listen to my body, and I do pretty good. I have pretty good blood work as a result.

Brendan [00:26:48]: What I'm hearing most of the health practitioners or let's say health educators that seem to be nondenominational as far as diet—they don't have a particular ideology necessarily, or they're open and flexible that those might change from time to time—that they seem to basically say we need, and this is kind of Michael Pollan's words, we need to "eat, mostly plants, not too much". Different order, "eat food, not too much, mostly plants." But it doesn't mean all plants. Most of these people are saying the healthiest populations in the world they typically ate fish. It's very common for those populations. But it wasn't necessarily like pounds and pounds of fish every day, probably not. I don't know the specific amounts, but that seemed to be it. They ate high quantities of plant-based foods and then they had some seafood.

Wendy [00:27:44]: Yeah, I think it's roughly about 15% as like the basic guideline for animal protein, and I find that's kind of what I naturally gravitate towards, but everybody is a little bit different. We all have a different genetic background, different digestive fire, and capacity and everyone's just different.

Brendan [00:28:04]: You mentioned digestive fire. I'm curious, do you anything Ayurvedic. When I hear digestive fire I think of … agni, the Pitta Dosha digestive fire. I'm a part Pitta, part Vata. Do you use that?

Wendy [00:28:26]: No. I don't. No.

Brendan [00:28:27]: Okay, let's skip that. So, one of the topics that's come up a lot in this event is the toxin glyphosate. What I haven't heard yet is—so Dr. Zach Bush has a way of defending and repairing the body from glyphosate—but as far as maybe its bioaccumulation and detoxifying, I'm just curious if anybody has any experience and insight into what's the best way to detoxify glyphosate.

Wendy [00:28:56]: The best way is bio-energetically. It's very difficult to do physically because it's just so pervasive in our environment, and there's really not a lot of research on glyphosate. I mean certainly taking binders … I mean there's not a lot of research on how to detox glyphosate, and I think taking binders like PectaSol-C is a great thing to do to absorb it I think. No matter what protocol you're doing, whether you're doing saunas or a physical detox, or IV chelation or whatever you're doing bio-energetically, you still have to take binders. Everyone has to. You can take ZeoBind or charcoal or PectaSol-C. Binders are where it's at to absorb metals and chemicals. Overall, you can get rid of glyphosate in 24 hours from your body by doing it bio-energetically. It's no joke. I mean there's Dr. Doug Phillips, Dr. Lee Cowden. Dr. Lee Cowden is incredibly well-respected functional medicine doctor. He is the one that developed this protocol, and he's Dr. Joe Mercola's personal physician. And he does a lot of training. He was at the last training I went to for NES health and bioenergetic,s and he does a lot of bio-energetic medicine at his AICM conference [probably meant to say "ACIM"], he talks about every year. I had a friend presenting in bioenergetics at his last conference. (also) Harry Massey. And so bioenergetics it's where it's at. You'll be hearing more and more and more about this in the alternative health community in the coming years. I have a podcast actually called "SuperCharged" where we explore a lot of different modalities and bioenergetics and bio-energetic concepts and how our body works quantumly. You know, we're not just mass, we're energetic beings, and if you work in the energetic spectrum and the energetic field, it's the main way our body communicates, and it's just far more effective, and fast and cheap and easy. You can do it at home. This is the way you want to be working with your body, and in a lot of different ways, not just physically, but you can help your body mentally. You can help yourself spiritually, emotionally, etc. by working energetically. And that sounds kind of weird, but you know a lot of different metals and chemicals have different emotions attached to them, so a lot of people find when they start detoxing they'll have anxiety or depression, or other kind of emotions tied to those metals. And I've definitely found this to be true in doing my own detox and working with clients as well. Back to detoxing bio-energetically, that's really the easiest way to detox glyphosate. There's more information on the SuperCharged podcast about that.

Brendan [00:31:57]: People can check that out if they want to learn how to access that technology.

Wendy [00:32:03]: And on the Heavy Metal Summit coming up, we'll be talking about that as well.

Brendan [00:32:06]: Awesome. You know I think it's really fascinating, your approach is unique in the world of what I've seen so fa, and I haven't, I admit I haven't been exposed to the bioenergetics. And you do this mineral ratio testing. It seems like the way to go about detox is individualized and so getting tested first, seeing what's going on, combining all of these elements, is really going to be the way to go for detoxifying.

Wendy [00:32:34]: Yeah, absolutely, and you don't have to get tested first. There's lots of things you can do just get started. You can take a binder. You can take Biosil. You can do infrared saunas. Just get the ball rolling because it takes time to detox, at least physically. Bio-energetically you can get detoxed very, very quickly, but you still have to maintain it, and you still have to take binders and things of that nature. But just get started, doing something, adding something to your regimen, and then at some point you can do some testing.

Brendan [00:33:02]: Very good. Well I really appreciated you being here with us and sharing those insights and wisdom. And thank you for your partnership in the Eat4Earth community.

Wendy [00:33:12]: Yes, thank you so much for having me.

Dan Kittredge Interview
Minerals, Spiritual Attainment, and a Technology to Measure the Nutrients in Your Food

Brendan [00:00:00]: Welcome to the Eat4Earth event. We're exploring how you can heal yourself, your loved ones, and the planet, with food. This is Brendan Moorehead, please join me in welcoming our guest right now, Dan Kittredge. Dan is a lifelong organic farmer, and he is the co-founder of the Bionutrient Food Association. Dan's mission is to increase quality in our food supply as the foundation and organizing principle for creating the reality that we want to see. This core strategy can be summed up in the simple statement, "When the people lead, the leaders will follow." The Bionutrient Food Association holds an annual conference called Soil and Nutrition and has a game-changing concept for technology that would empower consumers to know the nutrient content of our food and exactly what we're getting when we purchase food. This would open the door to a whole new era of true food transparency. So Dan, I'm really glad to have you here today, and I'm looking forward to learn more about this.

Dan [00:01:01]: Thank you for having me.

Brendan [00:01:03]: So, as we know, for decades now the nutrient quality of our food supply has been declining in very close association with changes in our agricultural system like mechanized plowing of soils, chemical fertilizers, pesticides, herbicides, fungicides that kill the soil organisms that make nutrients available to us, so our ability to develop normally from the moment of conception, and to replace cells with healthy cells throughout life, and neutralize the toxins we're exposed to daily, including through our food, is highly dependent on the nutrient content of our food. The nutrient content of our food basically has never been more depleted than it is right now, and never more important to our health, the full expression of our human potential, and even the survival of our species. Yet we as consumers don't really have a way to know the nutrient content of the food that we're buying. So tell us some more about this technology, where a consumer could point a hand held device at, say, a tomato or a bunch of carrots, push a button, and get a reading on its nutritional content. Why is getting this in the hands of consumers so important to you?

Dan [00:02:20]: I think, a lot of the things you said in your introduction factor into it. It seems that the way we treat the soil has a lot to do with the health of our plants, and the health of our plants has to do with the health of our bodies. And it correlates nicely to the health of our ecosystem and our culture. There seems to be a really nice connection between all these different things, which is really not that much of a revelation, except that we haven't been working strategically to address it. There's this topic, epigenetics, which refers to how environmental conditions affect genetic expression. You can have two carrots with the same genetics that are grown in different environments that basically, one grows well, one grows poorly. And it's not because of the genetics. It's because of the environment, and I would suggest that for the past two-three maybe four generations now, we can say most Americans, at least, have been eating food that was grown in a very unnatural manner. And functionally, because of that, the food has had dramatic insufficiency of nutrition, and through multiple generations of humans eating food that does not have enough nutrition in it, and we start to break down. Epidemic levels of degenerative diseases are becoming more and more prevalent, especially in the younger generations. And there seems to be a really nice correlation between what is or what is not in your food and your functional health. The idea is certainly if you grow food well, among other things you sequester carbon from the atmosphere, you can heal the ecosystem, all these great, wonderful, sort of big, grand things. But that is not enough of a driver for most people. The driver we think is their own health and the health of their children. The idea basically is that we can give consumers the ability to choose which bag of carrots off the shelf, which bag of flour, which burger, whatever it is you're buying, if you can choose the one that is most nutritious, it happens to be the most flavorful, it's the one your child is most likely to eat and it actually has the nutrients in it -- which make it a medicine. There's this old aphorism from Hypocrates, the father of modern medicine, he says among other things "Let food be thy medicine". I would suggest that most of what passes for food these days is not medicine because it does not have the nutrients in it that it needs to function like medicine. So we're working on this open-source technology, spectroscopy technology, to give consumers the ability to literally flash a light at a bag of carrots, or at a beef patty, or whatever it is, and discern relatively how good it is. And if you've got choices in the store, if you've got three different bags of carrots to choose from, you can choose the one that's most nutritious and let your money that you use to buy your food incentivize the supply chain to focus on quality as opposed to volume and aesthetic.

Brendan [00:06:00]: That would be so extraordinary. And will be so extraordinary.

Dan [00:06:05]: We're moving right along. It's not a future tense for much longer.

Brendan [00:06:09]: It sounds almost too good to be true because it's so … I mean, the implications are so extraordinary. How would you envision this influencing the food system and our food supply and so forth?

Dan [00:06:25]: When I was first trying to put these pieces together, five or six years ago, and understood what spectroscopy was and how it could be used., I mean, just for the audience here, functionally this could be a capacity of your smart phone in a couple of years, and I think I've been told, although I haven't checked it out, the iPhone ten has some of the tools in its camera now to be able to do this. So literally you take your camera on your phone, and you flash a light at the carrots, and you've downloaded the free app, and it says beep-beep 18 out of a 100, beep-beep 40 out of a 100. It literally gives you a reading in real time with a flash of light from your smartphone. So that's basically what we're talking about. The first couple of generations are probably going to be stand-alone things that cost a hundred bucks or a hundred and fifty bucks and fit in the palm of your hand. But once we get enough sort of momentum, I think it's entirely plausible that this capacity could be a functioning app on your phone. But the idea is, basically, when I was putting this all together, I remember I was talking to some—not totally muckety mucks—but some pretty high-up people in Whole Foods about this idea, and Whole Foods say they want to have … they're producing, you know, providing superior quality food, and I'm like. "This could be a market advantage for you guys to actually formally show that you have better quality than your competition." And the response from the person I was talking to was, you know, "There's not a chance that we're going to help you with this project, but when you're a couple years out from having this capacity, please come tell us, because we will tell our growers that they have two years to meet standard." The idea is basically that when the supply chain knows that the consumers can tell how good their food is, then they will work with the farmers to make sure the food is actually good. And they know that it's not, and they know the consumers can't tell. And it's too much of a hassle for them to deal with it. So really it's enlightened self-interest. Only when the consumer has the ability to test the quality of their food will the supply chain focus on improving the quality of their food, will the farmers actually apply the practices which produce high quality foods, which also sequesters carbon, can reverse climate change, can obviate the need for agrochemicals and all kinds of other really, really systemic issues.

So it's just transparency and enlightened self-interest. That's the basic strategy. But foundational to this is we are a non-governmental organization. We're a non-profit educational organization. All the research, all the engineering, everything is in the commons. It's open-source. It's not black box. It's not proprietary. We're not taking this information and marketing it. We're coordinating a big, open, collaborative research project basically.

Brendan [00:09:26]: You know, there actually is a precedent for markets and consumer demand shifting markets. There's a food chain in South Africa called Woolworths, and they're vertically integrated from what I understand, or at least they have a lot of influence over their growers, and so they've adopted the Nutrition Farming approach from Graeme Sait and his Nutri-Tech Solutions. You're familiar with that.

Dan [00:09:54]: I know Graeme and Arden was there for a while too, so yeah, there's a few people, a few of the bigger sort of consultants in the farming world that know how to do this stuff, have been working in South Africa with Woolworths and other companies. There's hot spots around the world where this is actually happening in large measure. It's not like this is revolutionary information. It's been proven. There just hasn't been an economic driver for it to shift the supply chain at large.

Brendan [00:10:21]: Right, yeah, this device would just take it to another level. But what they have, even just based on the difference in taste, Woolworths has grabbed market share from competitors that are now trying to catch up, from what I understand. You should tell Whole Foods maybe the same thing if you have another conversation say like, "This is already happening. This is what you're facing if you don't lead."

Dan [00:10:44]: Yeah, well, I mean, they say "Speak softly, and carry a large stick." I think that was TR (Theodore Roosevelt), but you know, you could go to them gently and say, "Here's a good idea, and in two years consumers are going to be able to test." And they'll be like, "Oh, that's a good idea". The large stick is this threat of empiricism and transparency, and until it's a viable possibility, I don't think this is going to go anywhere near as far as it could.

Brendan [00:11:19]: And I'm curious, have you spoken to Natural Grocers?

Dan [00:11:22]: I have spoken to Natural Grocers, and I'm going to be out there in Boulder in a couple of weeks, and I'll probably see them. I think they're out there. So yeah, I think of all the chains in and around the country they're one of the most allied.

Brendan [00:11:43]: That's my impression. So can you explain, in terms that most of us would understand, how this device works. What is spectroscopy?

Dan [00:11:55]: What is spectroscopy? Let me see, I like to use the example of a star. Alpha Centauri is a star that's I think five or six light years away, maybe eight light years away. It's a decent ways away, and if you ask any astronomer or astrophysicist about what Alpha Centauri is made up of, they'll tell you with great confidence that Alpha Centauri is 51% hydrogen; it's 48% helium; it's 1% other gases in these levels and ratios. We know exactly what Alpha Centauri is made up of, and we have never sent any probe out to Alpha Centauri to test it. How do we know what Alpha Centauri is made up of? We know because everything in chemistry like copper, or zinc, or protein, or carbohydrate vibrates at a certain speed. It's a thing in chemistry, but it's a vibration in physics. Spectroscopy is basically reading the vibration of things, and you know, light is vibration so you basically just point this little … you flash a light at something, and then you read the light that bounces back off of it, like a radar gun or something. And if you have the right sensors, you could basically figure out what something's made up of. You can discern its spectral signature, what its component parts are. So, a little bit heady, a little bit science-y, but …

Brendan [00:13:33]: I think that's pretty straightforward for most of us to understand. So where are we at with prototypes let's say?

Dan [00:13:44]: Well, here it is October, and we took this project on in August of last year, 2016. As an organization we said it's time for this. It looks like the technology has gotten to a point where we can do this at a consumer price point, which was our biggest issue. Before we could do this it might cost $10,000 or $30,000 to have a tool and might weigh ten pounds. Looks like now we're down to something that's half a centimeter by a half a centimeter square. That's a square quarter inch. In a year or a year and a half the whole gizmo is going to be a quarter inch square.

Brendan [00:14:22]: Wow.

Dan [00:14:23]: And maybe cost twenty or thirty dollars to manufacture. I don't know what the numbers are, but with the advances in technology, what cost billions of dollars twenty years ago and cost tens of thousands of dollars a few years ago might cost a couple dozen dollars in a year or two. This past year we raised enough money to build a functioning prototype, or we've got a few prototypes. This tool is a couple inches by four inches or something. It's not a quarter inch square. It's a couple inches by four inches, and we'll be taking it to a lab to build calibrations in about ten days. So we're hoping to roll it out at our annual conference in November and launch our Real Food campaign. People can preorder the prototypes in the crowd funding campaign-type endeavor. In 2018 we're going to have at least the research prototypes out there for people to have access to. Probably 2019, maybe 2020 we'll have the extremely small handhelds for consumers. It might even be in the smartphones by then. But we're looking at a couple year time frame basically to be in the market viably doing this.

Brendan [00:15:53]: Wow, that's encouraging.

Dan [00:15:55]: Yeah, it's kind of exciting, I've been thinking about it for like eight years, so …

Brendan [00:15:59]: Finally catching up.

Dan [00:16:00]: Feels good to be getting somewhere! (laughing)

Brendan [00:16:03]: Are you at liberty to share how it's being funded and even who is funding it?

Dan [00:16:10]: Donations, yeah, we're a non-profit. Everything is in the commons. Nothing is for sale here. There's no stocks; there's no shares; there's no controlling interests. This is all being done open-source in the commons. We've gotten donations from, you know fifty, a hundred dollars, to ten thousand to twenty-five thousand dollars, nothing more than that at this point. So it's really a bootstrapped operation. But luckily, with where technology is at and with the allies, the sort of people who are working of common interest, we can really synergize and leverage already existing efforts quite well.

Brendan [00:16:54]: Sounds like maybe it's costing a little less than you initially anticipated.

Dan [00:16:59]: Well, I mean, a first generation prototype is not a consumer tool.

Brendan [00:17:05]: Sure, sure. What do you still need, and how are people going to be able to connect with the opportunity to support you?

Dan [00:17:15]: We're going to be launching this campaign in the end of November at our conference, and we're hoping to have a significant media, social media, presence about it at that point. We're offering first generation prototypes of the tool at this point for three hundred dollars. So it's a crowd funding campaign, basically. We're hoping to sell at least a couple thousand of those, which should bring us to the level of being able to get those out to the first generation of users within a year. There's all kinds of work we're doing, it's not just the tool, I mean if you want to go into the depths of what we're up to—what is quality? There's all kinds of claims about how this is high quality etc.. There's nutrient density. There's all these, there's these terms, people throw around. Local people say their food is higher quality. Permaculturalists say their food is higher quality. Organic people say their food is higher quality. What is quality? We actually don't have a definition of quality because it's a complicated question, and so a much more significant endeavor for us than building a tool is actually figuring out what quality is. And that requires thousands of crops to be run through expensive machinery and lots of data points to be put together and algorithms devised. There's a whole bunch of effort. Money is needed for that. And then, really, we actually want to be able to give farmers best practices recommendations. We don't just want to tell them after they harvest their food, "Look, it's pretty much junk". We want to be able to tell them at the beginning of the year, or during of the year, "Look, these are your limiting factors, and if you just did this one little thing, things would work much better." And so that requires a big open-source, multifactor, epidemiological style research project as well. There's a few pieces to this puzzle, and the handheld tool is—I call it "the hook". That's sort of the thing the people get excited about and say, "Oh my God, this is going to be amazing". But if we actually want to pull this thing off properly, there's some serious thoughtful, collaborative work that has to be done to really have it be not just hot air in marketing, but really serious. I mean, I can happily say we need millions of dollars, and we're going to do a hell of a lot with whatever we've got. [Laughs] Feel free to give us money if you like. We're not offering controlling interest in anything.

Brendan [00:19:51]: It sounds like you've thought it through to quite an extent, including the backend for communicating to growers what they can do to improve and stay competitive.

Dan [00:20:06]: Which would be to become more economically viable, to sequester carbon, to obviate the need for agrichemicals, to really positively affect the eco-system because a lot of farmers are out there … they know that the things they're putting on the ground are no good. It's not that they don't want to do the right thing. They just don't have access to the tools and the information. And so the more we can support people in doing the right thing, as opposed to giving them a hard time for doing the wrong thing, I think the more rapidly the transition can occur. It's really exciting the level of degenerative disease on the one side, and climatic cataclysm on the other side. I think people are starting to wake up to the fact that there's some serious problems here, and if it's as easy as just buy the food that tastes good, that will heal my children, I think a lot of people will jump on this bandwagon. I think we've got a serious shot here of really doing some pretty powerful good stuff.

Brendan [00:21:05]: Yeah, and in terms of let's say the resolution of the nutritional analysis, at least in the first generation, what are we looking at? And is the goal to get to where we'll see parts per million, or however it would be measured, of individual nutrients and even phytonutrients, and vitamins? Or what are we looking at?

Dan [00:21:27]: Yeah, I mean, we're going to be taking the prototypes to the lab in ten days, and I'll be able to tell you then what we can and what we can't see with what we've got right now. I mean we've got what we've got right now, which we've built for very small money, and we've got conversations with big multinational corporations that can build these little chips. It's an iterative process. First generation looks like we can definitely see the correlations. We can definitely say this is better; that's worse. Second and third generations will probably be able to say yes, parts per million. Parts per billion, probably not. You might have to spend a thousand dollars for a tool that can say parts per billion instead of fifty, or a hundred, or hundred and fifty parts per million. But the thing about biological systems, living systems, is there's these patterns, and you don't have to be able to tease out every single detail to see roughly where things stand. And even if it's only as simple as a red/yellow/green scale. We should easily be able to do that with where we're at right now. Depending on whether you're a researcher or a consumer, you probably don't care if it's twenty-six parts per million of antioxidants. That doesn't matter to you. It doesn't mean anything to you. So, depending on what the use case is, I think different … all the information is there. We're not trying to hide it. We're not trying to control it. The question is how much do you care about?

Brendan [00:23:03]: Yeah, and maybe there could be … well, I'll develop that thought a little further before I go to another thought. With minerals being so central to human health, obviously we … there's been a lot of research showing how connected mineral nutrition is to so many diseases, but in your interview with Dave Asprey, the "Bulletproof Executive", a little while back, you raised something really interesting that has my interest. It was that I guess when you were in India, you were pursuing your spiritual practice or development.

Dan [00:23:49]: I was a twenty-year-old on a quest. Exactly, up in the Himalayas.

Brendan [00:23:52]: Oh, it was that long ago. Okay, like five years ago. [laughs]

Dan [00:23:56]: Twenty years ago. Half my life ago. (laughs)

Brendan [00:24:01]: So, you've said something to the effect that you were finding that your body was challenged with holding the higher frequencies of consciousness, something like that. I wonder if you could say more about that.

Dan [00:24:14]: As part of what my personal agenda is in doing this whole project?

Brendan [00:24:19]: Or just relating it to minerals because what I heard was that you were saying somehow it was connected to your feeling that you didn't have a mineral sufficiency to handle that.

Dan [00:24:29]: Just because I felt it doesn't make it true either. (laughing)

Brendan [00:24:33]: Right. I just have an intuition that there's reality there. I've had the same kind of thought.

Dan [00:24:35]: I think there might be something here, I'm not sure if I can convey it properly, but yeah, earlier in my life got the esoteric bug. I was like, "Wait, there's a whole eastern half of reality. This Western culture isn't all there is". I'd been asking questions through my childhood, in high school, and in college and never felt like my questions are being answered to my satisfaction. So when I came across the wisdom of the East, I felt compelled to go and investigate, and yeah, ended up in the Himalayas and living in ashrams and meditating and being an ascetic, basically. I spent a couple of winters up there and by the end of that stint had applied enough of the practices to my own body to be able to activate, in the Sanskrit terms, the chakras and the nadis and all that kind of stuff. There's a whole subtle physiology. There's a whole science to it. It's really quite brilliant I think. But at any rate, I was experiencing things that were certainly not part of my Western rational experience. They were predicted by the texts I'd been reading, and I basically got to a state where I felt like there was so much energy running through my body, so much current, that I was going to fry my circuits, you know, you put a hundred amps through a twenty amp circuit, and you literally melt the wire. So I felt like that's what was going on. My body couldn't handle the intensity of that consciousness, that prana, whatever the word is you want to use.

And so, I was brought up on an organic farm in a homestead. My parents are back-to-the-landers, they've built a passive solar house with a wood stove and a root cellar, and we had a milk cow, and orchards, and had a CSA, and raised all of our meat and our vegetables, and ate whole grains. I mean I grew up eating really well, physiologically in pretty good shape, and my insight there up in the Himalayas was if my body can't handle consciousness, and I basically had the blessing of a really good nutritional foundation, then I shouldn't judge other people for not being able to tune into their higher nature. For me to move forward in my practice I need to get my body to a higher level of function, so it can handle all this intensity. And maybe if I want culture to improve, if I want people to be able to tune into their higher natures, something I can do is to help their bodies become more coherent. I studied a lot of physics and things in college, evolutionary biology and quantum physics and organic chemistry. I was actually accepted to university as a music major, so the language of music made sense to me, but as I understand it, every compound in your body, every DNA strand is vibrating. It's vibrating and basically putting out a note, like a guitar string that's been struck. Every hormone is vibrating. It's putting out a note. Every carbohydrate is vibrating. All of the things in chemistry are actually vibrations in physics. We all have a vibe. We're actually vibrating, and if your DNA is broken because it's missing certain minerals, then it's vibrating out of tune. I like to use the metaphor of an elementary school band concert. If you've been to an elementary school band concert, usually not all the trumpets are in tune (**Brendan:** "I was!"), and usually there's a couple clarinets that are not quite in tune (laughing), and there's this really grating sound. And it's totally sweet that they're all there sitting playing their instruments, but it really, it's like fingernails on a chalk board. It's called dissonance. And my thought is if our hormonal imbalances are stemming from the fact that we don't have the minerals necessary to build the hormones completely. If our degenerative diseases are stemming from the fact that we don't have the minerals present for our DNA to replicate properly, on some foundational level, these compounds that our bodies are build out of, are vibrating out of tune. And if you want to go into the quantum mechanics and talk about dark matter, and dark energy, I say, I mean, according to the scientists, 95% of reality is on some frequency range we can't find. Dark matter and dark energy are 95-96 plus percent of reality. It's called dark because none of our tools can find it. Microscopes can't find it. Telescopes can't find it. Radar guns can't find it. None of the tools of Western science can find 95% of reality.

My thought is, Eastern science which teaches us that we have multiple octaves of reality in our bodies, you know, our bodies are tools for perceiving reality, and in the same way that an elementary school band concert is often times a dissonant experience, an acapella choir may be a harmonic experience. Have you ever been to, listened to a four part harmony choir that's exquisitely in tune. There can be four notes that are being sung and a fifth note that is sounded. I's called the harmonic, or overtones. It's like the keyboard, the piano keyboard, you've got your low-low C, and then low C, and then C, and then high C, and then high-high C. There's different octaves, and basically when one octave is vibrating perfectly in tune, then all of a sudden the other octave notes are sounded. It's called harmonics. It's a well understood phenomenon. So, my thought is that if our bodies, our physical bodies, are vibrating in tune because we have all the nutrients we need for all of our biochemical compounds to be built properly, then it's much easier for us to tune into our higher natures. I would suggest that all of the, not all, but a lot of the dissonance that's going on in culture, where people are having a hard time holding a coherent thought, where there's this apparently disparate perspectives, and Congress, and the media, everything is sort of a jumbled mess, I would say because we have been eating food that doesn't have minerals in it for three generations we are vibrating out of tune, and our culture is symptomatic of that. And so, if we actually want to solve these things deeply, if we want to address this underlying dissonance that's occurring, getting the basic minerals into our food that are what our bodies are built out of, would be a holistic, systemic solution. That was maybe a bit of a longer answer than you were looking for.

Brendan [00:32:30]: I think it's profound. I think it's something humanity needs to look into seriously because ... as another implication of mineral sufficiency and even what Graeme Sait would call luxury levels of minerals, you know, because we can have sufficiency—sufficiency isn't the right word at all—because we can survive, even deficient, and sufficient we live better, but maybe there's a luxury level that maybe existed five thousand years ago, two thousand years ago, when the great seers that underpin all of the world's spiritual traditions, they were able to ground the tremendous spiritual energy. And we haven't seen ... I don't know if we've seen anybody like that in thousands of years, and maybe, maybe there's a correlation with our nutrition.

Dan [00:33:21]: With agriculture and yeah, what was being done, what Native Americans were doing here on this continent was a much more sophisticated version of agriculture than any of us is practicing. The level of vitality in the ecosystem, the level of food that was freely available everywhere. Go all the way back to Africa, however long ago you want to go. There's a really good book called *Left In The Dark* which talks about the synapses and the pathways, and basically, if you look way back in our evolutionary history, we were eating high levels of these secondary metabolites, these compounds, these flavor compounds, fruits in the trees and all that kind of stuff. And if you have a diet based on all these amazing riotous flavors and colors, you actually have the spectrum of nutrition that facilitates the left brain and the right brain functioning together, and when you have a diet based on grain, which is pretty rudimentary as far as secondary metabolites are concerned, then these synapses aren't firing. They say we're using 10% of our brain. It's because the pathways don't function without the circuitry. You need the enzymes there that come from the nutrients that come from the food stuffs, and so yeah. I like to tell the story of when I was in college and I took organic chemistry, and I mean people talk about taking organic chemistry ... I started off in music and ended up in history, so what the hell was I doing in organic chemistry? Anyway, my final grade was something like 34, and I got my report card, and it was a D, and I was like, "I definitely did not deserve a D," but everybody else did horribly also. And so the professor said, "The only time in my entire life that I graded on the curve" was when we were all failures. And I was given a passing grade even though I had abjectly failed the course. My understanding, if you talk to plant geneticists is that the functional yield, not nutritive yield, but actual just pounds per acre that we're receiving on crops in this country, is something like 5 to 15% of genetic potential. Our plants are so weak and so sick that the actual amount of food that's being produced is something like 5 to 15% of what's possible. That means 85 to 95% of the yield potential is being left on the table because the plants are so sick.

Brendan [00:36:19]: And this is with all the chemical fertilizers and GMOs...

Dan [00:36:22]: This is conventional corn ...

Brendan [00:36:24]: And all that supposed beneficial technology.

Dan [00:36:26]: The potential of our field corn is a thousand to twelve hundred bushels per acre. Average yield's about 150-160. You do the math. So yeah, what is sufficient? If everybody else is doing a horrible job, then normal is horrible as far as I'm concerned.

Brendan [00:36:47]: Well, I guess they're getting graded on the curve.

Dan [00:36:50]: If we're all really sick, and we're operating at a low level of vitality, that's considered to be normal. But what is sufficient? What are we looking for here? Are we happy with a rudimentary level of function, or are we striving for optimal function in ourselves, in our families, in our communities, in our culture? And what are the environmental conditions that must be present for us to operate at that higher level? I think these are the deeper questions, and it's really wonderful to have an interviewer who's teasing them out. It's great.

Brendan [00:37:21]: It's my pleasure.

Dan [00:37:22]: Thank you, yeah.

Brendan [00:37:24]: I like to dig, and digging in the dirt is the best place.

Dan [00:37:30]: It's great to be playing in the dirt very regularly if possible. It's good for you.

Brendan [00:37:35]: So I see this, the question of human nutrition as an opportunity to look at upgrading our specifications as self-actualizing beings, and if we look at it like a computer, what's the speed of our processor? What's our random access memory capacity?

Dan [00:38:04]: Exactly, yeah.

Brendan [00:38:05]: And our storage, and our robustness, durability and so forth.

Dan [00:38:14]: Yeah, you can use whatever metaphor you want, but that's a pretty good one. In all honesty we're operating at a functioning embarrassingly low level. There's this whole thing about doctors and health care, and you know, "Everybody needs health care, because everybody needs to go to the doctor." As I understand it, you only need to go to the doctor when you're sick, and there shouldn't be a reason to have to go to the doctor if you're not sick. So, this whole conversation about health care, and I'm not saying that people shouldn't be able to go to the doctor, because they should be able to go to the doctor, but if everybody has to go to the doctor all the time that means everybody's sick. That is the state of our culture, physiological dysfunctions, psychological dysfunctions, emotional, biochemical, hormonal. We are literally falling apart. The more we abuse the Earth, the more we should expect to fall apart ourselves. The correlation is direct. Only when the food we eat, that builds our bodies, was grown in a deep and profound manner, biologically, synergistically, only then should we expect ourselves to function well. To separate, "Okay, I'm just going to buy cheap food because I can afford to", well, you know, it depends on how you define "afford". I mean these things are all really actually kind of self-evident, and what's exciting to me is being someone who goes out and talks about them, and people are like "Yeah, that makes sense." And I'm like, "Yeah, it makes sense." It's all kind of obvious. It all kind of makes sense. So the question is, how do we work together, how do we collaborate to achieve this future we hope for. And I don't think we achieve it by trying to maximize profit out of each other. I don't think we achieve it by trying to hide information and control each other. I think we achieve it by collaborating. We get to the solution by behaving in the right manner, and that means we share; we're open; we're collaborative; we're not trying to control and profit off each other; we're trying to empower each other. Most of my work in my life has been as a farmer and working with farmers, so I can tell you that all that stuff about "Mother Earth" and sacred, and all that stuff, whatever language you want to use, the happier the land is, the more vital the ecosystem is, the healthier the plants are, the better your economic viability is, the fewer pests you have, the fewer diseases you have, the better your yields are. The more you're working in harmony with Nature, the more you understand how Nature works, and the more you can work with Nature, the more well it all works. So, it's really exciting. It can be philosophical; it can be metaphysical; but it's also extremely pragmatic and empirical. All of these things can overlay. It doesn't have to be one or the other. They're all really the same thing. They're different lenses for seeing the same reality.

Brendan [00:41:30]: I'm curious because you're a soil farmer, we're talking about revitalizing the planet with soil farming, but for people who are …

Dan [00:41:41]: As opposed to not soil farming??

Brendan [00:41:44]: Right, well here's where I'm going with this …

Dan [00:41:46]: Don't call it farming buddy. You're going to cross the line [laughs]

Brendan [00:41:50]: Yeah, good point there. So we've got cultivating soil, we also have I guess cultivating food via technology-based methods, you've got hydroponics, aquaponics, aeroponics …

Dan [00:42:04]: That's industrial agriculture. That is literally the industrial system, that's a factory system.

Brendan [00:42:13]: I totally agree. What's your take on the food quality? If we were to just look at it, just head on in terms of food quality, what do you take as the differences in food quality between soil- grown and hydroponics, and … Some people get really excited about growing stuff, and we can definitely grow things in cities and so forth, it's not going to do a lot for the planet …

Dan [00:42:42]: People do this, people have cultures in cities. Have you heard about this thing? People live in little boxes, and they go to work in little boxes. And they stare at screens. You call that human civilization?

Brendan [00:42:55]: I think we can change how cities manifest themselves, but on a food…

Dan [00:43:00]: I think we're animals and we belong in Nature.

Brendan [00:43:02]: I agree. Let's bring Nature back into cities, too. That's another conversation.

Dan [00:43:14]: Yeah, sure you can grow plants in boxes. You can grow people in boxes.

Brendan [00:43:19]: I'm just curious if there's a difference in the food quality. Have you seen a difference in the food quality coming out of aeroponics and …?

Dan [00:43:30]: What is quality? I mean if you want to actually have a serious conversation and not get me all worked up. It's a continuum, and there's plenty of people that are growing crops in "soil" in the ground, that are doing a really horrible job. It's not a sort of simple, binary, dichotomy kind of conversation. It really misses the broader point. There's organic farms in Florida where they till the living daylights out of the soil, and it's basically a sand dune, and they're basically doing hydroponics through drip tape, in a sand dune, and that's called soil-grown. And there's probably proper hydroponics in a box somewhere that's better than that stuff. So it's a big conversation. It's a big continuum. I say it's original research. We don't know the answers. And that's what's so exciting about what we're doing is we're trying to frame this whole conversation transparently and work it out collaboratively and openly and see what the answers are. But it's a really important question. What is quality, and what are the environmental conditions that correlate with quality. I think that will really help clarify this broader conversation about hydroponics. I've got plenty to say on that topic.

Brendan [00:44:57]: Well, let's talk about one last thing just to give people something to run with. How can people tell, right now, until your device is available, how can people assess the nutrient qualities of their food. There's the Brix meter, but that might be too cumbersome for people. There's taste. I'm just curious if you have thoughts on how people can identify … I know I can tell the taste differences.

Dan [00:45:24]: The most sophisticated nutrient monitoring device you're ever going to have is your tongue. We're never going to be, I mean, maybe, I doubt it, ever going to be able to build a tool that will be as good as your tongue. So in the same way people focus on the flavor of wine, or the flavor of chocolate, or the flavor of beer, or the flavor of coffee. It seems like the drugs people pay attention to, the flavor differentials, and they have, they've trained their palates to know the difference between a good beer and a bad beer, good coffee and bad coffee. Well, the best way to do it is with your tongue: "That's a good carrot, and that's not a good carrot". The refractometer which measures Brix is a really wonderful, simple, inexpensive tool that you can use to get an empirical number if you want to be operating that way. I think those are probably the two simplest, best things you can do right now.

Aroma. Certainly your nose is another sophisticated nutrient-monitoring device, you know, how do things smell. If you pick up a bunch of basil in the grocery store, and you rub the leaf, and you don't smell basil, it's probably got nothing of value in it. If you pick up a cantaloupe, and you can't smell cantaloupe, it probably doesn't have any value to you. If you pick up a tomato, and you can't smell tomato, it's probably no good. It's better than a Jolly Rancher, it's better than Doritos, but nutritionally it's basically devoid. So, yeah, it's a continuum, and what's unfortunate is that many people live in cities or city-type lifestyles. They don't grow their food. They work to earn money to buy food, and the food that's available is of really rudimentary caliber. And so, until we can implement a system to improve quality in the food supply systemically, the only real option is to get out there and try to meet farmers who are doing a good job or grow your own food. And that's not going to work for the general populace because that's just not plausible in the short term. So, I'm sorry, but you've got to wait for the tool. I mean we're going to be launching it at the end of November. You can buy a prototype. You can order your prototype in six weeks, so that's not too bad.

Brendan [00:47:53]: That's better than I think we expected just six months ago, and that's amazing.

Dan [00:48:58]: It's moving along real fast. It's really quite exciting, yeah.

Brendan [00:48:01]: And Dan congratulations, I really appreciate how selfless you've been in dedicating yourself to this project and open-sourcing it. It's just going to mean so much ultimately to humanity and the planet. I just believe that the moment this technology becomes widely available, it will be one of those epic watershed moments in human history.

Dan [00:48:32]: Well, there's some work involved. It's not just the tool. We've got to figure out what quality is, we need the open-source collaborative data platform for identifying best practices and the feedback loops so we can support the farmers in doing a good job. We've got to do the media work to get the word out there. We need to coalesce our social movement. We can expect that this is not going to be taken up by the *New York Times* and the USDA. We can expect that this is going to have to come from the grassroots. We've got a serious social movement organizing project to do, and there's not many of those that have been successful. Getting people on the same page to work together and not bicker, and not dissipate, is a heavy lift. So, if we can pull this thing off, it's going to be quite impressive, and I think we've all got skin in the game right now. And I think it's entirely plausible. I don't think it's going to be a cakewalk either. [laughing] There's some effort involved. But the more people that get it, the more people that want to help out, the more people that support it … if you want to figure out where else you can put your energy, whatever energy you've got, you know, time, money, relationships that can have such an effect, I don't see anything better to do with myself and anybody else who feels that way, I welcome you to come help out.

Brendan [00:50:06]: Yeah, it will definitely be a process and that's why everybody that learns about this tool should, and the whole bottom up movement to shift our food system, should put their weight into it. Anything else that you would want to transmit to people as a message to people that care?

Dan [00:50:24]: Transmit [laughs]

Brendan [00:50:26]: It's just the word that came out of my mouth.

Dan [00:50:29]: I think I've been doing some transmitting. It's a great conversation. I really appreciate it. I really enjoy, you know, the caliber of the conversation is often times limited by the caliber of the interlocutors, so when you've got some people who get it, you can have some really exciting conversations, and it's just fun to talk about this kind of stuff. So thank you for being on the level, it's great.

Brendan [00:50:57]: Thank you for your leadership and your contribution to all of us here in the Eat4Earth community today.

Dan [00:51:04]: Thank you very much.

Robert Van Risseghem
Minerals That Heal & How to Increase Food's Mineral Content 10X

Brendan [00:00:00]: Welcome to the Eat4Earth event. We're exploring how you can heal yourself, your loved ones, and the planet, with food. This is Brendan Moorehead, and I'm speaking with a man that has extraordinary nutritional information to share with us that I've never before encountered, and his name is Robert Risseghem. Robert has developed unique methods of manipulating metal ions, including the family called the noble metals that have amazing roles in the human body. His background began in industrial and oilfield waste water management and treatment, and his research on the noble metals and the refining techniques associated with them led him to wonder how ancient civilizations had the ability to recover vast amounts of gold and silver without chemistry or machinery. His research ultimately led him to a book called *Noble Metals in Biological Systems* and learning of the high levels of platinum being found in the outfalls of the US sewage treatment plants, which demonstrated that people are losing platinum from their bodies. After seven years of testing, he developed the Soil Solutions product line designed to address mineral deficiencies associated with the most common health conditions, and he also founded his company Naturally Noble, Incorporated. Robert, I am so eager to hear what you have to share with us. Thanks for being here.

Robert [00:01:20]: Thank you for having me.

Brendan [00:01:22]: When it comes to human nutrition, it seems like the phytonutrients like the curcumin and the spice turmeric tend to hog the headlines, but I have a sense that minerals have a more foundational importance to human health. What would you say about that, and how would you describe to me, an average consumer, how to think about minerals and their role in relation to other types of nutrients like vitamins, phytonutrients, essential fatty acids, amino acids, and so forth?

Robert [00:01:54]: Well, you know, when you speak of turmeric, when we look at turmeric from India, we see lower incidences of Alzheimer's and diseases associated with the brain. And turmeric, because it's out of India, it isn't just a plant; it's the soils. India has a high level of boron and yttrium in the soil, and because of that, it delivers through that plant the phytonutrients that it needs. I use a book, *Natural Healing*, and I'll give you the references and cite all the sources at the end of this here, but in that book it does the greatest job of explaining how the amino acids, the vitamins and the minerals all play a part in our nutrition. B6 is important for liver function, but it doesn't happen unless we have magnesium in it. So if you're just having the vitamins without the minerals, we're lacking the key ingredient for cell processing, for amino acid processing. Going back to the vitamins, there's only one vitamin that utilizes a mineral, and that is B12; it utilizes cobalt. All of the other minerals that we see in our foods, because they've become so depleted, we're lacking that ability to utilize even our vitamins and amino acids properly. When a plant can take up a mineral ... and the unique part about that plant-based mineral is the particle size. That particle size is the exact size that we need for uptake into our body to actually make amino acids, to make the proteins. That particle size is ten times to one hundred times the size of an atom. That's very, very small, but that's the building block size that we need. When we look at colloidal minerals, colloidal silver, or we look at mineral supplements, our bodies can't break down those large particles down to size that we can properly absorb, and for that reason plant-based minerals is the only choice that I can see that we need for good health.

Brendan [00:04:33]: So we've got to get those minerals back into the plants, and to do that, the minerals obviously have to be in the soil and available to the plants. You mentioned that the turmeric from India has yttrium and boron. Are you saying that perhaps soils in the United States are not as rich in those minerals, or it's just not being made bio-available because of maybe poor microbial activity in the soil? We're bombarding it with so many chemicals and so much plowing and so forth.

Robert [00:05:09]: Well, microbials just die off when we're using synthetic fertilizers. That's our biggest problem.

Brendan [00:05:28]: Let me just ask you quickly ... so yttrium, probably very few people have heard of that mineral. Is that one of the noble metals?

Robert [00:05:37]: No, yttrium is one of the ... it's almost a rare-earth metal, but it doesn't fall under the rare-earth category. According to Dr. Olree, in our diet we just do not have it in any abundance in the United States. I've seen it a little bit on a few samples on bindweed where the roots go down twenty, thirty feet. It's able to pick up some yttrium, but (in) on our top soil I'm not seeing any yttrium in any levels, at least in my testing to state that we have enough yttrium in our diet. What happens, according to Dr. Olree's work is yttrium will displace the aluminum, or aluminum is used in place of yttrium in our diet, and that's why it can affect so much in our brain function. Yttrium is also one that we age faster because we don't have it in our diet because our body has to metabolize additional steps to make the aluminum work. In Dr. Rydell's book, he talks about a soil study that was a report that had come out in 1941. This report actually was compiled from the 1910's, 1920's, and it talks about how we are losing all of our nutrients in our soil and all the health conditions that were going to be associated with it. Back in 1912 we didn't have tractors. Most farms were ... they might've had the tractors but no implements. We didn't have the chemistry to solve this problem, not until World War II that we had a chemical revolution. So what happened was people invested in pharmaceuticals. Now we have the capability to correct this problem. Now we have farm implements. We have chemistry that we can bring these trace minerals back into the soil and address the health conditions through the farm rather than through pharmaceutical methods.

Brendan [00:07:55]: You said 1910 there were folks that were already concerned about the mineral content in our food. Is that what you're saying?

Robert [00:08:02]: Yes.

Brendan [00:08:03]: Wow, so it's been going on for a while, and actually if you look at what has happened since 1910 to our soils and the mineral content of our food, it's scary. I'm curious, in terms of minerals, are there any particular illnesses that are worth talking about, perhaps like cancer where mineral deficiencies may play a role, and that restoring some of these rare minerals as well as others, might make a difference for preventing or maybe even treating cancer?

Robert [00:08:45]: A great source for this is the Dr. James Duke database, which is a .gov site. Dr. James Duke worked for the USDA for forty years, and in this time he had studied how plants play a role, their chemical phytonutrient effects that the plants actually manufacture. And it also talks about how there's 23 different minerals in chemical activities that are beneficial to our health. Everything from cancer to Parkinson's, to psychiatric problems. They're all addressed on that database. It's a database that I recommend anybody go to. If you just google Dr. James Duke database, you'll see it right off the bat. In that database he talks about selenium and the ability for selenium to have an effect on different types of tumors, different types of cancer. It even goes so far as to give a dose. If you have breast cancer it will tell you the recommended amount of selenium. If you have brain cancer it will do the same thing. But this is where the disconnect is. Why we can't use that for healing up until we develop these minerals in a consistency in our foods because if you were to take selenium … and we manufacture selenium cheaply by using yeast. If you take a yeast selenium, chances are that yeast is still going to grow in your stomach. I don't know this for a fact, but I've asked manufacturers at different expos on whether or not the stomach acid can kill the yeast, or the yeast keeps growing and gathers more selenium and strips it out of your body. Studies have been done around the world where they've looked at the highest incidences of cancer, and they found where the lowest incidence of AIDS and cancer has the highest bio-available selenium in the soil. One of those locations is Senegal, Africa, a tribal community which is no different than Kenya where AIDS runs rampant, but they have the lowest incidence by percentile of AIDS and cancer because the selenium provided to them through their diet, through an ancient sea bed that's found inland. Another area is Bolivia. Their highest export is selenium. They have a low incidence of cancer. Anything about selenium, and this is an important point, is a lot of people will look at the Dr. Duke's database and see the highest plant content of selenium is in Brazil nuts. And that Brazil nut, according to the Dr. Duke's database could be three parts per million, or 497. A study was done…

Brendan [00:12:01]: 497, what would that…

Robert [00:12:04]: Milligrams per liter, parts per million. But there was a study done on Brazil nuts, and pardon me for not having that in front of me.

Brendan [00:12:19]: Oh, that's fine. We're just talking.

Robert [00:12:26]: They had studied Brazil nuts grown in different regions, and surprisingly in Bolivia it was only eight micro-grams per Brazil nut. We're talking a different unit here. But if you looked at the east end of the Amazon forest, that was the highest level, and you're up around two hundred micro grams, or if you were on the west end it might be about a hundred sixty. I'll cite the source so people can actually see the number, because it's that important to know when you're buying a food with the phytonutrient or mineral content in there that you're trying to treat a cancer, you need to know the dose, and you need to know exactly what that plant is able to give you. That's what my work is all about is we can bring the consistencies of these minerals back into our diet so when somebody is trying to treat themselves naturally—which I believe most of our illnesses can be treated naturally, because the symptoms are caused by the deficiency … well, some of our symptoms now are caused by bad drugs and we get into the cycle that catches us—but without rattling on about selenium, that's just one of them. For esophageal cancer there's molybdenum. And we look at molybdenum as an esophageal cancer ... the studies were done in China, had the highest levels of esophageal cancer. But when we study and go backwards, what causes esophageal cancer? It's acid reflux. What causes acid reflux? It's poor liver function. It just happened that I stumbled on by buying some precious metals, ruthenium, for lung cancer, we were growing plants within it. It takes eighteen months from the time that we started the test until we realized the ruthenium that was sold to us had impurities of molybdenum in it. A gentleman with lung cancer was looking at the ruthenium value. He had liver cancer. He had stage four liver cancer. His bile counts were up in the high teens. Within two days his bile count started dropping down. Within two months his stage four liver cancer was a fully functioning liver. Now that isn't a full medical study, but we have medical results from that. We believe that molybdenum showed those values and changes, but it's yet to be proven. So I have to ... I hate putting testimonials out there thinking that this is the answer for all people.

Brendan [00:15:27]: Yeah, we can't make any claims here, but you're noticing some interesting patterns, and molybdenum is quite an interesting mineral. I'm using it a lot right now, because I learned that it's very important for sulfur metabolism, and I had symptoms that indicated I was not handling sulfur very well, especially from the vegetables that contain a lot of thiol groups, cruciferous vegetables, and so forth, and certain greens. I have been on a lot of molybdenum, and now I'm tolerating them better. It's extraordinary. So, is there anything else to say about molybdenum because I find this really interesting. In fact, I think from another conversation, you told me that molybdenum helps empower other minerals like chromium and vanadium, which of course help insulin regulate blood sugar and so forth. Am I recalling that correctly?

Robert [00:16:25]: Yes, that was a conversation we had. You know, the molybdenum has ... let's first look at how we lose molybdenum because that's a critical component to what we're talking about. Because if we just say, "Well, we need to bring this into the diet, we need to bring that into the diet" ... we need to protect what's already in our body, and how we lose molybdenum in high levels is oxidized sulfur. This is different than sulfur that comes in through the food, but oxidized sulfur has the ability to leach minerals out of our body. We will talk about sulfur maybe further down the road, but we'll switch out back to molybdenum. How we lose the highest amount of molybdenum is the sulfurs in our food preservatives are leaching them out of our bodies. We see this in cattle feedings that are fed distillers grains. They're sprayed with an oxidized sulfur to stop molding, so the farmers won't feed their cattle molds. But they just stop all enzyme growth because they sterilize it. When it goes into your liver, it will leach the molybdenum out of it, but it will stop enzyme growth, which are so important for metabolizing chromium and vanadium. So when it goes out into the blood stream, it can attract the sugars in the way that our bodies intend to do it. Molybdenum has a very unique ability for liver health, and the liver is where you're building all the enzymes. You're taking proteins up that are plant-based and animal-based, digesting them; they're going to the liver, and they're reconstructing into enzymes and protein that are going out to our body to benefit us. Without that, we have what we call the Leaky Gut Syndrome. We have an immune system breakdown because we have particles in our bodies that we couldn't process properly, which I believe the immune disorders are because of our poor liver function. It's so important that we take care of our liver; we take care of what we put into our stomachs. We shouldn't treat our stomachs any different than what we treat our gardens. You wouldn't put garbage in your garden. Don't put garbage in your gut, and that includes GMO foods. Until we test our GMO foods to make sure that ... they're designed to kill weeds in your garden, they're made to withstand weeds ... so what's saying that those genetically modified foods are not having an effect on the way we process those? Do they have a resistance to being broke down? There's so much that we need to look at and reevaluate in our food system to ensure that what we're doing to ourselves isn't damaging.

Brendan [00:19:47]: Yeah, I just learned that apparently each time a GMO organism goes through a modification in the lab, or however it's being done, there's a lot of different ways to modify the genes of a genetically modified organism, but that on average it introduces 5% novel proteins, in other words proteins that have never existed on the planet before, or borrowed from another organism. But I think what it was saying is novel proteins. It's certainly proteins that have never been in our diet, and that's what can certainly lead to new allergies because the body is like, "Okay, we haven't seen this before, what's going on? Err on the side of caution. Attack!" So, that's what it does, and many times it encounters proteins that don't match things that the body has encountered and has discovered are safe and even nutritional vs. human proteins that the body knows. "This is self. Don't attack. It's self". But yeah, these new proteins are a serious concern that we should be looking at.

Robert [00:20:56]: Well, even when we look at wheat, and we're seeing more and more, because we're seeing soil depletion we're seeing less of a protein value in our wheat. And for good quality breads we have to have a higher protein, which gluten is a protein. And so most of our breads right now … they're taking refined gluten and adding it to the milled flour. So you're only getting part of a whole food, but you're getting an added refined portion of another food. So you're not given everything that you need to properly break and manage that food within your biological system.

Brendan [00:21:37]: And gluten being a protein that humans don't digest very well, if at all, and needing microbial support if the right species are there. The microbes may be able to help with breaking it down in the gut. But you brought up another point, is that new proteins and GMOs, or engineered proteins and GMOs, may actually be hard for the body to digest. If we can't break them down then that makes them potentially more allergenic, and as you mentioned they're designed to either produce pesticides within them or to resist high applications so that we can go Roundup-happy in the garden or the farm to annihilate weeds, and then the soy is still growing. Typically we're not growing soy in our gardens, but anyhow … You mentioned that oxidized sulfur is leaching molybdenum from our bodies and that this oxidized sulfur is commonly in the preservatives that are added to food. Can you explain … give us some examples of this type of preservatives that may be common and how we can find out which foods they're in.

Robert [00:22:54]: Well, there's a number of companies that sell sulfur test strips to test the oxidized sulfur level in foods, and we see oxidized sulfurs since the petroleum revolution, it's a by-product from petroleum refining. So it's made its way into the market because they're looking for any of these by-products from petroleum refining to utilize in different ways. But oxidized sulfur, sodium metabisulfite, sodium thiosulfate, sulfur dioxide as a gas … they're all used to do a number of different things to our produce.

Brendan [00:23:39]: Oh, so they're added to fresh produce, or are they only in let's say jarred and canned and maybe pickled goods.

Robert [00:23:47]: Some pickled goods, you'll find it, you know, olives, you'll see the sodium metabisulfite sometimes on the labels.

Brendan [00:23:55]: Does it have to be listed, or is there like a threshold under which they don't have to list it.

Robert [00:24:01]: It all depends on how they use it. I've seen back in, I believe it was 94, the EPA gave approval to use it as a pesticide, and they don't have to declare it on the food. It's a real tough situation. Let me break it down, what I see, when it entered into our food chain, what it does to us. First of all, we talked about molybdenum and how it leaches out of the body. We talked earlier about platinum. The highest levels of marine sludge levels containing platinum is at the outfalls of US sewage treatment plants. The highest level of silver in a marine sludge is at the outfalls of US sewage treatment plants. Also gold. And these aren't just a little step up numbered. These are extreme numbers. If you look at thiosulfate, it was Eastman from Eastman Kodak back in the 1780s, I believe. He had a patent for leaching silver out of rock, using a thiosulfate. Within ten years after that, it's such an effective leach, we went off the silver standard.

Brendan [00:25:19]: Oh, because silver's value plummeted or...

Robert [00:25:21]: Yes.

Brendan [00:25:22]: It became too easy to obtain from rock ...

Robert [00:25:25]: Yeah, it was too easy to obtain. You weren't just finding a specific ore source and smelting it. Now you could actually leach it in a pure form. But when we look at ... besides the noble metals, and all of those noble metals, and I probably didn't talk about it when we talked about the cancer. Cis-platinum was developed in the 1970s, and it was very effective for testicle cancer and throat cancers, some tumors, but it was very promising. Back in the 70's they tried to put platinum back into foods and were unsuccessful because they took shortcuts. They went with a platinum salt that shut down the plants. We also have ruthenium. The only place that we find ruthenium in our body is in our lung tissue. So when we look at our chemotherapy drugs, they use that as a way to deliver these minerals back into the system. Reality is we're losing these minerals out of our bodies from these oxidized sulfurs which give us a higher risk of cancers. When we breathe in hydrogen sulfide gas—and you can get that from tooth decay and stuff, the halitosis—when that hydrogen sulfide makes contact with our lungs we end up converting that to a thiosulfate so it's going to leach these minerals out.

Brendan [00:26:52]: Oh my goodness. So you tooth decay, or a tooth abscess or something, could produce microbial activity in the mouth, hydrogen sulfide, then we inhale that gas in our lungs, and it gets converted to thiosulfate.

Robert [00:27:10]: It becomes an oxidized sulfur on the surface of the lungs, yes.

Brendan [00:27:14]: Oh my goodness. What about in the gut, because I've come to understand that if certain dysbiotic bacteria, unhealthy bacteria in our gut, if we have them, if we have an imbalance down there, may produce hydrogen sulfide, so the same thing could happen in our gut, and also leached metals down there as well, the precious ones that we want to keep?

Robert [00:27:42]: I don't know on the gut as much...

Brendan [00:27:45]: Maybe because there's not as much oxygen, whereas obviously in the lungs you're going to have oxidizing reactions.

Robert [00:27:51]: Usually when it passes into the intestine, that's where it converts to the, we have the gasses so to speak, and some of them could be a hydrogen sulfide from the different microbes in our stomach. Potatoes when they rot or are compost, the only gas that a potato puts out is a hydrogen sulfide gas, it doesn't put out the CO_2s or other things that we see, and there were some really neat studies on different things breaking down. But potatoes is one that when it breaks down in the compost pile, it will just manufacture hydrogen sulfide as a gas. But let's go back to the oxidized sulfur in our food preservatives. Besides the noble metals that we talked about that it leaches, I believe it leaches out the non-noble metals: lithium is a big one, silver which is a noble metal, and molybdenum, copper. All of those, are in addition to the noble metals, and all of those have an important role in the, you know, where the deficiencies will show as symptoms of one of those minerals. I think what we're seeing in society today with the amount of lithium being leached out of our bodies, we're seeing more mental illness then we've ever seen before. And we shouldn't look at mental illnesses any different than another symptom like diabetes or anything else. They're all a symptom of our diet. They're all a symptom or mineral depletion from our soils. Plants can't make these minerals. They have to come out of the soils. If we're looking at replenishing these, we have to put them back in the soils, but we also have to take out these oxidized sulfurs as food preservatives. To me there's only three preservatives: there's canning; there's freezing; or there's dehydrating. Any other chemical preservatives, I call those embalming chemicals.

Brendan [00:30:10]: What about fermentation, isn't that a valid preserving method?

Robert [00:30:14]: I believe it is, yeah...

Brendan [00:30:17]: Lacto-fermentation.

Robert [00:30:18]: Yeah, I don't know enough about it to speak to it, but yes, it is. It is a way of preserving foods.

Brendan [00:30:28]: They keep breaking … I guess you can't stop the fermentation process, but ultimately it's not going to keep things in a static state as long as the other ones that you mentioned. So those are more true preservatives, safe, natural, or at least semi-natural in the case of canning methods.

Robert [00:30:49]: Well, wine is a great example of how this has creeped in to our diet with these oxidized sulfurs. You never see a bottle of wine at a high value, or when's the last time you opened up a wine and it converted to vinegar? The reason being is, the processing of wine … all of these vineyards now are using, or most of them … I could find a few vineyards with sulfite-free wines...

Brendan [00:31:23]: My understanding is that organic wines do not include sulfite. They can't add it.

Robert [00:31:31]: You're absolutely right, if it's listed organic. But most of us aren't buying organic wines so...

Brendan [00:31:38]: Should be.

Robert [00:31:39]: You should be, yeah.

Brendan [00:31:42]: Or biodynamic.

Robert [00:31:45]: But that many …

Brendan [00:31:50]: Are you hearing that sound?

Robert [00:31:52]: I am.

Brendan [00:31:53]: That's odd, that shouldn't be coming through. Go ahead.

Robert [00:31:58]: When we look at wines and how they changed their processing to use sodium metabisulfite, what that gives the winery is the ability to bottle on demand. They don't have to have massive amounts of warehouses of bottles. They can keep them in plastic vats where they won't mold. They don't have to bottle on a specific day, the way we used to manufacture wines. But bringing that into our diet, what it does to the liver. You know we used to say wine is good for us, and it should be, so we're doing more damage to our liver by stripping out the molybdenum by the oxidized sulfurs than we have any value in the wine at all.

Brendan [00:32:44]: And speaking of vinegar, as you mentioned that a minute ago, my understanding is that a lot of vinegars, not all, but have sometimes added sulfites or maybe a metabisulfite, I think. I think it's more common in the sort of distilled vinegar variety. Nobody should quote me on this at all, but it's something I looked into briefly, and I'm not sure I sorted it out.

Robert [00:33:13]: There's an easy test if you don't want to buy the test strips because they are expensive. If you have some old X-ray film, even if it's developed X-ray film, putting that into any of your food products or solutions, if you want to test your wine, if you leave it sit there, it will dissolve it right down to, you know, take either the negative or the silver chloride out from it, depending upon if it's developed or not. I've used that quite a bit before I found these readily available sulfur tests.

Brendan [00:33:51]: This is really important. I mean it seems like a very non-trivial matter to look at how oxidized sulfur preservatives are leaching key trace minerals from our bodies, which are so important in so many processes, including the immune system and so forth. I have actually started looking for products where I can be more confident that the vinegar that might preserve the olives, let's say, that I buy, does not contain sulfite. So I've been asking, when I buy something on Amazon, I'm asking "Hey, does this contain any added sulfites?" And I believe that there are some sulfites even in wines where it's not added, I'm not sure. So there may be some amounts in there. Do you know anything about that?

Robert [00:34:49]: I know that they naturally produce sulfites. It's when they're adding it to it to prevent a mold or to prevent something to go sour. Just keep in mind what that's doing. It has an anti-microbial effect on both your gut and also affects your enzymes and your liver. That's a number one thing that you have to protect. The chemistry, I'm probably not the right person to speak to the chemistry because my background is once again water treatment, making soils., and a lot of testing. I've done a lot of testing. But when we look at whether or not, or who should test these effects, of these preservatives, I go back to the Pure Food Act back between World War I and World War II. The government developed the Pure Food Act for one reason. At World War II we had so many young men that couldn't pass a military physical, and they were looking and researching what was the cause of the poor health for these draftees in World War II. What they found was ... the only two things that we did ... we pasteurized milk and we refined flour. And both of those had an adverse effect on our health. The Pure Food Act studied that. They decided we need to add vitamin D to our milk, and then we also needed to enrich our flours after milling.

Brendan [00:36:37]: And the vitamin D that they are adding to milk is it in the vitamin D2 or vitamin D3 form typically?

Robert [00:36:44]: Now pretty much it's all Vitamin D3.

Brendan [00:36:48]: So they upgraded that.

Robert [00:36:49]: Yeah, you know, now we're smarter [laughs], hopefully what we're doing is smarter. But yeah, I'm one that runs with a vitamin D deficiency constantly, and I couldn't get the levels up with shots, with doing everything until I took dairy completely out of my diet for a while. Now it's back in my diet, but my vitamin D levels are up to a level that I can manage. What I'm saying is, what our government did with The Pure Food Act, we should be requiring (of) any preservative. Any time we process food, if it's not a 100% whole food, if it's not preserved through whole food canning, whole food dehydrating, or whole food freezing, then if it has a process, it's a chemical reaction, it's a chemical compound that we're putting into our foods, we need to see the effects that it has on our diet. And The Pure Food Act, to fire that back up is the right way to go.

Brendan [00:38:01]: You say fire that back up. Forgive my ignorance, but is it ... did it go out of effect?

Robert [00:38:08]: No, it's still there, but I mean to expand...

Brendan [00:38:11]: Just being neglected or not fully utilized to its full potential.

Robert [00:38:15]: Yeah, just enable them to have, you know, don't say you solved a problem, and then you're just a government agency. We have additional problems that we need to address.

Brendan [00:38:29]: Definitely. In terms of getting minerals back into our soils, in our previous conversation you mentioned something about cobalt that was quite extraordinary. Can you get into that for a moment?

Robert [00:38:45]: Yeah, I'd love to. Cobalt is an amazing mineral. When we look at cobalt and what it does when we manufacture B12 in our gut ... our cobalt, it bonds to carbon and nitrogen in our gut, and when it bonds to that carbon and nitrogen in our stomach, it allows us to absorb many other additional minerals. Dr. Olree's book discusses that. I think there's 11 different minerals, all critical minerals for absorption. But when we see it in the soil, we see the same effect. We the rhizome area of the plant manufacturing the equivalent of the B12. A carbon and nitrogen triple bond is a cyanide. When we have carbon and nitrogen with a cobalt, it's a stable cyanide. It's not a triple bond. It's not reactive to that same way, but it has the ability to leach these minerals, make them bioavailable for the plants and...

Brendan [00:39:53]: So this is good leaching, in other words not taking it from our body but taking it from inert places and making it bio-available.

Robert [00:40:00]: Up until I had seen what cobalt did in the soil in the rhizome region of the plant, I thought we're doomed because our soil depletion is at such extreme right now that we will never be able to get our minerals back from our soil. When we see this leaching in the rhizome area, what we've seen on our control samples vs. our treated soils, we see 22 different minerals with a tenfold increase. That means there minerals had ten times the delivering power, these wonderful minerals, and we'd never seen them in our controls before. I had used that same control gardens soil for probably the last five years. And we grew kale in it, we grew radishes in it. We've seen increases of ten, twenty, thirty-fold across the board on kale. Kale by itself is a super food. You add cobalt to the soil, you have a magnificent super food. And it didn't take a lot of cobalt. I believe when we look at cobalt and the ability to put it back in the soil ... I only use pure refined minerals, and I do conversions to get them in there, but we can buy reagent grade minerals with that purity on the world market to make it a cheap enough soil amendment to solve a lot of problems. Cobalt is one that's water soluble. It's easily leached out of the soil, just like boron is.

Brendan [00:41:41]: You mentioned that ... oh boron, that's another one I wanted to talk about. Say that again. What was the last thing that you said that included boron?

Robert [00:41:53]: Well, boron is one that's easily depleted out of the soil. It's a very water-soluble mineral, but it's one of the easiest ones to put back into our soil. We have the ability to take boron, and ... Can you hear that?

Brendan [00:42:12]: Yeah, it's not too loud. Don't worry about that.

Robert [00:42:16]: Alright, I'll start over on boron. We can take boron and easily put it back into our soils. Reagent grade Mule Team Borax is an excellent source of boron, very water soluble. When we look at boron, and going back to turmeric, what we first started on, turmeric I believe has four different compounds that it manufactures using the boron metal ion, or element. These are so critical for brain function, it's so critical for maintaining the magnesium level in our body, so we're not excreting our magnesium. And also if you're having problems with vitamin D3, boron is a building block for the calcium to bond on to and to bring all of this to a natural state, There's almost a triangle level, everything has to be perfect. If you're out of balance you'll leach these minerals, but if you're there you'll maintain them and utilize them properly.

Brendan [00:43:24]: Yeah, you mentioned the term the "rhizome" part of the plant, which is part of the roots, and you mentioned cobalt operating in that realm, the rhizosphere, making other minerals available to the roots. I recall from the course I took from Graeme Sait at Nutri-Tech Solutions in Australia, his course called Nutrition Farming, and he said that one of the things he learned through the fathers of biological farming, was that cobalt is like mother's milk for the soil bacteria that fix nitrogen and do other things down there. So that's another fascinating thing about cobalt as far as making either directly or indirectly various minerals available in the soil. Also in biological farming, they refer to calcium as the "trucker of all minerals" and "boron as the steering wheel", and I don't know if we fully deconstructed that in the course. I'm just curious—I have my sort of intuitive understanding of what that means or maybe I'm just forgetting some of it was covered in the course—but I'm curious if you have any comments about that as far as trucker and steering wheel as functions that may be mirrored in the human body as well as the soil and plant interactions.

Robert [00:44:55]: Well, you know, when you're using those metaphors, one of the things that I've seen with calcium … you know, we look at organic wheat … the problem with organic wheat is thistle growth and bindweed. And what we found in some of our test gardens … the ones where we had a higher level of calcium, calcium was actually toxic to those minerals [probably meant to say "weeds" not "minerals"]. You know, here we are using glyphosate to kill these, and if you're an organic wheat farmer, and you have bindweed all through there, your harvests are going to be diminished. Eventually you can't sustain that farm without taking that field out of circulation, spraying on glyphosate, and then going back into your organic certification for the next three years. So when we look at calcium and its beneficial effect, it also has a toxic effect to some of the weeds. And so when you look at the balance between the calcium and then also the cobalt, the cobalt is …

Brendan [00:46:22]: Is that going to deep down the rabbit hole?

Robert [00:46:24]: It is a rabbit hole.

Brendan [00:46:27]: We could skip it for this conversation.

Robert [00:46:30]: Let's go ahead because I wasn't really prepared for it but …

Brendan [00:46:34]: Well, I know you have some great information prepared that we'll make available and maybe those charts as well, showing the effect of cobalt. Let me ask you this, how could somebody that's let's say a home gardener or a farmer, how could they make minerals more bio-available in their soils to their plants and ultimately to their bodies? What are some of the things they could do?

Robert [00:47:02]: The best thing to do for home gardeners, first know where you're starting. When we look at what is bio-available in our soil, that's the starting point. The soil test won't tell you bioavailability. It will tell you when you take a cup of dirt, dissolve it in acid, what those minerals are made up of. It doesn't mean they're bioavailable. So what I recommend, Activation Labs up in Canada, and I'll have a link to that site. We'll make it available for viewers of this video. Activation Labs have the ability to do a green leaf tissue test, or an ash leaf test. I recommend the green leaf tissue test. Just go to your garden, even if it's in the dormant stage, or if it's spring of the year and it's time to gather the weeds, just pull those weeds in, all of them, regardless what type of plant they are. Dehydrate them in a dehydrator, or put them in a brown paper sack to allow them to naturally dry. Once they're dry, mill them. Take about two tablespoons maybe, not exceeding a quarter cup. Put it in a plastic bag, and submit it to the lab up in Canada. If you have a thousand-square-foot garden, do two or three samples. If you have an acre, do ten samples. Keep them separate. If you're using a variety of weeds, weeds take up different minerals. It gives you a good snapshot of what's bioavailable to start out with.

Brendan [00:48:40]: Interesting.

Robert [00:48:42]: And this is the scary part. You know, for years we've had a lot of gasoline. If you're within a 100 yards of the road, check for lead. It's important. If you're in a mining area which has a high mineralized area, you might want to check for mercury. You will know all of these things from that test. And we've got to quit eating in the blind. Our biggest problem with our food supply right now it's, it's a liability. Our food supply isn't an asset. It's a liability because we don't know what's in it. If we take the time and actually test our foods properly, we can turn that liability into an asset. We can get rid of the fields that are delivering poor nutrition or we can amend them, or remediate them. But we truly, truly have to take … you know, I wouldn't get into a car without checking the oil. When you're eating foods, check the nutrient content to know that it's going to sustain you to the next meal. There's no reason in the world now, with the ability to lab test, to not ensure we're getting the daily recommended amount of minerals.

Brendan [00:50:04]: Yeah. Is there anything else that let's say the average consumer that's not a gardener or a farmer can do as far as keeping certain things out of their diet and making sure they get what they need in their diet. Of course, we all probably should be gardening, we should be using your products to get some really amazing things happening in our soils. But short of that, any other closing thoughts for what the average consumer can implement in their life right now.

Robert [00:50:39]: Well, you know, buying organic is good. I think until we...

Brendan [00:50:44]: And I'll throw in "and biodynamic".

Robert [00:50:46]: And biodynamic, yes.

Brendan [00:50:47]: Although I don't know how to find it in my own area actually. Not too common to be found in the marketplace.

Robert [00:50:52]: Well, you know, the Rodale Institute and the Patagonian group, when we were at the Regenerative Earth conference, they were talking about a new certification on regenerative earth. In our comment period, I put in that we need to look at the nutrition and the human health. We no longer should be eating in the blind, we should know the mercury, lead, and cadmium levels in our food.

Brendan [00:51:17]: Absolutely.

Robert [00:51:19]: I think because we have … pardon the pun of draining the swamp … but we need to take politics out of our food supply and out of the FDA. We need to put men with credentials and credibility in those positions, and they should never become politicized. It should never be how much money it takes to get an additive past the FDA. We need regardless what political affiliation we're with, we need to all stand together as consumers to demand a better quality food. We can't even trust our nutritional panels on our food. They're all from a database. Nobody's testing it. I have eleven different food products that I have labels on and I sell as a 100% foods. When I try to find a lab to test the sugar content, the fiber content, none of them would accept a sample. They would generate it for me at a price of a fee from that nutritional panel.

Brendan [00:52:27]: Right, which is based on some other product, tested at some other time, probably decades ago when there was more mineral in the soil.

Robert [00:52:40]: And it's accepted by our FDA or our USDA rather. Our USDA and FDA are kicking a can down the road. Eventually we have to open up and see the nutritional value of our food and be able to ensure that we're not running with deficiencies in our body anymore. To address to the average consumer, I'd say grow a garden, know exactly what you're eating. And we're not eating for the masses. Know exactly what you're deficient in. Interview the rest of your family. Find out what symptoms they have. Look at the Dr. James Duke database and see what mineral deficiencies may be causing those symptoms. Adding them to your food, your garden. I have a diabetic garden, our soil amendment. You know, we don't have to eat off from that 24 hours a day. One radish grown out of that garden according to the last set of tests that we did, a three-quarter-inch radish will give you the daily recommended amount of chromium, 170% of the daily recommended amount of chromium. It'll give you 280% of molybdenum, it'll give you all the vanadium you need for diabetes. That's within a quarter-inch radish.

Brendan [00:54:00]: That's amazing! That's like, yeah, this is the best tasting supplement you can use is grow some of your own food.

Robert [00:54:13]: To grow or to achieve that same amount of chromium in our control garden, unamended garden, it would take 57 and a half radishes.

Brendan [00:54:24]: Wow.

Robert [00:54:25]: So when we look at our diet and we try, you know, I'm pre-diabetic. Most people with diabetic issues have weight problems because their brain is saying you need more minerals to process the minerals that you have or the toxins that you have, but reality is we can feed people on less, we can bring the nutrient level back into our foods. Looking at that selenium report, when you see that, if you buy Brazil nuts in the highest-level region, on the east side of the Amazon forest, you'll see that it has 27 times the value of selenium that you find in Bolivia. So identifying … it would be a lot easier for each food producer to actually have their foods tested and sold by their nutrient content. If you have a higher value of chromium or selenium, market it. Get your value out of what you're delivering to that market. That way the consumer out in the market will be able to know exactly if they're meeting the daily recommended amounts. What I see out of our gardens is, once our data base is large enough, we'll be able to go to a phone app. If you're harvesting tomatoes and onions and are making a salsa out of the diabetic formula, and you know exactly how much you're growing out of it, because their soils are so consistent their plants are consistent. Our diet and the nutrient value will give you consistency, so you can use that in integrative medicine setting, or you can use that for your own personal garden. And you wouldn't have to do all the testing if you had the exact same soil or nutrient content. And that's what we try to provide.

Brendan [00:56:22]: This is really the future of food as medicine. This is amazing, and it's going to tie in very nicely I believe with the device that the Bionutrient Food Association is developing. And I've got a great conversation in this event with Dan Kittredge about that. Robert, thank you so much. This is groundbreaking stuff, your contribution to humanity is profound in bringing this to light and bringing out practical applications and products that we can use and buy. So I just want to thank you for that, and thank you so much for being with us here in the Eat4Earth community.

Robert [00:57:11]: I thank you for what you're doing and putting the summit together, and I appreciate the opportunity to share what I can bring to the table. Thank you.

Jeffrey M. Smith Interview
Newly Discovered Ways GMOs Can Harm You

Brendan [00:00]: Welcome to Eat4Earth. We're exploring how you can heal your body and the Earth with food. This is your host, Brendan Moorehead, and we're speaking with Jeffrey Smith of the Institute for Responsible Technology. He's the pioneering consumer advocate that has done so much to reveal the risks of genetically modified food organisms to the world. Jeffrey, it is wonderful to have you here. You are an important part of this event.

Jeffrey [00:22]: Thank you Brendan.

Brendan [00:24]: I am wondering if you can start off with letting us know how you got into this, where you came from, your background, and how this became the focus of your life for over 20 years.

Jeffrey [00:39]: Well, I went to a lecture by a scientist in 1996, and he explained the details of genetic engineering because he was a genetic engineer. But he was also aghast at the fact that companies like Monsanto claimed that it was safe, safe enough, to put GMOs in the food supply, or even release them outdoors. Because he was aware that the number one result of the process of genetic engineering was surprise side effects, and that once you put it in the food, you affect everyone who eats, but also when you put it outdoors it cross pollinates and becomes part of the gene pool, and we have no technology to reverse that self-propagating genetic pollution. We just let that species carry that gene pool until it is extinct. So, the only thing that lasts longer than gene pollution is extinction.

So, I realized that this was an A+ level priority that the biotech industry was essentially replacing Nature. And I found out later that they intended to replace all commercial seeds with GMOs, and now they want to go after insects, livestock, and grass. Basically, everything that has DNA. But at the time that I realized this is an A+ priority, and the scientist can talk science, but he wasn't necessarily conveying it in a way that would do anything, that would convince anyone, that would have a strategy.

Because I have a background in strategic communications and education and marketing, I realized that this needs to be handled carefully, and we need to make sure that this information gets out to the right people. We need a plan. And so, it wasn't like an activist looking for something to work on. I was just a chronic do-gooder doing, you know, working on things, and then this came up. And I went, "Oh, this is A+ priority. I'll kick in a little time." And "a little time" resulted in … I worked at a GMO-detection laboratory for two years, and they paid me to become more of an expert. And then I wrote a book, *Seeds of Deception*, and that became the world's best-selling book on GMOs since that time. That sent me around the world, and now 45 countries in 22 years, 1,000 lectures, and 1,000 interviews later, we're winning. But it wasn't that way in the beginning.

Brendan [02:50]: Gotcha. You know, in this event, we're exploring both how our agriculture systems are affecting our bodies and the planet at large and really discovering that it may be the number one priority of humanity, number one focus of generations alive today to transform our food system. And GMOs are such a massive cog in that machine that is eating us alive, eating our planet alive. So this topic is very foundational. And it goes deeper than I think a lot of us realize. Before we plumb the depths, I am wondering if you can give us a foundation in understanding the various ways that genetic engineering occurs, because I think that helps us understand what the implications and consequences are.

Jeffrey [03:43]: The traditional form of breeding is sexual reproduction. You can do selective breeding where you select a plant that is tall and another plant that resists disease, in the hopes that some of those offspring will get the genes from both parents to have tall, resistant results. With genetic engineering, they'll take one or more genes, or genetic material, from one plant and artificially force it into the DNA of another. I'm talking about plants, but it can actually be animals, it can be insects, it can be anything with DNA. In fact, they cross the species barrier. They will put bacteria and viral genes into plants, or plant genes into humans. That's the transgenic; that's where you cross the species barrier, or even the kingdom barrier, from one to the other. Most of the GMOs on the market are transgenic.

Then there is what we can call "gene-editing", where you go in and you manipulate the order of the genes. You knock out a few genes here and there. The biotech industry is claiming (and that is just another one of their lies) that it is not genetic engineering. Of course, it is genetic engineering. And they say that it is predictable and safe, which is what they said about GMOs. That wasn't true then, and it certainly is not true now. And they are trying to overcome even having to tell the government or the public that they are putting it into our food supply and into Nature, which is very dangerous.

There are things called "RNA interference", where you insert things that will then re-code or re-control the gene expression. There are things called "synthetic biology" where you use transgenic technology. You put a gene into yeast or bacteria, for example, and then that becomes a factory. And that also has side effects. So, in the 1980's, a company called Shoyodenko in Japan did that to a bacterium to produce L-tryptophan, which is an amino acid which can be sold to reduce stress, and insomnia, etc. They genetically engineered the bacteria to produce some components that they were normally having to add by hand, so they wanted to do it more economically. They ended up creating contaminants that killed about 100 Americans and caused 5,000-10,000 to fall sick. That was almost certainly the process of genetic engineering that caused those contaminants. So, these are some of the ways that they are genetic engineering now, and basically, it's not sex; it's not sexual reproduction. It's an artificial technique done in the laboratory, prone to side effects, massive collateral damage, increase of allergens, toxins, carcinogens, anti-nutrients, and other surprises.

Brendan [06:23]: So, in other words, if it's not sex, don't do it! [laughter]

Jeffrey [06:26]: I'm glad you said it not me, but yeah, that sounds good. [laughter]

Brendan [06:30]: So, gene-editing would be like what they are calling CRISPR.

Jeffrey [06:31]: CRISPR is an example of gene editing that is cheap. You know, I did an article in Huffington Post last year where they … when you do a CRISPR you knock out … you have some scissors and you send those scissors in to look for a particular sequence and then it cuts. And then, when it recombines, sometimes there is a deletion there, or an alteration there. But you are targeting one particular location, but that same sequence is all up and down the genome. So, you are going to end up cutting in different places. And so what they do as part of their "risk analysis" is they look at a computer program and say, "Hmmm, where are those scissors going to cut? Well, we think it is going to cut here and here. Can we live with that? This is what we do know about that sequence. It doesn't look like it's in a gene, or it looks like it's in a gene that's not so important, so we'll let it go, and we'll call it safe and precise."

So, most of them just look at this computer-generated model. Well, this group did a CRISPR cas edit on mice, and they actually sequenced the genome after they did this and found, "Oh my God, most of the stuff we were looking at was not predicted by the computer model." In fact, there were 1600 mutations that were completely missed, the point mutations, any one of which can be deadly and cause disease or whatever. And so, the actual looking at the genome instead of doing it by assumption, showed that this thing has massive collateral damage. And then, there were two other research studies done in 2017. Same thing. They found different ways that they totally wouldn't have predicted. And still there are people out there saying, "CRISPR is so precise that it is better than sex. It's better than … it shouldn't be called a GMO." And that is basically what the Trump administration is going along with, saying, "We don't need to … just look the other way, there's nothing here." And that's very dangerous.

Brendan [08:31]: Yeah, it sounds like it. You know, you mentioned the RNAi, RNA interference. I heard about that a couple of years ago from Jonathan Lundgren. He was at the USDA. I know, I believe you have interviewed him.

Jeffrey [08:45]: I have.

Brendan [08:46]: And that is when I heard about it, and he was actually being harassed about what he was revealing in various ways about different things, including that. So, I am wondering if you could just give us a quick explanation how that works so we understand what the implications might be.

Jeffrey [09:01]: Okay, so, there's a lot of arrogance in the field of biotechnology that seems to linger and take new expressions. Originally, it was, "Well, we know what genes are. And we figure, it's one gene is one protein, and anything that is not a gene is called 'junk DNA'. So, 98% of the DNA, we don't see how useful it is, so we'll assume it's junk." Well, they got everything wrong in that equation. It wasn't one gene producing one protein. It wasn't "junk". And they figured RNA, "Well it goes from DNA to RNA to proteins, that's how things get created. RNA is just a waystation, and it just goes in one direction." They got that wrong as well. The RNA can regulate gene expression. The double strand is double-stranded RNA, it's in a helix, and then it produces a single-stranded RNA, but that can also go around and then regulate other places in the DNA, creating more RNA, etc. There is a big circle. It's very complicated. It's not rocket science; it's much more complicated. So, it turns out that they discovered that there is a little strand called 'double-stranded RNA' which rolls back on itself. And it is like the hunt-and-destroy method. It goes along the DNA, and it finds something it matches with, and it will latch on to it and it will silence that gene. So, it is primarily a gene-silencing technique. It can silence a gene that regulates many other genes. It can change dramatic numbers of other genes. Now, they fed some mice some double-stranded RNA and it re-programmed a gene in their liver. And this was actually a revelation a few years ago. First of all, they said, "Oh, RNA is destroyed during digestion." Well, it's not; it actually got into the blood stream, got to the liver, and it re-programmed the expression of the liver in a mouse. So, it means that actually, it turns out, we know now, that food is not just vitamins and minerals and phytochemicals; it's also RNA. It can program the gene expression. So when you eat a piece of broccoli, or you eat a piece of cauliflower, they actually can affect which genes are expressed and how much of it because of this constant communication inter-species, and also inside of us. With the double-stranded RNA technology, they used it on apples so that they silenced the gene that normally 'browns' the apple. You can slice the apple, and it stays looking white or yellow for the life of the apple until it dries out. And they have a similar one with potatoes. Now, what do they do? They put in double-stranded R. So people call it 'the botox apple' because it lies about its age. [laughter] It can have terrible nutrition at that point, but it's not brown! So they use it in pre-sliced apples sold in supermarkets. Not all of them, but some of them. So, Jonathan Lundgren realized, "Wait a minute, there is a lot of evidence that double-stranded RNA, if we consume it, it can re-program our genetic expression." There is one article that I write about, a Huffington Post article, another one I wrote, showing that these honeybees were given one single meal of double-stranded RNA in larva stage, and over the next few weeks about 10% of their genes, over 1400 genes, changed their levels of expression, because of that one single meal.

And so Monsanto says, "There's nothing here. Look the other way. RNA is destroyed during digestion. It doesn't have any impact, and we can use it safely in these things." They have an insecticidal corn that they have it in. Intrexon has the Okanogan Fruit Company. This is really a dangerous thing because it is actually in the market now. And the concept is that if you eat the apple, or if you have the potato, it will match up, theoretically, with our DNA, two billion base pairs long, and this little double-stranded RNA is like 22 nucleotides long. It just has to match somewhere, and the chances of it matching somewhere … you know, in terms of is there a match that exists? It's 100%. Many, many ways up and down the DNA. If it happens to match, and then it happens to silence it, we are playing Russian roulette with our own genome. And so, I strongly recommend if you know that you're looking at the Arctic apple or the Innate potato, don't eat it! Don't let friends eat double-stranded RNA from genetic engineering!

And Jonathan raised this point and said, "We don't have a technology to do risk assessment at the USDA. We cannot evaluate it." I met him at a conference on biological diversity in Mexico, a UN conference, and I was at a side event, and he was giving his story there about how he recommended doing an analysis of the genome of all the different species that might largely come into contact with the double-stranded RNA to see if there is a match. It was sort of like he was soft-pedalling it. What was so obvious from his discussion was, "No! You cannot put this in the environment! There is no way! At our infant understanding of what is going on in the DNA, to put in something that might silence something almost at random!"

And now we know that it might silence something that is not an exact match, but silence things that are similar. It is a complete disaster. He wrote an article as a USDA staff member. People from the EPA wrote an article saying pretty much the same thing, that we don't have a technology for risk assessment. And the USDA went ahead and approved the Artic apple and the Innate potato, in spite of their own scientists raising these points, knowing they didn't have a proper risk assessment situation in place, and putting us all at risk. Not just us, but also all of the target and non-target insects. Insects, birds, whatever eat these things, fungus, everything is at risk, because now you have regulatory elements going around doing their thing, and chopping things away, silencing things at random, being pumped out in large volumes in these apple orchards and potato fields and who knows where else. And Monsanto even wants to create sprays using RNA interference, so they are spraying pesticides so that they silence the crop. And their thinking is crazy. It is like, "We can spray it on a crop. It will get absorbed into the crop and change the gene expression, but it shouldn't have any effect on the gene expression of humans who eat the crop, or get the spray sprayed on them.

Brendan [15:48]: Well, hey, they never got that wrong in the past, right?

Jeffrey [15:54]: No, not at all! [laughter]

Brendan [15:56]: One of the things I remember about Jonathan Lundgren's talk, where I met him, is he mentioned that for every pest species of insect, there are 1700 beneficials and predatory, and, of course, that is just a general, not a precise figure, but that was probably a conservative estimate. There is literally at least 1700 times as many beneficials and predatory insects, predatory on pest species. So this idea that we've got to focus on the pest species is ludicrous because all we have to do is create agricultural systems where we make homes for the predatory and beneficial insects and the pest species barely have a shot to even show up.

Jeffrey [16:45]: Case in point. I mean, the BT. The main reason they genetically engineer crops is to create those crops that are herbicide-tolerant, most popularly, Roundup-ready. Roundup-ready crops, produced by Monsanto, can be sprayed with Monsanto's Roundup herbicide and not die. If you don't have Roundup-ready crops and you spray the herbicide over the top of the field, everything dies. Here, it is very easy to weed; you just spray the crop, the entire field, with Roundup, and all of the weeds (biological diversity) between the rows, die. So, that's the main reason they created genetic engineering.

The secondary reason is BT toxin. It is a natural soil bacterium that produces a toxin that breaks open little holes in the walls of the guts of insects to kill them. They take the gene from the soil bacterium, make millions of copies, shoot it with a gene gun into a plate of cells, clone those cells into plants. Now every plant that is from that process has a gene-sized spray bottle that creates the BT toxin. The BT toxin is selected to target the corn root worm or the European corn borer or the cotton weevil. And so what happens is, it may kill until they develop resistance, which they're doing. In India, for example, it is killing the bole weevil or the cotton weevil, and now there are all these other pests that are coming in because they have taken over the niche of the one that was killed. And now people are spraying many, many times what they would normally spray. So, they're not actually saving anything, they're spraying, they're exposing themselves to the toxic chemicals, and the BT toxin is dangerous. And we can talk about that too. You don't want to eat BT corn, for example. You do not want to eat BT corn because there are a lot of reasons for that. Yes, when you look at the system of Nature, it is so complex. And here, they come in, you know, looking with half an eye at one little thing and messing up everything else. Same thing with the soil. The soil is so diverse. What happens in an ecosystem after a Roundup-ready crop, it is just disaster. Or BT, it is a disaster.

Brendan [19:04]: That's actually one of my questions for you in regard to the soil. One of the big focuses in this event is we've got to rebuild soil. It's the foundation of the nutrition in our food. It is the foundation of our health, and it's, we're discovering, the only way we are going to realistically have a chance at stopping and even reversing climate change and keeping our oceans from perishing.

Jeffrey [19:30]: Yes. Let me explain what happens to the soil under the wrath of Roundup. Most people don't know about what I'm about to say. It is very interesting how Roundup kills plants. So what I'm going to do is do it in the terms of a puzzle. If you spray Roundup, or glyphosate, its active ingredient, a glyphosate-based herbicide, onto a plant in sterile soil, you will stunt the growth of the plant, but you won't kill it. Same plant in field soil, you spray the plant, it will kill it. Now, that's the puzzle. Why is that the case? Here's the answer. Plot spoiler! I'm telling you right now. So, if you want to think about it, turn it off, think about it, turn it back on. [laughter]

What happens is, Roundup's active ingredient, glyphosate, was originally patented as a descaler to clean boilers and pipes. And the reason why it cleaned boilers and pipes is because it was a chelator, patented as a chelator. A chelator grabs onto, in this case, minerals, all the metal minerals, scaling it off of the walls of the pipes. That's calcium, zinc, selenium, cobalt, magnesium, manganese, basically, the minerals that we know and love. And when you spray a plant, then it grabs all the minerals, making them unavailable. Very few minerals get into the plant, and even fewer travel through the plant, and some of those minerals are bound up anyway, so they can't be used. Minerals turn out to be the center point of many reactions in the physiology of the plants and humans and animals. If you don't have a certain mineral, an entire metabolic pathway just hangs around unemployed until it gets it. So, you basically have disabled a lot of the functions of the plant. In this case, you have disabled the ability of the plant to defend itself against toxins. Now, that's one thing that it does.

Glyphosate is also patented as an antibiotic; it kills bacteria. But it doesn't kill all bacteria uniformly. It kills the beneficial bacteria very easily, but not the nasty stuff. And that's both the case in the soil and inside our own microbiome. In the soil, it will kill the bacteria that do two things. One, they take the minerals from the soil and change their form so that they can be used by the plant. They're gone. Now fewer minerals are available in plant-assimilable form. So now, you have two reasons why the plant is devoid of minerals: the bacteria are not handing it off, and whatever is handed off can be bound by the glyphosate molecule. The bacteria also have the role of keeping in check, meaning lowering the population of, the soil-borne pathogens, particularly the fungus. When you kill those off, which glyphosate does, the soil-borne pathogens are having a party. They eat the glyphosate for breakfast. It actually literally grows certain fungal pathogens.

This was determined by a USDA scientist, who then got, you know, suppressed and kicked out, so to speak, because that is what happens when you come up with a danger to Monsanto's products and you work for the USDA. Because the USDA and Monsanto are marching hand-in-foot, or lockstep, or however it works. Anyway. [laughter] So what happens is, the reason why the sterile soil doesn't kill it is because, okay, now you've weakened the plant, but there are no pathogens to kill the plant. In the field soil, the pathogens go crazy, the plant has an immunosuppressing—it doesn't have an immune system, but it has a defense system— that's all suppressed, and now it kills the plant.

What's happening is there are dozens of soil-borne pathogens that are on the rise throughout the United States because of the vast acreage that is being sprayed with Roundup and glyphosate-based herbicides. There are things like Goss's Wilt that in a small location in the Midwest for corn. It's all over the place because it is fed by glyphosate. The same thing with Sudden Death Syndrome for soy. Same thing with so many other things. At the same time, it kills the beneficials, and it compactifies the soil so the soil doesn't get enough water. So, if you were in the Midwest after a rain, and you have two cornfields, one with Roundup-ready corn and the other just plain natural corn, the Roundup ready corn has puddles on it. The other one—it is absorbed into the thing, and so it gets washed off. And so you end up with a disastrous lower biological diversity.

Then you have the BT toxin, which remains in the soil because it gets expressed from the roots. It binds with clay. You have a pickup of some of the microorganisms of the soil, of the DNA of some of these concoctions, and you have a completely altered ecosystem. You wash that BT toxin into a river; it kills the Caddis fly, or it causes a reduction in their viability, that creates an environmental disaster in that environmental economy, and you end up with a situation where you are killing below and above. And then the glyphosate gets washed into water, and so, it ends up getting evaporated. It is now in the air, and it's in the rain, and it's in the water, and it is also in our animals that are eating Roundup-ready crops. It's in our bodies. It depresses our minerals, and that is just a little bit of what glyphosate does for us. We can get a little more into that in a minute. If you are looking at the environmental impact, I haven't even mentioned that BT toxin is designed to kill one insect, but it will kill or maim other insects that eat the corn, or eat the insects that have eaten the corn. So, you have ladybugs, lacewings, and other things that you want, and they are being destroyed.

And then you have glyphosate's effect on honeybees. It can starve the honeybees for a number of reasons. It can misalign their navigation system, so they can't get back to the hive. It damages the Lactobacillus. It easily kills Lactobacillus, which is what happens in their gut. The Lactobacillus is used to digest, so they could starve, even though there is plenty of food around. So, it is a complete disaster, and it works along with the neonicotinoids to cause Colony Collapse Disorder, according to many people. There is one study that just gave regular environmentally relevant levels of glyphosate around bees, and there was a suppression of the bee population by about 30%, I forget the exact number. But it's like a smoking gun. And an article was just released last week. More smoking gun that the bees are being damaged.

And then the Roundup is sprayed on the cornfields. The cornfields have the milkweed normally there. The milkweed gets wiped out. The milkweed is where the larvae from the Monarch butterflies go, so now the Monarch butterfly population is being decimated because of the biodiversity. So, it is a very complex situation. They have just a couple of poisons they put in there with 300 million pounds a year, which is a huge amount. It is now in the rain, the water, the air, on the fields, in the soil, and it is decimating our natural civilization.

Brendan [26:46]: In other words, it is no longer enough to just think about, "Well, I'm going to buy organic, and I am going to take care of my own", and this kind of thing. Because this stuff is raining down on everything. There is now glyphosate in the rain that is landing on organic food and getting into our organic food chain. And of course, how is organic agriculture going to survive if honeybees are dying? Obviously, honeybees are not confined to one particular field. They are moved all around the country. They are getting exposed via many routes to whatever they are getting exposed to.

Jeffrey [27:15]: Right.

Brendan [27:16]: I mean, we are literally cutting off our lifeline to the planet. And, you know, you mentioned soil organisms. I heard something recently, and I don't know if I am interpreting it correctly … it was just in passing as I was monitoring out of one ear an interview. And it sounded to me that they were saying there is some kind of soil organism, at least I think it was some kind of soil organism, that is apparently perhaps behind the rising infertility crisis—young people in this country can't conceive as long as they are eating GMOs. They go off GMOs; they reduce their exposure to glyphosate, and whatever else is getting into their food from that part of the food chain, and they are being able to conceive. But apparently there was some evidence that there might be an organism associated with it, and it was some strange combination; it was sort of like a fungal organism, sort of like a virus, sort of like a bacterium, or something. I wonder if I am describing anything that is happening?

Jeffrey [28:18]: Yes. There is a huge problem with fertility, in humans and in animals, livestock for example, dairy cows. I'm putting out a film with Amy Hart called *Secret Ingredients,* and it is about how families and individuals heal from serious conditions when they switch to organic food. We have kids with autism who are no longer autistic and people with cancer who are recovered. Serious stuff. The doctors are explaining that this is typical among a percentage of their patients and that this can happen just with a change in the food, and the scientists explain why.

We visit one chiropractic clinic where they put their infertile couples on a normal organic diet as part of their treatment, and they have had a 100% success rate in having infertile couples have children. And it is nearly 100 couples now. No failures.

Now, what is it about a GMO, or Roundup, that might be affecting fertility? If you look at the animal feeding studies, mice that were fed GM soy had damage to their sperm cells and damage to their testicles. The female rats that were fed GM soy had altered hormonal balance and changes in the uterus and ovaries. There was a rat study that found that more than 50% of the offspring of the rats who were from mothers who were fed GM soy died within 3 weeks, compared to only 10% when the rats ate non-GM soy. And there are other studies that show changes in testicles as well. And there is demonstration that Roundup can affect placental cells, can change aromatase, which is important in the estrogen/testosterone balance, and that it can cause changes in the sexual development of certain animals when exposed. Also, it is linked to a lot of birth defects and miscarriages. In fact, a study just came out showing that when there is more glyphosate in the urine of pregnant women, they tend to have shorter pregnancies. So, there is a very high correlation there, but the mechanism is not clear. But that is also new information. There are more miscarriages in areas where farm workers and farmers are being exposed to glyphosate and other toxic chemicals, as well as cancer, too.

Cancer is another piece of the glyphosate puzzle. What Don Huber, who is a professor emeritus from Purdue University, found is another reason that might be affecting fertility. He wasn't sure what it was. It was some kind of very small organism that he thinks is more like a prion-type protein. Prions are implicated in the Mad Cow Disease and other issues. When they sprayed glyphosate, or fed the Roundup-ready crops, there was a lot of these prion-like organisms, or prion-like proteins. They replicate, an interesting combination. When they were able to isolate it, it did kill the egg inside the chicken. And then they were able to isolate it afterwards. So, they did go through the causal steps to show that this thing does cause problems. And when they fed organic and non-GMO feed, it was in lower numbers. And, all of a sudden, all the fertility problems on the farm or ranch were reversed. Because some of these places had terrible fertility; the animals weren't getting pregnant or weren't holding pregnancies. There is a lot of concern that this prion-like protein, which may be in high quantities, especially where Roundup is sprayed, may be promoted like in the same way that it promotes fungal growth. We don't know, but that is one of the reasons. Now, glyphosate also binds with minerals like manganese, and manganese affects sperm motility. There are so many reasons why. It could be this particular prion-like substance. It could be the chelation. It could be the hormones. It could be an aspect of genetic engineering because the process of genetic engineering itself causes problems, not just the two toxins we have talked about, the Roundup and the BT toxin.

Brendan [33:02]: Right. We've got all these novel, allergenic proteins. They seem to be things that are punching holes in the gut and contributing to systemic inflammation, and the whole cascade of cancer, heart disease, Alzheimer's, dementia, you name it, autoimmunity, that can come from there. It sounds so complex, and it is. I am wondering, what would be the most important thing for any of us to understand about this whole constellation of problems, so that we can just get really clear on, "Okay, I draw the line. I don't cross the line and support this system." Because I sometime hear people, even in interviews, where people are advocating that people … or they are basically saying that, "Yeah, GMOs are a problem." Yet, they will bring up the cost issue. I can't imagine that paying a little bit more, or even twice as much for organic, is a problem compared … which it generally isn't. Sometimes I pay less for organic, which is shocking …

Jeffrey [34:06]: I know.

Brendan [34:07]: … and encouraging and exciting. But, what would be the most important thing for people to really get, so that there is no doubt in their mind that they do not want to support this system, no matter what the cost? They will find a way, even if it feels like a pinch, or it just seems like it. Because, really, it is just a conceptual thing. "Oh, it costs a little bit more per pound in this situation." But it is costing far less. and it is delivering so much more. Also, as far as in the context of, "Look, I want to know how to communicate this, and I don't want to overwhelm somebody, how can I tell somebody: 'This is important for you to pay attention to. I care about you. You are complaining about your skin right now. Tell me what you are eating. Okay, here is something you should think about.'"

Jeffrey [34:51]: So, we have many websites that are Institute for Responsible Technology, and one is NonGMOSImproveHealth.com (this website may or may not be working). And on there you will see two links right in front of you. On the right is a deep, 21-page peer-reviewed article that I wrote, and on the left is the article summary. Do yourself a favor; just look at the summary. And there is also an interview I have available there with Michelle Perro, a pediatrician. Now, the article is about a survey we did where 3,256 people who had switched to non-GMO and largely organic foods reported getting better, and in many cases, completely recovering from 28 different conditions. The number one improvement was in digestion, with 85% reporting an improvement. And of those, for 80% it was either a significant improvement, a condition that was nearly gone, or completely gone. So, we are talking about dramatic change. And then, increased energy. And then, reduced weight, for those who were overweight. And then, brain fog. And then there were types of pain, anxiety, and depression, and allergies, and gluten sensitivity, and autoimmune disease, and on down to autism and Parkinson's and diabetes, all sorts of things. But, essentially, we're talking about most of the major diseases that we all know about, that we all know someone who has one. For some of these people, the change in diet was so dramatic and so clear-cut, there's no mistaking it.

And in the film, *Secret Ingredients*, we interview some doctors who say many of these patients, they get completely better or dramatically improved on a good diet. And then they "cheat". They either slip completely or they take, in some cases, just a single meal. And those conditions start coming back! And this helps them recognize just how sensitive they are to eating GMOs and Roundup. It's unmistakable. I know some people who in a single meal, they'll hit the fan, and with other people it's a longer process.

And I originally did not believe when people told me they could tell the difference between eating GMOs and non-GMOs until I had been speaking to doctors for many years. They were prescribing non-GMO diets, and then each of them had more patients converting to non-GMO than all the rats and mice put together in all the GMO research studies. I talked to one woman. She said "5,000 of my patients, non-GMO, they all get better." And I was like, "What?" Then I went to the clinic, and I interviewed a lot of those patients and, sure enough, within 3 days some of them had this thing and that thing, and whatnot. And it was shocking! And then, at the same time, I started interviewing the farmers who switched their livestock to non-GMO, and they were reporting the same problems getting better. And then I talked to veterinarians who deal with pets and pet owners, and the pets were getting better from the same problems. And then, I looked more closely at the problems that we we're seeing in the animal feeding studies, and there they were! You know, those problems, or their precursors. And then, if you look at those types of diseases, and you see their incidence in the United States on graphs, and you chart the increase use of GMOs, or the increased use of Roundup on those GMOs, they fit hand-in-glove! They fit like. In some cases, the correlation is astounding!

Now correlation alone is never what you are going to build an argument on. It's just not good, proper science to say that if they happen together, that one causes the other. But when you have all of that other information, both the peer-reviewed, and also the anecdotal, and then when you look at the modes of action of what is it that Roundup does, what is it that BT toxin does, what actual changes occur from the process of genetic engineering. We can go into that if you want.

We mentioned a little bit about Roundup, but there is a lot more. If we look at those, we could predict these changes. I asked Dr. Seralini, who has done more research on GMOs and Roundup than any other scientist. I said, "If you just look at what happens in laboratories, what would you predict would happen?" And he said, "Well, yeah, you would have the problems with the organs, you'd have problems with the hormones, you'd have problems with the digestion, That would come first." And he was basically describing the results that the doctors are now seeing because there are now thousands prescribing non-GMO diets.

And go to www.nongmosimprovehealth.com and listen to the interview with me and Michelle Perro, who prescribed non-GMO diets and sees the changes and sees it even when that is the only change that her family members make. She may be treating one member of the family who has autism, giving that kid many, many things, but then the rest of the family is just switched to organic to accommodate her prescription, and now the father's kidneys get better, and the daughter's ADD gets better, and the mother's respiratory situation gets better. And everyone is losing weight. And they go, "Oh my God, this is the panacea!"

Now, coming to the dollar figure, the dollar figure and the access, because people are in food deserts. They can get into one of these online buying clubs. But irrespective of access, the money itself … I first of all recommend switching to organic ingredients, rather than the processed foods, because that will be cheaper and healthier. But I talked to one family, a family of six, and they had a $18,000 average health bill each year. When they switched to organic, the next year it was $9,000, and the next year it was $3,000. And they said, "We're spending a lot less than what we are saving."

You'll see in the film *Secret Ingredients* about families. The kids just don't get sick anymore, and they don't go to the doctor. So, there is a savings there. But there is also a savings in terms of the quality of life in terms of increased energy, reduced depression, reduced anxiety. So, my bottom line is: "Change your diet and take notes." Write down your symptoms. Write down your energy level. Write down what you eat. Do it every day. Try it for a month, and see if you are one of the sensitive ones. Usually, if you have a digestive system, you are. Some people say they are not sensitive, but I say most people will notice a difference. And then let us know at www.responsibletechnology.org. Tell us your story, either sending us an email or going to our Facebook page.

Brendan [41:22]: So, this would be a place for me to send people if I am talking to someone. Maybe I will print up a little business card that says www.nongmosimprovehealth.com.

Jeffrey [41:30]: Well, typically, we have a lot of doors into our world. We have www.responsibletechnology.org, that's the 'mother ship'. You can sign up for our newsletter to see our regular reportings. We have www.petsandGMOs.com if you have pets. They are also affected. We're coming out with a short film about veterinarians and pet owners saying what happens when the dogs and cats get on organic food. It's remarkable. It's predictable, and it's remarkable. We have https://responsibletechnology.org/nongmoshoppingguide.pdf to help people make the transition by knowing if they can't buy organic, which is the number one recommendation, at least get non-GMO and here is what you can look for. So those are some of the ways into my world, and it depends on what your world looks like.

Brendan [42:20]: I think it might, as you were starting to say, it might be worth mentioning some of the other effects of glyphosate briefly. For example, since many of us here are very health-oriented, we know how important it is to detoxify, and yet glyphosate interferes with our detoxification pathways. And then, we have also got the endocrine disruption, which is very counterintuitive when you look at the U-curve. I wonder if you could explain those two. Also, for those of us who really want to get involved with this movement, how do we communicate to others? One of the other things would be the birth defects. I mean, it is a horrifying thing. I think that birth defects are a very emotional implication of all this, and we should understand that that is happening.

Jeffrey [43:06]: So, I am going to do this in a colorful way. Imagine you have set up an experiment where you have a certain amount of chemical, maybe it's glyphosate, maybe it's whatever, and it is dripping in at a higher concentration, then lower concentration, then a lower concentration. And it's killing cells or it's killing animals, or it's killing insects. And every time it gets dropped in, some die, and then a lesser amount goes in and fewer die, and then few die, and it takes them a little longer for them to die, and it gets lower, and lower, lower, lower. At a certain point, you go, "Okay, we're safe. At this point it is safe, it's not having an effect." And then the scientists leave the room, but the drips keeps happening. And it gets lower and lower and lower, and as the drips get really low, all of a sudden, the reaction gets higher. And it's not necessarily the same reaction. It's a different physiologic reaction that starts to go haywire, and as you get lower and lower, parts per million, parts per billion, in some cases, parts per trillion, the amount of its impact goes up. But the scientists are outside the door. They are missing it. And what they are missing is what's called "the low dose effect", which occurs a lot with endocrine disrupters. As you say, it's counterintuitive. Why, you may ask, why? Ask …

Brenden [44:32]: Why?

Jeffrey [44:33]: Thank you.

Brendan [44:34]: Tell us, Jeffrey, why is this happening? It's so counterintuitive. [laughter]

Jeffrey [44:38]: I don't know. But there is a mechanism where when you get to the smaller number of molecules in the system of this, it has an effect, typically on the hormone system. You can have low-dose toxic effects. But on the endocrine system, it has a higher impact the less there is. It's called the U-curve because you have a high impact at low levels, and as you increase the levels and the amount goes down, it bottoms out. Now the scientists enter the room, and they are seeing it go up this way. So, you look at the EPA, the Environmental Protection Agency—they left the room. Scientists have known about this endocrine disruption at low doses for 12-15 years. It is well-documented. It is standard science. But the EPA says, "We just believe that the dose makes the poison, and we just ask Monsanto and other chemical companies to only do their own research (the EPA doesn't do the research) on higher doses. So, we are going to ignore any potential endocrine-disrupting effects. And on the basis of these higher doses, we are going to come up with an Acceptable Daily Intake, the ADI."

Now, they will also make the Acceptable Daily Intake for an average male adult, so forget about the women and forget about the babies, and forget about the thin people, but that's the ADI. It turns out that the ADI for that reason, and many others, is so much higher than it should be. First of all, they only require the active ingredient to be tested. The glyphosate is what Monsanto declares the active ingredient to be, but the so-called "inert" adjuvants can be up to 10,000 times more toxic, and they also have endocrine-disrupting effects and also toxic effects. So, when you put them all together, Roundup can be up to 125 times more toxic than glyphosate alone. The EPA says, "Don't tell us that. We don't want to know that. You just test glyphosate, and we'll believe you." And then, it doesn't look at anything in terms of the low dose. We know that there was a study that was done in Europe where rats developed non-alcoholic fatty liver disease because of the glyphosate put in their water. And the amount of glyphosate was so low that by contrast on a per-weight/per-day basis, which is like this Acceptable Daily Intake concept, what the EPA allows in the water supply in the United States is 437,000 times more than what the rats were drinking to give them non-alcoholic fatty liver disease.

Brendan [47:21]: Wow!

Jeffrey [47:22]: That is a precursor to cancer and also other types of liver diseases in 25% of the US population struggling with some level of the non-alcoholic fatty liver disease. So, it's an absolute disaster. Now, you asked what are other things glyphosate can do. Glyphosate is a mitochondrial toxin. The mitochondria are now being implicated for so many more diseases than originally thought. Otto Warburg, who won a Nobel Prize, believed that cancer was a mitochondrial disease. But mitochondria, they create the energy for the cell. But many, many diseases are now linked to mitochondrial dysfunction, and now you have that. Glyphosate, when put it into a test tube with human cells, causes the cells to break apart. The tight junctions get wider. That's a form of leaky gut. Leaky gut is linked to cancer, heart disease, Alzheimer's, Parkinson's, autism, allergies, autoimmune disease, inflammation. So that's another mode of action. I mentioned that it damages the microbiome because it is an antibiotic. So, the microbiome is involved in detoxification, in digestion, in protecting against the gut wall being porous. It's involved in the immune system. And it can be damaged when you have an antibiotic, like glyphosate. When you have gut dysbiosis, where it kills the beneficials and allows the negative and nasty stuff to grow, that's linked to another whole list of diseases, and also causes leaky gut. The glyphosate is also a probable human carcinogen, a Class 2A carcinogen, according to the World Health Organization, for humans. For animals, it is a definite cancer-causer. Why is it definite for animals and only probable for humans? Because they don't have enough studies on humans. Because it is not ethical to give a bunch of humans glyphosate to see if they are going to get cancer. So they did that with enough animals, and so they say, "It causes cancer in mammals, and it probably causes cancer in humans." So, there is another reason to avoid glyphosate. We mentioned that it is a chelator. We mentioned that it is an endocrine disrupter, not necessarily at low levels. We have to get some more data, but it is certainly so at medium levels. We mentioned that it can break apart the gut walls.

There are other things, but I think at this point, you get the sense that it is not the beneficial weed-killer that it is safe to put into your garage and spray on your lawn. When you end up spraying it on your lawn, and your dog rolls in it, it gets absorbed through the skin, and it gets absorbed through the paws, and it sticks around.

The half-life, where the amount of time it takes to break down into just half its quantity, can be months or years or decades, depending on …

Brendan [50:09]: In your lawn is what you are saying. So, it is there. Every time your dog is going out 3 times a day or whatever to relieve him or herself, they are getting a dose of glyphosate through their paws.

Jeffrey [50:21]: And that is why one laboratory, who was doing analysis of human urine for glyphosate, did a couple of dogs and found that it was 50-fold! We tested the pet food and found that the pet food had higher levels of glyphosate than human food, but not 50 times! But the urine was up to 50 times higher, and so that means they are getting a double dosage from the food and from the environment.

Brendan [50:47]: No wonder we have … yeah, I mean, that could be the cause of the pets' cancer epidemic.

Jeffrey [50:50]: One out of two dogs! It's the mammal that has more cancer than any other mammal on the planet, and it gets glyphosate on the lawns and in the food, and the increase has happened, coincidentally, or not, after glyphosate has been pedal-to-the metal and been used so much more on our food and in our environment.

Brendan [51:10]: Yeah. I encourage people to check out Parents for a Safer Environment. They teach people how to get their communities onto integrated pest management instead of …

Jeffrey [51:24]: And I have another website for you.

Brendan [51:25]: Ah, you've got one. Perfect. We've got to get our communities to stop spraying all these chemicals in our children's playgrounds and so forth.

Jeffrey [51:33]: Yeah, www.rounduprisks.com. Rounduprisks.com is a website that we created where we have a training program based on three successful community models that got glyphosate kicked out of city use, or county use, and in some cases homeowners' associations, in schools and stuff. And it turns out that in some cases it's a single phone call followed by an email. So, we give you the phone call and the email to send. It should be easy, for some. For some.

Brendan [52:02]: You and I met briefly at the Soil Not Oil Conference, which, as you know, is a part of the grassroots movement for regenerative agriculture. And I see potential alliances between the GMO movement and the movement for a fully regenerative agriculture system, which would be not just an absence of GMO and not just organic, but actually making sure that the agriculture is actively building soil. Because, even organic, as you know, not all organic is created equal. Some are tilling too much because they are not using chemicals. So now they use tillage, plowing excessively to control weeds, instead of using biodiversity and feeding the soil with compost teas and so forth to really build that diversity under the ground too. Which suppresses all the diseases, and then you have healthy plants getting all the minerals they need, and that suppresses the pest populations. And, of course, if you have corridors of hedgerows of plants that the predatory and beneficial insects hang out in, you just are not going to have a problem, like Elizabeth Kaiser showed in her presentation here in this event.

I am just wondering what you think. Obviously, the GMO movement is being phenomenally successful, and this is what we need for the movement for regenerative agriculture to take everything to the next level. I'm just curious what you see as the possible alliances and things we can learn.

Jeffrey [53:30]: Well, you know, it is interesting. I get very excited when I see the lectures with the research showing the sequest … sequestration – I can't say it …

Brendan [53:42]: Just say 'carbon capture'.

Jeffrey [53:43]: There you go, the 'cc'. The carbon capture. It's very exciting. I originally in *Seeds of Deception* said, "I'm going to write a book on the environment and agriculture and explain how we can get an alternative, so people won't say, 'Oh, we need GMOs to feed the world.'" Well, that's a lie, and we have shown that that is a lie, but let's look at the alternative. But I realized that I hadn't yet gotten the word out to enough people on the health dangers, so I focused on that. And my second book and my four movies are all about the health dangers, and that's my wheelhouse because that is what's driving the needle in the marketplace.

But I think that, as people realize the whole systems approach, they're going to realize that, yes, this is what to avoid and this is what to choose. Organic is the basis of what not to do, but it doesn't tell you what you need to do.

When it was originally being created, Fred Kirschenmann, who was one of the fathers of it, he and one other person in the committee wanted to have levels of organic, so that they rewarded higher levels of organic certification if you did more things for the soil. And they got overruled, and so it became the bottom line, with the lowest common denominator: don't use synthetic chemicals, make sure that the animals have access to pasture, etc. Fortunately, there are no GMOs allowed and no Roundup allowed.

What's interesting is, Roundup— and I am getting a little bit off topic, but I need to say this—Roundup is not just sprayed on GMOs, Roundup-ready soy, corn, cotton, canola, sugar beets, and alfalfa. It's also sprayed on many non-GMOs like wheat, barley, rye, oats, potatoes, sweet potatoes, sunflowers, kiwis, citrus orchards, hops, grape vineyards. It is in *a lot* of foods. But Roundup is not allowed in organic products, nor are GMOs. So, if you want to avoid GMOs and Roundup, buy organic. If you can't buy organic, at least buy non-GMO so that you are not exposed to that overdose on Roundup-ready crops, plus the dangers of the GMOs.

So, I do think that regenerative agriculture provides a way forward. I am cutting the weeds of what we should be avoiding, and I think that what's interesting is, the reason we have been so successful is that we have educated people enough about the health dangers, that more than half of Americans are seeking non-GMO. They don't always do what they say in these surveys, but a significant percentage are, such that the food industry is now moving away from GMOs big time in the United States. We have achieved the beginning of the tipping point that I have been working towards for 22 years.

So, I would say that this series that you are doing can help generate a tipping point towards regenerative. My suggestion is this: before I started all the other non-profits and NGO's we were just talking about the environmental impact of GMOs and the agricultural impacts and the patenting, I had in my mind that that some Greenpeace person was going to be crop-pulling and then celebrating in a pub, eating corn chips that are genetically engineered. And that there would be a disconnect between fighting Monsanto and what they are putting in their mouths. So, I made sure to say, "You put that in your mouth, you are having a BT toxin that can poke holes in human cells, shown in a laboratory. You have Roundup that can do all these things. It might turn your intestinal flora into a living pesticide factory." Watch *Genetic Roulette* if you want to understand what I just said. So, it became absolutely imperative, especially for parents, to avoid eating GMOs because they wanted to protect their kids.

So my suggestion is, do research on the health impacts of properly raised food, on the minerals, on the phytochemicals, etc. Because we know that when something is raised properly, with good soil, it is more mineralized. And so you can get many times the amount of minerals in one, compared to many of the others. So, I would suggest that, yes, you are going to have people watching this who are going to make choices based on how good it is for the Earth, and because it is this altruistic understanding of all future generations and we're the stewards. Yes, but the percentage of people on Earth that feel that way is smaller. Most of those people will go, "Oh, you mean I might get cancer if I don't have these particular minerals, and if I can have these have minerals; I'll go for that." Or people who actually have these things actually get better from something. So now we have the evidence showing that's the case with organic and non-GMO. Hopefully, the movement will generate that kind of data for regenerative as well.

Brendan [58:14]: Well, it is a good thing that we put a lot of focus on that in this event. If you get a chance to check out some of the interviews, we went in some depth about exactly what you just described as far as what is going on when our soils are damaged, when we've got these chelators, and sucking the minerals out the food chain. And then the downstream implications of that healthwise. I actually came across some fascinating information.

Jeffrey [58:42]: Beautiful! I'll look forward to it.

Brendan [58:44]: Yeah. Very unique, some of it, like some that I had truly never heard, and I've been around this for a while. Now, I got a request or two, at least recently, from people who said, "I want to learn how to communicate about this. Like, really, like put on talks, and so forth." I believe that you have a speaker training or something like that. Can you say something about that?

Jeffrey [59:06]: Yes. There is a speaker training on our site at www.responsibletechnology.org. I think 1500 people have taken it, either online or in person. It tells people ways that they can communicate in a 2-minute conversation or in front of an audience with a PowerPoint. In fact, in 10 minutes I'll be doing a talk on Facebook Live, so I should probably have a Facebook Live training as well! [laughter]

But I would say one of the hints ... I go through the five pillars of an effective communication for behavior-change messaging. Because our focus is behavior change. You know, how do we get people to want to avoid eating GMOs, and then, for some, to get involved. And it's, first of all, you have to dismantle the credibility of those that are saying GMOs are going to feed the world, and they're safe, and all of that. And that is easy. Monsanto and the FDA left themselves so wide-open; they have such clear evidence that they are not telling the truth. You have to use third-party evidence to demonstrate that the products are unsafe; paint the big picture that this affects all of us who eat, all living beings, all future generations, and then suggest what they can do about it. We give information to fill in all those five pillars. It is pretty systematic and very easy. I always start when I am doing it live, I say, "Turn to a friend and tell them about GMOs." And people are floundering, and they don't know what to do. And then at the end I say, "Turn to someone and tell them about GMOs." "Okay." And then they have a very specific framework and it's like, "Ah, I feel so much better." The other thing is, even though you may have a strong emotional situation about it, I explain in it that if you go, and you start battering people, and speak melodramatically, it may not be effective. What you're saying is so melodramatic. It's so intensely melodramatic. You're telling a woman that her child's suffering may be because of what she fed the child. You don't need to sound melodramatic. It already is. You can be optimistic and say, "And guess what? People have gotten better from these things when they switched to non-GMO and organic." And give that person hope. But the information is powerful, and we share how to do that on the talk.

Brendan [01:01:22]: Excellent. Well, I really want to thank you for being here with us. It has been a huge contribution to our understanding here in the Eat4Earth community. So, thanks again for this time.

Jeffrey [01:01:34]: And I want to say, it is interesting that with this community, unlike the rest of the world, you guys are more in touch with being stewards for the planet. And so, I leave you with this big picture. Monsanto said that their stated goal was to genetically engineer 100% of all commercial seeds in the world and patent them. And their consulting company worked backwards from that goal to create the strategy and tactics to achieve it. They were slowed down by consumer rejection, but the goal remains the same for Monsanto, but it is expanded with the whole biotech industry releasing GM insects and fish, and basically, everything that has DNA. So we're at a pivotal point in history. If we allow this to happen, and they're replacing the products of a billion years of evolution with designer organisms, they're replacing Nature. And we know that with the side effects, that means a disaster multiplied and multiplied and multiplied that is irreversible. Because you can't then recall the mosquitos. You can't recall the contaminated genes in corn. It is a permanent change that we bequeath upon all future generations.

So, if you are thinking about getting active about something; you're thinking about it getting real; you're thinking about looking for some other excuse to avoid eating GMOs, for this community watching this, this may be more important than health. Because, right now, we are being forced to be stewards, we are being forced to stop a juggernaut that has the support of governments like the United States government. If *we* don't do it, if *we* don't take responsibility, then the *rest of eternity* on this planet may be contaminated by our folly. As long as those species exist, the contamination will occur, unless some future science fiction way to clean up a gene pool comes along. But right now, it's a permanent equation. So, I want to appeal to people to get involved. Go to www.responsibletechnology.org. Please sign up for the newsletter. We will let you know as new things come out. We will keep you informed. And we will give you ways that you can help others get the message out, so that we can stop this travesty and protect the food supply and all living beings.

Brendan [01:03:46]: Thank you. I couldn't agree more, and that really speaks to my mind in the sense that I don't know how many other people share this, but I actually value the health of the planet and all future generations far above my own. And so, that is my motivation, and I suspect that there's a few other people out there too. And thank you for leaving us with that.

Jeffrey [01:04:05]: You are most welcome. Safe eating, everyone.

Kelly Kennedy Interview
Why Lymphatic Drainage Should Your First Step In Detoxification

Brendan [00:00]: Welcome back to the Eat4Earth event, where we're exploring how you can heal yourself, your loved ones and the planet with food. This is Brendan Morehead, and I'm here with Kelly Kennedy, and Kelly is a biological holistic nutritionist, and she has studied with many pioneers in biological medicine and is on the board of advisors of the Bioregulatory Medicine Institute, which you can find at BRMI.online, a website you definitely want to check out. Kelly is an expert in lymphatic drainage therapies. And she also specializes in Computerized Regulatory, Thermography and pleomorphism. And as you know, in the Eat4Earth event, we focus a lot on toxins and detoxification, but unfortunately, much of the information out there on detoxification completely ignores, or at least overlooks, a very important piece of the puzzle in removing toxins from the body. And that is the lymphatic system and lymphatic drainage. And that is Kelly's wheelhouse. So Kelly, what exactly is the lymphatic system and what does it do?

Kelly [01:06]: So, first of all, thank you for bringing this conversation up, Brendan, because you're right. It's not talked nearly enough about, and I so appreciate platforms like yours that are out there, truly educating people about how their world works, which is their body that they're born with and leave with. And that's the only thing we can actually control in this world is this. And the lymphatics ... why I became the lymphatics expert isn't because I set out to be the lymph expert; it's that through the school of medicine that I studied in Europe and in Germany, we really talk about the terrain versus germs. So it's a very different platform for understanding how the body works. And I know you talk about terrain concept as well because it's the environment in which we live that is conducive to health. And so all the things that you're cleaning up is changing their environment and inside our bodies, the same thing because we have three times more lymphatic fluid than we do blood.

Kelly [02:03]: So I'm gonna repeat that. We have three times more lymphatic fluid in our bodies than we do blood. So we're basically a bag of lymph with some cells inside it. And those cells are Kelly Kennedy cells. And when you pull my blood and spin it and look at it, you can look at my red blood cells. That's great, but my red blood cells live in this soup. And this soup is this fluid that is housed in the fascia, which is underneath my skin. Is this other cellophane-y-like layer called the fascia. And the fascia goes from my head to my toes around every organ and every tissue, and it houses this lymphatic fluid and the lymph fluid is our toxic waste stop. It's where all of our garbage is taken out. And if for some reason, the garbage doesn't get taken out because the lymph, instead of being like fluid, gets thick. Why does it get thick. Sedentary lifestyle, chemicals, and metals, exposures, and ingesting them, as well as scars on the physical body, emotions, and stress thicken the lymph.

Kelly [03:12]: And then we have the WiFi, the radiation, and all those exposures. And it's always a combination of those things that makes us sick. But as those things start to build that lymph fluid also starts to get thicker and thicker. And instead of like fluid, that should be easily circulated throughout the body when we move, because the lymph system does not have its own pumping system ... our circulatory system has a heart that pumps ... we know that, right? And then it circulates that blood through the heart, through the lung, and then it takes it through the rest of the body. We excrete out the gases. Well, the lymphatic system drains into the cardiovascular system, and the lymph system's job—they're blind ended capillaries—it's a network of vessels, much like your circulatory system, and these little nodes, which are little organs, and some are bigger and some are very big.

Kelly [04:09]: Some are little and some are bigger. The bigger ones are found at your deeper joints, like in your arm, pit in your inner elbows, in your pelvis, around your neck and around your tonsil area ... tonsils are the gatekeepers to the lymph. And the lymphatic system is this amazing network. This ecosystem, if you will, of its own, which is basically to say, "Okay, I'm going to identify everything in here. I'm going to pump it through to the node. The node is going to identify if we need to create a white blood cell based upon whatever the body's up against, whatever interleukin is that a B lymphocyte or a T lymphocyte. These are different types of white blood cells. And then the body will generate those white blood cells at the level of the node, because it wants to address or attack that exposure, whether that's a metal, a chemical, or an immune challenge, like a bacteria virus, a fungus, or a mold that's in the body that's outgrown. So the lymph is your fluid. It's your toxic waste dump. And it doesn't have its own pump. It only moves if we move. And so sedentary lifestyles affect it. Tight fitting clothes affects the lymph. The WiFi and all the exposures and the emotions because the lymph on part two of this .. part two of what we're going to talk about ... is that the lymph is about letting go. The lymph isn't just about the physical body. It is also about the emotional body because we have ... you cannot separate the physical and the emotional, right? The mind, body, spirit concept isn't that I walk into practitioner and because they're mindful, they're now treating me mindfully. And so they're treating my mind, body and spirit. Well, every single person is ... you're responding to the mind, body spirit aspect of whatever they're kicking out, whether they're intentional and conscious of whatever they're kicking out is the question.

Kelly [06:05]: And hopefully the answer for you is your practitioner is mindful of what they're kicking out, and you like what they're kicking out, because that vibe of whatever practitioner, whether that's to handle your health, your finances, your, your legal aspects of your life, whatever it is that they have to resonate with you to have good, good vibes and good vibes out. Right? And so the lymph is about letting go of not only the toxins, but of also the emotional components. So the lymph is this network that allows the body to rid it, of its toxic load, as long as it works well. And the lymph system has in it, not only your tonsils, but your spleen is your largest lymph organ. Your thymus gland, your appendix, which stores, your probiotics, are all part of your lymphatic system, as well as your Peyer's patches, which are inside your small intestines. And, and, and, and! There's a lot to know about the lymph system. But the primary thing to understand for people is that your toxic waste. So when people talk about detox, you know, they want to talk about, Oh, I want to get more out of my bowels, which is great. That's why most people think of detox. I want to open up my bowels. That's great, but I will tell you right now, you're going to detoxify more through your lungs than you will any other organ in your body. Your lungs are your largest organ of detoxification. By just taking a deep breath, not a shallow breath, but a deep breath, a belly breath. When we take that big breath, there's a lymph vessel in the middle of our abdomen called the cisterna chyli. And when we take a deep breath, we pump that cisterna, and it drains all the lower body.

Kelly [07:51]: Lymph gets pumped up to that cisterna, then it drains up to my left thoracic drain, and then all the lymph drains from my upper, above my clavicle, above my collarbone down into my cardiovascular system. And so we will breathe out more of our toxins. Then we will also poop out, pee out, and sweat out. And if you're still of the age to bleed and you're a woman, then you will bleed out your toxins as well. That's how we get toxins out. It's not just the bowels number one. And number two, the body's job is to detoxify. There's three detoxification pathways that are elicited through your liver. Your liver is in charge of all the detoxification in the body. It's the captain of the team. It knows exactly what to do, and when to do it. A Lot of clients come to us and they go, "Oh, I'm on a detox protocol." And I'm like, "Well, what, what's the goal?" "Oh, I want to dump the toxins." "Okay. Do you sweat?" "No." "Do you poop?" "No." "Okay. Well, before we push the toxins around, cause that's all you're doing, you're pushing them around. How about we open up the pipes to drain them out first because you cannot drain anything, you can't detoxify anything, rather, if there's no drainage pipe to get it out." And this is what I think a lot of people are missing. They think that doing a detox is going to open up their bowels. The definition of detox is intracellular detoxification. Well, that only happens at the intracellular level. That only happens at the cellular level. And the cells are only about a quarter of the body. Three-quarters of the body is the lymphatics. So I want to get the lymphatics to drain and then allow the detox to occur because the body's not dealing with all the garbage that's in the lymph because it's drained out now there's room; there space. Now the body can deal with what's in the cell. And when it comes out of the cell, there's all these pipes that are open to take it out of the body. That's how the body should work.

Brendan [09:53]: It seems to me that's going to have a really a big impact on whether somebody has what people sometimes call a Herxheimer reaction, something like that, when they're detoxifying,

Kelly [10:05]: Thank you for bringing that up. Ever since I started working in the lymph, we don't get Herxheimer's reactions. When I first got into biological medicine and was trained in it, we went to the clinic in Switzerland, and we did our internship, and we had three clients that week that had Herxheimer reactions. And these were clients that were walking around, doing all sorts of crazy bodily uncontrolled movements. And my husband is very good. He does this vibrational technique, and he taught the practitioners, the docs over there, how to do what's called "break a reaction". And so he was successful at helping that, but I remember distinctly going, what do we do so that our clients never have that happen? Because if we weren't in a facility with seven medical doctors and 47 or more nurses and all that supportive staff, I would have been like, "What the hell is going on for this client?"

Kelly [10:58]: So what I realized is, as we did more with the lymphatics—I mean, they do a lot at the clinics in Switzerland for the lymphatics—we had just found some other ways that were a little bit stronger, I feel. As we started to work more and more on lymphatics, the concept of the Herxheimer reaction went away because you're exactly right. Brendan, what a Herxheimer reaction is, is I cleaned out my basement this weekend, and so all my trash cans are full. Now I'm going to go clean up my attic. Good luck. Where are you gonna put in all the trash? A Herxheimer reaction is my basement was cleaned out, but nobody took the trash out. Now I'm going to go clean out my attic. No, you need to go get the trash taken out from the basement first. Then you can get the attic cleaned out and it won't be this overwhelming mess that stinks and is gross for days, attracting all these bugs until the trashmen come---trash people.

Brendan [11:50]: All right. So I would love it. If you could show us a couple of questions about what does it look like? How do you know if you're congested? and how can you ... I think you have some self-massage techniques to show us, but you've also got this contraption in the background, and I believe you have a victim that we can give an experience on that while we're going to the self-care techniques. Tell us about that behind you.

Kelly [12:21]: Yeah. So the lymphatic system, like we said, doesn't move unless we move. And what we have found is that in all the work we do is the goal for us is to get the parasympathetic nervous system, which is our deep healing capacities, to encourage that, to incite that, to engage that if you will, to get that to turn on more than the sympathetic, which is this fight flight mode. When the body goes into the parasympathetic mode, the lymphatics start to want to start to be mobilized. Okay? So the goal number one is to get the body in that relaxation state. And so I'm going to get one of our assistants to come in and help me by putting them in the suit, but we call it affectionately the suits. And it's a suit that hugs you all over the body. Perfect. Look at that. She heard the cue, like she was walking outside. [Brendan: And who doesn't need more hugs?!], Exactly [Brendan: Even if they're mechanical] Even if they're mechanical hugs. Yes. So it really assists the body to go into that by hugging the body. But the lymph drains right here on the top of your clavicle, this is where it ends. So we always want to start opening that. Now this is a woman who's worked with us for quite a while. I know that her lymph is open. We just need to encourage it to move more, which is why we use this. If she was ... her first session, we would assess her first, make sure she doesn't need any manual stimulation. But one way to tell which none of us are dressed appropriately to show you this, is there's a difference between an armpit and an arm puff, but we are recording this in January, and it was 21 degrees Fahrenheit when I walked outside my house this morning. So you did not get to see my pit this today because it's just too darn cold out. But it's the concept. And maybe we can show some pictures, Brendan, I don't know. But some concept of, if you open up your shirt and underneath here, it doesn't look like it's going in, and it looks flat, then you have lymph stagnancy. You don't have to have lymphedema. You don't have to have big, swollen lens, really different in size to have lymphedema. Typically how people know that their lymph is stagnant is ... ready? They have headaches, constipation, improper cycles from their menstrual cycle. They don't sleep well. And joint pain. Those five things are indications that your lymph is stagnant.

Brendan [14:38]: That sounds like everybody.

Kelly [14:39]: Well, that's the thing. And, and why we got involved with the lymph was because we found that, "Oh, you do lymph before you do anything else. Oh, wait, you do lymph in the middle of everybody's cases. Oh, wait, you do at the end to ensure that they maintain their health. So wait, you do lymph from the beginning, the middle and the end." So, okay. So your whole life, you just gotta move your lymph. Well, yeah, the goal is can I move my toxins out faster than they're coming in? Right? The things you're teaching for instance, are teaching people how to stop them coming in, how to clean up my lifestyle and clean up my nutrition. So I stopped putting the toxins in, and now we have our lovely Julie to show us how to get the toxins out. [Brendan: Sounds good]. Back this up a little bit. Okay. Thanks for assisting us.

Brendan [15:24]: While you're doing that, I'm just going to mention to everybody listening that I wanted to look and see what the science showed about lymphatic drainage, and I didn't look exhaustedly, but I came up with, very quickly, a review article that was published in 2009 and looked at research from 1998 to 2008. And they said that, some of the many things that can cause lymphatic congestion include overexposure to adverse chemicals, food allergies, or sensitivities. And of course there's a lot more. You gave us a really big download of 10 minutes ago. And just to see that on pub med, just an authoritative review article saying, there's all these studies out there on this. This is not some flaky, backwaters theory about the lymphatic system. There's people researching this, and they're documenting this, and I find it interesting that food allergies and sensitivities is part of that.

Brendan [16:41]: And you were describing all these things that thicken the lymphatic fluid. And one of the things that I think is part of that very often—I think you've said this in other venues—is dairy. And so I have some questions about that. Like, is there a difference between cows dairy and sheep dairy? And let's say in the absence of an allergy, because anybody that has allergy ... any food that's allergenic to somebody is obviously going to cause a problem, but let's say somebody does not have a sensitivity to dairy. Is there still going to be potentially an issue with cows dairy? And is it different from sheep and goat dairy? And is it different if it's raw versus pasteurized, et cetera. And A1 cows versus A2 cows? Do you happen to know?

Kelly [17:23]: A1 versus A2, no, because here's what I do know about cows, and I come from the land of dairy farmers. So know that I'm [Brendan: Right, that's Pennsylvania.] sacrilegious as I say this to all of my family members. [Brendan: All the Amish are going to come with their pitchforks!]. Yeah. I mean, I'm from Western Southern New York. I went to Cornell University, and I was an animal science major, studied agricultural farming and pretty bad. Okay. Know a little bit about farming. One thing I realized when I was at Cornell University is they wanted to put me on the birth control pill because I started getting ovarian cyst one month after my car accident. So their solution was, "No problem. We are the ones that figured out the birth control pill stops ovarian cysts because we discovered when we tried to get our cows to produce more milk that if we put them on the birth control pill, we fake their bodies out to think that they were pregnant."

Kelly [18:12]: It reduced the ovarian cysts, but it did increase their cancer. But you know, "They're just cows, and they're just producing milk, and it's okay if they get cancer because they produce a lot of milk for us. And so that's okay." [said with irony] So right away at literally I got on the birth control pill before I went to Cornell University for acne and the cyst started to occur more, and they wanted to up my dose. And I wanted to talk to a doctor about why they were upping my dose. And it happened to be somebody who was involved in the research at Cornell on the birth control pill. So I was really like, "Wow, this is very interesting. I don't think I want to do this anymore with a pill." And as I started to research it, I also found that a hip injury or a scar can influence the ovarian to create cyst.

Kelly [19:03]: And all my cysts occurred on the left side. I had 30 of them burst in 10 years on the left side. When I was in the car accident though, I ate cow dairy all the time. I mean, cow dairy was my breakfast, lunch and dinner. I didn't eat meats, but I ate. cow dairy like it was my job. Well, a cow's DNA strand, I mean, a baby calf is born more than most humans will grow to as an adult, like they're born at like a hundred, 150 pounds. Then they grow to be a thousand pounds. How many of you listening or watching want to be a thousand pounds when it's all said and done? Well, that's the protein that they use as their building blocks. Proteins are the building blocks of life. Protein is the most basic substance of every organism on the planet. So if you need a lot of protein to build a huge cow, yeah, you need a really long stranded DNA, protein base, that's really long. And that's a cow. Goat's and sheep's (protein) are much smaller protein strands, much like the human, and coincidentally, a goat or a sheep at full capacity is at about 150 to 200 pounds. Much like the average adult under six foot is probably going to be, right? So their DNA, their protein, rather, is more similar to our protein. And so it's easy for us to digest their protein versus a cow protein. At the end of the day, you can only digest 60 grams of protein every single day. It doesn't matter. So if you're eating 128, your body store in 60 grams, and where is it storing it? In the lymphatics. And this is just going to make like bricks laying in your body that your body just has to move all over the place. Bricks moving here, bricks moving there, thickening up, creating dams, creating walls, where fluid can't go into now.

Kelly [20:54]: And so you're creating this whole scenario where you've got thick mucus. I could go on and out about cow dairy, but the bottom line is we're the only species that sucks the tit of another species ever, ever in our life. Once we've weaned off of our mom, why do we think we need to do this? This is the question. I love cheese. like the best of them. Like you have no idea how much I love cheese. Julie, do I like cheese? Yeah. I mean, I've got a cheese sheet I hand out the clients just to give them the sheet of cheese that they can [have]; it's all goat and sheep. All of it. And a little Buffalo mozzarella once in a while. But cow, one, it's how they're industrialized here in this country. Number one, you know, all the chemicals, all the metals. And even if you get a free range cow, it's free range next to all the carbon monoxide that it's breathing in from all the cars.

Kelly [21:46]: It's few and far between ... like I grew up, like I said, in Southern tier Western New York. And we were up there just a few weeks ago during the holidays. And we were driving around at all the farms and we were like, "Wow, look at those actually on the side of the mountain. I'm like, "Yeah, but right inside that barn, right there, is all the syringes full of all of the hormones and all the drugs that ... at least they're breathing cleaner air. There's no doubt. Then, you know, next to the city here at Philadelphia, but it's still, there's huge injections done because most of those farms up there now are owned by Land O'Lakes. They were not owned by Land O'Lakes when I grew up. But the average farmer can't survive now unless they're doing this high production, and that high production yield is only based upon the amount of chemicals and drugs they give those cows.

Brendan [22:38]: But you're saying it's okay if it's or somewhat okay, if it's goat or sheep or ..?

Kelly [22:43]: Yes. Goat or sheep. I mean, I love cheese. I do. And I do find that yes, raw cheese is going to be better than pasteurized cheese enzymatic production. Right? But the goal is that if you eat really well, you eat good greens. You've got good enzymatic production going on. Your hands are in the soil. You're grounding appropriately touching your hands and feet through ground. You expose yourself to the elements, to the trees, to the grasses that are not chemically treated. Your body's going to absorb. Absorb ... not absorb ...

Kelly [23:14]: That's not the right word, but [Brendan: Assimilate?]

Kelly [23:18]: Assimilate! Thank you. That's a better word. It's going to assimilate all the proper ecosystem here so that I can eat the things in variation and in variety and in spice, right? Like Julie and I—I will say I've known her for seven years or so—one my best friends ... listen, we like to eat certain foods, and then we find ourselves in ruts, and then we get sick of that food, and we find ourselves enough food, but we both changed so much in the last few years because we've tried to vary our diet, so we don't fall into these ruts. Right? We do it out of convenience. The woman's got six kids for God's sakes. And while I only have one child, I feel like I have 47 kids because of what I do for a living. So I'm busy; I'm on the go a lot.

Kelly [24:00]: And so we end up ... we were just talking earlier about, protein bars that we used to eat that we don't eat anymore because we get sick of them. Right? And we're always looking for faster ways to get good dense nutrition in our bodies because we both love to eat. And neither one of us could cook another meal in our lives, and we would be okay. [laughing].

Brendan [24:21]: So what is going on over there? You want to tell us anything about this before we dive back in?

Kelly [24:26]: Yes. So I've got Julia hooked up here. She's ready to go. She's like, "Yes. Please hit play." So she's all ready to go. I'm just going to hit my machine here, get her on her appropriate settings. So otherwise I might squeeze her to death. Hold on one second. Sorry. I just have to push a couple buttons to get the proper signs. Okay. We're good now.

Kelly [25:01]: So what's happening is there's air compression. That's increasing, releasing, increase, release, increase, release, increase, release, and it creates this nice little sequence, this flow in her body. And then it starts over. So compress release, compress release, compress release, and there's nine chambers. So it can all be customized from the hips to the abdomen, to the lower arm, to the upper arm. And then on the back, there's some, it's not going to compress, but it's just going to push a little nudge to go, "Hey, relax your shoulders." And that's where the PEMF technology pieces, which it's located at the level of the thoracics. So what the suit is doing is heating her whole body up with infrared. There's these other thinner cables here that are controlling the infrared, which on my computer system that I have, it will control the temperatures bilaterally and the compressions.

Kelly [25:56]: It goes on a scale of zero to 20 for the compressions and from about 95 degrees. So about 125 degrees Fahrenheit on the infrared, which most people start at 95 and end at about a hundred 'cause it's very ... it's that deep heat. So it feels very warm. So what this is doing is when we do it in a proper setting, I cover her eyes; I give her some essential oils; I cover her ears and give her some affirmations of self-love; and this soothes her body into a lull of parasympathetics while the compression and the deep compression is not only causing the sympathetic nervous system fibers to relax, which is allowing the healing capacities to increase, allowing the gut, which is where we have about 80% of our lymph is in our gut. So it's allowed that to all start to take better effect and allow that to take over, allowing those parasympathetics to engage, and allowing her own healing capacities to be stimulated.

Kelly [27:00]: And then the actual compression is moving the lymph. And so this is allowing her body to drain out toxic load today while she's essentially sleeping while on a talk with us, but it's very soothing. Most people fall asleep, as you can see, she went into it fully clothed. If you were in a situation where COVID is a concern for you, you can wear a mask while doing it, or the person that's putting you on can wear a mask. But what's beautiful about this is that nobody has to get undressed. You're in a room by yourself while you're doing this. It's a 40 minute session. And whether you do this at your own home for you and your family, or you do this in a clinical setting, it takes very little training for me to teach you how to do this.

Kelly [27:50]: It helps everybody sleep better. Helps the state of relaxation helps the body go into this parasympathetic state, which can help anything. It has been helpful for headaches, for allergies, for digestive issues, for anxiety, you know, for so many things, because it essentially engages that system to heal and allows the drainage of the toxic load to come out. The one side effect I would caution everybody to, is you have a great bowel movement typically right after it. And you have to race to the bathroom as soon as you're off, because it's moving a lot of that fluid. You had asked earlier, how do you know if you need lymph, or if you have lymph stagnancy, so some people will actually get a little excess fluid at different areas of their body, and it doesn't have to be huge.

Kelly [28:38]: It can be very negligible, but if it's noticeable to you, then it is edema of some sort, and you shouldn't have a edema anywhere in your body. So I noticed when I look at my before picture 'cause I ate cow dairy all the time, I just look like a little inflated, like somebody just like bwhoop bwhoop. And in all honesty, when I see pictures of myself and my family that I biological family come from, I can see the person who has stopped eating cow dairy and everybody who hasn't stopped eating cow dairy becomes very, very obvious because I'll just look a little swollen and a little inflamed. Well, yeah, go back to think about those 60 grams of protein. If you're eating a lot of cow dairy, you're getting a lot of excess proteins that your body can't break down and digest. So it's storing them. It's making thicker fluid. And now that thicker fluid is swelling, and the person just looks a little swollen a little bit everywhere.

Brendan [29:32]: Okay. Well, while she's getting the treatment, maybe you can show us how we can do our own self-massage.

Kelly [29:43]: Yeah. So the manual pumping. So the thing to understand about the lymph is it's just below the surface, you know, it's an eighth of a millimeter below your skin, so it's just below your skin. So when I teach how to pump the lymph, I try to teach—and hopefully the visuals so people can watch this—it's very much a slight pumping. I find a lot of people want to do this. It's not a pushing down. You know, we're so used to, "Oh, my shoulders are tight." Go ahead and squeeze them. You know? Okay, that's good for muscles. That's great. But your lymph is above the muscle just below the skin. So you just want to stimulate its movement by gently pumping it. Goosebumps, right? Everyone has goosebumps are. They have a very cool name. It's called arrector pili cause those are muscles. Goosebumps are actually tiny little muscles just on your skin that when you get that feeling, the arrector pili are contracted, and you see what show up as goosebumps. By creating goosebumps at our neck, that actually is enough to move your lymph. It's hard to create goosebumps on yourself, but if you had somebody else like tickling you or something, and you create little goosebumps, that's enough to start the stimulation of the superficial lymph. So you have superficial lymph and you have very deep lymph, and our goal for those of you that want to drain out your toxic load, is you want to get clear out the superficial lymph. That's great. But what you really want to get to is that deeper lymph. And you want to really do a fascial dumping of the nodes and get that lymph fluid to really flow.

Kelly [31:21]: And you'll see that evidenced by: I'm sleeping way better; I lost a little bit of weight, like three to five pounds. As I started to do this, my sinuses are draining. I have a lot of postnasal drip, all of a sudden, because you're going to start to move your lymph, and how you do that is you take typically these two fingers. I use my ring finger and my middle finger. I cross over my body because it's just easier to do it that way. And above my collar bone in this little like nook right here where it makes this little triangle, I placed my fingers in both those little sections.

Kelly [31:55]: Hold on, are you okay? Over there? She's like finally, "F I'm relaxed."

Kelly [32:00]: So I'm going to place it here. And I'm just going to gently pump it in a circular fashion toward my back. And it doesn't have to be a lot of pumps, like five to six pumps. And it's going to be in alignment with my ears. So I wore these earrings specifically so people could follow my line a little bit better. So right there is where you're going to pump. I think a lot of people are too far forward. They're like up here. You gotta go back here a little bit. Can you see that okay? [Brendan: Absolutely.] Okay. Okay.

Kelly [32:34]: And then the next area you do is up here at your tonsils. So just under your ears, under your jaw, just place your two fingers. And you're just going to gently again, I call it a roll pump. So it's like I'm pumping in, but I'm envisioning it rolling down my neck. A pump and a roll, a pump and roll, because once I open up the end points ... so the way that I look at the lymph is you have a highway, right? Which is your lymph. And there's a toll booth. And the toll booths are right here. And those toll booths have to be open for all the traffic to drain out. So you gotta start with the toll booths first. A lot of people teach dry brushing online, and I completely disagree with how they teach dry brushing from a physical physics perspective of how the body works. Please listen to this video or go to notmeds.com to my other website and check out the video there, complete with a PDF that you can receive when you sign up for our email. Because if you do not drain your lymph first, and then you go to push your lymph, you're doing the same thing you did with detox. You're just moving your toxins, moving them not removing them. You're moving them to another area of the body, not removing them.

Kelly [33:55]: If you push your lymph without opening up the end points, you're doing the same thing. You're just moving the toxins around, not out. Because the first thing you have to do is get the openings to open. So if the toll booth has 50 cars lined up behind it, I don't push the 50th car in the back and start honking. That doesn't do any good. I push the first car through the toll booth. And now the second car can [go through]. Now the third car can go through and now the fourth car can go through. So much like dry brushing and manual pumping.

Kelly [34:27]: I start here at my end points. [Brendan: This is the front of the line, right?] The front of the line, the toll booths, right. Then I get my tonsils to drain. Then I get this area here. It's called your apical node. It's right where a woman's bra strap will lay. So it's right here because your armpit will drain here. And then your rest of your arm including your inner elbow will drain to your armpit. Your armpit will drain here. So I open up this, I get this open. Now I move stuff into it. I get this open again. I move stuff in here. I open it again. Now I move this in. So how do I do that? I put my fingers right inside my armpit, close my armpit. And now I'm pumping in there. To show everybody that motion. That's what I'm doing. Okay. On the PDF, it kind of looks like we're pulling .. [It's] very hard to figure out how to show that on a one-dimensional page, but essentially what you're doing is pumping. And there's a quick video on that same notmeds.com website that you can watch in addition to this.

Kelly [35:39]: And please share it with everybody whom you know, who's trying to regain their health, or is already maintaining their health, get them this information. Or maybe they're trying to overcome something. Move their lymph. The answer, I mean, I hate to be the one pony trick show or whatever that sentence is, but I'm telling you, lymph is a key to so many cases. And when you open up your toxic load, because anything can cause anything. And it's just like a glass of tap water. You, those listening, know that when you pour a glass of tap water, it's not that it's [just] chlorine in the water. It's the 7,000 chemicals, and the pharmaceutical drugs, and all the crap that's in the water that we're concerned with. Individually, yes, but the combination of them all together is what we're really concerned about.

Kelly [36:28]: We have no idea what that really does, and we don't want you to be a lab experiment. So please stop drinking tap water, and drink purified good or alive spring water that's clean and active, right? [Be]cause you don't want all those interactions. Well, that's, what's happening in your lymph. There's all sorts of stuff going on in your lymph. And it's all interacting. As you drain that out you have no idea how good you can actually feel. I would like to say that number one. And number two, as you drain that out, you'll be amazed as this list of symptoms starts to really [home] in on what an actual issue is. So if you have a real chronic issue, it'll continue to show up. Then you can seek the advice of a practitioner. Go, okay, here's this one thing that I have left.

Kelly [37:12]: But so many of you listening to this, as you start to move your lymph, you can eliminate going to a practitioner because you have this on your own.. And you have the capacity to do this on yourself and on your kids, your loved ones. So you're going to pump here. You're gonna pump here. You're gonna pump here. You're going to pump in your armpit. And you're going to pump in your inner elbow a little bit. It's just gentle; takes about five minutes. Then you're going to pump right in that cisterna [cisterna chyli] in that inner abdomen area we talked about. Then you're going to pump in your inguinals. The sun is really coming in. So I'm on my leg, not on my hip. So if my leg is bending, I'm on my leg part, and I'm going to pump it here. I'm going to pump in my inner thigh, behind my knee, and in the middle of my calf. And then I will always go back and repump my openings to make sure that those tollbooths, now that I've moved the 50th car through, still stay open, so the hundredth car can keep going through.

Brendan [38:10]: So that's kind of the reverse order of what people are talking about when they're showing brushing techniques. 'Cause you're usually starting at the extremities and going towards the ... what do you call the part here?

Kelly [38:23]: The clavicles. The termini. And a lot of people teach that. And I have no words for that. I don't really know why because once I learned about lymph, my friend Desiree DeSpong, who created this wonderful, amazing device called FLOWpresso, she taught me so much about the lymphatics. I had worked with other people that had done her training for a year or so prior to meeting her. And once I met her, we started making videos and so forth because I was like, "I don't understand how this got misunderstood out there." Like how is everybody else on the planet doing lymph the wrong way? Like what you said and what I know now about the anatomy makes complete sense. You can't push against 50 cars. It's not going to go anywhere. You've got to open it up and allow the pathway and then things will start to move and move out.

Kelly [39:14]: Now, the other thing I think of, Brendan, is it's like a dam. So if my, if my lymph is dammed up, I've got to unplug the dam first. But I don't want to unplug it with a sledgehammer that creates a Herxheimer reaction. I'm going to unplug it with a little pin hole and allow it to start to come out, just ever so gently. And then it will naturally open up larger and larger. So what people notice when they start doing lymphatics, the way we do it, is they first go, "Wow, I slept better. I pooped better. Oh, wow. I'm pooping every day now. Wow. My cycle really changed. Wow. My cycle's a little heavier now. Wow. My cycle normalized." This is over the six month period, let's say. "My headaches are reduced. Wow. Instead of getting that anxiety and living in it 24/7 at a ten, I'm living in anxiety two to three days a week at about a three or four, unless this situation occurs.

Kelly [40:06]: So they gently start to drain out their toxic load. If I don't know the person;, they're chronically ill; they come and I go, "Okay, you're going to do FLOWpresso every day for five days. They're going to come to me after five days and be like, "Dude, all the crap that was in my body for 25 years just came out, and I've had diarrhea and rashes. And I'm throwing up, and I'm nauseous, and I'm dehydrated. And I feel like crap, and I'm anxious and I'm moody." You could do that in five days if you have a tolerance for it. Or you can do it over a slower time and allow the body to get better. The body didn't get sick overnight. Allow it to heal at the pace that it got sick—slowly, gradually. It's not to be fast and hard. It's supposed to be slow and gradual. And that will win as long as you keep feeding the right things in and let it come out faster than it's going in. And this is a wonderful way to do it. And as you can tell that, even though we're in the room talking, she's barely moving because she's almost asleep because it puts you into a deep parasympathetic state. Would you agree Jules?

Brendan [41:15]: So does it make any sense to combine brushing in some pattern with the massage?

Kelly [41:26]: Yeah. So what I recommend is do the pumping first, then do the brushing second. And the process should take you 12 minutes, six minutes of each. Don't make a big deal out of it. I could do it in the car a lot. Like if I'm a passenger in the car, I'll do it. If I get stuck in traffic, I'll do it. You know, I don't honestly dry brush that much anymore, to be honest with you, because I do so much of this. I don't need a lot of dry brushing these days 'cause I get on this at least once a week and I do my manual pumping whenever I need to. I don't need it as much as I did five years ago, where I'm at today.

Kelly [42:00]: My clients, however, and the people that I work with across the country, I do recommend that they do manual pumping. If not once a day, at least twice a day, until they sleep five to seven hours a night and feel rested when they wake up; until they have two to three bowel movements every day, because they ate two to three times that day; until their energy level, when they wake up, they have good energy, they have natural lulls, they go to sleep and they're tired. As long as they don't have headaches or any other symptoms or rashes, then we know that their lymph is moving. I have no symptoms outside of, I drive people crazy 'cause I don't sleep a lot. And I have a lot of ideas and questions and you know, a lot of things to do. Outside of that, I don't have symptoms in my life.

Brendan [42:43]: That's interesting you should say that because I've noticed recently that I've needed less sleep. And there's, you know, many things I'm doing, and I've gone through cycles of that. But one of the things that preceded that was starting to do lymphatic self-massage. I also sleep five inches elevated with my head up, not my head up, but the head end of the bed elevated five inches compared to the foot end.

Kelly [43:06]: To allow gravity to work for you, to allow gravity to pull lymph. If your head is flat, your brain won't drain. And the whole game is for the brain to drain. If the brain isn't happy, while the heart sends more signals up to the brain, the brain is kind of in charge like the master electrician up there that's making sure everybody's getting what they need. So you gotta make sure the brain is fed and, and drained from its toxic load so that everything can work properly up there. And you do that at night when you sleep, it naturally drains out, particularly when you give that elevation. Or if you notice Julie has a pillow, an extra pillow. Typically, we have two pillows under her head, but you know, just for demo purposes, I didn't give her the extra pillow.

Brendan [43:50]: What is the advantage of using a machine like this versus just self-massage?

Kelly [43:57]: So self-massage is going to open up the pin hole of the dam. This is going to assist the body to move more out and allow that pin hole to open up gently. There are other compression suits out there. I'm biased because we worked with engineers. My friend Desiree did to create something that was specific and ideal for the lymphatics. It's a wellness device that's determined for the parasympathetic state. In all honesty, that was not what we set out to do. That was the side effect, but it became the primary because we know when you get the body into the parasympathetic, everything else gets better. Now the side effect is it also mobilizes your lymph when it's there. We also have a second program on the same unit that also works the fascia. So it's more compress ,hold, compress, hold compress, hold, compress, hold. I'll switch programs real quick. Not that you can necessarily see that, but we'll let Julie speak to the difference. I have to turn everything down by one, because otherwise the compress-hold, compress-hold, compress-hold gets too tight. So she just needs it to be—and now it's like holding her whole body and then it'll release in one fell swoop. So the benefit of doing this over the manual pumping is: the manual pumping for me is a good way to start to get yourself some good relief from sinus congestion or something else, but it's not going to necessarily be enough to unplug and decongest the lymph at the pace that you need it to. Because here's the point. If you've been getting congested for 20 or 30 years, and we finally open it, it's going to take a day or two to get your level down once it's open. So you want to be committed and devoted to getting that down as fast as possible.

Kelly [46:01]: So it's cumulative what you're doing. Otherwise, I'm pumping out what I took on today. I'm pumping out what I took on today. You and I probably eat a very clean diet, very live organic, all that, really good. Really great lifestyle. We're not exposed to chemicals and metals. All of that. Still 10 to 15% of our diet is going to have Roundup in it. Still, we're going to have mercury and aluminum in our diet. Still, we're going to have pharmaceutical drugs in our diet. So as good as we can, it's still the onslaught that we have. So if you're just manually pumping, that's probably just maintaining today's input, not going to be enough to get to the chronic issues that are going on in the body. Whether you're dealing with chronic symptoms or not, there's still chronicity going on in the body if you haven't manually gone after to move the lymphatics. Because, I don't know if that was true, Brendan, a hundred years ago. But in the last 70 years, that's certainly true. Since really industrialized food came in, and we weren't working out in the fields as much, gathering up, and we're not as active, we're sitting around televisions and radios and listening and podcasts. The most active person today is probably not nearly as active as a hundred years ago as a person who is active. That's just the way it is. And so by the nature of how the organism is living, we are more stagnant. And then we have things that are causing that lymph to clog. So I do believe in the future, you're going to see FLOWpresso's, that's also part of my mindset, is you're going to see these on every corner. Like you see now Starbucks and Massage Envy's. But we're going to need to see FLOW's because we need these everywhere. So people can sleep better. They can heal better, they can poop better. They can allow their body to go in that healing capacity and they can drain out that toxic load so that they're staying ahead of the curve before they actually get sick. True preventative illness, true wellness, huh? Yeah. Didn't even mean to say that, but the name of my center is the True Wellness Center. I didn't really mean to say it.

Brendan [48:15]: You know, it's a shameless self-promotion [joking with her].

Kelly [48:19]: It was. My husband came up with the name, and he's brilliant because it really is. We're trying to get people to help achieve true wellness. And that is not a destination; it's a journey that you decide to do every day. But this is why I love FLOWpresso because this is something that encourages the body to be in this state of relaxation and also in connection with ourselves, which is hard. And I mean, let's just be honest. It's hard for people to stay connected with themselves. They're connected with this [holds up phone]. They're connected with their social media platforms, and they're connected with their neighbors, and they're connected with everybody. But ask them, when was the last time they looked in the mirror for five minutes or spent five minutes alone in a room by themselves just being. And unfortunately for the majority of people walking in Western society, that answer is "few and far between". And that's one of the things we need to shift in 2021. We need to spend a little more quiet time by ourselves and be. And FLOWpresso helps them do that in addition to moving their lymph.

Brendan [49:22]: So maybe it's kind of like a float tank, but with additional benefits.

Kelly [49:26]: Exactly. It's kind of like a trifecta. You've got the infrared, you've got the ... we do the deprivation 'cause we cover your eyes, cover your ears. And then we put you in this like floating. [Talking to Julie on the FLOWPresso table] Have you done program two before? How do you like program two versus program one?

Julie [49:47]: It's way more intense.

Kelly [49:48]: Yeah. Yeah. Is it too intense for you?

Julie [49:50]: No, no, no, no. The first program is more of like a light flow, I guess. And this one is just like, you feel like it's the compression-holding and then like a, aah. Yeah.

Kelly [49:55]: A big release. And so CrossFit queen here, but she's no longer CrossFit queen, thank God, because she learned her ways that was killing her fascia. Right? That's why a lot of people that do CrossFit get injured so often because they're overusing and they're causing their body to be in sympathetic mode all the time. She's gaining her health as she's doing less CrossFit because she's allowing her body to recover more. And that's what the sport mode is, recovery mode for somebody like Julie who does work their fascia so hard, who does heavy, awkward lifting and moving because that's really good for your cardiovascular system. Tough though on your fascia. So you need to accommodate both. [Talking to Julie] I'll switch your programs.

Brendan [50:46]: So how would somebody find one of these and maybe even get one for themselves?

Kelly [50:54]: So, we launched last March out of New Zealand and here in the United States, and we just got into Canada about a month ago. You can access myself. I'm actually one of the two distributors here in the United States, I'm very blessed to say. And that's available on our website, which is notmeds.com. They are used for both home use and professional use. They're $8,400 including shipping, and taxes, depending upon what state you live. And the training we do over the internet. It takes about an hour the day you get it and an hour a month or so, or a week or so, down the line, depending on when you need it, for understanding the protocols and what is occurring, and that kind of stuff. Because when you start to move your lymph, it's not that your lymph is moving. It's what's in your lymph that's moving that you might need to address. So if you've done years of healthy living, and you move your lymph, like you, Brendan, then you're just going to be like, "Oh my gosh, I'm sleeping better." I actually noticed when you signed on, your eyes look brighter. I didn't know why. I thought maybe it was just a different part of the day than when I saw you the last time. But you know, you're just going to generally feel better. If you haven't lived this way, and you start moving your lymph, you may feel a little crappy in the beginning because it's going to start moving out your toxins, and it's going to be like, "Ooh, that feels like crap". That's okay. That's just motivating you to stop putting that crap in your body or exposing yourself to that crap. So you don't have to get it out next time.

Kelly [52:21]: We're all about making sure you don't put it in, so you don't have to get it out later. But bottom line is you've been putting stuff in for a long time, for as long as you haven't known what you know now. And so now that you've stopped that leak, now you can start to clean it up. It might get messy in the beginning. But as you start doing this—I'm not kidding you—over three to four weeks. If you get really diligent, and you really do this, if you found a location has FLOWpresso, and if you go to our website—-there are some locations listed there—-or you can reach out to me. Some of the personal units might be willing to let you try it. If you link up with me, I can help you figure that, or my team can. And you may want to do this once a week and get a much better shifting in the tissues, and shifting in what's happening in the terrain than if you do manual pumping. You know, manual pumping you're going to have to do week-in, week-out to get the same effect that this is going to make in one session. So it's just a matter of how fast you want to go. But [for] some bodies, this is the best way to start to build up to do something like this.

Brendan [53:27]: Gotcha. I think it also has had, I mean, it's really hard to say what causes what in my own experience because I'm always doing different things, but sort of a brightening of my mood. You mentioned brightening of my eyes, but brightening of my mood overall has occurred recently. And I'm like, "Where did that come from?" Instead of being, a little bit of like kind of a blah, just a little bit brighter, a little bit more optimistic, less irritable or more cheerful. I think I'm always optimistic, but anyway ... So I think that could be coming from the [FLOWpresso], I'm pretty sure that if you clean out the junk that's not getting out, you're going to be less irritated.

Kelly [54:08]: Well, yeah, because most of what is in the lymph is metals and chemicals, which are hormone disruptors and hormones are affecting your mood, obviously. The deep compression that she's doing right now reduces your cortisol by 31%.

Brendan [54:28]: That's huge. And that's going to be really big for weight loss for certain people where their stubborn weight gain is related to cortisol issues, just chronic, that chronic stress just bumps that cortisol up a bit.

Kelly [54:40]: And it thickens your lymph. And when, when Desiree set out to find something that was different, 'cause we had some other pieces of equipment we used for the lymph that were good, but they weren't quite hitting all the marks that we needed to hit. And so she, as a researcher, set out to find something on the market that she could enhance. And what she found was something that was great for weight loss, that was great for cellulite, that was great for body sculpting. So she changed it and upped it. So now it does all this other additional stuff. But yes, what stores in the fat is the toxins. So when your body has a pathway to get the toxins out or let the fat go with it, and when the toxins aren't in the fat to disrupt your hormones, you're going to feel better in general. But yes, this reduces your cortisol and increases your oxytocin and your serotonin by almost 30%. So it decreases your bad hormones by 30% and increases your good hormones by 30%. This is 60% shifting your hormones with a 40 minute session. You can see why I'm so passionate about getting this out there to everybody on the planet right now. We need more relaxation, more happiness, and more connection than we've ever needed ever in our lives. And this is one way to do it, a quick, easy way. And it also gives you the great benefit of moving the lymph and helping your body drain out its toxic load.

Brendan [56:01]: Cool. Did you say it also reduces cellulite?

Kelly [56:04]: Yeah. By the nature of moving the lymph, yeah. Should we drop the suit and let her [Julie] say how she feels?

Brendan [56:19]: Sure. And for everybody watching, I'm going to have a link for you to download to the right page on her website to download. It's notmeds.com, right? So yeah, just go straight to notmeds.com. You can download her guided two-page guided self ...what is it self therapeutic ... what's the term?

Kelly [56:46]: Self-pumping.

Brendan [56:48]: Self-pumping. There's another term I was looking for, the one in the literature. What was it? It was ...

Kelly [56:55]: The one in the literature?

Brendan [56:57]: Yes. In the research literature. They call it manual lymphatic drainage, I think is what they call it.

Kelly [57:03]: Yeah. Just different. I interchange all the time. Hey, Julie! She loves being put on the spot and loves speaking in front of large groups of people. That's her favorite thing to do.

Brendan [57:17]: Well, thank you for being willing to get on there and show us how it's done. And for being here with us.

Julie [57:25]: Yeah. It put me in such a parasympathetic... It's hard to actually get back.

Brendan [57:31]: She can't be verbal right now, folks.

Kelly [57:33]: Yeah. Exactly. But you can see the glow coming off that smile that it's excessively fun to do. Thank you very much.

Brendan [57:45]: Any last good words?

Kelly [57:50]: Drop the cow dairy. Move your body. And don't worry about what you heard today. Take the step one step in the right direction; start to move your lymph. And two months, three months, six months, eight months, 10 months from now, you're going to notice such a change in your life. I promise you, you'll notice it right away. It'll start to work right away, but continue with it, and you'll see such a benefit in all your healing and all the other things you're doing. You'll be so thankful you did. And thank you for listening and sharing this information. Because it just makes me so happy that people are talking about the lymphatic system and that they're getting the results that they deserve from doing all the other work they're doing because their body's own ability to heal and drain has been encouraged and engaged to, to let that go. So thank you.

Brendan [58:40]: And thank you, Kelly, so much for showing us how to do lymphatic drainage. And this is so missing out there in the world of health and teaching about detoxification. It's really the first step and just takes two minutes a day. You can go to notmeds.com. That's notmeds.com to download Kelly's two-page guide to what she just showed you. And I also recommend watching this video again to see her demonstrate it again. And thanks again, Kelly, so much for being here with us.

Day 6 – Finding the Right Diet for Your Body and the Earth

Reversing Heart Disease with a Plant-Based Diet
Caldwell Esselstyn, MD
What You Will Discover

- What exactly happens in a heart attack
- Dr. Esselstyn's formula for stopping or reversing heart disease
- The substance in balsamic vinegar that can help open arteries in the heart and block the formation of a certain carcinogen in your gut

Calling All Real Food Movements to Come Together for the Earth
Michelle Norris
What You Will Discover

- 3 Common myths about the "paleo" diet
- Why the health crisis is everybody's problem even if we ourselves are healthy
- What will happen to us economically if current health trends continue

Live Longer, Slow Aging, Super-Power Your Brain, and Save Your Life with Your Primal Fat-Burning
Nora Gedgaudas **Blueprint**
What You Will Discover

- The evolution of our taste for fat
- The enzyme that some people lack for converting plant-based omega-3 fats into the form that we need and use in our bodies
- What has happened to the human brain in the last 10,000 years since adopting agriculture-based diet

Kale vs Cow: The Case for Healthy, Sustainable, and Ethical Meat
Diana Rodgers
What You Will Discover

- A fresh look at the ecological, nutritional, and ethical issues around meat
- The difference between "blue" and "green" water, and the actual water consumption of pasture-raised cattle compared to crops like rice
- The deep flaws in the research that maligned meat as an unhealthy food

Planetary Eclectic Herbalism and Finding Your Own Perfect Diet
Sarah Wu
What You Will Discover

- The history of "planetary eclectic herbalism"
- What it's like to live in a tropical forest
- Sound advice for finding your own perfect diet

Caldwell Esselstyn, MD Interview
Reversing Heart Disease with a Plant-Based Diet

Brendan [00:00:00]: Welcome to the Eat4Earth event. We're exploring how you can heal yourself, your loved ones, and the planet with food. This is Brendan Moorehead, and it's my honor and pleasure to welcome our guest, Dr. Caldwell Esselstyn. Dr. Esselstyn is the Director of the Cardiovascular Disease Prevention and Reversal Program at the Cleveland Clinic Wellness Institute and has led a career of prestigious physicians at the Cleveland Clinic. Twenty-three years ago, while Chairman of the Cleveland Clinic's Breast Cancer Taskforce as a general surgeon, Caldwell Esselstyn grew disappointed in the way he and his colleagues were treating cancer and heart disease. Research studies had been suggesting that the culprit for heart disease and many cancers was the Standard American Diet. Targeting heart disease, Dr. Esselstyn and his wife adopted a plant-based diet cutting out oil, meat, fish, fowl, and dairy. Cleveland nutritional consultant, Chris Napier, attributes some of the success in Dr. Esselstyn's research study to the time and personal attention that the surgeon devotes to the patients.

Dr. Esselstyn, it's not many physicians that are as committed and generous as you, and it's truly an honor to be speaking with you today.

Dr. Esselstyn [00:01:13]: Brendan, thank you so much. I'm delighted to be with you.

Brendan [00:01:18]: Dr. Esselstyn, you know in the United States heart disease is taking the lives of one in four people. How do Western diets initiate cardiovascular disease?

Dr. Esselstyn [00:01:29]: It's almost an embarrassment to think that here in the West, we have created a billion-dollar industry over an illness that does not even exist in half of the planet, though that tells you right away, I hope, a lot about how you deal with this disease causation. I think that in the area that all experts would agree is where this disease has its initiation, its inception, its onset, is when we progressively injure the lifejacket and the guardian of our blood vessels, which happens to be that delicate, tender innermost lining, the endothelium. And the endothelium manufactures a truly magic molecule of gas, nitric oxide, which is really the salvation and the great protector of all of our vasculature because of its numerous and really quite remarkable functions. For example, nitric oxide makes certain that all of the cellular elements within our bloodstream are flowing smoothly, like Teflon rather than Velcro. It keeps things from getting sticky. Number two: Nitric oxide is the strongest blood vessel dilator in the body. When you climb stairs, the arteries to your heart, the arteries to your legs, they widen, they dilate with nitric oxide. Number three: Nitric oxide prevents the wall of the artery from becoming thickened, stiff, or inflamed, protects us from getting high blood pressure or hypertension. Number four, and this is the absolute key: A safe and adequate amount of nitric oxide will protect you from ever developing blockages or plaque. So literally, everybody on the planet, whether in Colorado or whether they're in Denmark or Yugoslavia, anybody who has cardiovascular disease has their disease because by now in their life they have so trashed, injured, and compromised that the capacity of their endothelial cells to make nitric oxide, they simply don't have enough to protect themselves and now ... I'm sorry, I'm going to mess you all up because I just had a Labrador Retriever who wasn't at all interested in what I was saying. He just wants to be petted.

Brendan [00:04:02]: We can keep going.

Dr. Esselstyn [00:04:05]: Be brave. So, the fourth point, number four: Nitric oxide in an adequate and safe amount protects you from ever developing blockages with plaque. So literally everybody on the planet, whether its Colorado or Denmark or Yugoslavia, have their disease because by now they have so sufficiently trashed and injured and compromised the capacity of their endothelial cells to make nitric oxide they don't have enough to protect themselves from making blockages or plaque. Now, the thing that makes this so exciting though, this is not a malignancy. This is a completely benign, foodborne illness. Not your genes, not your stress. It's a foodborne illness. A toothless paper tiger. So, once you can get patients to understand how, over the decades, eating all these Western foods that every time it has passed their lips they have taken a hit to their endothelial cells, once they get that straight, and they never again put something through their lips that is going to further injure an already train-wrecked endothelium that they present you with, the endothelium begins to recover, and it makes enough nitric oxide so the disease progression is halted, and we often see significant reversal. I hope that answers your first question. Now, you probably are asking what are the foods that pass through your lips to injure the endothelial cells. Well, although I occasionally have been known as a taskmaster, I am also told that I'm not as mean as I look so, alright, what injures the endothelium? Any oil, any drop of any oil: Olive oil, corn oil, soybean oil, safflower oil, sunflower oil, coconut oil, palm oil, oil in a cracker, oil in a piece of bread, oil in a salad dressing. Oil injures the endothelial cells as does anything with a mother or a face: meat, fish, chicken, fowl, turkey, and eggs. And anything that is dairy: milk, cream, butter, cheese, ice cream, and yogurt, and you gotta go very easy on sugar, sugary drinks, cakes, pies, cookies, Stevia, agave, excesses of maple syrup, molasses, and honey.

Brendan [00:06:43]: What is it about those food substances that causes the injury? Is it that they tend to be pro-oxidants, creating oxidative damage?

Dr. Esselstyn [00:06:54]: Well, there is no question that when you look at a plaque, it is an absolute caldron of oxidative inflammation. So it's a combination of things that happens. Once you increase the amount of free radicals, you injure the endothelium, so that now there are fissures and cracks and openings. So what is otherwise a completely benign molecule of LDL cholesterol circulating in your bloodstream, it now becomes problematic when it finds itself suddenly in the subendothelial space because there it then becomes oxidized by these free radicals, many of which are from our food. And once you have the LDL cholesterol as a small, hard, dense molecule in the subendothelial space, the subendothelial space then calls upon our swat team or white blood cells, which come across into the subendothelial space and begin gobbling up, gobbling up, gobbling up all of these small, hard, dense LDL cholesterol molecules until that macrophage becomes so chockfull of these, its now a foam cell. And the foam cell is truly the Darth Vader of this sequence of events because the foam cell elaborates or manufactures the enzymes we call metalloproteinases like stromelysin, elastase, collagenase, myeloperoxidase. What do they do that is so bad? They progressively erode the cap over the plaque so it gets thinner, and thinner, and thinner, and now these smaller inflamed plaques, usually between 10% blockage of the artery and up to 50%, when that cap gets so thin the shear force of blood running over it tears it. Now that's the key moment because once you have now ruptured, once you have ruptured the plaque, there is now the oozing out of, if you will, or the extravasation, of plaque content into the flowing blood, which activates our clotting factors and platelets. And suddenly now, where that rupture has occurred, we begin to get the formation of a thrombus, a clot, which is in and of itself self-propagating, so in a matter of further minutes that partial clot has gone "boom" all the way across the artery. No time for months and months for the arteries to develop collateral. Suddenly, all of the downstream heart muscle, which has been deprived of its oxygen and nutrients because of the blood flow cessation, and that part starts to die, and there is your classic 90% of heart attacks.

Brendan [00:10:01]: Wow. You know, I have never actually been given the full sequence of events to explain that particular case, which I guess that's the most common one. Is it? Is that the most common way that heart attacks occur?

Dr. Esselstyn [00:10:16]: Yeah. I think the reason that I'm so fussy about making that clear, is that if I've got somebody in the room who has cardiovascular disease, and they've had a heart attack; they don't want another one. Or they've been told they have to have a stent; they don't want to have it. Or they've had a stent; they don't want to have any more. Once they get their arms around the fact of how it is that they produced this themselves over four, five, or six decades by hammering away with these horrible foods and injuring the capacity of their endothelial cells to make nitric oxide, and when I suddenly realize we are empowering them to absolutely annihilate this disease by giving them the opportunity to stop the foods that are further injuring this train wrecked endothelium and getting it to come back and recover, it's pretty exciting stuff. And then it's very hard for them to want to cheat. For instance, it's always a lot of fun, after I've counseled somebody I say, "Well now, how often do you eat out at restaurants?" "Well, not very often." "Well, let's try that again. How often do you eat out at restaurants? "Well, maybe once or twice a week." I say, "Okay, let's look at that. That means that on 104 days out of the year, you are already further trashing that destroyed endothelial system with more and more restaurant food. I grant you, you can if you work on it, you can get a safe meal at a restaurant, but if you don't specify about avoiding oil, there you go, you are injuring your endothelial cells again." So, oh, the answer is usually, "I didn't think of it that way."

Brendan [00:12:11]: Right.

Dr. Esselstyn [00:12:14]: They say, "I'm good all during the week. I can belly-up to the trough on the weekends." "Whoa. Hey, wait a minute. That means if it's Friday, Saturday, and Sunday, that's 156 days that you're trashing the endothelial cells."

Brendan [00:12:28]: You know, when it comes to oil, I think about, aren't there healthy oils like flax oil, which has got anti-inflammatory properties. I believe it's got high omega-3's. What would be the problem with a flax oil that has, let's say, rosemary extract that counters the oxidation in the oil to keep it from going rancid? Would that be an exception?

Dr. Esselstyn [00:12:53]: You know, the minute you begin to get reductionist, I'm gonna come after you.

Brendan [00:12:58]: Yeah, please.

Dr. Esselstyn [00:13:01]: I have no problem with flax seed meal. I don't want the oil. I don't want injury to endothelial cells, but a flax seed meal, Chia seeds, I'm with you.

Brendan [00:13:14]: So as long as the oil is not extracted from the whole food, you're, it's absolutely fine with you, and should not present a hazard.

Dr. Esselstyn [00:13:23]: Look, our approach is not a no fat diet at all. We know the importance of omega-3 and omega-6. Nobody will ever be deficient of omega-6.

Brendan [00:13:37]: No, probably not.

Dr. Esselstyn [00:13:39]: But you want to be sure you're getting your omega-3 so, you know, on your cereal you need a couple of tablespoons of either Chia seeds or flax seed meal and plenty of green, leafy vegetables, and you're not going to be short on omega-3. Have you ever heard of anybody who went to an emergency room and said, "Oh my God, help me out. I'm deficient in omega-3."

Brendan [00:14:02]: Well, I haven't, but I have heard that many people are deficient in omega-3. Do you believe that, let's say, many people on a Western diet have a deficiency of omega-3?

Dr. Esselstyn [00:14:13]: I haven't seen that study.

Brendan [00:14:15]: You haven't seen it. Okay, great, and I can't quote any either. It's just my understanding that there is deficiency in that regard. Maybe it's just a case of imbalance that's what …

Dr. Esselstyn [00:14:27]: But you're not going to have it. You're much less likely to have imbalance if you're eating this way because the foods that I've asked people to give up, namely the oils, the meat, the dairy, and the sugar, then the omega-6 is way down.

Brendan [00:14:47]: Yeah.

Dr. Esselstyn [00:14:48]: Because what are you going to eat? You're going to eat all of these marvelous whole grains for your cereal, bread, pasta, and rolls, and bagels, and 101 different types of legumes, lentils, and beans, and all of those marvellous red, yellow, and green leafy vegetables and some white potatoes, sweet potatoes, and perhaps some fruit. And, my gosh, there you've got the whole food plant-based nutrition, which is now increasingly the nourishment of professional athletes. Why? Because they find that they have much better stamina and the recovery time is less, and matter of fact, the strongest human being on the planet, a German by the name of Baboumian, is totally plant-based; 1,200 pounds that he can lift.

Brendan [00:15:33]: Wow! Wow! You know, a moment ago, when you said you hadn't seen this study, were you referring to omega-6's or omega-3's? You hadn't seen a study showing any deficiency.

Dr. Esselstyn [00:15:45]: I haven't seen a study where they are deficient in either.

Brendan [00:15:49]: Oh, in either. Okay, great, just wanted to clarify that. Now, what are progenitor cells? I've seen you write about progenitor cells, and apparently that's a pretty important part of this.

Dr. Esselstyn [00:16:00]: Yeah, this is sort of a new kid on the block, but not to be underestimated. The endothelial progenitor cells derive from our bone marrow, and they replace our senescent, injured, worn-out endothelial cells. Now if I happen to draw blood from somebody in front of me who happens to be obese, who is diabetic, who is hypercholesterolemic, who is a smoker, who is a couch potato, the endothelial progenitor cells are going to be kind of low. And if I take somebody who is the antithesis of that who is active, nonsmoking, not diabetic, not obese, and not hypercholesterolemic, they'll be higher. But for my patients I truly want the endothelial progenitor cells to absolutely sparkle. So, we got information on that from a wonderful peer-reviewed scientific study from Okinawa where they took the healthiest human being on the planet, the Okinawan woman between the ages of 17 and 34, and half of the group got, were the controls, placebo, and the other half were consuming 5x a day different green Okinawan vegetables. When they concluded the study and they tested them, the endothelial progenitor cells were strikingly higher in the group that were having the additional green leafy vegetables. About six years ago, for our patients we've incorporated the following so that anybody who has cardiovascular disease when I'm first seeing them—especially those who have angina, were a little bit, really rickety—I asked them to imagine getting their head inside that coronary artery that is filled with plaque and what they would see would be an absolute caldron of oxidative inflammation so we need antioxidants. No, do not go down to the health food store and buy a jug of pills that says 'antioxidant' because it won't work, and its probably gonna be harmful. They're gonna get their antioxidants from food. Okay, what food? Food that is high in what we call ORAC value. O. R. A. C., oxygen radical absorptive capacity. So, if they're having raspberries, blueberries, strawberries, and blackberries on their oat cereal in the morning, that's a terrific start, but nothing can trump the antioxidant value of green leafy vegetables. So, I want these patients to chew 6x a day a green leafy vegetable roughly the size of their fist after it has first been boiled in water 5.5 to 6 minutes so that it's nice and tender. Then I want them to anoint it with several drops of a delightful balsamic vinegar. Why? Because the acetic acid in the vinegar has been shown to restore the nitric oxide synthase enzyme that is responsible within the endothelial cell for making nitric oxide. So they are going to chew this alongside their breakfast cereal, again as a midmorning snack, again with their luncheon sandwich, that's three; midafternoon, four; dinnertime, five; God I adore it when they have that evening snack of kale, that's six. What are they doing? All day long they are basking and bathing that horrible oxidative caldron of inflammation with Nature's most powerful antioxidant, and this is why you often will see those with angina getting really much relief within 7 to 10 days.

Sometimes it has disappeared. Now, what are the green leafy vegetables I am talking about? They are bok choy, Swiss chard, kale, collards, collard green, beet greens, mustard greens, and turnip greens, Napa cabbage, Brussels sprouts, broccoli, cauliflower, cilantro, parsley, spinach, and arugula, and asparagus. Now, the top six would be kale, Swiss chard, spinach, arugula, beet greens, and beets.

Brendan [00:20:43]: Got it. Well, I had some beet greens last night, a lot of them.

Dr. Esselstyn [00:20:49]: How about this morning?

Brendan [00:20:51]: No. I'm not on the five per day plan yet, but let me ask you this.

Dr. Esselstyn [00:20:56]: You don't have to do that unless you have heart disease.

Brendan [00:20:58]: Yeah and fortunately, I don't have the evidence of heart disease. I'm curious because I think its Joel Fuhrman, believes that we benefit if we blend on a high-speed blender, I guess like a Blendtec or something I'm not sure what his preferred machine is. But, greens so that it breaks up in the cell wall, and I actually, after, actually it was kind of a sauté in just water, had sauteed some red kale the other night. I had put it in a blender with romaine lettuce, I think some beets, raw beets, blended it up, threw in some balsamic vinegar for taste, not even thinking about, not even knowing about your method there and the reason for it, and I had that, along with my meal. I'm curious what your method, how you would compare chewing to blending. Is there an advantage one way or the other?

Dr. Esselstyn [00:21:59]: I don't know that it's ever really been tested. They probably are both going to be okay.

Brendan [00:22:04]: Umm-hm.

Dr. Esselstyn [00:22:05]: I'm just a little nervous about some of the things that, the rumblings that I have heard, not a peer-reviewed scientific study, but about when you blend on high speed maybe you compromise the fiber effect. And also, I guess I'm a little concerned that...I have no problem with somebody eating an apple or an orange, but if you throw an apple or an orange and other fruits into the blender to take away the tartness of the taste, that has now been separated.

Brendan [00:22:40]: Well, I'm referring to a blender, not a juicer. In other words, not a juice extractor, but a whole food blender where you're getting all the pulverized everything, pulp and everything.

Dr. Esselstyn [00:22:49]: I understand.

Brendan [00:22:50]: Okay, great.

Dr. Esselstyn [00:22:51]: And I just think that once you separate it, the fructose from the fiber...

Brendan [00:22:57]: Okay.

Dr. Esselstyn [00:22:38]: The is like a rocket going off in your stomach because sugars coming in that rapidly can injure the liver, glycate protein, and injure the endothelial cell. So that's just a ... I haven't really seen the hard science on that, but that's somewhat my concern. Also, just from the convenience standpoint, you can of course pour the smoothy and refrigerate it and so forth. On the other hand, for these people who are working in the midmorning and the midafternoon, if they take some spinach with them and a little balsamic, they can perhaps chew it. I don't think there's a great deal to choose between those two.

Brendan [00:23:43]: Okay. You mentioned...oh, go ahead.

Dr. Esselstyn [00:23:48]: Well, we're just very happy with the results that we've been getting so far with that, yeah.

Brendan [00:23:52]: Wonderful. I'm going to try that just to, you know, see what it does for what ails me, which is not heart disease at the moment. In regards to antioxidants, there is a class of antioxidants called polyphenols, and I believe you've had some, you've done some research at the Cleveland Clinic involving polyphenols from fruit pulp and their impact on the microbiome, the bacteria in our gut. Could you say something about that?

Dr. Esselstyn [00:24:23]: No, I don't think that I've done any of that research.

Brendan [00:24:25]: Okay.

Dr. Esselstyn [00:24:26]: What was done at the clinic on the microbiome has mostly been pioneered by Stanley Hazen. What Stan was looking at was primarily the molecules of carnitine and choline, lecithin. Those are largely found in meat, fish, fowl, eggs, dairy, seafood, in other words people who are omnivores. And he found that when the omnivore eats a lamb chop, for instance, and you measure the blood, there will be a spike in the TMAO, trimethylamine N-oxide. And trimethylamine N-oxide is a nasty molecule in terms of injuring your vasculature. So when he took somebody who was totally plant-based, gave them a lamb chop, measured their blood, no spike in the TMAO. Why? Because those who are totally plant-based do not possess the bacteria in their microbiome that allows them to metabolize into TMAO. Now, if you keep giving that plant-based person a lamb chop for four days, then they are going to convert their microbiome and they'll be in trouble.

Brendan [00:25:57]: Okay, and there was also the effect, I believe, that these polyphenols for people that did have the bacteria that were generating TMAO from the choline ... that it (the polyphenols) actually paralyzed the bacterial enzymes, rather, the polyphenols paralyzed the bacterial enzymes that were converting choline to TMAO? Was that part of the research?

Dr. Esselstyn [00:26:21]: I'd have to review the paper that you're referring to, but I do know that DMB, dimethylbutanol, which is found in things like balsamic vinegar, can block the formation of TMAO.

Brendan [00:26:46]: Okay, that must be why ... I mean, I love balsamic vinegar. I think most people do. Now, I'm curious, you know, when it comes to people taking on the plant-based diet and using your approach, does it need to be cold turkey off of everything or are there other paths to transition? Is it easier to transition gradually? How does it usually go?

Dr. Esselstyn [00:27:13]: I think that if the patients totally grasp what you and I had been discussing earlier about the endothelial cell and the fact that they so trashed their endothelial production of nitric oxide— that's why they have active cardiovascular disease—it's very difficult for me to embrace the concept of having them continue to destroy their endothelial cells at a less aggressive rate, which is what happens if you don't do it cold turkey. Now, the other thing that I think obtains here is the Monell Chemical Senses Center in Philadelphia did an interesting study where they took patients, and they put them in three different levels of fat: 34%, 20%, and somewhere around where we are around 11%. One of those groups, at the end of 12 weeks just totally lost their craving for those fat foods, and that's the group at 11%. So if you don't do it aggressively it seems to me that you're … here's what you're running up against: you don't downregulate the fat receptors or the sugar receptors rapidly. If you don't downregulate the receptor, the craving is there. And if the craving is there and the misery of not having it, and then you have failure and recidivism. So I think we're much better off. I have a chapter in my book entitled, "Moderation Kills".

Brendan [00:28:48]: That's brilliant. That's a very, very important insight, it strikes me. Now, so with every program, every eating program, every healing program, some people stick with it, and some people drop out. What kind of compliance rate are you experiencing?

Dr. Esselstyn [00:29:05]: In our most recent paper, let's see, July 2014, *Journal of Family Practice* there were some 200 patients, two were lost to followup, that means we had 198 that there were 177, 89.3%, almost 90%, were compliant, and there were 21 who wandered from the flock. That's about 90%, and I'm anxious to even make it better because the … I think the way you get numbers like that is you try to show the patient respect, and the only way that I know to show respect is to give them our time. So when patients see us in consultation, I usually limit this to groups of 10 or 12, always with their spouse or significant other there. You try to do this without the spouse … they have to understand what you're asking them as a couple, and it's so much more appreciated when the spouse is there to hear the rationale and understand the science behind this as well. So right now, our present program is … because about 85% of our patients come from outside the state of Ohio, we very well can't ask them to stay for days at a time, therefore, I get one day with these people, 5.5 hours. It's an intensive seminar. And always about 10 days beforehand my secretary will give me a list of who's coming with their phone numbers, and I personally insist on calling everybody so that I can get my arms around their story and at the same time, they have an opportunity to ask questions of me so that coming to the seminar we have a strong platform from which we can all move forward. And at the seminar, they are going to learn all about the behavior that they have had that created their illness in the first place. They are going to learn how they can be empowered as the locus of control to halt and to reverse this disease. *And* they all get a very hefty notebook. And in that notebook is a copy of every PowerPoint slide that I use, several of our scientific articles, a 44-page handout with many additional recipes that add to the 240 in the two books that we provide, and there is a marvelous hour and a quarter presentation from a woman who has had 30 years' experience acquiring and preparing plant-based foods, with reading and foods, travel and restaurants. And then everybody receives a DVD of the entire seminar, which I have filmed from an earlier one. So should they go home and get forgetful or rusty they can flip this on and get themselves back up to speed. And then, we have, we always have three local or regional participants that have previous successful experience share their story with those in attendance who can then say to themselves, "Listen, if he or she can do this, I can do this." Then, we answer all questions, have a delightful plant-based luncheon, and stay in touch as necessary through email or a phone call. And I think that that's really how we get the close to 90%. It's really very exciting to see these people begin to walk away from their disease and their drugs and those procedures, which, with all due respect to my cardiovascular colleagues, none of the drugs, none of the procedures, and none of the operations have one single thing to do with the causation of the illness. And I think the reason we do so well with the patients who comply is that ever since the days of Hippocrates, there has been a covenant of trust between the caregiver and the patient, that whenever possible the caregiver will share with the patient what is the causation of the illness. And sadly today in cardiovascular medicine that's not being done, not because of malice of forethought for heaven's sakes, but because cardiology is very candid about the fact they never get any nutrition training either in medical school or in their cardiovascular training, so they have really never had an opportunity to learn the causation of the illness which they have been designated to treat.

Brendan [00:33:57]: You know, I'm so impressed with your commitment to health and healing and people really, really winning and overcoming heart disease. And I really want to thank you for that contribution to humanity, and I have one more … go ahead.

Dr. Esselstyn [00:34:16]: No I'm just stating, I guess, it's been 16 years since I retired from surgery, and the reason I guess I'm so passionate about medicine today is that we are truly on the cusp of what could be the seismic revolution in health because when we treat these patients, it's not only their cardiovascular disease that goes away, but hypertension goes away, diabetes goes away, obesity goes away, and risk of stroke goes away, risk for vascular dementia goes away, and colleagues and others, and anecdotally in cases we've seen, Crohn's disease goes away, ulcerative colitis, rheumatoid arthritis, lupus, multiple sclerosis, allergies and asthma, and renal disease. And, my gracious, it's as if the heavens have opened and said to the medical profession, "Hey! How do you like this?" Whole food plant-based nutrition. There's no extra cost to the patient. There's no hideous side effects. And the results endure. And the result is you're empowering these patients to absolutely annihilate chronic illness. What could be more exciting than that and do it so simply?

Brendan [00:35:40]: Absolutely. And, you know, I'm curious because the soils in this country—I'm speaking of the United States, but truly it's across the entire planet—our soils have been quite abused and nutrient levels have declined, and we've got declining levels of nutrients in our foods, even organic foods are not the same as they were 100 years ago. Of course, we didn't have an organic certification and pretty much all agriculture was organic 100 years ago. And I'm just curious, do you direct people to seek out the highest nutrient values in the food that they purchase, perhaps organic over conventional, biodynamic, regenerative agriculture in general?

Dr. Esselstyn [00:36:24]: Well right now, I think its just a little bit unfair for the patients who perhaps can't afford the cost. They know that organic are perhaps unquestionably superior, but even if you can't eat organic, if you're eating whole food, plant-based nutrition, it's not going to stop you from liquidating this disease, shall we say.

Brendan [00:36:47]: That's good news. But let me ask you this, do you mention it at all and would you be willing to mention it in order to support the growth of a regenerative food system that restores soils and higher nutrient values to food across the board, organic and conventional? I mean, it wouldn't be as pesticide-laden, and pesticides would not be necessary if we were rebuilding our soil and having strong plants. We probably would not use pesticides or inorganic fertilizers any longer after a time.

Dr. Esselstyn [00:37:19]: I'm all for it.

Brendan [00:37:21]: Beautiful. Well, thank you so much for being here, and I really appreciate your time. It is wonderful to speak to somebody who is so articulate and passionate, and it has been a joy.

Dr. Esselstyn [00:37:34]: Brendan, it's been my pleasure. Have a good day, and don't forget your greens.

Brendan [00:37:39]: I certainly won't.

Michelle Norris Interview
Calling All Real Food Movements to Come Together for the Earth

Brendan [00:00:00]: Welcome to the Eat4Earth event. We're exploring how you can heal yourself, your loved ones and the planet, with food. This is Brendan Moorehead and our next guest, Michelle Norris, is as passionate about food and health as I am. Michelle Norris is a former corporate warrior, trained chef and multi-potentialite whose previous health issues and an extended battle with traditional medical advice inspired her to up-end the way the world tackles health, wellness and prosperity. She soon became one of the most outspoken Paleo evangelists and then co-founded and is now CEO of Paleo f(x), the largest paleo health and wellness event in the world. Having survived the death of her twenty-two year old daughter, Michelle knows what it's like to fight back from paralysing loss. She used tragedy as a catalyst to follow through with her vision of leaving the economic status quo behind and becoming a self-made entrepreneur. Her belief is that you can always find beauty among the ashes. Through the paleo lifestyle she can show you that your inherent stone age genetics can be unleashed and coaxed to thrive, without having to sacrifice the benefits of modernity. Michelle, it's so awesome to have you with us today.

Michelle [00:01:12]: Thank you so much for having me Brendan, I appreciate it.

Brendan [00:01:15]: Yeah, you and I have been through hell in the health department. I don't know all the details of your journey, but we both found an approach to food and health that could be called be called paleo, primal or ancestral. *Ancestral*, just so it doesn't sound like incestual or something. What do you think makes these approaches to food different from other approaches out there?

Michelle [00:01:46]: Well first of all, going back to my roots, and I have a lot of connection to that, with that fact that our deceased daughter had a tattoo that ended up becoming part of one of my endeavours. It ended up becoming the logo for one of my endeavours, my catering company. And the tattoo actually basically said, "It is good to go back, and look at the past and then learn from it." And the thing is, is that we learn things when we look back and we see that our ancestors didn't have all these diseases of modernity, and the reason that they didn't is because they didn't have access to these hyper-palatable foods we call Frankenfoods. Things that are actually technically not food, they are created in a plant or a manufacturing plant, if you will, instead of coming from a plant or coming from an animal. And you know our ancestors didn't eat this way. They didn't eat hyper palatable foods. They were opportunistic eaters, and so it's really good to go back and take that. And that's the approach that paleo, ancestral, primal gives us is going back to that template of saying okay, if we could not have dug this up or taken it off of a bush or a plant or a tree or something like that or we couldn't have hunted it, then it's probably not something we should be eating. So, all of these processed foods, removing all of that, removing some of these inflammatory foods from our diets is a really smart move because it creates health. It doesn't just create health, it creates optimized health. Especially when you think about paleo and primal as an actual lifestyle and not just a diet or a nutrition template, because that's really what it is.

Brendan [00:03:51]: Yeah, and you know when it comes to paleo, primal, ancestral, whatever we're going to call it, you know it seems like there are possibly some misconceptions out there about what it is, what it entails. You know, you described it as basically what our ancestors ate. There is potentially some debate about that itself. People in the vegetarian, or let's say vegan camp, might differ in their opinions as far as what we ate and so forth maybe. I don't know if we are going to tackle that one head-on or not, but I am curious to know what you have encountered as far as the perception of what paleo is about and how people see it and experience it.

Michelle [00:04:41]: Well, you know it's interesting because you know at one point ... actually because of this issue, because there can be this road block or kind of you know a closed mind mentality towards paleo, because there is a lot of myths and misconceptions about it and a lot of people believe that it's all meat, or that it's all bacon. I've heard that one, and that one cracks me up because man cannot live on bacon alone, I don't think. But it's weird to listen to some of this. One of the big things that I've heard probably the most is that they think that it's a raw type of diet, and I find that interesting because you know, cooking is one of the ... you know, there is scientific studies about cooking ... it's one of the ways that was able to actually help us grow our brains. So, kind of funny to hear all that, so it's just real interesting to see people's road blocks. So we were actually looking to change the name of Paleo f(x) because we had so many times where there were people that just had this pre-conceived notion of what paleo was without having any of idea of what it was. So we thought, you know, the problem is that we want to make sure that what we are doing at Paleo f(x) is continuing to reach the masses, continuing to reach the people that are not already singing from our hymn book and that need it, that don't have any idea that there is this whole way of eating out there that doesn't including taking any pills, doesn't include having to go to the doctor on a constant basis, doesn't include all of the things that most people think are normal now. So for us it's a mission to just really get the word out, so for us, we actually looked at changing our name to Health f(x) and we decided against it ultimately. But it is interesting because I think that a lot of those myths and misconceptions are out there and a lot of them have been created by people who are trying to scare people away from it and everything, and the simple fact of the matter is that it would have been much easier if we hadn't called this paleo or we hadn't called this primal and we called it you know, your Grandparents Diet, you know what I mean. Because this is really, most of our grandparents ate this way because they all mostly ate locally. They mostly ate from the farms that were around them. They didn't have processed foods. They didn't have a lot of sugar. They didn't have all of this. So it would have been good to name it that, but after a few generations that wouldn't work anymore. I think that it's interesting that there is so much misconception out there, but the problem is that's where we get into that place where people don't take responsibility for their own health, and they don't take responsibility for learning and really truly understanding. We are a very, you know, kind of a fly by the seat of our pants kind of people at this point in time. We are on the go all the time. We are in a hurry. We get our news and information in snippets, or in bullet points, or in now fake news, and so that's how things go down now. And so you have to have ways of being able to educate the public where they don't technically or necessarily know that they are being educated, but getting the information that they need so that they can make important decisions. And the thing is that it would be great if everybody just took responsibility for themselves and would do the work and do their homework, but that's just not where people are.

Brendan [00:08:50]: Well, you're really helping people I think by making the information more readily available and making it ... it's exciting. When I attended the Paleo f(x) in 2017 it was the best health and food event I have ever attended, and I learned a ton. The level of cutting-edge, science-based content was just off the charts, and I think the issue that comes up most saliently when it comes to paleo is the whole, "Is it all meat?" and "should humans be eating animals?" And people fall on different sides of that camp. Personally, I have wanted to, since college, not eat animals or didn't want sentient conscious beings to die for my food, but all the evidence and my personal experience say that at least my body is going to thrive better if I have some animal products, especially proteins ... the proteins and the fats. And it seems like that works for most people better than veganism, but I think that veganism can work for a certain number of people, I just don't know how long. Sometimes they run out of steam on that, and then eventually go back to adding animal products. But what I'd like to see is people of all persuasions no longer arguing about it and just coming together and say well let's find what we do agree about. So, you know, it's interesting you brought up the cooking issue, and there is you know some information online from vegan sources saying that you know its cooking starches, tubers, that contributed to the development of the human brain, and whether it was that or the meat or both, I don't necessarily think it was one or the other. I think that we are omnivores, and I think that the evidence is that we're omnivores, and therefore I see this approach to eating—the paleo, primal, ancestral—as scientific omnivorism. And so I think it's what's going to work for most people, but ultimately there is a lot of variability in my experience between people as far as what they need. But any other myths that you find ... you mentioned taste, and people being on the go all the time. So people are pressed and the hyperpalatable food comes in hyper-convenient packages and you know, people are just struggling to survive out there in the economy and in their lives and their families and so forth, and then maybe the idea of eating whole natural foods seems inconvenient and maybe boring. I'm just curious what you have found. Is that one of the myths?

Michelle [00:11:59]: Yeah, well I think, honestly, I think it is an excuse. So lots of people are out there ... they don't want to give up the foods that they are ... and I'm not preaching at anybody ... I'm talking with ya, because I was there. It was really difficult. So my speciality as a chef was Italian, so imagine, I made my own pasta and my own pizza dough and all of that. I had to give up the foods I loved the most and that I also was part of my repertoire and everything, in order to be healthy. And so the thing is that I understand that that can be very difficult. People have emotional ties to their food, and so when you start talking about taking things away from them they start kind of coming up with all kinds of excuses why that that doesn't work for them or that's never going to work, and it's just not convenient, and "Oh that's boring." And my thought process around that is focus on what you get to have, not on what you don't get to have because when you focus on those things, actually the food can be quite entertaining and can also become a challenge to create new stuff that you may not have ... I see it as building skills and building a new repertoire of foods that you can now get kind of those skills underneath your belt. So I look at it as more a challenge to make something that I would normally have thought ... Brussels sprouts for instance...

Brendan [00:13:39]: Oh I love them.

Michelle [00:13:41]: Brussels sprouts, never in a million years would I have ever thought that I would love Brussels sprouts. How boring is that food? You hear about that; it's even been in movies and stuff as we were growing up. The punishment is eating your Brussels sprouts, or you can't leave the table before you eat your Brussels sprouts, or you can't have your dessert before you eat your Brussels sprouts. Well now the Brussels sprouts recipes that I have, I prefer the Brussels sprouts over dessert. You know, that's something, that's just something that you build with playing with them. And I think it's an opportunity to go into the kitchen and unleash your creativity and actually play and have fun and find what are the tastes and flavours that work together.

Brendan [00:14:45]: I have no … yeah.

Michelle [00:13:47]: I find it a lot easier to eat this way than it is to eat the other way, and a lot of people … the other excuse is that it is expensive. Quite frankly, I can't say I agree with that because it's expensive to buy all of these you know snacks, and whatever. And you're eating so much, not to mention—and a lot of people forget this—you're paying in your health; you're paying ultimately down the road in your quality of life. Not just your quality of life now, but your quality of life down further on the road, and the thing is that my quality of life, yeah was eating this food and stuff, and I enjoyed it, but my life sucked. Because my health sucked, because I didn't feel good, I had pain, I had chronic inflammation, and I had horrible headaches. And so, how do you … you've got to be able to quantify that in some type of cost as well. And a lot of people look at this as a cost instead of an investment, and your health is an investment.

Brendan [00:15:56]: Yeah, I totally agree.

Michelle [00:15:58]: Yeah, and when you start eating this way, too, this is also helping the environment, because when we start getting rid of some of these hyper palatable foods … because this is the deal: if you stop spending money on them, they will stop making them, which ultimately down the line means the manufacturing processors and that type of thing will turn to something else, something that you want, something that you need. And so that's why you are seeing this surge in protein bars and in jerky and in meat bars and in all of these things. It's because people are wanting them. And so you will see manufacturing turned to that instead of Doritos, Fritos and Cheetos. Which I don't know about any of you, but I find it oddly weird that all of those end in "tos". It's crazy to me, so I'm like what was the thought process around that. Doritos, Cheetos and Fritos. But anyway, I digress. I just feel like this is a way to sustain our environment and our planet too. We need to be able to contribute in that, and that's part of what we're eating. When we're eating foods that are not serving our bodies they're definitely not serving the planet.

Brendan [00:17:14]: Yeah, it just so happens that both of those are … it's one and the same when you look at it. When you look at how food is being grown right now, the kinds of foods that's producing, even the fruits and vegetables just are a shadow of their former selves, the real food. I mean we can still do a lot by switching from, you know, Doritos to avocados or whatever, and of course we can make chips. We can still have chips in a different way, we just do them in a dehydrator or something if we are going to try and avoid the hydrogenated oils and the high temperature cooking and so forth and the GMO corn and all of that. But you know I think the hyper palatability issue deserves a little bit of … here's what I want to say about that: it turns out that we basically crave what we always eat, so our bodies get adjusted to it. That's why a lot of these diets out there are called resets. Because that's what happens is your tastebuds get reset. So if you go and just quit the Hagen Das and quit the this and that, there are tastier substitutions that are so much more enjoyable and good for the body and good for the planet, but you have to go through the reset. So you do have to give up the Doritos, for that you know, duration of three days to three weeks, depending … and then they're not going to be so appealing anymore. But if you start to indulge frequently, guess what, they are going to be real appealing again because they do have that hyper palatability factor. They've got the salt, the sugar, the fat, things our bodies really want and need. The sugar is a signal of mineral density in the natural world out there, but we've managed to make absolute cardboard sweet and salty and have the fat that our body is always looking for. And also, umami, right, that newly characterized flavor that we find in mushrooms and cheese and so forth. Of course, cheese is not considered a paleo food. So when you get pizza together, where you've got mushrooms and cheese and wheat, the umami factor is off the charts, and so that's like a perfect food that will cause over-eating like it did to me. When I was twelve I could eat a whole large pizza and did every time, until I developed intolerances to all of the ingredients. So in terms of this approach to eating, I think that what we can do in the kitchen, whether we put junk ingredients in there or fantastic highly nutritional medicinal ingredients, we can create the same kind of, roughly the same kind of flavour combinations, right? I mean you're a chef … it's just that the flavors could pop even more I would think minus the Dorito factor. Maybe we haven't mastered paleo Doritos, or have we?

Michelle [00:20:25]: Honestly, I got to say I find that the meats and fruits and vegetables in the most simplistic ways, are truly the best. Because you really get the flavors of whatever the foods are. I particularly … one of my favourite things ever, is just to mash up avocado, put a little bit of coconut oil in it and a little bit of sea salt—or I generally will use pink Himalayan—and that to me is the best snack ever, and just with a little bit of celery or cucumbers or something like that. Or there is some really great paleo friendly snack chips and stuff out there that all come to Paleo f(x) and I love those with it. But I find that sometimes the less you do to foods, the better they taste because you are getting the whole flavor of what they are. So it doesn't have to be complicated to be really super delicious. And you know you can always get into the sauces and stuff like that. And the thing is people feel like they're missing out on something, and in all honesty you're missing out less being paleo than you are on a SAD Western diet. You're getting everything that you need, what your body needs for satiety, for you to feel good and to have energy and all of that when you eat this way. It's just the way it is.

Brendan [00:21:58]: Totally. You mentioned Brussels sprouts. Recently I've gone on Brussels sprout binges where I have them … I eat them cooked. Most people probably do. And when you cook vegetables that are grown well, and say like mushrooms and green onions and Brussels sprouts and maybe some spices, some Italian spices, and that's more— oh my god, the flavors—you can do anything with it. It's so tasty, it can be so, so rich and nuanced and Doritos don't hold a chance, I think, once you've actually tried to actually eat real food. And if you season it well you can get amazing subtleties there, I mean amazing complexity there, let's say. But then just back to avocado, lime and salt, oh my God that's just to die for. I love it. So, anything else about paleo, since you are the Paleo f(x) woman? I'm just curious is there others ... or anything else to say about it as far as, you know, how you want it to be understood out there?

Michelle [00:23:13]: Well, this is the thing, one of the reasons that we created Paleo f(x) is to empower people in their health journey. And so the thing is, is that most people, we grew up believing that doctors were all-knowing. They were kind of gods. You do what they say. You don't question them, and quite frankly, that's really not the American way either. You're probably broadcasting this all over the world, but the majority of people that come to Paleo f(x) are Americans, and they don't question these people. And the thing is, they're humans. They aren't gods. They aren't all knowing. In fact, unfortunately, because the way the system is rigged against our doctors, our doctors don't have time to continue their education in the way that they need to, to stay up on the latest science and everything. And I can tell you, my current doctor who is wonderful is not as knowledgeable about nutrition as I am. And the majority of the people that I know and run with, most of the doctors that I know, don't know anything about nutrition. You know, the thing is that they get about 6 weeks, if they're lucky, of nutrition in a twelve-year to fifteen-year school education period.

Brendan [00:24:33]: I thought it was more like 6 hours, if that? I don't know.

Michelle [00:24:36]: My, well mine, I do know some doctors that got about 6 weeks. The thing is that they can be ... they're lucky if they get 6 weeks. It can be a whole lot less, they get a lot more on pharmacology than they do about nutrition and really, nutrition is the basis of all health. So one of the things that we have done at Paleo f(x), is we've put this into place, because we want to empower people to understand that it's not only their right, it is their obligation, to society, for them to take their own health in their own hands and become their own health advocate. The thing is, is that you have that right because you don't, you shouldn't just go in and blindly do anything that a doctor tells you to do. This is why you have second opinions, because men are fallible, and that's just the way it is. And I don't mean men, like as in just men.

Brendan [00:25:28]: Oh yeah you do. [chuckling]

Michelle [00:25:29]: Opinions are fallible, we are fallible humans. We make mistakes. We are totally not infallible, and so the thing is that unfortunately doctors kill people by pure accident, not by intention, because they are not able to keep up with the education that they need in order to make sure that they make good decisions for people. The thing is that we are never, ever going to get to the bottom of everything in health. It's just it. There is always going to be more to learn and more to learn and more to learn. And the more we learn, the more we are going to know we don't know. And so, the thing is that that means you need to be diligent in going in and understanding what is going on with your body and start listening to your body. That's the other thing is we can kind of tap out and go, "Okay well this seems ... this is normal. I have headaches every single day, I have chronic pain in my knee. My stomach hurts every single time that I eat. My back hurts. Oh it's just normal. It's just part of getting older." That's bullsh_t. The simple fact of the matter is that we were not designed to just have this slow decline into death. That's not how we're designed. Our bodies are miraculous. Our bodies are designed to heal themselves. The problem is, is that you have to put the right fuel into your body for it to do that work and what it was designed to do. And the thing is that when you do fuel your body the way that it's designed, it will run. It's kind of like a car, okay. So you want to drive a Ferrari, but you're treating it and putting in the things that you would put into a Volkswagen. No offence to anybody that's driving one.

Brendan [00:27:20]: I grew up with one, hey.

Michelle [00:27:21]: Alright, but if you want to perform like a Ferrari you don't treat yourself like a Volkswagen. That's just the bottom line. And the thing is, that it doesn't have to cost what a Ferrari costs. You just need to do the right things, and you need to learn, and you need to listen to your body. And when your body is giving you signals like you have knee pain, or you have back pain, or you have stomach pain, or you have headaches, they are all signals. Those are all signals to tell you "Hey, hey, hey I've got something wrong, can you please address it?" And instead, we go to a doctor, and we get a pill and then take the pill and then what it does is it damps down and it masks those symptoms to the point where we don't have the symptoms anymore, so voila, we're happy and we're good. While, all the while, there's this turmoil, this hurricane and volcano that's brewing underneath our skin that is going to erupt at some point, and then that's when guess what? You have this long, slow decline, painful most of the time, painful decline into death. And that's not how we are designed. We are designed to live until we die. And we are supposed to ... how people think is normal is for us to go like this and then go like that. And that's not it. We are supposed to be born; we are supposed to live; we are supposed to die. That's it. That's all. Born, live, die. And you're just supposed to drop off at the end, there is not supposed to be this long, slow painful death that's also costly. Because you talk about all of that, so the other part of it is all the cost factors that go into having poor health and not taking your health into your hands. Which is a drain on society, it's a drain on resources, it's a drain on your personal resources, it's a drain on your family, it's a drain on everybody that loves and cares about you because it's painful to watch somebody die a long, slow, painful death. So you owe it not just to yourself. You owe it to society. But you owe it mostly to the people who love you and care about you, your friends and your family. And so, like I say, I believe it's an obligation to research, to know what your, what are your symptoms. I mean that's the big thing. Become your doctor's partner, because he gets what, five minutes with you, maybe, maybe, in his office. Make those five minutes productive. Come in there with your questions ready. Go in there knowing what you've got going on. Go in there knowing your ideas, your thoughts around your health because that's the thing— they're in there for five minutes. They can't come up with ... "Okay, I have knee pain, I have back pain, I have stomach pain, I have headaches ..." whatever the case may be .... "I have all of these things going on," they can't do enough research to figure that out for you. So what they are going to do is, "Okay, well you know, you might need ..."—and one of the things that I find too is that for a lot of stuff they just start throwing them into these syndromes they don't have answers for, and so then you start getting on medication that actually may be detrimental to one of your other symptoms. And so, you end up in this cascade of taking a pill here to take care of this thing and then you have to take a pill here because that pill now causes something else. And it just goes into this downward spiral. My thought process is, get educated about your own health. Start tapping into what your body can do for you because your body can tell you what's wrong. Then you can start figuring it out from there.

Brendan [00:31:07]: You know, I totally agree. The body can tell you what's going on. The tongue is amazing. That's part of you know, the reset idea I think, which is you know, once you do some kind of reset back to real food, your tongue starts to tell you what you need in the moment and what is real food and what isn't. But if you've been only providing yourself with engineered foods, it doesn't really know. It's just going to choose what tastes good, what's the saltiest, sweetest and fattest-tasting thing, because that's typically in the natural world a signal of what the body needs.

Michelle [00:31:47]: Or the other part of it too, is when you start putting that on, it's kind of like a drug. So your tolerance keeps going up, so you need more. Going up, need more, going up, so you need more. So it's and quite frankly I honestly believe that sugar should be categorised as a drug because it's addictive, and it's much more difficult to get off of sugar than it is to get off of some drugs. So, for me, that's the best analogy, is, you have to think of these things like drugs. They are just increasing in tolerance so then you need more, and your tolerance goes up, and you've got to have more. And that's the way drugs work. And so when you have a system that's set up like this, this, there's no question why obesity is at all-time highs. In our entire history of the world, obesity is the highest it's ever been. Heart disease, highest it's ever been; cancer, highest it's ever been; diabetes, highest it's ever been. And it's starting to affect our children. That is what is scary as all get-out, is to watch and see what's happening to our children. Some of these kids don't even know what real food is, have no clue that when you eat, you know, chicken nuggets, that that actually comes from an animal. They have no clue. So it's kind of scary to see what's happening, and so when people don't recognise that these are all the parts of your body that work this way intentionally for your good and you just ignore them, it's a problem. And that's the other part of this too, is that ultimately damps down all your, all those senses and everything. So, I know people that are, will have something so incredibly sweet to the point where it makes my teeth hurt, makes my stomach kind of hurt, and they're like, "Oh no, it's not sweet," and I'm like, "Oh my God how much sugar do you need?" Or same thing with salt. I am super sensitive to salt. And the thing is we need salt. We have to have salt for vitality and to live and part of our energy source, but some people get crazy there, and that's because all these things have damped down their taste buds so they can't taste that either. So it'll go both ways. They've got to keep increasing their salt intake, and they've got to keep increasing their sugar intake. It's awful. Awful.

Brendan [00:34:26]: Yeah, you know you mentioned the cost and like people thinking that a real foods diet is just too expensive. But, actually, people like Diana Rodgers and Nora Gedgaudas, have put, they've looked at this, and they've analyzed it. And I'm sure there are others as well. I'm just mentioning two people in this event that people need to listen to, if only to hear the numbers on that. It (a processed food diet) costs more. It just does. The most exhaustive study I've heard of or analysis was done, was commissioned, let's say, by Nora Gedgaudas. She had somebody else create that analysis, and it costs less to eat primal than to eat chips and this and that. It can cost more (to eat real food), but in her analysis given the assumptions she is using, it costs less or similar. And the bottom line is, yeah the bottom line is …

Michelle [00:35:26]: You can buy all grass-fed all the time 100%, whatever, and you can buy the best and whatever, and yeah, like you can buy fillet mignon versus you know buying some hamburger. Of course, that's going to be ... cost less ...

Brendan [00:35:39]: Yeah, it's different sure, absolutely, each item. But, and as far as you know—this is something I think we all need to look at—and you brought up a really good point. As far as, you know, people love you. Do it for them if you're not going to do it for yourself. Do it for them. But also on the macro scale, our economy is under stress. I think 20% of GDP goes into health care cost. Well guess what? By 2040, it will, I don't know what percentage of GDP, but the prediction is that by 2040 our entire federal budget would be allocated, under current trends, it would be allocated only to health care. Nothing left for military, nothing left for whatever. Whatever people think is important that the government does, and so it's totally untenable. If we love our country, then let's eat healthy. If we love our siblings and parents and children, let's eat healthy and help them eat healthy and turn them onto this information and get them a free ticket to Paleo f(x) or whatever. Yeah, so that's my, that's my diatribe on cost. So, on...

Michelle [00:36:58]: The other thing, they don't relate the costs of, okay they think of the here and the now. But ultimately down the road, this is the thing ... with health care being where it is right now, and honestly nobody really knows where it is, like nobody knows what the system is that we are going to ultimately have. And like Obamacare ... if Obamacare is going to stay the way that it is, if it's going to change, if it's going to be completely dismantled, whatever the case may be. We don't even have any concept of what that system looks like. We don't have any concept of what's coming down the road. My suggestion is, make damn sure you don't need to be part of it. And the way to make sure that you don't need to be part of it is to be healthy, to get yourself healthy and to stay that way. The thing is, is so we don't know what that system is and so generally, when you don't know what something like that is going to be, it's going to cost us a lot of money. And under even just the circumstances of right now, if we just went based off of costs for right now for health care and for hospitalization and all of that, it is unbelievable how much it costs just to go to a hospital, even to go in outpatient. But if you had to go into a hospital for long-term care because you're sick, your quality of life needs to be taken into account and the cost of that ultimately on you and on your family. Are you going to leave your family a legacy, or are you going to leave your family in debt? And the simple fact of the matter is that right now, these people that are all really super unhealthy and that are in their last, on their last leg of life and are going through all of this process and believe that life is that long downward slog to death, the problem is that those people are spending their entire, everything that they have, their savings and everything to just be kept in this state of disease and "comfortable", whatever that means, until the moment that they die and they leave this Earth. And so, the exorbitant amount of money that is, in my opinion, wasted because that's a waste because it's preventable. If it wasn't preventable, it is what it is. But the majority of deaths in this country are related to nutritional issues that could have been prevented. And so, when we don't do that, we again tax resources. We tax our family, friends, all of that stuff. We deplete our, whatever, our legacy or what we could leave behind for our family, as far as any type of inheritance. We totally screw them all over. And so it's just a big burden to everyone. And I don't know ... the thing is like I said, that most of this is preventable. Heart disease is preventable. Cancer is preventable. Diabetes is absolutely preventable and reversible. This is the big thing: preventable and reversible. Now Type 1 right now is not reversible, but you can bring that down a whole lot. All of this stuff, the majority of these things, are completely preventable.

Brendan [00:40:25]: Preventable and reversible, yep. And it comes down like you said, to responsibility. And you know, I want to acknowledge paleo, the paleo movement and the vegan movement, for both being big on planetary stewardship, responsibility for the planet. Of course, there are disagreements and it's unfortunate that all animal products have been associated uniformly, universally with the factory farming system as if that's the only way animal products can be produced and therefore are evil. But, as far as planetary responsibility, I also see within vegan and paleo movements that sometimes that responsibility, in the planetary sense, is actually not fully implemented. I would love to see people really take that on because that's where food really comes back to life is if it's truly being grown in a way that's supporting the soil, biodiversity, water resources. And it just so happens that it can restore a lot of, restore landscapes, ecosystems and planetary cycles that we need to rebalance. And, if we just go halfway on the planetary ethic we are not going to get there, we are not going to make the difference. We can make a huge difference. And as omnivores—let's call ourselves omnivores as a substitute for paleo, primal, ancestral … there are subtle differences in there, among the three perhaps, or maybe none—but it seems to me that whether we are omnivorous or vegan we can actually be supporting tremendous … we can be the most regenerative or the most destructive force on the planet—because agriculture has that power—even vegan diets grown with conventionally grown grains that are still destroying soil, even in organic systems, many of them. So I just want everybody to get that these two movements have something in common. They don't have to agree on everything, but that thing in common is something that I want to see everybody embrace even further, which is let's take our food back to its full potential as medicine for bodies and for the planet. I'm just curious what your thoughts are on paleo and any other food movement as a potential consumer responsibility, consumer-driven antidote, to the public health and planetary disasters that industrialized agriculture has unleashed.

Michelle [00:43:19]: Well, I can tell you that we have attempted to get some people that are vegans to Paleo f(x), mainly for our sustainability panels and stuff, because I believe that we need to bridge that gap. The thing is, is that we agree on far more than we don't agree on. We both agree on good animal husbandry and respect for the environment. And the thing is, is that I know that we are categorized sometimes by vegans as just wanton carnivores, and that we are part … we don't … none of us believe in CAFO's. None of us believe in that.

Brendan [00:43:59]: Let me just define that for anybody who's new. "Confined animal feeding operation." CAFO. C-A-F-O.

Michelle [00:44:05]: So I, you know, we don't believe in them, so we all believe in farming responsibly. And, I don't know if your viewers have ever seen Allan Savory's TED talk on desertification. He goes into that and how we need to get back to doing things this way and go away from the factory farming, so that we can replenish our soil, so that we can bring our Earth back because we have really destroyed it with—you're completely correct—in some of the crops that are being grown that vegans eat readily are very destructive to the soil and very destructive to the planet. And the thing is that if they are done at this monocropping is what's happening, and it's destroying everything, all the soil. It's destroying the nutrient value of our soil, which ultimately it destroys the nutrient value in our foods in our fruits and our vegetables. And so, if we don't start doing something about it and get back to a type of farming that's not the monocropping, but is the crop and the soil rotation and the things that our Earth needs, we're going to be in a world of hurt because we're going to see more and more people sick because these CAFO's turn out meats and by-products of that that are not healthy and that are completely nutrient shallow. I don't know how else to say that. They just don't have the nutrient density that they need to have to sustain us as individuals. And so I would love to be able to have us come together as different "real" food movements because that's really what we believe in. Both of ... I believe both of our movements believe in that. I don't know how much vegans care whether or not it's processed because my understanding is that they do eat a lot of processed food.

Brendan [00:46:25]: Well, I don't think we can generalize. You know, I think there are different camps both in, yeah.

Michelle [00:46:29]: Oh yeah, so I don't know. I don't really know, but I would love for us to be able to sit down and talk about that and say, "Hey processed food is really not that great for you, and it's also not great for the planet," and then ultimately you know, on down the road, us have those discussions where we can learn from each other. But the thing is that at the end of the day, we have our government, particularly in the United States and in several governments around the world, that are trying to control our food. And this is the thing, that whoever controls our food, controls us. So, if we don't have food freedom, if we don't have the opportunity to choose how we want to eat and we are told how we are supposed to eat and then we are only given so many different types of things to choose from, the simple fact of the matter is that we lose power. We lose a lot of power, and the thing ... there's, there's legislation that's trying to come down now that will control a lot of different things. And it's a lot better if us as the real food movement, the vegan movement, the paleo movement, all of these movements come together and start working together because we have power in numbers. And the thing is that individually we won't have as much power as we would together to be able to stop some of that and to also start making sure that we start trying to pull away from this factory farming. The thing is that's all coming down because Big Ag and Big Pharma and all of the big Corporate America stuff, is coming down because they want us to be dependant. They want us to be controllable, and so it's not you know, tin foil hat. Let's be honest, if we haven't all noticed our freedoms, and particularly in America, are being diminished pretty regularly at this point, and we're allowing it to happen. And this is one of the biggest things we can never allow to happen ... that we are never, ever told what we can and cannot eat. And so, I think that it behoves us to come together as these food movements and start working together to ... and set aside our disagreements, such as, "I believe you should not eat animals," or whatever the case may be. We've got to stop all of that and come together because our numbers will be powerful to be able to stop that from happening.

Brendan [00:49:05]: You know that is so true, this ... you know what you said about, we are being controlled, and we don't necessarily realize it. And so in some ways Kraft American cheese is the most un-American thing if it's un-American to allow your government to control you with your food choices, what's available to you, now it's grown, and subsidizing a way to grow food that impoverishes the body and the Earth. So thank you for calling that out. Because eating can be not only a medical act—right, you can heal yourself with this stuff—it's (also) an economic act where we're sending our vote through our pocket book out into the market place and ...

Michelle [00:50:00]: It's economic and political.

Brendan [00:50:02]: And political, yeah, that's what I was getting to next, and that makes it ... yeah, it becomes political. So eating, that's where it all begins in a way. There's a lot more that springs from our food choices than we actually necessarily realize until we really examine it. It's like, whoa, it spreads out. So, thank you for calling that out, and I want to encourage everybody, as much attention as you are now going to pay—and I know a lot of the viewers already do pay a lot of attention, right—we're all paying a lot of attention to our health, some of us more than others, and I just want to encourage everybody to realize that understanding how food is grown is the next dimension of that, like really getting as fascinated about that as we do about phytochemicals, let's say, and polyphenols, you know, things that we talk about in health circles. So, that's all coming from how food is grown, and of course how our food is grown is affecting many things out there in the world, not just the planet, but economic systems, political, refugee crises and so forth. It's, anyway, we'll leave that for another conversation, but thank you for bringing this kind of information, the paleo information, which you're going to rebrand as Health f(x). You have other events as well now called Health f(x), smaller events. Say something briefly about that, like what is that about?

Michelle [00:51:40]: Yeah, we have Health Entrepreneur f(x), which is an event that is skewed towards entrepreneurs in the health and wellness space, who we're trying to make sure that they get the type of support and information that they need to be able to grow their businesses. Because when they do, it actually helps all of us. And so that's one of the events that we have. We do have Health f(x) as that's an entire IP that we purchased several years ago to start creating a place for us to move to. Like we needed to get away from the paleo moniker, and so what our intention around that is going to be is probably creating some smaller events around the country and around the world, where we can get people used to paleo that might otherwise kind of have a closed mind or a pre-conceived notion about what it is, and so that we get them introduced to paleo and then ultimately into Paleo f(x) and then understanding what the movement is about, so they can really, really, understand what true health is about.

Brendan [00:52:54]: Beautiful. It's such a noble mission and thank you for that and you're just such a great example for anybody who's suffered and come out victorious and also for anybody who has, I guess, felt trapped financially. You've created a growing entrepreneurial empire that fires you up and heals people, so thanks for all that you do, and thank you for being here with us in the Eat4Earth community.

Michelle [00:53:31]: Thank you, appreciate it.

Nora Gedgaudas Interview
Slow Aging, Super Power Your Brain, and Save Your Life: Your Primal Fat-Burning Blueprint

Brendan [00:00:00]: Welcome to the Eat4Earth event. This is Brendan Moorehead, and together we're exploring how you can heal yourself, your loved ones, and the planet with food. Our next guest, Nora Gedgaudas, is a widely recognized expert on what is popularly referred to as the paleo diet. She's the author of the international best-selling book, *Primal Body, Primal Mind: Beyond the Paleo Diet for Total Health and a Longer Life*. She's also the author of the bestselling e-book, *Rethinking Fatigue: What Your Adrenals are Really Telling You and What You Can Do About It*, and her latest book, which I'm totally in love with, is *Primal Fat Burner: Live Longer, Slow Aging, Super-power Your Brain, and Save Your Life With a High-fat, Low-carb Paleo Diet*. Nora is an experienced board certified nutritional consultant and clinical neurofeedback specialist, speaker and educator, widely interviewed on national and international radio, popular podcasts, online summits, television, and film. Nora, you are an extreme powerhouse of information. I can't wait to get into this, and thank you for being here!

Nora [00:01:07]: Well, it's an honor, Brendan. Thank you so much for having me.

Brendan [00:01:11]: So yeah, I'm excited because I've just started to tap into experiencing ketogenic metabolism. I'm not sure that I'm fully adapted yet, but I started to see some differences. It's awesome. I mean it's just like ... it's amazing. You know, in your book, *Primal Fat Burner*, what's fascinating to me—'cause I just geek out on everything—but you present some amazing evidence about human fat in the human diet and in our evolution. And I'm curious if you could just kind of give us a bit of the evidence. Are you saying that humans are essentially lipovores, in other words, fat burners?

Nora [00:01:54]: Well, what I am saying ... there are a couple of sort of unusual hypotheses or sort of unprecedented, I should say, hypotheses in my book, *Primal Fat Burner*, which sounds like a weight loss book, which, you know, that might be somebody's favorite side effect, but that's not the focus. It's really about adopting a fat-based metabolism as opposed to a sugar-based metabolism. But it forwards the hypothesis that dietary fat, including dietary animal fat and fat-soluble nutrients, are not simply arguably central to human health, but they're literally central to what made us human in the first place. And as a species early on or as an evolving species, we developed an unprecedented—insofar as other primates go—taste for animal fats that was not really shared by other primates to the same degree. This was evident in some of the first hominins, you know, the evidence that we have from some of the earliest hominin sites where they found stone tools that were used to cleave the meat and marrow from the bones of animals, for instance, that either they were scavenging or possibly even hunting.

[00:03:14]: And one of the things that's true about dietary fat is that it's certainly a lot more calorically dense than either carbohydrates or protein, and that nutrient density ... because it also tends to be very high in fat-soluble nutrients ... it's not just about energy, but it supplies us with ... you know, I think we figured out that fat ultimately means survival for us, that when we consume fat, it's satisfying for a longer period of time. It's something that we developed a taste for very early on in a way that was kind of unprecedented in the rest of the animal kingdom. Now, mind you, even obligate herbivores, like ruminants, for instance, and other herbivores, even though their diet is extensively based upon carbohydrate foods, right, and in order to meet those dietary requirements, you know what herbivores do. Their faces are in the grass and into the bushes and the trees and whatever else, and they're eating more or less constantly during their waking hours in an effort to meet their nutrient requirements. But interestingly, where they're getting at least 70 percent of their calories is not carbohydrates, but is in fact short-chain saturated fats from the bacterial fermentation of all that fiber that they consume all day long. And it's those big vats of bacteria in their guts that are responsible for their digestive process and are responsible for extracting all of the nutrients from those foods to basically nourish and fuel them. And so, even herbivores are actually designed to rely on fat as a primary source of fuel. We as supposed omnivores … and I say "supposed" … yeah, we're omnivores. That doesn't mean that everything we consume is equally beneficial or nourishing for us, everything that we're capable of consuming. But we actually have a hydrochloric acid based digestive system as opposed to a fermentative one.

[00:05:41]: Now, even the chimps that, you know, chimpanzees that are supposedly our closest primate cousins … For one thing, all great apes hunt and consume at least some meat, with the exception of herbivorous gorillas, which by the way have a brain about a third of the size that would be expected for a primate of their size. But chimps have a much longer fermentative section to their gut than we do. The fermentative portion of our digestive apparatus is, you know, our colon, makes up only about 20 percent of our total digestive tract. We have a much longer small intestine, much shorter large intestine, than even other primates, much less other animals that are designed to eat a plant-based diet. And we also have ample gallbladders, right? So, we are really, truly designed to get fat, not from bacterial fermentation, but from animals that we consume that have synthesized those fats for us in a much wider variety than would otherwise be available in, say, raw plant foods and what have you, or even through fermentation. So yeah, we have this … you know, chimps, on the other hand, the fermentative portion of their gut makes up at least 52 percent of their digestive tract. And you know, chimps look like they've got beer guts. They have these big barrel guts, gorillas especially, they look like they've been drinking beer all day. And that is because they have a diet that is much higher in fibrous plant foods. And it's sort of interesting when you consider that a chimp has a brain that is a third or smaller of the size of the average human, and that brain hasn't really changed in its morphology or its capacity or its size, for that matter, in about seven million years. Well, why is that? Because really, they haven't really changed what it is that they're consuming. You know, they're still kind of swinging in the trees and eating all those leaves and bananas. You know, we had an intrepid ancestor that swung out of the trees, decided to stand up on two legs on a, presumably a very drought-stricken African Savanna, where they could see longer distances by standing up on two legs and develop opposable thumbs, able to grasp and create tools and implements. And they began a process of scavenging, probably initially, and later hunting. And by 2 million years ago, you know, it's pretty well established now within the peer-reviewed anthropological literature that we already had an established hunting economy as an evolving species by then. And that was the very first, you know, hominin of the genus Homo … Homo Erectus was already pretty much a full-time hunting animal. We have a brain that has more than tripled in size in this relatively brief span of time. In terms of evolutionary biology, it's truly unprecedented in all of the animal kingdom. And one thing that characterizes us versus other animals, and particularly even other carnivores, other hunting animals, I should say, is that ... well, let me put it this way, because I've spent time working with wild wolves, right? I spent time living in the High Arctic, less than 500 miles from the North Pole, with a family of wild wolves. That's a whole other podcast, you know, that's a whole other deal.

Brendan [00:10:02]: Quick comment. I read the book *Arctic Dreams* a long time ago.

Nora [00:10:05]: Yeah, Barry Lopez. Yeah. I know him, actually.

Brendan [00:00:00]: You brought that book right back, and I was just, you know, that book deeply affected me. Just reading a book about the Arctic was amazing.

Nora [00:10:18]: Lopez is just about my favorite natural history writer. There's just nobody that can touch his eloquence. Also, his wife was an archivist. So, I mean he had access to a tremendous array of literature to create from. But what an immensely creative man. He also lives here in Oregon. And yeah, I was pinching myself the day I finally met him because, you know, he influenced me a lot actually. He wrote a wonderful book called *Of Wolves and Men* as well that I thought was just really a profound piece of literature. But yeah, *Arctic Dreams,* I actually had a copy of that with me while I was up on Ellesmere Island, so that I could really more fully appreciate my surroundings. But at any rate, one of the things ... and of course, I bring this up now because I'm making the case for the fact that I've observed this first hand, that when a predator hunts its prey, for the most part, they're going after the weak, the sick, the infirm, you know, the very young, not because they prefer that kind of meat, but mainly because that's easiest for them to catch. It just stands to reason that they can only run so fast, and all that kind of thing to go after. And it's extremely risky to hunt animals in their prime. It's very difficult and it's very risky to hunt animals that are better able to defend themselves and harder to catch and whatever else. And so ... but we developed this unique capacity as a species. We developed a capacity for technology, and we developed an ability to be able to create hunting implements that allowed us to more selectively choose what we hunted.

And mind you, the other thing that we kind of forget, because I think that a lot of people look at the natural environment out there, and they assume that it's very similar to what prehistoric humans faced as an ecosystem and environment when, in fact, for one hundred thousand generations or so, it was an extremely different planet. And we shared this planet with at least 120 more species of enormous herbivores that we call megafauna. And usually, the larger the animal, not always, but very often is the case with the larger the animal, the higher the body fat level of that animal. Now, we know woolly mammoths, of course, is sort of the stereotypical megafauna that we all think of when we think of the majority of the Quaternary Ice Age. You know, the whole Pleistocene scene ... which was an animal we definitely preferentially hunted, but there were so many others, so many others. But just as an example, woolly mammoth they estimated had roughly 50 percent body fat—and they're extrapolating this from what we know about elephants, which also primitive humans would have hunted—and had roughly four inches of subcutaneous fat beneath their hides that we would've gobbled up along with the marrow and the brain tissue and everything else. And you know, you take down a fat and sassy woolly mammoth and you've got about a week's worth of family barbecue to come. And we were able, with the technology that we had and the smarts that we had, to be able to selectively hunt these animals and bring them down where, you know, wolves and lions and things like that would have had a much more difficult time bringing down something that huge. They were bringing down smaller, typically more fleet-of-foot prey, that they were designed to go after. But you know, we were able to be more selective, and it turns out all the observations of human hunting—and I cite a lot of this in my book, and I have a lot more citations than were able to actually make the book—but we were quite selective in the way we hunted animals, based on how fat and sassy they were.

Brendan [00:14:40]: How did we …. I'm curious, you know, because I read a book, a very popular book, recently that I love. I love a lot of parts about it, but one of the assertions there … and I actually haven't looked at the… it was audiobook that I was listening to, and I haven't looked at the print book to see what citations were attached to it, but it basically said that this idea that we hunted woolly mammoths and ate all this big game and lots of it was either not supported or was not properly interpreted or something. So, I was just curious. What's the evidence?

Nora [00:15:13]: Actually, there was a recent article published in *Science Daily,* pretty recent, saying no, what mainly what we had on our plate was woolly mammoth meat, fat, and vegetables. That was actually what has shown up. And we have stable isotopic analysis now from the Max Planck Institute for Evolutionary Anthropology in Leipzig, Germany … has done decades now of stable isotopic analysis of the human bone and collagen remains of our ancestors from all periods of our evolutionary history and have found consistently, even in the Mediterranean regions, where you would guess that they might have preferred seafood, that our preference was nearly always for extremely large terrestrial herbivores. And in many places where woolly mammoths flourished, those would've been a major item on the menu. A lot would have depended, of course, upon the specific ecosystem that humans were hunting in, but there's no question that we had a preference, in any case, for extremely large terrestrial herbivores, the majority of which would have had high levels of body fat versus … you know, once we arrived at the end of the last ice age, where there was just a very sudden and cataclysmic climate change, and there was an extinction event, effectively, that rivaled that of the demise of the dinosaurs. At least 120 species of megafauna just vanished in like the blink of an eye. And you could see there's just a huge spike in extinction, and all of a sudden now we're left with … and I'm sure human populations probably bottlenecked during that time, too. But we were left with a much smaller array of prey to hunt that was much more fleet-of-foot and harder for us to catch, more challenging.

And it's not that fat was any less important. It just, in fact, it became all the more precious. And it's known that human hunters, you know, kind of more Neolithic hunting populations and things that have been observed, were observed to have hunted preferentially for fat by being able to observe the curves of an animal and just … You know, they went for fat, and they hunted most aggressively during the times of the year, like in the fall, when the animals would be fattest, right, and have the most fat on their bodies. Now, even though the meat of younger animals is more tender, they always went for the older animals that would have had much more fat. Even aboriginal hunters in the Outback, because this isn't just about cold climates, if they, say, killed a kangaroo, if that kangaroo was overly lean, they would just leave it in the sun to rot and go after a fatter and sassier one.

Brendan [00:18:28]: Interesting!

Nora [00:18:30]: Lean protein is not necessarily our best friend in huge quantities. And this is where I actually run a little bit into odds, shall we say, with perhaps what is the majority of the so-called Paleo community out there of people promoting Paleolithic diets. You know, just because our ancestors did something, and we did consume a lot of lean meat along the way, isn't necessarily a good enough reason for me to want to do exactly the same thing now. And ...

Brendan [00:19:04]: I suppose that could play the same way for eating so much fat, right? I'm just thinking in terms of all this thinking that, "well, fat is the enemy", but what I what I'm gathering from all of this is the picture that's emerging for me is, okay, if we originated from a largely herbivorous primate species, we were getting most of our calories from saturated fat as a result of the ...

Nora [00:1933]: Well, from animal fat, only a portion of which is saturated, right? It's not just saturated. I mean, if you have a steak on your plate from a grass-fed animal, I mean, close to half of that fat might be saturated, but the higher percentage is actually going to be unsaturated fat, monounsaturates, polyunsaturates, hopefully a good amount of omega-3s in there, which are highly polyunsaturated. And you know, it's not the absolute amounts of any one kind of fat that is at issue. It's the relative balance, right? Saturated fat in and of itself, I think, is among the most neutral of fat sources. In other words, it's neither good nor bad. It just sort of has a role to play. It's certainly protective. It gives our cell membranes integrity and allows for a certain degree of permeability of our cell membranes. It also helps to preserve some of the more delicate polyunsaturated fats and transport them to places in the body where they can be safely incorporated into our tissues and utilized, helps us digest protein. So, saturated fat has a number of beneficial roles to play. It's not the be-all -and-end-all of fat. And I would never say that, but I would also never ... Yeah, go ahead.

Brendan [00:20:56] Herbivorous primates, you mentioned that they were getting a lot of their calories, not directly from the plants, but from the ... I suppose butyrate, propionate . . .

Nora [00:1933]: Yeah, short-chain saturated fats.

Brendan [00:21:10]: Well, ironically, our potentially more herbivorous ancestors might have been getting a higher percentage of their calories from saturated fat, but I don't know. But maybe as you look at the ... if you summarize the whole evolution of our lineage, we found a way over time to go more directly for fat, potentially as a result of climatic changes, reduction in forest cover where now we're out in a more open environment ... which might explain why we still have vestiges of an herbivorous digestive tract, because alkaline saliva, and we don't have the slicing, crushing, you know, structures in our jaw and teeth that what we call normal carnivores have. Yet we've evolved a higher stomach acid and a shorter digestive tract, but not a totally smooth digestive tract. So, it's kind of like gotten part way towards a carnivore, but not all the way. So, we still have vestiges of ...

Nora [00:22:21]: Well, our digestive system has way more in common with carnivores than herbivores, right? We don't have the capacity that an herbivore does to extract all of the available nutrition in plants.

Brendan [00:22:31]: Yeah, definitely not.

Nora [00:22:33]: But in theory, there's calcium and there are all these minerals and things in certain plant foods, but what gets kind of lost along the way is that fact that in humans, it actually takes the presence of hydrochloric acid in sufficient amounts to be able to ionize those minerals, for instance, to make them absorbable by us. And we're designed not to synthesize nutrients the way that herbivores do from bacterial fermentation, but to get them directly from animals that have synthesized those nutrients for us. It's a much more efficient way of getting nutrition. We're designed to eat a far more nutrient-dense diet. And the evidence also shows—and I cite this in my book, and in my talks—I actually show a nifty little graph that you just look at the graph and you know. Unfortunately, the publisher didn't want me publishing scientific graphs, which really bummed me out because I was excited to share it. But anyway, but that showed that among all primate species that we have an unprecedented brain size that is directly proportional to the nutrient density of our diets. In other words, the proportion ... what they call the high-quality diet that is based in meat and especially fat calorically. And again, when I talk about eating a diet that is mostly fat, I'm talking about calorically speaking. Fat has twice the calories per gram of protein or carbohydrate, and it actually takes a lot less fat to equal the caloric intake of either of those kinds of foods. And so, it doesn't take a lot to actually be satiating, to be satisfying. The idea is to get those fats from as wide a variety of sources as we can to meet not just our energy requirements, but to meet our structural and immune requirements.

And also, you know, we have a rather unique brain, not just in so far as how large it is, but the composition of our brain is quite different. The dominant fatty acids, for instance, in the non-human primate brain that's responsible for its cognition are largely omega-6 based. For us, it is predominantly omega-3 based. And so, the two fatty acids that are most responsible for human cognition, out of all of them include both arachidonic acid and also docosohexaenoic acid, both of which are found within the diet exclusively in animal source foods. And we can't make DHA from plant-based omega-3 fats at all. Arachidonic acid, an argument could be made that we would be able to synthesize some arachidonic acid from plant-based fats. But if you're lacking a particular enzyme that is involved in that elongation process—it's called delta 6 desaturase—which if you're of northern European descent, Celtic descent, native descent, you may not produce that enzyme at all. You may have a zero capability. But one thing's for sure, that if DHA is not in your diet, it's not in your brain. And our ancestors got the majority of their DHA from the fat of the animals that they hunted, fat of animals that had fed upon foods that were natural to them, in other words, natural green forage. If you're eating feedlot meat, you're probably not getting any DHA there, either. And you're probably getting excesses of omega-6s that are more likely to be pro-inflammatory than anything beneficial. You might get arachidonic acid, but docosohexaenoic acid is supposed to be more predominant. So, we're unique that way. We're unique that way, and our brains are constructed—our unusually large and sophisticated brains, maybe with some exceptions, but I'm not naming names —are constructed from the very fats that we supply them with, with what it is that we choose to eat.

Brendan [00:26:50]: I'm curious how you would explain the fact that some people … and I don't know what the percentage is. I mean, I know that there's plenty of people that bomb out, crash out, fall out, whatever, of vegan diets, and I was one of them. I mean, I didn't really try it for that long. I tried vegetarianism for eight years. But there seem to be some that do it for a long time, remain passionate about it. How do you suppose they're surviving, and of course, a lot of them are—not necessarily, of course—but a lot of them are advocates of a starchivore hypothesis for the evolution of a sugar-burning brain. And so, given that some of them seem intelligent and can carry forth a good conversation …

Nora [00:27:41]: Yeah, I mean, your brain is amazing in its capacity to compensate for things. And the fact of the matter is that an estimated less than two percent of the population is vegetarian or vegan to begin with. And out of that, you know … I mean, that's still a fair number of people, but there are at least a few different studies that have shown anywhere from 75 to 85 percent of all vegetarians and vegans end up abandoning that way of eating, usually within a decade of starting, mainly or predominantly due to health-related concerns. So, I think the people that are most passionate about their vegetarian and vegan lifestyles are the ones that have been at it for not a very long period of time.

Brendan [00:28:29]: There are some doctors who have been doing it for 30 years, let's say.

Nora [00:28:34]: Well, if you're talking about some of the doctors that I'm thinking of, I wouldn't necessarily want to emulate their disposition. Dispositions are … you know, I mean, again, I think that what we're talking about is a relative capacity to tolerate certain things. There are some people, for instance, that appear to tolerate grains better than others, but there's no one for whom grains are an optimal food. This is not something that the human digestive system and the human immune system was ever designed to put up with, certainly not as a primary source of nourishment, but there are people that seem to do okay on those foods for a while, until they're not doing okay anymore. And so, usually the most passionate proponents of these things, those that seemingly do okay long term—and again, we're talking about seemingly okay long term— are going to be a radical minority.

Brendan [00:29:42]: What would you make of the oft-cited—I don't know how oft-cited—but there was a discovery that stone tools from about 105,000 years ago in Mozambique indicated that the early humans of that time were collecting sorghum grass seeds and grinding them and eating them?

Nora [00:30:09]: I will point out that by 200,000 years ago, we already had our large brains. So, certainly we would not have … and then about 10,000 years ago, our brains started shrinking in earnest. And we've lost roughly 11 percent of our brain volume in the last 10,000 years since we adopted agriculture and more of a carbohydrate-based diet. We adopted agriculture because we understood the fact that some of those foods were edible, right? But just because those things were edible doesn't mean that they were optimal foods for us, right? And again, some things we did just because we needed to survive, because it was convenient, it gave us calories, in the face of maybe a lack of other things that we might have preferred to consume. And …

Brendan [00:30:59]: Wasn't that the point where just before that when the megafauna had … there were several extinction events, but wasn't the final blow … let's say, was … maybe culminated about 12,000 to 13,000 years ago, something like that?

Nora [00:31:21]: Yeah. Roughly in there, yeah. The really cataclysmic … I mean, you're right. There were a series of things that happened where things were just rocking back and forth climate-wise. And so, yeah, at that point, we were forced to come up with something else. And we had observed animals gnashing on grass seeds and thought, I wonder if we could make use of that food, and figured out we could mash it up and, you know, kind of make a porridge out of it and eat it. It doesn't necessarily mean it was ever an optimal food for us at all. And again, one of the things that characterizes my work … and like I say, I'm not wed to doing something just because our ancestors did it. You know, our ancestors weren't necessarily trying to live the longest possible life free of disease and whatever else. They weren't going for longevity. They were going for survival. They probably understood more about what was healthy for them than we do, but they didn't have science, for instance, to be able to evaluate the nutritional content of the foods they consumed.

Brendan [00:32:30]: You know, it strikes me that … kind of what you alluded to earlier is that you have an approach that's different from maybe other paleo approaches …

Nora [00:32:40]: Yes, yes, yes.

Brendan [00:32:43]: You call it "beyond Paleo". I'm just curious, how…

Nora [00:32:46]: That's where I was going with this, it was the human longevity research, I'm using human longevity research, basically, to evaluate what…

Brendan [00:32:54]. Right, just because we want what's optimal, you know. We want a long life, we want good cognition, and we want to look good in our jeans. Okay, boom. What do we need to do, right?

Nora [00:33:04]: We know what's important. Yeah. So, what longevity research … So, for instance, the Paleo thing … You know, the foods that would've been available to us as an evolving species the most consistently would have absolutely served to establish our basic nutritional requirements and our physiological makeup. And I think that's the only rational starting place we have, is really looking at what our ancestors did as a general litmus of what is it that we're actually genetically adapted to consuming now. Right? What's in alignment with our human evolutionary and genetic heritage. What longevity research allows us to do is to take a look at those fundamental principles of, so-called Paleolithic principles, and then evaluate them for, you know, how well they're able to keep us optimally healthy long enough to be able to lead a longer and healthier life. And so, what we know from the 100 years or so of longevity research now is that there are two primary factors that seem to be kind of the rate-limiting factors for our health and longevity.

One is that we know now that the less insulin we require over the course of our lives, the longer we're likely to live and the healthier we're going to be by far. And since dietary sugar and starch are the primary impetus for the production and secretion of insulin in terms of what dietary factors are going to stimulate its release, in any case, and because there is no such thing as an established human dietary requirement for carbohydrates in any form by science, not in any medical textbook or any textbook of physiology, to me it's kind of a no brainer. Let's leave out the sugar and starch to the extent possible to minimize our production of insulin along the way. The other thing that we more recently discovered was the fact that when we consume protein in excess of what we need for our maintenance and repair, that triggers certain reproductive mechanisms that stimulate cellular proliferation.

Now, if you're pregnant or wanting to become pregnant or you're a baby, child, or teen that is growing and needs to make new cells, well then eating a higher amount of protein makes sense. But if you're not growing or reproducing and you're not really … you know, you have had no need to do that, when we consume protein in excess of what we need, we're triggering metabolic pathways that have greater odds of triggering things like cancer. You know, you take a mutated cell—and God knows we're exposed to so many mutagenic substances in modern life that our prehistoric ancestors weren't exposed to—but you take a mutated cell, and then you give it a proliferative impetus, as with over-consuming protein or excessive insulin, you're basically creating much higher odds of creating cancer.

And so … but the interesting thing is that when you limit that protein to just underneath that threshold, and it's through a mechanism—there is a protein sensor that we have metabolically that's known as mTOR, which stands for "mammalian target of rapamycin", and when we limit our production or release of mTOR, what we instead do is send a message that, "you know what, there's not quite enough nutrient availability to reproduce right now." So—and I put this in modern day economic terms that people can kind of relate to—it's too expensive to build a new house right now. So, let's fix up the one we've got. And what gets fixed up is you. Your body goes into a repair and regeneration mode instead of a making-new-cells mode, which is a very expensive thing to do. And by doing that, it literally has an anti-aging effect. But the two mechanisms for aging and for degenerative disease and cancer and whatever else, from that standpoint, are really relegated to protein and carbohydrates.

Dietary fat is not really included in that equation, in that same equation, in that it appears to be a free fuel insofar as we can consume as much of it as we want. It's not going to trigger these adverse metabolic pathways. If we're consuming fat, for instance, in the absence of high carbohydrate foods, or like sugar and starch, it does not have the same deleterious effects and in fact supplies us with a fair amount of energy and also nutrition because there are a lot of fat soluble nutrients in fatty foods of high quality. It creates for us an ability to go longer without eating, allows us to eat less protein without feeling deprived, allows us to not have to rely on a carbohydrate-based metabolism, which I sometimes refer to as a state of metabolic enslavement.

Brendan [00:38:39]. Yeah, I can relate to that because … God, I mean, my whole life, sugar burner. And you know, I have tried … Even when I was doing intermittent fasting for the last two years, I still was not … So I'm still a sugar burner. I would have to reload on carbs every few days. And so, just recently really started to break into some ketogenic metabolism. It's a different world.

Nora [00:39:05]: It is!

Brendan [00:39:06]: Carbohydrates don't even … They still taste a little bit attractive here and there. And then I have a few bites, and it's gone. Like a few bites, I'm done, and its no longer … [unintelligible] I'm like, "I think I need some fat now." And so, I'm curious, though, because there's so many recommendations for fat out there. There's 0.4 grams per kilogram lean mass all the way out to …

Nora [00:39:]: Oh, you're talking about protein.

Brendan [00:39:06]: Did I say fat? I meant protein, yeah. Excuse me. So, 0.4 grams of protein per kilogram lean mass is the lowest-ish I've seen all the way up to 0.8 grams for kilogram of lean mass or ideal body weight, which is how you do it.

Nora [00:39:50]: Right. I do it that way because the majority of the researchers have used relative to lean body mass. Well, how many people are going to go out and figure out their exact percentage of lean tissue mass. It's a difficult thing to do. You know, it can be a little complicated to do, and the average person simply isn't going to do it. When a person estimates their ideal bodyweight, most people idealize their weight when they're lean, right? And that's going to… it's going to be closer. It's going to be closer to reflecting lean tissue mass.

Brendan [00:40:29]: [unintelligible] See, if I use … from one book, my ideal protein consumption is only 29 grams a day. That's too little for me. I mean, I've tried it. I can do it for a few days, in fact, being keto makes it fine for a few days, and then I start to feel the backlog, and I start to wind down, feel weak, don't want to exercise, stuff like that.

Nora [00:40:51]: You know, what I did was I did a guesstimate, right, based on … So, a lot of the early researchers said, okay, one gram per kilogram of body weight of lean tissue mass. Well, okay, I'm going to say 0.8 because it's easier to estimate that from an estimated ideal body weight. Right? It comes a little closer to being in that ballpark. Now, the 0.4 grams per kilogram might be quite appropriate for somebody who's been, say, either at high risk or had been diagnosed with cancer. I would definitely go down to that level. But here's some of the relative concern with the lower amounts of protein. The point is well taken when it comes to going a little lower on that, but the problem is not everybody digests well.

Brendan [00:41:41]: Yeah, and I have an issue with that.

Nora [00:41:43]: Right. And so, if you have issues generating sufficient hydrochloric acid to be able to break the protein down, or your pancreatic enzymes aren't up to snuff or whatever, for whatever reason, and there can be lots of reasons. There are lots of things to interfere with this. We could do a whole podcast on just that. Then …

rendan [00:42:00]: You do in your book. I mean, your book is such a resource. I'm just going to plug it. It's such a resource. You cover all of this in so much depth. But go ahead. What were you going to say?

Nora [00:42:10]: Yeah, yeah. So, I was going to say that if your digestion isn't optimal, then you may ... you know, the idea is that you want to be able to extract all that you can from the nutrition you consume, especially if you're moderating your protein intake. This is not a high-protein diet that I'm advocating here. It's a very moderate protein diet. You know, if you looked at my dinner plate, you might think I was a vegetarian at first glance because there'd be all these vegetables and whatever. And then you'd be like, "Oh no, look, there are little bits of meat in there." And then if you did a calorie analysis of what was on there, you'd see the majority of the calories were actually coming from fat, from a variety of fats. But you know, to look at the plate, you might not know it kind of a thing. So, it's not like everything is floating in grease or anything like that.

It doesn't take that much fat to dominate calorically a plate of vegetables. You've got a smattering of calories, and protein has roughly four calories per gram, and the majority of the protein that we're consuming is really going to go to meeting our kind of regeneration and repair needs. It's not there to be a source of energy production for us, which would be glucose production, anyway, for the most part. A certain percentage of the amount of protein that we consume in excess of what we need for maintenance and repair gets converted to glucose. It's a laborious process. It doesn't spike your blood sugar, but it would get used ultimately the same way. But you know, dietary fat is just inherently satisfying. But it's important when we're moderating our protein intake for these purposes, that our digestion be as optimal as possible. And unfortunately, it isn't in a lot of people. So, I erred on the side of slightly more than some people suggest, but I also qualified that, I believe, in the book, at least in the original manuscript version of it, I did, saying that if you've been diagnosed with cancer, you may want to go lower. You may want to cut that in half.

A lot of people who are really ... their book is focused more on longevity. Those are the ones that like ultimate longevity, and they're not addressing that nuance. Like, hey, this might or might not be for you if you have really poor protein digestion, but they're basically saying, look, get down to these lower ranges eventually. That's going to be the best for longevity. But it's a process to actually get down to that efficiency with protein.

Nora [00:44:42]: Right, and the idea is that you really don't want to be consuming more than about 20 grams or so of protein in a particular meal, either. You know, this is one of those few instances where the RDA actually has it about right, 44 to 50 some odd grams or whatever of protein a day relative to your body weight. It's kind of about right. And we're talking about something that is smaller in the amount of protein that you're consuming per meal than the palm of your hand. We've got really small amounts that are able to meet our requirements.

rendan [00:45:21]: It's not what you see on the cover of a cookbook, then?

Nora [00:45:24]: Oh, yeah. Well, a lot of paleo cookbooks are like rife with desserts or huge slabs of meat, you know, and whatever else, as tasty as that looks ...

Brendan [00:45:36]: Paleo-approved [inaudible] that may be not optimal. I mean, this really … what we're edging towards is, you know, talking about ketogenetic metabolism and how that's different. But just one last thing before we leave the evolutionary side, why animal fats?

Nora [00:45:55]: Because that's what we would have … that's where we would have gotten the majority of our fats.

Brendan [00:46:01]: What about all the evidence, so-called evidence that saturated fat is a problem? Is there a difference between the epidemiological research that seems to suggest that saturated fat raises cholesterol and that cholesterol is a problem, or is it more nuanced than that and there are experimental studies that revealed that actually maybe saturated fat is doing good things for cholesterol and that cholesterol is not the problem itself?

Nora [00:46:28]: Well, again, you know, we have to talk about what kind of saturated fat are we talking about. Some of … there are two things about the early research that we have to be really clear about. Number one is that a lot of … when heart disease began emerging—and it emerged like in the early 1900s as a going concern—f you graduated medical school in 1910, you never heard of coronary thrombosis. In 1911, the first four cases of coronary thrombosis were published in the Journal of the American Medical Association. Had we all of a sudden begun eating saturated fats? What was happening at that time? Well, there were two things. Number one, we were consuming more polyunsaturated fats from vegetable oils. But number two, we were also beginning to consume an unprecedented level of carbohydrates, and particularly refined carbohydrates. And the sugar industry, we now know … and there were big headlines about this time last year in the *New York Times* saying, "Oh my God," they uncovered all these documents to show that it was the sugar industry that was actually paying off researchers at Harvard and other places to suppress the emerging evidence that it was actually dietary sugar that was the source of suddenly this rampant runaway problem of cardiovascular disease and other diseases, metabolic diseases, and instead turn the blame on saturated fat and particularly animal fat. But the other thing is that a lot of the early research concerning saturated fat didn't distinguish between artificially saturated fat and naturally saturated fat, right? And you know, a lot of …

Brendan [00:48:09]: So, they were throwing margarine in with beef tallow and butter and …?

Nora [00:48:14]: Right. And the other thing that is never, you know, the other things that are oftentimes not really looked that closely enough is what other things were also being consumed. Were these fats being consumed in the absence of sugar and starch or in tandem with high sugar and starch diets? You hear, "Oh, well high-fat diets are really bad." Well, where are you getting that? Well, because look at fast food. Well, fast food, for starters, I promise you is really high in carbohydrates. Number one source of fat calories right now in the American diet is actually partially hydrogenated or esterified soybean oil and canola oil. Number one source of calories overall has been identified as like high-fructose corn syrup.

So yeah, it's no wonder we're in a mess. The problems associated with saturated fat … dietary fat in and of itself is not problematic. Dietary fat in combination with sugar and starch very much can be problematic. And we have to look at also the quality of what we're talking about. You know, are we talking about … the health of the meat and fat we consume is going to directly correlate to the health of the animal that meat and fat came from, right? Now, one more evolutionary comment before we move on from that subject is that … I don't know how many of your viewers are familiar with Weston Price, right? He's often talked about today as an early nutritional pioneer. This was somebody that studied diets of, gosh, almost innumerable primitive and traditional cultures in the 1920s and 1930s throughout the world and evaluated their diets and their health against that of people who were eating a more modern, you know, from the more modernized food supply, more industrialized food supply.

And one of the things that he discovered was that, of course … Well, invariably, wherever a people group was consuming their traditional diet, they were far more apt to be optimally healthy. They had excellent skeletal structure, dentition, mental and physical health as compared to people consuming a more industrialized diet. But among the optimally healthy primitive and traditional people groups that he studied, there were two things they all had in common. Number one is that they all consumed as many animal source foods as were available to them. In other words, there were no vegetarians or vegans among them at all. And he sought that out. I mean, he really looked for that. He tried to find a primitive culture that was like a vegan culture or something. And he was quite disappointed that he wasn't able to find that. He found that wherever people appear to be optimally healthy, they were consuming as many animal source foods as were available to them.

But the second thing they all had in common is that by far and away in all of those healthiest cultures and people groups, the most important food, the most venerated food, the most sought after foods were consistently those foods that were highest in fat and fat-soluble nutrients. And so, even among more Neolithic people groups that were consuming a more primitive or traditional diet, dietary fat never lost its central importance in the equation. And it's only in modern times that we've created this experiment where now … you know, the United States Department of Agriculture's Food Pyramid, right, telling us that we should be basing our diet on carbohydrate-based foods. There's no human people group in the history of the human species that has ever eaten a diet remotely resembling what the US Department of Agriculture Food Pyramid—no conflict of interests there—suggests as optimal. This is a modern day experiment, and it's one that has gone awry.

[00:52:27]: And even the data that has been used to evaluate what these things have been doing to our health … And I write about that in my newest book as well. And I provide the citations there for studies that actually looked at, "Well, how have these dietary requirements been affecting our health since the 1960s?" It turns out the more closely we have followed those guidelines, the worse our health has become statistically. And now, I can't think of a single—you know, I mean, let's call it what it is—there's not a single multinational corporate interest on planet Earth that would not be absolutely committed to promoting carbohydrates as a primary source of nutrition for human beings because it's incredibly cheap and easy to produce. It's immensely profitable. There's no way that you could make a 5,000% profit on a grass-fed steak like you can a box of cereal, and it keeps whoever is eating that way more or less perpetually hungry.

So, fabulous for Monsanto. Also fabulous for the oil industry, because their number one customer is big agribusiness. Fabulous also obviously the food industry and for the chemical industries that supply the chemicals that are thrown on agricultural lands, for the biotech industry that's creating all the GMOs, for the fertilizer industry that is strip mining the Earth for phosphate and whatever to create artificial fertilizers or whatever to do all of this. And by the way, 95 percent of what passes for agriculture isn't, you know, fresh vegetables. It's basically mono crops. It's grains. It's legumes. it's like soy and whatever else. There has never been a more destructive force on planet Earth than agriculture, and it's understandable why these things would be so heavily promoted. And by the way, I mean Bill Gates right now owns the lion's share of so called "vegan meat products."

Brendan [00:48:42]: Oh!

Nora [00:54:44]: Oh, yeah. And so, these things are being promoted in earnest now by various media sources and things like that, because there's a lot of money to be made with these things. Natural animal fat, it can't be made proprietary. It can't be like, you know, patented and packaged and whatever and then sold for a huge profit the way carbohydrate-based foods can. And this is why the food industry became interested in carbohydrate-based foods, because it's a boom for them, you know. And heck, undertakers and Jenny Craig are making out like bandits, too, in this equation. What do they feed to livestock to fatten them up? Grains and legumes. Well, human beings could take a hint from that.

Brendan [00:55:32]: Right. You know, what I'm hearing as we wrap up is quality matters, too, whatever we're eating, and especially when it's … especially when it's anything really, but animal products, whether it's vegetables, quality matters a lot because, as you mentioned in particular with regard to animal products, it's a totally different animal, so to speak, if it's been grain-fattened, because you can fatten and finish …

Nora [00:56:09]: Right. It's bad for human health. It's bad for the planet. It's bad for everything, you know.

Brendan [00:56:14]: Yeah. Whereas, the other side we're learning from many of the other speakers in this event, holistically managed pastured animals can be one of the best things for the planet, if used in the appropriate landscape.

Nora [00:56:25]: Well, also feeding vast human populations in a nutritionally superior fashion. But of course, Monsanto has nothing to gain from this, right? And maybe three percent of all the meat and fat produced is produced in that manner. It's up to us to create a greater demand for that. It's up to us to make the decision. We vote with our food dollars. It's the only kind of voting we do anymore that's worth anything, that actually has an impact at all. But of course, you know, what industry is doing is increasingly eroding what it means to buy grass-fed and what it means to buy organic and whatever else. Laws don't favor human health and well-being and protecting human beings. The laws are largely designed to protect the interests of industry. So, increasingly now, this is eroding as we move into a corporate-dominated political structure throughout the world.

And we really have to be … you know, it sucks, but we have to be vigilant. We have to pay attention. It pays to know directly where your food actually comes from. I have relationships with the farmers that are doing the right things in the right way for the right reasons. And I prefer to give my money to them as opposed to, you know, who knows who, doing who knows what, and claiming whatever. Increasingly, I'm less enamored with buying my food from grocery stores, and I'm trying wherever I can to either grow it myself or come into contact with people who are able either to hunt or produce that food in a way that is uncompromising. And the dietary approach I promote really is about consuming … basically I'm advocating a very low carbohydrate ketogenic approach to eating that is in alignment with our human evolutionary and genetic makeup and is also of uncompromising quality, meaning that it comes from animals, for instance, that have been allowed to eat a diet that is natural for them and optimally healthy for them as a source of nourishment for us. And that ends up being a better thing on so many levels that it just isn't even funny. But of course, multinational industry is not going to look kindly upon this movement. It's doing what it can to trick us into looking at it differently. And we have to realize that a lot of the rhetoric that gets either put in ridiculous documentaries or gets headlined, you know, either on the evening news or online articles or whatever else really are … if you understand all of this really well, you understand that there are hidden agendas involved that are designed to steer us toward a way of doing things that isn't necessarily in alignment with our best interest as it is with someone else's profit.

Brendan [00:59:46]: Yeah, and you know, I really respect you for getting very specific in your research and your understanding of things and in your talks about what's really happening in our food system and in our bodies, because when you tell the unadulterated truth, you cannot be popular with everybody, in fact, perhaps only (with) the deepest truth seekers out there. So, you definitely have your following that's absolutely enthralled and passionate with you, but like you said, not all people in the paleo movement embrace you, and certainly, you know, because it's not popular to be at all at odds with commercial trends, let's say, that are driven at least some, you know, compromised by marketing and appealing to mass tastes or whatever.

Nora [01:00:46]: Right. I'm not interested in telling people what they want to hear. I don't have any hidden agendas. I really, truly don't. Look, I spent 20 years, more than 20 years, as a very full-time practitioner working in a clinical capacity with people who were suffering in a variety of ways. And I am deeply passionate about suffering, human suffering as well as animal suffering. I've worked on behalf of animals a good part of my life as well. Those things matter to me. There's a cycle of life and death of which we're a part, whether we like it or not. And I think so many of these trends toward vegetarianism and veganism, although I appreciate the emotional impetus that goes into those things and the beliefs that go into the adoption of that way of eating. I mean, I shared it at one point, too. I shared those same ideas.

It's not what, you know, what these people think it is at all. It's oftentimes the opposite of what they think it is, but it's made popular because it is so potentially profitable. But so much of this is also just so symptomatic of how far removed we have become from the natural environment that we evolved in. And we have our rightful place within the cycle of life and death. There is no such thing as a karma-less diet, right? All living organisms in this world have to kill in order to eat, even a vegetarian. We're just talking about the relative value of the life of a plant versus the life of an animal, which is an arguable thing, especially from the plant's perspective, right? And there's quite a bit of evidence now to suggest that plants have their own unique form of sentience that's very real. So, you know, nothing is bad or evil because it has to kill in order to eat. All things have to kill in order to eat. It's a matter of the attitude and the sense of stewardship that we bring to that and the consciousness we bring to the process of creating the food that we consume, or procuring the food that we consume, that ultimately speaks to our, you know, our level of higher consciousness, right? Our ethics as a species, as a human being. And so, I would submit that, look, I understand the objections to factory farming and CAFO operations, feedlot kinds of operations. I'm right there with the average vegetarian or vegan with a pitchfork and a torch, you know, wanting to put an end to that method of food production.

But the alternative to that isn't necessarily, doesn't have to be veganism. In fact, it's better if it's not. We're not designed to be herbivores at all. I mean, we're not designed that way, and it's not like … you know, there are some people that have the idea that, well, as omnivores, they're … certain diets are better for some people than for others. Look, there isn't a different book on anatomy and physiology for everybody watching this. What defines us as human beings is not our differences. It's those things that we have in common. And this whole everybody's different thing is nutritional politics. Yes, there are nuances that differentiate us biochemically and whatever else. Somebody might have to take more of one particular type of supplement, and one person might do a little better if they increase their vegetable intake than another person, or whatever.

But fundamentally, again, what defines us as humans are not those nuanced differences. It's those things that we share in common. And we all have a hydrochloric acid base digestive system. We all have a fundamental requirement for certain fat-soluble nutrients, many of which can only be gotten from animal source foods in a form that is readily utilizable for us. And you know, you can't fool Mother Nature, you know, by claiming something different. And so, the fact of the matter is it's not a black and white thing that, well, because conventional meat production is a horrible, horrible, unsustainable thing does not mean that we all need to become vegetarians and vegans. What it does mean is that we need to make different decisions about how we go about producing the food that we consume. And there are ways of doing it that are not only much more sustainable and much healthier for us, but also have the potential to reverse a lot of the environmental destruction that we've created on the planet and restore—I mean literally reverse things like desertification that's occurring across two-thirds of the Earth's land mass right now—and restore healthy watersheds and eco-diversity in places in ways that can't be accomplished any other way other than by putting ruminant animals back on the land en masse, the way it has always been. For tens of millions of years, there were tens of millions of these ruminants that thundered across the landscape. We've removed them from the landscape. Now we sequester them into corrals, and we kill off their predators and we changed … we've radically changed the landscapes. Ruminant animals and grasslands co-evolved. You take them off the grasslands, the grasslands die. And they just begin to desertify, and the soil begins to erode. And then you start plowing the soil, and you radically accelerate top soil loss and erosion. You also create more kind of climatic instability, because you have more extremes of heat and cold on a parched piece of ground than on one that is lush with vegetation. And by putting our focus on animal source foods that are produced in a way that mimics natural systems, again, through something like Holistic Management, we can turn all of that around in a way that literally no other technology we have available to us can. And it doesn't cost us anything. We know how to do it now. And it's just a matter of creating the demand for that method of food production. So ...

Brendan [01:07:34]: I'm so happy to see that there's organizations like Hunt Gather Grow and there's people that are from different dietary persuasions, even people that don't eat meat, that ... You know, people are getting together just changing the food system. We don't have to agree on everything. People will find their own way. We just have to not destroy the soil in the process.

Nora [01:08:01]: You raise a good point that I really want to expand on a little here. It's the whole idea that, you know, there are going to be ideological differences between people who choose to eat meat and vegetarians and whatever. But I would submit that we actually have much more in common between these perspectives than not. The little ideological difference about whether what you have for dinner had a face or parents are not, right? We all care passionately about our health and the health of those we love. We care about sustainability and care about suffering of humans and animals. You know, we care about the idea that multinational corporate interests are co-opting our food supply and polluting the heck out of the planet and everything else. I mean, all these things tend to matter to these seemingly different passionate groups of people, but really we have more in common and more that we need to be working together on than we need to be at odds with. And the degree to which we focus on what we don't agree upon is the degree to which, you know, multinational corporate interests get to operate with impunity and sit back and laugh about us basically eviscerating each other while they get to go off and keep doing what they're doing, which is undermining us and undermining everything that truly matters. Look, I'm not saying the other aspect of the debate doesn't matter. We can always do that over drinks sometime, you know, in a padded room, if need be, but our priority should be those things that matter that we have in common, that we can join forces together and make a real difference. We have to be focused on what is positive about the things that we have in common and focus on that, because with that ... if everybody directed their passions toward that, instead of all the nit-picking that goes on, I mean, we would have the power to move mountains. And that's almost literally what we have to do, you know, if we want to turn things around at this point.

Brendan [01:10:19]: Yeah. I just want to thank you for being such a high integrity and courageous leader in this space and for all the former vegetarians and vegans you're repairing at a physiological level in your clinical practice.

Nora [01:10:35]: I get a lot of emails, a lot of very grateful emails from people like that. Yes. And I'm, you know, I'm a recovering vegetarian, vegan myself. I mean, a lot of us have been there.

Brendan [01:10:49]: We love the Earth, and we just ... unfortunately, we'll have to continue eating animals as much as we ... It's not so unfortunate really. I mean, it's like we're giving them a great life if we choose to get them from sources that are operating entirely according to the principles of Nature and combining that with humane slaughter. I've said it several times. I would submit my own life to be cared for, tended for, fed, and slaughtered humanely in an instant. But anyway ... So, there probably will be more suffering in my own life. But anyway, you were saying something else.

Nora [01:11:33]: Oh, well, I just said, you know, we all end up serving as food for something else when it comes down to it. That's the nature of life on the planet. And again, you know, we've lived away from our natural environment for such a long period of time, we've forgotten what that place within that cycle means. Look, Native American cultures, which are frequently sort of idealized and venerated, right, even among vegan groups, because they love the Earth and whatever. I think they had a deeper appreciation for living things, for life itself in all of its manifestations, than anything we can begin to comprehend because they lived in direct contact with that all the time. And yet it didn't make Native American people groups, or aboriginal people groups anywhere around the world, vegetarians or vegans. What it did do was it gave them a sense of the sacred in the process, and that's something that we're lacking today. We buy our meat shrink-wrapped in a way that is removed from having had any part in the process at all or any realization of where that food actually came from. And I would submit that that needs to be part of the equation, is restoring that firsthand knowing of where food comes from and restoring our natural place within that cycle of life and death in a responsible way that reflects a certain stewardship that I think is our legacy as the supposedly most evolved species on the planet. We need to start acting like it with our behavior, and it's not that hard to do.

Brendan [01:13:20]: And it feels so good to have abundant energy and not be tied to an eating routine that I have to eat every three, four, or five hours. I can skip meals, if I want. So, I'm loving it. And I love fat. Who doesn't love fat? I mean, that's what the body seems to be oriented ... I mean, there's not a single person ...

Nora [01:13:42]: Right. Well, we love sugar, too. A lot of us like the taste of it, but we realized what it meant to our ancestors when they ate sugar, like a ripened fruit in the late summers and things, they did it to make themselves a little bit insulin resistant, right? Because that sugar rapidly converts into body fat, which at one time served a purpose to kind of help us a stave off famine, right? To become a little bit insulin resistant, you know, in the fall so that we had better odds of surviving the time of year where food might be more scarce or where the climatic conditions might be less hospitable and may require more fat to keep us warm. And so, the degree to which we used to crave sugar, you know, we didn't have access to carbohydrates the way we do now. Today, carbohydrate-based foods dominate our food supply, and we're nowhere near designed to weather that tsunami of insulin. We're not designed to do it, and it's compromising us, but that's not necessary. We don't have to be reliant upon so volatile and damaging a source of energy as sugar and can instead rely on fat as a primary source of fuel, which makes infinitely more sense. The slimmest person watching this has 100-150,000 calories of fat on their bodies that they could be drawing upon as a source of energy to keep their brain and their body and their organs working like a well-oiled machine, so to speak, even in the absence of regular meals. It's a stable even burning source of energy. And doesn't that make much more sense as a primary source of fuel than something that is doing this all the time along with your energy and your brain function and your mood and everything else. But it's nowhere near as profitable for the powers that be, and so, we're going to continue to hear a lot more that promotes carbohydrate-based diets than what we're talking about. But if you look at the body of literature, you look at the available scientific evidence from independent sources that are not being paid by corporate interests, you will find that there is an inherent superiority to a fat-based metabolism, and one based on animal source foods of uncompromising quality than anything that could possibly be gotten from eating according to government guidelines.

Brendan [01:16:24]: Yeah, I love how you call it the American paradox that the closer you adhere to the U.S. food pyramid, or whatever the latest guidelines are, the worse your health gets.

Nora [01:16:35]: It's true, yeah.

Brendan [01:16:40]: On that note, thank you for joining us here in the Eat4Earth community and for having brought the unaltered truth.

Nora [01:16:47]: Yeah, you're welcome. And actually, thank you for doing what you're doing by bringing this whole subject matter to light, right, and really putting a focus on the quality of the food that we consume and how that actually can lead to greater sustainability in our food production. It's a wonderful thing that you're focusing on, and I hope it gets seen far and wide.

Brendan [01:17:16]: Nora and I had two other full-length interviews that go into greater depth about things like essential fat-soluble nutrients, like vitamin K and a whole lot more, and these are included in the Eat4Earth Upgrade Package.

Diana Rodgers Interview
Kale vs. Cow: The Case for Healthy, Sustainable, and Ethical Meat

Brendan: [00:00:00]: Welcome to the Eat4Earth event. We're exploring how you can heal yourself, your loved ones, and the planet with food. This is Brendan Morehead, and I've been looking forward to this conversation with our guest, Diana Rogers. Diana is a real food licensed Registered Dietician, nutritionist and nutritional therapy practitioner. She lives on a working organic farm, west of Boston, and she has an active nutrition practice where she helps people get on track with diet and lifestyle. She also is an author, a host of the "Sustainable Dish" podcast, and the mother of two active kids. Diana speaks at universities and conferences internationally about nutrition and sustainability, social justice, animal welfare, and food policy issues. She's also the consulting Dietitian to several gyms and also to Nom Nom Paleo, Whole30, Dr. Kirk Parsley, The Farm to Consumer Legal Defense Fund, and Fresh Advantage. She's also a board member of Animal Welfare Approved. She's a staff writer for Paleo magazine, contributes regularly to several blogs, and her work has been featured in the Los Angeles Times, the Boston Globe, Outside magazine and in Mother Earth News. Diana, this is going to be a very interesting conversation. Thank you for being with us today.

Diana Rodgers [00:01:14]: Thanks for having me.

Brendan [00:01:15]: Yeah, so Diana, when I was in college, I started working at being a vegetarian, even a vegan for short time, because I wanted to eat what I thought would be the most planet-friendly and humane diet. But after eight years I wasn't thriving, so I went back to meat eating. But I continued to be concerned about the planetary impacts of my meat consumption and like myself, many people have been drawn to a plant-based diet, believing that all forms of animal agriculture are ecologically inefficient, and unsustainable. I also wondered whether all animal products might be inherently unhealthy. I wanted to stop killing animals for my food. Then I started encountering evidence that caused me to question these ideas and realize that they might actually be harmful to at least some people, to me personally—the dietary decisions I was making weren't working—but also harmful to the planet. You've analyzed these issues quite a bit and are working on a film called *Kale Versus Cow: The Case for Better Meat* that will tackle at least some of these issues. Why were you inspired to create this film?

Diana Rodgers [00:02:30]: So, there's a bunch of reasons why I'm working on this film. I think that there's a lot of confusion out there. There's a lot of people that assume that plants are cleaner, healthier, cause least harm and are environmentally better for our planet than eating meat products. And unfortunately, because so many people are disconnected from how our food is produced and living in cities and just not familiar with regenerative farming techniques, the idea of just going to the store and buying some kale or spinach and seeing so many celebrities pushing this diet for health reasons, seeing so many documentaries and other media propaganda that's showing only factory farming of animals and not showing regenerative farming, it's really easy to buy into this idea. But because I have spent the last 15 years of my life living on a working farm where we use regenerative techniques, and we do organic vegetable production, but then we also do pasture-based livestock—we do sheep and goats eating grass; we do pigs that run through the woods; we do chickens that are in these mobile houses that we move all around the farm—I've seen the benefits of pasture-based animal agriculture on our land firsthand. I've really studied the benefits to overall biodiversity of animals on pasture versus animals in factory farming. So, I'm not advocating for factory farming, of course. I think that's, you know, incredibly misguided and unfortunate that that's how most of our food is produced. Just because grass-fed beef is a small percentage of our meat that we can get in the grocery stores today doesn't mean that we need to completely give up all animal products from our food system in order to be sustainable. Because there's actually, if you're looking at this from a least harm perspective, there's actually quite a bit of harm that comes from plant-based agriculture as well.

Brendan [00:04:53] Yeah, I've actually started to look at that and been very surprised. It just had never occurred to me to look into that. I think maybe we'll touch a little bit on that in this conversation. So, the question of sustainability of animal agriculture obviously involves multiple issues. You've got land use, greenhouse gas emissions, the quantity and type of water used, and then from a humane perspective, how many animals are being killed, and how are they being killed, and how are they living? So, you know, the movie *Cowspiracy* made some assertions about things like water and land use that have been questionable and found to be possibly inaccurate, based on certain assumptions that deserve more investigation.

Diana Rodgers [00:05:42] Exactly.

Brendan [00:05:42]: Is there anything that you would call attention to in that regard?

Diana Rodgers [00:05:46]: Yeah. So, I do like to break this into, you know, nutritional arguments, environmental arguments, and then ethical arguments. So, with the water argument that's really in the environmental arguments. We've got water use; we've got feed use; and we've got land use; and then greenhouse gas emissions. Those are sort of the main complaints that people have against cattle specifically when it comes to the environment. As far as water goes there's different ways of measuring water, and a lot of the numbers that are thrown out there are looking at green water use instead of blue water use. Green water use is water that would naturally fall from the sky, the rain water, things like that. If you look at a cow on grass, they're calculating the rain that falls on that grass as water that goes into cows. They're also not looking at the fact that cows pee, right? They're not just exploding bubbles that suck up water, and it's gone forever. Blue water is a much more accurate way of measuring water. That's from groundwater, water in lakes and rivers and aquifers, so water that we need to use for irrigation or to suck up from the ground and use to give water to animals. It's really important when you look at the water numbers, how are they measuring water? Is it precipitation or is it water that we're using for irrigation or for watering animals?

Brendan [00:07:31]: I think there's, oh sorry.

Diana Rodgers [00:07:31]: No, go ahead.

Brendan [00:07:31] I think I saw some figures, might have been on your blog, about what it actually takes in grain-based agriculture for each pound of meat. Of course, these are average numbers, it's not hard and fast. It wasn't quite the same as what *Cowspiracy* came up with. I think it was a lot less. Then, if you look at grass-fed, I guess I'm not sure if that figure for just grass-fed included blue and green water or just green water, which, of course, like you said, the cows are peeing, so it's going back into the soil. It's going into the soil; it's fertilizing the soil. Urine is one of the best fertilizers in appropriate doses, and then it's part of the water cycle again. It's not leaving it. So I'm just curious, do you have any of those numbers with you handy?

Diana Rodgers [00:08:25]: A pound of rice requires about 410 gallons of water. Avocados, walnuts and sugar are similar. That's about how much water that UC Davis calculated in blue water is required for a typical pound of beef. That's a cow that is finished at a feedlot. I should back up too because a lot of people think that cattle spend their whole lives on feedlots. Just like, when you see factory farms, chicken or pork … now those animals are in confinement situations their entire lives. Typical chicken, typical pork are under fluorescent lights in crowded environments their entire lives. Cattle do not spend their entire lives, even typical cattle that end up at feedlots. They start out eating grass, and then if a cow is finished on grain at a feed lot that's only a portion of their life. That's not their whole life. Another thing that we have to look at is the entire cycle. So if we're looking at this in a reductionist way, yes, there's water that goes into cows, and you can say that it gets lost, and it doesn't get peed out, but we also have to look at the fact that cows grazing on land, if managed well, so not in an overgrazing way, not a poorly managed way where you would have a cow eating the same patch of grass for its entire life, but moved around frequently, they're actually improving the water-holding capacity of the land. So they're making that land much more able to hold onto rain water instead of it flowing away. There's a lot of different ways to look at it and when we started looking at it in a more "holistic systems" approach instead of a reductionist way, which is how I like to look at nutrition and ethics as well, cows are actually a net gain for the environment. And the same can be said for the greenhouse gases as well. So when cows are producing manure on the ground, that manure is actually fertilizer. It's not waste. It's the way Nature actually gets inoculated with healthy microorganisms in order to help the grass grow stronger. The roots actually have a beautiful relationship with the microorganisms from the cow poop, and it actually can help sequester carbon. So when we're looking at just net cow farts, that's one way to look at it, but when you actually have cows that are not over-producing too much manure in one area, and are moved around frequently, so intensive grazing, holistic management, those types of practices, so constantly moving the animals across the land, and their manure is spread out nice and evenly, it can hold onto water better, and it can actually help sequester carbon. And then we get into land use as well, so a lot of numbers will say, well cows take up so much more land, and we could be growing grains on a much smaller piece of land. But that's assuming that you can actually grow grains and soy everywhere, which you can't. And so the croppable landmass on Earth is a much smaller percentage of our land mass than what we can effectively graze cattle on. And so when you are using pastureland, which can't be cropped, for animals that are eating grass, which we can't eat, sequestering carbon, and providing a nutrient-dense protein for humans, it's a win-win.

Brendan [00:12:30]: Yeah, and this was incredibly big news to me, as somebody who had been reluctantly eating red meat because it was the only thing that was balancing my metabolism, my energy, my ability to think at all for quite some years, because I went through chronic fatigue and all this stuff, meat became a staple. And I was at odds with that internally. I'm like, "I'm getting off this (meat) at some point." Then I, you know, saw Allan Savory's video on a TEDx and dug in. I went to as many conferences as I could and wanted to know, *is this real*? *How does it work*? It's extraordinary. That just by mimicking how ruminant herbivores used to roam and get chased around ... they didn't hang out, they got to moved quickly. They were in close bunches and so forth. I won't get into explaining it, because I'm not a trainer of Holistic Management or similar methods. But interestingly enough, it brings back biodiversity. One of those things is dung beetles. Dung beetles will make a cow dung patty disappear in less than 24 hours and increase the water infiltration rate right there so quickly. It's amazing. I've seen that even in Australia. A cow dung patty on a dry dirt road that was like cement. They turned it into soft earth right under the cow dung patty overnight. It was just amazing. You also mentioned the methane issue. I just thought I would pipe in that in one of my conversations with Walter Jehne, who's part of this event as well, he mentioned to me that in addition to methanotrophic bacteria, which live in healthy soils and digest methane, there's also photooxidation of methane. So when you have moist soils that are transpiring moisture from the ground up into the air, and you've got the sunlight coming in, the sunlight breaks some of the water molecules in the air into a hydrogen proton and an oxygen radical. Then that oxygen, excuse me, hydroxide radical (Correction: hydroxyl radical / hydroxide ion) with a negative charge, that's very reactive. It breaks down methane. So, there's a lot to be researched there to see if methane is really an issue. Because, you know, we had like 70,000,000 bison on this continent, plus another roughly 40,000,000 smaller herbivores, according to the numbers I saw, in North America. We now have 30,000,000 beef cattle and 10,000,000 dairy cattle. So that's a lot smaller number of herbivores and if they're on pasture, chances are they're healthy pastures and regenerated grassland ecosystems, not in forests where they don't belong, but in the appropriate ecosystem, you're not going to be emitting, I don't think, more methane than twice as many animals. And again, if those mechanisms of methanotrophic bacteria and photooxidation of methane are actually happening, then maybe methane is a moot point. And it's really been harped on. We need the research to see what's really happening before we dismiss that issue, but certainly on the carbon side it's very clear and becoming clearer all the time that, you know, cows can actually grow soil. And that's a good thing.

Diana Rodgers [00:15:55]: Yeah. And then when we look at plant-based agriculture and the land that needs to be cleared in order to make a huge soy or wheat or corn field, the plowing that has to happen releases tons of carbon. A lot of the agricultural lands that we have left, if we all gave up meat and went for a plant-based diet for the rest of human population, we'd need to cut down a whole lot of forest in order to convert the leftover land that we have into crop-based agriculture, which will destroy ecosystems for all the animals that live there, convert the whole land to one crop, which is not increasing biodiversity. It's decreasing it. And then you've got all the chemicals used in chemical agriculture. So how are you going to fertilize the ground? You can either do that with oil-based chemical agriculture, or you can do that with animals. We can use things like manure and compost in an organic system, or we can use chemical ag. Chemical ag is obviously not great for the soil biome. It's not good for the insects, which we're losing tons of every day. And then you've got tractors running through decapitating little bunnies and chipmunks and mice and all the things that will live in a field of soy. So when you're looking at it from a net death perspective, if you're trying to actually cause the least amount of deaths for the food that you're taking in, one large herbivore on grass can provide about 470 to maybe 500 pounds of meat. That feeds a lot of people for a really long time. Compared to how many little animals are going to die in order to make that block of tofu. So from a least harm perspective, I would definitely argue that eating large herbivores is actually causing least harm.

Brendan [00:18:13]: You know, I saw a very convincing article on that. I read several articles and looked at the different arguments both ways, and the only one I've found convincing *at all* was the one that—well, I'd say there were a couple that I've found convincing but one version of the argument that was better-documented. So basically, the bottom line they came up with was when you look at all the mice and reptiles and birds and so forth that are killed in the field—in this particular example, the number might have been swayed a bit higher because they were including mice being poisoned—that every time when you have grains you've got mice plagues, at least in Australia where the numbers were coming from. So, they're killing lots of mice every year with poison. I suppose if there was some way to avoid that and not poison mice, you'd still have a lot in mice and a lot of rabbits that are getting hit. Farmers talk about it all the time where they see these animals going right up into the combine, boom, boom. So maybe there's a way to avoid that. Maybe there's a way to minimize that.

Diana Rodgers [00:19:22]: I live on an organic vegetable farm and death happens there, too. So, we've got, you know, you'll harvest a piece of lettuce, and there's a snake curled up often in that head of lettuce. There's a lot of life on an organic farm, but there's also death that happens on organic farms, too, and again, how are we as organic farmers fertilizing our soils? It's with animals. We have a large compost pile, we take in horse manure from local horse farms. But then we're also composting animals that die on the farm from a coyote kill or something like that. They're all going in, and they're all turning into soil food.

Brendan [00:20:10]: Yeah, absolutely. And I will mention this. I mean, there is an approach called veganic, and I think that you can do good farming without animal manure. Singing Frogs Farm is part of this event as well with Paul Kaiser. They essentially now have a veganic technique. I don't know that they call it that. They just don't have animal manure, and they're doing great things with soil, so just wanted to mention that.

Diana Rodgers [00:20:39]: I've seen them present, too. I think they do import compost from off-farm.

Brendan [00:20:44]: But does it have animal manure in the compost?

Diana Rodgers [00:20:45] I'd be interested to see with their technique. It isn't a totally closed loop that they're working with there, so if we are trying to do a completely closed loop system because Earth is a closed loop, right? So, I think the goal of every farm should be as closed as possible.

Brendan [00:21:07]: Sure.

Diana Rodgers [00:21:07]: So it would be interesting to me to see if maybe that's an awesome system. But, I think with our farm where we are incorporating animals into the mix, we can actually improve our soil really well by using animal products as part of the mix. I don't think that you can really have a totally sustainable farm without any animals at all. They're definitely incorporating, of course, earthworms and, and other smaller animals. So whether or not it's a larger goat manure or horse manure, they're still using beetles and worms and soil microbes in order to help produce their vegetables.

Brendan [00:21:55]: Yeah, while we are on the issue of animal welfare, ethics, morality and so forth, first of all, I thought I'd just mention or complete my thought on the Australian analysis. So they were looking at average beef production when it's grass-fed per acre or hectare and comparing that to grains. They came up with, per hundred kilograms of protein from grass-fed beef, it was 2.2 animals that would die, literally because there were slaughtered. And in the fields with mice and all the other animals it was 55, so a 25-fold difference between the two. I thought I'd just mention the numbers because it's extreme. You could discount that all the way down to a lot less, and it's still a difference.

Diana Rodgers [00:22:54]: Yeah. When you get into numbers, I think that's where a lot of people will try to challenge you. That's why I try to look at it. Are we talking about Kenya? Are we talking about Vermont? Are we talking about … ? There's just so many different soil types where you can get better or less returns depending on the humidity of the climate and all this. So, it is, it is … I find that people get really hung up on numbers and challenging numbers because that's an easy one to attack, but I mean, if you just use common sense and think about it from a whole systems ecology perspective, it just makes sense to have larger ruminants as our main protein source. Certainly, from a nutrition perspective, you've got iron and B12 so strong in red meat compared to … you know, we're eating so much more chicken now than ever before, and we're seeing iron deficiency anemia is the most common nutrition deficiency worldwide. And so, really red meat is, even if you go to the Academy of Nutrition and Dietetics websites, you know, standard government websites, they will say that red meat is the best, most bio-available source of iron that you can find.

Brendan [00:24:17]: It's also a great source of zinc.

Diana Rodgers [00:24:19]: Yeah.

Brendan [00:24:20]: And it's kind of a hybrid issue I'd say between ethics and morality, and nutrition in that perhaps we should expand our look at welfare of sentient beings to include humans?!

Diana Rodgers [00:24:36]: Yeah.

Brendan [00:24:41]: And there's people around the planet who need these nutrients, and they're on landscapes that are only good for raising livestock. And they can regenerate their watersheds by doing so if they're doing it appropriately, with the methods we kind of discussed before. And so, maybe we should look at … should we be trying to turn them into plant-based diets when their landscapes are not going to support it, or it's going to get degraded, or it already has been degraded by that kind of activity? I mean animals are the only solution both nutritionally and ecologically for them, from sustainably and for them to make the turnaround to come back from famines.

Diana Rodgers [00:24:41]: Yeah, regional reliance, regional food systems are the smartest way to go moving forward, and exactly what you just said. If you were to go to the Masai and say, "I know your health is awesome, and I know cattle are a mainstay for you nutritionally. I know that soy doesn't really grow that well in Kenya, but you know, I don't really want you eating cows because it disturbs me, and so I think that you should just let us provide you with all the grains, even though they don't grow in your country. We'll just provide them for you." I think that's really, ethically, a big challenge for me to look at it from that perspective. So when we look at traditional diets, what we see commonly is lots of organ meats, lots of animal fats, lots of animal proteins and really healthy populations.

Brendan [00:26:16]: Yeah. And obviously, that's very contrary, that observation is very contrary to the kind of message we hear in the mainstream about meat products and have been hearing since the United States vegetable oils and grain-based oils lobby got going in the fifties to vilify saturated fats and tropical oils at the time that dominated our vegetable oil market. But anyway, I'm just curious what you would have to say around these issues of red meat, saturated fat, cholesterol, different types of studies that seem to impugn it as a health hazard for cancer and heart disease. I'm just curious what you know, you've obviously looked at this a lot.

Diana Rodgers [00:27:01]: Yeah. I have absolutely no problem with animal saturated fats or with animal proteins at all. I think the studies that are vilifying red meats … there's a bunch of different flaws I find in them. Usually what they're doing is they're looking at vegetarians compared to someone on a standard American diet, so there's a lot of lifestyle factors there that are not accounted for in these studies. When you separate out the confounding factors, things like exercise, smoking, drinking, overall lifestyle, overall vegetable intake, when you separate that out and just look at a vegetarian diet or a vegan diet compared to a healthy-ish diet where someone's eating a lot of vegetables plus eating meats, there's no difference in mortality at all. So, there's no benefit to being somebody who excludes meat from your diet. If you're trying to reduce your overall caloric intake and increase your protein, which is the most satiating macronutrient, which can help us balance our blood sugar, you can either do that with meat which is very efficient at delivering protein for low calories or you can do this with something like peanut butter, right? So you can get 30 grams of protein from about 700 calories worth of peanut butter or about 130 calories worth of fish. Right? Red meat is, has a little more calories than fish per ounce, but that's because it also has some healthy fats in there. There just is not a plant-based protein that's as bio-available and calorically efficient as animal proteins.

Brendan [00:28:55]: You mentioned that healthy fats, I think it's definitely worth a quick, quick look at the differences between grain-finished cattle and grass-finished cattle, cattle that have spent their whole life on grass. What differences do we see there?

Diana Rodgers [00:29:11]: Well, we do see some differences. I've been presenting frequently lately at a different health and also grass-fed beef conferences. A frequent a claim by grass-fed beef producers is that they have more omega-3's if they're produced on grass than finished in a feed lot. And while that's true, it's not really … beef is not a significant source for humans of omega-3's. So even though it does have double or triple the amount of omega-3's, it's still a relatively small percentage of omega-3's. So you would still have to eat like, I think I calculated, and it was like eight or nine pounds of grass-fed burgers in order to get the same omega-3's you would get in a small three-ounce piece of fish, say wild salmon. So, salmon is just going to beat beef every time for the omega-3's. When we look at grass-fed dairy we do see a significant difference, because we're eating a lot more fat from the animal in full-fat dairy products, so full-fat fat, grass fed milk has a lot more omega-3's, and it is a significant to human health difference. We also see a lot more CLA; we see a lot more fat-soluble vitamins in grass-fed milk. So even though in grass-fed beef there is an increase, the benefits to us for eating grass-fed beef are really in least harm of animals and least harm to the environment, and not as much direct if you were just to take a grass-fed steak and a feedlot steak and really look at them because we're eating relatively low-fat pieces of meat there. There's not a huge, huge difference in the nutritional quality from the research that we have today. Now there's probably a lot more micronutrients, but those aren't typically measured by the USDA database. I have seen anecdotally from some producers much higher selenium, much higher zinc. That depends on soil type and the grass that they're eating and all that kind of stuff. We're still looking at better research for that, but as far as nutrition goes, not necessarily a healthier product to humans, but that doesn't mean we shouldn't be eating grass-fed beef.

Brendan [00:31:51]: Well, again, there's the issue of how, if it was organic or conventional feedlot beef, If you're eating the grain-fed version because obviously in the conventional model, they pump them full of antibiotics, and you're creating the whole antibiotic resistant organisms …

Diana Rodgers [00:32:09]: Right.

Brendan [00:32:10]: … cauldron there, and getting some of the residues of those antibiotics in the meat perhaps. Also, maybe hormone residues if they're giving them hormones. There's also a big difference between conventional grain-fed, organic grain-fed, and then maybe the more subtle differences there you're pointing to between …

Diana Rodgers [00:32:25]: Yeah. The biggest challenge with antibiotic resistance is really the environmental factor there as well. So, is it being sprayed on our spinach, this cattle manure from CAFO farms with antibiotic resistant strains? That's a big difference. It gets into our water supply, it gets into the air from feedlots and different confined animal operations. Not so clear on if you eat antibiotic-free meat and cook it well. Not that clear research yet on whether or not that's really getting into our bodies. The bigger concern is the environment that these strains are getting into and then onto our food and into our water and into the air that we're breathing.

Brendan [00:33:24]: Yeah. I've been listening a bit to some authorities on that antibiotic resistance. They are saying that the issue that we're seeing in our whole human population is being generated largely through these feedlots. But, of course, there's the over-prescription of antibiotics to humans.

Diana Rodgers [00:33:41]: That's all I'm saying is it's not necessarily getting to the meat we're eating. It's more getting into the environment, and then getting to us that way.

Brendan [00:33:52**]:** In terms of proteins, I do very well on animal proteins. and as I mentioned I've tried to make plant proteins work for me, and they have not worked so well. Refined pea protein seems to work alright for me, I think. But I think it's worth mentioning that some people have, a lot of people, have challenges with lectin, plant lectins. I shouldn't say "lectin" singular, because there's so many plant lectins. There's lectins in carrots. There's lectins in milk. But a lot of the plant lectins are harder for some people, many people to deal with, especially with a damaged microbiome and gut. So, I think it's worth mentioning when people are ... the way I look at this whole picture is I want people to understand that we can raise almost any kind of food in a way that works for the planet, but we're not doing it, by and large, but people can find what food is going to work for them. And then I really want them to look for how they can source that food and not be destroying the Earth. In your practice, do you encounter people that are maybe like me, that were sort of recovering from a damaged gut and could not, I still am, and can't yet tolerate a lot of plant proteins? I love the taste of beans. I can't eat them.

Diana Rodgers [00:35:16]: Yeah. I think everyone's on a spectrum as far as what plants they can tolerate. I have a pretty destroyed gut from celiac disease. My husband, on the other hand, seems to do really well even with gluten and lots of plants. I don't tolerate plants as well personally. I think a lot of people are sort of somewhere in between. Plants can't run away from us, so their only defense is to kind of try to harm us a little bit as they're going through our system because their entire goal is to be in the ground growing. So, seeds and nuts, the reproductive portion of the plant really wants to try to get through your system as intact as possible so that it can be transported by your body to a new location to be planted in the ground and growing. And so some people are just a lot more sensitive to that than others for a lot of different reasons, from gut problems, different viruses, things like that, that sort of induce some gut issues. In my practice I tend to see people with IBS-type symptoms who are also looking to lose weight. They're either a combination of both of those things or one or the other. What I find time and again is that going back to a meat and vegetables-type diet that's low in grains, for some people need to be very, very low in carbohydrates, other people can do a little bit more carbohydrates than others. But focusing on animal protein, healthy fats, and for some people with a really destroyed gut, vegetables just aren't going to work for a while. We have to focus on broths and well-cooked meats for a little while before we can then start introducing some softer cooked vegetables. Other people can jump right into raw salads and top it off with some animal protein and they do fine with that. So it really all depends on the level of gut problems that we're dealing with. Of course, I get in supplements with different types of probiotics and things like that. That can kind of help restore the gut to a healthier biome.

Brendan [00:37:44]: That's the path I have found myself on. In light of what we've discussed in terms of sustainability, potential sustainability in the right context, of livestock that can be a very regenerative force on the planet, I think it's a counterproductive for people to argue about veganism or omnivorism. I want people to thrive, and I want the planet to thrive, and both can happen at the same time regardless of what food you choose. So we may disagree on morality issues that may continue to persist as a disagreement. I don't know, but it's my hope that people will kind of unite around a common vision of a healthy planet with healthy people and dietary diversity, biodiversity in our food cropping systems. I took some, of the things that I have wanted to see more of ... I want to see animals, if I'm eating them, I want them to be slaughtered as humanely as possible, more humanely than an animal getting pulled up into machinery on a row crop field or something. And I saw your film, the short film that won the real food, or was it ...

Diana Rodgers [00:39:19]: Real Food Media .

Brendan [00:39:20]: Yeah, Media Contest 2015, this woman, Mary Lake, who is, or was a vegetarian who was just in a situation where she ended up working in an abattoir that was using the Temple Grandin method. And I watched them like, "Oh my God! this, this pig is getting affection all the way up until it blacks out". I thought, "That's how I want to go!" Unfortunately, I may not have that blessing. I don't know how I'm going to go, but I can feel a lot better about that. You know when the animal gets stunned before anything violent happens to it, neurologically stunned. Anyway, it's a whole kind of a creepy thing to talk about I guess. But I think it's important to acknowledge ...

Diana Rodgers [00:40:07]: No, I think it's really important.

Brendan [00:40:09]: ... that we are a part of a system, and we're going to kill something. Everything kills something to eat something. We may think that by eating plants, we're not killing animals, but chances are we are. Some of us just don't need to trash our own health, if we can't survive on plant foods. I have not been one that could do it yet. But I have succeeded recently in reducing my consumption of certain things that I'm not sure are as sustainable as I would like them to be. But anyhow, I really appreciate this conversation. Let's all stop eating factory farm meat. If we're going to eat, meat, let's make it a holistically managed or rotationally grazed. There's going to be some labels coming out like "Land to Market" where we'll be able to see just how good that grass-fed methodology is. I'm looking forward to that, and I'm just wondering, is there anything else you might want to say? You've got this film coming out. That's going to be exciting. But anything else you would say in wrapping up?

Diana Rodgers [00:41:16]: Yeah, just touching briefly on what you said a second ago about humane slaughter. I think that if we're looking to reduce suffering, a lot of people will say that, well, you know, animals, that's great. They're good for the land. They can improve it, but can't we just let them live out their lives and die a natural death? That's something that I've really explored a lot, too. That natural death doesn't mean dying in your sleep. That's not how life happens in Nature or death happens in Nature. They can be hunted and killed by coyotes and wolves or eaten alive by hyenas. There's a lot of different ways to go. I think one of the main problems is that us humans don't like to talk about death. We don't even like to think about our own deaths and how we'd like to go, like you mentioned a second ago. I've worked in long-term care. I've worked in hospitals, and I've seen people suffer at the end, because they weren't prepared to really face their own death and have a plan for their own death. I certainly hope that when it's time for me to go I have a button, and I can just die in the least harm kind of way. I think that, if we're really looking when people think about their pets, do they want their pet to suffer a long agonizing death? Do they want their grandmothers to suffer a really long time before she goes, or do you want it to happen really quickly? I think when we're looking at least harm, we would like things to die pretty quickly, hopefully not even knowing that it's coming. And so, it's a bigger thing that people don't like to talk about, but I think that, again, it just comes from our disconnection from the fact that we are Nature. We're not on top of Nature. We don't control Nature. We are animals ourselves. We have the ability as humans to be humane about how we kill the animals that we eat for food, and it's our obligation to do that. I feel very strongly about that. As you mentioned, I'm on the board of Animal Welfare Approved, and we try very hard to make sure that there's humane handling standards that are above and beyond at the slaughter houses that we work with. That's pretty much it, I guess, on that topic. I do believe that red meat is nutritionally an important food for humans. I believe environmentally if managed well, it can actually improve the land and be a lot less harmful on land than plant production in a lot of ways. And I also think that from a least harm perspective, red meat from large ruminants is actually quite a good choice for people who are trying to be ethical about the food that they eat. People can more about all that stuff on my page, "Sustainable Dish". Click on the "Film" button if they want to know more about the movie I'm working on.

Brendan [00:44:43]: Wonderful. The only thing I would add to that, it occurs to me to say that if we eat meat that is grown, if we just specify livestock that are raised in these ways that build biodiversity back and soil back and potentially even help mitigate climate change, then our meat eating can be a regenerative force on the planet. Given the state of our food system, how is it going to change if we don't eat meat and vote with our dollars for the type of meat? That's just one thought. I don't know.

Diana Rodgers [00:45:18]: Yeah, I mean definitely giving up meat and opting out of the system. I mean there's definitely people I know that have opted out of society, and they live in the woods. That's not really going to make much of a big change in the overall system. That's definitely a way to avoid the conversation, or you can choose to actually try to make a big change through your purchases and actually just eat better meat instead of completely avoiding it.

Brendan [00:45:50]: Yeah, just be a vocal, outspoken consumer that votes with their pocketbook. Diana, I really appreciate that you're willing to take on these controversial issues head on. What I really appreciate about you is you're a rigorous thinker. You're sensitive to the issues. You don't go out too far on a limb. You know, you're conservative with talking about numbers and so forth, holding back that … hey, there's a lot of nuances here. So, here you're a nuanced intellect, and I appreciate that.

Diana Rodgers [00:46:50]: Yeah. Thanks.

Brendan [00:46:34]: You're working on this documentary called *Kale Versus Cow: A Case for Better Meat*, and I can't wait to see how that comes out because *Cowspiracy* does deserve an answer. And you with your fine arts background, in the past, I guess, I know you're going to do a great job. It's apparent through everything you do in your website. It's beautiful, one of the most beautiful websites on the Internet. I believe that this is going to be an important film for this ongoing conversation about animal and plant foods and eating sustainably, regeneratively, humanely. Thank you on behalf of myself and the Eat4Earth community for being with us today.

Diana Rodgers [00:46:17]: Thank you.

Sarah Wu Interview
Planetary Herbalism and Finding Your Perfect Diet

Brendan [00:00:00]: Welcome to the Eat4Earth event. This is Brendan Moorehead, and together we're exploring how you can heal yourself, your loved ones, and the planet with food. Our next guest is Sarah Wu, the current Director and Educational Curator of the Punta Mona Center for Regenerative Design and Botanical Studies, leading trainings and workshops in herbal medicine, Permaculture design, tropical Deep Ecology, field-to-the-plate, holistic nutrition and women's retreats. She is a clinical herbalist of 17 years, practicing planetary eclectic herbalism with a foundation in Traditional Chinese Medicine and Wise Woman Reclaiming philosophy, focusing on food-based healing and local ethnobotanical traditions. She's a passionate mentor and educator. Sarah is the co-founder of Medicines from the Edge: A Tropical Herbal Convergence and co-producer of Envision Festival. She loves cats, books, plants and soup. Sarah addresses personal and environmental issues with strategies that are specific to individual constitution and bioregion. So, we're going to be talking about some of the many ways in which each one of us is unique nutritionally and in so many ways. So, Sarah, this is going to be fun and fascinating. Thanks for being here.

Sarah Wu [00:01:16]: Yeah. Thank you for having me. I like, I like hearing the intros. Kind of fun to have someone else read about yourself.

Brendan [00:01:25]: So, Sarah, a major undercurrent that, I've tried to create in this event is the idea that there's no one right diet for everybody and that there's no one right planet-friendly way of eating. So, you call what you do "planetary eclectic herbalism" and there's probably another term I could throw in there. Could you unpack that and talk about how you view human individuality when it comes to food healing and living in general?

Sarah Wu [00:01:53]: Sure. Well, just to kind of unpack what "eclectic herbalism" is, is that actually comes from a group of herbalists, predominately male actually, who were around from the early 1800's until the beginning of the 1900's in North America. And so, these were doctors who were classically trained and in the most kind of modern technology of the time, but what they didn't believe in was the reductionist philosophy and the treatment of people with poisons such as like with mercury and bleedings and or those kinds of things. And so, just to kind of define "reductionism", it means that, it's a very kind of typical way of thinking that all the different parts of the whole have no interaction with each other. And so, it's the opposite of holistic perspectives. And so, the eclectic herbalists, you know, they were coming from Europe, or they were born in North America, and again trained in the European kind of style. But what they were doing is they were pulling from their traditional roots as well as looking to the people, the native peoples of North America, to learn about them their healing traditions from their plants, from the bioregions themselves. And so what "eclectic herbalism" refers to is pulling from many different traditions to treat the individual. And so, we're not looking to just say the Chinese system of medicine or just Ayurvedic system of medicine [unintelligible], or the Latino traditional herbalism or Caribbean or whatever it is. You know, it's like every different area around the world has this traditional system of medicine. It's traditional, kind of cosmic vision of the relationship with the human body with the heavens, with their gods, et cetera, their views on the relationships with each other, and with, with their bioregions.

And so planetary eclectic, it refers to, you know, this kind of global population that we are now as a global community, global society. And we're able to learn from many different traditions from all over the world, you know. It doesn't mean that we're using those plants from all those different bioregions. You know, we're going to try to focus on our closest bioregions, but we're going to take those ideas and merge them together to help the individual. And so that's kind of what eclectic herbalism is speaking to. And so the second part of the question, how do I view human individuality when it comes to like food and healing and living in general. I think it goes back to that. And it's, you know, if we put this umbrella over us as a species, *Homo sapiens*, we haven't been the only *Homo* species out there, you know, we just somehow became the dominant one over the past, like, few hundred thousand years in particular. And so, you know, we lived amongst other, again, *Homo species*, and all these other species of plants and animals, et cetera. And so, you know, we co-evolved along with them and along with the plants and in response to the external environment of our bio region, you know, and that shaped our worldview and it shaped for some of us our physical form, possibly our blood types. There's all kinds of different theories about that. It dictated what foods we are able to consume, foods we were able to grow, what animals we were hunting, et cetera. And so thinking about our individuality, I think starts with where we were in our respective bioregions as we were evolving and not traveling very far from home. As we came out of East Africa, it took us a long time to migrate around the world, and as we started to settle again, like depending on the seasons, we were hunter gatherers for a long time. So, we, we roamed around small territories, it's like the way that we move today, even just a hundred years ago, people would never have traveled like we do and it was a very rare few set of people that really traveled around the world. So that, that kind of ... I would hope that answers the question in full.

Brendan [00:06:17]: Anything with the word "eclectic" in it speaks to me because there's so much wisdom in so many places, and we don't tend to find it all in one place or to get a comprehensive picture of anything. I think any inquiry in any domain of knowledge or human experience has to be eclectic. And so, what you're saying makes total sense and mirrors exactly how I view human evolution as well. So, because we do find a lot of metabolic diversity, a lot of differences between what kind of dietary approach works for different people. And unfortunately, we've got a lot of people out there ... it's like the warring of the points of view ... it's this way ... it's that way ... and everybody finds their evidence to support it. And they're all right to a certain degree. The only time they're wrong is when they're saying somebody else is wrong.

Sarah Wu [00:07:10]: Yeah, exactly.

Brendan [00:07:12]: Finding a piece of truth that it is somewhat relative. I mean because it applies to the people that it worked for, and I believe in kind of empiricism. I mean, like, if it works consistently, it's true, even if you don't understand. And if you find exceptions to it, well, OK, it doesn't work there. That doesn't mean it's not true because it's clearly working here.

Sarah Wu [00:07:35]: And with empirical evidence, which is how a lot of herbalists operated as well, is that you know, you'll see it working in a handful of people, or a few handfuls of people, or just in one person. And then that just gives you the bigger picture to the story behind what, what those plants are effective for or what that diet's effective for, but not getting hung up on that this is going to work always, you know. And it's always those times when things don't work, when we get the negative feedback loop from the plant that tells us, or from the diet that, that tells us, "ah, OK, there's something here that's individual, and I have to really think more and dive deeper and experiment more on what's going to work." And especially with our global community that we live in right now and people being of all kinds of mixed heritages, we can't just go back to our heritage diets or heritage plants anymore, unless you're the same as you've been since your ancestors have lived in their respective communities. And so, you know, it makes the decisions and the treatments tricky to figure out now. But that's, I guess a part of the fun of it.

Brendan [00:08:50]: Yeah, it's so experiential, basically. You mentioned the Ayurveda, which is something that a lot of people find very helpful as a lens or a method or system or something which you can overlay on any type of diet, and it works—I don't know how universally, but it seems to be pretty universal, which is fascinating to me—and there's sort of a science in there that explains how it works. And I'm curious if you could, I guess first give us what are some of the systems that you, or lenses or whatever words you might apply, to describe these different approaches to understanding individual constitutions.

Sarah Wu [00:09:34]: So from my perspective? What I'm using?

Brendan [00:09:38]: Yeah. So Ayurveda is one.

Sarah Wu [00:09:40]: Well, not really, actually. I have a very basic understanding of Ayurveda. I'm very basic about the doshas, and I do apply some of the herbs into my, what you call your Materia Medica or materials of medicine which is essentially your apothecary or your toolbox. And so, my foundation is actually through traditional Chinese medicine and then what we call ... which is another whole system of medicine which has had its own evolution throughout time, through 6,000 years and you know, Ayurveda and TCM, like to kind of fight over who's older. Yeah, it's one of those like funny kind of things in the herbal world, and then my other lenses would be through what's called the Wise Woman tradition, which comes from what we would call European witchcraft, kind of like the head witch, the healers of those communities, which has also evolved and is in a renaissance right now.

And then, the other perspective because I'm also a Permaculturist and live off the grid for many months of the year and have lived off the grid for years at a time and really close to Nature, is what we call Deep Ecology, which goes into the belief that the Earth is a living, breathing, feeling, responsive super organism. And that we're not just a bunch of different parts that constitute the Earth, but it's a whole being that we are a part of. And so, it goes into like the kind of interconnected web.

Brendan [00:11:20]: Like the Gaia theory.

Sarah Wu [00:11:42]: Yeah, very much like Gaia theory. And so, I'd say like those are kind of my three perspectives, you know, and merging together because it's eclectic, you know. And then I love learning about other traditions too, you know, like living in Latin America, like learning about the Latino traditions and some of the indigenous traditions. And again, like diving a little bit into, swimming at the surface of Ayurveda and my rudimentary understanding of that. And so, you know, I like to pull from different traditions. I would say that the main scope of my lens is through TCM and Wise Woman tradition.

Brendan [00:11:57]: OK. And, you mentioned something in another conversation we had recently, I think you said people sleep differently, they dream differently, communicate differently. So what are some of those realms or functions or processing that are individual, including ones maybe we're familiar with that, "OK, yeah, I get that everybody has a difference there." What might you be able to say in more depth about how we sleep differently and even other domains which I haven't mentioned?

Sarah Wu [00:12:31]: Sure. That's what we would call the individual constitution. So, we can put this umbrella over *Homo sapiens*. We are, right? And then we can divide ourselves into the two-gender group space and how you're born based, not based on your identity, but your physical, your anatomy and your physiology. What allopathic medicine and reductionist perspective do is: "OK, well you all have heart, lungs, liver, eyes, nose, ears, mouth, arms, legs. You know, you have all the same stuff. You're just male and female. And so therefore you should process everything the same. And therefore, our assessment of you and your treatment protocol is going to be the same across the board." So, when we're looking in holistic perspective and also from a constitutional perspective, which all systems of traditional medicine do touch into, using some different language for it is that, you know, yeah, that's true. OK. So, we're umbrella *Homo sapiens*. We're male, female through our anatomy, but again, like the, the way that we metabolize our food, where we carry our body weight, our bone structure, our skin color or eye color, our hair color, the texture of our skin and the texture of our hair, how our teeth sit in our mouth, you know, how we, again metabolize and eliminate our waste products. You know, the foods that we're drawn to are the foods that we're averse to, the foods that cause us, an imbalance. You know, we're always looking at in balance and out of balance, and trying to keep things from going like this and to keep things more like this (holding her two hands level with each other, or in balance), where our emotional highs and lows are, how we sleep, how many hours a night we need to feel vital, our dreams, how we communicate, the sound of our voices, how we think and process, how we see that is a big issue in the United States. I'm a little US-centric because that's just where I come from -- and in the echo chamber of my social media news, mostly the US --but you know, when we look at the education system for example, that kind of industrial system putting children through the same standardized tests and those kinds of things. People learn differently, you know, like some learn by doing, through seeing, through reading. Some have to have a kinetic experience, moving through the learning experience. And so, all of those little things are different for every single person. And some people will resonate more with others. When we look at say, at TCM and the five elements or we go into the Dosha, you do embody all of those, but you have dominant traits within you.

So, just like we have dominant genes that made my eyes and your eyes brown. But maybe we do have ... like I have a blue gene, maybe you have a blue gene, but we still hold on to those things, but it's like what actually is what we're born with, what we inherit from our parents, from our ancestors that make us this constitution that we are. And then what are the external environments that then manipulate our constitution, you know, like kind of the nature versus nurture thing. And so, you know, the external environment can benefit your constitution. It can also really make it a challenge. And some people have had, you know, traumas or things happened to them from early on that all of a sudden to them is normal, like going throughout their life.

You know, where really maybe that's just their constitution out of balance. And so actually like digging down into well, what is your true constitution? And what can we tweak a little bit, to put you into a state of peak vitality? So that's also where things are a little tricky trying to figure it out like, well what, what am I, you know, going through it all. Like what elements am I? What's my predominant Dosha and where am I out of balance? And so it takes time, you know, to dig down into somebody and just asking a lot of questions. You know, that's what's so beautiful about like the kind of patient intakes when you're practicing holistic medicine is they're hours long because there's so many layers to things that you're trying to ... it's like the onion, you know, just trying to an unpeel it all and figure out where, where you are at the root.

Brendan [00:16:55]: Right. I'm curious what your thoughts are as far as you know, how individuality applies to things like a plant-based diet versus an omnivorous diet with animal products. And 100% raw diet versus partially cooked, partial raw diet.

Sarah Wu [00:17:06]: Yeah, I mean that, that brings up so much because some people are so diehard about their diets, and they'll fight like actually to the end, you know, to defend their diets and sometimes can get really judge-y about it, which I feel is like really unfair because what it can do is hurt people that way. And I think when we go into, again, it's going back into the constitution. There again there is kind of the theories about blood types and our evolution in what we co-evolved with, with the animals and the plants. And so, I, I don't believe that that's the whole picture, but I think it's an interesting part of the picture. You know, I'm not like an expert in that by any case, but I always like to ask people, you know, as a part of their intake - do you know your blood type and what is your ancestral heritage? Where did your people come from?

Because, you know, again, when we think about where did people evolve and the bioregion that they had to respond to I think has a lot to do with it. And so, you know, if we look at, I know like with the raw kind of argument is that, well, human beings, we didn't start cooking until x number of years ago. and so we were eating raw foods, and how have we changed, how have our bodies evolved since that time, or not? And I think what it comes down to a lot with all the various diets is what makes you feel the most vital without your self-judgment, without your judgement of your peers, or from your mentors or your students, whatever, who have their philosophies on food. It's like when you eat x, how does it make you feel?

And really going into that kind of ... no guilt or intellect about it, but really, are you eliminating better or worse? Is your energy increased or decreased? How's your skin feel when you eat this way? What is your breath like? Are your eyes clear? Are your nails stronger? And so, it's evaluating when are you your most vital, and really paying attention to that. Like I know ... sure, like I do best, for example, on a lean protein and greens and fruits diet. Essentially, I'm Paleo. And that's like this hip kind of thing, talking about Paleo Diet, you know? And it's not because like I'm into that diet, but it's what makes me feel vital. And I know for myself that like, yeah, I crave cookies. If someone puts a pack of cookies in front of me, I will eat all those cookies. How's it going to make me feel afterwards? I know it's not going to make me feel good. You know, like I'm not going to feel guilty about it. Like I don't guilt myself about food, but you know, I know that it's like, I'm not going to eliminate the best. Maybe it's going to make me moody, and then I'm going to start craving more. And so I know those things about myself because I'm self-aware enough to realize what's happening in my body when I eat food. And I think that's like so much of what it comes down to, but people when they choose their diet, it's like we can again guilt trip ourselves and go into all the intellectual reasonings why we should be doing things. But what does it actually make you feel like? You know, and I, I think that so many people are so void of their mind/body connection. Like they don't put it together, like my terrible mood probably has to do because I drank a soda an hour ago. Or you know, I'm really low energy right now because I drank four cups of coffee in the morning because I went to bed really late, and I was on social media or was playing video games or was watching TV, whatever. And I couldn't shut my mind off, so I couldn't go to bed. So, I didn't get fully rested because my alarm clock went off after five hours of sleep. And I'm downing all this coffee, and then I have these peaks, and a lot of people don't put that together. So it does take a level of self-awareness to choose the best diet for yourself.

Brendan [00:21:16]: And of course, it's a two-way street in many of these regards, so not only does what we eat affect how we feel, our stress level, our sleep and so forth. But our stress level and our sleep affect what we're going to crave to eat, and so forth. And there's an intermediary in there which is another super organism that basically constitutes part of our super organism, the super organism that we are. And that's the microbiome. And we're discovering so much about our relationship to the world through the microbiome inside us and outside us. And I'm curious to know if you have anything to say about that. We're involved in these very interesting milieu of organisms, some of which we took into our body, into ourselves. We call it mitochondria. Of course, that was before there were even multi-cellular organisms. But then as we evolved, we obviously evolved in different bioregions with different plant foods and animal foods and fungal foods and different microbial strains and so you look in different parts of the world and some people's microbiome is more skewed towards one species array and in other parts of the world is skewed towards another. Just curious what you might have to say about all of that.

Sarah Wu [00:22:33]: Oh, yeah, well, for me as when you think about just where our world came from and how it came into being the world that we know of it today is all because of bacteria. You know, it's like in our oceans when our world was this kind of scary gaseous volcanic inhabitable place, we had these oceans. And some of the theory is like how did the bacteria is even get formed in the ocean, like lightening striking and all those kinds of things. And over millions and millions of years the bacteria is living and dying and evolving. And in our oceans eventually cyanobacteria form, which was the bacteria that was able to photosynthesize. And that photosynthesis started to change the planet as we know it. It started to take in the carbon dioxide and release oxygen, and eventually those bacteria started to make their way onto the earth and become terrestrial bacteria, which some of the ancestors of that are like our algaes and stuff. And they literally transformed our Earth. And so, I deeply believe that the plants are our ancestors, and that we came from that evolution of the cyanobacteria onto planet Earth and through all this time of the bacterias responding to their external environment. And so, I've heard those cool statistics (that) there's more bacterial cells in our body than human cells. And if we clumped it altogether, it would be bigger than our human brain and those neat kinds of things, like we're actually walking bags of bacteria, which is kind of funny.

Brendan [00:24:16]: We provide them with food, transportation, and entertainment. We're like a cruise ship for bacteria.

Sarah Wu [00:24:21]: Exactly!

Brendan [00:24:22]: I'm borrowing that from a scientist named David C. Johnson.

Sarah Wu [00:24:24]: I like that. Yeah, I like that. And we see all this evidence of the sterilization of our world and all the issues that it causes from antibiotics in our animals to fungicides and pesticides and bacterialcides that we're spraying on our soil and killing our soil, which is like the strata of all life on our planet. And even comparing things of children who grow up on farms versus children who grow up in sterilized suburban or city environments and the effects on their immune system. And so, you know, I think what's really important for people to understand is to not be bacteriaphobes, you know, and so how can we ... we can give people plush animals. Like when I was a kid growing up it was plush animals with pandas and bald eagles to get us excited about those kinds of things to get them off endangered species list. So, it's like some of our bacteria is endangered too. And so, it's like, we're not going to make plush animals out of bacteria maybe, or plush animals to look like bacteria, but it's like, how do we get people excited? And one of the things that I do is I love geeking out about soil and just like trying to blow people's minds about how amazing soil is, to give them an emotional attachment to it, because bacteria, for a lot of people, are scary and they equate bacteria with one thing, which is a disease or an illness, not realizing that bacterias are so critical to our life.

Sarah Wu [00:25:59]: And it goes into like all these different relationships that we find, you know in Mother Nature, which is, you know, symbiotic relationships, cooperative relationships, predatory, parasitic, contractual parasitic, and neutral relationships. It's like we have those relationships with all these different kinds of bacteria. And so people will take probiotics to be well and all this kind of stuff. And some of the things, I say to people is don't wash your produce. You know, like if you're getting produce from your garden, like don't like kind of shake it off, like I don't wash my produce unless there's obvious like animal poop on it, like a bird or something.

Brendan [00:26:48]: You have to make sure it's soil (that) you know. It could be soil that got a dose of cow manure from a CAFO facility where they're breeding antibiotic-resistant, flesh-eating bacteria or something you don't want ...

Sarah Wu [00:26:55]: But the food that's coming from my garden, if you're, if you're growing food in your own garden, like by all means, unless it was like, you know, some toxic waste on it or something or it's the garden bed that your cat also likes to poop in, and it's like you want to be mindful of those kinds of things. But I, I think a lot of it goes down to is like trying to just get people inspired about how amazing that co-evolution is between us and the soil itself. You know, and how we actually did evolve from bacteria. I know that challenges some people's belief systems. So, finding like gentle ways to get excited about it, you know.

Brendan [00:27:40]: What's amazing about soil and soil health is that in a healthy system, you basically have many, many species present. But the healthy ones are predominating. There could be pathological ones there, but they don't exert an influence, a (unintelligible) soil from a healthy soil system. And there might be pathogenic bacteria there, but they're out-competed. They're outnumbered. And it really comes ... this is David C. Johnson saying something like this ... he said basically every, everything's everywhere. It's just a question of what's dominant. I'm paraphrasing, hopefully accurately. So if a system is obviously healthy, you don't have to worry about, "Oh, but could there be some bad bacteria?" Yeah, there are some bad bacteria, and they're marginalized by the healthy bacteria. And when you have healthy bacteria in your gut, they marginalize any intruders, and the intruders don't have a chance to ...

Sarah Wu [00:28:40]: We have the bad bacterias on us right now, so to speak. It's that dance of in balance out of balance. So right now Staph infections and antibiotic resistant-Staph is an issue, you know. There's over 300 strains of Staph. You have a lot of staph all over your body right now, you know, underneath your nails, in your nose, in your armpits, in the webs of your fingers and the webs your toes, under your toenails. It's there. But yeah, like you said, when your immune system, when the healthy bacteria of your microbiome is diverse, it's going to stay in balance. And somewhere that staph bacteria is filling a niche, like in the ecosystem. Everything has a place in time and in space somewhere interacting with other things. And so, what does that Staph bacteria feed? Why does it live on our body? And there's a reason why it's there. And when it gets out of balance is when anti-bacterial soaps or nasty cuts that you don't get clean, or maybe that you're in an environment where you're stressed out all the time, and that wound opens up, and then the Sstaph comes in. Or in places like hospitals with the rampant antibiotic use, the bacterias are evolving too fast that we can't fight them, and it's become this war against bacteria, which is really dangerous. And so, I think so much goes to maintain healthy microbiome, goes into diversity in our diets as well. You know, like we've been monocultured for a long time now, like thousands of years. Our society has moved into what we call monoculture or just one culture, and it's moving even faster now. You know, with industrial farming, with suburban sprawl, with colonialism. And we can look at it from many different perspectives, but the monoculturing of our diet I think has drastically affected the health of our microbiomes and the lack of diversity in food in that our healthy bacteria thrives on eating fruits and vegetables, and if you're only consuming a corn-based diet or you're only consuming a wheat-based diet, which a lot of people are, or you look at places that are protein deficient, malnutrition where they're just eating yucca, or they're just eating rice, or they're just eating tortillas and beans. It's not enough diversity to feed the diverse bacterias as well. And so, when I think when we were hunter gatherers, you know, one, we are probably consuming soil, but we're also eating diverse foods that fed the diversity of bacterias as well. And so, I think one of the important things to nourish our microbiome is getting back into what some of our heritage and diverse bioregional foods are. You know, not depending on super foods shipped in from faraway places, or eating strawberries in the middle of winter. It's like really going into the seasons and, and re-shifting towards the local diet, and finding your co-op or the small organic farmer or the CSA that's holding on to the heirloom seeds still because I think that's one of our biggest struggles right now is keeping the genetic banks diverse because there's a lot of stuff working against us trying to monoculture everything into the most productive or the prettiest.

Brendan [00:32:22]: And losing a lot of times the nutritional value with that.

Sarah Wu [00:32:27]: Yeah. Yeah. And when we're eating foods from faraway places, even California to New York, those foods are harvested before they're at their peak vitality, so they're harvested really green so they can survive shipment, and then they're ripened in cold climate within a supermarket, underneath artificial light in air conditioned, weird filtered air. So, they're not getting living air and living water and living soil and sunshine to help them come to their peak vitality, which is where we get the most nutrition. And you can see that from like the tomato you buy at the supermarket, to the one you grow in your garden. There's a huge difference, even if it's the same seed selection.

Brendan [00:33:13]: And I think it's important for people to realize if that produce is not organic, it's often been irradiated. Something that a PhD soil microbiology student told me is that what they're seeing in some of the research is that what you get on the surface of produce has been irradiated. So, there's beneficial soil bacteria that you would find on the head of cabbage that you could turn into sauerkraut simply because there's enough soil bacteria right there on the cabbage that in a matter of days gives you delicious sauerkraut. If it's been irradiated, the soil bacteria is probably dead. And they do that to extend shelf life of produce because they don't want the bacteria to start to break down the produce. So, what you end up with as the microbiome of an irradiated head of lettuce is something more like the sum of the microbiomes of the hands that handled your food before you bought it. The hands that touched it after the irradiation and prior to you buying it is what you're getting. So that's just another big reason like, whoa …

Sarah Wu [00:34:26]: Well, and that's how we get outbreaks of Salmonella and those kinds of things because the sad reality …

Brendan [00:34:33]: Somebody went to the bathroom and didn't clean their hands.

Sarah Wu [00:34:36]: The working conditions, you know, like they're not provided with adequate sanitation or time to even to do that. And so, it's a sad state that we're in right now. And then you also think about the animals who receive massive antibiotic treatments. Those antibiotics travel through their waste stream and then you know, through their manure, which then goes onto conventional crops or it gets washed into our water systems and then those antibiotics are being placed right back into the system, like they're not going away, you know. And so, it's a big issue and a hard thing to tackle because sadly the industrial food complex is affordable to most people. And so how do you tell someone like, "Oh, well, you're hurting your microbiome by eating that hot dog," when maybe that's all that they can afford, you know? And so that's like a really hard part of like the kind of socioeconomic disparity between those of us who want to be vital and well, and it doesn't mean that those people don't want to be vital and well, but it's like who can afford to be vital and well and to have access to the information? And it's not being taught in schools, you know, maybe touched on in some good public schools or whatever. Some private schools are touching on it, but it's not like the focus. It's like if you can afford to go to a cool alternative Montessori farm school, then you're going to learn about it. But again, there's that gap, you know? And so just starting in something so simple like our conversation about microbiome, it opens up a whole can of earthworms.

Brendan [00:36:25]: You know, one of the things that concerns me most about our food supply and our planet is just the fact that we're destroying ecosystems. We're losing plants, species, medicinal plants. We don't know what they are yet. How many species are … you mentioned the term Materia Medica, which is I guess herbalists' Pharmacopoeia. Like how many plant species do humans know of collectively?

Sarah Wu [00:36:58]: Whoo, that's a big question,

Brendan [00:37:02]: I think I heard you say 80,000 once.

Sarah Wu [00:37:04]: Well, 80,000 medicinal plants have been cataloged since humans started writing about plants. And so that's going back to referencing like cuneiform, which was the first written language in ancient Sumeria. It's looking at ancient Chinese texts; it's looking at that's looking things written in the Bible and the Torah; it's looking at things written in Egyptian. And so, we know about 80,000 medicinal plants. Right now, what is known to our human materia medica is about 35,000 medicinal plants only. And so, thinking about foods like … (looking around her room) I could go grab it … I have like a net geo over there that talks about food. A few years ago they did every issue of the year about our food system. And there is some statistic about like how we've whittled our diversity down to like nothing and you know …

Brendan [00:38:03]: Research shows that we were eating like 250 plants; we were traveling as hunter gatherers or whatever. So, we evolved with a lot of diversity that agriculture whittled down to like a few dozen species.

Sarah Wu [00:38:18]: A few dozen species. Yeah. I mean, think about your supermarket. What do you see in your supermarket? You know, like two or three varieties of tomatoes, one variety of bananas, you know, one variety bananas and the supermarket where it's like at our farm we have like 40 varieties of bananas, you know, but there's one that looks pretty on the shelf, you know? And that's like, the sad part is …

Brendan [00:38:40]: I can tell you the best ones are small and stubby with color.

Sarah Wu [00:38:42]: And brown. I love that rise of like the ugly food stores, but that's just to keep food out of the waste stream. But that's not even talking about diversity in food. I don't even know where we're at right now actually.

Brendan [00:39:01]: Well, you know I think worth mentioning (that) it's not just the plant world either because … enter stage right or left depending upon the mirror effect going here (holding up a jug of brown liquid) … so this has both plant and fungal foods. So this has got some of the chaga mushroom, which I love and you know, gosh knows how many fungal species maybe are in the tropical forest that we don't know what they might do for our consciousness, our nutrition, our mental performance.

Sarah Wu [00:39:28]: All over the world.

Brendan [00:39:29]: ... for our mental performance ...

Sarah Wu [00:39:36]: The majority of plants depend on multiple fungal species to survive, the majority of which are in the soil. We have fungal species above the soil, and we'll see their fruiting bodies above the soil. But fungus, mycelium, is critical for plant health, you know, and that it helps the plants to retain water, to metabolize sugar to, or their starches, to prevent invasion from other species. And the mycelium helps the plants to communicate with each other below the soil, you know? And so ...

Brendan [00:40:08]: And mind-blowing things.

Sarah Wu [00:40:10]: Yeah. Yeah. Fungus is critical to plant health ...

Brendan [00:40:16]: I'll just mention briefly, because I have mentioned just because I have mentioned tropical forests as this vast biodiversity, but temperate forests ... also huge resources we've lost most of, and that's where chaga comes from. Temperate forests.

Sarah Wu [00:40:33]: It does. Just be mindful on your chaga consumption. It's one in every 20,000 trees has a chaga mushroom on it. Yeah. And it does. Yeah. And it doesn't reproduce very ... it only releases spores between 12 and 24 hours a year. So just be mindful on how much chaga you're consuming. Right? Even though it's amazing. Yeah. There is a glut of global demand. And unfortunately—there's an organization I'm a member of called United Plant Savers, and chaga is on the threatened species list.

Brendan [00:41:02]: I didn't know that!

Sarah Wu [00:40:05]: Yeah, yeah. Sorry to burst the bubble. But I believe Paul Stamets, who's our mycelium wizard out there ... I believe he is manufacturing chaga in a lab. And so, you might want to, probably a little bit more expensive, but you might want to think about that one.

Brendan [00:41:28]: Right. So, you know, one of the things that I see happening in the world is people are moving from a possession-based economy to an experience-based economy. We're realizing that the greatest ... what we all seek as humans is experience. We don't really seek possessions; we think we do because we want the experience we think that possession is going to give us, and some of the best experiences available come from plant foods, fungal foods, but also just being in the environment that produced them, as much. And so, I've had the most amazing experiences of my life ... and everybody, if you think about it, most vacations are booked to go to somewhere beautiful. And you know, except for those excursions to Dubai or something. But I do like dancing crazy to some electronica sometimes, but I've done that in a forest environment before and nothing beats that. So, the question I want to ask you is you live in a tropical forest, south east corner of

Costa Rica, the Mona facility there. I'm just curious what you like, what you like most and even least. There's pros and cons to everything about living in a tropical forest environment.

Sarah Wu [00:42:57]: Yeah, definitely. You know, so through my evolution as an herbalist and as an environmentalist, I came to Costa Rica in 2001, 19 years old and really had my head cracked open. I grew up in a rural suburban environment. And so, I always had a connection to Nature. We're one of those generations still that, you know, we remember times before computers. My first cell phone was when I was 20. You know, like we remember those times still when it was like, you played outside. And so I always had this special connection with Mother Earth, and it was one of the things that really stimulated me to become an environmentalist as well as become an herbalist. I started studying plant medicine at 19 years old as well. And so, when I … the majority of my twenties was in a city in Philadelphia and learning herbalism there, and not living and being with the living plants was hard, you know, it was a lot of like tinctures, teas, pills. I was working with the medicinal plants that way. And so, for me, when I relocated to Costa Rica in 2009, and started living directly with Mother Nature, it was probably the most humbling experience in my life, you know, it really took us from—took me from—this anthropocentric world that revolved around my experience, you know, and the experience of my friends and colleagues and peers, to centering myself in this inner … it's the interconnected web. It's not just something I call it, you know, I got that from David Suzuki. I Love David Suzuki. I read him a lot, and that interconnected web and this concept of the declaration of interdependence was just like really stimulated in me from living in the jungle. And the jungle is quite different from temperate forest in that everything is expedited. You know, like growth. You'll see these trees sometimes that you're like, "Whoa," you know, and if you're in the northern climates, like where I grew up in upstate New York or Philly or something, it's like that tree would be like hundreds of years old, and you're like, "Oh yeah. It's like, you know, 50 years old or 14 years old." It's like these young trees that just … when you have that much sun and that much water, it's like the elemental things that they need to just like explode into life. And they don't go into that winter pause. There's that which you're just amazed by. And then there's the other part that they die really fast and that they break down fast. And so, you see just the growth and the death process, and the composting and how important the death cycle actually is and how it just feeds all new life. And so for me, living in the jungle is just … it's one of the most beautiful experiences because you really are, you feel your inner connection with everything and taking it out of the anthropocentric world into the ecocentric world, and "eco" just means "home", like really going back into home and the whole concept of like when people say "one love"—we live in the Caribbean—that's what that is for me, is that ecocentrism, and that I'm no different than the dolphins or the coral reef. They're right in my front yard or this plant or that fungus or that toucan or that toucan, my chickens or these other human beings that I'm living with. And so, the tropics for me is just … it's the greatest, greatest teacher. And it's all beautiful, and it sounds really romantic. And the hardest part of it is that there are exponentially more bugs than human beings on this planet Earth. Whether they're under the ground, they're at knee level, they're at eye level, they're up at the sky. There's a lot of bugs.

And the fungus … the tropics, where we live in Punta Mona on the southern Caribbean coast, only about seven miles from the border of Panama is … we get three and a half meters of rain. OK? Most people count their rain in inches. We count ours in meters. And so, when you get that much rain a year, literally, like things are rotting.

Your books smell. If you have leather, good luck. Your clothes are going to get all stained. And so, the hardest part has been living with fungus and just the bacterias and the wildlife and the bugs and everything. Nothing is dead, ever. And that's another really beautiful lesson that like, even though you think it's gone, it's not. It's been transformed into something else.

And so that's the hardest part, but it's also some of the most important lessons, especially about like materialism. Like you're saying, we want actual experiences; we don't want material objects, and we've just been kind of marketed to believe that. And so, it really helps you to let go of your attachments to things, whether it's the tree that you were in love with that fell over in the tropical storm, or whether it's your favorite book or your favorite pair of shoes. It's a transient place a little bit, too, because we're an education center, and we do volunteering. Whereas the person who just became your best friend just left. And so, those were the beauties and the challenges of it, you know, is that we're not at the top. You know, I really believe that we're somewhere in between like dolphins and fungus evolutionarily, and our intelligence and everything. So just somehow, we became dominant. We're just very dexterous.

Brendan [00:48:55]: We're pretty intelligent as beings on Earth go.

Sarah Wu [00:48:57]: Yeah, we are.

Brendan [00:49:00]: So, you said something in our first conversation on a Skype call, and you said two things that kind of summarize for me what this event is about. Number one, you said, "There is no panacea." And basically, you were saying there was no one diet which we've kind of talked about. And then you also said, "If our planet is not thriving, we're not. If our planet is in collapse, we are." And that's just kind of sums it up for me. I should have you on my copywriting team, so thank you for that. It sums it up beautifully. Anything else you would add? I know that you teach people things in your world there. People come there and take courses, or they stay and live there, and I'm not sure how it works, if they get a home there, or they homestead. What would you say in concluding?

Sarah Wu [00:50:02]: Oh Gosh, well, I'd say in conclusion that yes, there is no panacea, and so learn everything you can, you know, whether it's about diets or it's about food or it's belief systems, and then formulate for yourself what makes you feel the most vital physically, psycho-spiritually. I would suggest that. And then also in conclusion is that like always ask why, and question everything. I think that's how we also come to our own conclusions and opinions and really kind of formulate our experiences and what we're able to then reciprocate back out to the world. I believe in mutually beneficial relationships, and I think if we're not asking questions, and we're just taking in what we're being told, then we're not able to really give back our own experience and in a mindful way. And so yeah, there's that. And is this like a time for props or shout outs or whatever? Self-promotion?

Brendan [00:51:16]: Yeah, how do people work with you individually?

Sarah Wu [00:51:18]: Yeah, I do some individual consultations, and we can do this online, in person if you're in Costa Rica, but what I'm really excited about, which goes much in line with what we're talking about today is this curriculum I'm writing, which is a pretty unique, called Permaculture for the Herbalist Path. And so I'm also Permaculture teacher. Permaculture for those listening who might not know what it is a set of principles and ethics and modality, a design process, for living in line with the natural systems, depending on your individual bioregion. So, it's all about like strategies for lightening our footprint on the Earth and really ... not being stewards to say like we're not responsible for the Earth to thrive, but we're a critical part in it. And so, Permaculture, it's really beautiful, and it can be applied to many different things, whether it's farming or social justice or education, or your office. And so, what I'm doing with that is merging it with herbal medicine. And so, it's looking at that, like how the state of our planet and the health of our bioregions regions, the health of our air, water and soil is all directly related to our human vitality and our human experiences. And so, what we're going to do is in merging those together is see how does herbalism apply to this, whether it's how we're looking at community health care or global health care, your family ... how our bodies mirror our environment, et cetera. And so that's this March, and hopefully it'll become like an annual thing and eventually a book is what I'm hoping for. So, I'm really excited about that. So, you can go to our website, which I'm sure it's going to be in your info.

Brendan [00:53:08]: I can't wait to see that because it's not that many people out there doing an eclectic, multidimensional approach, and it's so needed in the world. Thank you for your thought leadership in that regard. And thank you for being with us here in the Eat4Earth community.

Sarah Wu [00:53:21]: Oh absolutely. And thank you so much for putting this summit together and taking the time to talk to me today and inviting me. So, thank you.

Brendan [00:53:29]: It's been great. Thank you.

Day 7 –Regenerative Food Systems: Should Animals Play a Role?

Biomimicry, Healing the World's Grasslands, and Reversing Climate Change with Holistic Management
Victoria Keziah
<u>What You Will Discover</u>

- Savory Global's "big, hairy, audacious goal" to help reverse climate change
- How "biomimicry" harnesses Nature's time-perfected systems to grow better food and heal the planet
- How the "super-organism" "interface" role of plant-eating animals can make livestock a regenerative influence on the planet
- The key difference between the "Land to Market" "Ecological Outcome Verified" program and certifications like "Organic".

Cows from CAFOs vs. Cows That Reverse Climate Change
Allen Williams, PhD
<u>What You Will Discover</u>

- The staple vegetarian food that emits high levels of methane
- How cattle can rapidly grow soil carbon
- How methane from cattle gets handled in natural systems
- Why friends don't let friends eat beef fed "dried distiller's grains"

Did We Get Agriculture Wrong 10,000 Years Ago? Regenerating Grasslands with Livestock, Grains, and Cover Crops
Colin Seis
<u>What You Will Discover</u>

- How a devastating fire and drinking too much beer turned out to be a good thing for agriculture all around the world7
- The crazy idea that enabled Colin to revive a natural grassland and never again have to buy $80,000 of chemicals every year
- How Colin grows vegetables in a restored grassland ecosystem that also produces grains, animals, and native plant seeds
- Why Colin gets no pest attacks despite not using pesticides for over 20 years.

Cow Curious, the Hunt for Carbon Cowboys, and the Potential Redemption of McDonalds
Peter Byck
<u>What You Will Discover</u>

- The surprising benefits of intelligently managed livestock to bees, birds, and other wildlife

- A focus on soil as the vehicle for farmers and ranchers to get out of debt
- How certain grazing systems are reducing livestock stress and infections, and giving them a good life
- What McDonalds has done for the study of planet-healing livestock management

Transforming Agriculture & Food's Nutrient Density with "Tree Range" Chickens
Reginaldo Hasslett-Marroquin
What You Will Discover

- Why the chicken was chosen to "take over the world" for regenerative agriculture
- The world's first humane poultry production system designed in collaboration with the chicken themselves
- How this system captures "free" ecological energy to out-produce conventional agriculture 4-8 times while reducing consumer cost per unit of nutrition
- Simple design innovations that enable chicken production throughout the Minnesota winter without high energy inputs

Victoria Keziah Interview
Biomimicry, Healing the World's Grasslands, and Reversing Climate Change with Holistic Management

Brendan [00:03]: Welcome to the Eat4Earth event. This is Brendan Moorehead, and together we're exploring how you can heal yourself, your loved ones, and the planet with food. Our next guest, Victoria Keziah is a brand and business strategist with 25 years of commitment to serving organizations that are leading the way toward positive change. With experience as a strategic planner in the New York advertising world she founded and built one of the world's first boutique branding strategy firms, Kendrick Keziah Incorporated, which grew to house three divisions with offices in Boulder and New York, and a roster of Fortune 500 companies. In 2005 she sold Kendrick Keziah to senior management and devoted her work to full time to sustainable and social innovation exclusively. She views her work with clients in many sectors of the green economy and her current focus on regenerative agriculture through the Savory Institute as the greatest work of our time, healing the land and our relationship to it. Victoria is a certified biomimicry specialist and a Master's Degree candidate in biomimicry at ASU (Arizona State University). She brings her understanding of natural systems and evolutionary fitness to the rollout of the Land to Market program at Savory, the world's first verified regenerative sourcing solution. She lives with her family in Boulder, Colorado where she spends every possible moment in the great outdoors. Victoria it's awesome to have you and your luminous presence with us. Thank you.

Victoria [01:30]: Oh thank you Brendan. So great to be with you.

Brendan [01:32]: My pleasure. So what is biomimicry, and how does it relate to our food, our health and the planet?

Victoria [01:39]: Yeah, well, biomimicry is defined as "the conscious emulation of Nature's genius." And then I typically append that with "in human designs and systems and strategies." So, Nature has essentially an encyclopedia of wisdom just outside the door that's available to us all the time that provides to us -- if we're willing to take the time to observe and receive it -- the patterns, the strategies, the forms, the processes, and the relationship structures that have facilitated long-term evolutionary success for tens of millions of species over billions of years. And so biomimicry is really our chance to step back out of our existing mental model and expand that to consider ourselves as humans, as participants in our wider ecosystem, and understand how we can best fit in again, and remember ourselves to the planet on which we depend for our health.

Brendan [02:48]: That is so beautifully stated. I love that. And I'm curious, how does this relate to you as a branding strategist?

Victoria [02:57]: Well, actually I had a little bit of a turning point in my own career where I was working in very conventional markets, building brands, and that I learned a lot about how to create community around an idea and how to stimulate acceptance and trial of new products. And that was tremendously instructive in the early part of my career. And then at a certain point I realized that the way that I was approaching all of that was through this sort of industrialized ethos of pursuing infinite growth at all costs without thinking about the unintended consequences of that … of assuming that competition is king rather than collaboration. And of really accepting and prioritizing the extraction and exploitation of resources for the sake of profit as really the definition of success. And all of that was embedded in my work as a brand strategist and was kind of the only way that I could look at a client's challenge. And when I pivoted my work to focus on sustainable and social innovation I realized that those clients were less concerned with some of those parameters, that they really wanted to focus on how can we be better participants ecologically, economically, and socially? How can we actually prioritize collaboration over competition? And how can we not extract resources for profit but actually contribute to the ecosystemic web, the food web, if you will, that we're a part of? And so I needed a new mental model, and that's how I discovered biomimicry. And I would say that most biomimics work in kind of the form side of the business, so, you know, mimicking the, I call it "the what of the it". Like for instance, the bullet train that's modeled after the beak of the King Fisher bird for its aerodynamics and efficiency. And what I do is more mimicking the "how of the whole", so looking at Nature essentially as a whole system and life as a process that's ongoing and trying to apply that to organizations that really want to be leaders and participate in the regeneration of our resources.

Brendan [05:11]: Awesome. And how does biomimicry relate to the Savory Institute and what's going on with what the organization has been doing for so many years in producing the counterintuitive results that you can actually raise more cattle if you do it in a certain way certain whether well, any kind of livestock and regenerate landscapes as opposed to the way livestock is often grazed that destroys landscapes?

Victoria [05:37]: Yeah. So that was what drew me originally to Savory Institute was I read the story of Allan Savory, the founder of the Savory Institute, and essentially that the epiphany that he had when he essentially quieted his own analysis of the bush in Africa where he was working and he just allowed himself to really observe both the signs of degradation and regeneration in that region. And he realized … and this was the conventional perception at the time was that any sort of livestock or any sort of grazer, wild or domestic, was depleting the grass beneath their feet simply because they were consuming it. And so there we're actually cullings of wildlife in order to rejuvenate those landscapes. And what he realized was that the presence of those animals was actually performing an ecosystem function. And that was the birth essentially of Holistic Management which allows a land manager, a farmer or a rancher to view their operation, their ranch, as a living system. And so essentially what Mr. Savory discovered, and what Holistic Management teaches, is that there is a fundamental, inevitable mutualism, interdependency, between grassland and grazer. And that's on many, many levels. At the landscape level, a herd of herbivores or ruminants, when they're under threat of predation or some sort of pressure to have them move as a herd, they actually perform sort of landscape gardening, right? Because their hoof action turns up the soil which makes it more receptive to rain water. It actually grinds decaying matter back down into the soil so that it can be turned up into useful nutrients again. And then the act of them feeding on the grass … the digestive waste they leave acts as fertilizer. So at the landscape level, there's this interdependency between these herds that, originally through migratory behavior, and now that we mimic through Holistic Management, creates that necessary disturbance for the grasses to regenerate. And then the other interesting interdependency that I learned through biomimicry and that we don't talk about as much is that there's also an interdependency at the microbial level. So grasslands themselves tend to be very brittle, which means that they receive only seasonal precipitation. That means that the soil under the grass actually is a less hospitable habitat for a whole host of bacteria that would perform what's called the "interface function" of turning decaying matter back into useful nutrients. So that interface species over these millennia of coevolution and developing mutualisms actually reside in the gut of the grazer. So again, there's this tremendous marriage really between the grass and the grazer that is both at the landscape level and also all the way down to the cellular level in the bacteria. So it's really fascinating stuff. And what we do is empower farmers and ranchers all around the world essentially regardless of context, meaning what is their ecological set of conditions? What sort of rainfall do they have? What sort of land requirements do they face? What sort of social conditions are they under? We allow them to just reenact this mutualism in context.

Brendan [09:40]: So it's kind of like they're roving composters of grass and depositing compost everywhere.

Victoria [09:47]: Yeah. It's sort of like they're like a roving landscape crew, so they, they like aerate the soil. They turn it up. They grind that decaying matter down, and yes, they do fertilize with their digestive waste. Actually, when we look back at the dustbowl in the US, we humans actually facilitated that. That wasn't really an act of Nature or an act of God. It was really our act in essentially culling the natural herds of Bison and then colonizing the land and laying out fences so that even if livestock were there they were essentially dispersed and just able to kind of roam without any structure. And what Holistic Management does again is it mimics that herd movement of a super organism through mobile paddocks so that aggregate hoof action really takes effect in the soil.

Brendan [10:41]: How is that different from, I guess more laissez faire forms of grazing that are actually destructive with even fewer cattle? Far fewer actually.

Victoria [10:53]: Yeah. Essentially, and again, it's not about the number of cattle. I know we often go off track with that discussion. It's really about we again, and this is where the whole discussion about biomimicry comes in. How we as humans participate in the ecosystem through our management of those livestock. So in a traditional ranching operation the livestock may be turned out into sort of a section of the ranch, and then they're allowed to essentially eat their favorite foods that their discretion, their favorite species of grass at their discretion, not necessarily at the right time in terms of the growing season of that plant and not necessarily for the right reason in terms of how that disturbance that the cattle creates actually facilitates the regeneration of that grass. So it is complex, but once a rancher understands that for their own region and that they can use a herd as a tool like, like we've said, to regenerate that landscape it starts to really sink in and make a difference. And then the cattle aren't dispersed. They're managed as a whole.

Brendan [12:07]: Would it be accurate, if I'm trying to understand it most simply without understanding all the interactions, does it -- and this is oversimplifying it -- but is it largely a matter of duration? In other words, under what I was calling laissez faire. You know, just letting the cows out into a pasture not so planned. They stay too long in a certain area, overgraze. Whereas you could have a lot more cattle going through, but for very short duration. It actually creates a positive ecological impact that's very different from. So is it partly that?

Victoria [12:42]: That's exactly right. Yeah. So you're already getting it. So what the farmer or rancher does and what are our hubs around the world train them to do is create a whole plan where they actually look at different sections of their ranch as individual paddocks, and they plan exactly when they're going to put their herd on that land according to what species of grass are emerging and where the grass is in its lifecycle, and also other concerns around migratory behavior of other wildlife and other factors about precipitation. But then essentially those that herd is placed there at that specific right time for the right reasons and for the right amount of time so that the disturbance actually creates regenerative rather than degenerative outcomes on the land. That's exactly right. Yeah.

Brendan [12:42]: Ok.

Victoria [13:28]: Yeah, and that's about as much as I know because I'm not a rancher. (laughs)

Brendan [13:36]: (laughing) You're not the lead scientist for this organization. Do you have any photos you can show us? So we kind of get a visual of what it does on the landscape ... Ok, I see your screen.

Victoria [13:47]: Good. Yeah. So this is just a great example of ... we call these our fence line photos where you see a landscape that is degraded. There's a tremendous amount of desertification and bare ground. The native grasslands are not regenerating, and then after just a couple of years or sometimes even less of Holistic Management. Which simply means that the livestock that may have already been on the ranch as we've described have just been dispersed ... when they're managed as that whole herd and that disturbance happens that the grasses actually do begin to come back. And that's the only thing that changes. There isn't a change in bringing in any kinds of fertilizers or any additional moisture, anything. That is the only thing that changes is using the livestock as a tool. So that last slide was Namibia. This here is a similar example from Mexico, and then here's one from Australia. Exactly the same landscape, but just with the change that Holistic Management can beget.

Brendan [15:00]: Wow, that's amazing.

Victoria [15:01]: Yeah, it is. And it is, it becomes, you know, really empowering and intuitive for the rancher. It obviously allows with that increased forage of the grass ... it does allow them to, if they wish, to increase their stocking rates, which increases the productivity of their ranch. They also can bring on additional species and continue to sort of build complexity on the land. So it's a win win.

Brendan [15:38]: Yeah, and the term tool makes a lot of sense because a tool can be used well or misused, and that's kind of the way I see it.

Victoria [15:41]: That's such a good point. That's one thing that we talk about a lot is that our opportunity as humans is we're such good tool users, right? I mean, that's a huge component of how we have survived thus far and succeeded as a species. You know everything from spears to atom bombs. We build tools and we can look at cattle as a tool as well, or livestock could be sheep, could be goats. And we can actually think with that tool mindset about how to facilitate regenerative outcomes.

Brendan [16:14]: So even though livestock can be tremendously destructive as we know in various ways, basically we don't want to throw out the baby with the bathwater. If grasslands in fact evolved as they did with ruminant herbivores … just have to restore the right ecological relationships.

Victoria [16:31]: That's exactly right. And the opposite is also true. If we remove that interdependency, if we deprive the land of that marriage that it had with these large ruminant herds, then the land will not be able to facilitate its own regrowth because of the ecosystem function that those grazers performed.

Brendan [16:52]: That's what my understanding is of Allan Savory's TED talk. Where I guess they thought, "OK, we need to cull elephants." He loved elephants, but they culled elephants, and the land got worse not better. So they realized, "Uh-oh, it's totally different than what we thought." It's counter-intuitive.

Victoria [17:12]: That was a big part of his learning process for sure and something that I think still lives very close in his heart was, you know, we all have certain suffering that actually leads us to hopefully do better with our lives. And I think that was a real turning point for him. And now what we're learning in biomimicry is so interesting. We assumed that the relationship between predator and prey was always antagonistic. But what we're learning is that there's interdependency often built into many predator and prey relationships. So I don't know if you've heard the example of the whales and their krill that they feed on, but blue whales essentially facilitate the regrowth of their own food source through their digestive process as well. So they give off these … it's kind of gross, but they give off these fecal plumes of their own digestive waste, which then rises to the surface of the water that feeds the plankton, which then ultimately feeds the krill. So one of the things that the fisherman found as they were … the krill fisherman found was when they got rid of the whales, which they thought were part of the problem, they lost their krill source. And when they brought them back the krill came back. And so the same can kind of be true for us. It's a little bit more metaphorical. But when we think about our own food and as the consumers of it, how in consuming it can we contribute to its regeneration? How can we not assume that it's just this linear "take, make waste" model? But how can we actually participate in the regeneration of our own food sources? And Holistic Management and the livestock and food and fiber supply that we're creating is one example. But there are probably many others across different categories of food as well.

Brendan [18:59]: I love that example of the whales. I've seen the video narrated by George Monbiot and he calls them poo-namis … fecal plumes that fertilizes their own food source. And that's what cows do they fertilize their own food source. So how broad is the usage around the world of this particular method?

Victoria [18:59]: Sure.

Brendan [19:27]: So hectares, which is two and a half acres.

Victoria [19:34]: Yeah. So Savory has 30 regional hubs or affiliate sites around the world that are producing these outcomes across all habitable continents around the world. Wrapped up within that network, we call it our network is about 20,000,000 acres that are currently converted and under influence and producing we believe are producing regenerative outcomes. We're getting ready to actually prove that with science. And then I would say there's a legacy load that actually precedes the formal creation of the hub network, which was launched in 2012. All of the acreage that was just effected through trainings and workshops and influence that Allan and his early founders created. And that legacy load takes us up to more like 50,000,000 acres around the world.

Brendan [20:20]: Wow. And you goal is?

Victoria [20:24]: Our goal, our big hairy audacious goal, thank you for asking, is to affect 1,000,000,000 hectares of land around the world. And we think it's going to take us about a hundred hubs to get there or some other similar kind of acceleration model. But at that point we will have reached a tipping point in terms of the ecosystem function that grasslands can actually provide. Grasslands cover one third of the earth's surface, but about a fifth of them are degraded and desertified. If we can continue to bring them back then, even at the meta level we can be absorbing carbon and providing climate and water and food security and get back on the right side of history in terms of our carbon footprint as a species.

Brendan [21:17]: Ok. You know I've heard and there's speakers in this event that have given some of the quantifications of their beneficial impact in terms of increasing soil carbon, a percentage of organic matter in soils under their herds. And I'm just curious if there's any quantification that's happened anything you could share as far as the impact of this, of a Holistic Management in your network?

Victoria [21:42]: Yes. We're right in the throes of that, and that's a piece of Land to Market which is the component of it that I'm helping to bring into life. But we're developing something called the Ecological Outcome Verification. And that is a scientific protocol whereby our hubs actually go to producers in their regions. They lay down what we call transects. They keep, they collect some initial data around key criteria that together with some academic institutions we've developed as indicators of land regeneration. So those include biodiversity, water infiltration and retention, and ecosystem function. So some of the things we've talked about before -- the mineral cycles, the cycling of carbon, the cycling of water, the cycling of energy -- all of those things get wrapped up into what we call a Land Health Index. And then what we do is we track and trend it over time with annual monitoring. And a given farm or ranch that chooses to participate in the program and get verified would then be able to say that their land and therefore the products coming off of it are serving to regenerate that landscape. So Ecological Outcome Verification is something that we're developing right now, and we'll be talking about a lot more in 2018.

Brendan [23:10]: Ok. And the Land to Market program, as I understand it, is a certification. Is that correct? And can you tell us what that is?

Victoria [23:16]: Sure, so actually what I just described as the certification, it's actually not a certification because it's not really a top-down bureaucratic vetting model without any consideration for the farmer's stake in that outcome. It's much more a bottom-up movement where the farmer or rancher seeks to become verified for their own learning, to compare that learning to that of other ranchers and farmers in the network. And then yes, to receive some differentiation in the marketplace for the fact that whatever they're doing on the land is actually producing these outcomes and biodiversity and ecosystem health and water security. So the, the Ecological Outcome Verification is actually the label that will ultimately come out. Land to Market, I view as the community. And that is a multidisciplinary community, all of whom are joining in this movement. So it's the farmers; it's the ranchers; it's our hubs; it's brands; it's retailers; it's Savory; and it's consumers, all of whom want more information and want to know that they're really having an impact with their food and fiber choices and purchases. And the Ecological Outcome Verification is really the "Intel inside" for that. It's where the rubber hits the road and where we can say this product came from a place that is regenerating.

Brendan [24:38]: Ok. So what was the name again of the actual certification that we would see on a, on a package of some kind of product?

Victoria [24:45]: Sure, it'll be Ecological Outcome Verification or EOV for short. And yeah, it's a little wonky, but we want it to say what it is so people know that you actually can measure outcomes on the land. You know, historically, these verifications or these certifications have been practice-based. So they've looked at what is the farmer or rancher doing or not doing? Are they organic or not? Are they tilling or not? Are they cover cropping or not? This is much more about not the farmer or rancher saying or providing testimony to their practices. It's giving the land literally giving the land a voice to see how it's responding to us being on the land. So it's a little bit of a new step. And we're really excited about giving the land to voice in this way.

Brendan [25:30]: And a really important step. I mean, goodness, I mean, that's really what I want to see in all certifications is what does this actually doing for my planet and for my body. And so what types of products will this apply to mean anything across the board or is it just livestock?

Victoria [25:47]: Well, our core competency, as I said, is those 20,000,000 acres of grasslands around the world, and they tend to be livestock operations. So we're talking about food and fiber. Primarily meat, dairy, wool and leather. And then within the meat, you know typically, it would be beef or sheep and potentially goat as well. That's where we're going to begin with the program. But in many cases these farmers and ranchers also have crop operations. They might have other species of poultry and other meats that could come into the program. So we're going to start with our core competency and measuring outcomes on grasslands. And then we'll try to build alliances and partnerships to expand the dialogue beyond that.

Brendan [25:47]: Ok. That makes a lot of sense.

Victoria [26:32]: But essentially it'll be meat, dairy wool and leather to start.

Brendan [26:35]: Ok. And now let's say if I'm, if I buy that type of product or friends do, and I want to encourage them, "Hey, get EOV. Don't just buy that feedlot livestock." When would I and my friends expect to see this on the shelf?

Victoria [26:53]: Yeah, we're actually in beta right now with some key early partners, working out some of the kinks and actually bringing our supply into the market place. So I would say you will hopefully be able to see something no later than fourth quarter 2018. And definitely by 2019 early.

Brendan [27:18]: Ok, great. What, I mean, I'm definitely hearing a big difference between this and potentially any other certification because it's, it's essentially results based. Is there anything else to say about it that's different from other certifications that are out there?

Victoria [27:29]: You know, I think that's really the key—that and the fact that it's really meant to be a learning that ... to create the sense of learning across the practitioner network of farmers and ranchers. And then also for consumers, for us to start thinking about what do we really mean when we say regenerative? You know, it is the next step beyond sustainable, and we need to not just treat it as sort of a greenwashed new badge that we can wear. We really need to understand that what we mean by regeneration is creating conditions conducive to further life again and again and again through facilitating that, those cyclic processes. So understanding things like the importance of biodiversity. Understanding the importance of things like carbon absorption and water security. You know, we hope that it can be also a source of education for the consuming public.

Brendan [28:25]: You may have essentially already answered this question, but is there any particular guarantee, any particular criterion or criteria that I know are met if I EOV on food?

Victoria [28:38]: Well, essentially it's the, and this is where the magic of Savory comes in. This isn't a one size fits all methodology. It is referenced against the contextual parameters within a given region. So we lay down reference areas that are within a certain ranches region. So I won't be able to say it's, you know, it's absorbing x amount of carbon every time or x amount of water. But the point is that the Land Health Index, which is the aggregation of all of these criteria will be on the rise. The point is that we'll be seeing progress and improvement on the land.

Brendan [29:18]: You know, there's a particular issue that comes up with regard to raising livestock here in the United States. And that is livestock that are grazed on public lands. And from what I understand, I haven't researched it in depth, but the USDA has had a program that is now called Wildlife Services and it is, one of the things it does is it culls predatory wildlife. In other words, wolves and bears and mountain lions that may be a quote unquote "threat", or that could be, you know, maybe to human populations nearby the habitat or something, but apparently also to protect wildlife, or excuse me, livestock that are grazed based on a lease or some agreement that the grazer has with the United States government that actually owns this public land -- Bureau of Land Management land or something like that, maybe even National Forest land. And so that's a big concern if there's a ... to me anyway, and I think a lot of other people, if those livestock are used as a reason to kill predators, predator populations. So I'm just curious if you know anything about that, and is that in any way an issue or subject or addressing the way through the certification?

Victoria [30:40]: Yeah, I mean I can, I can give anecdotal, an anecdotal response to that not knowing exactly what the scientific sort of paper trail behind it would be because I am a little bit new to this, this conundrum. But I can tell you that biodiversity, as a component of Ecological Outcome Verification is front and center of consideration to us. And so what our farmers and ranchers are doing is they're tracking biodiversity both below and above ground. So both sort of the whole host of bacterial species that would be churning and burning in healthy soils and then above ground both domestic and wild species treating that ranch as a habitat for biodiversity, which ultimately begets the kind of resilience that a healthy farmer ranch would have. I know specifically that we have farmers and ranchers that because they've managed their land well they see wildlife come back. In my experience, they welcome it even if it's a threat to their own domestic species because they do see that as a bellwether of the fact that that land is functioning at an optimal level. In certain places around the world outside the US it's actually desirable because so many of these endangered species that is their habitat. There's nowhere else that that can be their home. And so they want to see, these large sort of emblematic species of the region come back also for tourism purposes. So I would say, you know, anecdotally that there's a reception to, and a welcomeness, to having those predators come back if it's an indicator of the wider complexity in the environment.

Brendan [32:27]: I've witnessed that in every conversation pretty much I've had with, with the producers, the ranchers that have this regenerative ethos. Part of the love of their work is what it's doing for the planet. I'm not saying that's true of every single producer that happens to have pastured animals, but certainly the ones I've met through the community of producers that are using a Holistic Management or similar type of planned grazing approach. So it's wonderful. And I'm curious. What are the, I guess, what are the challenges in implementing this certification? Is it you just need more ecological data, and you have to get that done and by fourth quarter, 2018? Is it PR? I mean, I believe that there's perhaps a PR challenge with any kind of livestock related certification in the wake of *Cowspiracy*, the movie.

Victoria [33:39]: Well, I mean, I think it's … so first of all, again, I'll just say that we do prefer to use the term "verification" than "certification" just for the sake that it's not going to be bestowed from on high. It's really going to be gathered and internalized from the ground up. But the barriers are similar to the barriers you have faced with any sort of systemic change that you're trying to beget. Right? So it's education. It's awareness. It's having the right alliances in the right places. It's scale and availability of what you're trying to adopt and sell and bring into the marketplace. All of those things are moving targets or plates that we're spinning all the time and trying to manage pardon the phrase, but manage holistically so that we can develop this healthily and sustainably over time. But yeah, we need to certainly educate the consuming public about what regeneration is. Why it matters. Why it's the step that needs to happen that goes beyond sustainability. You know, we obviously need to develop partnerships and we're really excited about some of the partnerships that we've already formed, with some brands and retailers that will be sharing publicly in 2018. We're finding that there are businesses that really want to walk the walk and put their money where their mouth is and create the world's first verified regenerative supply chain for their own access and for the access of their customers and even their competitors because they really want to see this shift. So we just need to keep kind of doing our work, building alliances, generating that awareness and forming the partnerships that, that make the most sense.

Brendan [35:25]: Well, I'm very much looking forward to hearing about who the partners are and which companies I can trust a lot more as a result of being part of this alliance. And I'm always in awe of anybody who has marketing and branding skills and of course applies them to good purpose in the world.

Victoria [35:25]: Let them be a force for change.

Brendan [35:55]: Yeah, I mean communication is a superpower, and you have it in spades. And I'm just curious if you could give us a lesson of … is there anything that if I want to see this kind of thing grow, and I mean this, whether I consume animal products or not, I want to see this happen, and I actually for a long time wanted to minimize the amount of animal products that I eat. Through a ketogenic diet that's happening now, astoundingly, but even if I become a vegetarian, which I was at one point, I will always want to see landscapes being regenerated and livestock being used in the appropriate way. So I'm just curious if you could give us a lesson so that I, regardless of what I'm eating, can try to influence other people to make the right choice as far as where their livestock and their animal products and any other products that go through this verification process, how they're sourced. How they're raised.

Victoria [36:57]: One thing I like to think about is the notion of expressing instinctive behaviors. And this does tie back a little bit to biomimicry as well. But essentially what we do when we industrialize agriculture is we prevent those species be they botanical or animal from expressing their instinctive behaviors of contributing to that landscape. So I think that's a nice lens to look at it through whether you're a meat eater or not. Whatever it is that you're choosing, do you feel like that particular organism actually contributed to its system in the way that it was really intended and put on the planet? Now we know that ruminants were put on the planet to regenerate grasslands. But you know, pigs were put on the planet to route through and aerate the soil through their snouts. And poultry were put on the planet to scratch the surface and spread bacteria around. I mean it just goes on and on. And I think us sort of shifting our lens and thinking about those creatures as having those instinctive attributes can be really instructive and then thinking about ourselves. So then what is instinctive to us? And it differs for everyone. So your choices of how you contribute or participate in the food web will be different from mine. But what's most instinctive to you? And then how can you bring that to life on your plate?

Victoria [38:26]: And then in terms of communications I think you were also asking me a little bit about what's a lesson that we can learn about communications. Is that right?

Brendan [38:35]: Yeah. Like how can I apply this to everything in my life because I wanna be a better communicator. But I definitely want to hear specifically how I can do it with a verification program like this. Yeah. But both.

Victoria [38:49]: In terms of with a verification program like this, I think for us we always err on the side of transparency even maybe for lack of glitz and sexiness and sizzle, because for us we really just want to tell the truth and make that truth available. So the whole point of Land to Market is to allow consumers ultimately to, if they look below the hood at any time they can see that this leather or this wool sweater or this piece of meat traces all the way back to this plot of land that is regenerating. That's the promise of the program once we scale it up and really get it going. So to me it's less about sort of telling and more about showing. And that's really the ethos that I try to bring to my communications work is that it's always about just demonstrate, just exemplify, just stand for something rather than using a big bull horn to claim your cause. I think showing is much more important than telling.

Brendan [39:53]: Yeah. I think we're all so ready for that in our world and our culture after so much so much of the other approach, so much that ended up as greenwashing and so forth. Obviously, we want to avoid that. And this program is all about it not being green-washed, but being for real.

Victoria [40:14]: No, I think that's an important component of this Brendan that you bring up is we've done some study of millennials and what really is important to them attitudinally. And there's a global survey of millennials of the top 10 things that concern them. Thousands and thousands of millennials around the world. The number one thing that concerned them was planetary health. And then there were a series of things fanning down to the very least important on a scale of 1 to 10 was their economics, security and opportunity. And this was not a study that we did. I'd love to pull up the slide to share it with you while I'm talking, but essentially what we're hearing from millennials is that their definition of their own health, their definition of their own vibrancy and of their own potential to thrive is deeply tied to Nature health and to climate health and to water health and to ecosystem health. And now they know that, and I think that feedback loop is just getting tighter and tighter with every generation. And so they're even placing their own individual concerns well behind the collective concerns that they face as a generation and the planet that they and their children will call home. So that's just an important lens to look through as we continue to communicate.

Brendan [41:56]: I'm really glad you showed that. I'm in shock and awe and gratitude that this is the case.

Victoria [42:00]: Yeah, yeah, absolutely. It's gonna be a really creative time the next several decades. I err on the side of hope and think that we're up to the challenge. And I think we have an opportunity to be benevolent participants rather than extractors from our home habitat. And if we just continue to move the conversation in that direction, regardless of what we eat, regardless of what our opinions are about that, I think we'll all be moving in the right way forward.

Brendan [42:33]: Well, I am such a huge fan of Savory. Savory seems so astute and able to hone in on exactly what is the most, what actually makes the most sense, what works and so forth. So I guess it's not surprising that Savory has come to the conclusion that we need a consumer revolution. So consumers are going to have to drive this. We can't wait for somebody else to do it. Hey, it's just not happening unless we drive it. And so I'm really appreciative that Savory has got all of that under the hood. And any last words as far as what we as far as me as a consumer driving this?

Victoria [43:26]: Not really, no. I just want to thank you for what you're doing here to just stimulate this dialogue and put it into a format that people can sort of take at their own discretion and participate in. It's clear that you're on your own journey in terms of sharing the insights that you've developed over time and then opening the dialogue to include not just your own health or an individual's own health but the health of our planet. And so I just really wanted to thank you for that.

Brendan [43:55]: Oh, it's my pleasure and my obsession. You can count on it. Thank you for bringing your obviously amazing branding and strategy experience from the New York advertising world to the most important place that you could bring it to bear, and that is regenerating our planet and our human health and so forth. Thank you for doing that. And for being here in the Eat4Earth community with us.

Victoria [43:55]: Thank you Brendan.

Brendan [44:26]: I love how Victoria introduced us to regenerative animal agriculture through biomimicry and the Holistic Management approach to grazing livestock.   Next we're going to see some examples of the amazing soil building benefits of this type of approach. It's really mind blowing actually when you see it. Plus, combining it with row crops as well as a model using "tree range" chicken.

Allen Williams, PhD Interview
Cows from CAFOs vs. Cows That Reverse Climate Change

Brendan [00:00:00]: Welcome to the Eat4Earth event. We're exploring how you can heal yourself, your loved ones, and the planet with food. This is Brendan Moorehead, and I'm very happy to be speaking with our next guest, Allen Williams, PhD, and that's because it's very vitally important that any red meat that any one of us consumes is 100% grass-fed because of what it can mean for the health of the planet, the health of our farms and ranches, and of course, our personal health. Dr. Allen Williams is a sixth-generation family farmer that uses regenerative agriculture as the framework for whole farm and ranch planning. He currently serves on the board of directors of the Mississippi Sustainable Agriculture Network and the Grass Fed Exchange. He is also a core team member of the Pasture Project, coinvestigator for Team Soil Carbon, founding partner of Grass Fed Beef, LLC, and of Grass Fed Insights, LLC, and is a partner in Joyce Farms, Inc. Dr. Williams considers himself a recovering academic having serving 15 years on the faculty at Louisiana Tech University and Mississippi State University. He holds a BS and an MS in animal science from Clemson University and a PhD in genetics and reproductive physiology from LSU and he has coauthored more than 400 scientific and popular press articles and is invited as a speaker at regional, national, and international conferences and symposiums. Dr. Williams is featured in the Carbon Nation film *Soil Carbon Cowboys* and *Soil Carbon Curious* and has a recently released book coauthored with Teddy Gentry called *Before You Have a Cow*. Dr. Williams, it's a great pleasure to have you with us today.

Dr. Williams [00:01:40]: Well, it's good to be here.

Brendan [00:01:42]: So Dr. Williams, beef production, as you know, is an extremely controversial topic for health. Actually, I hear that you didn't know until recently just how controversial it was, but it's very controversial in certain circles for health and environmental reasons especially after the movie *Cowspiracy*, but you have a different story to tell about the potential planetary benefits of cattle and other livestock. And a growing body of evidence in science supports this alternative approach. What is it about this approach that makes it distinctly different from how most livestock is currently raised, both on feedlots and finished on grains, and also pasture-raised livestock out there in general?

Dr. Williams [00:02:25]: Well, it's all predominantly about management to be honest with you. You know, it's how we manage our livestock that makes a profound difference in what happens in terms of soil health, our ecosystem health, and, of course then the nutrient density and healthfulness of the food products that we're consuming. So, what we do is we focus first and foremost on the soil. We want to make sure that we're treating the soil right, that we're building that soil microbial population, and what I call the livestock under the ground. So we focus first … instead of focusing on the livestock above the ground, you know the cattle or sheep or anything else that we may have, we focus first and foremost on the livestock below the ground. And that would be the microbes, the earthworms, the soil level insects, pollinators, those types of things, that are vital to us and to our ecosystem. So all of our focus is centered on that, and we call that building the foundation. So we want to make sure that we're implementing practices that we call "adaptive management practices" or "adaptive grazing" so that we are building that foundation for the ecosystem, using our livestock as a tool to do so.

Brendan [00:03:50]: And is there a way of describing how that's done just sort of in broad strokes for a general audience? How would they distinguish between what you're doing and, of course, you know there's labels that help distinguish that and we'll get into the certifications, but if they were to look at what's happening on a field, what would be different about what you're doing and a typical grazing operation for example?

Dr. Williams [00:04:14]: Well, what we're trying to do is create ecomimicry and biomimicry, so we utilize grazing methodologies that simulate the way that the large, wild ruminants used to move across the landscape. We have taken a look at how did the large, wild ruminant populations of the world, both historically and for those that still exist currently, how did they move across that landscape on a daily basis. What is the impact that they make on that landscape? And why is that impact important? So here in North America, the obvious choice is trying to emulate the movement of the bison. And, you know, they were the large ruminant of choice here across the plains of North America and actually existed from the Atlantic to the Pacific and from south of the Arctic Circle all the way down to the Gulf Coast. Bison were a large grazing ruminant that had a profound impact historically for thousands of years, building the tremendous fertility that the early settlers encountered when they first moved across this continent. What our grazing looks like, in order to emulate that, is that we graze them under higher stock densities or what we would call "mobs", just like the bison moved across the prairie. You know the bison were kept fairly tight because of the influence of large apex predators like wolf packs and things like that that followed them around and shadowed them everywhere they went. So, the predators had a profound effect on how the bison moved across the landscape, the type of unit that they moved in, and those units were under what we call higher stock densities that created a lot of trample of the plants in their path. That trample creates brand-new soil. Soil organic matter breeds and produces a much higher population of soil microbes. So in essence it feeds the soil, that's the easiest way to say it. So what we do … and those bison moved every day, right? They didn't hang out in a location. First of all, they had to eat everyday, and secondly they had predators pressuring them, so they were moving every day. And so we do the same thing with our livestock. We no longer have the wild predators that are going to pressure them so we use temporary poly wire fencing, just single strand poly wire fencing with temporary posts that's super easy to use, and we can move the cattle across the landscape under these higher stock densities just like the bison moved and again, simulate what they did and recreate the building of the soil, the building of the microbes and the pollinators and all of these other things that the bison influenced in the thousands of years that they were here.

Brendan [00:07:34]: Most grazing operations that I see, let's say from the highway, driving by, you know the cows are just ambling about, and it's kind of "*laissez-faire*" looking. What's different about the two of these approaches and the differences in their ecological impacts?

Dr. Williams [00:07:51]: The vast majority of grazers in North America use typically one of two different grazing methodologies. One is what we call "continuous", or "set-stock grazing", and that means that their livestock basically have free run of their entire farm or ranch year-round. They can go anywhere they want to go on that farm or ranch year-round. And what that does is that actually creates slow degradation and compaction of the soil. And it allows those livestock to be highly, highly selective in what they eat every day, and that actually has a very detrimental effect on our plant species, diversity, and complexity. It will trend our plants in those pastures towards a monoculture or a near monoculture or reduce the total number of plant species there and create a lot of weed problems. What we do actually does exactly the opposite because the cattle are moved every day from paddock to paddock throughout a farm or ranch so they are only grazing a portion of it in any given day. And because they are in these mobs, then they are far less selective in what they are grazing, so that encourages a much broader array of plant species, diversity, and complexity. The other method that most grazers use is what we call a "slow rotation", which means that they move their livestock from pasture to pasture across their farm or ranch maybe once every two weeks, once a month, something like that. And when we look at the research and the actual results on the ground for farms and ranches, what we have found is that the slow rotation is not any better at producing positive results in terms of soil health parameters and plant species diversity compared to the set-stock grazing.

Brendan [00:09:57]: How interesting. So obviously, this is doing a lot for biodiversity and for the soils, but what about the issue of methane? Is that still a problematic issue with cattle and their belching up their cud and chewing it?

Dr. Williams [00:10:17]: Okay, so the first thing we have to ask ourselves … and I get this question a lot … the very first thing that I ask somebody is, "Well let's consider the historical context, and tell me what the massive herds of wild ruminants did." They're still ruminants so they still belched as well. They ate and digested their forages exactly the same way that domesticated cattle do. So if we look at bison, if we look at wildebeasts, if we look at any of the other large, wild ruminants that have been on the surface of this Earth for thousands of years, if they created a methane issue then we've had this issue for many thousands of years, and we actually need to get rid of all the wild ruminants as well. Now when I make that statement we know that that's a ridiculous statement. Obviously, they were profoundly good for this Earth and they produced very positive results. As a matter of fact, most of the land area of this Earth evolved under the influence of a multitude of wild grazing ruminants. So we know that they had a profound positive impact. So, if that's the case, and it is, and they produce methane just like the cows do, then what is the difference? Well, here's the difference. If we have healthy soil, what else is healthy in that soil? Well, it's the microbial population, right? So if we have a very healthy microbial population that includes microbes such as methanotrophs that have the ability to be able to digest the methane that is being produced by these wild ruminants. So in other words, it was a system naturally that sustained and supported itself. Now, when we degrade soil through poor agricultural practices, and we significantly reduce the population of soil microbial species, including the methanotrophs, then we have a problem. So it's not a problem of the cows, it's a problem of our management, how we manage those cows and how we manage that soil microbial population. I'll say one more thing on that, is that in our research that we're doing currently, one of the things that we have found is that we are seeing much more methane being released in row cropping operations, so the growing of our crops. Now why? Again, we have to ask the question "Why?" We've known for years that rice production, when you flood rice fields and you have rice production, rice fields produce and emit huge amounts of methane. As a matter of fact, they're one of the major methane emitters in agriculture in the world. Why do they do that? Because we've flooded the fields and we've created anaerobic conditions in that soil. What we have found is that with constant tillage in our other row cropping operations, such as growing corn and soybeans and wheat, we have actually created an ever-increasing degree of anaerobic conditions in those soils, and therefore they are now emitting higher levels of methane. So, the methane issue is not simply an issue with mismanagement of livestock, it's also an issue with mismanagement of row cropping operations.

Brendan [00:14:17]: That's an important revelation right there because obviously the soil under row crops that are being managed in that way probably does not have methanotrophs to take care of the problem because it's very degraded soil whereas under the type of grazing that you're doing, it's quite possible that those methanotrophs are taking care of all of the methane from those ruminant herbivores. I recently ... I believe it was Christine Jones, I'm not certain, I read somewhere that, or maybe it was in a conversation, that around termite mounds, which are extreme emitters of methane, there is so much methanotroph activity because there is a constant source that the ambient methane levels around this huge emitter of methane is actually lower than in other area further from the termite mounds. So, if the same kind of situation applies to livestock then the methanotrophs might actually consume all and more of what the livestock are emitting if the livestock are revving up methanotroph activity. I'm just curious, does that make sense and have you seen anything like that?

Dr. Williams [00:15:30]: That's precisely what's happening.

Brendan [00:15:32]: Okay.

Dr. Williams [00:15:34]: Let me give you just a little bit of data here. I always hesitate to throw out a lot of data because that sort of bores people, but this data is important and it really illustrates what we're talking about here. We've measured soils all over North America both from farms' row cropping operations and from grazing operations, and what we have found is that the average soils—whether we are talking about pastures under continuous grazing or farms that are row cropping and cultivating routinely these fields, you know, plowing up these fields routinely and not planting cover crops, by the way, in between their cash crops, that the soil microbial population as expressed in total biomass, in other words the total mass of microbes that's in that soil and we express it in nanograms per gram of soil—what we're finding across North America on a majority of farms and ranches is that they have less than 2,000 nanograms per gram of soil microbial biomass. That's pathetic, okay? Most people won't relate to that, but that's very, very low. In our operations and in operations where we have implemented these adaptive practices, what we have found is that microbial population of the soil has now increased to above 10,000 nanograms per gram of soil, and on many of these farms and ranches we're above 15,000 nanograms per gram. So that's an exponential increase in the amount of soil bacteria, fungi, and protozoa and so forth that is supposed to be there in that soil. So to answer your question, yes, it has a profound impact and it can totally mitigate greenhouse gasses that are being emitted. To prove that, we've actually put out a series of flux towers on farms and ranches where we are right now actively measuring greenhouse gas emission from these farms and ranches to be able to validate the statements that I just made.

Brendan [00:18:09]: Wow, that's quite something. That's going to be exciting to be able to see that because we need to know this because if this kind of grazing management is actually a highly beneficial planetary activity, then people need to know that because there is so much negative propaganda that's just applied to all animal agriculture across the board.

Dr. Williams [00:18:33]: Absolutely.

Brendan [00:18:35]: Now, you might be interested to know or maybe you already know this, but when I was speaking with Walter Jehne from Australia, who is a soil microbiologist, he said that there's a process called photooxidation that occurs with methane as well and that it only occurs when there is a good transpiration stream of the moisture in the soil being drawn up through the plants like the leaves and the grass and other forage species and going up into the air and creating that humidity, and then the water molecules are split by photons from the sun into hydroxyl radical and hydrogen proton, and the hydroxyl radicals, the 'O' for the oxygen and the 'H' with a negative charge on it, the 'H' for the hydrogen, highly reactive and splits the methane into carbon dioxide and what the other byproducts would be. I'm just curious, have you looked into that at all? Is that a possible mechanism that's also occurring only when animals are grazed on healthy pastures with moist soils because it has the organic content in those healthy soils to hold water, pretty much year-round probably.

Dr. Williams [00:19:51]: Yeah, that's correct. What we're finding, first of all, we call that the principle of compounding. The principle of compounding is basically this … and I teach this in our workshops to farmers and ranchers. We always have compounding effects in nature, in biology, and they're either negative or they're positive. They're never neutral, so whether they're negative or positive is solely up to us and the way that we manage those soils, the way that we manage our farms, the way that we manage our livestock and our crops. If we manage to protect the soil, protect those microbes, protect the soil moisture, protect the soil temperature, and keep living roots in the ground year-round, as long as we possibly can, then what we have found is we create very positive and exponential positive compounding effects. And that includes the things that you were just talking about. And so we have a multiplicity of interactions going on here in Nature. It is simply Nature at work doing what she was supposed to do, and that's precisely what we're doing. So in our grazing for instance, we never allow the livestock to graze the pastures down tight, to take off the majority of the forage. We want a lot of forage left so that we are shading and protecting the soil from the sunlight. We're preserving, just as you said, preserving the soil moisture. We're protecting the soil temperature, and we are therefore protecting and feeding those microbes so that they can continue to grow and function and create those impacts and include the transpiration, the evapotranspiration process, the liquid carbon pathway process, all of that. We're feeding and facilitating all of that at the same time. And when that happens, then we have very positive things going on in our entire ecosystem, and our livestock are a critical tool to help us achieve those positive impacts.

Brendan [00:22:28[: And with soils being degraded to the tune of 75 billion tons of soil every year around the world, 7-billion tons of that, maybe about 10% just in the United States alone, and USDA says that farming is likely to collapse within 30 years if we don't turn this around, farming in the US, so we need to be very serious obviously. Can you quantify how much soil is being built in your operations, and how much soil is being created instead of destroyed like in all these other systems?

Dr. Williams [00:23:06]: Yes, we can. We have quite a bit of data now to validate and substantiate how rapidly you can rebuild soil. And the good news is we have found we can rebuild it much more rapidly than we ever thought. And as a former academic, the truth is, I thought when I was a formal academic, and when I was teaching college students, that it took hundreds or even thousands of years to rebuild even a miniscule amount of topsoil. And we're finding that's not just the case at all. As a matter of fact, what we have found is this—and again, we've done this in multiple regions across the US and Canada and even Mexico and have data on this—that we can rebuild organic matter at a pace of anywhere from 0.5% to 1% annually for at least the first five to six years. After that, the pace of increase will slow down to a smaller, incremental increase, but we can still continue to increase it. We've been doing this for 20 years now. We haven't hit a threshold yet, and that's the good thing. To give you a few examples, on our own farm we were able, for the first four years of implementing high-level adaptive grazing practices, to increase soil organic matter at the rate of 1% annually. So we added 4% soil organic matter in just four years. Now let me tell you how impactful that is in terms of water. For every 1% organic matter increase per acre, that acre can hold an additional 25,000 gallons of water.

Brendan [00:25:04]: That's amazing.

Dr. Williams [00:25:06]: It is. So that meant that over four years, we increased the water holding capacity for every single acre by 100,000 gallons. Now, what that does is that mitigates the impact of drought and the impact of flooding. And I'll mention this, I've done a lot of work with farmers and ranchers in south Texas around that greater Houston area. We all know what happened earlier this year with Hurrjcaine Harvey, and we know the catastrophic flooding that occurred in that region. You're going to flood if you get 30 to 50 inches of rain, but the question here is the severity of that flooding. And what we have found is that on the coastal prairie surrounding the greater Houston area to the East and North, the West and the South, those coastal prairies have been degraded so much in their soil organic matter that the majority of them now have less than 1% and many of them less than 0.5% organic matter. So that means that for every inch of rain that falls, those soils can only infiltrate about two-tenths of an inch for every inch. Now think about that. If they had been restored to their more historical level of soil organic matter, 5+%, now every acre of soil could have infiltrated eight-tenths of every inch of rain that fell. If that would have been the case during Harvey, we would have still had flooding, but the reach of that flood and the catastrophic activity of that flood would've been greatly reduced.

Brendan [00:27:16]: That makes me wonder if insurance companies might be an unusual ally in all of this. Have any conversations begun in that regard because five years to 10 years max, I guess, under these intensive conditions, you could turn this land around so that it can actually capture that and reduce these devastating floods.

Dr. Williams [00:27:36]: Well actually I've been contacted, believe it or not, by several entities in that area because obviously now they're wanting to throw billions of dollars at solving that problem so that this catastrophic flooding doesn't happen again. What most engineers are looking at is the obvious. They're looking at, well let's build more waterways; let's build more reservoirs; let's channel more water into these reservoirs that are going to hold these flood waters and hope that that relieves the flooding. Well, I call that a band-aid on a gushing wound. We're not solving the flooding issue at all. We're just trying to figure out a way to hold the flood waters and keep them from devastating communities. That's all we're doing when in essence, we can actually solve the root of the problem by doing exactly what you just said, by working with the farmers and ranchers in that region to significantly improve their soil's water holding capacity. That is the real solution, and that is the solution that we're trying to get an audience for right now to present to the powers that be in that area.

Brendan [00:18:53]: Wow. I'm really looking forward to hearing about that for sure. Now, in terms of growing soil carbon, we've been speaking in terms of percentages. How does that translate into tons? Is it possible to make a general translation from, let's say, if it's half a percent (0.5%) per year, how many tons of carbon per acre is that?

Dr. Williams [00:29:13]: What we have found is that with our adaptive grazing practices, and it's going to vary a little bit depending upon the region of the country obviously, and the amount of rainfall, the amount of total forage growth annually, how many grazings you can get annually, but what we have found is that in the majority of the US that with adaptive grazing practices we are able to sequester between 4 and 7 tons per acre of carbon.

Brendan [00:29:43]: And what range of percentage organic matter would that be? Is it possible to say?

Dr. Williams [00:29:47]: Well, actually it has far more to do, as we increase organic matter to 3% and above, that's where we have the most profound impact, but it's really more relative to the amount of forage or plant growth that we can produce annually and then the grazings that we can get because every time that we can go in and graze that growth, then we stimulate brand-new growth activity out of those plants and that stimulates, in turn, a more rapid grabbing of the carbon out of the atmosphere and putting it back into the soil. And so what we have found, if you want to compare that to a typical southern pine forest, a typical southern pine forest is sequestering less than a half ton of carbon per acre per year.

Brendan [00:30:47]: Is that just in the soil or is that also in the wood?

Dr. Williams [00:30:51]: That's in the soil and then, for course, in the roots, the liquid carbon pathway, the whole bit. So, they're doing about a half ton per acre annually of carbon sequestration in terms of a pine forest. So we can greatly outpace that with our grazing. Now compare that to a typical row cropping operation, and a row cropping operation is going to sequester somewhere in the neighborhood of three-quarters of a ton to one ton. So again, we're four to six times greater than any of these other systems.

Brendan [00:31:33]: Aren't row cropping systems typically putting carbon actually into the atmosphere on a net basis, so three tons of carbon or even more per year into the atmosphere rather than a net capture of carbon?

Dr. Williams [00:31:49]: Yeah, and of course that all depends on how you're row cropping so yes, you're more conventional row cropping operation is actually putting a lot of carbon back out into the atmosphere because you've got a lot of passes that you're making over these fields every year with your cropping operation. And then the majority of them … you know, less than 5% of all farms in the US are actively planting and growing cover crops in between their cash crops, so what are they doing instead? They're going in and after the cash crop they're turning the soil over and leaving it exposed and bare for the rest of the year all through the winter until they go back in the next spring with their next cash crop. And that very act itself burns up a lot of carbon into the atmosphere.

Brendan [00:32:44]: Somewhere I saw that the average row crop operation in Wisconsin is averaging about three tons of soil per acre lost each year.

Dr. Williams [00:32:57]: Yes, that's correct. And unfortunately, in many other regions of the country that's even higher.

Brendan [00:33:04]: Now, given what you're accomplishing, is the academic world taking notice? Are you in touch with anybody like Rattan Lal?

Dr. Williams [00:33:15]: I'm not in touch with Dr. Lal. I'm very aware of Dr. Lal, but I will tell you this, that there are a lot of other people that I'm working with that are still with the universities and, of course, I'm a scientist with Team Soil Carbon, so even though I'm no longer affiliated directly with the university, I still am a scientist and we still are doing research. We're doing collaborative research right now with a number of scientists from different universities including Texas A&M, University of Arizona, Michigan State University, University of Wisconsin, and a handful of others. So with this Team Soil Carbon Project we are actively looking at this. We're making paired comparisons around the US between farms and ranches that are managed adaptively versus those that are managed conventionally. So those paired comparisons, including measurements of soil biology, physical structure, chemistry and so forth along with flux towers being set out. We're also doing pollinator sweeps, insect sweeps. We're working with Dr. Jonathan Lundgren as well, a world-renowned entomologist, to do this. Also, we've done work and I've collaborated with people like Dr. David Montgomery who wrote *Dirt: The Erosion of Civilization* and *Growing a Revolution* and Dr. Christine Jones out of Australia. So there's a host of people globally that we're working with, well-respected scientists that are seeing and understanding this. Now, that being said, there are still the vast majority of the scientists at our land-grant institutions that basically want nothing to do with this research at this point in time. They're still heavily focused on very conventional research and conventional methods of production and don't have much at all to do with those of us that are looking at this type of research angle.

Brendan [00:35:33]: Okay. You know one of the angles of looking at this that has been put out into the, I guess you can say popular media by the movie *Cowspiracy*, was the idea that if all Americans ate their average of 209[1], there's variations on that statistic, but 209 pounds of meat for each American using grass-fed beef—and they used certain assumptions—that it would require 3.7 billion acres and that compares to only 1.9 total billion acres in the lower 48 states. I'm just curious, if we were supplying that much meat to Americans, I mean that's how much they're eating now, it's just mostly out of feedlot finished animals, and if it was done in systems like yours, how much of our grazing land and/or agricultural land would that take and would it take over South American and, you know, what would be required?

Dr. Williams [00:36:32]: Yeah, I can directly answer that question. First of all, I will have to say that their statistics are absolutely wrong. That is completely incorrect, so let me give you the real statistics here. First of all, every year in the US, there is between 28 and 30 million head of fed cattle that are slaughtered or harvested each year for human consumption here in the US and then for the export market. That number is important to remember relative to what I'm getting ready to tell you. So, in other words, right now to supply the American consumer demand for beef, plus the export demand, we're harvesting 28 to 30 million head a year, okay, in the feedlots. Now, we have run the numbers and that includes me, Jim Gerrish, and a host of others. We have gotten together and run these numbers and here's what it would take to grass finish all of those in terms of acres and so forth. Actually, we found that there's three primary sources of grassland acres that we can utilize that would not interfere with anything else whatsoever. First of all, across the United States we have tens of millions of idle grassland acres, completely idle. Nobody is using them. They're owned by farmers and ranchers and or absentee landowners, but they're not being used. Crops are not being grown in them, they're not in CRP, or in the Conservation Reserve Program, and they're not being grazed. They're just sitting there completely idle. So we have found that just on idle grassland acres alone in the US, and using only 50% of those, we can finish 15 million head of grass-fed cattle a year just on those. Now, the second tranche is we have the intermountain region of the US, and we have a lot of acres available there for grazing under adaptive management in that intermountain region. If we properly use those, that would add another six to eight million head to that already 15 million and then if we just took out 15% of the land currently used for growing row crops, and guess what that 15% is? It's the 15% that is producing the row crops for the feedlot industry.

Brendan [00:39:24]: Okay.

---

[1] The figure of 200+ pounds of meat consumption per year per American actually consists mostly of poultry and pork, not beef. Americans eat approximately 55 pounds of beef per year.

Dr. Williams [00:39:26]: So, if we didn't have the feedlots, and we replaced those with grass finishing and we instead returned those acres to grassland rather than row crop production, which, by the way, would be far better for our ecosystem anyway, right? So, if we returned those 15% of corn and soybean acres back to grassland and grazed those for grass finishing, then all of those three added up equal 42 million head a year of grass-fed cattle that we could harvest in the US. Now remember, I said we're only harvesting 28 to 30 million, so the fact of the matter is that just here in the US, without having to find acres and manufacture acres somehow or take away from anybody else, we could already out-produce the feedlot industry in the US on grass alone with only 50 million acres of grassland - only 50 million.

Brendan [00:40:32]: Wow!

Dr. Williams [00:40:33]: Only 50 million. Now the figure thrown out by *Cowspiracy* was what, 3.7 billion? Right? No! No sir. We only need 50 million acres, and actually we don't need that. We only need 35 million acres to produce the current number of cattle that are being harvested in the US today. Just 35 million acres of grassland properly managed under adaptive grazing would allow us to accomplish that.

Brendan [00:41:06]: That's just amazing. You know, in a conversation with Daniela Ibarra-Howell at the Savory Institute, they, I guess did a study of their own, and they looked at what it would take to grass finish all the livestock or at least the beef in the US, and it would only increase the stocking rate about 30%. And yet what has to happen for that kind of management system, theirs and yours, which have strong similarities if not practically identical, we won't dive into that right now, but the bottom line is stocking rates have to be increased dramatically more than 30% to actually get the beneficial impact on the land and so a 30% increase is, in general and no over-generalizing, but 30% increase is trivial compared to what they typically do in order to implement this management system where you get more cattle out of the same land and a much better impact, meaning a beneficial impact of the land. Just another way of looking at it, another organization's analysis.

Dr. Williams [00:42:26]: You're absolutely correct. The fact is that if we manage our domesticated livestock properly using these adaptive principles, then we actually need more of them because of the very positive impact, just like you said, the very positive impact they have on our soil and our entire ecosystem because again, remember, our ecosystem has evolved around the world under the influence of large, wild grazing ruminants, and all we're doing is recreating that, simulating that with our domesticated livestock.

Brendan [00:43:04]: So, if eating 100% grass finished beef and other livestock is potentially a way to "eat for Earth", so to speak, how would somebody know for sure that they're getting livestock raised in that way?

Dr. Williams [00:43:19]: Well, you have to look for, first of all, it needs to say …

Brendan [00:43:26]: I said 100% grass finished, that doesn't mean it's being done with adaptive management like you are. Just to be specific, 100% grass-finished using methods like Holistic Management, using methods like your adaptive planned grazing and so forth.

Dr. Williams [00:43:43]: Yeah, that's where the consumer needs to do their homework and they need to know who their sourcing from, who produced it, and how they're producing it. So the consumer is not released from an obligation here. They have to take responsibility as well for the foods that they purchase and who they support with those food purchases. Obviously, the bottom line is this: Us farmers and ranchers are less than 2% of the entire US population now, so we don't exactly hold a lot of sway here in terms of majority. We are the vast minority, and so the consumer holds all of the power. They're the other 98% of the population. They hold all of the power, and therefore if they vote with their food purchase dollars what they want to buy, that will have a profound impact and influence in the way other farmers and ranchers manage those farms and ranches. And that's what I want. I want the consumer to become more educated to study who they're buying their food from. And we want to make that easier for them. I have to admit, it's been confusing so far because there's a number of different certification programs out there, which by the way, almost none of them have any consumer awareness whatsoever. If you ask the vast majority of consumers, "Do you know who AGA is? Do you know who AWA is? Do you know who Food Alliance is, or Certified Humane or any of these others?" they would say, "Never heard of them." That's our fault, okay? We've got to do a much better job, and we're actually working on that right now, to develop a uniformed, streamlined program with the brand awareness campaign that will hopefully create awareness very similar to other very successful labels and brand awareness campaigns like the Fair Trade. You know, the majority of consumers to recognize Fair Trade and understand what that means. They do recognize Rainforest Alliance, and if they're buying electronic appliances, they do recognize the UL label and know to look for that. That's what we're in the process of trying to create here within the pastured protein sector where we have a single seal that identifies to the consumer that if you buy this product, no matter whose brand—because there's still a bunch of different programs out there and we need those different programs—but no matter whose brand you buy, any brand as long as they follow these standards and protocols and submit to the certification, can qualify for this unifying seal. Just like there's multiple brands of coffee and cocoa that can be labeled fair trade, it's not just a single brand that is labeled fair trade. We want to create that same deal so that all we're telling the consumer is to look for something and right now for lack of a better term let's call it "pasture pure". We want to be able to tell the consumer, "Look for the pasture pure seal of approval, and if you see that than you can be guaranteed that it was produced by USA family farmers and ranchers following these minimum protocols and standards."

Brendan [00:47:26]: Now are we talking about the certification, the AGA certification that you already have or are we talking about something in addition to that that would be perhaps … go ahead.

Dr. Williams [00:47:36]: Well, right now we're really, and again, I'm not on the board of directors or a decision maker for AGA. You know I'm on the board of directors for the Grass Fed Exchange. So those are two entirely different organizations. The Grass Fed Exchange, we're an educational organization and not a certification and policy-making. Now, the AGA, or American Grass Fed Association is the certification and policy-making organization, but right now we don't have that with the AGA as of yet. So we're working through all of the programs that currently exist to try to unify these standards and create that one seal so that we no longer confuse the consumer with all of these different seals and certifications that, once again, they have no awareness of. We're not helping ourselves by doing that, so we want to have the one unified seal that any branding program can qualify for as long as they follow adaptive management practices and procedures and meet the minimum standards. That takes away the consumer confusion. It also alleviates the issue that we have right now of imported product that is sold in our retail grocery stores labelled product of USA. Because of the lack of country of origin labeling for beef, imported beef, including grass-fed beef from other countries can be brought in. It's all run through a USDA processing plant and repackaged to be sold in the US and legally once that happens, that packer can stamp produce of USA on that package. That's terribly confusing to the consumer because they see grass-fed and then product of USA and then what do they think? They think it was raised by us, American farmers and ranchers, and it was not. So they're wholly unaware they're buying an imported product. So this seal would alleviate that problem as well. It would assure them that this product was produced by real USA family farmers and ranchers.

Brendan [00:50:05]: At this point, do we know what the name of that will be, that certification, or is that still in the formulation phase and when it might be available?

Dr. Williams [00:60:15]: It's still in the formulation phase. We are hoping to have that available by 2019. That's what we're hoping.

Brendan [00:50:25]: Now, in terms of nutrition, what can you tell us about the nutritional profiles and the effect on the human body of grass-fed versus grain-fed and maybe even amongst different styles of grass feeding or forage feeding, pasture feeding animals? The reason I ask is in the little bit of research I've looked into I see some variability in results even contradictory results in terms of impacts on HDL cholesterol and on the ratio of omega-3 fatty acids to omega-6 fatty acids.

Dr. Williams [00:51:02]: Yeah, we've done a lot of fatty acid profile analyses and we've looked at different regions of the country, and we've looked at finishing in different seasons of the year and different types of forages and so forth and the impact on that. As a matter of fact, we just did a big study with Michigan State University where we looked at a couple of thousand samples, and that study will be released here probably second quarter of 2018 and be made public so we'll have that data and those results available. But bottom line is this ... are there differences in the fatty acid profile depending on the region of the country that they're finished and even the time of the year that they're finished? Yes, yes, but likewise, so are there between all of the different feedlots. I think it's a misconception among the consumer and even among producers, ranchers, that all cattle that are feedlot finished are uniform in their nutritional profile and their fatty acid profile. And that is wholly incorrect, and here's the reason why: Every feedlot feeds a ration that is what we call "least-cost formulated" so that means that their nutritionists are constantly formulating rations to include the lowest cost ingredients to reduce the cost of that feeding. And so for different regions of the country that means that these feedlots are actually finishing cattle on very different rations. Some are finishing them more on a corn silage-based ration or a steam flaked corn. Others are finishing them feeding a high-degree of dried distiller's grains or DDGs that are a byproduct of ethanol production. Others are feeding, for instance in the pacific northwest, those feedlots feed a high percentage of beet pulp and potato waste from the beet and potato production. So all feedlot beef is not equal in nutrition and the nutritional panel. They're widely different as well, but here is what I can say: Every comparison that we have made between feedlot finished beef no matter that ration, whether it was DDG-based, corn-based, potato-based, or beet-based, every one of those compared to the grass-finished, the grass-finished fatty acid profile is always significantly better in omega-3s, omega-3 to omega-6 ratio, CLAs, and antioxidants. So it's always significantly better, but what we do have to remember is there is going to be variability, and that's natural. That even happens in the natural world. So when the Native Americans were harvesting bison, those bison didn't have the exact same fatty acid profile year round. By the way, neither does salmon or tuna. It will be a little different depending upon the time of the year and the exact composition of that diet. That is natural. That's part of Nature. But the point is, is that the fatty acid profile is always much more highly favorable. Now, the thing that we are finding, and we're getting ready to release data on this, is that this dried distiller's grain, the DDGs that are being fed from the byproduct of ethanol production, those in the ration are producing very unfavorable omega-3 to omega-6 ratios in that meat. As a matter of fact, what we're finding is that those ratios can be anywhere from 1:35 to 1:55.

Brendan [00:55:09]: Holy cow!

Dr. Williams [00:55:11]: Which is terrible. You don't want to eat that, okay. You don't want to eat that. That's a terrible omega-3 to 6 ratio. Now compare that to traditional grain-fed beef. The grain-fed beef that Americans fell in love with decades ago where those cattle were eating conventional corn, not GMO corn and no DDGs or any of this other stuff, right? Cattle that are on that diet, the omega-3 to 6 ratio is 1:11 so we go from 1:11 up to this 1:50 to 1:55 when you're incorporating DDGs and the thing about it is, is these DDGs are also heavily incorporated into the diets of dairy cow, vertically integrated pork operations, and vertically integrated poultry operations, so the DDGs are impacting that fatty acid profile of virtually every protein that is being produced right now. In my opinion if we can do one thing, it would be to take the DDGs out of these animals' diets because of the very negative impact it's having on that omega-3 to omega-6 ratio.

Brendan [00:56:31]: I think it's also important for people to consider the fact that if they're eating grain-fed animals or DDG-fed animals, anything where the feedstock is from conventional agriculture that's likely to be GMO agriculture, which is designed to take really heavy doses of glyphosate, in other words...

Dr. Williams [00:56:51]: Glyphosate.

Brendan [00:56:53]: Yeah, and that bioaccumulates in the fat and ... I believe it does, doesn't it accumulate in the fat...

Dr. Williams [00:56:58]: Yes.

Brendan [00:57:00]: ... in the animals, but also in the meat and that that's traceable to a mother's milk in humans and, of course, to our bloodstream, pretty much all of us have that in our bloodstream. It's even being rained down from the sky, 65% of rain. One of the important vectors of that, of these chemicals, would be through eating grain-fed livestock. Also, another thing that most people probably really haven't considered is the level of lectin sensitivity, plant lectin sensitivity, in the human population now with our destroyed microbiomes and so forth and, of course, it's not getting helped by all the antibiotics that we're getting from so many sources and there are some traces in these meats from conventional feedlot operations where they get doused with antibiotics that, because of the crowded feeding conditions and also simply because it's one more way of adding weight to an animal more rapidly, so the combination of these things, and I'll just mention the plant lectin issue as in Dr. Steven Gundry and his book *The Plant Paradox*, he points out that the worst patients that don't get healed by anything else, they come to him with autoimmune disorders, cancer, heart disease and so forth, inoperable heart disease, and one of the things that seems to be the last ditch effort that makes a difference is when they go off of grain-fed animals of all kinds—chicken, pork, lamb, beef, and so forth, that seems to remove lectins that are getting into their diet from meat, and I'm talking about plant lectins because obviously there's animal lectins, but it's the plant lectins in general that seem to be an issue for more people and especially lectins from grains and legumes and especially ones that have novel forms of those plant lectins because they're genetically modified. That's another thing, I think, for people really consider about grain-fed animals and that just switching to grass-fed, aside of the fatty acid profile, might relieve a tremendous burden on the body from those plant lectins, (and) from the antibiotic residues, the organic phosphate residues that are coming through the meat.

Dr. Williams [00:59:11]: Yeah, we've actually had a lot of customers that have told us that once they started eating grass-fed beef and quit eating grain-fed beef that a lot of the digestive discomfort and disorders that they had been experiencing have gone away, and I can tell the difference myself. If I eat a grain-fed steak at a restaurant, I seriously regret it. I know within 10 minutes, you know, from the gut feeling, and it's not pleasant at all. Whereas when I eat, you know and the only thing I eat here at home is grass-fed beef, so when I eat our grass-fed beef I never have any issues whatsoever. You know, you're always left with a very good mouth feel and gut feel, and you have proper digestion, the whole bit. So that is the case, and again, you know, very early on I mentioned the principle of compounding, and I said that those impacts are never neutral, they're always positive or negative. What you're speaking of now is the negative consequence of the principle of compounding, and we're seeing a host of negative compounding effects including our own health. What we're experiencing is a steady and slow deterioration of our health. And if you trace it over the last several decades, we have seen a significant rise in heart disease, strokes, diabetes, various forms of cancer, and various neurological disorders and dementia. All of those have increased significantly in our population. Now, as you know, I am a geneticist by formal training, and I will tell you that from a genetic standpoint that is not happening due to normal course of mutations in the population. That's impossible for that to have occurred at that rapid of a pace. Rather, it is the result of these negative compounding effects creating negative epigenetic impacts within our human population. And that is why we are seeing the ever-increasing incidents of a whole array of human disease and disorders.

Brendan [01:01:56]: Yeah, and I can't see how we could possibly say that, let's say, eating animals is the cause because we've been eating animals for so long, and not too many decades ago is when all of this began. And did meat consumption suddenly escalate? Not really. It has gone through several ups and downs over the past 50-60 years, as I understand. Well, Dr. Williams, this has been amazing, and I think I have one more question for you, which is, with the consumption of grass-fed, pasture-feed beef and other livestock increasing very dramatically right now, I guess it presents an economic opportunity both for existing ranchers and farmers to switch over. Apparently there's a potential higher profit margin and also some mission-driven folks, career changers and so forth, that are getting excited about and feeling patriotic about the idea of, "Hey, let's rebuild our soils with livestock and integrations with livestock and row cropping like pasture cropping, and so you've consulted with more than 4,000 farmers and ranchers in the US, Canada, and Mexico and South America on operations ranging from a few acres to over a million acres so you've pioneered many of the early grass-fed protocols and forage-finishing techniques and spent the last 15 years refining them. What would you say to anyone that is possibly considering the idea of changing the existing operation or getting into the business from scratch?

Dr. Williams [01:03:38]: You know, we do this every day, and so we're constantly travelling North America, talking, speaking, doing workshops and so forth to introduce farmers and ranchers to this, to the adaptive management practices. And so what we do tell them on a daily basis is that if you want to be truly profitable, truly sustainable and not just sustainable but regenerative in what you are doing, and you want to restore the quality of life that you're now missing, this is the way to manage your farms and ranches because this is exciting. It's a continuous road of discovery, and what we have found is that our quality of life, our enjoyment out of life has gone up immensely, not only because we have helped many farmers get out of debt and experience high levels of profitability and productivity, but also because most farmers and ranchers in their hearts are still stewards of the Earth, and they want to be good stewards, and it hurts them when they see the soil degrading, when they see the loss of life within our ecosystem, and they see water quality declining. It hurts them to the core. So they really … its like they're rediscovering themselves, they're rediscovering their soul. Right? They want to be a part of this, and when we give them the way, the path to go down to be a part of this, they get real excited, and they get energized. And that's a beautiful thing to watch.

Brendan [01:05:38]: That's so awesome. It's making my eyes water because all you have to do is mention the word soul in conjunction with the Earth and I start getting all weepy because I just feel very close to the Earth, and it feels good to know that we can, as consumers, help farmers and ranchers really reconnect with their core passion as stewards. Thank you so much. This has been so eye-opening and mind-blowing really, and you're giving so many people a path to turn animal agriculture from an extraordinarily degenerative and destructive practice to one that is regenerative, revitalizing and so thank you so much for your leadership in regenerative agriculture, regenerative animal agriculture, and for being here with us as a participant in the community we call Eat4Earth.

Dr. Williams [01:06:41]: Well, thank you. I have immensely enjoyed it and thank you for what you're doing because what you're doing is also critically important. You're helping us get the word out and we deeply appreciate it. Thanks.

Brendan [01:06:56]: Thank you.

Colin Seis Presentation

Regenerating Grasslands with Livestock, Grains, and Cover Crops

Brendan [00:00:00]: I'm here with Colin Seis, a fifth-generation farmer from Australia. His claim to fame is that he is actually the originator of pasture cropping, which is a very unique regenerative agriculture method that he's now teaching all over the world. He's been developing this over the last 20 years at his family farm that is probably one of the most researched farms in the entire world. Colin, it's great to see you again.

Colin [00:00:27]: Thank you.

Brendan [00:00:29]: Yes, so, go ahead and tell us what it's all about. What is this and, I see your first slide here, how did we get agriculture wrong because I think a lot of us know that we did and we're scratching our heads wondering how do we recover.

Colin [00:00:47]: That is true. I'm going to talk today about that, about how we got agriculture wrong or pose the question, "Did we really get agriculture wrong?" I'm going to present some methods that I've used on my farm to regenerate my farm, but not only regenerate the farm and soil and soil ecosystem and farm ecosystem, but produce healthy food off of it as well.

Now, I'll just start with where I am. I'm obviously in Australia, as Brendan said, but about 200 miles northwest of Sidney, which is in southeastern Australia. Myself and my son, Nick, are on the farm. There's 2,000 acres here, and it's granite soil. It's not a very fertile soil, but it's okay soil. 26-inch rainfall, and now it's a restored native grassland, but we don't have any irrigation as well so we've had to do this with natural rainfall and the soil type we had. Just a bit of an idea of the enterprises we have, we run 4,000 Merino sheep here, which is for wool and meat production; some trading in cattle, as in we have cattle on the farm during different seasons. I grow about 500 acres of crops with what is normally called small grain crops, which is wheat, oat, cereal, rye, those types of crops. They're all grown using the pasture cropping methods that I developed in 1993, and I have been growing them that way since that time. Also, a major part of our enterprise is harvesting and tilling native grass seed, which we harvest off of our grasslands here. We also run one of the largest working Kelpie dog studs in the world and sell dogs for sheep and cattle work around the world. Another part of our enterprise mix is the sale of Merino rams to other sheep and wool producers.

Now, if we look at agriculture and why and how it started or the agriculture methods that we use now around the world, it started in Mesopotamia over 10,000 years ago. And it started then with the Sumerian people harvesting many of their native seeds from their grasslands at the time. Their native seeds happened to be wheat and oats and barley, which are the crops that have been developed over time that we grow in many parts of the world now. The people of Mesopotamia also domesticated sheep and goats around that same time, about 10,000 years ago. The plow was developed about a couple thousand years later, 8,000 years ago, and then oxen and cattle were domesticated in trying to pull the plow. Egyptians and then later Romans fine-tuned these agriculture techniques, and then that was adopted in Europe. And that is really the birth of modern agriculture. But that form of agriculture has created deserts around the world, not only created deserts, but major salined areas and poor dysfunctional soil. One thing it has done is destroyed grasslands all over the world. So we need to really ask the question, did our ancestors get agriculture wrong, and are there better ways to grow crops, and are there better ways to graze animals, and simply are there better ways of doing this? I would suggest that there certainly are better ways of doing it. We have to find better ways of doing it. We can't continue with the agriculture methods that have been developed up until this point in time. So, were the methods of growing crops and managing animals wrong from the start, and are there better ways of producing food and fiber? To answer that question and give you some idea of my history and how I developed the methods that I've developed, we'll just go back in time a bit to the 1860s when my great-grandparents started farming here and settled this area and bought the original settlement block on this farm. They started with Merino sheep and wool, which is very common in Australia. Merino sheep are the most farmed animal breed really, whether sheep or cattle. And they started growing wheat in 1868. Obviously, horse teams were used to sow wheat in that era, and up until the 1920s horse teams were used until my father adopted industrial agriculture in the 1930s. My father started with horse teams, but then started using tractors, and he started growing wheat. And in the 1930s, he was still running sheep as well. Wheat growing in the 1930s was very profitable, so my father grew wheat continuously during that era. Here's an interesting thing, but also important—my father didn't need or require any fertilizer to grow wheat crops in the 1930s. The photo I have here of him standing in front of a wheat crop (that) is a good wheat crop in any era. And now we need huge amounts of fertilizer to grow wheat crops all around the world. We need to ask the question, why can't we do that now? And really the answer is because our soils are now dysfunctional and lacking nutrients and minerals to grow crops. My father, because there was good money in growing wheat during that era, he continually grew wheat through the 1930s and did major damage to the farm and the soil. Because he was plowing the soil, he destroyed the grasslands quite quickly and then had major erosion problems. In the photo you can see on the right-hand side here—it's actually a photo that my mother took of one of big eagles, which is like the American eagle with a big, 6-foot wingspan—but the photo isn't about the eagle. Really, it's about the erosion behind it. And that happened about five years after my father started farming. So he did major damage very quickly. But because he did that damage, it was of great concern to him, and he fixed the problems within the next 20 years. And he was very much a pioneer in what we now call industrial agriculture and adopted many of the methods that we now call the Green Revolution, which started from the 1940s and 50s on. He fixed the problems he created by sowing the whole farm down to introduced pastures of clover and rye grass, but those pastures needed fertilizer so he was fertilizing them and cultivating soils and then in the 1960s and 70s using high rates of pesticides and fertilizers. And that's the form of agriculture that I grew up in, and I started to adopt some of those methods in the 1970s as well. That whole input method of agriculture was very productive in that era, and it worked very well. However, no one knew at the time the damage it was doing. We had lost our perennial grassland, and it was replaced by annual introduced pastures. The farm became more infested with weeds, became unproductive, and even with all those weeds and being unproductive, it was costing us over $80,000 annually to maintain this farm. And that was mostly related to fertilizer, artificial fertilizer, phosphorous fertilizer primarily.

Now, we can take that form of agriculture all over the world. If we look at the form of agriculture my father was using, that was adopted all over the world, but it started to crash here on the farm on Winona in the 1970s. Fertilizer costs became too high. Costs of sowing pastures became too high. Soils became hard and compacted. So many problems. Trees dying. We were going broke and we were going broke because it was costing us too much money. But around the world for the last 60 years, this form of agriculture has been adopted even though it started to fail in the 1970s. And it's been influenced by the use of monoculture crops, supported by high rates of fertilizer, and pesticides . And it's been an ecological disaster. It's been a total failure, yet this form of agriculture still gets promoted, and that form of agriculture is crashing all over the world because it doesn't function in an ecologically sound way, and no one looks at farms as ecosystems.

Now, if we look at what's happening in agriculture, we have reduced soil carbon levels, which requires more irrigation, reduced soil fertility, more artificial fertilizer, increasing insect attack, which is more insecticide, increasing crop disease, and more fungicide. There's a bit of a pattern developing here; we need more and more inputs for agriculture to function, which I love to call "more-on" agriculture. It requires more and more product for agriculture to even function. but very few people seem to be realizing that this is a disaster, and that it has failed. Farms should function as ecosystems, and very few people ever look at that. Ecology and agriculture really have to be put together in the same sentence. To expand on that, we're often told that it's only possible to feed 9 billion people in the year 2050 with the use of more inputs of chemical fertilizer, pesticides, and now genetically modified crops. I do not have enough adjectives to describe how angry that makes me feel. Well, I have plenty of adjectives, but I can't use them in this presentation. That is potentially a disaster. That is not only not going to work, but if we want a planet for us humans to live on, we cannot possibly go that way. Agriculture is supposed to be about food, but there is something fundamentally wrong because not only is our food now full of pesticides and herbicides, but it doesn't have the minerals in it that it used to have. And just this slide here and the next one is from the United Kingdom and its Ministry of Agriculture, and we can see from the reduction in minerals like copper, calcium, iron, magnesium, potassium, and now it is possible to buy an orange today that contains zero or no vitamin C at all. If we go on to meat, it's the same story—iron, copper, calcium, magnesium, all of those—all our meat has got reduced nutrients in it. So it is no wonder that we need to take vitamin tablets all the time; our food does not have the minerals in it that it used to have in 1940. If you look at the screen, the last work that's been done—this is in 1990 and 1991, and I would bet that in the last 20 years that those minerals have depleted even more, but it's very hard to find that information. Most of this decline in nutrients is related to a serious decline in soil health and soil carbon. Poor quality food is caused by poor quality soil, and it is that simple. So, when we look at all of what my family did and what's happening around the world, why and how did I change? It's been suggested that I'm probably a lunatic, and that could be right, but during the 1970s the cost of farm production was becoming high and unprofitable. In 1979, we had a major bush fire or what people in the US call wildfires, and it destroyed the whole farm really. It destroyed our homestead and the house, all the infrastructure, the shearing shed where we shear our sheep. 3,000 sheep were killed out of the 4,000 we owned, and many of the surviving ones were burned as well. All the buildings were destroyed; all the fencing was destroyed; and we were instantly broke with that fire. So how do you survive that? What I did was look at low input agriculture methods in the 1980s. No one was looking at low input agriculture, which it had to be more than low input agriculture methods for me because I had no money in the 1980s. So I stopped using pasture fertilizer and pesticides. I couldn't afford them. I focused on groundcover, 100% groundcover, and I adopted holistic planned grazing in 1993, developed pasture cropping in 1993 and combined the two, which is where I really got great results in 1995. But what I really focused on was restoring Winona to grassland or prairies or the original native prairie or grassland.

Just a little bit on grazing management and what we do here—and I won't be long—its only one slide. With our 4,000 Merino sheep, we run most only in two mobs and rotate them. When we have cattle, we include them with the sheep. We have 75 individual paddocks, and we work on plant recovery. So we try to get three to four months and even five months plant recovery, and the animals or the sheep are very much an important part of preparing our areas or our paddocks that we plant crops into. Now, this slide here, a very important slide, and that's a photo of an Australian bottle of beer, which is very important in that a good friend of mine, Darryl Cluff, and I developed pasture cropping in 1993 after about 10 or 12 of these beers one night (laughing) because you had to be drunk to think of something so stupid because we've always killed everything to plant crops and what we thought of or noticed after 10 or 12 beers is that we were killing our native perennial grasses to plant a crop. Those grasses were dormant or went asleep for the winter, and that was when we were growing our crops. Why did we need to kill those grasses? So, we thought about this, and then within a couple of weeks we did zero tilling while planting crops into those dormant grasses, and it worked the first time. So alcohol, or in our case bottles of beer, were very important in the development of this technique, which is unique around the world. So what it is, is a perennial cover cropping technique where annual crops are zero tilled into dormant perennial grass or grassland without killing the perennial grass. And if we look at it, for 10,000 years we have killed grassland to grow crops. And pasture cropping is the first cropping technique developed where perennial grass is not killed, and crops are planted into living dormant grassland. So zero tilling of crops is the technique we use. I'm not going to dwell on this; I don't have time in this presentation. We don't plow; we never kill perennial plants; and with zero tilling we primarily manage by creating large quantities of thick litter and by using good grazing management of livestock. We can especially when people first start, use very, very careful use of very selective herbicides, but most people move towards almost an organic system over time, as we have here. There are very few herbicides used here now at all. Just quickly, what pasture cropping will do … it allows grazing … we still graze these pastures, in fact, we use our animals to create mulch and litter that we plant the crop into. We can produce very good crops for grain and/or forage. It does improve soil structure. It does improve soil organic carbon, improve nutrient cycling, certainly reduces cost, and it restores the farm ecosystem. So, when we look at that, and why all around the world we put cattle into feedlots and feed them grain when these animals are herbivores … they should be eating grass. How do we get cattle out of feedlots? We don't need them in feedlots. It is a disaster, and its part of our industrialized agriculture model, which has been a major disaster. Sheep and cattle can be fattened on good quality pasture and/or species-diverse green crops.

So how to produce extra quality forage for grass-fed animals while doing all of this, while restoring grassland or perennial pasture or prairies, reduce fertilizer, reduce herbicides, reduce insecticides, improve soil structure, soil health, and soil nutrients. We need to ask the question, why are crops grown in monocultures of single species, and why have they been grown in monocultures for thousands of years? Ease of harvest, ease of weed control, and the need to separate different seeds, but the main reason is that we've always done it that way—and we humans are supposed to be intelligent—but we seem to always just copy the things we've always done. Just a few slides here on the sequence of growing a crop. Starting here now with a grassland, which has 50 or 60 perennial Australian native grassland species in it—next slide—we harvest native grass seed off these areas also, which is a major part of our income. Then we plant with zero tilling a crop into that, a multispecies crop now into that, after it's been grazed and mulched with sheep or cattle. Next slide shows that effect, we've planted a crop into that. That's all mulch of the grassland that the animals have mulched onto the soil. We haven't used any method other than animals to put that material onto the soil surface. Now we're planting a multispecies crop, which in this case is oats, forage brassica, vetch, radish, clover, field peas, turnips, it can be more than that, but this is what we've used here. That's just a photo of multispecies crop showing a field of pea and oats and radish, and the dry material in there is the dormant grass that is asleep for that winter period in amongst that crop. A mix of species sown into a grassland does produce superior quality and quantity stock feed, vast and very fast improvements in soil health, soil structure, carbon and nutrient cycling. We can add nitrogen with legumes. It does create weed control. It does create insect control with flowering plants, which attract beneficial insects, and we can still harvest the crop after it's grazed. That grazing of that crop does produce better quality diet, healthy diet, faster fattening of livestock, faster growth rates and more feed. Now we can, and I do, add vegetables like turnip, radish, peas to that crop as well. So it is possible now, and I'm doing it here, to grow vegetables in a grassland as well as cereal crops, so it opens up the potential to do many, many things. We don't necessarily need vegetable farms that will grow vegetables. We can do that within a grassland, and that further improves soil, and it certainly produces far better quality food for human consumption as well as animal consumption in that now-improved soil.

So, just a photo here of a crop that we had in 2015, which had oats, barley, vetch, radish, pea, turnip, clover, and forage brassica. We harvested that crop; this photo, sorry is taken at the same place, that crop has been harvested there. We harvested the oats off that or the mix of species off that, primarily oats, and you can see all the green material underneath the crops, some of the brassica species primarily there. We grazed that after the crop was harvested. This is a photo of the grain that we harvested, a mixed species grain. The darkest, smallest seed in that photo was hard wheat. We separated the small seed from the large seed from it. So we harvested a multispecies grain crop off that. Now, that grass then is grazed after the crop is harvested, and we then harvest native grass seed after the crop is harvested. That seed is sold for re-vegetation and, in the future, it can be sold for human consumption. Native people all over the world, including our aboriginal people here in Australia, a lot of their diet was seed from our grasslands, which they made into a form of bread, and so that can be a great form of food for human consumption in the future as well. We just need to rediscover a lot of what our native people did around the world. This is a photo of that same area six months later, a functioning, growing grassland again. So, over that 12-month period, the paddocks have produced grazing from the grassland, grazing of the crop, grain from the crop, and vegetables, grazing of the grassland after harvest, and native grass seed. All of those are in a 12-month period on one area of land; huge production off this. We don't need all that industrialized form of agriculture to be very, very productive. I would challenge that this far more productive than a single mono-species crop. While it's done that and produced that huge amount of food or crop off that area as well as feeding livestock, it has improved soil structure, soil health and nutrient cycling; it has had great insect control, reduced on our fertilizer, no insecticide, no fungicide, and no plowing of soil. That also has restored the grassland and soil and produced healthy, nutrient-dense food.

So, what were the results on Winona? I'm going to present some data here from some research organizations and universities in Australia that have done work here, but it has restored the grassland or the prairie. When I started with this 25 years ago, 23 years ago, it was annual weeds and it did include a few native species, but only a small percentage were grassland species, 10%. Now, there are very, very few annual weeds, and there are 60 species of native grass, forbs and herbs with 84% of our grassland species. So, we have planted no perennial grass; none of those perennial native species have ever been planted. What we've really done is created the conditions for the seed that has been sitting in the soil for 50 years to germinate. The pasture cropping technique, when overlaid with the grazing management, holistic planned grazing that Allan Savory developed, a combination of those two things have been shown to stimulate the growth of perennial grass seed that has sat in the soil for years and years. No insecticides have been used here for 20 years, and we get no insect attacking in crops or pastures. That is supposed to be impossible. Now, some work that was done by an Australian National University student, Elise Wenden, showed that insect numbers have increased by 600% on the farm here, and insect diversity has increased by 125%, but we no longer have insects attacking crops or pastures. The reason why we get no insects attacking crops or pastures is that most of that insect increase has been predators like spiders and predatory wasps that control the crop- damaging and the pasture-damaging insects. There has been no fungicide used here for over 20 years, and there is no crop disease or pasture disease. How is that possible? Industrial agriculture uses more and more fungicide. In fact, it's rare that you can grow crops without it. My crop tests have shown huge increase in soil microbiology or soil microbes. Fungi have increased. Bacteria have increased. Protozoa and nematodes, and that huge diversity of soil life is controlling crop plant disease. No fertilizer used here on pastures for over 30 years, and crop fertilizer has been reduced by 70%, and now we're using more and more organic fertilizers. How is that possible? How can we grow crops with very little fertilizer? Living, growing plants are the drivers of soil health, soil structure, and nutrient cycling. Plants add dead and decaying material to the soil, which feeds soil microbes, and plants secrete sugars through their roots, which feed soil microbes. It's plants that drive soils and soil health, and plant diversity, especially perennial plants, but also the plants that we're using in our pasture cropping mix, and multispecies pasture cropping is driving this improvement in soil health and making nutrients available to other plants. This is a photo of my soil and my neighboring soil. These were only taken about 15 minutes apart over a fence line. There is over two feet of soil built on the one on the left, and the neighbor's soil only has about four inches of topsoil on it. That soil has over 200% more organic carbon than the one on the right. It has sequestered almost 60 ton of carbon per hectare, and over a 10-year period that has removed over 200 ton per hectare, about 100 ton per acre of carbon dioxide from the atmosphere. If we can get more farmers doing this type of farming—growing more plants is really all it is, and plant diversity—

we can remove much of our carbon dioxide out of our atmosphere. We can, that is farmers all around the world, can be the cure for a lot of our climate change, global warming problems that we've got by simply removing carbon dioxide out of the atmosphere and storing it in our soil as carbon. It is very simple, and it can be done. The other benefits of that are that now this soil holds 200% more water, and all of the nutrients including trace elements have increased by an average of 162%. That is relevant because those nutrients are now available in the food we're consuming from these soils and also the nutrients are available in the animals now that are grazing these grasslands. Is it profitable? Obviously, this is very important from a farming point of view.

[00.33.29] And yes, it is very profitable. Annual income is higher, compared to when I was farming with the industrial type of agriculture. Crop yields are similar to what they were then. We're running more sheep and cattle. Now, we harvest and sell over 1000 kg of native grass seed annually, and that's significant because that seed is 70 dollars a kilogram, so it's high-value seed. Soil organic carbon levels are increasing. Soil phosphorous, calcium, nitrogen, pH, magnesium, and trace elements are all increasing. That's not just in availables, but the total is increasing as well. Now, all of this has been possible with $80,000 less inputs and far less labor. Far less labor is required on the farm now, so everything is far easier than it used to be. Industrial agriculture is destroying our farms, soil, and our planet. How can we produce more food without destroying our farms and our planet? If we look at primarily what I've been talking about—vertical stacking of farming and grazing enterprises—in other words, we can stack enterprises on the same area. We can grow different enterprises on the same area of land, and I'll explain that. Now, if we look at what I've just spoken about, on a given area over a 12-month period, we've produced grain, sheep meat, cattle, wool, vegetables, native grass seed—and also that can be native grass seed for human consumption—and I really haven't mentioned carbon sequestration when trading in carbon. So all of that can be done—and I'm doing that now—and we can add to that. It can be greater as well. By including vegetables in a multi-species mix we can produce vegetables for human consumption as well as produce a grain crop. Those vegetables can brassica crops like turnip, kale, and peas. And we can also do a summer crop as well. All of this can be done while we restore grasslands, recycle nutrients, and improve our soil ecosystem.

The enterprises in a vertically stacked enterprise mix need to be ecologically compatible. The reason it works is because they are ecologically compatible. They complement each other, in other words. They complement each other ecologically. They complement each other financially. And if they're ecologically compatible they will regenerate the farm, and they will be more profitable. So to sum all this up, agriculture and sound ecological practices should function together. Agriculture doesn't have to destroy farms, ecosystems, and the planet. Good agricultural practices can produce vast amounts of good quality food, far more than the industrial model. We can produce far more food, using these methods. We can also regenerate our grasslands or our prairies. We can restore our soil ecosystems, supply and cycle soil nutrients, control insect damage and plant disease. In other words, agriculture can be more profitable, regenerate our farms, ecosystems, and the planet. But agricultural practices need to function closer to how Nature had it originally designed. Thank you.

Brendan [00:37:25]: Wow, that was amazing, Colin. Thank you. It's the second time I've seen your presentation, but it never ceases to amaze me, what you've accomplished. And from what I understand, part of the reason your operation has been researched so much is that people didn't believe what you are doing was possible, is that right?

Colin [00:37:47]: That is correct, yes, especially when I was getting early results here of being able to reduce fertilizer, people thought that was impossible. And when I was saying we no longer got insect attack— remember this is 15 to 20 years ago that these results were starting to come through—no one was thinking about this, that it was possible to be able to manage things naturally and without all of these pesticides and fertilizers that we've now had forced upon us. So, I challenged the scientists to come and do their own research, and also Dr. Christine Jones, who has been a wonderful supporter of mine and really was the science brain behind a lot of the development of pasture cropping and what I've been doing on this farm. She also challenged her fellow scientists to do the research on the farm here as well.

Brendan [00:38:58]: Also, from what I understand, organic agriculture used to have more of a focus on multispecies cover cropping. I'm not entirely certain of that, but what's your understanding because I think that organics might ... obviously, pasture cropping didn't exist as far as combining grazing and planting into dormant grassland and so forth— that's what makes this so unique and moving our agriculture systems more toward an ecological model—but you've been around all of this a lot. Were you familiar with how organics was conceived, and was it more similar to this in any regards than it is now and how it's practiced now?

Colin [00:39:41]: Yes, organic agriculture has been very, very close to having it right, but one of the biggest problems with organic agriculture is plowing. Plowing soil is very, very destructive no matter how you do it. Turning soil upside-down is extremely destructive and kills soil microbes and destroys soil structure. The organic people have done a wonderful job over the years of removing pesticides and working out how to get soils functioning closer as an ecosystem but could never really get a handle on how they could grow crops without plowing, especially without using herbicides. Now, what's happened recently with cover crops—and Gabe Brown is probably a very good example of what's happening with this—as we grow, we can grow annual cover crops with multiple species. And what happens there, as it does with my pasture cropping, the more species you get in there the faster it drives soils and soil health, cycle nutrients, and control of weeds. So now we can grow crops in a very degraded system, a multispecies cover crop, get it on the ground with either rolling it or, better still with animals, mulch it onto the ground, and then plant crops into that. That is very similar to what I'm doing, except mine's a perennial system. I don't need to plant the covers because the perennial grasses cover the ... what I'm doing, which is perennial cover cropping, is the reverse of annual cover cropping in that my multispecies crop is my crop. It is not the cover, if you understand that. I don't know if that's confused everyone or not.

Brendan [00:41:50]: Ah, no, I understand. Oh, by the way, is Gabe Brown the one who figured out that by having cover crop mixes that included species from five different families, I think it is—brassicas, grasses, legumes, cereals, and chenopods, is that the five?

Colin [00:42:13]: Yep.

Brendan [00:42:14]: Was it him that discovered that?

Colin [00:42:16]: No, Gabe would say that the main driver of the multispecies mix or the main person was David Brandt in Iowa, and Gabe would also say that ... but Gabe is taking it to another level and also incorporating animals in it where Dave hasn't been incorporating animals. But David Brandt, I guess, is the pioneer in the US of multispecies cover crops. Where I developed multispecies mixes, I was growing oats and single species into my diverse grassland here. I spoke at No Till on the Plains Conference in 2012 and met Gabe and Dave and all of these guys that were doing multispecies cover crops, and the penny dropped with me in that I realized then that a multispecies crop would move my soils even faster in the soil's health and nutrient cycling. And so, what I've done here is combined what I originally developed with pasture cropping and combined it with what Gabe and Dave have been doing and sort of overlaid the two of them.

Brendan [00:43:40]: Got it. What I find absolutely fascinating about that five species mix ... or is it families, five families?

Colin [00:43:50]: Yeah, we need at least four or five and there's a grass species and brassica, a legume, one missing here somewhere ...

Brendan [00:44:13]: Chenopod?

Colin [00:44:14]: Yes, as many in there as we can possibly put in there. Now, if you relate that to just a wheat crop or corn, in that they as a monoculture, they're a single-dimensional root system. If we mixed all of those species together, then we have a three-dimensional root system, and that's why we're starting to drive soils and soil health and carbon and all the wonderful benefits. And it shouldn't be a surprise to us because that's what Nature does. Nature never has anything as a single species. The original grassland here and your prairies, had 200 or 400 probably in the US prairies, 400 species, in that original grassland or prairie so why are we growing crops as a single species? It's just madness.

Brendan [00:44:58]: And I think one thing here that's so counterintuitive, but we're seeing that the more roots you have in the soil, the richer the soil gets, and yet we've sort of maybe been conditioned to think that roots only take things out of the soil, but they put so much into the soil that, you know, the sugars and so forth that they exude to feed the organisms, and then your organisms create their little home out of those sugars and build complex carbon structures and the whole thing as they then go out and mine the parent material of the soil with their organic acids and enzymes and make minerals available to the plants. The whole thing just grows and becomes more complex and more stable and so forth. It's totally counterintuitive from a mind that has been conditioned to think of roots as extractive.

Colin [00:45:50]: That's exactly right, and we've been told that with the industrial model that if we have a plant growing or plants growing, they are removing nutrients, and then when they've removed nutrients you've got to replace them with fertilizer. That's the biggest lie we've ever been told. That's dreadful information. All a plant does is cycle nutrients round and round. It doesn't remove nutrients. Okay, if we totally remove that plant, you will remove some nutrients, but we have never looked at the benefits that plants do. I guess if you're selling fertilizer, you don't really want people to know that information either—that we're cycling nutrients and bringing nutrients up from depth, and not only that, we're releasing nutrients from the original soil particles or the particles in the soil.

Brendan [00:46:49]: Yeah, and the other thing about this that's interesting is we're used to thinking of plants as competing with each other for scarce resources, whether its water, minerals, and other nutrients in the soil. And I suppose maybe there are some rare instances where there is competition, but what we're seeing with these multispecies cover crops and many other poly-cultural instead of mono-cultural systems is that the plants actually get more done when there is more of them. And I guess with these five species, or the five families, represented in a cover crop, you have all of these phenolic compounds being exuded into the soil, is that it? And, the microbes then get stimulated and go into a supercharged metabolism and build soil even faster or something like that.

Colin [00:47:49]: Yeah, and I guess we don't really know exactly what's happening under there, and it's only an emerging field really, soil microbiology and soil ecosystems. We're really only just starting to look at them, but in the past we've certainly got it wrong in the way we've gone with agriculture with our single species and need for fertilizer. We've known in gardens for a long, long time that many plants are complementary, and we've done that in gardens, and we've also put litter or mulch on gardens to conserve moisture and control soil temperature. All of this we've known in gardening probably for a thousand years, but we've never applied it to agriculture. The organic people have to a degree, and we need to move that organic system even further, but the organic people have had it really close for a long time.

Brendan [00:48:53]: And you've increased your soil carbon how many percent?

Colin [00:48:58]: It's over 200% now, and we've seen the benefits of that. One of the first things is increased water-holding capacity in our soils, and our crops just do better in dry times. Or our pastures and grassland grow a lot better in dry times. We don't need the rainfall that we were dependent on before. We get huge, huge benefits in many ways by increasing soil carbon.

Brendan [00:49:31]: So in other words, by having more species rather than competing, they're creating more soil carbon … rather than creating scarcity for themselves with the water, they're actually creating a soil that holds more water so there's more to go around for everybody, I guess.

Colin [00:49:50]: That's right, yes, yes. It's really quite amazing. Well, it shouldn't amaze us, I guess. Mother Nature developed it over a million years or more, or billions of years, sorry, so we shouldn't be surprised that yes, as soil carbons increase and everything associated with that, everything has just become healthier and healthier to a point now, as I said in the presentation, that the nutrients are also increasing. The average increase has been 162% increase in all the nutrients. That's trace elements and the major elements as well. They're all increasing. That is not supposed to happen, and some soil scientists will argue that that's impossible, but I'm not the only person doing this. The people that move in this direction all report from their soil tests that nutrients are increasing. If we get it right ... if we get agriculture right, we can do it for thousands of years into the future. If we get it wrong, which we have now, I suggest we're going to struggle in the next hundred years. If we get it right, because it's regenerative, if we get this right, it regenerates the soil and soil ecosystem and farm ecosystem so it will continue to constantly improve.

Brendan [00:51:21]: I was listening to Christine Jones speak, and I believe she was speaking about your soil, and she mentioned that she sent off soil to the lab and had it assayed for the available minerals. With the information they sent back to her, she calculated the total quantity of minerals. She knew that she had sent off soil that had a certain bulk density that would equate to almost 8,000 kilos per hectare in the top 50 cm of soil, and so it should be 7800 kg that they send back if they're analyzing all of the minerals, well 97% of that, because I guess your soil was at about 3% organic content, much of which is carbon, and so the other 97% should have added up to, I guess, 97% of the roughly 8,000 kilos. And they sent back an analysis that showed a total of 200 kilos. And so she called them up sort of tongue-in-cheek, I guess, and asked them for all of the available totals, "So where's the other 7800 kilos that's not accounted for here?" [Colin is laughing] and they said, "Yeah, that's right, the soil test is only going to tell you about 1.5 to 3% of what's in it." She said, "Well, what is the other 97%?" He said, "That's your minerals." And she asked if those other 97% minerals were available to microbes. He said "Yes, but we don't test for that. We test for what's readily available." So obviously, there are a lot of minerals in the soil that aren't going to show up in tests and aren't going to be showing up in our plants and in our food if we don't have the microbes because it's their job to make it available. And the more active the soil gets, the more those minerals will show up in the tests of the soil and in, of course, our food.

Colin [00:53:44]: Yep. That's exactly right, and in those tests that I showed I didn't include nitrogen in that. And nitrogen has more than doubled in there, but it's organic nitrogen, now that the microbes are there, is more available to plants. So, yes, there's so much that we not only don't understand but is not even tested for in our soil tests. There's a lot more for science to learn about this. And many people that are adopting regenerative agricultural techniques are seeing these types of results, are seeing it in their plants, seeing it in their animals, but it doesn't always add up in the tests. There's something else going on that science yet can't measure, I guess.

Brendan [00:45:45]: Yeah, well, Nature is far more powerful than we have fully realized up to this point. So, is this a lot of extra work for you to produce so much? There are so many things going on. You've got native grasses; you've got sheep; you've got stud sheep; you've got Kelpie dogs ... what am I missing? Multiple crops, multiple incomes. Isn't this making you a little too busy?

Colin [00:55:16]: No, it actually makes it a lot easier than what I used to do. There is a lot less work on the farm than there used to be. The reason why is—and I didn't talk about it in this presentation and I probably should have—but to be able to generate more production, or produce more food is a better way of describing it, more food off a given area, off an acre, if we stack those enterprises vertically on top of each other, in other words, if those enterprises, like the animals grazing, the crops growing, and native seed, all of those are complementary, if they're ecologically compatible and complementary, they support each other so there's actually less work to do because it's being driven naturally, and everything is complementary. And so that's how and why we can generate more food, more production off a given area with less inputs, less costs, and far less money to drive it. And not only that, it'll keep regenerating so it's about enterprise stacking, and Joel Salatin actually does a lot of that type of thing. He describes it a little bit different than the way I describe it, but Joel stacks enterprises that are also complementary ecologically.

Brendan [00:56:58]: Yes, he's got quite an operation.

Colin [00:57:02]: Yep.

Brendan [00:57:04]: So, where does this type of farming work? I mean, this can't possibly work everywhere, I imagine. In what types of locations and climates can this work?

Colin [00:57:22]: The broad principles of it can work pretty well anywhere. Now, pasture cropping in itself relies on a grassland or the majority of the species that are becoming dormant at a particular year, and then the crop we're growing or planting into it is actively growing when that perennial grass or grassland is dormant. And that's the original concept that I developed. However, now this thing just continually evolves as I learn more, and especially with animals, we can manipulate that grassland so that we can create a niche, an ecological niche where we can plant things into even the living grassland so we can manipulate it more, and we can manipulate it, again, without herbicides. You could use a herbicide if you wanted, but we can do it without that. And we can do that either with grazing animals, we can do it with things like mulching machinery to mulch that material, anything to suppress that grassland to create a niche to grow things in. It's as broad as our imagination will allow it to be.

Brendan [00:58:50]: Could you have achieved the same results without animals?

Colin [00:58:55]: I don't think so, although in saying that, David Brandt's doing a wonderful job without animals there and getting wonderful soil and healthy improvements. But no, the animals are a very essential part of this because I'm using large mobs of animals on relatively small areas to mulch that perennial grass down or, in my case, mulch the cover onto the soil surface. They're adding nutrients in manure and urine onto that soil surface which the plants then use so that's producing a lot of our fertility or a lot of our nutrients for our crop that we're planting. In my case, the animals are very important. They're doing some weed control, and we're manipulating that grassland with the animals and creating a niche for the crop to be planted in. So the animals are a very important part of it, more so also, as well as doing all that, a very, very important part of overall farm income. We're not just growing a crop, but we're grazing animals as well.

Brendan [01:00:12]: Is there a role in all of this to make it even better with GMOs? I'm not sure how that would work because I haven't seen GMOs accomplish a whole lot, but do you see any role for GMOs?

Colin [01:00:27]: Am I allowed to answer that question by swearing? [laughing] I don't think there's any role for GMOs at all. I think they're a disaster, and all they are, is … Well, the original grain revolution failed. The GMOs are being developed and often being promoted as the next "Green Revolution". Why would you want the next Green Revolution? The last one was a failure. No, GMOs have no place at all. We don't need GMOs. There is enough diversity in Nature to select, as we've traditionally done. We don't need GMOs. All they're doing is allowing the use of herbicides, pesticides, and insecticides on a crop. No, there's absolutely no place for GMOs at all, and we don't need them anyway. They're making multinational companies wealthy and sending farmers broke and making people all over the world very unhealthy and sick and dying, I'd suggest.

Brendan [01:01:40]: Yeah, it's amazing, the research that has come out from professor … is it Huber? (Professor Don Huber)

Colin [01:01:50]: Yes, yep.

Brendan [01:01:51]: … who has discovered that at least part of the way that Roundup works, that glyphosate works is it's a chelator of minerals and nutrients [**Correction:** Glyphosate was patented as a chelator—this is not what Professor Huber discovered.], so it's blocking these nutrients from being utilized by the plants, and so they develop plants that can survive on fewer of those nutrients or something. I actually have to look into that further myself, but I thought it was interesting you mentioned that the first step that you help farmers get through is to move toward other herbicides first, is get off glyphosate as sort of the first step and an essential step to stop killing the soil and stop tying up the minerals.

Colin [01:02:40]: Yep. It's interesting when I do workshops and talks around the world on this and to get people started and that transition from industrial agriculture, moving it more towards a biological system is important. To transition from an industrial form of agriculture to organic agriculture in one go is a recipe to go broke. People do it, but you can transition off that gradually, which is a better way to do it. It's no point in wanting to be green and going broke. So I transition people and get them onto, I guess, a softer herbicide if there is any such thing, and then gradually show them how to wean off many or all of those inputs over time. And then you can transition off that and still be very profitable. Your income is still flowing and then gradually wean off those inputs.

Brendan [01:03:52]: How do you teach this to people, as far as lectures, courses, and do you have anything in development so that more growers can learn from you?

Colin [01:04:03]: Yeah, I've been developing—and hopefully it'll be out soon—an online course so we can get our message out to more people around the world. I get to the States almost every year now. I was just there in July doing workshops. I was in Kansas, Oklahoma, and California last time. So yes, hopefully we'll get this course up and running in the next few months, online course, which will get the message out on how we can do this. A lot of this is very simple. There's nothing very complicated about pasture cropping and my work. It can't be very complicated for two guys drinking beer all night can dream up … It is actually quite simple, and really what we're doing is mimicking Nature very, very closely. We don't need to reinvent anything. Blueprints have already been written. We need to just mimic natural systems a lot closer.

Brendan [01:05:17]: Yeah, that's a beautiful way of summarizing it, and I think it's pretty instructive that you guys came up with the idea by simply not having the money for inputs any longer and you said, "Well, we've gotta figure out something that doesn't require all of this extraneous …" I mean, you didn't think of it as extraneous I suppose at the time, but you didn't have the money for herbicides, so, "Let's just plant it right into the dormant grasslands and see what happens," and it worked.

Colin [01:05:47]: Yes, that's exactly right. We simply didn't have the money, and often change happens because of a disaster. And in my case that's certainly the case, but change often happens that way because then people are forced, as I was forced, to do it a different way because I didn't have the money to continue with the methods I was using.

Brendan [01:06:10]: Yeah. Beautiful. Well, thanks again, Colin. This has been great.

Colin [01:06:16]: Okay, thank you.

Peter Byck Interview

Cow Curious, The Hunt for Carbon Cowboys, and a Possible Redemption of McDonalds

Brendan [00:00:00]: Welcome to the Eat4Earth event. We're exploring how you can heal yourself, your loved ones, and the planet with your food choices. This is Brendan Moorehead, and it's my honor and pleasure to welcome our guest, Peter Byck. Peter is an award-winning director and editor. His first documentary film won the South by Southwest Film Festival. Peter is also a senior sustainability scientist at Julie Ann Wrigley Global Institute of Sustainability and also a professor of practice at the School of Sustainability at Arizona State University. His AMP research project seeks to produce whole system science data surrounding use of adaptive multi-paddock grazing for carbon sequestration in soil, water retention, plant and microbial biodiversity, and human well-being. Other arms of the project include rancher and farmer outreach and education and agriculture policy development. Peter, you are a true renaissance man and it's my pleasure to have you here today at the Eat4Earth event.

Peter [00:01:00]: Well thank you, Brendan. I appreciate it. It's a great series that you have started.

Brendan [00:01:04]: So how did you get from filmmaking into science and research and now you've got these very audacious goals with this AMP project.

Peter [00:01:14]: Yes, so my second feature film was called *Carbon Nation*, and in that we did a lot of research on solutions to climate change, and in that, our research and the folks were teaching me, the folks I was interviewing were all talking specifically about soils and that the soils do hold a lot of carbon, and they could hold more because a lot of our soils are losing carbon through erosion and misuse. Then, within then that world, it was the grazing world that caught my attention. It seemed like it could be maybe the biggest bang for the buck of getting more carbon back into the ground, back into the soil. So, the first film that was coming out of the gate once I got here to ASU was called *Soil Carbon Cowboys*, and in that film we follow three innovative farmers/ranchers who are doing what we're now calling adaptive, multi-paddock grazing, so AMP grazing where you put all your animals in one herd, and you put them into small paddocks, sometimes for a day and sometimes for a few hours. And you just let them eat what's going on in that small paddock, and it's a really heavy hit with their hooves, which is simulating seed growth, the manure, their urine, which is getting the microbial life fed. And then they leave that spot, and that spot gets to rest. It's that heavy hit and rest is the way the grasslands and the herding animals evolved over tens of thousands of years or more so these farmers are replicating that in a small scale on their land. It's kind of like the way the herds used to move across the Great Plains. The predators would come, and they'd move them across and that land would rest, maybe for a year or more on the Great Plains. And the Great Plains produced the deepest, richest soils, I think, we've ever seen on earth, I think, you know 15-feet deep of beautiful topsoil. And so as I was making the film and doing the research on the film, I was asking a lot of scientists, "Are these ranchers storing carbon?" And I was taught it was more complicated than that. "There's different pools of carbon, which have different periods of durability. There's the carbon that lasts for days, the carbon that lasts for decades, and the carbon that lasts for centuries, so what are you studying?" And I was like, "Okay," and then other scientists say, "Well you gotta get those greenhouse gasses; you gotta get the methane and the nitrous oxide and the CO2 coming in and out of the system." "Alright." "You gotta study the microbial life. You gotta understand what's going on underground, and then you gotta study the bugs above and below the ground. You gotta study the plants above and below ground. You gotta study how the water is infiltrating and being retained in the system. And what about the animal wellbeing. and what about the rancher wellbeing?" And so all of these scientists were teaching me their part of this picture, and it just seemed to me clearly that this was one picture. And a lot of them were thinking the same thing, so we formed a team to compare AMP grazing and conventional grazing and find out if indeed we can measure the differences and point at the method of grazing as the reason that it's different. And so it came out of the film. and I made a bunch of more films about these ranchers in different parts of the country. People will say, "Yeah, it might work in Mississippi, but it's not going to work in Kansas." So, I go to Kansas and film it in Kansas. Yes it works there. "Well, it's not going to work in North Dakota," so you go to North Dakota. Yep, it's working there. What about the southwest? So, we go to New Mexico, and film it there. So I'm seeing success stories amongst these innovative farmers and ranchers. I want to tell their stories because I want farmers and ranchers to do really well. I want them to make a lot of money. I want the people growing our food to not be in debt, and we're seeing farmers and ranchers who are focusing on soil health first, using any kind of way of grazing. We're just focused on one type of regenerative grazing, but hey, have at it. When they focus on soil health first, they're getting themselves out of debt and to me that's where the rubber meets the road. And why would we want farmers and ranchers to be in debt when they're producing our food? So that's what I'm learning. I came in at this through climate change, and now I'm coming at this as I want our farmers and ranchers to do well. And then I've learned that soil health is the North Star, and when you have healthy soil you have nutritious plants. And if you just eat the plants, that's great, and if you eat the animal that eats the plants, that's great too. At the end it all came from the short film and then from the bigger film before that.

Brendan [00:05:43]: And just for our listeners, I think it would be good to … you know how does this contrast from typical grazing? You touched on it, but I think it bears explaining a little bit so people get … it because we know that grazing can be quite detrimental, right? And in this case, it's actually regenerative. We're building soil, we're restoring nutrients into the system, so how is it different from degenerative grazing?

Peter [00:06:14]: So, I would say that every farmer and rancher wants to make their soils better and wants to make their land better. I think that there's new techniques that are being discovered now that can help them get there faster. So with conventional grazing, ranchers and farmers are allowing their animals to graze a very large area, even if it's not their whole farm, it might be a paddock that's a quarter of their farm or a fifth of their farm, and they let the animals graze that area at their own pace, going for the plants they want to get. And what happens is the animals go after the plants they love and overgraze those, don't go after the plants they don't like, and those take over so there is a lack of balance of what's growing. And a lot of times the fields themselves will be planted in mono-crops, just one species or two species because as one of our farmers tells me in the film, it's easier that way. So when you have just one or two species out in this field, you're sort of putting yourself at the mercy of a lot of invasive species of insects because you don't have a lot of plants for those insects to live off. The more variety you have of the plants, the more resilient the land is. And a lot of conventional grazing doesn't have a variety of or a plethora of diversity of plant forage material. Therefore, they're needing to put a lot of fertilizer on there or they might need insecticides or herbicides. And so the conventional needs help where what we're seeing with regenerative grazing is they're using Nature first. It's like giving nature a seat at the table as my buddy Russ Conser just said last week, and I'm like, "That's great!" It's also keeping the animals tightly in a small area for a short period of time. That's the big difference. AMP grazing does that, and conventional grazing just sort of lets them disperse sort of to the fence line, and that's not the way the grazing animals evolved, but that's the way we've evolved in our land use management.

Brendan [00:08:27]: Got it. Yes, my understanding is that when you just let them graze as they please, they take it all the way down to the stubble, and then the plant has a hard time coming back, whereas if you limit their time, you put them in there with all their buddies, and then they're chomping as fast as they can because it's all lush growth, but you don't let them take it beyond a certain point, like maybe 50% grazed, and then the plants have plenty of that leaf left to regenerate, and they regenerate, and in that process they regenerate vigorously.

Peter [00:09:00]: Yes, and they have that plant leaf left to still do photosynthetic activity. And you're right, a lot of ranchers and farmers are trained/taught to have these lawn-like pastures where it's short, and that's the way they want it, with no weeds or anything like that when actually, as Allen Williams says in our film, what's a weed? If it's nutritious and animals like to eat it, then I call it forage. So there's this issue of, "Your fields don't look right. You're letting it grow too long. You're being lazy. You're sloppy. You're not a good farmer by having your field up to waist-high." But there's a lot of really amazing connective benefits to the way these folks are grazing and the way they're letting their forage ... One, they're getting a lot of diversity of forage because a lot of times when these ranchers are changing from conventional to AMP, they're seeing plants come up that they didn't plant. The seeds are just in this latent seed bank, and they haven't expressed themselves because they haven't been treated in a way that they feel like expressing themselves, if I can be so bold as to give them feelings, but we're seeing that all over the place. There's all these different systems of plants that are coming up that they didn't plant, but are expressing themselves. You get this diversity of forage, and you let the weeds come up because they aren't weeds, and what's happening is the animals when they can graze forage that's this high or this high or this high—I don't know if you can see [gesturing over his head]—they don't have to bend over as much so its not as stressful for them. And a lot of problems with grazing is the stomach worm that the animals get. And the stomach worm lives near the soil surface, and so when animals graze on their own they don't go down much further than, like you said, halfway down. I think of it as like asparagus, I only eat the top part; I don't eat the bottom part. So, the animals are doing that as well. They know what to graze; they know what they need; they're very smart. There's some great science that's been done on how animals graze and that they know what they need to get, and they'll balance their own diet if they have the option, if they have the variety. So they'll eat down to a certain point, but they'll never get down to the surface of the, soil and so they don't get the stomach worm. Therefore, they don't need to get the stomach worm medicine, and what does that do? Well, the stomach worm medicine kills the worm; it also kills the dung beetles at the other end. So these folks are letting their animals graze to here, letting their forage grow up really high, are almost eliminating their stomach worm medicine bill, and then they're getting the benefit of these dung beetles on the other end recycling the manure like they've evolved to do and getting all that nutrient into the microbial life, into the subsoil quickly so that it doesn't release a lot of greenhouse gasses while it's just sitting there on top of the land. So by letting your forage grow high and letting them graze where they want, you're actually getting an enormous amount of benefits, and that's just some of them. So that's why in our science project we have the bug scientists; we have the water scientists and the plant scientists and the animal scientists and the social scientists and the carbon folks and the greenhouse gas folks because we look at it as a system. No, let me rephrase that … it is a system, and we're choosing to measure it as such. Now, that's not every bit of the system, but we're trying to get as much of the picture as we can, as we compare different grazing methods and so, you know, wish us luck. McDonald's has come on board for 4.5 million dollars to our research project. We need to match that, and if we match just a part of that this year, then we're out in the field in the spring. And so that's what we're working on right now is that funding. We've got a couple of irons in the fire, and that's kind of where my job is. I helped to organize this team; I helped put this team together. I am a filmmaker; I'm a communicator; I'm not a scientist. We have 17 scientists on our team, but here at ASU, we look at interdisciplinary, interuniversity projects with great gusto and the university support given to me as I've been building this team and building this project with this amazing group of scientists …

Brendan [00:13:44]: So … what's that?

Peter [00:13:48]: They teach me every phone call. I mean every phone call, I'm a layman …

Brendan [00:13:52]: It's a download of revelations, right? I mean, I've listened to these guys talk various times at conferences, and every time my jaw is just hanging open going, "Oh my God." And that's why I started this event. The vision for it came from hearing from these scientists and realizing everybody needs to know about this because it affects them very personally, right down to their food and their nutrient density that they're ingesting that either builds a strong, healthy child and their own body or not. But tell me, back to these natural systems … so by grazing in this way, there are seeds being recruited from this old seed bank that maybe have been dormant for decades. I know that's the case with Colin Seis in Australia. He's got these grassland species coming up that hadn't been seen for a very long time, and the seeds were just down there, and now it's another crop for him. He's selling these seeds, which may eventually become human food, but right now the seeds are being, I believe, marketed to maybe other ranchers so they can give their land a headstart if it's been too badly poisoned or something. This is very exciting. What else happens in the system when you get this plant biodiversity? What else are you seeing? Other forms of biodiversity? The insects, I guess, and wildlife? What do you see?

Peter [00:15:24]: Yes, all of those things build from that. Our working hypothesis—and there's a paper from Penn State that supports this piece of it—is that the more biodiversity of plant life you have aboveground, the more biodiversity of microbial life you have below the ground. It's a logical assumption, but they actually did the work to do the studies for that. The more biodiversity you have of plants above ground, each plant is attracting its own suite of insects, both beneficial and predator. But when you have a lot of different insects from a lot of different plants, then the predator of that plant is food for the insect that loves to eat from this plant. They sort of balance each other out so the insecticide bills on these ranches that we're studying have gone down tremendously. We'll be looking at that specifically. We'll be looking at the farmers and the ranchers and their books, if they'll let us, so we'll see exactly what their vet bills are, what their insect/pesticide bills are, all those things. We want to quantify it all because this has to be good business or its not going to happen. It has to be good business for the farmer, or it's not going to happen. So, we're seeing biodiversity of birds that are feeding on the insects; we're seeing biodiversity of the insects and different pollinating insects; and we're seeing wildlife coming onto these ranches. Allen Williams has a partner, and they bought this ranch near Starkville, Mississippi. People had put three hunting lodges on this thousand acres to make it a deer hunting place where they could sell the right to hunt the deer on that land and then have people pay for staying in those lodges. But it wasn't very rich with wildlife, and so they sold it to Allen and his partner. Allen then started doing AMP grazing on that land, and I filmed Allen on his fourth year after the transition, and in the county that Starkville is in or in the county where his farm is—I don't know if it's a neighboring county—that land just in four years of a change of grazing is now the hotspot for deer. So that company wants to buy it back. so they can do what they set out to do, which is the deer hunting. But Allen and his partner say, "No, we're keeping it as is." So the grazing management alone was the only difference, and it attracted wildlife—breeding birds, the ground nesting birds—and the way these folks are grazing their animals are going together really well, surprisingly so, and so its been pretty amazing on that front. I wanted to, if I may, connect what's happening with bees and grasslands. We're losing bee colonies, and there's all sorts of reasons for that, theories and science behind it. And our bug scientist, Jonathan Lundgren and I, we're thinking that we have all these different modules to our research. It's like, where are the people who want to spend money on the bug part of this? We have all these different parts and some people might be interested in the bird part, some people might be interested in the animal well-being or the rancher well-being, so where are the bug people as we're looking for funding? And so we were really digging into his knowledge base, and something I didn't know is the pollinating insects, the bees themselves … a lot of insects pollinate, but if you just talked about the bees, the beekeepers have to put their bees someplace when they're not pollinating, and the place they want to put the bees is where the bees naturally went, which is grasslands. And we're losing grasslands, just a tremendous amount of grassland loss just in the Midwest to folks plowing it up and planting corn and planting soy. It's astounding how much grassland we're losing right now. And so if we encourage regenerative grazing, what we're calling AMP grazing, then we give a place for those pollinating insects to be for the times that they're not pollinating. So then you connect grazing to food production. And what he was telling me was even when you have self-pollinating plants like wheat … I think oats right now are self-pollinating, and I think corn … even when you have the self-pollinating plants, if you have the bees nearby their productivity goes up by like 20%, he was telling me. So even then, so the bees and production and grazing, we're making those connections, again systems thinking, so that we can then find funders who might not even think about grazing as part of their business, but might not realize how grazing is enabling their business to be more resilient and enabling their food supply chain to be much more resilient. Every day it's one more thing like this, and like you were saying, you go to conferences and hear these scientists speak, well, I get to talk to them on the phone and ask them every question and say, "What was that? I didn't understand that last part." It's an amazing journey and, you know, we want to get out in the field, we want to do the science, but it's been an amazing time just to know these people, and we're friends.

Brendan [00:20:43]: When you were speaking about the corn and wheat and some self-pollinating cereals, are we talking about pasture cropping? Something like that, which Colin Seis does when he's …

Peter [00:20:57]: We're just talking about conventional farming.

Brendan [00:20:59]: Okay.

Peter [00:21:00]: … and when you have pollinators in those fields when the plants are growing—I don't know exactly when the best time would be to have them there, I'll ask Jonathan that—but we're just saying that even in conventional farming those bees will help produce more food per acre.

Brendan [00:21:19]: Right, right.

Peter [00:21:21]: So regenerative grazing will still make other systems more resilient, more productive because you give the bees a place to rest and make honey.

Brendan [00:21:34]: Right, gotcha, so in neighboring land. We need these reserves of grasslands to support our other production landscapes of grains, but where I was going is what Colin Seis is doing. Yes, he's stacking. There's not this order necessarily between the grain growing land, the grassland, the grazing land, it's all one. He's got at least four revenue streams, four crops coming out of the land every single year, and the soil just keeps getting better to the tune of, an average I believe of 9 tons of carbon per hectare per year, and so that brings me to asking you …

Peter [00:22:16]: Nine tons of carbon?

Brendan [00:22:18]: Nine tons according to Christine Jones' calculation.

Peter [00:22:21]: Wow.

Brendan [00:22:22]: Per hectare, not acre.

Peter [00:22:25]: Richard Tiegs found three tons per hectare per year in a study funded by the Dixon Water Foundation in north Texas over about a 10-year period, and we've had many good soil scientists and earth scientists say, "That's way too much, we don't believe you." And that's at three tons per hectare per year. We did a pilot program up in Alberta, and we found comparing conventional to AMP grazing from about 1.1 tons of carbon per hectare per year up to 2.2 tons of carbon per hectare per year, more on the AMP versus conventional. So we saw those numbers, and then we have a couple of just drill sites we've done with one or two samples, and we've seen bigger numbers, but that's just one or two samples. We're seeing more carbon stored with the higher rainfall, and so we're thinking the southeast US would be the place to see the most carbon stored per hectare per year so that's why we're focusing on that for our first year of our field research.

And then we want to get to the upper great plains because it's a very different region. It's dryer. It's cooler. And so, like I said earlier, the "yeah, but" thing really does come to play where yeah, it works in Mississippi, but it won't work in Alabama, you know, going down that line. I've had a farmer tell me that not only is it state-by-state, but it's actually fence line. We filmed a guy named Michael Thompson in Kansas, and he studies Gabe Brown who is doing the row crop and the grazing all on the same land, cover crops as well, and so Michael's got really rich soil. He'd been doing it I think for about 10 years when I filmed him—I think about that long—and so he planted a corn crop right on this hill right next to his neighbor, and his neighbor was just transitioning to using cover crops, so his soil hadn't had time to make the transition. He was in his first year. Literally, Thompson's corn, when I was there in July, his corn was at least a foot higher. There wasn't even a fence, it was just corn here, and corn here based on the soil health, and his neighbor said that he must've gotten more rain, or another neighbor said that.

Brendan [00:24:51]: Yes, Christine Jones jokes about that, where you see a fence line, and one side is green and one side, she says, so you can see that it rains a lot more on that side of the fence when it's really, you know, the water holding capacity of the soil.

Peter [00:25:06]: There might be a little modicum of truth to that. Michael Thompson was telling me this, he watches the rain come in with a drooling mouth because he's in north Kansas, and it's incredibly dry. And he's seen rainstorms split and open and circle and not rain on these really dry, overgrazed, uncovered cropland, like they're creating a heat cloud that's actually splitting the rain. There are some studies on that. I haven't read enough about it, but the idea that a channel of heat coming off of really hot soil that's not cool from cover crop, you could see that pushing away water. So it might be that it rains less on those pieces of land.

Brendan [00:25:51]: That is amazing. That's, I believe, also referred to as a "heat wall" in the lingo of Michal Kravčík and other people that are following his water paradigm. There's people talking about how one of the ways we need to focus, as far as cooling the planet, is restoring the water cycles. And we've got to do that by restoring the plant biodiversity and the soil microbial biodiversity and therefore the carbon content of the soil, so that you don't have this "heat island" effect. That's another name for it. In cities, they call it a "heat island", so yes, these heat walls, heat islands, heat cloud I think you called it, and yes, that's amazing that you're saying they actually see clouds splitting.

Peter [00:26:37]: Yes, that's what Michael is saying, and then there's a scientists whose name I forget, but he's at Montana State University. And he was studying land that was under the CRP program. I think it's the Conservation Reserve Program. And so much soil was eroding and going into our river ways and then clogging up the Mississippi that the USDA's idea was, let's just get people to stop farming for 20 years, and see if we can get a handle on that erosion. So, there's a lot of land that's now coming out of CRP, but this guy studied CRP land, which was lands where plants did grow over it—it wasn't a great biodiverse amount of plants or diversity of plants—but it was cooler, and that's what he found. Even as the Earth has been warming over this last decade, he found that the land that had the plants on it was actually two degrees cooler. And so he was just proving that plant cover cools the land. And so think of all those millions of acres of plowed farmland that's just fallow or just has the soil. I don't know if you've been on farms when you can just sort of feel the soil where it's got a cover crop on it and a thatch, and then you feel the soil that's got nothing on it—it's just sunlight—and it's a huge difference in temperature. I think it could be like 20 or 30 degrees difference in temperature. And so does that soil heat up even more and how does that treat the microbial community, versus the cover crop? I'm circling around a few different things, but you were talking about stacking enterprises. We made a film on a guy who you should interview if you haven't already, his name is Will Harris. He's at White Oak Pastures in southwest Georgia right near Alabama and right near Florida, and he's fourth generation rancher—daughters are fifth generation now—and he's just had some grandkids so the sixth generation is now alive. Well, I don't think they're working on the farm yet, I think they're less than a year old, so maybe they are. Maybe they are working on the farm with Will. But he grew up raising cattle just like his dad did and on down the line four generations back. And now he's raising 10 different types of protein on the same land, so he's stacking protein production. So he's not growing his row crops as feed, but he's still getting a lot more production out of the same amount of land just because he's focused on soil health first and let all his decisions come from that. And so that was a great experience filming him, and that film is called *One Hundred Thousand Beating Hearts*. It's on our website. I don't know if you're going to show the website anywhere, but that would be cool if you did.

Brendan [00:29:20]: Yes, in the resources I certainly will have that. It's amazing that so many ranchers are keying in on soil health and really, like you said, all farmers and ranchers are concerned about soil health, just some of them may have been educated in the system, maybe most of them educated in the system, that the way to do that is actually damaging the soil with the nitric fertilizer and the pesticides and herbicides and so forth.

Peter [00:29:51]: I do believe it's unintended, but it's still happening.

Brendan [00:29:55]: Yes. Now so how does this play out in terms of global impact? You've got some pretty big goals for this project, and so how does it play out at scale with certain numbers of hectares of land? Where is that land and whatever your estimates are for annual carbon sequestration ... how does that calculate out, and how much is that mitigating our emissions and so forth from fossil fuels, that is, and other forms of ...

Peter [00:30:25]: It's all about the scale. I mean the emissions are from agriculture too, the methane, the CO_2. Some people think that a fifth of the CO_2 in the atmosphere is from soil, carbon from soil that's now oxidized and gone back up into the atmosphere as CO_2. So I think agriculture has a huge part to play in solving climate change. When we deal with what we think the scale can be, you know there's a big caveat and that is, we're doing science right now to see if our hypotheses and our early data is accurate. Could grazing be a greenhouse gas equivalent sink? Could you store enough carbon in the soil to offset the methane coming out of the animals? Can you reduce the amount of methane coming out of the animals? The methanotrophic bacteria in the soil ... how much methane does that uptake? So there's a lot of questions about the nitrous oxides coming off the system, and if you're using a lot less nitrogen fertilizer, would that mean you're having a lot less nitrous oxide coming out of the system? So, we're going to ask all those questions, and obviously, no science is definitive, but we want to make it comprehensive enough that we really help educate us and hopefully a lot of other people. If our science comes back in the positive that these ranchers tell their story. You know, this is only going to work if ranchers and farmers want to do this, and one of the biggest issues is perceived risk, or risk. A lot of times, Christine will tell you—Christine Jones has taught me this and other folks as well—when you change your system you might have a dip in productivity for two or three years before it then comes up and goes higher than what you had. And so is there a ranch transition finance mechanism that we need to develop to help people over this hump? Could the USDA play a big part of that? That's where the policy comes in. Can we have USDA policies that really focus on soil health as the goal? That would be huge. If we get to scale, if we get all these pieces together, if the science proves it, and we get a lot of momentum, and we get a lot of people who are skeptical right now think, "Hey, you know what, maybe there is something to this" and then they start researching it themselves, they start finding out for themselves and it builds to scale, we think on an annual basis the US agricultural community could be storing a billion tons, a gigaton, of CO_2 annually. And the amount of land it would take, if we use Richard Tiegs' number of three times per hectare per year, then we'd need about a quarter billion tons [he meant "acres" not "tons"] of grazing land, basically about, I'm sorry not a quarter billion a quarter million tons [acres] …

Brendan [00:33:18]: Do you mean hectare?

Peter [00:33:21]: I'm saying 250 thousand acres (he meant 250 million), I'm sorry, I'm sorry. My numbers, I'm looking at this chart. It's 250 million acres, and that's about 100 million hectares. That's what it is. So we'd need about a quarter billion (he meant to say million) acres of land, and that's about a fifth, I believe, of the grazing land in the US right now so it's not even all of it. Then if you start thinking about integrating … and these numbers are not even back of the envelope; they're based on just big assumptions. So I'm not going to the bank with these numbers, but it's the kind of big picture that we're looking at if we can get to scale, that big numbers of carbon could be sequestered in the soil, we think. And how durable is that carbon. That's part of our science? You know, which carbon pool does that go into most? Even if its decades as opposed to centuries—you know, the different pools of carbon—that would still be pretty amazing, give us a leg up, help tone this thing down if we can get to scale, help slow down climate change. So then, if you look at integrating row crop production with livestock production—which is happening, you know, and folks like General Mills are pushing that, so big players are starting to look at this stuff—then you're doing even more to reduce the carbon output because you're integrating on the same acres. And so we hope to be part of the knowledge base that's growing about regenerative agriculture so that we can help push this to get to scale. Scale is our goal, and I know when I've been talking with McDonald's and their support for our work, scale is their goal too. They're not just in it for a science project; they want to see this scale. If the science comes back positive … we're all at that 'if' place. We need to have these answers. And they want to see this scale as well, and then you start getting big players involved, and you could see how the scale could happen.

Brendan [00:35:28]: Right, and I think it might make, as one last thing to touch on, it might make sense to address the methane issue. You mentioned methanotrophs. What are methanotrophs, and how do they play into this because most people who've heard about the risks and the impacts of animal agriculture—you know, we know that methane is 23x the power as a greenhouse gas as carbon dioxide and then we've got all this methane belching that livestock do—so what's different in a grazing system like this, versus other places where cows are belching methane?

Peter [00:36:10]: One of our hypotheses is, would a healthy soil system uptake a lot of methane and methanotrophs or methanotrophic bacteria that we're hypothesizing would be in this healthy soil system? It's not just a hypothesis. People have been measuring this part of this and our scientist that's leading this is Jason Rowntree at Michigan State. His work is looking at how much carbon does the system need to uptake and store to offset the methane coming out, so greenhouse gas equivalence. In a paper that he put out, I think it was a year ago, it was between one and two tons of carbon per hectare per year needs to come into the system to balance the methane, and then anything past that would be drawing down more carbon than the methane equivalent, you know than the methane warming that is happening. So that's one study. And so we're going to be looking at that. We're going to be measuring the greenhouse gasses coming in and out of the system. And so we don't know the answer to that right now, but we want to help find out the answer to that. I don't know the validity of the stuff I was just reading, but people are talking about it, that feeding livestock seaweed is reducing the methane coming out of the livestock by large amounts. I was just reading this stuff. I've read it before, but I was just rereading it and learning more about it before you and I spoke today, so who knows, right? I was talking to a farmer in Alabama about this. He's our AMP grazer in Alabama, and he was just wondering, you know, since all of this land used to be under the ocean, could some of the microbial life that's in our soils be evolved from the microbes that were under the ocean and could that be a connection to the rumen of the animals, and then the seaweed is helping the animals digest their food more efficiently, therefore less waste. Methane would be waste, I would think, from just a systems perspective. I don't know the answer to that, but I just emailed Jason Rowntree about it, and he hadn't really looked into it, but I want to find out. That might be a huge thing.

Brendan [00:38:29]: Well, that's fascinating because, you know, in a healthy soil you have algae growing, and so maybe when you have healthier soils you get some of that algae and maybe other organisms that, you know I don't know, but it's just where my mind went real quick.

Peter [00:38:45]: Yeah, I mean, a lot of bacteria and the fungi in the soils, I haven't heard much about algae in the soils from our team, so I've got more to learn.

Brendan [00:38:54]: And Christine Jones—I believe it was her—I hope I'm not misquoting, but somebody—I believe it was her—said that there was evidence that, looking at termite mounds, which are huge emitters of methane …

Peter [00:39:06]: Right.

Brendan [00:39:07]: Around termite mounds, according to this source, whether it's Christine or somebody else, at least in one study or another, that methane levels were lower around the termite mounds than they were in the air further from the mounds. In other words, there's methane in the system from wherever it's coming from, from the termite mounds and so forth, but the interpretation that might be possible from that is that methanotrophs, when they're close to the methane source, actually are so fired up that they're consuming more methane than is being produced or at least … yeah, so you have this reduction in methane concentration.

Peter [00:39:55]: I've got to look at that, right? We've got to know more about that because methane is a critical piece of this puzzle, and if we ever were to suggest that grazing was a greenhouse gas sink, we have to have the answer to that, and to nitrous oxide, we have to. And so that's a key element to our research because we want to start measuring that in detail.

Brendan [00:40:20]: This is really important work, Peter, and I really appreciate your leadership in this, in quantifying the potential of this type of land use to help restore soil, landscapes, wildlife, water resources, a stable climate, more nutrient-dense food for all of us. And so, on behalf of myself and the growing Eat4Earth community, I thank you for your contribution to all of us and to this vital of research and for your contribution today here at the Eat4Earth event.

Peter [00:40:51]: Wish us luck on our fundraising so we can actually do the science, and thank you for your kind words. I appreciate that. I'm part of a team, and you're just seeing me today, but there's 18 people on this team directly and then the support, everyone's teams around them. So it's definitely a team here, but today I get to do this and be the front person, so it's fun. Thank you.

Reginaldo Haslett-Marroquin Interview

Transforming Agriculture and Food's Nutrient Density with "Tree Range" Chicken

Brendan [00:00:00]: Welcome to the Eat4Earth event. We're exploring how you can heal yourself, your loved ones, and the planet with food. This is Brendan Moorehead and I'm very, very excited and impressed with what our next guest has created. His name is Reginaldo Haslett-Marroquin. I'm just going to call him Regi. Regi is the Chief Strategy Officer and principal architect of the innovative poultry- centered regenerative agriculture model that is at the heart of Main Street Project, which builds regenerative food and agriculture systems that deliver social, economic, and ecological benefits in the United States, Mexico, Guatemala, and Honduras. A native Guatemalan, Regi received his agronomy degree from the Central National School of Agriculture, studied at the Universidad de San Carlos in Guatemala and graduated from Augsburg College in Minneapolis with a major in International Business administration and a minor in Communications. He has served as a consultant for the United Nations Development programs, the Bureau for Latin America as an advisor to the World Council of Indigenous Peoples, a founding member of the Fair Trade Federation, and as Director of the Fair Trade Program for the Institute for Agriculture and Trade Policy, as a key player in the startup and launch of Peace Coffee, which is a Minnesota-based fair-trade coffee company.

Regi, you have something really amazing that you've developed, and you have a way of thinking about agricultural systems that is fundamentally different from the structure of our current food system, which produces pollution, malnutrition, and even poverty. What's the key distinction between these two systems?

Regi [00:01:42]: Thank you for this opportunity. I really appreciate that introduction. Well, to begin with, when we want to end up with different results, we have to start by engaging a different process. You can't expect the same thing out of the same process, right? I mean I think that's pretty well established. The first thing is, starting with the right team. You want to align yourself with individuals who are willing to think from a different starting point. We're going to talk about poultry today because poultry is at the center of our modelling system and at the center of a much larger-scaled system that we designed around energy cycles, and this energy mainly depends on how you integrate animals back into the landscape. So, from that understanding, our team right now includes those folks directly with the organization and those folks outside of the organization. And you can see in the photos we have from left to right on the top is Lindsey and Julie, Bob, Craig and Linda who own a new farm that we just purchased and then sold it to us and stayed part of the farm. And then in the middle on the left is Cliff, who is one of our entrepreneurs. In the center is Neil, and then center right is Wilber. He's got data from Zamorano Agricultural School in Honduras. Then you have, from left to right on the bottom is Rocky who runs our production operations, myself, and Paula on the right, who, together with Lindsey run Ecological Designs, which is a consulting firm that is now intrinsically connected to us. Now, this team came together to be able to take poultry, in this case studying and understanding poultry as a jungle fowl. This is the first thing that makes us different, different from a lot of folks who are working in poultry today. We did not decide whether poultry was a pasture animal, a grain confinement or anything. What we said was what if we were to design from the standpoint of how poultry evolved over millennia, over geological time, in other words. What if we were to take the genetic blueprint that evolved over all of those millions of years and started from that departure rather than from what we people, people-centered, homocentric approach to designing and engineering a poultry system. You will see at the end of this presentation that we ended up with a system that is centered on the poultry, but it is not about poultry, and that is one of the fundamental things that makes this different. Most engineering happens, whether it is about soybeans, and you end up with soybeans; corn and you end up with corn, and in the process of doing that, we reduce and diminish the creativity in the engineering process. Our departure point is one of natural blueprint. When you start with the natural blueprint of the chicken, then you unleash creativity instead of hindering it. Those are just basic departing points that give you a pathway from which you engage people, markets, science, technology, and all of that to deploy large-scale change in, in our case, centered in poultry because of the fact that in regenerating a landscape you have to incorporate animals. For us it was more important to select a livestock that would allow us to engage the most people around the world and in the social context, nothing beats a chicken really. Chickens are a common denominator to most of the farms. If not 100%, it's very close to 100% of the small farms under 10 hectares around the world that produce, according to the United Nations, approximately 70% of all of the food that we consume in the world today. That's the foundation of why poultry and then where did poultry come from as a foundation of them saying, okay, now we got a departing point. So the next thing is to think about, how diverse is that departing point, and for us the nice thing about poultry is that it's still one of the most diverse livestock that farmers have access to around the world. If you want to create a revolution of farmers, it's very easy to do it on the backs of the chicken, meaning most of the time you're gonna find that the farmers already have the breeds, already have the resources, knowledge—and especially women and the elders—they have the knowledge to manage poultry, but they may not have a blueprint that is scalable, that can replace or that can substitute conventional confinement animal production systems, but if provided with that design, they normally will have most of what it takes to then redeploy their own poultry systems. And that was another really important departing point for us. Once you look into that, then you go into the engineering process, and this is where it gets very exciting because this is where we get to apply natural sciences to that departing point that I was so carefully trying to describe. If you start with an alternative perspective, you are more bound to end up in a new destination point.

Brendan [00:07:21]: And God knows, we don't need any more confined animal feeding operation models, right?

Regi [00:07:28]: Exactly, and we don't need to keep talking about pasture poultry either because poultry, by design, is not a pasture animal. So, if we were to look at it from the poultry perspective, what the chicken says is something like this, or at least the way Nature designed this process is more like this: first of all you have energy. In the case of a poultry unit, the energy comes in in the form of feed. That energy is then put to work as food for this poultry inside a fenced area where chickens roam free within that still defined area, but big enough so that there is no exact confinement. We call it free range because chickens are able to range as much as they want, but then the fence allows us to create a perimeter, and that perimeter was not defined by us, it was defined by the chickens. We first had them without fences to watch them roam and behave and all of that. And it's a lot of science behind how we came to this point, but inside that space you get to capture a lot of what we call free energy. In Nature, about 80% of the energy that is visible to you in the form of cellulose—in the form of plants and eggs, meat, carrots, whatever—about 80% of that energy did not come from the soil, it came from the air. And so what we are doing is now bringing that original energy into the paddock and then taking that energy and using it to capture more of that free energy floating in space, in the air. What it does is it starts to reproduce, in other words, regenerate those cycles of energy. Instead of creating a linear equation now, we are creating circular hundreds and hundreds of circular cycles where energy is the common denominator and the currency. Now that energy then goes into the paddock. From inside the paddock we can harvest. First of all, we get meat, eggs, hazelnuts, elderberries, you know, to point out how that perennial canopy or that jungle where the chicken came from gets built, and yet each one of those components in the paddock is a productive component. So in this case, hazelnuts and elderberries form the canopy that then protects the chickens from the sun, from the wind, from the predators especially, and also maintains the conditions of the soil in a stable manner. So, meaning temperature is stable, humidity is stable, organic matter goes up, and that is the foundation for that regeneration process that we are talking about, but also is the foundation of efficient energy transformation in this case. And remember, energy transforms itself in many ways, based on the laws of thermodynamics. You can't destroy it, you can't create it, so the only thing we can do is transform it. And when we think linearly about production systems in agriculture, then we are most of the time wasting most of the energy that goes into the system. And that waste is what shows up in the form of pollution not only of the air, the water, the soil and all of that, but also now is coming directly into polluting our bodies. So, when you go to the store, instead of buying nutrition, you're actually buying pollution. Most of it, if you actually do an analysis of most of the conventional so-called food that we buy at the store, what you're buying is a lot of pollution that then costs you a lot of money to cure yourself from. That's really where the real cost of traditional food, conventional, corporate foods is hidden. On the other hand, if you measure the nutrition, the nutrition of these eggs and meat and these hazelnuts and elderberries coming out of this more integrated energy cycle, it's actually more dense; it's a higher content of it. If you were to measure the nutritional farm products against the nutritional conventional products, you will find that our products are probably half the price in nutrition as conventional industrial products and have no contaminants that could degenerate your health, on top of being less expensive on the basis of nutritional units. So that's what we are getting out of this first harvest. The second harvest is the organic matter, all the byproducts that we can harvest out of a paddock. In this case, we are looking at a space under that canopy that allows us to sprout grains on a larger scale. Those grains then become part of absorbing some of that energy from the soil. So the chicken has taken the energy from the beginning as it came into the system as food, and then a lot of that food turned into manure, turned into other things, and those organic compounds then allow for the biodiversity of the soil, fungus, and bacteria to develop in a more healthy way and balanced way, which allows the system inside the paddocks to capture more of that free energy that then gets turned into this organic matter, which then allows us to create the conditions for sprouting grain and other things that are very valuable for the poultry, but also valuable for us at the end when we eat either the eggs or the meat. At the same time, the sprouting systems are able to take some of the energy that was then deposited, whether it came from the leaves of the hazelnuts, the leaves or the stems of the elderberries, that got into the flora of the soil, and then, combined with the manure of the poultry, the sprouts are able to absorb very nice, clean energy again. And we're talking about sometimes multiplying the value of that grain by six to seven times than what it was originally just as grain. If we were to grind that corn or that seed that we are spreading under that canopy, we will get only one-seventh of its value and none of the nutrients that it absorbs out of the soil. That's what we call regenerative, where the cycles of energy continue to grow, regenerate, and most of what they grow on is the free energy that they harvest out of the air, that 80% I was talking about. So in general, if you look at this, the other thing you have is that you get excess energy out of the first harvest in the form of say manure, giblets, feathers and stuff that you are not going to just throw back into the paddock, but rather you move this out of the paddock and start growing non-paddock-based is what we call this. When you look at one unit of production of poultry at 1.5 acres and you can take four, five, or six acres where there are no chickens, but yet the energy that came out of the production unit is giving you all of this, what we call non-paddock or landscape-based production. When you again get another harvest, that harvest is again alley crop vegetables between hazelnuts and elderberries again, perennial crops, food crops, annual grains, perennial grains to the point that some of those grains go back in the form of food into the same system again. When you really look at this, what we are doing is putting ourselves as farmers in the rightful place as we were sort of intended to be to begin within historically, and that means we are not producers of stuff. We are managers of energy, and if we do that right, the energy balance on those products we produce not only is highly nutritious for the consumer, it's highly regenerative for the landscape we grow them in. Now that's where we are at. That's what makes us so different, and this is the departing point that I see so many people refusing to adopt in their engineering processes. So, what we have out of that kind of design is more or less what you see in this photo—an endless cycle of capturing energy and recycling it. And as we recycle it, we take that 80% growth that we're talking about of the new energy coming in, we harvest some of that plus part the energy that we put in, and what you end up with is a system where you are only harvesting about 30% to 40% maximum of the energy that this system is producing, which means you are leaving up to 60% of the energy that was generated in the system, leaving it in the ground to continue to regenerate the capacity of that space to continually increase and improve its efficiency and its productivity rather than robbing Nature of the very foundation that made it regenerative and made Nature what it is to begin with. This is massive, massive in terms of how different our engineering processes are, how different our entrepreneurial building process is. If you think of this picture, you have the higher canopy producing one product, one enterprise level here, perennials. In the case of Minnesota it's hazelnuts, oaks, sugar maples and you've got the elderberries. In other places like in northern Guatemala, it's up to seven stories, seven different canopies with up to eight or nine species grown where the poultry provides the animal disturbance, and the animal gut so that we can inoculate the microbiology of that space on the floor of that canopy. This is the rightful place for poultry, not in a pasture, not in an open space, but in a fully integrated vertical production system where the poultry is just the beginning of it. And that's why I said, we're gonna talk about chickens, but it is not about chickens. They are just the center of the system. The system is really way more than that. But if you go into the more specific pieces, for example, in our design, we know we need to have a shelter because without the shelter the chickens are exposed to predators and other things of night and the elements and so on. This shelter changes based on the region where the system has been deployed. In Guatemala and Mexico where we get longer light hours and where the weather never gets to 30 below like it does in Minnesota, it's very simple structures that provide the same exact function—manage the light, manage the elements, manage the space where chickens are protected at night and all that. All of the units have two paddocks. Both paddocks in every unit are planted with perennials. What perennials? It depends on the ecological blueprint of the area where the system is being deployed. So in the highlands in Mexico the higher canopy is being provided by olive trees, but in between those olive trees while they develop, just the same way as we do in Minnesota, we alternate corn and sunflowers. One year is corn. Another year is sunflowers. So we still create that canopy without the developed perennials. Once the perennials develop then we don't need the annuals anymore, but then we have a full space where we can sprout grains and improve that nutritional value of the food that is coming to the chickens, but also eliminating to a certain extent the need for ground feed, which is critical because ground feed is between 60% and 70% of the cost of raising a chicken. So you see the incorporation of economics, really fluid energy flows as a way to make the economics work, restoration of a landscape as a way to make it more attractive for young farmers, for people who are interested in the sciences and all of that rather than just going out there and producing things. This makes it very attractive for visitors too, highly marketable. The products sell themselves as a result of all that design. So it's not just talking about production of chicken. Whenever we engineer systems, we have to engineer all the way across the board, from producer to the market and ensure that all of that alignment is put into that process. So that's what one of these units does, but also allows us to then go and manipulate the unit based on the ecological, social, and economic conditions back to the triple bottom line. It allows us to then manipulate this and build technology and build experiences and history and data bases and all of that so we can then track and improve continuously on the basis of that production unit. You know basically this is another way for listeners to look at the different components of that unit in case you had any more questions there. The way we did this work was, you know, not only did we engineer the units and the production and all the energy cycles that you heard about, but also develop a standard. And this standard was developed not only by consolidating information from five global standards that are out there for poultry today, but also incorporating all of our learning because most of those systems don't incorporate canopies and especially the sprouting systems and all of those other things that we put in. Then we modified that to accommodate high intensity production without creating at any point any saturation of nutrients or anything like that could degenerate the space.

So, these are some of the facts. We use 42 square feet for meat birds on the outside, so 21 square feet per paddock. The total ranging area of paddock is 31,150 square feet roughly. They don't have to be square. This could be a circle, could be a triangle, rectangle, whatever. The landscape is going to define what it looks like, but the square footage cannot be compromised, at least to the extent that we already defined what that square footage will be for a specific area. In Minnesota, this is standard. Northern Guatemala we can put more chickens because there is year-round production. There is more rain and all that than in Minnesota. San Miguel de Allende in Mexico for example is dry—so semi-desert area—so we cannot put as much density because the space doesn't regenerate the same way. So it changes. The density per square foot is going to change depending on which one of those areas we're working on. The key is with the foundational design already in place, then we can develop and modify those standards. The main standard we can modify to the local conditions to meet their regenerative capacity of that specific ecology. So what you're looking at is the standard for Minnesota or for a place that gets similar precipitation, has a similar ecology, similar soils and so on.

This is a photo of chickens under the corn rotation, and you can see the size of the ears of corn. We have some unique quality corn this year when we produced it. This is another example here. We produce top quality corn, about 25% production above the neighbor growing GMOs, and yet that was a byproduct of our system. It wasn't a main product. Corn has a high nitrogen cycle so it really thrives on the poultry manure. You also see that there is no exposed soil. That's part of that standard. Chickens are always walking on grasses or greens or something like that. You take that unit, and then you move it up to a farm level, and here's what you see is the design of five production units on the bottom part of the farm, and then all of this other landscape where the manure is going to be circulated on the rest of the farm to improve the productivity of the overall farm, on top of producing more per acre of this space.

So to address the issue of how much more production can we achieve while regenerating the landscape and all of that, right now we have calculated that the first few years we can outproduce a traditional monoculture system up to four times as an average per acre, and over time we can outproduce a monoculture system up to eight times.

Brendan [00:23:27]: Wow.

Regi [00:23:28]: That means adding all of the high- density production from the poultry and also averaging it with the lower density production where there is no poultry roaming but still have poultry byproducts feeding the rest of that space. So if you average—in this case we're talking about 42 acres—and if you average total income for the 42 acres, you will be around eight to ten times, you know over time, what a conventional monoculture farm can produce. And, at the same time, you are only harvesting only 40% of the amount of energy that you capture, which means you are regenerating that space significantly, building soil and so on.

Brendan [00:24:09]: Also you're not generating these piles of animal excrement that the animals are walking around in and generating disease and needing antibiotics just to stay alive and creating that whole disaster with antibiotic-resistant bacteria that those other models produce. So this is groundbreaking for sure.

Regi [00:24:38]: What happens is that when you interfere with Nature you have to make up for it. And what happens is when we interfere with Nature we become very inefficient energy transformers, so to speak. And as we do that we have to make it up somewhere, so we start bringing in more inputs into the farm, and we have to manipulate the environment where the chickens live. When you put them in confinement you have to start putting antibiotics to keep them from growing infections, also all kinds of other drugs. I don't know if you have seen the latest releases out of the government. They were forced to release some of the lists of the drugs that are being put into confinement poultry, and it's just disgusting. I mean seriously, no wonder people are getting sick with conventional poultry. None of that is necessary.

Brendan [00:25:29]: Yes, the conventional poultry apparently is one of the biggest influences on the health challenges, especially on the obesity side. It's been heavily linked to generating obesity because of, I think it's possibly the arsenic that's used in conventional poultry. Even though many of the forms of arsenic were outlawed, there's still some that are allowed, and that's probably just one of them. I mean, there's so many things that are going into that poultry, but it's something that not many people are aware of and, of course, obesity generates the whole host of inflammatory cascades that lead to heart disease, cancer, and the rest of it. So anyway, go ahead. Just something I thought I would say.

Regi [00:26:22]: Well, of course. The whole saying that we are what we eat isn't really that far from the truth. It's actually exactly the truth. When we eat food that has been produced with such high level of contaminants, from antibiotics to arsenic to [unintelligible] drug to all of that that the poultry industry puts into confinement animal production systems, it is no wonder that at the end we have such amount of diseases. It is calculated now that there are over 80 diseases that are attacking us on a mass scale. Most of them are directly connected to the food we eat, and some of those you already mentioned—obesity, diabetes, colon cancer, liver cancer. Things like that that are massive profit-making ventures, which also happens that the companies behind the food industry are also the companies that are behind the medications for some of those diseases, and they're making money on one end selling us the stuff to make us sick and on the other end are creating the cure. This is why we have to change the way we think about food. And this is our contribution to changing how we think about food, but also not only from a consumer perspective delivering high quality, high nutrition, very inexpensive nutrition if you compare it to the conventional system. Our products, even though we are still doing the research, we have been reading the documentation from the USDA that shows that production that happened before the industrial revolution, products from before, whether is was a carrot, a chicken or whatever or an egg. It was about three, four, five, and six times more nutritious than the same product produced by the industrial system today, and the reason that happens is because we have eliminated nutrition as the factor of food products and included instead mass, biomass that we sell. That's what we sell ... we don't sell products; we sell nutrition.

Brendan [00:28:27]: They sell weight, and so they get to inject poultry with up to a third of the weight apparently with saline water, salt water, to increase the weight, diluting down the nutrient density. Which is, you know, the nutrients per calorie is one of the most important things that we should be looking at if we want to thrive as humans. [Of course, injected saline water does not reduce nutrients per calorie; it reduces nutrients per unit of weight and the consumer's cost per unit of nutrition.]

Regi [00:28:53]: Exactly. I mean we don't regenerate our own bodies when what we are putting into the body is degenerative to begin with. See, that's another difficult thing to understand. Also, when you go to the store, what do you buy? Are you buying lettuce, or are you buying food? Because if you are buying food, it means you are buying nutrition. And if you are buying nutrition, don't buy the conventional lettuce because there is very little nutrition in that, even though it looks like it. If it's cheap, nutritionally speaking it's twice as expensive as our lettuce even though our lettuce costs twice as much for the same head of lettuce. The nutrition in it is half the price of conventional lettuce.

Brendan [00:29:37]: In other words, it's twice the price, but four times or more the nutrition.

Regi [00:29:41]: Exactly. And that's what we are buying. So, if you are just buying something to fill yourself with and make you sick with, by all means by cheap food. If what you want is to nourish your body, regenerate your molecular structure so that your body doesn't degenerate, so your joints don't degenerate, your liver doesn't degenerate, your kidneys, all of that, and so that you don't end up with neurological interferences because of all of this stuff, especially the chemicals that are coming into your food … if you don't want that, then buy the less expensive, highly nutritious foods that show in the market about twice the price per unit as those other products that claim to be cheap. Nutritionally speaking, products that are not conventional, like our products, are about half the price [per unit of nutrition] than the conventional products.

Brendan [00:30:33]: In other words, half the price for the folate you're getting if its lettuce, half the price for the chromium in the chicken breast or whatever it is.

Regi [00:30:42]: Exactly. And we will be producing this data. So far, the data we have collected thoroughly and methodically is the nutritional input to the poultry. So we know that there is more nutrition because science doesn't lie to you. If you are what you eat, so is the chicken. So, the chickens that we are raising have a really broad spectrum of minerals, nutrients, and all of that coming into their body, and they also have a natural environment where the body of the poultry then can fully incorporate all of that broad nutrition. You can take all the pills you want and have all the nutrition that you're supposed to take, but taking pills doesn't replenish eating the food that goes through your intestines and that actually mimics the way Nature designed you and me and then the poultry, to process food. So, you could put all the supplements you want in the feed in a confinement animal poultry production unit, and you will never achieve what we achieve because basically you have to have the natural environment and the proper systems in place for that diversity of nutrients to actually find its way to become a diversity of nutrients and density, whether its in the muscle of the chicken we eat and the broth from the bones and all of that or the lettuce or the hazelnut and so on. And, we have taken indicators of the other parts, like the Brix value of even the weeds inside the paddocks and outside the paddocks and all that, so we have indicators that we have really highly nutritional garlic and vegetables that we have been growing. This coming year, because we also had to allow some of these paddocks to mature, this coming year we'll be taking samples out of the grocery store and out of our fields and sending them over to the lab. We know it's going to be a huge difference. We calculate it to be at least twice, and then we can calculate that on the basis of weight because highly dense, nutritionally dense products weigh more. And we know that because our products weigh more. I bought a pound of beans the other day at the store, and then I took a container of beans out of my harvest, put them together, and mine weighed at least 0.5 more than the beans from the store. These are the same exact beans, black beans, right? So the nutrient density makes a huge difference, and it's well established that a bushel of anything is not just a bushel of anything. Not all of them were created equal. If you have a bushel of GMO corn that was grown conventionally, it weighs way less than a highly nutritious corn that you grew in a system like ours.

Brendan [00:33:38]: I suppose that the reason for that is higher mineral content because minerals would probably be some of the most dense components of any foodstuff. So minerals, you know the mass per volume, or something like that, of minerals would be among the highest, and so it might be an indirect measure of the overall mineral content.

Regi [00:34:02]: Well, exactly. Honestly, it's the carbs are not going to weigh that much more. The proteins, maybe because they incorporate other kinds of nutrients, but especially, if you think of it, where is the nutritional value of food? And it isn't really on the carbs and the fats and all that. It is actually on the microelements, the stuff that has been robbed from our food, and that's what makes it lighter in weight, and that's what makes our system, our products heavier in weight. So, it's a pretty straightforward equation. We don't have to do too much digging to know that our products will have more nutrition, and at least they will be twice as nutritional, but that's a low ball. I know the results are going to show way higher, just the same way as the sprouts. The sprouts, for example, if you put the same mixes we use right now in the field, you take them and sprout them in just water, the result is nothing compared to the result that we achieve in the field where the poultry is ranging. That much we knew from the start, and this is what's guiding some of our assumptions and our hypotheses as we go forward. What we need to do now is collect that information.

Brendan [00:35:20]: So, before you go there, to this next slide … so the sprouts are pulling minerals up from the soil, is that correct?

Regi [00:35:28]: Exactly.

Brendan [00:35:29]: Because you're sprouting them in soil in a natural system as opposed to in a tray, devoid of soil.

Regi [00:35:36]: Exactly. Now in Minnesota, you know, we have winter, and winter is pretty brutal here. So one of the things we can't do in the winter is sprout the grain in their paddocks. So right, here you see a paddock; so you see the coop here, and then you see these are hazelnuts, and these are sunflowers in the middle. This is a patch of corn. And so in this space we can sprout a lot of grain during the summer or during the warm season, and sometimes it goes into the fall; we can sprout large amounts of grain in that space. We mix them based on how we want to … well, let's put it this way, one single grain, even if you sprout it here, will produce a different nutritional profile if you pair it with other grains that can supplement its bio. So, even that kind of combination we have been experimenting with here and researching it carefully to see which grains go with what. So because we can't do that in the winter, we now have created this enriched water system where we put nutrients, lots of nutrients, in the water itself so that the sprouts can absorb them out of that. It doesn't work the same way as it works out in the fields, but at least gives us a tremendous competitive advantage for winter production. Basically, this solarium as we call it, which we incorporate into our design in cold climate, this is where we distribute most of that sprouted grain. So they're still getting sun, they're still absorbing some of that energy and then transferring it into the poultry. The insulated area is where the chickens sleep at night so that we can close it, and if we need to, we can heat it a little bit, although for egg layers we never needed to heat it because they produce their own heat.

This is the process of building one of those units. You can see here the perimeter already for the solarium. This is the insulated part that is being built. This is a system we use here in Minnesota to create a solar heat recovery system. So, in the solarium, we spread this perforated pipe on the bottom. This we will bury two feet, one foot with gravel and then another foot with the same soil we took out we'll put it back in. And we'll cover all of that so that when it's done, you can see this is now filled back. The end of the pipe is here. So, on the top of this, there will be a big 10-inch diameter pipe that is going to be around 55 feet long. And then inline fans on that pipe, which then blow the air through this pipe underground. It heats up the rock and that rock then releases that heat very slowly into the soil up here. And then in the soil up here, we can put a lot of grain, presoaked and pre-enriched grain, we can throw it in there, put grass over it, and when the chickens come out of the night shelter, then they can absorb some of that extra energy that they wouldn't have otherwise. So, this is how we have gotten around the winter issue to still produce highly dense, really healthy products, even during those months when we have those limitations in this climate where we live. In Guatemala, Mexico and all those places where it doesn't go below 40 degrees, we don't have to worry about this part. But, just to give you an idea, we have to be creative in every way. We can't just talk about one thing. The engineering process is extremely intricate and requires a lot of science, especially the proper application of thermodynamics from physical energy that we're manipulating here to bio and chemical and physical energy that we manipulate out in the fields to create this environment where then we can have this poultry that can really outproduce, outcompete almost anything that we have seen out there. And that was our objective to begin with.

The meat birds and the egg layers, the big difference between the two is that the meat birds, we don't feed them indoors. This building, if it was for meat birds, it wouldn't have the water, the feeders, or the nesting area. It would just be a space with perches because we still want the meat birds to perch. That's natural to their behavior. That's the way they sleep. They relax more, and they don't suffer from chest infections and feet infections and stuff like that when you put proper perches. The food for the meat birds is especially important to not be indoors so they do not attract mice and other rodents, but also so the birds will range because they won't range if they have food indoors, at least most of them won't. The egg layers, it doesn't matter because they like to be outside and with the canopy. It really pulls them out of the buildings. They just lay their eggs, eat, drink, and get out and spend the whole day outside. And so this is the way we avoid having to go into the coop to collect eggs. Eggs are collected from the back here. Chickens live in this area, and then they climb up here to lay their eggs. So, this is just to give people an idea of how deliberate we are about not only avoiding work, because this eliminates a lot of work, makes it very efficient mechanically, but interferes absolutely nothing, absolutely no interference, with the natural behavior and especially the daytime natural environment where the chickens spend most of their awake hours anyway.

Brendan [00:41:20]: This strikes me as a very, very humane system. And that's beautiful.

Regi [00:41:28]: That was the objective. The objective was to create a humane system not because we say so, but because the chickens like it. If we watch a chicken that is going around like the nests or it doesn't leave the coop, or if we had had any number of them that do that, instead of trying to push them out what we did was try to figure out why were they not leaving. Instead of thinking about the humane part, as into what we want them to do, look at what we were doing wrong. Look at it as a chicken-centered rather than a human-centered view of what was going on. And that's how we ended up actually solving a lot of those really important issues that have to be solved if we're going to grow animals in a way that is really humane. It's not about us. It's about the animal. Let's put it that way. It's not about no cages. It's not about a door for them to go outdoors. It's not about them going outside. It's about what they want to be doing, and chickens especially don't want to be in the open space. They don't like the sun, and they don't like forages like the ruminants do. They do like tenders, they do like bugs, and they do …

Brendan [00:42:42]: What are tenders? You're muted. I can't hear you right now. There we go.

Regi [00:42:54]: Sorry. So yes, tender shoots. I mean the tender sprouts, the new stuff coming out of the ground. That's what they go for. When the grasses grow beyond a certain point, they trample them. They don't eat them anymore unless you force them, unless you starve them, unless they have no choice. This unit was built by the Pine Ridge Native American Reservation down in South Dakota. This is the centerpiece for their agronomical or farming training. We will be training Native Americans on how to grow their own food and also, again, expand beyond their historical foods to accommodate in a way that is regenerative to the new foods basically because they have been on the short end of the stick of degenerative foods. Not only foods conventionally are produced in a factory-like linear way, which makes the end product truly degenerative to our bodies, but Native Americans and poor communities around the country get even the most degenerated of the degenerated foods. So this is one way to turn that completely around and bring the production right into the reservation, right in the hands of the Native Americans who live there. The young people know that and train them on how to do this and stop that importation of cancer and all the other things that they are importing right now in the name of food. The fencing we use is pretty straightforward.

Brendan [00:44:26]: Let me ask you … I'm going to interrupt for a second again. I wanted to ask, are you, by chance, measuring changes in the soil, like increase in soil carbon or anything like that? Because obviously one of the things we're looking at in regenerative agriculture is capturing carbon in the soil to draw down carbon from the atmosphere and also of course to rebuild the soil sponge, the soil carbon sponge. As the soil gets more and more organic matter, it holds more water, and so it infiltrates rain better and recharges aquifers and drives the local water cycles stabilizing local regional microclimates and so forth. And it all adds up to macroclimates as well. So, just curious if you're measuring increases in soil carbon growth.

Regi [00:45:22]: Yes, we have, and mostly we're just using two indicators right now. We went from 2% organic matter in some of these places. This one we're looking at, this is a new farm. We're just setting it up. It was one year just sitting there because we wanted to let some of the detoxification happen. So we put (in) cover crops and this year we built the fences. So we are starting with around 3% to 4% organic matter now. It was like 2% the year before, and this will go to …

Brendan [00:45:55]: Wait a minute. Did you just say that it went up 1% or 2% in a year?

Regi [00:46:01]: Yes, and the reason is because we are bringing in organic matter into the space.

Brendan [00:46:05]: Oh, okay.

Regi [00:46:06]: But in spite of the regenerative process, you gotta help the land out because it's being depleted so bad that if we just let it fallow it will take years, many years...

Brendan [00:46:19]: So you boosted it, okay, so you boosted it and you imported some carbon so it's not just carbon from the atmosphere through better microbial activity, at least in that year, in that period. But of course it is going to lead to more carbon being drawn down from the atmosphere as well.

Regi [00:46:35]: Exactly, because we are starting too low. If we come into a space where we encounter the organic matter, say at 3%, we know that within one season, the microbiological systems will repopulate that space, and there is some food, even if it's polluted, for them. So, in that space, we would just rely more on the natural regeneration where that 80% growth that I was talking about will become part of that landscape. In the original paddock where we have the prototype, the original prototype that I showed before, we went from 2% organic matter when I moved in there in 2006 to 11% organic matter last year.

Brendan [00:47:14]: Whoa, and how long was the period?

Regi [00:47:17]: Well, it was 11% four years later, but it is significant because what happens is, to manage the poultry correctly we are bringing in not only sprouts, but also they're putting manure out into the fields. It's not a lot because most of the manure is accumulated inside their buildings. And that manure we don't put over in the paddocks because we don't want to overload that space. But we also have straw that we have to put in for them to scratch on and for the sprouts to happen properly. So we're bringing in sometimes in excess of 60 to 70 bales and up to 100 bales of straw into the paddocks for the chicken environment to be properly managed. So that disappears within a year. It gets absorbed into the soil by the worms from the second season, and that's why the organic matter shoots up so significantly. But, in the fields where there are no chickens, we're still bringing in that manure. The manure comes in with wood shavings, which is a lot of carbon. And then we add aged wood chips for at least one year. We keep the piles of wood chips, and then we mix that with the manure we are harvesting from the chicken coops. And then we bring that out and put it into the alleys between the perennial crops. And so we are also bringing a lot of organic matter into the fields. Once you have that seeded back up, it takes very little every year. And using some of the most sophisticated, especially the cold composting process for manure, we also don't need more than 150 pounds, maybe 125 to reinoculate those fields every year. So beyond that initial regeneration, it's self-sustaining from then forward. And then the fields can restore their own organic matter with their own production.

Brendan [00:49:13]: 11% is quite an achievement. So you went from 2% to 11%. There's no way that really a significant ... I mean, I'd be curious to know what the math is, maybe you've done it and maybe you haven't, how much of that increase from 2% to 11% in only four years was imported and how much of it had to have been from the atmosphere.

Regi [00:49:35]: Oh right, no, in fact, in those four years most of it was imported because our perennial crops that you see now were just barely getting established. They were not dropping leaves every fall like at this point. There is very little that we are bringing in now because the system is now maturing, and we have a lot more organic matter being captured and dropped into the ground right there on the space. But think about it, we only have hazelnuts, and we're already starting to see a lot of that organic matter generating itself right there. Once the oaks and the vast woods and the sugar maples grow, especially the sugar maples produce a lot of leaves, and all of that ... and we have to manage these trees because you can't just leave them hanging out by themselves, otherwise they will kill everything else. There's a lot of organic matter we're actually harvesting and putting it in there.

Brendan [00:50:27]: Wait, my ... sorry ... what you might find though, if you analyze the numbers entirely, you might find that there's more carbon accumulating in the soil than you can account for from the organic matter you're importing and the organic matter that drops from leaves, which would be hard for you to measure. There's the liquid carbon pathway as well, which is these plants are secreting carbohydrates largely in the form of sugars, and so that's how a lot of the carbon gets into soils once you fire up the ecosystem, the agricultural ecosystem. Then the plants and the organisms in the soil do their little dance, and the plants feed them with root exudates. I think that's one of the things that is commonly forgotten or is not fully conscious, even in regenerative agriculture, is that's where a lot of the carbon is getting into the soil. At least that's what Christine Jones has really brought out, and I think people are recognizing that because that's the only way you can account for so much carbon accumulating in the soil.

Regi [00:51:46]: Right, and remember that a lot of that carbon is coming out of the atmosphere.

Brendan [00:51:50]: Yes, that's what I'm saying. I was just making the point that it's not just the leaf litter that's being absorbed into the soil through the microbial action and the worms and so forth. It's also there's a direct pathway from the leaves photosynthesizing and creating carbohydrate and a certain percentage of that is going down out through the roots to feed the soil organisms and barter for minerals and so forth.

Regi [00:52:14]: Totally. I mean, bottom line is one reason we're not measuring much yet—because honestly we don't know what to measure yet—we weren't just going to go out there and see what people were measuring and start measuring that because the bottom line is that most folks out there are not measuring whole systems. They're measuring just components of a system, and for us it's not about what we report. It's really how the system works better because we know what's going on. So from that perspective, not only do we want to measure carbon, but also nitrogen, many other components in the soil. And not only that, but just like the sprouts don't sprout the same way in isolation, those nutrients don't behave the same way. Even if you were to import, say organic fertilizer into the space and put it on the ground, it won't behave the same way that the nitrogen that will be produced by the plants themselves because that nitrogen fundamentally followed a very different biophysical and chemical pathway. And that pathway is more in alignment with Nature than something we imported. So there is so much more to consider here so we've just been taking indicator samples, so organic matter and Brix in the weeds and in the plants so we know that we're on the right path. Starting next year, we will have, like this unit we're looking at is new, we have some brand new ones that haven't even gone through one year of restoration. And we have a new 100-acre farm in Main Street Project that we are launching now that will give us a lot of raw data from what the space looks like before any of our systems go in. And we also have the 8-year-old unit that will give us a look of the future of these other farms. Then we're going to start being able to make much more informed decisions as to what is exactly going on because right now I don't think scientists can actually fully explain because unfortunately for us most scientists in agriculture never worried and never had the reason to actually look at the full system. They were mostly trained by industry to look at linear equations, and there is nothing linear about what we do.

Brendan [00:54:28]: Yeah, you get so much synergy there, and so what I'm wondering here is, if we want to take over the world of food production, the world of agriculture and claim it for the regeneration of human health and the health of our planet, how is this model going to help accomplish that? Just as sort of maybe some closing comments to just sort of wrap it up, like, how is this going … this is a small model, and one critique might be, somebody might think, "Well, it's only a couple acres. How is it going to really influence the whole world?"

Regi [00:55:05]: Well, here's what we know about historical world changes. They all start with a well-designed idea, but that idea has to also be in the context of ripple effect. So, you can have a great idea, but if when you implement it, it doesn't have a ripple effect, normally it doesn't change anything. It doesn't make the whole thing vibrate and shift places. So what we knew was that by starting with the poultry, if we can design a system that starts with the unit of production so a farmer can understand it— and here's one of those flocks coming into the building—then you take that flock and put it through a process that was well thought out, you know, in a way that delivers high quality regeneration and absorbs water, and all that to your previous question, in ways that no system that is not fully regenerative can do, like in this case, in this rain event, we had seven inches, and we did not have standing water outside.

Brendan [00:56:07]: Wow! That's huge. I'm sure people living in flood plains would love to see this model deployed in every single place that it could.

Regi [00:56:08]: Well, we're actually next to a wetland so this should be flooded by now, and yet the water is flowing through. It's getting absorbed, it's getting stored, and then it lasts longer too because its getting retrieved in a different way than if you didn't have it covered, you didn't have organic matter, and the water was just shooting right back up through what we call capillary water, and then you lose it within a few days. In this case, not only do you absorb immensely more water, but then it gets retrieved slower, and it lasts in the field a lot longer. So it makes the space more drought resistant and so on. Also, a lot of the water ends up in the aquifer instead of down in the Golf of Mexico, full of nutrients and all of that. Regeneration is also really critical as we do this because this allows the farmer to produce more income than just what they can get out of the chicken, still producing high quality chicken that can be sold just the same way as the conventional system sells chicken, now with the difference that we are selling nutrition. And this chicken, even though it may be the same weight and everything, delivers a lot more nutrition for the price that people pay for it, making it highly competitive on the price of nutrition with the conventional products. And you also have all of the derived products, like in this case we got more sunflowers than we know what to do with. All of them were just cut and fed back to the chickens right there on the spot. That's recycling of energy, which makes the farm more profitable for the farm owner, and in the case of corn, same thing. Hazelnuts come out of the same space, which is income for the farmer too, and then biomass that we can put back into the space to restore the carbon and the fertility and the environment so the chickens can do better in the next season and all of that.

What happens is, back to your question, how can we take this … well, we have to win, but we have to win big in one specific area first before the rest of the system is going to change. We propose that we can do that on poultry because it's what engages the most people around the world. You could change cattle production, pig production, and it still wouldn't change the food system because fundamentally most people in the world, number one, don't eat beef and pork. Number two, those species are not adapted to most of the world anyway. Chicken is. So on the basis of that, we decided on this sequence where we can take the proof of concept, which is what I showed you, over to the farm level, which also I can show you in a slide right after, moving it to regions of production so we are no longer looking at a few chickens. Every farm, every production unit maybe. But a farm has say 10 production units, say 40,000 to 50,000 meat birds per farm unit, like in the case of the farm I showed you before. Now put it together as a region, and you have a system that can compete in terms of numbers of birds, going out with any large producer. And then you institutionalize it so we make sure that universities are teaching this so that we get a stronghold in the area where right now all the scientific knowledge is being produced for conventional industrial foods. We start incorporating these systems into that channel too, so new generations of farmers can scale this to the point that we can take over the whole system. That's really how it goes, you know. The prototype that I showed you in this with the hazelnuts, sunflowers, and corn … all it shows is how a farmer is supposed to get started. But it really isn't just about that, it's about how then the farmer organizes that production within the larger farm, how they become, you know … this is a different farm that is producing the same exact thing with a different design because of the landscape and because there' s more water here and so on. You take that and move it into a regional deployment, and then move it into a region of states, like the Midwest, especially because this, all the way down and from the east from this line here, is hazelnut and other various territory, so we don't have to even redesign the system for that whole region. And then put it through a process that allows us to methodically and scientifically move people to the process of discovering their space, discovering their farm's possibilities, developing their business plans, gaining the capacity, launching the operations, growing their operation so that that process can align with a larger scale deployment, and then building all the infrastructure around those farmers so we can then grow to whatever it is that the system is going to allow.

So fundamentally, to go to the next level what we did was develop a standard on the basis of principles, criteria indicators, and verifiers of which you've already got a taste of it because you saw the principles ecologically, economic, and social are pretty consistent toward the PowerPoint presentation even though I did not isolate them. Criteria, you already saw the criteria on how poultry is raised and all of that. The indicators are the carbon, the sugars, the nutrients and all of that. And the verifiers are just the methodology that we are now developing so that we can verify that all of those things are being met in that larger scale landscape. You move that into the principles again—you know, the resiliency, the health of the product, the environment and all that, financial transactions, transparency, and especially economic sustainability. Sustainability, by the way, has nothing to do with natural ecosystem management; ecosystem management has to do with resiliency. We manage for resiliency, not sustainability. You can make something sustainable that is not resilient, but something resilient is always sustainable. That's how we move into this area where we then consolidate this into a triple bottom line impact design, which is what you just saw in the design there, and then you bring it into a triple bottom line enterprise integration where you take the meat, the chicken, the egg, the meat poultry, the meat processing, the grain processing, grain production, manure management, perennial nuts and all of that, and instead of thinking of them as farms, you now think of them as components of a new industry. Once you think about it this way, then we win, then we transform the system. Then we take it back and make it regenerative.

Brendan [01:02:42]: Awesome. You know this is so exciting because not only is it so well thought-out, I mean, it's an ontological approach almost. You began with the very foundation, questioning everything and seeing what makes sense, what works, where the free energy is, having it be in line with thermodynamics instead of the thermodynamic nonsense that we so often engage in with our agricultural systems. And I love that this is, as you've said in another context, I think you called it "tree range" chicken—even though chicken is not necessarily, I mean its the center, but not necessarily the focus—it kind of captures something there, so this is "tree range" chicken.

Regi [01:03:27]: Well, Tree Range is our brand.

Brendan [01:03:29]: Ah, it's your brand. That's where I heard it, okay.

Regi [01:03:30]: Well, its one of our brands. We expect people to come up with creative things like that to name our chickens.

Brendan [01:03:35]: Yeah, I've already got mine actually. I'm not going to … I don't want anybody else to take my brand name. [laughing] I need to go see if the domain name is there. But I hope that people listening here are going to take this and go seek it out, go ask for it, go introduce their farmers to this model, and say hey, "Check this out. It works. It's really profitable. I'm going to do it if you don't." So hopefully the other folks listening too that will take this and run with it as a livelihood. We didn't have time to get into the numbers. I've seen them though, and they're impressive, and you can actually earn a pretty good living. I mean, you're not going to be Bill Gates, but then again Bill Gates is not necessarily doing as much for the planet with what he's doing with chickens. Just real quick, how is this different from what Bill Gates is doing with chickens around the world? It's the difference between handing a man a fish and teaching him how to fish …

Regi [01:04:32]: Well think about it, rich people got fetishes. We need solutions to our hunger, and I grew up hungry. That's the difference. I'm seeking solutions not fetishes.

Brendan [01:04:42]: (laughing) Okay, nice. Well, thank you for developing this, for your precision with it, your passion, and thanks for sharing this and being with us here in the Eat4Earth community.

Regi [01:04:56]: Awesome. Thank you.

Day 8 – Grow Great Food and Earn a Living Regenerating the Earth

6X Veggie Harvests, 4X Soil Organic Matter, and $105,000 per Acre with No-Till Farming
Elizabeth Kaiser
What You Will Discover

- Her secrets for $105,000 of revenue per acre on a vegetable farm
- 4 key practices that quadrupled the organic matter in her soil
- How the USDA helped her create a natural pest control system

$7-Figure Regenerative Edible Landscaping Business
Erik Ohlsen
What You Will Discover

- The "lenses" of Permaculture that empower you to transform your world
- A key attitude you must have to be successful in building a regenerative design business
- Your 3 next steps if you're considering starting a regenerative business

Grow Your Own Food, Make Your Own Medicine
Marjory Wildcraft
What You Will Discover

- How Marjorie treated a snakebite would without going to the hospital
- How to create and use a poultice to heal a wound
- Which vegetables are easiest to grow

Grow and Eat "Beyond Organic" Raw Plant Foods
John Kohler
What You Will Discover

- The personal health crisis that drove John to radically change his diet
- John's issue with the definitions of "organic" and "vegan"
- What John adds to his compost, and how he grows "beyond organic" food

A Passion for Plants: The Perennial Diet
Stephen Brooks
What You Will Discover

- Perennial vs annual crops and foods
- The next superfood coming from Africa

- Essential lessons from permaculture to build the life of your dreams

Elizabeth Kaiser Interview

6X Veggie Harvests, 4X Soil Organic Matter, and $105,000 per Acre with No-Till Farming

Brendan [00:00:00]: Welcome to the Eat4Earth event. We're exploring how you can heal yourself, your

loved ones, and the Earth with food. My name is Brendan Moorehead, and I have the distinct pleasure of welcoming our next guest, a true innovator in regenerative food cultivation, Elizabeth Kaiser. Elizabeth is a Public Health nurse with a Master's degree in the science of nursing and a Master's in Public Health from Johns Hopkins University. In 2007, Elizabeth and her husband, Paul, founded Singing Frogs Farm in Sebastopol, California. Singing Frogs Farm is a unique, no-till, ecologically beneficial, highly-intensive vegetable farm in Sonoma County, California. Through innovative, regenerative farming systems, including no-till soil management, Elizabeth and Paul have more than quadrupled the organic matter in their soil in six years, producing more nutrient-dense food and over six times the state average harvest revenue per acre per year while bringing back tremendous healthy populations of pollinators, beneficial insects and vertebrates that serve as natural pest control. They use less water to produce vegetables because of their super-charged soil organic matter. They use no sprays of any kind – not even organic sprays. They have created living-wage jobs for an awesome crew of year-round employees that have job security. And they've done all of this while raising two children! Elizabeth, I'm so happy that you're here with us today, and I think that what you're going to show us might blow some minds and inspire some action.

Elizabeth [00:01:36]: Oh, Brendan! Thank you so much! And thank you so much for having me. These are all topics that really excite me. So, thank you very much.

Brendan [00:01:43]: And, before your presentation, I first want to add some additional context for what you're about to show us. Throughout this event, we're learning just how important soil organic matter is to nutrient density in food, to human health, and to restoring the water cycles that can help stabilize our climate and oceans. So, I'm very excited about what you're doing because even the most, uh...even the best organic tillage systems, meaning farms that use plowing, that were studied at the Rodale Institute have only raised soil organic matter by 25% over a period of 30 years. But at Singing Frogs Farm, you use a no-till organic system, beyond organic, that grew soil organic matter 400% in six years, which is about 56 times faster. And this has HUGE implications for human and planetary health if methods like yours are used on farms around the world. Seventy percent of the world's food supply is grown on small farms and, in 2014, United Nations stated that "Only small farmers and agroecology can feed the world." So, with that, I'll let you get into your presentation.

Elizabeth [00:02:52]: Well, thank you very much and maybe we can talk about the differences between different types of models later. So, first of all, thank you very much again. Let me get into the beginning of this. Fantastic! So, I wanted to give you a little bit of a context. First of all, where we're located. As you just said, we're in Sebastopol, California. That's in Sonoma County. It's about an hour north of the Golden Gate

Bridge of San Francisco. And I pulled up this satellite map to give you an idea of something that we went through recently. You can see the Bay Area here, San Francisco right here, and this is our Sonoma County up here when we had such horrible fires here in our county. And, for me, this was really, really important because I see it as the direct impact of climate change on us locally, and I think everybody has their own direct impact by climate change. And, as you will see, climate change is something that is very important to me and very linked to our farming processes and why we want to share about them. For us, specifically, it was because, in California, we are having a lengthening fire season, a lengthening dry season, that is. We had the wettest year on record last winter. So lots of extra biomass was grown. And then the five years prior to that, we had drought. And then we had these incredible winds, all of which are climatically related. So, for me, this is very important and I just want to bring you into my personal local context. Oh my, there's something in the middle of that. Pardon me! So, ignore the word in the middle of that screen, but I wanted to share with you a little about my farm.

So, this is my farm. This is about 80% of the fields. And a little bit about our farm ... So, we're in the valley bottom. Our property is about 8 acres, and about 3 acres of that production is intensive vegetable production. This picture was taken two years ago, end of October. So, this is as we're getting ready to go into winter. You might think that we're in California, so, easy for us to grow year-round. But I will tell you that we do get quite a lot of frosts. So far this year, we've already had about seven light-frost mornings and we will hit 10 degrees usually once a winter. So, not deep frosts, but it does impact. So, we have a very small farm but super-intensive. About 40% of our produce goes to our CSA (Community Supported Agriculture) so we have a direct relationship with those consumers for the long term. About 50% of our produce goes to farmer's markets and about 10% goes to restaurants. So, this is just to give you the idea that we're super-local. All of our produce is sold within 15 miles of the farm, and that's something that's very important to us.

Now, there's three things that make our farm unique and I'm calling these the "tenets" of Singing Frogs Farm model. The first one is that we do no tillage of any sort. The second one is that we're very intensive. And the third one is that we are very ecologically based. So, I am going to talk about all of these as we go through. But first I'm going to start with the basics, with soil and soil organic matter. This is taking things super-simple but when you look at soil, what you're looking at is about 95% minerals, air and water and the last, about, 5% (and we'll talk about that in a minute) are soil organic matter. Now, that is important to us because soil organic matter is the one thing that allows us to take death and turn it back into life. That is where our microorganisms are contained. That is where our roots are. That is where all the functions are happening that will give nutrition to our plants and vegetables and even our meat. And it's also important to note that about 57% of soil organic matter is carbon per weight. Now, as I'm sure you've heard in other lectures, and maybe you just know this, but we've had tremendous changes in soil organic matter both nationally as well as globally. They believe that, historically, top soils in the U.S. (and it's similar world-wide) had about 6-10% soil organic matter and that's now 1-3%. In fact, in California, the CDFA—the California Department of Food and Ag—about 18 months ago came out and said that it's as low as about 1% in California where we are producing a very large portion of the vegetables for the United States. Globally, about 2/3 of our planetary soil carbon has already been lost from cultivation. This comes from Ohio State and tillage is one of the major practices that reduces the organic matter level in the soil. And this is from the Food and Agriculture Organization of the United Nations. This is not new. We've known this for a very, very long time. And I'm gonna talk a little about how that happens. So, how it happens is this: When you do tillage... and it doesn't matter if you're using a horse and plow, a rototiller or really big John Deere tractor ... it's all gonna be the same. You're turning over the soil, you are breaking it up, you are breaking the aggregates or the clumps of soil that are in the ground, and you are increasing the surface area in proportion to the volume. And you're bring oxygen into contact with more soil by doing that. So, what happens then is a couple of different things. First of all, the oxygen will join with different compounds, soil, and the soil organic matter and become CO2. That's where you really get the loss of carbon and the loss of organic matter into the air. It's that very simple C plus O2 equals CO2.

But at the same time, you're also having other things happen. You're also having a great loss of nitrogen with oxygen becoming nitrous oxide. Now, those are your two most potent greenhouse gases. But, as a farmer, as a gardener, those are two of the things that are most important for us. Carbon for our soil structure, nitrogen for our plant growth. So we want to keep them in the soil. That's where they belong. We don't want to put them up in the air. And then, it's not only these nutrients that are getting volatilized. There are also all sorts of micronutrients and other minerals that are getting volatilized. And it's been known ... and one of the reasons that farmers have continued to till is ... just after tilling, when you put in your next crop, a lot of minerals are much more available to plants. But, it creates a rush and then a crash of these minerals. And it's actually very similar to, like, a sugar crash. You'll get a rush of energy and then a crash. So we don't want to break up those systems and bring in that extra oxygen, which is really like a supercharger on an engine or bellows on a forge or something like that. So, physically, that's what's happening with tillage. Then, tillage is also very bad for the microbiology that's in the soil. Not only are you destroying the carbon in the soil and volatilizing it up into the air, but you are also destroying the ecosystems where the microbial life is living by breaking up the aggregates, by bringing in the oxygen and then sometimes just through manual chopping, be that of your mycorrhizal fungi or your larger to you earthworms or your snakes and so forth. In fact, we love this quote from the USDA, "Tilling the soil is the equivalent of an earthquake, hurricane, tornado, and a forest fire occurring simultaneously to the world of soil organisms. Simply stated, tillage is bad for the soil." So, I get a kick out of that quote and, really, that's what's happening at that level.

And, yet, there is a lot of hope. This came out of some studies out of Europe that, not only is agriculture a large part of the greenhouse gas emission, however, it has the greatest potential to mitigate that. And I love this slide because you can see all sorts of other areas like industry, waste, energy, refrigeration, and so forth. And what it's showing down here is the mitigation potential in terms of tons of CO2 equivalent and the cost to sequester that. And you can very easily see that agriculture has the ability to mitigate far, far, far more at a far-reduced cost. So that makes it really exciting to me and I really want to get the idea out that we need to reduce, and even just completely stop tillage, and get the carbon back in the soil. And how are we gonna to do that? The same studies have found that 89% of that potential of for greenhouse gas emission (meant mitigation) is very simply from soil management, crop land management, grazing management, restoring organic soils and degraded lands. So, taking this to a more global view, they believe that a two-percentage point increase in the carbon content of the planet's soil could even offset 100% of the greenhouse gas emissions going into the atmosphere. So, this is really exciting and this is what makes me want to share this information. If we treat our soil right, we have the ability to put the carbon back where it is and reverse a lot of the carbon that is in the atmosphere right now.

So, let me transition to our farm and to some of our practices. One of the things that we found is, talking about soil, it's easy to talk about it in terms of general soil health principles. And there are many different sets of these principles. They are all very, very similar. We've taken them from the USDA. The USDA actually has good science. Maybe not the best policy, but we like these because they're really basic. And we think about it on our property when we make a change or maybe we move into a new area. And then we'll also think about it when we're working with new farmers and gardeners who have a slightly different context, a different soil type, or different crop types they're growing, different climates, something like that. So these are really important and I'm going to go through them step by step. So, the first one is, "Disturb the soil as little as possible," and this is pretty easy. Don't till it! Just leave it in place. And I've already given you the reasons for that. But a couple of images to show ... so, on the left here, we have some soil in a bed and this was taken right when somebody harvested a head of escarole. You can still see the stem of escarole is the white patch in the middle. And you can see all the surprised earthworms going, "Oh! Wow! Where did that head of escarole go?" But this is very active soil! I do not want to go into this and till again. People do like tools and, if I'm gonna tell them not to till with their Rototiller or their tractor, people like to know, "Well, what can I use instead?" One of the things that we used at first was a broad fork, which is what you see my husband, Paul, using on the right side. It's not a tillage mechanism but it opens up the soil a little and aerates it just a little bit. This is something we used as we transitioned to no-till and it is something that I definitely recommend that new farmers, who are transitioning or starting their farms no-till, utilize. At this point, our organic soil matter is high enough that we don't use it on our own farm, but it is a usable tool and people like tools. So, that was the first principle.

The second and the third we'll actually group together. So, let me read them both first. "Grow as many different species of plants as practical," and "Keep living plants in the soil as often as possible." So, keeping living plants in the soil as often as possible ... that is really the solution to the problems that I just presented you with climate change and with tillage. How are we gonna reverse that and get the carbon back down in the ground. This information was put together by Dr. Christine Jones and I just love the simplicity of thinking about this. So, I'm gonna take you back to your middle-school biology class and talk about photosynthesis and what's happening there. When a plant is photosynthesizing, what they're doing is they're taking minerals, sunlight and water and they're capturing CO_2. They are taking that carbon atom off, releasing the O_2 (the oxygen) and then they're taking that carbon and they are creating your most basic carbon-based building block of life, which is gonna be glucose. Step number one. Step number two, they're gonna take glucose and they're gonna resynthesize glucose into a myriad of other carbon-based products. More complicated sugars and carbohydrates and amino acids and proteins and waxes and fats and so forth, and so on. Now, here's the exciting part, and this is called exudation. Only about 40-60% of the products of photosynthesis is that plant going to utilize for its own growth and development, and that depends on the season, the type of plant and the researcher that you look at. The rest of that 40-60% isn't utilized directly by the plant, but it's pushed out as exudate by the roots into the soil to feed the microorganisms and the symbiotic relationships that they're having. These relationships are extremely important and the microbial life in the soil ... we are just barely, barely, barely starting to understand the relationships between the millions and billions of different organisms. But we're finding that, as you have more organisms, you have healthier plants. It boosts their immune system. They help move water around. They actually help plants communicate. If there's one plant that has a pest attack, he will communicate with other plants via mycorrhizal fungi, for instance. What else? It's going to help pull out minerals from inorganic states into states that the plant can utilize and bring it right up to the plant. So, it's actually very exciting to me that a lot of the relationships we see between plants and the microorganisms that they work with are very similar to what we're learning about our own body and the microorganisms that are in and on our own body, in our GI tract that help us we now we're finding out about our mental health, and with our immune systems, and so forth. There are very similar correlations there.

Okay, and then back to the four basic steps of drawing down carbon dioxide. The last one is called humification. So that is really the creating of the humus, putting that carbon down in the soil and creating soil organic matter. So, this, I love! This gets me really excited. This is the answer, to me. This is the answer to climate change. It's the answer to having healthy plants, having healthy soil, having resilient farms, having profitable farms. I can just go on and on and on in that. So, once we have that feeding of the soil, this is a different take. A little more focused on the soil food web. This is from NRCS (National Resource Conservation Service). You are, again, seeing the plants creating organic matter through their exudates and, immediately, they are feeding bacteria and fungi, but then those bacteria and fungi are feeding protozoa and nematodes and arthropods and then we get up into bigger animals here. So, this is what we want. We want a healthy soil food web for healthy plants, healthy humans, healthy ecosystems, and I could just go on and on. So, on our farm, this is actually a picture from several years ago, but you can see here, keeping green living plants in the ground as often as possible and a diversity. So, you've got over here some pepper plants. You've got some Brussels sprouts plants with some fennel in between. You've got some eggplants, and you've got some new transplants in there. So, lots and lots of different things going on. Here's another shot. And you'll see a bunch of pictures of our farm, one thing after the next. And soon as one is done, the next healthy new plant is going to be put in. So, because of this, we are able to do three to eight sequential economic crops in any one bed in a one-year cycle. So, right now you have bok choy and lettuce in the foreground. And that may have been beets before that and cabbage before that and broccoli before that, and we will just rotate through. One plant is done, get the next one in there right away. So it's very intensive management.

Okay, then, back to our principles for soil health. I've gone through the first three. The last one, then, is keep the soil covered all the time, so that you're not having a little bit of volatilization and also so that you are helping mediate the temperature of the soil. Soil does not want to be heated up in the day and then very cold in the evening. But if you have plants covering it ... some sort of mulch covering ... it's going to mitigate against that. And so, ideally, what kind of cover do you want on it? You want green photosynthesizing plants as your cover on the soil. And if you can't do green photosynthesizing plants, our second best would be a mulch, you know, like a straw mulch or leaves or even wood chips. And if we are not able to do that, well, sometimes we do an artificial mulch but I'll say, honestly, that happens less than 5% of the time on our farm. Here's another example of green cover on the soil, as much of the soil having roots in the ground, photosynthesizing plants feeding the soil, feeding the microorganisms. Here, again, the same. And one of the ways that we will do that is we really focus on using large, healthy transplants. So, having really nutrient-dense soil in our nursery to have very large plants going out to the field so that one photosynthesizing plant is coming out and the next photosynthesizing plant is going in. So, here you have some baby bok choy heading out in the field. Here you have some lettuces just being planted. Here, on the left, is some summer squash. On the right is some kale. Crops just came out of those and immediately the next crop is going in. Sometimes, additionally, we will actually plant two crops at the same time in the same bed. One of the things we like to do is Brassicas. When they go in, there's a lot of soil visible so we'll put in, not 100%, but about 60-70% crop of something fast, usually a lettuce, in the same place. So you have 100% cover of your Brassica. Your Brassica, in this case, is a cauliflower but it could also be broccoli, Brussels sprouts, and then you also have the lettuce. The lettuce will come out far before the Brassica has finished growing but you are getting an extra half-crop out of those beds at the same time you are feeding the soil. You are covering the soil and so we see this as a win-win. Here's a couple of other examples. Leeks and another lettuce. This is a before and an after shot. Tomatoes and lettuces, or escaroles in this case. This is just when they went in. This is when the lettuces are ready to be harvested. And so, in that way, we try our best to follow those four steps of soil management.

Now, I want to give you a little bit … that's all the theory, why we do what we do … I want to give you a little bit of how we do what we do in terms of transitioning a bed from one crop to the next. I know this isn't a farm school, but I also know that many of you have gardens, and people just like to see how that happens. So, I'm actually not going to read through this 'cause I have it on the next slides. So, the first thing we're going to do with a crop that's done … and this was a kale crop that, although it was flowering, had really luscious kale on it a couple of springs ago … but we want to clear the bed, and we do not want to pull those roots out of the ground. We do not want to pull the plants out because that's essentially tilling. And, not only that, but because the plants have been feeding the soil, the area right around their roots is called the rhizosphere because it's got the densest amount of microorganisms right around them. We do not want to pull that out of the ground and disturb that ecosystem. So, we will cut the crop at the ground level and take all the green above-ground matter to the compost pile.

Next, we'll prep the beds a little bit and we might do the broad forking, like I mentioned before, and then very, very, very occasionally, beds will need to be reformed a little bit, which is what you're seeing him doing. And then we may apply some organic fertilizers or compost as needed. As a farmer, I'm in the business of exporting nutrients off our farm and the sunlight and CO_2 and all the relationships with all the microorganisms are going to bring a lot of nutrition to the plants. But I do need to bring a little of it back and compost is our favorite way. We make about half of our own compost from the green, above-ground mass from the prior crops but we also purchase in compost from our community because we believe strongly in cycling and re-cycling those nutrients in our community. Then we do use a couple of fertilizers. A very low concentration of nitrogen in the form of a chicken feather meal and, in the past, we've also used some calcium in the form of crushed oyster shells. So we try and go for renewable resources that are going to help keep the beds mineralized so that we have healthy plants going in there. And then the very next is going to be transplanting. I had to get a picture of my daughter in there. It's one of her favorite activities. But we'll transplant the next crop right in and then we're going to water it in and really let it get settled into place. And then, as needed, we will cover our crops and we'll cover them for a variety of reasons. This is for cold 'cause I think this was a January or February shot. But it might also be for pests and pests might include deer or birds. This is bird and deer netting. So, I just explained all those steps, and I would now like to show them to you in the form of a video. So, we've got here four beds. They're all about 85 feet long and we've got three people that, in 45 minutes, are going to transition this over from the crop that you see. There is a broccoli that was just finished being harvested and there was an Asian green that bolted. This was about March last year. So you see these three people? They are clearing the crops. They are cutting it all. The wheel barrows ... they are taking it all to the compost pile. Next, you're gonna see they're just gonna take the irrigation lines off. They're gonna be applying a little bit of the two fertilizers that I was just telling you, and they're covering it with a bit of compost. Now, it looks like a lot of compost because of the color differentiation. We do have a tractor on our farm, but it is our compost machine. It's a lot of work so you need a little bit of a coffee break. And then you can see they are immediately transplanting right back in. And we do have a double crop that's going in here. We've got a Brassica and a couple of different kinds of lettuce. So you can see they did the Brassica first, and now they are going through with the rest of the lettuces. They are watering in and done! So, I hope that helps you sort of understand what this looks like in a practical way, but it was short and very intensive. Uh, it is skilled labor, but it's very enjoyable. We have a lot of fun out there. Okay. So, just to recap all of that: All of the carbon and biology that these plants helped put into the ground without soil disturbance is going to help the next crop or these plants thrive. And this is sort of the key to what we're trying to do.

Brendan [00:28:11]: That looks fun! (Laugh)

Elizabeth [00:28:15]: It does look fun that way! (Laugh) You know, it is really good work, and we have a fantastic crew. And, I talk to some farmers and farming can be very isolating and, on our farm, it is not at all. There are times when you're working alone, but most often people are working in teams, and it's great! You learn what you're doing, you get your hands into it, and then you have a fun time while you're talking and working really hard.

So, I wanted to transition to sort of the third tenant that I was telling you about that is key to our model. So, just recapping again: The first one being no till, the second one being intensive and the third one really including ecology. And that is definitely a focus on the ecology in the soil but also about the above-ground ecology. We have actually dedicated quite a lot of our space on our farm to perennials. Early on on our farm ... we've been farming for almost 11 years now ... and about nine years ago, we got some USDA grants through our RCDs (Regional Conservation District) to put in 3000 Sonoma County native, pollinator-friendly, perennial plants. Since then, we have continued to add perennial plants. So, these are some native dogwoods and roses in the winter time. You can see frost on the ground. This is another row. We call these hedgerows. Hedgerow is an old British name for a row of hedges or a row of bushes. We have them in rows on our farm. We also have them in clumps and triangles and circles and things like that. And they're really important to us for a variety of reasons but I would have to say that beneficial insects is really key amongst those. There are a lot of studies out of different California agricultural colleges and universities that have shown that your beneficial insects prefer your dense, branched perennial bushes, and your pest insects prefer your annual plants. And they are going to be feeding off of your annual plants. And just to bring it down to a really basic level, I love this analogy. "Your beneficial insects are really your predatory class of insects and your pest insects are the prey." Some of their relationships are very similar to other predators and prey. So, think coyotes and bunny rabbits. For me, that's a really easy one. So, bunny rabbit is smaller. (It doesn't necessarily always have to be.) It has a shorter lifespan. It has more progeny more frequently, and it doesn't need a lot of wild space to live in. Now, the coyote, on the other hand, has a longer lifespan, fewer progeny less frequently, and they need more wild space to live in. Well, the same is true for your beneficials and your pest insects. One of the pests that we have on our farm is the aphid. For crying out loud! They are born pregnant! You know? (Laugh) They have a lot of progeny very quickly! As our hedgerows have developed on our farm, we have seen a tremendous reduction in pest pressure on our farm. We do still have pests. In fact, we have all the pests that all of our neighbor farms have. And we need to have that to have food for our beneficials. But this is important for us because we use no sprays of any sort and so, as this has grown along, we've just had a much more successful system. Now, not only does it provide ecology for insects, but also for other animals. This is Miguel, who has worked on our farm for several years. He's from Oaxaca, and I would like to point out that a Oaxacan is holding a snake and smiling! When he first moved on our farm, he was petrified of snakes. They have become his friend. One of our pests on our farm are rodents ... field mice and voles and gophers. Up here in northern California, we have a lot of gophers, and this is a gopher snake. And what we have found is that the hedgerows are someplace that the gopher snakes, as well as some of the other snakes that we have on our farm, really feel safe and so they will make their burrows in there and then go hunting out into the fields. And so, we love our snakes and, as we have stopped tilling and increased our perennial ecology, we have increased the snakes on our farm tremendously and we love that. But, it's not only snakes. It's also birds and many, many other things. So, just having that diversity and living with Mother Nature, working with the cycles of Mother Nature rather than against her, can be tremendous. And I feel like that is what we have found and that is what we aim to do. Here's another picture of a hedgerow in the winter with our crops covered and this is a wild area with a series of hedgerows that is all of 15 feet from our intensive cropland. So, we have space for both of them on our farm.

So, coming back to soil organic matter, when we started...here's a picture of one of our beds in 2007 or 2008. Not very productive. You can see the soil is very light in color. You can see where the drip irrigation has been going. It has really formed a crust almost concrete-like. We started out doing tillage and so this was in a tillage field. As we have transitioned our processes, you can look over at a bed on the right side. This has got tomatoes and then a multi-crop that is a panisse lettuce. You can see the soil has a very different quality. So we have gone from a soil organic matter of 2.4% to a soil organic matter of 8-11%, depending on the fields. We have about 13 different fields on our property, and each of them is managed the same, but yet each bed is managed a little bit different, and we are able to do that because we are so intensive. We do test our soil organic matter, not on the top, because we do surface apply a little bit of compost on the top after most crops, about 80% of the crops, so we felt that we needed to test it down where the roots are at a depth of about 6-12 inches. I showed you the slide at the beginning of the talk, "Changes in Soil Organic Matter," historically where they were and where they are today. And I bring this up for two reasons, again, and one of them is … you just noticed that I said our organic matter on our farm is now 8–11%. Well, gee, it's actually very similar to historically where it was before we did large-scale agriculture with a lot of tillage. It's where Mother Nature had her fertile soils. And what we've realized in the last couple of years, or what we hypothesized, I should say, is there is just some balance in that area. Mother Nature knew what she was doing. You get your soil organic matter to that area, and it provides enough ecology for the microbiology to thrive and have a good food web and things just get easier. We actually have had a couple of our fields get up to a little bit above 11%–13%, and we didn't find any added benefits. So, we think that Mother Nature knew what she was doing!

And I'm actually going to talk a little about nutrition right now, and I'm sure other people will as well. But, as you saw here, historically, our soil organic matter went down tremendously. Well, what has also gone down is our minerals in our vegetables. I got this from a study in nutrition and health from, gosh, almost 15 years ago but we've had a tremendous decrease in a lot of the nutrients, and, of course, that is because of the relationships that are lost when you are losing that soil organic matter, and the health of the plants and, therefore, the health of what they are producing. Our model is very, very, very intensive. Like I told you, we only have three acres of crop and, because I live in northern California where the cost of living is very high, that was one of the things that really drove us to be intensive. So, I just wanted to share a relationship with other types of farming. We are very intensive, and we realize some of these are extensive. So, if you look at the average gross revenue per crop acre, so, that is the money that is brought in. That is not profit, that is gross revenue. If you look at all California vegetable farms, it's about $1,900 per acre. Now, if you go to organic, it almost doubles—$3,700—and that is because there is a higher price for organic, but not always doubled. So they definitely have better practices, they are definitely going to have cover crops, and so forth. Then, if you jump to California small, diversified, direct-market vegetable farms, which are mainly organic, these are the people you really see at the farmer's markets. These are our competitors. The average jumps up to about $11,000. Now, I live in Sonoma County and we are in wine country and for many years people said, "You gotta get rid of vegetables. You gotta put in vineyards 'cause vineyards will make money." So we had to throw this in! Sonoma County vineyards are about $11,000-12,000 average per year. Now, some studies out of the UC Davis showed economic viability for small, but diversified, organic vegetable farmers. They believe they need to be making about $14,000 or more per acre. And two of our best university teaching farms do definitely do that. But with our intensive method, we're able to sort of blow that out of the water. We're able to get about $105,000 in gross revenue per acre. Now, that is not to say that I'm profiting all of that. Seventy percent of that goes to pay for people to work on the farm but, to me, that is a really good thing. I would rather pay people than pay tractors and John Deere. I would rather pay people and make compost than pay for artificial nutrients to be added to our soil. So, the point in this is, a lot of the farming up here is extensive on larger amounts of space, and so what you might have as a comparison is that we're producing as many vegetables on our three acres as most other farmers are going to be producing on 30-50 acres. And this is the result of it. This was our crew last summer. We have a lot of people. In fact, we have never been able to get a picture with everybody because we have a lot of part-timers, and it's a really vibrant crew. We have a lot of fun, and a lot of people go off and start their own farms. This is actually from last year. This couple here was just learning from us. Over the summer they started a new farm in Melbourne, Australia. This guy's starting a farm in France. She's currently working in New York City on rooftops. So, we have people going off and doing lots of things, which is great.

So, just rounding it back together, the three things that we think are most important to the way that we farm: First being no till. Second being intensive. And third being ecological. All of them being very important. I don't think you can separate out and just do one of those things. This is Nina with a couple of heads of very healthy broccoli. We have a lot of people who are very interested in what we are doing. We definitely do have people come work on the farm for a period of time if they have experience farming. But one of the best ways to learn, aside from, you know, coming to presentations and listening to presentations like this, is we've started doing some one-day intensive trainings. We do about seven a year, four in the spring and three in the autumn. These dates have passed already because we've finished our autumn dates for the year, but this is a great way for people to come out and get their fingers in the soil and give it a try while we all share and talk about it. And about one-half of the people who come through are farmers or new farmers and the rest are just interested parties and gardeners. And we have a lot of fun. These are great! And then I also wanted to share that there are a lot of other farms that are starting this. The two people I just showed you from Australia—they are Mossy Willow Farm. We have Handlebar Farm in our community. Tuff, which is down in Fresno. It is very hot and dry. Ten Mothers is in North Carolina. Two Roots and Tierra Vida are both no-till, intensive farms up at 9,000 feet in Durango and in Carbondale. Red H Farm is here in our community. Hillview Farms is in the foothills of the Sierra at about 3,000 feet elevation. Very tough clay soil. They started out on just ¾ of an acre. They have now purchased more land. I believe they're up to three acres. Nye Ranch is up in Mendocino. Woven Roots did not learn from us. They, and we, have developed our own systems. They are in Massachusetts, but we love sharing because there are a lot of similarities. And here are a couple of pictures. So, this is from up in Carbondale. As you can see, it looks very similar to our farm. This is from Durango, CO. A farm up there. This is the farm up in the Sierras. This is another farm here, locally. And then our Singing Frogs Farm. And that is where I'm going to leave it! Thank you all for your interest, and let me know what questions you have.

Brendan [00:42:21]: That was so amazing! Thank you, Elizabeth.

Elizabeth [00:42:25]: Absolutely! Thank you for having me again.

Brendan [00:42:28]: It's really great to see all the details, and I just want to thank you for your contribution to other farmers, to communities. Everything about your business is so worthy of emulation from beneficial ecological footprints to nutrient-richer food you are supplying to everybody to the socially just and equitable relationships with your employees and the community. And so I just want to thank you and Paul for being such beacons for the potential for regenerative agricultural. So, thank you for spending this time with me and with the Eat4Earth community.

Elizabeth [00:43:14]: Absolutely! And I'm excited that you and so many other people are interested in this topic. I, by no means, want to leave the impression that everybody needs to farm exactly like we are. I just want to share what one model can look like, and emulate it or make it make you think and crack outside of the box in some other way, or have other innovations, maybe on a different scale or with different crops or in different climates or something like that. I just think we need to share what has worked and go from there to create a better world.

Brendan [00:43:52]: Wow! What a privilege for us to learn from Elizabeth and her husband Paul showing us and the rest of the world what's possible. $105,000 gross revenue per acre, so one can actually support a family farming, putting all the carbon and more back into the soil, employing people and paying them well, and producing beautiful, nutrient-dense vegetables. Does it get any better than that?

Erik Ohlsen Interview
7-Figure Regenerative Edible Landscaping Business

Brendan [00:00:00]: Welcome to the Eat4Earth event. We're exploring how you can heal yourself, the people you care about, and the planet you love, with food. This is Brendan Moorehead and our next guest, Erik Ohlsen, is super passionate about creating businesses that help people and the Earth thrive together. Erik is a licensed contractor and the founder and owner of Permaculture Artisans, an ecological farm and landscaping company. Erik is a renowned certified Permaculture designer and certified Permaculture teacher, and has been practicing Permaculture and designs since 1998, when he co-founded his first non-profit organization called Planting Earth Activism. Erik has been teaching Permaculture design and implementation since 2001 and is known in Northern California as a premier teacher of Permaculture. He has taught courses in Permaculture and related subjects throughout the United States, Canada, and the United Kingdom. His engaging, energetic, do-it-yourself teaching style has captivated hundreds of Permaculture students from all over the world. Erik, it's great to have you here today.

Erik [00:01:04]: Thank you, Brendan. Great to be here and love what you're doing.

Brendan [00:01:09]: Thank you. I first met you at the Permaculture Voices conference in 2015. I was just totally blown away by your passion for helping people create a business that's good for humans and the planet, and you do that through Permaculture. For those who are not familiar with Permaculture, maybe you could define that real quick. There have been other speakers in this event talking about Permaculture briefly, but maybe you could give your definition.

Erik [00:01:36]: Absolutely. Everyone has their own definition because Permaculture is such a broad subject. But, I'd like to say Permaculture is a design science that integrates all the needs of the planet with the needs of humans. So, and we do that through mutually beneficial relationships. So it's the intentional design of human communities and human settlements in a way that aligns and integrates with the needs and resources of our environments and our ecologies. So, it's about regenerating our communities, our social systems, our economic systems, our lives while at the same time regenerating our environment.

Brendan [00:02:18]: Beautiful. And, since in the event, we're connecting human health with planet health through soil health. Why are you excited about Permaculture as a framework for generating green jobs and the regenerative economy?

Erik [00:02:34]: Well, first of all, Permaculture is based on a set of principles and those principles are design principles that are derived from Nature. So, it's how do we design our systems, our human systems, in a way that is like Nature? That takes into account relationships. That takes into account resource constraints and takes into account all of life. You know, all of living organisms. So, how do we take that approach to our gardens? To our homes? To our communities? How do we design these things in a way that fully align with Nature? And so, what's so powerful about aligning these principles, is how it affects our food and our soil and our water and our health is that we are learning about how to be in a place. We're learning about how to live in the places that we are. If I live in the desert, I'm going to have a completely different approach to growing my food and living aligned with that environment than I would be if I lived in a tropical environment. So, Permaculture gives us the observation tools and principals that allows us to understand, observe, and relate to whatever place we are at so that we can be in the best alignment with that. It's part of that decision-making process that helps us identify what are the appropriate plants for my climate? What are the appropriate soil-building techniques for my soil type. And, you know, it just goes on and on. So, I think it's very powerful in that if we're truly applying the principles of Permaculture, then we are hyper-local in our decision-making processes and developing a deeper understanding of our place.

Brendan [00:04:20]: So, in other words, it's not about cutting and pasting corn, soy, wheat, and [laughter]. And it's, basically, each location generates its own design.

Erik [00:04:45]: Yeah. And I think it's a key point that often gets missed is that it's not about what works in one place works everywhere. That's kind of missing the point of applying the principles of Permaculture. And what we know if we are settled in environments where people have settled for thousands of years and indigenous communities have settled in many places that humans are. You know, like cities. Places where we are in high number now. That there is a certain type of relationship with those climates, with those soils that can be sustainable and ecological. And so we have to be humble ourselves to realize that we don't know everything, and that's what Permaculture leads us to ask the right questions that will guide our activities, our implementation strategies in a way that is truly in alignment with those ecologies.

Brendan [00:05:47]: Are there any other differences worth pointing out between a Permaculture approach and conventional agriculture when we're looking at growing food? Obviously, Permaculture is about a lot more than just growing food, just looking through that lens.

Erik [00:06:00]: Well, you know, as we look through the Permaculture lens, we don't silo out parts of the system so we wouldn't just focus on agriculture, you know, one part of the system. We would create agricultural systems that are integrated with the social systems of that community, that are integrated with the economic means and the relationship needs of that community. So, we think systematically. And, with Permaculture, we're whole system designers. So often what we like to say is we're not designing things. We're not designing the vegetable farm. We're not designing the water harvesting system. What we're designing are the relationships between water and soil. We're designing the relationships between sun orientation and our planting beds. We're designing relationships between the human community and what their needs are and the type of crops that we're growing. So, Permaculture is really about relationship design and not just design of the elements themselves. And sometimes we get a little bit lost in technique. And we focus too much on technique with a disregard to dynamic relationships. That's where I think Permaculture is very different … is that when you start making decisions about your farm. You start making decisions about the crops you're going to grow. You do that through the lens of community, economy, climate, and all of these other layers, which is the real world that you're living in. And I think as well, because you asked the difference between

Permaculture and conventional agriculture. And then, of course, that there's an ethic that we, Permaculture designers, apply which is care-of-Earth and care-of-people and reinvest the surplus. And so with that in mind, if you apply the principles of Permaculture through the ethical lens, then the kinds of decisions that we make we won't choose farming practices that are going to destroy the biosphere. We're going to choose practices and techniques that are actually supporting the watershed, that are enhancing the habitats of birds, and amphibians, and reptiles, and other wildlife. And so, that in and of itself adds a decision-making tool as a way in design that, when we have an ethical intent, is a sea change, honestly, from the kind of industrial agricultural systems that are plaguing our world today.

Brendan [00:08:43]: There's a question that might come up in some people's minds, certainly if they have a conventional agriculture background and that might be "So, okay, but I'm going to grow food with … that's my goal. That's what my business is." So how, and I didn't prepare you for this question at all, but I'm just curious, what kind of examples might you be able to give of, let's say, systems that actually are productive, that is some way that can be compared, because productivity is sort of this thing that I think that conventional agriculture seeks, but they optimize for one species and actually the way it's being done we're not getting to any kind of efficiency overall at all, and actually the corn yields are pathetic on, in our conventional agriculture system. So corn is—I won't pass judgement about whether it's a desirable product or not—but, the actual genetic potential of corn is far under-tapped in the conventional agriculture system and just, overall, my perspective is you get a lot more overall productivity in this system that might include corn but is more Permaculture designed, or just in general polyculture, even if it's not specifically a Permaculture system. And the overall yields and the overall profitability of those systems often far exceed, even by several multiples, of what you get out of a conventional system. Just curious, can you give me any examples. And one of the speakers in this event is Elizabeth Kaiser. Obviously, she and her husband, Paul, just blow it up. You can't compare anything to them [laughter] except other people that are doing something very similar. So, I'm just curious what you might have to say about that idea. "Well okay, but we can't feed the world on organic" and "We definitely can't feed the world on Permaculture" or whatever somebody might come up with.

Erik [00:10:47]: The thing is we have to first understand the current context. And I think that as we get clear about the context we're in today, it gives us a better sense of the kind of changes we need to make. Because our context today is that our industrial agriculture system has become dependent on chemical input, upon fossil fuel technology, and that to go to these farmers and to say, "Well, you need to change overnight. You need to stop applying all of these chemicals. You need to stop mono-cropping, stop treating the watershed and the soil this way." Of course, they're going to throw their arms up because now you have more than one generation, now we have multiple generations, that have been steeped in this industrial agriculture model. And those families are completely dependent on the systems that they have. And, like you printed out, while they look like they're efficient because they are quote unquote "productive", they can grow a lot in … they can do these multi-thousand-acre farms and harvest hundreds of tons of yields and all these things with low human inputs because they have fossil fuel inputs and all this. It looks glamorous to the farmers that, "Oh, technology has made this easier for us. To have high productivity and high efficiency." But the truth is it's very short-sighted, and it inevitably will collapse. It's already collapsing as we see around the world through top soil loss and the loss of arable land. Land that has the capacity for food and care for people is becoming less and less available because those lands are becoming overly polluted, or they're becoming salinized or there's no water because all the water has been used up to irrigate these systems. So, it's almost the time frame that we're talking about. So, that's sort of like the question. What is the time frame that we're talking about? If we're talking about the next ten years, then what farmers are doing now might seem the most efficient and productive, but if we're talking about more, multiple generations of sustainability of food production on that same level and that same landscape, those same soils, well then, we absolutely have to look at the carrying capacity of those landscapes, the soil health, and the water health, and habitat health. And so, the example is that if we focus on soil health over pest management, over plant growth, right? Because a lot of industrial agriculture is looking at growing plants really, really fast, shortening the growth times so you can get quicker harvests and then mechanizing those harvests. Now if we focus on soil health, it's going to look slow at first. It's going to look more inefficient because we have to now repair all the damage that we've done, and that restorative time-frame is going to be a transitionary time-frame. And so the folks who have a short-sighted view of agriculture are going to say, "This is less productive. This is more expensive." And that is often the excuse and the argument that we hear when we have conversations about ecological agriculture versus conventional agriculture and this whole thing about which one can feed the world or what not. It is that it's a short-sighted view that the industrial agriculture system today can actually provide food for everyone or the planet. And that if we get stuck in that short-sighted view, we've missed the thing entirely, which is that soils have to be able to sustain that kind of activity, that kind of growth, that kind of extraction. And the only way for soils to be able to sustain that sort of production, is if they are alive with biology. If they are sequestering carbon every year and have an increase in organic matter every year, like Paul and Elizabeth Kaiser, they're actually two properties that way [points to his right], so they're good friends. Yeah, I could almost throw a cucumber and hit their property from where I'm sitting right now. So they're good friends of mine.

Brendan [00:15:06]: Throw it this way. Yeah, I love cucumbers.

Erik [00:15:08]: Yeah. Okay.

Brendan [00:15:09]: Don't waste it.

Erik [00:15:11]: Well, they'll be coming [unintelligible] my way.

Brendan [00:15:12]: And I actually just had one an hour ago. [Laughter]

Erik [00:15:15]: It's really about a time-frame piece, and I think that we see more and more examples like Paul and Elizabeth Kaiser. I mean not exactly like their system, but we see more and more polyculture, smaller scale ecologically sensitive farms cropping up every single day because the other part of the issue is that we have this globalized agriculture market and, again, we can't flip it overnight. It's going to take time, but going back to local is an ultimately more long-term solution. People are producing where they live and purchasing and consuming products close to where they live. That is, honestly, the only multi-generational ecological agriculture model that I believe will work over time. Now we have this bloated economy and this bloated industrialization where we're transporting goods thousands of miles to get to people's dinner tables. And so it's going to take time to transition from that, but we see a really positive trend in the small organic farm movement, through community supportive agriculture, through farmer's markets. These are actually growing and increasing every year. You might have the study, I'm not sure, but I know there was some study recently that was like organic farming is growing at a massive rate compared to the agricultural endeavors and is one of the fastest growing markets at least here in the United States, probably globally as well. Usually those are smaller scale, so we see some interesting things happening like say with Amazon buying out Whole Foods and with Walmart trying to go organic and so we see some of these big corporations now actually investing in their version of organic, which is kind of a watered-down version of organic agriculture. It's still monoculture. It's still highly extractive. But they're limiting synthetic use of chemicals and fertilizers and such. So there's some gains there. But, ultimately, it's the more diverse, ecologically situated farms that are truly the way of the future. That are focusing on soil health. That are focusing on water health, focusing on habitat.

Brendan [00:17:52]: And to me, all the examples I've seen is that what generates productivity and, yeah, there might be a transition period. But the examples I've ever heard of are just blowing conventional agriculture out of the water like the Kaisers, like Gabe Brown, things like that. Colin Seis, you know he's also in this event. It's mind-blowing. So I'm actually going to read a quotation from Bill Mollison, founder of Permaculture. Bill Mollison said once, "There's one and only one solution and we have almost no time to try it. We must turn all of our resources to repairing the natural world and training all our young people to help. They want to. We need to give them the chance to create forests, soils, clean waters, clean energies, secure communities, stable regions, and to know how to do it from hands-on experience." So, you're providing that opportunity for people to regenerate their local environments and produce food. I'm just curious if you can get into how your training works. How do you make this available to people as a planet friendly, planet loving, planet-celebrating lifestyle.

Erik [00:19:12]: Well, I absolutely love that quote. I really appreciate your sharing that because I think it really speaks to the kind of situation we're in. And the answer to that about the work we're doing and how people can create livelihoods from repairing the Earth and give opportunities to our young people, to everybody to do this work. The answer is that it's going to be different in every community, so again context is really key and applying the principles of Permaculture to our movement-building is really, really important. And what we've discovered we're in the United States is that we have some really serious challenges in terms of people being able to do this kind of work. And here are some of the challenges. One, is that there aren't a lot of jobs or career paths or economic opportunities for people to do ecological landscaping, regenerative farming, or to get into this work as a career, and that's a huge problem in the United States, especially because people don't have access to large areas of land anymore because of private property and in the way that our communities have been designed. So a lot of folks just can't even get on to the land because of private property issues and land access issues, and they can't take the time to just work the land and be in relationship because of the burden of the economic system that we're currently living in where people are striving to just get health insurance or healthcare, or to pay their rent or to transport themselves to their jobs or what not. So, what we've done, and I'm the Director of the Permaculture Skills Center, and we've been around since

2012, and the reason why I started the Permaculture Skills Center was specifically to address this issue because I've been doing Permaculture since I was 19, so that's about 20 years, and in that time, through applying Permaculture in a lot of different types of ways, through activism, through non-profit work, through community volunteerism, through farming, through landscaping, through business, I've applied to all these different kinds of realms, and one of the things that's been very frustrating is that, for many people, this work is a hobby, a hobby that they do on the weekends because they're tied to their jobs. Because they're burdened by the economic system. Because they don't have access to a lot of land where they can, say, grow a farm, or create some kind of economic income. That for a lot of people, it's become a hobby, and so what we've done at the Permaculture Skills Center is we've been strategizing and designing an economic model using the principles of Permaculture that train people to become professionals in ecological design, in regenerative farming, and all the sub-categories that fall into that. Because there's a lot. You could operate a nursery. You could grow and create herbal medicine. You could be a teacher. You could do worm composting. There's all kinds of micro-businesses and economic potential within the realm of ecological restoration. But there's not a lot of training to not only learn those techniques but then to market them effectively, to build a business plan, to have a thriving business. So that's really the piece. Because I own five businesses. I have Permaculture Artisans, that's the landscaping contracting company. I've got Forsyth Mapping, that's a digital mapping company, and I've got Permaculture Skills Center. That's our vocational training school and farm incubation training center. And so as we work these different edges, what we're trying to do is create as much economic opportunity for folks to get into the restoration economy. I've had this vision of, "What if everybody, for their career, were actively restoring the planet?" Because you've got folks unhappy in their jobs. You have people doing desk jobs or they're working for huge corporations. They're not happy but they need that income. They need the money to take care of their families and a lot of people work really, really hard to just provide basic income, basic need for their families. So what if the work we did was building soil, was catching and filtering water, was growing organic food, was providing herbal medicine, was taking care of people, providing emotional support and social community support for people. What if those were career paths that folks could step into, and that we actually create an economy around restoring the planet? Because here we are in this day and age. We've lost hundreds of millions of tons of top soil. We've polluted millions of gallons of water. There's so many issues with climate change, and you could pick any one of the ecological crises we have today and you can see that it's a huge problem. So what if we built an economy that actually repaired the systems, that actually regenerated all the basic processes that provide for healthy living communities and a healthy world. So that's what we do at the Permaculture Skill Center. We kind of have two tracks. We've got the farming track so people who want to actually get into food production as a business. And it's not just farming. There's distribution. There's marketing. There's how to build, how to create a business out of it because now-a-days that's how small farmers are going to make it. It isn't just because they grow really great carrots, or they have the best pastured eggs. I mean, having a high-quality product is important, but that's not what's going to make a farmer successful in this day and age. It's going to be, are they able to build relationships with their customers? Can they provide consistently? Can they at least break even so they can have a livelihood out of it, if not actually make a profit so they can invest in themselves and their families? So these are the kinds of questions we're asking at the Permaculture Skill Center. And ecological landscaping, in my opinion, happens to be a huge potential for developing career paths in all of these realms because many people, at least in the United States and in many countries in the world, have some kind of landscape. I mean, in 2016, it was a $72 billion industry in the United States. Landscaping was. And I always wonder, and I don't have the metrics on this, but how many of that $72 billion of landscape projects in 2016 was chemical intensive, water intensive lawns versus drought tolerant or edible gardens or carbon sequestering landscapes. So that's an industry that I feel has so much room for people to create career paths becoming ecological landscapers. And within becoming ecological landscapers we're designing people's homesteads. We're connecting people back to their food. Literally. I'm designing and building kitchen gardens for my clients where they're now harvesting all of the vegetables they need. They're getting eggs from their chickens. Some of them might even have some cows. They're getting milk, they're making cheese. They're in relationship with their land because we do have this private property issue, and so people who are buying and stewarding lands and stewarding landscapes. Well if we can get to those people, and we can …. If our message can be, "You can have a beautiful landscape that meets all of your aesthetic requirements, but at the same time, has all of these ecological benefits of catching and storing water, building soil, sequestering carbon, enhancing habitat, of growing food so you can, in a way, have your beautiful landscape and eat it too." And so, that's one of the things that we've been focusing a lot at the Permaculture Skill Center is how do we train people to become professional ecological landscapers and farmers and build career paths so, like I said, its way more that technique. It's way more than knowing how to prep a bed. It's way more than knowing how to plant a fruit tree or put in a rainwater harvesting system. It's how do you build relationships with those clients. How do you market your services? Where do you get your materials from? How efficient can you be in your implementation strategies? What's your follow up plan? And a lot of these are business skills that we don't teach in the ecological community. We're often focused on technique and design and not necessarily business acumen. So what we're trying to do is bring business organizational structures, understanding and training to augment the ecological training that's out there and help people actually build livelihoods, full-on livelihoods and careers doing this work. And, of course, it's going to look absolutely different depending on where you are. If I live in Oakland versus rural Sonoma County. I'm going to have a much different approach to creating my ecological business because the community I'm in, and the environment I'm in, the climate I'm in. So it's how do we train people to have those assessment skills? The assessment of their community. The assessment of their demographics. The assessment of the issues that are happening in their community that they want to solve. Because, ultimately, you have to start with solving the problems of your community, and doing that in an ecological way. If you can identify what the problems are in your community and then come up with solutions, ecological and social solutions to regenerate those communities and those landscapes, then people are going to flock to that solution and support it.

Brendan [00:29:35]: Can you give me some examples, maybe, of things you've done? I have this vague recollection from how many years ago? I guess it's almost three years ago. At Permaculture Voices. And it seemed to me you were giving examples of something. Because you started out by giving a lot to your community and that was actually, like kind of your marketing. But it was so fun for you as I recall because you're very socially oriented in all senses of the word. So, just curious if you can give some examples of identifying community problems in the community, solving them, and having that grow your business.

Erik [00:30:14]: Yes, absolutely. So in our community, and this is a simple one which is really rampant not just in California, but other parts of the world and the country. So, first off, we've been in a pretty significant drought here in California. Last year was a very wet year, but proceeding that, were three very dry years. We're still fully in a drought. This might be another drought year, this season 2017-2018 season. So one of the issue that came up. There's a whole series of issues. So you had first the drought, then you have lack of funding for our municipalities and our County government to actually care for their public landscapes. So people can't afford to irrigate, so farms are drying up because there's no water. Folks can't even water their lawns because it's too expensive, or there's only so much water you're allowed to use. There's rationing. So there's all these issues related to water, and that affects landscape. And then people still want to live in beautiful landscapes, and they still want productivity. So how do we solve this problem? So a few different things have happened in our community. People who would never really get involved in Permaculture, ecological gardening or farming. Folks who are just conventional, regular people all of the sudden their wells have dried up. All of the sudden, the water's too expensive or they're rationing. So they actually start calling my company, Permaculture Artisans, because they need a rainwater harvesting system. That's the only way they're going to be able to have water to use to even grow a few plants outside. Even if they want beauty, not even talking about edibility or other functions. Just aesthetics. Someone even just wants a drought tolerant native aesthetic garden, you still need some water to establish getting all that. So the drought has been a huge problem that has impacted a lot of communities, not just ecologically-minded communities. Everybody's impacted by this. And so people start getting attracted to the same exact solutions that we've been providing for decades. The same solutions that folks have been using around the world, homesteading people and ecological designers for generations, which is water harvesting storage. And even in a drought, water harvesting is still one of the most viable ways to get to secure water because here we've got 20 inches of rain. That's a drought year for us. And 20 inches of rain can still harvest tens of thousands of gallons of water off the roof of my house in a drought year and store that and have that to use for irrigation. So that's one of the problems we've been solving is helping people with their water systems and their water security, not only in the catchment and storage of rainwater off of structures and storing it in tanks, but also designing their landscapes in such a way where they don't need as much water. I mean to a lot of people just the idea of mulch is a new idea. And putting mulch down on a landscape will reduce irrigation by 30%. So, it reduces evaporation and everything. So even just getting people's landscapes mulched, designing contour water harvesting systems in their landscapes so that when it does rain, their landscapes hold water rather than drain water away and then creating storage systems. So that's been a huge one. And so then on top of that you have municipalities and county governments that are trying to figure out how to care for their public lands. And so one great example is that we worked collaboratively, in our town here, Sebastopol, along with an amazing organization called Daily Acts, who are cutting edge leaders in providing these kinds of solutions in a public sphere. And so Permaculture Artisans, together with Daily Acts, together with the City of Sebastopol, we redesigned our whole city hall and library. Our city hall and library are right next door to each other. So we redesigned that whole landscape to be a water harvesting, edible food forest. Now what's really interesting about this, and something that I think that is worth mentioning, is that sometimes in order to get a client or a community to buy-in to an ecological concept, you have to sell them on some other ideas that they're really excited about. So here's the example. When we were designing the city hall library, it was a group of folks from the community, master gardeners and artists and volunteers from the community were coming to meetings where we were designing, planning, and organizing this project. And it took us two years of planning. I think I gave about $5000 worth of design time away for free. Permaculture Artisans did professional designs, and we didn't charge anything for that. Out of that community process, people wanted historical context in the garden. They wanted education. They wanted a whole set of different functions in that landscape other than just reduce the water needs. And other than just having some public edible gardens that people can … So what we did was we integrated all that, and that's the beauty of applying the principles of Permaculture is that we accept and integrate feedback, and we look for those relationships where the sum of all the different parts is greater than each individual piece because we're systems designers. So what we did was, we created a cultural history garden. So the garden was broken into four different sections, each representing a different era of our region. So there's an area devoted to indigenous native plants that the indigenous people of this area, the Pomo, have used for millennia. So we have a whole area that's dedicated to that era. Then we have, we're a very agrarian community. People have settled here and have grown crops for a couple hundred years. So we had the agrarian sort of settlement era garden where we had apples and plums and figs and grapes and things that people have been growing. Luther Burbank. His base of operation is in Sonoma County. So we had the Burbank Garden, and then we had kind of the modern day ecological Permaculture garden. So part of why I'm sharing this example is because it's weaving in a lot of different pieces that came out of a community process, and I think that's really, really important that people do this work in the community. Is that we don't show up with all the answers. That we actually show up with listening ears so that we can be in a community process where everybody has a voice and then, as the Permaculturist, we look at integrating and organizing these different voices and this different input in a way that everyone can be happy and that we have an ecological impact. So now when people visit the city hall library, it's been a couple of years since we installed this food forest, they can actually walk through history and learn about the land relationship history of our region for the past hundreds or millions of years or even thousands of years just by walking through that garden and they can pick food and eat it and experience that.

Brendan [00:38:10]: That's beautiful. And you know some of the questions that might be on somebody's mind if they're looking at this, and they're like "Wow. This sounds like a great way to make a living and be a contribution in the world, but I've got a family of four. I've got to support". And I remember being at a business seminar quite some years back, and the guy that was speaking about his program, he had been a musician and you know, one of his jokes was "What's the difference between a musician and a pizza? And the answer is … a pizza can feed a family of four". [Laughter}.

Erik [00:38:51]: That's a good one.

Brendan [00:38:52]: And can one of these businesses that you help people design, feed a family of four, and how well? [Laughter] Hopefully, you get to eat better than pizza.

Erik [00:39:05]: Or they're eating wood fired oven pizza out in their natural oven that they built all with harvested toppings. So, yes, very good question. What's the viability of building an economy that restores the planet? What's the viability of creating businesses that build soil, catch water, grow food, connect people back to the land? And it's huge. You can make plenty of money. You can have an abundant life doing this work, but you have to be strategic. And I think that is where people get hung up, and this is where things get a little controversial, I believe, because you have a spectrum of doing Permaculture and ecological farming and landscaping. There's a spectrum, and where are you on that spectrum? If you're way over here and absolutely 100% pure ecological "I'm going to have no impact. I'm going to use zero fossil fuels. I'm going to only eat food that I'm going to grow". Then that's actually not a very economic model. That could be really amazing for a personal, someone who is very principled, and they want to have the least impact on the planet. Well, I absolutely admire people who are doing that. I admire them hugely. But that's a very isolated life where folks are essentially living off the grid, growing their food, operating their homesteads. But they can't really leave their homesteads because of the amount of work that's required. And that's not really a way to necessarily have an income. So the reason why I bring that up, is the truth is most people don't even have a choice to go live off the grid and grow their own food. That's not an option that is viable for most people. And while it's a beautiful, beautiful sentiment—I wish all of us could do that—it's just not the reality of today. And if we say that you can only practice Permaculture if you're pure like this, then we've essentially doomed most people on the planet because they literally don't have land access for that. So I bring that up because if you want to be successful, if you want to create a career, well then you do have to integrate in the modern day economy in some ways. So there's some sacrifices to be made. You might have to drive yourself to your jobs. You may work with client's, and you may have client's every now and then that are doing things that aren't great. They aren't spraying chemicals, but they want to build rock walls everywhere and where's that rock coming from? And they're making decisions around the house that they're building that you don't necessarily agree with, but you don't have the power to change their idea, but they really want you to create a water harvesting system to go along with their big, chemical intensive house. So there's a part to this which is that we can be in this transition phase where we help people transition away from extractive practices to the ability that they have the capacity to do that, to push people to their edges, but without turning them off so much that they're just going to write us off as a subculture hippie movement that isn't going to last and isn't actually relevant in today's economy, in today's world. So I think that's an inner thing that people have to reconcile with, and it's obviously all about context and where they live and the community and the demographics and all that. But, if you're willing to integrate with your community, whatever that is, even if they're not ecological, even if they don't have the same consciousness that you have and that you push with the values of your business, that is what I teach my students, is that … your message, the message that we use, the language that we use, the attitude that we bring to the table when we're working with clients, this is the make or break for any of these businesses. And if we show up, not in judgement, but in empowerment, where we're supporting people's visions, and we are pushing them in the right direction and providing as many ecological solutions as we can for them, then we can really have successful businesses that are pushing the edge of ecological solutions. And one thing that I've noticed is that, because I work with a lot of these clients, who are at that transition edge, once they get in, and you get them for the first time they grow their own tomato, for the first time they've harvested a carrot out of their garden or they harvested an apple from a tree that you've planted for them, that becomes an addiction for folks, like "Wow. That food … it tasted better. I saw it grow, and I have this relationship with it. I was watering it and I saw the birds landing on it." And there's this whole story now that you've connected people back to their place through, say, ecological landscape that you may have designed and implemented for somebody. And that is going to lead to new things. That's going to lead to those clients having more questions, hopefully, wanting to dive deeper, and it's a start. So, Permaculture Artisans, my company, we've been around since 2006. We sell over a million dollars of landscapes every single year. And I have over 15 employees. Everybody that works for me is getting paid a living wage or above. And some of these people, who are working for me, they're sending money back to their families in Mexico. There's dozens and dozens of peoples and families that are being totally taken care of through my company, Permaculture Artisans. And the people who work for me every day, they're designing and installing systems that are catching water, building soil, connecting people to the land, growing food. So this is possible. It is doable, and you can make a good living doing it. It's just what happens between the ears is actually where all the limitation occurs. So if we can open ourselves up, get out of our own way, then we can really see what's possible and implement these solutions at scale.

Brendan [00:45:51]: That is so exciting. There was an article that I read somewhere. You were quoted as saying "Imagine creating a business that catches millions of gallons of water, builds soil on hundreds of acres, plants hundreds of useful trees every year, restores native habitats, redesigns our cities or schools and new developments." And so I think that pretty much sums up the potential of eco-regenerative landscaping. I'm curious, do you have like top three tips for somebody creating a livelihood like this or maybe it would be better to ask, what's the game plan for somebody to start this? Obviously, there's a transition period. There's training. What does that look like?

Erik [00:46:41]: Great question. And so the top three tips would be, 1. Identify the problems in the community. What are the issues in your climate, in your community, that need to be solved, whether it's a drought, whether it's flooding, whether it's a waste issue, whether it's the forest is dying. What are the kind of catastrophes that need to be mitigated? Do you live in a fire ecology? Are there hurricanes? We just had this fire storm that hit Sonoma County just a few months ago, and this has opened up the opportunity to have a whole conversation about land management, about how do we live in a fire ecology? And this opens up, honestly, a whole bunch of potential ecological design markets for people in this community to support people in the regeneration after fire. In the remediation of the toxic runoff. In the management of our forest ecosystem so fires aren't so catastrophic. So these are the kinds of things you want to ask yourself about your community - What kinds of issues your community might deal with. And so that the more you can observe and assess, first your community context and the context of your environment. That should lead to a bunch of different ideas about potential services or products that one could offer. So I would say that step 1 is to do a deep dive assessment of the context of your community and your environment and the problems that need to be solved. Step 2 is an inner reflection. What makes you happy? You know what kinds of activities do you enjoy? Because this is, ultimately, going to be the make-or-break for most people. It's great to get excited about doing this kind of work and to see the vision, but if you hate it, it's not right for you. Now, if you're more of an educator than you are a farmer, that's totally okay. Then you want to move your business to more of an education angle than a farming angle. So you also need to have that inner context, your own holistic context about who you are, what interests you, what your skills are, and let that help guide that kind of business design. So then step 3 would be now bring these two together. You've assessed your community. You've assessed the context of the problems in the community and how to solve then. You've done some inner reflection about who you are and what makes you happy and the kind of work you want to do. Now, step 3 is to brainstorm what kinds of businesses where you can thrive in who you are and provide services or products that solve some of these issues in the community. So I'm going to add a step 4 here. So, there is those three steps. So step 4 is get out and start building relationship in your community. What other organizations or individuals or businesses that are already doing some of the things that you're interested in, that you want to do? It's okay. We don't have to think about this as competition. We can think about it as collective organizing and cooperation and community building. But go out there and volunteer for other people's organizations. Help other people's projects, because that is the network that will be the foundation for your new business when you start your new business. And step 5 would be to get the training where you've identified "Well, I need to learn these 5 skill sets in order to now be successful". Well, go get that training. It's okay if you don't have the experience. If you have the interest and the passion, you have a good model for what you're going to do, then you can learn anything. And if you're determined and passionate about it, you'll gain those skills, you'll get the right people on the team, you'll network with the right organizations and you'll have a real recipe for success.

Brendan [00:50:39]: Awesome. And so you're recommendation might be Permaculture skills. What's the full name of your company, again?

Erik [00:50:46]: The Permaculture Skill Center.

Brendan [00:50:48]: Center?

Erik [00:50:50]: Yes.

Brendan [00:50:51]: Awesome. Well it's been great to have you here, and you're so articulate and making such an impact and inspiring a lot of people. It always inspires me to hear you speak about this. To actually have a track, a path to run on. It's not just ideas up in the clouds. It's grounded. You've got students. They're doing what they're doing, and you have a whole teaching faculty. The Kaisers, they also teach for you, correct?

Erik [00:51:24]: Yes.

Brendan [00:51:25]: And they farm. And they're also active as teachers. I think I'm going to move to Sebastopol.

Erick [00:51:31]: Yeah, exactly. Come on out and get trained.

Brendan [00:51:35]: Let me ask you this. Let's say I'm not moving to Sebastopol, and I live where ever I live. How can I, if I wanted to, access training of this sort? How would I do that?

Erik [00:51:45]: We've come across this issue quite a lot the last few years, which is that it's difficult for people to come out to our training center and take our programs. Because people live all over the place and it's a lot of energy. So what we've done is we've now created a whole set of online programming. And that online programming (our first major program) is the Eco-Landscape Mastery School. We call it the ELM School, and that is a full step-by-step online training program where folks can learn everything they need to know to design, develop, build, and scale their own ecological landscaping business. And so folks can sign up for that. They can get the whole program all at once, and then every month we do live questions and answers. We have the mastermind group where we do have a lot of engagement and then we bring in experts from all over the world, kind of like your model here, Brendan, of bringing people in and having these conversations that augment and support people on their journey. And then we also work with our partners at Lift Economy. They're incredible business mentors. They've been business mentors of mine for many years. And so we've created a coaching package with them. One-on-one coaching for folks who want to get involved. It's pretty exciting because I actually want people to stay where they are. Don't come to Sebastopol. I mean if you want some hands-on...

Brendan [00:53:17]: That would defeat one of the principles, right? [Laughter].

Erik [53:20]: Yeah. Exactly. Reduce your carbon footprint. We do have a lot of hands-on training at our center, so that is beneficial if people come out for our hands-on training. Because there's nothing like getting your hands-on and learning that way. But, for the most part, you can learn in your own community and implement in your own community. What we're providing through the ELM School is a full mentorship, coaching, and support training program that helps people create livelihoods restoring the planet. And so we have our initial ELM School, and now we're also producing a whole series of short programs with experts from around the world. So we'll have Penny Livingston talking about regenerative agroforestry. We have Robert Kourik talking about drip irrigation and so on and so forth. Creating a whole set of mini courses so people who are like "Well, I really need to learn about irrigation", then we'll have a course just on that. That folks can get some engagement there. And we'll bring a lot of live sessions, kind of like the way we've done this, where we have video conferences, live video webinars and such that help people get more engagement, ask questions, get those questions answered, and such. So, I think, with the technology today, education is really changing and evolving and the more that we can utilize these online programs, like what we're doing here Brendan, is absolutely incredible to be able to get this knowledge, this inspiration, these tools, these techniques out to people all over the planet. In a way, you can be sitting in your home, in your pajamas, one weekend. Your kids can be playing in the background. And you can be learning and getting inspired and moving forward with your dreams. It's a beautiful thing and we're excited to be able to offer some of that too.

Brendan [00:55:11]: Awesome. Thank you once again for being with us here in the Eat4Earth community and your contributions to the entire planet.

Erik [00:55:19]: My pleasure. Thank you.

Marjory Wildcraft Interview
Grow Your Own Food, Make Your Own Medicine

Brendan [00:00]: Welcome back to the Eat4Earth event. We're exploring how you can heal your body, your loved ones, and your planet with food. And I'm speaking with Marjory Wildcraft today. Marjory is the founder of The Grow Network, and she's been featured as an expert on sustainable living by *National Geographic*. She hosts the annual Homegrown Food Summit, which reaches hundreds of thousands of viewers every year, and she's also best known for her DVD series, *Grow Your Own Groceries*, which has over half a million copies in use by homesteaders, foodies, preppers, universities, and missionary organizations around the world. Very impressive, Marjory, and I am so glad to have you here!

Marjory [00:43]: Thank you for having me on the show, Brendan. I sure appreciate it.

Brendan [00:47]: Yeah! So, Marjory, whereas my focus has been on driving consumer demand and pressure on the food system to change the food system, your focus is more on helping people opt-out of the food system by growing their own food and medicine. So, why do you believe that it's so important for each one of us to learn this?

Marjory [01:11]: Well, there are numerous reasons and, first of all, I would really like to acknowledge the work you're doing, and activism to change the food system is absolutely important. My main concern is that there's a timeline there. Right now, every bite of commercially-grown food that you're putting into your body ... GMOs, pesticide-laden and horrible factory-grown meat ... is doing damage to your body. *Right now*! And, yes, we really want to change that system, but it's going to take a lot of activism and a lot of time, and you don't have that time. You need to be eating healthy, good food right now! A lot of people go, "Hey, I'm eating organic food," and I'm going to tell you that organic standards really have been watered down. And, yes, you absolutely want to support your local farmer but, really, we can't have a local ... Another reason for this is that we can't have a local food system without a huge level of participation from backyard gardeners and backyard farmers. We just can't. I know a lot of people say, "Our local food movement is healthy and it's clean and safe," and, "Let's support our local farmers." And I say, "That's great but you know what? We cannot depend on a network of local farmers." There's just not ... Historically, it has never been possible for a bunch of local farmers to feed people. Everybody has to participate at some level. And, you know, the kitchen garden, the backyard flock, the backyard rabbitry, the pig you raise once a year, that kind of thing ... and we can go into why but it's absolutely vital ... a network of farmers could not survive without a supporting network of backyard producers.

So, one: You have to get going immediately. You can't wait, alright? Your health is in danger *right now*! The other is that a real, truly sustainable food system absolutely has to have ... I hate to use the word "army", but it really does have to be on that kind of magnitude or scale of backyard producers. And the third thing, you know, is we live in incredibly challenging times, right? This latest trade war and interest rates rising and, you know... The fact is, the United States government's bankrupt. It has been for a long time. I love that quote ... I think it was Roy Rogers who says that, "You go bankrupt slowly [unintelligible] suddenly." And there are many, many other threats or scenarios where we could have a lot of problems. The bankruptcy of the United States would ultimately be accompanied by massive amounts of inflation and hyperinflation. Of course, there's all these other ... and I don't like to get all gloom and doom, but the bottom line with almost any one of those scenarios is food becomes very difficult to maintain, food and medicine. So, having the skills to be able to grow or produce or wildcraft your own supply of food is like being able to print your own money. And it just is a level of insulation and security. People talk about wanting to heal the root chakra, and the way to do that is to have a garden and a flock of chickens. (Laugh) You know, really! (Laugh) And, so, people go, "Oh, but I could never ..." Listen, we have a product called, "How to Grow Half Your Own Food in Your Backyard in Less Than an Hour a Day." We show you how to grow half of your own food very simply and very easily, just in a backyard-sized space. So this is something that's very achievable by anybody and even, just, absolutely necessary.

Brendan [05:02]: You know, you also help people grow their own medicine, and I'm just wondering if you can give us an example, like, what does that mean, "Grow your own medicine?" And, I mean, food as medicine, sure, but anything else that goes beyond the regular dinner table food as medicine ...

Marjory [05:22]: Absolutely, yes!

Brendan [05:23]: ... with all the nutrient density that comes from growing your own and good soil. But what else is there? Is there anything else to the growing-your-own-medicine idea?

Marjory [05:30]: Yeah, there's a lot more, and I'm so glad that you acknowledge that the premier one is what you're eating. That is absolutely your first medicine. But, absolutely, I grow a ton of other medicines and, actually, quite a lot of them are just plants that are growing in my yard, or that I wildcrafted, that are just available. One of my favorite medicines is prickly pear. You know, you use the flowers of the prickly pear. It's a really, really good thing to make into a tea and it's very good for microcapillaries. I'm working on a project to improve my vision and, uh, vision is highly dependent on good ol' bloodflow from your micro capillaries in that whole eye area. I also use the pads of the prickly pear for poulticing for treating all sorts of things. Breaks, sprains, bites, injuries. Actually, all around my yard ... everywhere. I look at everything as ... You know, dandelions? Great! If you have any kind of digestive upset, that bitter really helps you. I often just eat a little bit of dandelion leaf before supper because that bitter will help get the digestive going. I'll get more nutrition out of whatever I'm eating because my digestive system is primed for it.

Um, you know, tons and tons ... Often when I'm travelling, I go to a gathering of people who are ... we practice and trade the skills of the Paleolithic era. It's kind of a hobby for me, and they meet up in the Sonoran desert. And, while I'm there, I harvest a bunch of chaparral, which is an amazing bush that is very, very good for treating sunburn or when you have too much exposure to the sun. It also, on a tonic-type of basis, is very good for helping support the liver and liver function. So ...

Brendan [07:18]: So is dandelion. I think it is a super-powerful liver tonic, really. For me, anyway. Some things affect some people more than others, but for me dandelion is very powerful for liver and gallbladder cleansing.

Marjory [07:33]: Yeah, so, you know, there's medicine everywhere. And I think one of the big distinctions between home medicine and this kind of medicine and, say, you know, the allopathic conventional medicine is, herbal medicine's very gentle, and it's often much more preventative, and it focuses on being preventative. You know, the allopathic is going to be the "wham, bam, thank you ma'am," you know ... antibiotics, surgery or, you know, some major thing. Whereas, herbal medicine is a lot more gentle and it's a lot more simpler and often, if you really do have something you're working with, you're not going to just take one herb. You're going to use two, three, or you're going to use them in a variety of different ways. So, it's often a much more holistic approach. But, yeah, you know, the two go hand in hand. The Grow Network is actually the premier community of people who are growing their own food and making their own medicine and becoming extraordinarily healthy. And we have an emphasis on both in the community, both herbal medicine as well as growing food.

Brendan [08:37]: Okay, and have you ever actually had a situation where you needed to use your medicine?

Marjory [08:43]: Many, many, many times, you know? (Laugh) So, I think one of the most famous incidents happened about two years ago. I was out in my tomato garden. I got this big, fat, big steak tomato. It was gigantic and I was so excited and I was barefoot ...

Brendan [09:00]: Now, was this in Texas or ...? It must've been in Texas.

Marjory [09:04]: Yeah, this was in Texas.

Brendan [09:06]: Not in your new home. Right now, we're talking to you in your new second home in Colorado. Your, I guess, farmhouse that you're renovating?

Marjory [09:12]: Yes, that's why my background here is looking kind of rough. But, I was in this tomato patch, and I just kind of threw caution to the wind because ... the first rule you should never do is, you shouldn't stick your hands or your feet where you can't see them. And I had this one tomato that was so big and I said, "Oh my God! I wonder if there's another one in there." And I just plunged into the patch and then, BAM! I felt this sharp pain on the top of my foot. And I looked down, and there's the tell-tale, two-puncture wound. I had been bitten by a snake and, just through the process of elimination, it became very quickly apparent that I had been bitten by a copperhead, which is a venomous snake. And it was a deep bite because when I jerked my foot back, I felt the fangs dig in even deeper, right? So, I know I got a good dose. You know this is going to be a trip! I didn't even think of going to the hospital. At this point in development, I've been using herbal medicine now for fifteen or twenty years and my husband said, "You want to poultice it?" And I was like, "The prickly pear patch! Go get me some pads of the prickly pear."

By the way, you could use a lot of other things. You could use chopped cabbage. I've used that to treat mastitis, a breast infection. You can use clay, a great classic poultice. You can use plantain leaves. You can use comfrey leaves. People very successfully have used chopped raw potato. I haven't had a chance to use that one yet. I will also just use raw meat. Once, I had a big eye infection and I just put a piece of steak on it and it felt so good! It was just drawing out all the...

So, anyway, we treated it at home, and it took a couple of days to overcome. And I could give you a tip. If you want to poultice something, the two keys to poulticing are ... there's two things you have to do. One is you need to make the poultice much bigger than you think. So, for example, on that snake bite, it was on the top of my foot, and my foot was swelling to about my ankle. We got big prickly pear pads. My husband took the spines off and put it in the blender and created this slurry. And then we put that in a plastic bag, and we encased my foot in this prickly pear slurry, the entire foot, halfway up my calf. And that's the first thing. You want to make it much bigger than the actual injury. And the second is, you need to keep it on longer than you think. So, we would have a prickly pear pad slurry on my foot for eight hours and then clean it all off, put all that in the compost pile, and then put another poultice on of the same thing. So, we would change the poultice every eight hours. And we did that basically for two days. And then we backed it down to just having it on at night for eight to ten hours while I was sleeping. And really, within the first day, we could clearly see that this was having a really good impact. And by the second day, most of the swelling was gone down. And so, really, just the next couple of days and keeping it on in the evening was to just finish it off. But, it's almost magical, you know, the power of plant medicine and your own ... You know, the real difference there is I was willing to come out of this and take personal responsibility for my own health. And I had years of experience doing this on much smaller injuries or ailments or burns or scratches and scrapes, or whatever, so I was very confident in my skills and my ability. You know, I don't want anybody running out and thinking that they could go do that right away. And starting small is one of the steps to getting started. But that just gives you an idea of where you can go with it. I mean, that really is a venomous snake bite. It's potentially a lethal situation, so ...

Brendan [13:05]: Yeah, and back to the first kind of medicine just being food, growing it at home and taking care of the soil ... obviously, we can do a lot ... potentially exponentially higher. I mean, ten times higher nutritional content is quite possible. And it's documented, in fact, by one of our other speakers, what they were able to do from normal vegetables to vegetables that had been grown in a soil with certain mineral combinations that then ignited the ... this is Robert Van Risseghem ... it basically ignited the soil bacteria and then they made ... I mean, this is a hypothesis about how it works, but, bottom line is he showed that it worked. And it basically ... adding one mineral made twenty-two minerals available at ten times higher levels actually in the plants. Not just more available in the soil, but the plants had ten times higher ... across twenty two minerals.

Marjory [13:59]: I've got to watch that interview. Wow! That sounds really interesting.

Brendan [14:03]: Yeah, fascinating stuff. And he gets into ... well, we won't go down there. But he talks a lot about different minerals and their relationships between each other in the body as well.

So, I'm curious. You know, with your own growing, have you done any nutrient measurements? Did you use a Brix meter or anything like that and notice anything? Well, obviously you notice your vitality going up and you started skateboarding in your late forties or something ...

Marjory [14:26]: Yeah, right, isn't that crazy? Yeah, I need to get into those Brix meters. And that is something ... and also the bio-nutrient folks, Dan Kittridge ...

Brendan [14:36]: Yeah, I interviewed him as well. He's in the event.

Marjory [14:40]: Yeah, we're starting to get into that. I have not been as scientific about it. The other real indicator that I use is taste. You know, you can taste when a vegetable or a fruit has a high mineral content, and when it doesn't. And it's astonishing to me, like, in a kid's garden ...I was... For a while there, I was teaching gardening and botany to a local school. My daughter was going there so I had this other ulterior motive. But we had a little garden there, and I was shocked that a lot of the other kids there thought that breakfast was a Lunchable, right? And they had never eaten vegetables. And, so, I'm like, "Well, this is gonna be interesting, 'cause here we are growing all of this broccoli and kale and lettuce." You know? (Laugh) I definitely had the sweet peas in there and the stuff that I knew ... and the strawberries. I knew they'd go for those, but I was wondering about the other stuff. And you know what? Vegetables that are grown in nutrient-dense soil taste so much better. And then we had little cups of ranch dressing for them in the refrigerator of the classroom and on recess, they'd grab a little cup of this ranch dressing, and they'd run out to the garden, and they would eat fresh vegetables right out of that garden.

Brendan [15:53]: Maybe the reason kids are reputed to not enjoy vegetables so much, and I don't know when that whole pattern started, but maybe it's because vegetables started to lose their taste, and kids were like, "Well why ...?" Instinctively they know don't eat something without taste. Unfortunately, the hyperpalatable foods, so to speak, with all the salt, sugar, and vegetable fats, you know, to trick our taste buds into thinking that they're nutrient-dense, have taken that place.

Marjory [16:21]: You know, you have to go back a long time to find somebody who remembers what real food tastes like, other than people like myself who are eating it right now. Like, my brother's in his seventies ... I have an older brother and he's, like, "You know? You're right. Carrots and tomatoes just don't taste like carrots and tomatoes did when I was growing up." Yeah, I do want to get more into the scientific aspect of it. That's definitely a direction The Grow Network wants to go to ...

Brendan [16:48]: Well, since you're very hands on and practical and empowering people right and left with just the "how-to's" of it, can you give us some sort of ... Like, how should the average person start? Maybe some concrete tips on growing vegetables. Let's start there, and maybe if we have time we can talk about growing animals. But maybe just stick with vegetables for now.

Marjory [17:11]: Well, I would say, "Start small is the first thing." My first garden was huge, giant, and I just had a huge mess, huge weeds, and I couldn't keep up with it. So, really, a fifty-square-foot bed or a hundred-square-foot bed ... If you have a small yard, be grateful because that will limit you, alright? And the reason why is you're going to be creating a lifestyle change here, and doing it small and doing a little bit and having success is way more important than doing something big, getting overwhelmed, and having a large failure, right? So start small.

The other thing is ... grow things that you really like, right? That you really enjoy. And if that's sweet corn, if it's tomatoes, if it's cherry tomatoes, if it's, you know, bell pepper, whatever, grow something you really like.

And also, then the other thing is try to get connected with some other people who are growing. Expand your circle of relationships. If there's somebody down the street that has a garden you pass by and you don't know them, go bring them a little gift and talk to them. You know, hang out with them. Maybe go to a Master Gardener meeting or one of the ... you know, there's the gardening clubs. But, having other people that are doing it in your region ... and they'll tell you, "This variety is going to be better than that variety," or they'll give you some extra tomato plants, and say, "Why don't you transplant these in ...?" Again, you're talking about a lifestyle change, and not only is that going to be different behaviors for you, but it's going to be different circles of friends. So, start with those three. One, just start small. Two, grow something that you really, really like. And three, go find some people that are already doing it, that you could hang out with and help get some mentoring.

Brendan [19:05]: Are there specific ... so, obviously within the world of vegetables that people like ... are there any particular that are easier to start with than others? I've heard that tomatoes are not the easiest plant to learn how to grow. And a lot of people love it, but maybe it's good to get a base hit first. Get some easier wins. I'm just curious what your feedback would be.

Marjory [19:33]: I would agree with that. You know, everybody loves tomatoes. The National Gardening Association does all these surveys, and tomatoes win hands down, way above every other possible thing that you could grow. And, you know, I'm going to tell you, I do not successfully have tomato crops every year. Some years are great, and I just really haven't gotten tomatoes always down. You know, it's funny because I've been contacting a bunch of experts that are gardening experts and say, "Hey, I want to make this video all about growing tomatoes. Will you be a tomato expert?" and they're all, like, "Oh, no! We don't consider ourselves ..." And I'm, like, "Wait a minute, you're like ... whatever." (Laugh)
So, I think it's kind of a big secret that tomatoes are actually really difficult to grow, even though they're the most common. And sometimes they're really easy. It's crazy with tomatoes. But squash, cucumbers ... those kind of things ... grow really, really well. Watermelons grow really well. They might need a little bit more room. Beans are usually really easy to grow. Let's see ... some of my other favorites ... Now, I love lettuce, and I have a really great time with lettuce. That grows really well for me. Again, something that you really have a resonance with.

Brendan [20:50]: How about broccoli? Is broccoli hard to grow or easy to grow?

Marjory [20:54]: Oh, I love kale and broccoli and all the Brassicaceae family. Kale is another one of my favorites. And chard ...

Brendan [21:00]: That's easy right? And you can have a kale tree producing leaves.

Marjory [21:05]: Yes, you can. Those are pretty bullet-proof. And they'll even grow in partial shade, which is nice when you just have some ... I was just at a friend's and she goes, "I've only got four hours of sunlight a day! What can I do?" And I'm, like, "Go for the leafy greens." (Laugh)

Brendan [21:20]: Awesome! Now, if somebody's a little more experienced, are there any sort of, I guess, hitches that people will encounter in their learning curve with particularly popular vegetables or just in the learning curve, in general, where you could give a tip that would take them to the next level or might solve one of the common hurdles?

Marjory [21:45]: Well, you know there's always going to be hurdles, and there's always going to be challenges. I think the next advice I would give to anybody is, "Don't ever expect a hundred percent from your garden." Even all of our commercial growers, whether they're organic or conventional, you know ... a thirty percent loss every year is considered acceptable. So, just be prepared for losses, and don't let that phase you, right? Very, very rarely are you going to ever get everything from the plants. So, if that helps the person get over the next challenge, that's my advice to you there.

I think the next thing most people complain or issue, or wonder about is insects and pest damage. And I'll tell you, the fundamental key to controlling insects is soil vitality. So, just like you ... actually, I had a friend of mine call me up and she said, "Marjory, I got a ..." We were at this gathering together and she goes, "I think I got a cold from this other guy who was there." And I said, "No, you didn't get that cold from him." I said, "Colds are everywhere, right? You got that cold because your body ..." She lives in Durango. She'd been dealing with the threat of fire and her house burning down for the last months so a lot of stress there. And then she went on a trip to London because she'd won this big award and, then, now she was at this other meeting with me, and I said, "You're exhausted." I said, "You're going to catch a cold. Colds are everywhere. It's not because of so-and-so. It's your body." And the same thing is true with your plants. Like, when your plants don't have the nutrients that they need and they don't have the water that they need and they don't have what they need, they're going to get ... the predators of the plant kingdom are the insects, and the insects are almost always around. If a plant is really strong, they're able to fend them off. And if they're weak, then the insects will attack it. A friend of mine was an older organic gardener, and he showed me photographs he'd taken of a row of squash plants he had, and the weak one was completely devastated by the insects, and they left all the rest of the other plants alone. You know, when you've got a really good soil that's alive with microbiology and minerals and everything that that plant needs, they're going to be way healthier. And there's always some minor insect damage. That's not going to be anything, really, to worry about. And the great news is, as you eat those plants, you will get those minerals and you'll become a lot healthier, too.

Brendan [24:29]: I'm curious, have you ever done anything with fulvic acid? Because fulvic acid helps make minerals more available. It does a lot of things in the soil and for the plants, as far as facilitating mineral transfer.

Marjory [24:44]: Yeah, for sure. I love to make a compost tea and add a little bit of fulvic acid to it just to help really activate that tea and all the points you're making. It just helps the overall health of the plant. So, absolutely!

Brendan [24:58]: When you make a compost tea, are you using one of those, sort of, commercial-strength ... you know, those big reservoirs? And where do you get it? I mean, I've seen different sizes ...

Marjory [25:11]: You know what? You know, years ago I did a whole series of courses with Dr. Elaine Ingham, who was kind of the soil diva. The diva of soil microbiology. Amazing, amazing woman! And at these gatherings, she would have a "tea-off!" A compost "tea-off," where everybody would bring their compost tea maker, and we would let it brew over the weekend while we were taking the class and, at the end of the class, she would analyze all of the compost tea that had been made by all these different things. And they had this guy that pulled in with one of those big vortex machines, you know, and other people with big machines, and this is, you know, about five or six years ago and the technology has changed. You know who won? It was this guy with a five-gallon bucket and a couple of aerators with a fish tank air-bubbler. He kind of cheated, in a way, and kind of not. I mean, it ended up being a great lesson for all of us because they had given everybody the same compost to start with, and they had said, "Just use good quality water." Well, he had gone to a local pond and gotten some pond water. So, he was using the same compost, but that pond water had so much more vitality and stuff going on in it, too, that it gave this whole thing another boost. But, anyway, hands down, this guy with pond water and the same compost beat out all these other machines. So, we all had a really good chuckle over that, and it was just great. Because, really, for most home gardeners, you dilute this stuff generally ten-to-one, right? And, so a five-gallon bucket is going to give you a lot of coverage. So, really for most of us doing backyard food production who want a batch like that every now and then, it's plenty. We don't need a fifty-gallon thing of it, so...

Brendan [27:03]: That pond water idea is interesting. I was speaking to somebody recently about pets ... you know, food for pets, and so forth ... and they made the comment that pets often gravitate to the water in a pond, not the water you give to them. And you think, "Oh, don't drink that dirty water!" But it's got all this vitality. It's got good organisms. I mean, if it's not like ... it could be contaminated in certain situations, but ... especially if you're downstream of a confined animal feeding operation, then maybe it's going to kill your pet. Antibiotic-resistant microbes in there. But absent that, the water there is potentially very, very good for them, and that's why they're drinking it. You know, it's got all kinds of things going on that we could get into, even besides the organisms, but ...

Marjory [28:00]: You know, I saw that in ... So, I'm very interested in ... That's why backyard food production is so important, and real calories ... producing real calories ... and so I've always been a big proponent of raising rabbits in the backyard. And, for years, I've raised mine in cages like most people do. But I really ... the humanitarian ... like, I ... they really are ground dwelling animals, so I created this system, and ... I do a lot of research, you know, and it's been in existence. I'm not the one who invented it, but I worked on it and developed it ... raising rabbits in a colony, which is basically having them in a confined area that they could basically free-range in. And in my colony, I had a pond. A small, hand-dug pond just, you know. Like, three feet by five feet across, not a big thing, and a couple of feet deep. And when it got low, I would just fill it up with a hose or something. It wasn't any big pond. And then, of course, I had some fifty-five-gallon drums with feeders and waterers for them. And I found that the rabbits, from what I could tell, tended to prefer that little pond more than the waterer that I had placed, which had clean water in it. So, if you want to see that system, go over to Colonyrabbits.com, and there's a free video that'll show you that whole system. But I was really quite astonished to see the rabbits tended to ... I mean, I wasn't out there 24/7, but I hung out with them a lot. I like to go out and meditate amongst my rabbits. But I'd often see them in the pond drinking, instead of going to the other waterer, and I thought, "Wow! That's really interesting."

Brendan [29:38]: Maybe I was watching your video and I think my memory could be flawed. I might've actually heard … rather than having heard that in a conversation with somebody, I might've heard it or seen it on a video of yours. Maybe it was your video in the summit. I think that might've been what it was where you were talking about the rabbits. But so, anything else? Any other odd tips for getting started or getting to the next level before we move on? Anything else?

Marjory [30:06]: Well, the other thing I would say, if you're getting started … and this is at any level … if you haven't already started doing this, is start a compost pile. Because, really, fertility is going to be the key to everything you do. Start a compost pile right now. The scraps in your kitchen, the scraps from your yards, whatever … get it going because building your own soil and creating your own fertility is going to be hugely, hugely important. That's the other big tip, right? Making your own fertility by starting to compost.

Brendan [30:42]: You know, it also occurs to me to ask you about any obstacles that people … and most obstacles, you know … As we learn, as we go through life, most obstacles to doing things we want to do are right between our ears. But I was just curious … what do you find stops people … I'll out myself here. What stops me from growing right now is a). I live in an apartment, and I don't have my own deck, and I'm super busy. So, you don't have to necessarily solve my mental obstacles there. Or you could take one or both of those on. But, you know, what do you encounter as far as people's mental obstacles. The push-back, like, "I can't do this now, but I totally want to" …

Marjory [31:30]: For sure, time is definitely the biggest issue. Everybody goes, "I don't have time to do that," right? "I don't have time to do that." And, you know, I understand. But, how much time did you spend on Facebook or how much time did you spend watching Netflix or how much time did you spend on YouTube on those stupid cat videos? I love stupid cat videos. I do! I love them but, really, how important is your health and your vitality to you? I know a lot of people are going, "You know, I don't really want to do that," and I can totally get that. But that's also why we created that system of how to grow half of your own food in your backyard in less than an hour a day. To show people that, "Look, it doesn't take a lot of space, and it doesn't take a lot of time." And, you know what? That hour a day will become your most precious hour out of every day; that you will like to think you would not be able to live if you didn't get out there and get some time with your chickens or your garden. I mean, with gardening and being in an apartment, there are lots and lots of options. There really are! And I always say, "Where there's a will, there's a way." When you have an idea and you say, "I really want to do this," and you put that out to the universe, then it will be manifested. Some simple things are … you know … CSA. You can go and say you'd like to volunteer an hour, an afternoon a week or something like that. And a lot of times they'll give you the vegetables in exchange for the labor like that. And, there, you're learning directly about how they're farming, and it's almost like you're growing your own. And, of course, community gardens. And then there's … I believe it's called Shared Earth. There's a lot of different websites out there that are all about people saying, "Hey! I've got a backyard, if you'd like to garden here, let's work it out." And then there's just plain, old-fashioned, "guerrilla" gardening" of "there's a vacant lot. I am going to start planting it." You know? (Laugh) So, there's lots of ways to do it. It's really, you know, when is it going to become that important to you? And I would encourage you to do it now because it's the deep sense of security, that incredible nutrition, the quality of food and the whole enhancement in the quality of your life is so worth it. It's so worth it.

Brendan [33:55]: Yeah, awesome. You know, one of my other soapboxes that I get on in this event ... not as much as I talk about mineral deficiency and all that, and how we've got to get minerals back in our foods through soil health ... also, one of the things that's a disaster, possibly the worst disaster in our food system, or one of them, is the loss of seed and crop diversity. And it occurs to me that we've got to start building an army of people saving seeds, trading seeds and stuff, because we have certain other companies out there that actually want to make sure that we don't have access to that so they can control the food gene-pool. But it's impoverishing, not only our food but our genome because our genes were evolved along with the diversity of foods. We're made to get all of these things like RNA and so forth ... different messenger molecules and phytonutrients and so forth ... through our food and through the diversity. And when we chop out certain chunks of the food kingdom, we lose, in a sense, a part of our epigenome, or it's really our exosome, as they call it, that affects our epigenome. I'm just curious what you would have to say about that because I think you're pretty big on the issue.

Marjory [35:29]: Absolutely! I mean, at the very beginning of this interview you said, "Why?" And I said, "Well, because farmers cannot produce..." You absolutely have to have a huge participation by backyard producers and genetics is exactly the reason why. You know, people who are farming for a living do not have time to do experiments on varieties and what variety is going to be best. They do not have time to do a whole lot of plant breeding 'cause they're worried about commercial production. And, actually, historically, all of the vegetable varieties that we have now were basically developed by backyard gardeners. And one thing that I'm looking to reinstate through The Grow Network are the regional competitions. So, there used to be the regional competition where you won a ribbon for the best apple, or you won a ribbon for the best green beans, or there were prizes for the best tomatoes and what people brought in, and there was this great competition. Just a healthy regional thing, right? We have to have that because backyard producers, we have the time and luxury to experiment with things that commercial farmers, organic or whatever, don't have time to do. And that's absolutely essential for keeping it all alive. And there's been some studies that were done, and it depends on which ones you read as to whether it was ninety-seven percent or whether it's seventy-something percent, but we have basically lost almost all of the genetics that have been developed throughout history by humans. There used to be hundreds and hundreds and hundreds more varieties of different types of corn or squash, or almost any sort of vegetable or fruit that you can think of, that have been lost and gone extinct. We have already lost a huge amount of the genetics of our own food supply that had been developed over hundreds of thousands of years by our ancestors.

The same problem is happening with our livestock. One example are pigs. For the past couple of decades, we've all been on this fat-phobia thing. Nobody wants fat, so we've bred all these pigs that are really, really super lean. Actually, historically, all the homesteaders and people who raised pigs, they raised pigs for the fat. That is what they raised the pig for. The fat was not only calories, it was also soap. It was just an unbelievable, useful material.

Brendan [38:03]: It's very vitamin D rich, if it's pastured. Super healthy!

Marjory [38:09]: Yes! And all these varieties of backyard pigs we used to have. You know, pigs that were developed in the south that could withstand heat and would forage or the ones in the north that could withstand the cold. And the ones that produced the most fat were the ones that were most gentle-natured. There were all these varieties that are almost all now gone. We're really down to, you know ... We've still got some left, but that's the work of the Livestock Conservancy, which I have been a huge proponent of getting the word out about these different breeds, and saying, "Hey, if you're going to raise something in your backyard like rabbits or chickens or turkeys or pigs or whatever, raise some of these heritage breeds because we absolutely have to bring them back, and of course they're going to produce better for you than buying the commercial breeds of animals, you know, like the Cornish-Rock crosses for chickens. You're going to do way better producing with heritage breed chickens in a backyard scenario. It's similar to the seeds. We absolutely have to rebuild that whole network of backyard food producers that are breeding and exchanging genetics and developing the genetics and learning about it. And the long tail ... You know, to talk about the Ten-Year Plan for The Grow Network is ... So, initially we're building this rather massive ... I almost was stunned to find out that we actually are the largest organization on the planet now that's doing this, creating this network of backyard producers. And our mission is to get more and more people growing food. But, ultimately, we are developing products and services and information that, as you journey and as you age, ultimately you are becoming a breeder. You know, we'll have the Brendan corn, or the Brendan squash. You are a breeder of different varieties of the Brendan chickens, you know. You are creating varieties that are vitally important for the region that you live in. And that is a contribution. That's a legacy that you would be leaving for, not only your family but, your neighborhood and your community and your area. And that is ultimately where The Grow Network is going, is recreating this whole generation of people that are actually breeding their own varieties.

Brendan [40:38]: And to me it seems like it's not just an, "Oh, it'd be nice to have that." I don't know that humans can make it if we don't do that because the resilience of the seed, you know, the whole seed genome and the crop genomes ... it's all in the heritage. There's really no resiliency in the mass-produced stuff. They're more and more dependent on the chemical inputs. They no longer form mycorrhizal associations with the mycorrhizal fungi that deliver nutrients straight into the plant. We've built a very brittle food supply that can break. It'll break under the changing climate conditions and all that.

Marjory [41:24]: The main breed of cattle that they're growing for the commercial slaughterhouses cannot even survive on grass anymore They have been so over bred to only be dependent on grains that you can't put them out on pasture. They won't live.

Brendan [41:39]: The crazy thing about cattle, I mean ... They say, you know, sort of ... the conventional farmers have in their head that the cow will have to be in some warmed barn over the winter and this and that. And then there's people out there that are developing the genetics, resurging the genetics from the heritage breeds, where those cows could be out there in forty below, and they'd just huddle up like the calves in the inside and they're fine. You can have a natural system that produces more, at lower cost, of higher quality. And it's more in reach for the rest of us. We don't have to invest in all this stuff that has us wedded to annual production loans, and a certain way of doing things to qualify for the production loans, and this debt we can never get out of and all this extra burden of chemical inputs that everything in the system is addicted to and can't go without it.

Marjory [42:44]: Where you were going with that ... So the purpose of The Grow Network is to stop the destruction of the Earth and creating the premier community of people who are growing their own food and making their own medicine, and becoming extraordinarily healthy. Your body is a part of the Earth, right? So, the members of The Grow Network get that, and our catalyzing statement is ... so, everybody that works at The Grow Network ... you say, "Why do you come to work every day?" and they go, "Our statement is: Home-grown food on every table." So, everything we do is to really focus toward that. And sometimes we get people through herbal medicine, and then we go, "Hey, if you grow your own medicine, it's going to be more potent." And they grow their own medicine. And then I'm like, "Hey! You can grow your own food ..." So, we bring people in in lots of different ways, but, "Home-grown food on every table" is our catalyzing statement. And people can give me some real push back, like, "Marjory, that's ridiculous! You think about the grocery store and the beep-beep-beep every morning. They're like, "There's no way. This system is here." And I'm, like, "You know what, we're going back to home-grown food on every table one way or another. You can take the cliff, which is the way a lot of people are going ..."

Brendan [43:58]: The cliff that the lemmings run over?

Marjory [44:00]: The cliff, where you may not survive it! Or you can take the switch-backs down and start growing a garden. Start having medicinal herbs. Maybe having some chickens. Take the switch-backs down the mountain or go off the cliff, it's your choice. But we are going back to home-grown food on every table. (Laugh) So it's great to have a catalyzing statement that's inevitable. (Laugh)

Brendan [44:25]: That's awesome! So, what are some other ways that people can connect with these resources? You mentioned one which was the Colonyrabbits.com.

Marjory [44:36]: Yeah, Colonyrabbits.com is a great one. It's a short video that's just really inspiring. Like, you could grow rabbit meat in your backyard. If you go to Garlicmiracles.com, or miracleofgarlic, we have ... Your first home medicine is how to use garlic, right? It's just a great antibiotic, and you could prevent taking pharmaceutical antibiotics in a lot of situations just by this. It has a great little ebook. I believe it's garlicmiracles.com.

And just head over to thegrownetwork.com. We've got all these really interesting blog posts coming up and then the forums are some really amazing discussions. And we have a lot of people in The Grow Network who are home-working farmers. We've have naturopaths, herbalists, veterinarians, retired engineers ... a lot of really, really knowledgeable people who are coming to this and rallying around this idea that we really have to re-localize the food supply right back into our backyards. And I really have been overwhelmed and grateful and just sometimes almost brought to tears by the quality of people who are getting involved in The Grow Network and are furthering this mission. So, it's awesome! Head over to thegrownetwork.com and come check us out.

Brendan [45:59]: Awesome. Thank you so much for leading the charge to help us all re-establish food sovereignty, autonomy, and self-sufficiency. You're doing some really powerful work, and I'm excited that's it's growing so big and so fast.

Marjory [46:16]: Well, thanks so much Brendan, I sure appreciate the opportunity to get to talk to you and everyone else.

John Kohler Interview 1
Grow and Eat "Beyond Organic" Raw Plant Foods

Brendan [00:00:00]: Welcome to the Eat4Earth event. We're exploring together how you can heal yourself, your loved ones, and the planet, with food. This is Brendan Moorehead, and we're about to get real hands-on with our next guest, John Kohler. John is a public speaker, Youtuber, health coach, entrepreneur, gardener, and all-round health enthusiast. John was born with a variety of diseases and health conditions including allergies, asthma, dry skin, and eventually spinal meningitis, and eating a standard American diet in combination with unfortunate genetic predispositions left John with the option of either dying as a young man or changing his lifestyle. Fortunately, he chose the latter and in his twenties he began to heal himself predominately by eating a 100% plant-based and raw food diet. His YouTube channels are OKRaw, Growingyourgreens, which gets a lot of views, and Rawfoods as well. His website is Growingyourgreens.com. John, it's awesome to have you with us.

John [00:01:03]: I'm glad to be here.

Brendan [00:01:05]: Thank you. So, John, I really look forward to learning what you have to teach us about growing food, getting more fruits and vegetables in us, as easy and conveniently, and tastily, as possible, and even capturing carbon from the atmosphere in our own back yards and front yards, and even making money from it. You kind of cover the whole range of it in your videos. I'm curious, when you first started, when you switched to raw, was it an overnight thing or did it kind of take some time to transition?

John [00:01:38]: For me it kind of was overnight, I had a health crisis. I almost lost my life. I had spinal meningitis which the doctor said was caused by complement immune deficiency. I had also other auto-immune diseases as a child, you mentioned some of them, dry skin, eczema, allergies and what not, and when I got out of the hospital because the doctors had no cure for me, they couldn't treat me for anything because I had a viral version of spinal meningitis, which is a really nasty bug, that many people die from it unfortunately. At that point it was too late for me to do any kind of dietary intervention, and unfortunately that's how it is for most people. You get a heart attack, and you're gone. You don't get a second chance. That's what happens. Luckily, I was given a second chance, and when I got out of the hospital I said, "Well, doctors, why did I get sick?" and they said "You have what's called complement immune deficiency" which they said ...

Brendan [00:02:31]: What was it?

John [00:02:32]: Complement immune deficiency, which they said was defective genes that were just not strong, so I was not quite as bad as "the boy in the bubble" that 70s movie with John Travolta where you have to live in a bubble, and if you get any little sickness you could die. I wasn't that bad, but I wasn't like a normal person who had a pretty strong immune system. I was somewhere in the middle, and I just needed to figure out how I could build my immune system because the doctor said I could have a reoccurrence even though I got over this bout of spinal meningitis. I could have a reoccurrence and get it again or get some kind of other disease and then not be so lucky to make it out. And you know, being in the hospital as the last thing I'm seeing, just getting out of college, graduating college, that's not where I wanted my life to end. And I don't want that to happen again, I don't want to put myself in a situation, where I have some control in my life, and I could do things in my life to basically disease proof myself so that I don't get sick, I don't succumb to my complement immune deficiency because as later in time what we learned, there's genetic expression. And so what you eat determines your gene expression. Epigenetics is what they call it. And I learned that by eating better I could be a better person; my genes would be more fully expressed. I'd have a stronger immune system. I could have boundless amounts of energy. I could keep my youthful figure and my weight stable, unlike all my high school cohorts that are probably all overweight now and look like ten years older than me. It's like anti-aging, the diet that I've been on. So I just really went for it overnight because I'd read books and I learned information at the time, some of which was actually inaccurate information at the time, that I know now is inaccurate but it served me at the time. Like one of the things I learned was the reason why we shouldn't cook food is because of this thing called leukocytosis. And leukocytosis is basically when your immune system gets activated, when your white cells increase, it was said and I'd read back in the day that leukocytosis is kind of like "The boy who cried wolf", right? The boy who cried wolf … when the boy who cries and the wolf's coming, and then all the people, the villagers come and there's no wolf, and he does that a couple of times for fun, then when the wolf comes he calls "wolf", and the villagers don't come because they think he's playing. So that's how it is with our immune system. Every time we eat supposedly cooked foods, it activates our immune system, causes leukocytosis reaction, and basically it would wear your immune system down or this is what I thought, or what I had learned, and that's why I didn't eat cooked food because now my immune system could take a break and rest, and heal and regenerate, and then when I really did have some immune situation it would be ready to go, it wouldn't be boy-who-cried-wolf-ish.

But unfortunately, since that time I've learned different. It's not just any cooked food that causes leukocytosis. More recently I've determined that it's actually only cooked animal foods, so any cheese, any meat, any dairy, any eggs -- those foods cause leukocytosis raw or cooked because of the foreign proteins. And that's why if you get a liver transplant or a kidney transplant from somebody that has a similar kidney than you, you have to be on immune suppressive drugs for the rest of your life so that your body will not reject that kidney because it's foreign protein. And in plant foods there are no foreign proteins because our bodies are meant to and designed, we're designed in my opinion, to digest these plant foods.

Brendan [00:06:09]: Got you. And are you still a 100% plant-based and raw, and how long has your diet looked like that?

John [00:06:20]: So when I started in 1995, I went a 100%, or that was my goal in my head anyway. And I'm not perfect. I've slipped off the raw food bandwagon and had some baked potatoes or some like McDougal burritos like twenty years ago when I broke up with a girlfriend and had some emotional eating bouts. I'm over that stuff now, I don't need to emotionally eat anymore, like that anyways. I've tried meat like once or something and had some dairy a few times, but other than that, in the later years, like the past five, ten years I've been all plant-based. I mean I do do honeys so people that are vegan wouldn't call me a vegan, but I try to make sure it's ethically sourced because besides just being plant based or not, I think what's really important is how is the food raised, whether that's an animal product, whether that's even honey. In my opinion honey from the grocery store is atrocious. They're doing some crazy things to the bees. They're spraying them with bad chemicals, pesticides. They're mean to the bees, and basically the honey is just a commodity of farmers to basically extract money from the bees and take all their honey. But in the same token bees are required for 30% of some of the crops to be pollinated. So vegans that might chastise me for eating honey, meanwhile they're eating almonds, and what they don't realize is that those almonds have been pollinated by bees that came from south Florida or from some of the southern states, and shipped across the country in trucks with nets on them, similar and worse as pigs being trucked across the country to be slaughtered. And all these bees die in the process of coming across the country, and then these bees are enslaved in an artificial environment to pollinate these almond groves so that vegans can have their almonds, or peaches, or other fruits. But what's more important is that the bees are sustainably raised and taken care of in a proper manner and not abused. It's kind of like, you know, many people may have pets like dogs or cats, they love their dogs and cats. They're pets, and we take care of them. They provide us something; we provide them something, and there could be an even exchange in Nature like with bees. I've met compassionate bee farmers that have bees in addition to having not just monoculture but a variety of different crops for forage for them, and they don't smoke them when they need to grab the honey, they don't steal all the honey, they take just a little bit of honey but leave the bees plenty because that's literally the bees' food source. It can be done in a way where we're working with the environment, with Nature, instead of against them, instead of just basically raping and pillaging bees or animals or anything else on the planet like extracting all the oil and all the different minerals, and mining things from the planet. It's destroyed just for money.

Brendan [00:09:03]: You made a really good point as far as overall how is this food being grown, and I've heard you use the term "beyond organic" in your videos. I'm just curious what that means to you, what do you mean by "beyond organic"?

John [00:09:20]: I mean, I really like the organic standards, don't get me wrong, I buy organically raised foods, organically grown fruits and vegetables. I was just at the produce terminal on Monday, and I bought lots of different organic foods and I have actually produce haul videos showing how cheap organic food can be if you buy it properly and buy it right and get good deals on it. But the thing is, organic tells what you don't do to the plants or to the crops. Organic standards say "you could use these things; you can't use these things" and that's pretty much the rule. It's kind of like if you're a vegan it tells what you don't eat. It says if I'm vegan I don't eat animal products, but it doesn't say necessarily what you do eat. If you're vegan you could drink Coke and Oreos, and those are technically vegan supposedly, but it's junk food vegan.
Same thing with organic agriculture. It says what you can't do, it doesn't tell you what you should do or you must do to have high quality crops. And especially the vegans, a lot of people, most of them are using a fertilizer for organic crops that's actually coming from manure from factory farming, which in my opinion, I don't necessarily want the food that I'm eating growing from manure from factory farms, which is an industry which I actually don't believe in. And furthermore that industry is producing in my opinion contaminated feces, or poop that may have GMO remnants in there, maybe have heavy metal remnants in there, may have different herbicides or fungicides or whatever that's gone through the animal, or even worse like antibiotics, it's now going into the soil and affecting the soil, I mean that's what's being used normally on organic agriculture.

So to me that's at least something because it's better than conventional with the synthetics and all this kind of stuff which is actually really destroying the Earth bad. I like to kind of rise above that and do better. Not many farmers are into growing beyond organic, or using minimal, if any, manure. If you do use manure, I encourage people to use a trusted manure source like from their own cows, pigs, or sheep, or rabbits, or maybe even making human manure out of your own stuff. I'd rather use my manure than some random chicken's coming out of a factory farm, because I know what I've eaten. It's all clean stuff.

But what I like to try to use instead is actually plant material. You could compost plants that feed other plants. Compost woodchips, leaves, vegetable scraps, food scraps, everything out of my kitchen goes into my composters which then gets composted down to grow my plants, so it's basically all the nutrients the plants need because it came from other plants.

In addition I add other things, that they don't do in the organic standards, I like to add trace minerals. I could add rock dust which could add up to seventy different trace minerals. I could add ocean solids which adds up to ninety different trace minerals. And in standard agriculture, they're worried about three main minerals, and in some cases they worry about sixteen to eighteen minerals. But there's a lot more minerals that naturally should be occurring in the Earth's crust, in the Earth's soils, if we didn't degrade the soils by strip mining or by bulldozing and tilling, and all these crazy things that we've done over the years that literally destroyed the soil. And then furthermore even beyond that like, okay, in organic, you can actually spray "organic" approved pesticides, but let's face it, whether it's an organic approved pesticide or not, if it's organic approved pesticide, it's probably in many cases derived from some kind of plant, or flower, or neem tree, or some kind of essential oil extract, or soap. But the thing is, people don't realize that anything you spray, if it's going to affect the bad bugs, in many cases it's also going to affect the good bugs as well, so even better than spraying even organic pesticides, is maybe having and building soil systems so you have healthy plants that have a strong immune system so they can actually fight off the bugs, so that actually the bugs don't want to eat your plants, or have beneficial pollinator plants and native plants that will actually attract the beneficial insects. I've got a permaculture style moringa farm today, and they have basically all of these coconut shells and bricks randomly stacked in the garden to attract the lizards and other spiders and things that actually eat bad bugs. So really we want to kind of look at Nature's system and design that into our garden because Nature is a natural balancer. Nature balances things out automatically. That's how this Earth has been created over all these years. And now humans became evolved, and we've sprawled over the Earth and taken over and we try to dominate with our systems, or our chemicals we think that are better than Nature. And in my opinion it's not, and we need to really kind of get back to Nature. So, food could be a lot more nutritious. It could have a lot less sprays. It could do a lot less environmental damage to other creatures or earthlings on the planet.

Brendan [00:14:15]: Yeah, you're making a lot of good points and one I would love to call out right now just to underscore is the fact that first of all, I mean organic, while not perfect, overall it's an important standard. It's like one of the only things we have to discern between pretty good, to sometimes excellent food, really depending on how passionate and dedicated that farmer is to their soil versus only meeting the standards and only sort of ... I think it's Ronnie Cummins from the Organic Consumers Association, he criticizes organics himself, or at least how they're being implemented, in a sense that I think he calls it "organic by neglect", in other words, or even "organic by substitution", where you're not allowed all these pesticides, but you're allowed these, so there's still a lot of organic farmers, I'm not saying all of them but, are approaching organic farming in sort of the, I'm going to use a word that's not maybe quite accurate but, an allopathic approach, in other words, like the Western medical model applied to farming. If we do it in a conventional way it means we're using chemical fertilizers and chemical pesticides, while we make it a little better in organic, or even a lot better by eliminating pretty much all the chemical fertilizers and the vast majority, if not all of the chemical pesticides, while still allowing certain quote unquote "natural pesticides" that are still pesticides like you said. Another key thing about organic is there's still tilling, there's still carving up the soil in most cases, and sometimes erosion in organic farms is just as bad or worse as on a conventional farm, especially if the conventional farm is no-till, but the organic is tilling. We can't become complacent about organic if we really care about our health, and we really care about the planet. It's important I think that we all become aware and nudge, and push, and advocate for organic 2.0 and organic 3.0. People like Andre Leu from The International Federation of Organic Movements, he's out there talking about that. He's speaking with heads of state saying the next level of organic is to really bring in the regenerative, or bring it back. I mean, organic was founded on regenerative principles, regenerating soil, growing soil, because that's where the health of the whole system is founded, and that's what makes nutrients available for the plants, and so when the plants are strong, like you said, they're much less vulnerable to the insects. The insects will pass them over for the weak plants. Walter Jehne — he's also in this event, from Australia -- he's a microbiologist, worked for Australia's main research agency. He says insects would just fly right over healthy fields and prey on the unhealthy ones. It's extraordinary. So anyway, thank you for bringing that up, I just wanted to sort of underscore some of those things. Back to ... we're talking about food quality. What are some of the foods you recommend to people that are just dynamite nutrient powerhouses?

John [00:17:59]: Good question, that question kind of scares me on some levels because as people we always try to categorize things like "What's the best one, John?".

Brendan [00:18:10]: Yeah, good point.

John [00:18:12]: "What's the best pair of shoes?", "What's the best car?", and then it's just like you want to buy the best car and don't want to do the other ones, right? And as much as you want the best car, there's a lot of cars, and depending on what's important to you. I think one of the best cars is like a Tesla, because it's an electric car, it's hella fast. They're pricey, but you could power it with solar panels. But that might not be the best car for everybody. If you have a contractor, you can't be hauling two by fours and four by eights and all these stuff in a Tesla,. It's not really designed, it's like a family car that could hold like six people and that's great. Or if you're a single guy and you've got a sports car to try to pick up the chicks -- it depends.
But that being said, I would say that the healthiest foods or the foods on the planet that everybody should include more of, include the leafy green vegetables and herbs. Those are by far the best foods, and then I can take that further down to say "This is better than that", I mean of course I have my favorites, things like moringa. I was at a moringa farm today and that's a really powerful food, not to say that we should only ever eat moringa, but we should try to include all these different foods even in smaller quantities in our diets.

I like this one called ashitaba. It's from Japan. *Angelica keiskei*. There's a lot of research on that. It's a very anti-disease food. Let's see ... *Gynura procumbens* or longevity spinach, like Egyptian spinach. It's very high in nutrients. Basically what it is ... plants are little chemical factories, and they're not running on power from coal, or you don't have to plug them in. They're running on sun energy, and basically when the sun hits the plants, the plants photosynthesize. They make carbohydrates. They make other nutrients provided they have all the different vitamins and minerals and things in the soil and the micro life. They're basically pumping out different chemicals, and it's not for our benefit. It's for the plant's benefit, so that it could repel the strong UV rays of the sun; so that it could repel bugs from eating it. So I could to all these different things, and then when we eat those plants, we get these different plant metabolites or if you want to call them phytonutrients or phytochemicals. They have words from like lycopene, anthocyanin, zeaxanthin and lutein, all these different pigments and nutrients in the food that are good for us. Every plant has different ones. So in general I like to say the leafy greens.

Things like cannabis ... cannabis is an excellent food, and unfortunately people think cannabis, and they think "Reefer Madness." And they think stoned and high. And they think you're going to go mad and crazy. Cannabis to me is just another herb. You could juice it, I prefer actually the CBD dominant strains vs. the THC. I have a funny video actually where I juiced cannabis, and Dr. William Courtney talked about raw. He says cannabis is a raw foods poster child. If you eat it in its raw state, you don't heat it, you could never get high. So I'm like "great, I want raw foods, and I don't want to get high." I did that when I was in college. I won't lie. But I don't want to do that because I live on a regular high, an alkaline high from my vegetables and my diet. I don't want to be like a weird high from cannabis. And if you want to do that, that's totally up to you. That's not what I want to do, but I want to get the benefits, the cannabinoids, or once again plant chemicals that that plant makes and gives to me because it's shown that I have receptors in my body for some of the things in cannabis, that I may not be fulfilling with other foods, and I felt that I got to the next level when I started juicing cannabis and eating it.

I think it should be legalized everywhere, and I want people to know that it shouldn't have that stigma of drugs associated. To me it's just a food, and yeah anything could be used improperly, right?
Moving on ... there's so many other things, like watercress. Even watercress, one of the most nutrient dense vegetables in the Brassicaceae family. It's anti-cancer. On the ANDI scoring system derived by Dr. Joel Fuhrman, that's one thousand, where he ranks foods on their nutrient density vs. caloric density and all the different phytonutrients, vitamins and minerals as compared to the calories. The problem with Americans today and just people in general is they're eating very high calorie foods, and these foods are processed foods and have very little nutrients, whether that's a CAFO-raised animal, that is basically just fattened up so they could sell it and sell it for more money because it's fat, but there's not a lot of nutrients in there vs. grass fed cows that'll have more nutrients. But even blowing away the grass fed cows is the leafy greens because guess what, what is a cow? A cow is actually only a leafy green accumulator, and he basically concentrates the leafy greens by eating a lot of them, it gets all the nutrients in him, and of course makes other ones along the way. But if we just eat copious amounts of leafy greens we can basically by pass the cow and not have the animals, based on my research and my opinion. And actually what I've been doing now for the last 22 years, we could be extremely healthy because not only are we not getting the bad things like the foreign proteins from the animals or some endogenous toxins in the animals, we're just getting all the plant phytonutrients that actually you don't get second hand if you're eating from the cow. And these are the things that are actually, anti-aging, and anti-disease, so that's really where my diet and my life is focused throughout in eating these high anti-oxidant rich foods, and not just any particular food but all of them.

Today I was visiting an Aloe farmer, an *Aloe vera* farmer, *Aloe vera* is an amazing food. I made a video talking about *Aloe vera* and how people should eat more *Aloe vera*. And it's not just this one food but we want to include small amounts of all these foods and they give you amazing things. *Aloe vera* could ramp up your tumor necrosis factor, which basically it makes your immune system find and detect and kick ass over cancer. I hate to say just "eat aloe the rest of your life; go do an aloe juice fast, or an aloe gel fast". No, we want to include all of these different things. Every plant makes all these different phytonutrients, phytochemicals that could have positive effects in us.

Most people eat a standard diet, if you go to the grocery store, you have a shopping list; you usually get the same things every week. If you're just getting your Gino's Pizza Rolls, your bananas, your Cokes and your Oreos, and then every next week when you eat them all, you go back and get the same thing. And people don't rotate all the different things they're eating. I like to eat seasonally, so whatever I'm growing, it's in season, that's what I'm eating, so I'm automatically rotating my diet. Plus when I travel, fortunately I get to eat things that are in season in the place that I'm going, and so I really like to eat wide varieties and always trying new and different things, which is really fun.

Brendan [00:24:55]: Yeah, you're making a lot of wise points. A number of researches have pointed out that we evolved eating a diversity or hundreds of species and plants that were changing with the seasons obviously. So we weren't eating the same things all the time and there's probably some harm to that, and unfortunately, like you pointed out, the human mind's like "What's the Tesla of the plant world? I'll just eat that." And you have to eat it all. You've got to have the variety. If you only ate the Tesla, whatever that would be ... I don't know if that's the perfect metaphor, but I like it ... then ultimately certain things might not be happening in your body because there are other things that maybe aren't as sexy on the polyphenol fraction or something, but they have something else that's really important. Even if it just isn't as ... if our minds haven't grasped what it is yet. As you mentioned, there's so much.

One of the things I think is, when people eat really broadly from the plant world it develops diversity in the gut microbiome, and that's super important for people to understand and to develop. And over time, then as we develop the various strains in there, and high, high diversity corresponding with our highly diverse diet, then we get more out of the food, and we need less of it, and we get more energy. What I'm experiencing ... I'm shifting because I've been eating a lot of animal products for a long time. My microbiome had been decimated from antibiotics in my teens, and I could not digest. And it was hard as heck to build it back. I kept losing it, or I'd gain it and lose it again. And then I lost my appendix unfortunately, and that makes it extra hard.

What I found recently is that a combination of things, and as I really focused on eating a lot of plants, a lot of them raw, a lot of salads, I crave more and more salads. I'm living more and more on salads than anything in my diet these days, and it's actually blowing my mind because I used to just really need animal protein with every meal, and quite a bit of it, and now I'm like down to a few ounces a day of animal proteins and tons of salads, tons of avocados, olives. I mean my body likes fat. Your body might like less fat. I don't know where you're at with that, but my experience with metabolic typing suggests that some people need a lot less fat, and some people need a lot more. I'm one of the fat mongers. But anyway, thanks for bringing up all of those good points. Now, you teach people how to grow their own food as well. Why do you feel that's important?

John [00:27:52]: Yeah I mean, I teach about health and how to eat healthy and all these stuff, which many people may or may not know that I do. Many people know me mostly as a gardener because I teach gardening, and I actually have the number one gardening channel on YouTube. It's the most watched gardening channel. It has the most videos. And I don't think anybody because of my diet could keep up with the amount of videos and the content or the depth of content actually that I produce. I mean today I filmed two videos actually. I'm supposed to be on vacation, but me making videos is actually me on vacation because I love what I do, like this lights me up! I get to visit cool places growing cool stuff. I learn new techniques. I can share things. And more importantly I can educate people about healthy good food that unfortunately they're not going to learn anywhere else because I think I'm pretty unique in the world on what I do and what I teach.

But I think really the ... if you want to call it the raw foods end game, if you're a raw foodist, or even if you're just a standard person, I think we really need to take responsibility for our lives, whether that's for your health, don't put the responsibility of your health to your doctor when you get sick. You should be proactive with your health and do the right things now so you don't get sick, so you don't have to go to the doctor. And we should take responsibility for our food not to the farmers, not to organic farmers because of what we talked about a little bit earlier. In my opinion they're not really doing as good of a job as they could. I mean yes, it's better, and it's at least something, and we've got to start somewhere. But it could be done a lot better.

Always one of my core principles in my life is this principle of CANI or maybe in Japanese it's called kaizen. It stands for "constant and never-ending improvement" -- you know Tony Robbins -- you've heard of that before. I always hear like "Hey, John, I'm on a raw food diet. I'm eating high volumes of fruits and vegetables, how can I get my diet better?" One of the ways was to increase the variety. That was pretty easy, but the other thing was to increase the quality of the food I'm eating. And this was made apparent to me by my friend Don Weaver who wrote a book on soil re-mineralization. And he always talked about that to me, and I didn't quite get it until I was ready to get it. And then when I started tasting some rock dust mineralized food and how much more vibrant it was, how much more it lit me up -- it made me feel more alive -- that's when I was like, "You know what, I need to start growing my own food." And then along that journey it just kind of came like, "Well I need to learn how to do it on my own. And at the same time nobody's really teaching how to do this. Let's just make some videos for fun". I never thought it would go anywhere, and I just did it for fun, and pretty soon I just kept making videos and even though not many people would watch it. And then I'd get more and more views, and now my videos get lots of views these days.

I think it's really great, but really we need to take responsibility because the problem I see with the industry whether that's the food industry or any industry, there's a lot of trade secrets, and I don't want any trade secrets. I want people to know how their food was made. If you want to eat Oreo cookies, everybody has a right to eat Oreo cookies if they want. I mean I know what it could do to you so I don't want to. But if you do want to eat it, I want people to know like if on Oreo cookies you could press a little button, and there'd be a screen above the Oreo cookies that show how the Oreo cookies were made, like where did the flour come from? How much the flour gets processed? Where did that hydrogenated sugar fat stuff come from? Maybe it came out of this bag, out of this chemical factory. If you knew the process of how Oreo cookies were made and all the preservatives in them and where they came from, would you really be eating it?

If you saw animals in a CAFO being penned together and slaughtered, and dying, when you were to go buy a chicken, would you buy it? No, because it's easily, nicely packed. It's clean. They've taken away the blood. I mean that's what my cousin said "John I only eat the meat because it looks nice and pretty in the store. It's not all bloody, and I don't have to kill it myself."

I think the problem with society today is that people aren't taking responsibility to know what it takes to grow their own food, and we just work at jobs so that we could get money to buy our food, but why don't you maybe work less in your job and take some time to grow your own food? You get a higher quality foods that build your level of health higher, to grow a wider variety than money can buy, and also taking responsibility for the food you need to eat because we're taught to basically put blame or put responsibility for what we need in our lives to others. And we should be more sustainable on this planet, or even regenerative with our personal lives, and if everybody did that, the world would be a greater place. So, my gardening videos are just my outlet of creativity and also my message to the world to take responsibility and to give them a little piece of how they could do that if they've never done it before.

Brendan [00:32:28]: And I believe you brought up a really important point about minerals, re-mineralizing our bodies through our foods, through our soils. I think that's actually going to be one of the growing topics in the health arena. We've been aware of minerals; we talk about minerals, but I don't think that minerals have actually received quite all that they're due as far as attention because they're so powerful. They're so foundational. That's what enables plants to actually create all the different compounds that they create. In fact, in our bodies, we can't always even use the phytonutrients if we don't have certain minerals along with them. You mentioned rock dust ... I'm curious, was there a particular site? I mean, I don't think it's like any old rock dust. It's not like just granite or something. Is it paramagnetic rock dust by chance or ...?

John [00:33:21]: You know what, there's so many different rock dusts, and I'm not like an expert on rock dust or anything but I have interviewed experts about rock dust on my YouTube show. I've visited them and their place, and I've seen all the different rock dust they've collected. And I have my own collection. I've got a handful of different kinds of rock dust, paramagnetic, non-paramagnetic, granite-based, basalt based, clay-based, and there's different kinds. You can ask my friend Don Weaver who's like more of an expert on rock since he has studied it longer than me. Basically, he's like once again we're trying to do that "What's the best rock dust? What's the best vegetable? What's the best food? Because I'll just eat that, and I won't eat anything else." So the thing is, it kind of depends on where you're starting at, but in general what I think is, I like to mix a lot of different rock dust because each different rock has its own pros and cons and its own benefits, has its own spectrum of different minerals. And paramagnetic rock dust is one aspect of a rock dust but that's because it has magnetic properties of how certain minerals in there, but there's other kinds of rock dust that could be good and balancing out with that, so I like to mix rock dusts and blend rock dusts and then add that to my soil, so I've got all my bases covered. Actually, I met a company once that was going to source rock dust from all over and then combine them in the right amounts to make sure you have the right balance of minerals, and I don't know if they're still in business. I think it went under, but that was a really good idea to me.

Brendan [00:34:40]: So is rock dust your secret to so much energy?

John [00:34:45]: I mean minerals of course are very important for energy, but aside for that you talked a little bit earlier about microbiomes. That's really important also. Life force or enzymes ... I mean without enzymes reactions won't happen in the body, and that's one of the reasons why I eat raw foods, because they have more enzymes and are more enzymatically active than processed cooked foods that have been heat processed. So it's all these things.

Brendan [00:35:09]: [inaudible] so fast and easy. Even fat ... you would not believe how many avocados and olives I can eat. I actually had to clean out my liver before I could do it, but now they digest as easy as anything else practically. And sometimes I use some lemon juice with it because if I go overboard and have like four avocados ... But anyway, go ahead.

John [00:35:33]: Yeah, I mean just the plant foods that I fill myself up with and eating fresh foods. Most people don't eat fresh foods. If you're buying produce at the grocery store, Whole Foods, or Whole Paycheck, or wherever you're going. People don't realize that that food that you're buying, in the case of apples at this time, were picked last year.

Brendan [00:35:50]: I know.

John [00:35:51]: Not quite last year but maybe six months ago, or it could even be imported. They're months old; they've been in cold storage for months in an oxygen deprived environment. I wouldn't last too long in an oxygen deprived environment, but they can store apples in an oxygen deprived environments so they don't go bad faster, so they don't lose their profits. And when you get them they're soft and mealy and they have nowhere near the level of nutrition that they did when they were fresh picked. I mean even just something like broccoli, broccoli could be three weeks old by the time you get it, and it's hard and crusty, and it tastes horrible. And we've all eaten home grown tomatoes vs. the pink tomatoes that bounce at the store that have zero flavor. and when they have zero flavor that means they have close to zero antioxidants too because the flavor that we're tasting are the nutrients.

Brendan [00:36:34]: Yeah this is one of the big problems with getting all of your food from the supermarket. I mean some of it is going to be, you know, like Whole Foods they make their effort to buy a lot of local stuff, and so it's going to be a lot fresher, but especially that out-of-season stuff like you mentioned ... It's been in cold storage. A lot of times it was picked under-ripe, and then they ripen it with ethylene gas.

John [00:36:55]: Yeah, bananas, especially.

Brendan [00:36:58]: Yeah, and they're forcing a ripening but that just sweetens it. It doesn't add anymore phytonutrients, so we're getting a raw deal so to speak, on that.

John [00:37:08]: Faux food.

Brendan [00:37:10]: Yeah, so how much of your own food do you grow, and where do you grow it? Is this all just around your house, in the front and back yard, or how are you doing it?

John [00:37:20]: Yeah, it depends how you measure how much food do I grow. If it's by calorie it'd be pretty low unless it's like the summer day when my persimmon trees or my fig trees are going off or loquats or apricots or whatever fruit I'm eating at the time, or pineapple guavas, right? So caloric wise it's low, but nutrient wise it's really high. So nutrient wise dominates because I don't necessarily tend to grow a lot of … I grow some fruit trees, but I grow mostly the vegetables and the high anti-oxidant, high nutrient content foods.

I mean I go buy fruits because the thing is, if you plant a fruit tree, hey, planting fruit trees are great I encourage everybody to do it if you have a lot of space. But if you plant a fruit tree, it will fruit like, depending on the fruit tree and where you live, generally once a year. Fruit trees fruit once a year. So at that one point of the year you have lots of food that then you've got to either eat, preserve, dehydrate, juice, do something with, or it's going to go bad. And then all that space that that tree is taking up is basically not being used for the rest of the year. But if you plant vegetables for example, you can plant some perennial vegetables like my tree collards that grow into a tree that will grow 365 days a year, and I can pick collard greens that are anti-cancer, anti-aging, high in different phytonutrients, every day of the year. That's much better use of my space, and then I'll go buy good quality apples from a farmers' market or maybe go to a wholesale produce store and get them for super cheap. So on a nutrient basis, over 50% of my nutrients are coming out of my garden because they're coming directly, not from my garden actually but from the soil that I'm building, that my plants are being grown in.

Brendan [00:39:03]: Awesome. So I'm curious, is your diet mostly … are most of your calories coming from carbohydrates like fruits and so forth, or are they mostly coming from, like in my diet, even if I was a complete raw foodist right now, even if I was raw vegan, most of my calories would still roughly be about the same percentage coming from fat, which is like, I haven't measured it but it's probably well over 70%. And that's basically a ketogenic diet. And there's ketogenic diets that have some animal products, and then there's some people that do a totally plant-based ketogenic diet, where they have high nuts. I eat a lot of nuts as well. So I'm just curious, what works for your body? Is it more on the carb side, or more on the fat side?

John [00:39:55]: Yeah of course, so, my diet's changed over the years. In general my diet is predominated by carbohydrates and also in fats and proteins. So dominant carbohydrates, with probably more fats than protein calories if we're just looking at that. But once again, as time has gone on I've noticed I need to eat less, and I eat different things. I try to get most of my carbohydrates from vegetables predominantly, and that doesn't always work, they don't have a lot of calories so I tend to eat some fruit. And I try to focus on nutrient density.

Like what did I eat today for fruits? Oh, I had longan, local grown longan here in Florida. But I didn't even eat hardly enough of them because I was too hungry so I went to a raw food restaurant a little bit earlier tonight, and that was probably a more fat dominant meal because that's what they put in raw food restaurants. But normally I like to eat some percentage of fat so, I mean I give a range … I like to eat 20 to 30% of my calories from fat, mostly from carbs then of course some protein. Although I'm a "raw" foodist, I like to eat live foods as well. Beans is a category of food that I think people should eat and include more of, and so for me as a raw foodist, I eat beans. Because beans have toxins in them and things that should be cooked in most cases. So I could eat like sugar snap peas and even peanuts or jungle peanuts, raw, or carob is another legume that you could eat raw.

What I started doing is I actually getting fermented bean products. For example miso, I've been eating miso for a long time. Some of my favorite ones are nattos. Natto technically is cooked, but then you actually put a culture in there, you culture it so now it's a "live" food. The culture actually even more so than the cooking breaks down some of the bad phytonutrients, makes that more available to us, plus it now has the beneficial probiotics of the culture. And raw, unpasteurized tempeh, if you go to buy tempeh in the store, it's been pasteurized. It's really hard to find unpasteurized tempeh, or you've got to make it yourself. Same with the natto, I get organic natto, and also organic soy tempeh when I do get soy tempeh. Very important so yeah that's something that I'm trying to include more often than not are the beans or fermented beans.

Brendan [00:42:19]: Yeah, fermented. Fermentation is oh so important it seems to me. We've been rediscovering that. A lot of people have been talking about it over the last decade, increasingly so, and I actually have done best when I've been pretty intensive about it. I've gone back recently into more intensively cultivating fermented vegetables, eating them, and man is it delicious. I mean seriously, when you get into these things, you develop the craving for it, and you're just like "Oh my God, it's so good". I literally feel like I could live on sauerkraut. And you mentioned, gosh what was it? I'm blanking out. Oh, I was going to make a connection to something else. Fermented foods are kind of like the compost. It's kind of like compost. It's human compost, and you talk about compost, because it's feeding the bacteria in our gut … You're not quite following that one …

John [00:43:25]: I mean I get it, but I wouldn't necessarily use that analogy.

Brendan [00:43:29]: Go with me, go with me! It's just something that occurred to me in the moment.
So you teach people about compost, and it's very important in soils. We have to restore the bacterial life in the soil, so you teach about composting. And I saw something really interesting on your Growingyourgreens.com webpage which is the Boogie Brew, and I just had a chance to look at that briefly. I'm wondering if you have more to say about that because to me that's like a bacterial inoculant just like sauerkraut is a bacterial inoculant for people. So now can you go with my parallel?

John [00:44:06]: It's pretty good. Boogie Brew is just a product. it's basically just a compost tea product. Boogie Brew happens to be the brand that I like to use because I don't have to formulate my own compost tea. Somebody's already done it for me, and it's a really good kind of compost tea. They basically add a bunch of different items in there including fungal dominated compost made out of woodchips that adds the fungal matter into your mixture, then they've got things like worm castings which add a lot more microbiology in there. They add some sources of food, whether that's some kind of kelp or soil humates that increase nutrient uptake, or they put some sugar in there to feed the microbes, all different kinds of things in there. And then you basically take this; you put it in clean purified water, and you bubble it with an airstone. So basically you're brewing a whole batch of microbes that then you take these microbes, and then you pour it into your garden, spray it on your leaves. Now you're inoculating your garden with basically a probiotic supplement, kind of like a fermentation.

When you're fermenting you're creating more probiotics so that you eat them so that you could populate your intestinal tract with probiotics that do amazing things. Much like us. We need our probiotics and beneficial microbes and fungi in our soils. I mean literally probiotics help us digest food that really make the soil food web happen. I mean if it wasn't for the life in the soil, there wouldn't be good food, and unfortunately in a chemical-based system, they're subverting this whole process of Nature. And there could be different like disease suppression qualities from the compost tea. And the soil microbes basically break that organic matter and make it bioavailable for the plants. And the plants are working in symbiosis with the microbes. They're super critical, and I would say the compost tea is kind of more synonymous with maybe like a sauerkraut vs. like compost. I think of compost as rotting stuff, I guess it's kind of similar but maybe I have a little bit of a different analogy.

Brendan [00:46:20]: Isn't it all fermentation? I mean it's a certain type of rotting.

John [00:46:25]: Well, controlled fermentation, yeah I don't know if compost is always...

Brendan [00:46:28]: Maybe it's not always as controlled. But if you do it right....

John [00:46:32]: Well, it should be controlled to get good quality compost. There's no legal definition of compost. Somebody could put something in a pile, compost it or let it sit for two weeks, put it in a bag and call it compost and that's crap. It's mulch. I mean that's a whole big ... that's a whole other topic.

Brendan [00:46:52]: Yeah, I will leave that to Elaine Ingham. She's the expert on that, and she's in this event talking about things. We don't get too deeply into the compost aspect, but she's the queen of compost, and she has a lot to say about that and how to do it right, and how sometimes people don't. But I'm curious, if people are growing their own food, what are some other things that you teach that are foundational as well as maybe advanced or nuanced? What's important for people to learn?

John [00:47:22]: I think one of the most important things that is forgotten about when people are growing food is how to start your seeds. If you can't start healthy seeds, you're not going to have healthy plants because when the plants are seedling that's the most important time in the seedlings life or even for like a human baby, that's the most important time that you must nurture that baby very carefully, feed it proper or else it's going to grow up and be messed up. That's why I want people to get into sprouting, and growing micro-greens. These are the most nutrient dense food in the entire planet, even kicks ass over kale and big vegetables. It's these little micro greens or sprouts that you guys could grow in your own kitchen, and the cool thing about it is you don't even need a garden space, you could live in an apartment in New York City, and you can do it on your counter, next to your sink. You could have a stainless steel rack to grow them in your living room. Or if you're only renting a bedroom, put it up in there and grow them inside. We can be independent, we don't need to have an outside space to grow. Grow these sprouts and microgreens. And the cool thing about them is that they can be ready in as short as one day. I sprout whole buckwheat, and my buckwheat is sprouted in one day in Vegas in the summer, when it's nice and warm. And I'm eating them, and I grew it with my own two hands. Other micro greens could be ready in like ten days, seven to ten days sprouts and microgreens, depends on what exactly you're growing. But that way it's a quick turnaround time, you have instant gratification. And the cool thing is because it's a short time elapsed you have less time to mess up. So you don't have to ... like if you're growing a full size tomato, you have to grow that tomato sixty to ninety days before you even get a fruit. And a lot of things go wrong in those days. So grow microgreens. It's really easy, and I think that's really foundational to help people learn how to start and grow seeds. And we can go into more like, gardening stuff, but I think that's something that everybody should be doing on a regular basis.

Brendan [00:49:18]: It's so easy like you're saying, you don't have to start the composting. You don't have to have a soil patch to work on. You have some videos about making money at growing stuff. What's that all about? What are the models that you're talking about?

John [00:49:39]: Sure, I want to make America great again by everybody being their own boss, being their own entrepreneur, and not having to work for "the man" in a job you hate for money you don't need, to buy useless things that are going to end up in the landfill. I want people to create their own income and do something they're truly passionate about. I know a lot of my people that watch me, that are gardeners, they really don't like doing their regular jobs, and they want to find out how they could make some money by doing what they love. I want to excite people to do that. I'm a born entrepreneur, I started selling pencil erasers in the fourth grade, and by high school I was in a ROP program, I started my first company, doing computer consulting and building PCs back in the day. I want everybody to be empowered to do this. It's unfortunate that in our schooling system, we're not taught how to be our own boss and to have our own job and create and income for ourselves, and how we can live in service to help others to provide them something that is valuable for them that they don't want to do.

Especially in this day and age, I see a key role that microfarms on a small level that are taking care of just the city blocks around you, we could thrive. It's really cool when I get to visit ... because I don't necessarily make a living off what I grow. I grow for my own personal consumption. I don't sell my food. Everybody's like "John, you've got actually food that I could buy." "No, it's for me! I'm eating it! That's why I'm growing it. I'm going to dehydrate it if I can't eat it fresh, I'm going to juice it and go through a lot of produce fast." But I had the opportunity to visit so many cool people around the country. I visited a cool wheatgrass farm in the middle of Vegas, that actually the guy sells and it's his business. He made $60.000 dollars a year selling wheatgrass to the local Las Vegas area. I visited a microgreens farm in Baltimore Maryland. The guy makes a $100,000 dollars a year by selling micro-greens to restaurants. And of course this is inside inner city Baltimore where land is really expensive, and they've got those high end restaurants. And those chefs, once they taste the microgreens, they'll pay $40 dollars for a tray of microgreens, which is a lot of money because you guys could grow them yourselves for five or six bucks, and now you turn your five or six dollar investment in seeds and time and some lighting in to a forty dollar tray that you could sell to restaurants. And they order on a continuous basis. And you just get dedicated customers. He's figured out the system how to do that. I visited cacao farmers in Puerto Rico that want Americans that come down to Puerto Rico, buy some land, and it's actually probably really cheap now since they had the hurricane, which is sad, but now Puerto Rico has a second chance of rebuilding and having more infrastructure so that it could support itself and hopefully they take this path and encourage more farming because it used to be an agricultural place. And so America got involved, and that's a whole other topic. But anyway you could start your own cacao farm in Puerto Rico, which is American territory and make a lot of money that way. Whatever turns you on.

I have episodes of growing spirulina in a fish tank. You could grow spirulina in a fish tank and harvest it and sell it to people. Today I went to a moringa farm that the guy started growing moringa at a residential house here in south Florida, and he grows it and powders it, and basically he sells it for a hundred dollars a pound. His dry moringa grown, and now he's up to having multiple properties with trees, with 250 trees. I had Curtis Stone on my show who's up from Canada, and he actually uses OPL, other people's land, or OPP, other people's property, to grow micro farms in the inner city, wherever he is in Canada. And he harvests the crops off that, sells it to the farmers market, and makes quite a good income. I don't want to like claim anybody's going to make what these other people claim they can make, because I haven't verified and seen their tax documents, but it seems realistic to me when I kind of do the math in my head that it's about as much as you can make. And it depends on how much you work, and plus you're your own boss now.
And whether you want to start do vegetable starts and cuttings, like I got consulted with a guy on the phone the other day about growing these exotic, rare, perennial plants that you could grow by cutting. If you cut them, you put them in a cloning machine, and it makes forty of them, especially maybe when cannabis gets legal everywhere you'd be cloning cannabis plants and selling those for money, if it's legal. Don't do it if it's not legal where you live, of course.

There's many other plants besides cannabis that you could grow and propagate and sell to people that are in quite high demand like some of the ones that I talk about, like the longevity spinach for example, something very valuable even just herbs and things. You could start seeds for people. Seeds are cheap. You could start them and sell starter plants to people if there's no good places in your area where you could get good local plants starts and you have to go Home Depot to buy these imported Bonnie plants that are regional that they spray with things they won't reveal, which is kind of scary.

Brendan [00:54:45]: Indeed. I'm curious, what would you say if somebody wants to also build soil, capture carbon, any particular approach?

John [00:54:58]: Yeah, so building soil, capturing carbon, that's really important. Just the fact that you're gardening in your own backyard and doing it organically will do that, but there's even more steps you need to take to do it properly. Make sure your soil is always covered, right? Don't till your soil. Try to always keep something growing in there, right? You can add things like biochar which is actually carbon because that will directly store it in your soil, but actually woodchips are a great resource, that are normally going to the landfill. You could bring that on your property and let them decay over time, and that will really build a nice healthy soil. I visited a lady down in Costa Rica who's working on planting more trees because trees will suck up the most carbon but just the active growing plants on your property instead of having a rocked in backyard like my neighbors in Vegas where I have a full-on green backyard, it's capturing more carbon than not. And by composting and by doing healthy soil practices like some of the ones I mentioned, you just help the planet out. And it's going to take all of us to do this because unfortunately big companies and big agrifarms are not doing in my opinion what it takes to turn the carbon situation around.

Brendan [00:56:14]: Yeah, we all can play a part. And Graeme Sait, who's also in this event, you know him ...?

John [00:56:21]: Yeah, of course.

Brendan [00:56:23]: Nutri-tech Solution. So one of the things he's really talking to people about, really pushing is "Roll up your sleeves and garden." We all need the nutrient density we can create like you said, by growing our own food, have it be fresh, tending our own soils, making sure the microbes and the minerals are all bubbling away. But also in that process we can actually capture a significant amount of carbon, if we do it en masse, then it's going to add up. I don't know if he's done any exact calculations but he says the impact, you can have a far more than swapping out all of your light bulbs, and maybe even driving a Prius. There's so many benefits in doing that. I would love to see more people tossing out the chem lawn and putting in collard trees or whatever, is that what you called it?

John [00:57:18]: Collard trees, yes. I mean perennial plants by far...

Brendan [00:57:22]: Kale is like that too, kale will just keep growing and putting out more.

John [00:57:27]: Well it depends on the kale, sometimes they'll basically flower and continue to grow, but they're not really lush and big, so these tree collards make nice big huge leaves, and in general they don't flower depending on where you live, but in a stressful situation like Vegas they flower, but then when they're done flowering they just keep going back to growing. I've planted some trees, actually I have pictures, I was looking at my pictures on Instagram, I think I planted them like last December. And now they're like pushing six feet tall, from last December to this December. And they've been growing through the hot 110 plus degrees summers in Vegas, no prob. And now the winter time is the time I really love them because the leaves really get a lot sweeter.

Brendan [00:58:06]: Oh interesting. Well you know, I really appreciate your passion, you're so fun to talk to. It's just energizing as heck, and I know that's why you've got so many YouTube views because you're just like full on, bringing it and really turned people on to some of the most important things people can be doing. So thank you for that, thank you for being a leader in that, and thank you for being a part of the Eat4Earth community.

John [00:58:35]: Cool, yeah, thank you.

Brendan [00:58:38]: John and I recorded a second interview about different types of juicers and how to create a vacuum sealed blender to protect the nutrients in your smoothies and that's available in the Eat4Earth Upgrade package ("Day 9" bonus interviews).

Stephen Brooks Interview
A Passion for Plants: The Perennial Diet

Brendan [00:00:00]: Welcome to the Eat4Earth event. We're exploring how you can heal yourself, your loved ones, and the planet, with food. This is Brendan Moorehead, and I know you're going to love the passionate purpose of our next guest, Stephen Brooks. Stephen is the founder and primary director of Punta Mona Center for Regenerative Design and Botanical Studies on the Caribbean Coast of Costa Rica. Living in Costa Rica since 1995, Stephen observed the problems facing small farmers in communities in Central America, in Costa Rica, due to a mega monoculture agricultural practices and the loss of dynamic community. He strives to provide students and landowners, businesses and neighbors, regenerative solutions and strategies to increase quality of life. Steven is an avid and passionate ethnobotanist, plant collector, permaculture designer and educator, operator of environmental and botanical education tours, community developer. He implements permaculture gardens and food forests on home scale and multiple-hundred-acre scales. He is the cofounder of Envision Festival and Medicines from The Edge: Tropical Herbal Convergence. Stephen it's awesome to have you here, thank you for being with us.

Stephen [00:01:12]: Thank you so much for having me.

Brendan [00:01:14]: You know, I used to ... I visited Costa Rica...

Stephen [00:01:17]: It's so funny man ... before we started this the interview, you made sure I turned off all of my notifications, and I turned off my phone and my Facebook and all my things ... but I can't stop the howler monkeys, they're screaming. I tried to turn off that notification but I couldn't.

Brendan [00:01:37]: [laughs] Please, keep the howlers notifying.

Stephen [00:01:40]: [laughs] Crazy. Sorry about that, go ahead.

Brendan [00:01:43]: Yeah, no problem. Yeah, every time you hear them let's pause so we can ... well not every time necessarily ... there he is. So, I spent some time in Costa Rica. I was there in 1991 ... no 1990 was my first time there, and I kind of toured all around the country for three months. In 1992 I was there, and I did a little research project on the commercialization potential of various rainforest products that could create income streams to keep forests intact so that there's an economic incentive and a livelihood to support living, standing forests. That's my experience with Costa Rica, and well I've seen also the devastation where mega-monoculture bananas and so forth have just turned the rivers brown and killed coral reefs on the coast, and denuded the hill sides that are eroding. Well, bananas are typically more on the flats, but other areas where they've taken the forest off the hills, the hills are basically running into the ocean over time. And then I've seen the beautiful areas where the rivers are so pristine, and there's fish in them and all kinds of beautiful stuff. I'm curious, how did you end up on this path? I mean I mentioned a little bit in your intro but, how did you become a "regenesist"?

Stephen [00:03:09]: I like it, I'll take it. I grew up in Miami, Florida, had a very suburban, normal childhood in Florida. My dad was a dentist on an island on The Bahamas, so I was always really connected to Nature. I was an avid tropical fish collector, I had seven hundred gallons worth of fish tanks in my house, and everything in it I collected. I was really into that, I was really from a young age very much connected to Nature. In 1995 I came on Costa Rica on vacation and fell in love with the country, the beautiful beaches, and rainforests, and rivers, and the people. It wasn't until I got to the Caribbean side where I really fell in love. I felt like I was in Jamaica, but I was in Costa Rica and this incredible convergence of indigenous cultures: Afro-Caribbean culture, eclectic foreigners, Costa Ricans, and Nicaraguans—all living very interestingly harmonious. And one day while I was there, in March of 1995, I decided to go check out the town of Bribri. Bribri is the administrative center of the Bribri people, they are one of the largest indigenous cultures here in Costa Rica. And I'd read about it in my guidebook and I decided to go check it out, and was literally meandering through the most unbelievable of forests. There's this bridge you go over, called the Rio Catarata, where you stop your car, and there's a giant waterfall right below the bridge. And I was just buying exotic fruits that I'd never even heard of or seen, on the side of the road on my way to Bribri. Looking at the thatch huts and these beautiful indigenous people that had never really seen people that look like this, and it almost felt like the movies.

I felt something and then all of a sudden as I'm meandering on my way to Bribri, I come around this corner and as far as my eye could see were banana plantations It was almost like it was a mirage, and I turned around and the beautiful rainforest and the beautiful thatch huts to just like a never-ending sea of banana plantations. And way off in the distance I could see the Sixaola river which is the border between Costa Rica and Panama, and they just keep going, and there's no buffer. There's no borders in the corporate reality. Something triggered me, and I decided to turn my little rent-a-car and drove into the plantations. And all of a sudden out of the corner of my eye I watch this airplane just a few meters above the plantation, with a big stream of smoke behind it. Literally I thought it was about to crash, I was like "My goodness, I'm about to see a plane crash" only to realize that it was a crop duster spraying the banana plantations with literally neurotoxic chemicals. They flew right over the car, and I felt my eyes and my face burning, and then I watched it fly right over a playground full of indigenous children playing soccer and I was just like [gasp].

Brendan [00:06:02]: Oh Gosh.

Stephen [00:06:03]: Yeah, and it was just like "Wow, what is happening here?". I kept driving, and I got to this point where there was this metal cable thing that came down. And if you've ever lifted a bunch of bananas—they're really heavy. So, the way they move the bunches in the plantation is on these cable systems. And so I had to wait there, almost being like at a bridge that's up. I had to wait there ...
Oh my goodness, I hear a white ... it's one of the rare times I hear a white-faced monkeys and howler monkeys at the same time.

Brendan [00:06:30]: Ah, "cara blanca".

Stephen [00:06:33]: They might cruise right behind us during this interview, that would be amazing.

So anyway, I'm sitting in my rent-a-car, watching the bananas zip by. Just watching them, they looked so green and perfect and almost like they were plastic. And after like thirty-forty or fifty bunches, I'm sitting there, and I see this guy hanging from the same cable, moving them along. And he stopped right in front of my rent-a-car, and he was like, I don't know, maybe five foot one, thick and stocky and solid, and he stops right in front of my car and he stares at me. I'm in my little air-conditioned rent-a-car and he stares at me right in the soul. And I'm like, "Who was I? Why am I in this rent-a-car staying in the cool eco lodge, eating at the gourmet restaurant that night. While him and his family are being sprayed with neurotoxic chemicals even though they've been treating the Earth like it's an extension of their body for centuries. And who am I, and how is this happening? What is going on here?" It was like an emergency brake on my life. "How can we be a part of a system that's so broken?" And I started feeling so angry. "Who could be responsible for this?" And I realized I was. I realized I was responsible every time I sliced my Chiquitas into my Cinnamon Life cereal in the morning through my childhood, or my Cinnamon Toast Crunch. I was supporting a system that is destroying ecosystems and destroying people's lives and I didn't [inaudible] "Wow, oh my goodness, I'm 21 years old." I was just recovering from mourning the death of Jerry Garcia. I was a big "deadhead". His death was probably a big impetus why I was able to just leave US because it was something I was really attached to. I felt like I got catapulted up into the universe. I was just looking at this beautiful blue-green ball spinning, and like "How are we destroying harmony like this to these beautiful people, to this beautiful city." And what came to me was, it was just design. It was just design. Soon after I lived in Spain. I lived in this apartment complex with this elderly woman, and we would literally walk through ... so it was this apartment complex. t was like ten buildings in a row, and there were big roads on either side, but you could walk right through one building to the next. And all the buildings had commercial things downstairs—bars, restaurants, barber shops, cheese shops, food stores, everything. And you could go in, and you never had to go to the streets. You could walk right through the buildings. And I walked with my—I called her "abuela"—walked with her in the streets and everybody would be like "Hola, abuela", "Hola Maria", "Hola Pablo", "Hola abuela", "Hola Snuffelofagus". What is this freaking Sesame Street? Why does it feel like this? Why does everybody care about each other so much? And what I realized is that it was just great design. It was designed to foster community. So what I started to think, not because I knew anything—I'm a suburban kid from Miami—not that I knew anything about agriculture, but like, "Why are we growing just one thing like this? Why is it all so corporately driven? How can we be destroying rainforests and ecosystems like this? How could we be treating people like this in this beautiful culture?" And from that moment on I decided I was going to dedicate my life to try to find another way to design and merge where we live with what we eat, and merge that with regenerating ecosystems as we go.

Brendan [00:10:07]: Awesome, yeah design is the core of all ... I think it was William McDonough, the architect and eco-designer, who said that design is the first signal of human intention. It's what it comes down to. So do we intend to poison and kill children? Do we intend to destroy the planet? Do we intend to destroy our bodies? Probably not. We just have to kind of look at design again, which of course brings up permaculture, and you teach permaculture. For anybody who's not familiar with it, I'm just curious if you could summarize?

Stephen [00:10:49]: Yeah, absolutely. When I think about all the different philosophies and all the different ways to approach this incredible task we have of healing the planet, and healing ourselves and this broken ecosystem of everything. Permaculture just makes so much sense. It's an ecological design system. It has nothing to do with tropics or temperate or ... it has nothing to do with farming or agriculture. It has nothing to do with even "eco". It has to do with efficiency and intention. What you said about intention ... how can we merge efficiency and intention? The way I define permaculture is how can we meet our goals and use less energy. Now when I say to you "Do we all have the same goals?" and you might be like "Um, no" but in the end, on a macro level, we all have the same goal. We want to play more than we work. We want to eat well. We want to be safe, We don't want there to be an arrest or war outside our house. We want to be comfortable, and we want to live in a comfortable place, whether it's the temperature inside our buildings, outside our buildings. We want to be loved and cared for. Everyone has these, whether you're a Sri Lankan tea farmer, or creating an online course about wellness. We all have those same goals. And when I say, "How can we meet them and use less energy" what do you think that means? This is all energy, it's what are we taking in and what are we putting out. We like to call it EROI, energy returned on energy invested. "What do we need to meet those goals?" We need abundant diverse nutritious food, and we need to meet those goals. How are we going to set it up? How much energy is that going to take? Energy is not just like ... people think "solar, and this...", no. Energy is everything. "How much physical energy am I spending to do that?". Whether I'm out there planting and hoeing in the garden, and trying to grow my own food, or I'm buying it shopping at Whole Foods. I want to get organic good food. And then how much energy is it taking to get to the shelves of Whole Foods? How many tractors are going in and burning diesel. I'm using all of that metal to make the tractor. Or how many people are using oxen and running them to plow the fields? Or how many people are physically doing it?

I think what that brings me to, and I think really what I'm excited to show you today Brendan, is this concept of a perennial diet. It's like, how can we merge what we eat with our love for the planet? How can we merge our own health with the same love for the planet? I feel like the answer is ... and one of the things that permaculture really tells us to do ... it just tells us how to philosophize. To meet our goals of diet and health we want to grow perennial foods. And just in case anyone out there is not clear what perennial or annual is, those are the two ... it's either annual or perennial. Annual is something like a tomato or a cucumber, or squash, or beans, corn, or rice, or marijuana. These are things that we take a seed and we plant them and they grow a season, three-four months. They fruit or flower. We collect that. And then they die.

A perennial is something that's ongoing, and it's a tree, or a shrub, or a vine that lives several years. And what we think about and want in our systems is to create these food forests. We want to be intentional about the plants that we put in certain zones around where we live. And we want to find ones that really serve humanity in these zones close to home. We've got go figure out what are our needs, and then the rest of it we want to regenerate. and want to reforest, and want to revive broken ecosystems. Just some examples of perennial foods are things like ... here in Costa Rica my very favorite one is called "pejibaye" or peach palm. If I was sitting where I was before, I could've shown you, I could actually take the computer and show you one in my yard. Peach palm is ... if I had to go to a deserted island, it's the one seed I would bring. It's a palm that you ... it's where heart of palm comes from. If you've got a jar of heart of palm, it comes from the peach palm. What most people don't know is that same palm makes a fruit that you boil, and it tastes like almost avocado meets potato. It's super fatty and nutritious. It's like a palm fruit, like acai that became the craze, or coconut's so incredible. Palm fruits are often fatty, and oily, and rich. The peach palm is one of the greatest ones out there.

So we get the heart of palm, we get the peach palm fruit, and then the bark is an amazing building material. All from the same plant. You could make your floors, your walls out of it. It's incredible.

Other things are things like avocado, or mangosteen, or acai, or almonds, or cashews, or walnuts, or hazelnuts. I'm looking at my yard. Cashews I'm looking at right now, papaya, mango, ackee, acerola, surinam cherry, pulasan, jabuticaba, avocado. Oh my God the avocados are full of flowers right now. I'll show you in a minute. All of these things are perennial foods that we can constantly be harvesting. and we can create systems that work with Nature, rather than fight it. What's happening in industrial agriculture is we're like so yang and so agro, and so trying to kill the pest, and kill the funguses, and kill the weeds. As opposed to nurturing things in a way where they grew like they did in Nature. Everything that we use from every plant at one time grew wild, and it grew perfectly, and all we had to do was ... and now what we want to do is nurture the system where these things come from. It's just like "Duh". So much of permaculture is so "Duh". Do we want to work harder? Bill Mollison who coined the term permaculture along with his student David Holmgren, used to say "How can we design our realities to maximize hammock time?" I almost did this interview from the hammock, but the sun was bright and ... we tried it right before, but my hammock's right here. I actually could move into it. We want to maximize hammock time. That's really just a metaphor for spending more time doing what it is that we love to do. If we're too busy spending energy meeting our goals, we don't have the energy to be with our family. We don't have the energy to be taking care of ourselves. Self-care is also so important. We don't have time to do the things that we like to do for recreation, whatever they are. We want to be intentional with the design of our realities. We want to be intentional with the design of our agriculture and of our homes, and of our own lives. Many people spend their whole lives living in ... working in a place they hate, doing a job they hate, married to the wrong person because they don't even have time to stop and press pause, and think about it long enough to shift things. I think this idea of being intentional and efficient is brilliant. From the minute I heard about permaculture and this concept that just makes a container for all these things that we're striving for, we all want to help heal this broken planet. We all want to protect the ecosystems and endangered species. We all want to thrive and feel healthy. This is a design philosophy that promotes this regenerative renaissance.

Brendan [00:18:19]: Awesome. And what makes natural systems efficient is that all these relationships are doing things for you, and the total production in the system is way higher than optimizing for so called "efficiency" of producing one crop, which is what the mega-monoculture model is. Sure, you can get more bananas, more rice, more wheat out of a unit of land typically anyway, when you optimize for that particular product. But the amount of food total that you get pales in comparison of that system to a polyculture where there's biodiversity, and you're growing multiple things because you have an agro-eco system, agricultural-eco system. And that's what permaculture essentially is. It's an intelligently designed agricultural eco-system that takes care of you.

Stephen [00:19:05]: Another thing that I just want to bring up, it's that it's bringing it out of the farm and into the reality. We talk a lot in permaculture about the different zones. Zone zero is my heart, my soul, my body. Zone one is the area right around me. It's my home and the area right around it. Zone two is further off. Zone three is further off. Zone four is further off. Zone five is like the wilds. And the way that you interact and relate with those areas is the amount of energy that they take to maintain. How much energy do they need from you, and how much energy do you need from them? The things in your zone zero you want to be the most intentional and the most cared for, and with the most interaction between you and them. And then zone two less, and less. And same in our own social circles Zone zero is still yourself. Zone one are your best friends and your family that you speak to several times a day. Zone two are the people that you speak to once a week. Zone three are the ones that you ... maybe once a month or once every two months. Zone four are like maybe you send them a Facebook "Happy Birthday". And then zone five are the billions of people that you don't even know.

This philosophy of seeing everything as energy and seeing how we can be more efficient and intentional, and often pressing pause on the Google map of your life and zooming out, and zooming in, "Am I on track, am I on the path I want to be on?" Even when talking about health ... you know this is more of a program about health. It's like, "What can I do to start directing myself towards more optimal health?" And it's not like "From today to tomorrow I'm going to cut everything out." But it's being intentional. "Okay, I'm going to start cutting out dairy in February. In April I'm going to start cutting out this, and I'll see how I feel, maybe I'll bring things back if I don't feel better." And we can come up with a plan and a vision, and that's just for our own health. And then we can think about our job and our relationship like "Is there someone in my zone one that isn't serving me, that's a negative EROI? Maybe I need to stop that relationship, or maybe I have to shift it around a little bit so it's serving and it's creating a positive EROI.

Brendan [00:21:10]: EROI?

Stephen [00:21:11]: EROI, energy returned on energy invested.

Brendan [00:21:13]: Okay, got it. In terms of perennial vs. annual, what are some of the differences in the effect on the planet, on our body, or is it not possible to generalize?

Stephen [00:21:31]: What you have to understand is that the amount of energy ... if anyone out there has ever grown an annual crop, like a crop of corn, or a crop of rice, or a crop of wheat, or a crop of any annual big-field crop ... it takes a lot of work. You have to till the soil constantly, you have to prepare the soil, you have to go in and seed it. You're growing a field of corn whether using a big machine which they do now, which is taking a lot of machine and diesel, and research, years of figuring all that out and all the metal and the mining, all of it. You have to account for all of that. It takes a lot of energy to do that. The other thing that you're doing is, every time you're tilling you're just releasing all the carbon rather than keeping the carbon in the earth. It's like we're constantly just ripping up the ground to grow annuals. Where in perennials we're just tending a forest which is providing oxygen, and it's holding in soil, not causing runoff. It's keeping our rivers clean. It's providing a habitat, and it's providing food for wildlife.
My neighbor Patty, may he rest in peace, when I first moved to where I live in Punta Mona ... he's an elder Caribbean man ... he died at 84 ... we lived together for twenty years. He used to say, "You boy, you need to grow enough for the animal, for the thief, for the neighbor, and enough to put away." And I said yeah that's ... And then the other thing he used to say is "If you design things right boy, all you do is reap." All you do is reap. And that's what perennial farming is about. Your whole job is harvesting. There's a little bit of pruning, there's a little bit of tending, but once you set it up right, all you do is reap. And when Patty said that ...

obviously I didn't understand it at the time. It's a constant evolution of even understanding this. Imagine if all you did in life was reap.

Brendan [00:23:34]: Yeah, I mean, in annual systems we keep rebuilding the system every year, whereas a perennial system—you build it once, you tend it, you optimize, you manage, but you don't have to keep reinventing the system and re-disturbing the system like you said with all these expensive inputs. It's so destructive and not efficient.

Stephen [00:23:58]: Sometimes there's that whole concept of NIMBY—not in my back yard. As long as you don't see the indigenous children being sprayed, and as long as you don't see them mining the steel ... you know steel industry. If you don't see those things you don't really feel it. You slice those bananas in your cereal, and you don't really know what they're doing. You might kind of know. You know there's fair trade out there. You know there's children in Africa that might be working growing your Hershey's bar or your Snickers bar. You know that. That trip to Costa Rica with the banana plantations for me was so mind-blowing, and so eye-opening to my relation to these broken systems, and I don't want to be a part of it, and I want to help other people break their chains. That's the name of the book I'm working on right now, it's called *Break Them Chains: A Suburban Kid's Escape from The System.*

Brendan [00:24:49]: Sweet! I can't wait for that. What's the projected release date?

Stephen [00:24:52]: I don't know, I wrote 140 pages a few years ago, and then I just stopped. I need to start again.

Brendan [00:24:59]: Well I'm looking forward to that.

Stephen [00:25:00]: Thanks.

Brendan [00:25:01]: So obviously where you live, in a polyculture and in permaculture—you've got biodiversity. Biodiversity is so much more important than we realize. That's a rabbit hole we can go way down if we want. I'm just curious ... why are you so passionate about biodiversity and collecting plant species?

Stephen [00:25:20]: I just became extremely passionate about it. I'm a passionate guy, whether it's The Grateful Dead, or with the tropical fish, or all the different things I've been throughout my life. I think there's nothing more sacred than finding some plant, or cutting, or seed and bringing it back to your home and growing it and then getting to eat the first one and sharing it with your friends. And then going to their house and seeing them have it. There's some joy in sharing this abundance of whatever you want to call it, Gaia, Goddess, God, Hashem, Allah. This incredible creator that is just bestowing us. We can pray to our books, or we can pray in our buildings, but the only thing we know that this divine creation is putting these incredible plants that coexist with us, and I just think it's such an incredible ... incredibly holy act, to be able to share and interact with these incredible ... I'm so into plants, I literally dream about them at night, and I'm so excited. There's this one plant I don't have yet but I'm working on it. I actually got it for one of the projects I was working on. It's funny all the super foodies out there are always waiting for the next one. I think one of the new ones that we'll start hearing about is called safou, have you heard of it?

Brendan [00:26:40]: No.

Stephen [00:26:41]: S-A-F-O-U, or butter fruit. It comes from Africa, and it's this amazing, creamy, perennial fatty [inaudible, signal interrupted] you know, and it's hot off the press. It's male on female so you need to plant a bunch of them. I'm constantly getting okari nut. I just planted it. Java almond. I'm always looking for these new obscure nuts. Pili nuts from the Philippines. These are things that are going to start hitting our realities as we begin to wake up to this solution that is food forests.

Brendan [00:27:19]: Yeah, biodiverse food forests. There's so much richness there, and like you said it's a gift from the Creator, and like the pope says … I think he said something like, "The soil is as it were a direct caress from God". I love that.

Stephen [00:27:34]: I love that too. Who said that?

Brendan [00:27:38]: The pope.

Stephen [00:27:39]: Oh my goodness, for real?

Brendan [00:27:41]: Yeah, yeah, he's talking about soil. He said that I think two years ago.

Stephen [00:27:46]: I need to look that up and share, oh my God. I love him by the way. He drinks mate. How could he not be amazing?

Brendan [00:27:53]: What's that?

Stephen [00:27:54]: He drinks mate.

Brendan [00:27:57]: [laughs] Yeah, and you know chocolate, what an amazing beverage that is.

Stephen [00:28:02]: Chocolate, coffee, mate—these are all perennials. All perennials.

Brendan [00:28:08]: Yeah, and the Kuna people not to far from you, down in Panama … they were studied, and a cardiologist' studied them and determined that it was their high consumption of a coffee drink, they grew their own coffee, it wasn't some commercial hybridized coffee they bought somewhere. They grew their own coffee—excuse me I keep saying coffee— cacao. They grew their own chocolate, cacao, the basis of what we think of as chocolate. And they had blood markers of people in their twenties when they were in their seventies. That's what I heard.

Stephen [00:28:46]: Cacao is really amazing, and what's amazing about cacao …

Brendan [00:28:48]: As long as it's pure, right? As long as it's pure ... go ahead. I'll get to that.

Stephen [00:28:53]: I mean mostly cacao, you get ... if it's cacao, it's pure, it's just cacao. Chocolate is where you get a little bit weird. But what I think the most important thing about cacao is the fairness of who's growing it. I think that's what you really want to be careful about, and really connect with the brands that you support. I just had my friend Freddy ... he was staying here last night. He's the founder of Dagoba chocolate, which was really one of the first, kind of pioneers in organic, and fair trade, and connecting with source. It's like connecting with your brands, and connecting with where things come from. But cacao is just such a magical food. Last Saturday we did this event in San Jose, it was called "Una Noche de Soluciones", a night of solutions. Opening ... [inaudible – signal interrupted] it was mostly ... it was all Costa Ricans, literally a 100% Costa Ricans. We just sat around talking about ... we had four speakers that talked about what they were working on and change, and then we had a question and answer, and then we ate a bunch of cacao, I mean these truffles that I made that day from cacao that was grown by a cooperative of indigenous farmers, literally made with so much love and all the inclusions, the cardamom, the vanilla, and the cinnamon—a lot of it we grew. And then we had a DJ. It wasn't like getting drunk and dancing to a DJ or partying. We were celebrating cacao. And I looked around, and all the feedback we've gotten about the event has just been incredible. Yeah, I strongly recommend cacao. Also really, for me mate has just been such an incredible ally.

Brendan [00:30:33]: That's awesome. I've just started discovering that recently. I mean I knew about it twenty plus years ago, but I didn't actually start imbibing anything with caffeine until recently, because my adrenals had been shot long ago and for a long time, so I couldn't even tolerate caffeine. Now I just love it.

Stephen [00:30:49]: I love mate, and I love cacao.

Brendan [00:30:53]: The thing I'll mention real quick about cacao in case people aren't familiar with this fact ...

Stephen [00:30:58]: I could walk down to the tree right now.

Brendan [00:31:01]: ... is if you eat chocolate, there's one level of processing, but if you combine milk with the cacao or chocolate, the milk protein binds to the polyphenols, and you lose the benefit there. So it's important for people to realize. Same thing with coffee. The milk protein binds with polyphenols, so if you put milk in your... whether it's your green tea, or your coffee, or your chocolate, or cacao, you're robbing yourself of the miraculous benefits of those foods.

Stephen [00:31:37]: Amazing. Let me give you just a little glimpse of where I am. So, oh, I haven't even mentioned this, the place where I live right now is called La Ecovilla, and we're a community of three-four families from twenty-five countries. We started our own school here. We have thirty-five students in it. It's a community that's merging where we live with what we eat. We have roads made from recycled plastic. We have one of the largest methane digesters, meaning our shit, our septic, and our grey water goes into a methane digester making methane to cook with. It's an incredible Noah's ark style. I've brought all these nice species from Punta Mona here, and this is just our surroundings, and this is our yard which is just pumping with food and ... I don't know how this looks. Does it look okay?

Brendan [00:32:25]: It looks great.

Stephen [00:32:36]: Cashews and avocados...

Brendan [00:32:28]: Looks like the backyard of a friend of mine who lives in Bali, she showed it to me and I'm like "Oh my goodness". Unfortunately, the volcano evicted them recently...

Stephen [00:32:38]: Primary rainforest, that's [inaudible]

Brendan [00:32:42]: Wow.

Stephen [00:32:44]: Trying to find the monkeys.

Brendan [00:32:48]: I heard something.

Stephen [00:32:49]: I know, they're out there. There's howlers and white faced out there right now. Yeah this has been so fun. I mean it's just the tip of the iceberg. I really recommend anybody out there to take a permaculture design course, whether you do it in your own backyard, or you can come down to us and do it. It's not about the details, it's about the mind frame. And what I think what's so amazing with what we do at Punta Mona, with our permaculture courses is you're learning about all these different ways to design, and you're learning about macro-things, water systems, and food systems, electrical systems, and alternative currencies and decision making, while living in deep community, while you're living with forty or fifty people, off the grid. You're not on the phone, you're not in cell service, you're not going to see a car for the several weeks that you're there. You're going to sit around at meals and talk about change, and talk about ... and you're going to be eating food that most of it grew right there. It's just like a complete change of everything, and meanwhile you're learning all these things. You come out the other end and it's like you can't go back, things will never be the same.

Brendan [00:33:51]: Yeah. You mentioned in your permaculture ... my permaculture design course ... I didn't take the full design course, but I did take a shortened course. It was a weekend course. That was my introduction. I still need to complete my PDC, but one of the things we did was we actually used banana plants to process water waste, and producing food from greywater.

Stephen [00:34:20]: Where did you do that?

Brendan [00:34:21]: This was in Brazil.

Stephen [00:34:23]: Oh, beautiful.
Brendan [00:34:24]: Yeah in the Pantanal region in the southwest, a somewhat swampy area.

Stephen [00:34:31]: Was that with Ali Sherif?

Brendan [00:34:34]: No, no. But anyway. So bananas, we could grow them the way you described, or we can grow them in this entirely different manner and enjoy their fruits and have it be a regenerative plant. If we create an "Earthship" like Mike Reynolds teaches people to do, you can have bananas growing in your house, in any climate. It could be subzero outside, and you could have bananas growing in your... basically in front of your living room, in the solarium, and it's processing your grey-water and so forth. There's so much magic in just harnessing Nature's innate ingenuity and combine it with human ingenuity, and the sky is practically the limit.

Stephen [00:35:20]: Yeah man, it's amazing once we start getting creative and once we shift our... kind of like we shift channels. We shift gears to going from putting all of our energy into accumulating as much as we can, and looking so much at dollars and how much we're making to really focusing on the quality of our life. And really focusing on our health, and really focusing on where do we want to be in a year, or in five years, or in ten years, or in twenty years. And "What can I do now to get on a path where I'm going in that direction? What can I be doing in six months? And what can I be doing in a year?" That's kind of what permaculture is. It's planning. It's intention, and it's efficiency.

Brendan [00:36:01]: Does your permaculture design course have a particular ... some permaculture design courses kind of have a focus in one way or the other while adhering to the overall structure and conveying all the principles and so forth. I'm just curious what your course is like.

Stephen [00:36:20]: Our course is a very ... there's a curriculum and 72 hours that you have to follow. I would say living on that same land for 22 years, there's a lot that comes through that, even if I don't say anything. You're surrounded by more species and plants than you ever have been in your life and they're like bombarding you. So, all of these different things that we're talking about in the course, we can show you twenty examples in one minute of our classroom. I think that's a really unique thing.

The other thing is, my wife Sarah is an herbalist, and her dedication to health and to the connection with plants, herbal medicine. I think that combination and also her... she just is such an incredible teacher, not because she's my wife, but because she's constantly reading and incorporating. She's usually reading three or four books at a time, and she's constantly incorporating what she's reading into her classes.
And then what's also amazing is the dynamic of our ... our courses are pretty international. All of a sudden, you're living with people from seven or eight countries, and it's amazing what you learn... You learn a lot from Sarah and I, and our other teachers, but you learn a lot from the other people in the class. And then we do the design projects which are always ... every course I'm realizing that we're getting better as teachers because the design projects are just so amazing.

Brendan [00:37:47]: Awesome. So you mentioned you've got all these ... you've got tons and tons of plants around there. What is maybe your favorite plant of all? If it's chocolate, then maybe it's chocolate. But I'm just curious, what's your favorite plant, your greatest discovery? Or the greatest discovery, not necessarily yours but something you found out and you'd like to share with people.

Stephen [00:38:08]: Yeah, the peach palm, I told you the pejibaye. And then I love jackfruit, I love breadfruit. Breadfruit is like flour, like a potato. You can make flour out of it to bake and make pancakes with and it grows on a tree. It's abundant, it fruits three or four times a year. It's incredible.

One thing that's exciting about what's happening now is, here I sit in this freaking dream of a reality, and this is just the beginning. We're ready to keep [inaudible, signal interrupted] we're ready to invite 80 more. We're trying to create urban realities where we can create health food stores, and alternative health clinics and co-working space. One of the other things that we're trying to add on to this addition is we're really focused on ... we already started the school which is more of like a kinder-elementary, and now we're ready to start kind of the green middle-high school, boarding school. And the assisted living, as we get older ... we've got to take care of our children, but we also have to take care of our parents. They're getting older. We want to really try to take care of our parents in a way that they're not thrown into some old age home, but they're part of some incredible, healthy program and the most incredible and vital foods, surrounded by other freaks' parents who are also probably cool. I think it's time we start living the life of our dreams, I mean there's nothing that's holding us back. Together these visions are just happening and unfolding. If you feel like you're not sitting in the place that you want to be, if the life of your dream isn't unfolding, I think it's time to press pause and zoom out and get on course.

Brendan [00:39:47]: Beautifully stated. One last question. Since obviously you're in the tropics and you collect largely, if not entirely, tropical species, I'm curious, are there any let's say temperate species that you use or love to tell people about, or are some of the species you collect there that work in the tropics, would any of them also work in temperate areas?

Stephen [00:40:15]: Yeah, I mean ... I think we grow temperate plants, lots of them, and in the temperate areas we can also grow tropical plants, but again what we're doing isn't some ... what we're teaching in the permaculture is not about the species, it's about the relationship between the elements. The species are just the variables, they're just the placeholders. What we want to do is create systems that work together and flow, and that's what's most important to what we try to teach. Don't get attached to ... there's this whole concept of paralysis by analysis, and that happens when we're just trying to wrap our Western brain around everything. And it's like, "No, figure out the long term; figure out the elements; figure out the way that these elements are going to interrelate." Don't be too caught up on the species, or too caught up on the ... get clear on your criteria, what do you want your life to look like? Where do you want to live? Do you want to live in the tropics? Do you want to live in the temperate? Do you want to live in the city? Do you want to live in the suburbs? Do you want to live in the country? Do you want to be a farmer? Do you want to be a graphic designer? What do you like to do and how can you merge all those elements to meet those goals and use less energy, the planet's energy, your own physical energy, your mental energy, all of it? Get on path to figuring out optimum way of living.

Brendan [00:41:40]: So in other words, it's not about transplanting your tropical paradise into my backyard. It's about me learning how to design an effective system that works in the context of what I want my life to look like and where I am, and what grows there, and what works.

Stephen [00:42:00]: Exactly.

Brendan [00:42:02]: Well thank you so much for ... I mean what you've created there is so awesome, so inspiring, such a home for a growing number of people. I can't wait to visit myself, maybe live there, I don't know.

Stephen [00:42:16]: Yes, I like the sound of it.

Brendan [00:42:18]: [inaudible] there. So blessings to you, thank you for raining the blessings on us and all the planet, and being a Noah's ark for plant species and rocking it. So thank you again for also being here in the Eat4Earth community with us today.

Stephen [00:42:39]: And thank you so much for doing this and organizing this and finding people ... I'm not so organized to be out there doing what you're doing, organizing all these ideas and thoughts, and I hope a lot of people watch this and take these lessons and incorporate them into their lives. And if you need help ...

Brendan [00:42:58]: You froze so, you said "If you need help ..." and then it froze.

Stephen [00:43:02]: We're here for you, we're here for you. You're not alone. If you're dreaming the same dream, you're not alone, and we're here for you.

Brendan [00:43:10]: Beautiful. Thank you. Have a great next Envision Fest, and if you want to say something about the Envision Fest real quick, that would be cool.

Stephen [00:43:19]: Yeah I should.

Brendan [00:43:21]: You said something, you're not organizing stuff like I am. Are you kidding me? You're organizing one of the biggest festivals in the world, and you've done it multiple times.

Stephen [00:43:32]: Our goal is to create ... we want to create experiences that change people's lives. I've been going to Burning Man since 2001, and I was so inspired by Burning Man that every year I started bringing my Costa Rican friends up to Burning Man. And then I was like wait a minute "Why don't we just bring a little piece of Burning Man down in Costa Rica?" And I joined up with a bunch of friends, and now it's grown into just an incredible experience that is mind-blowing, from the food to the speakers, to the music, to the yoga, to the ... just everything, the co-creation of community. It's like when people get to taste that for the first time, you never want to go back, man. It's just so sweet and delicious.

Brendan [00:44:11]: And is it always in February?

Stephen [00:44:12]: Yeah at the end of February every year.

Brendan [00:44:15]: Cool, awesome.

Stephen [00:44:17]: Excellent, thanks for making that plug! (laughs)

Brendan [00:44:19]: Again, thank you for being here today.

Stephen [00:44:21]: Thank you so much man, have a great day.

Brendan [00:44:23]: You too.

Stephen [00:44:24]: Peace.

Day 9 – Bonus Interviews

How to Transitioning to a More Plant-Based Diet, Microbiome Balance, Transmutation, Chernoble, and Fukushima
Zach Bush, MD
What You Will Discover

- The two main types of intestinal bacteria and how they affect health and disease
- The vegetable that reduces prostate cancer risk by 48% with just two servings per week
- The phenomenon of transmutation of elements (most scientists don't believe this is possible, but Dr. Bush discusses the mind-blowing evidence)

The Toxin Solution: Essential Keys to Safe and Complete Detoxification (Interview 2)
Joseph Pizzorno, ND
What You Will Discover

- The role of "single nucleotide polymorphisms" in your detoxification process
- Why it's important to balance "Phase I" and "Phase II" liver detoxification processes
- The three types of "Phase II" liver detoxification steps, including one related to risk of Alzheimer's Disease

Identifying and Resolving Mineral Deficiencies with Food
Robert Van Risseghem
What You Will Discover

- The 4 mineral deficiencies that Robert believes are related to prostate cancer risk
- How to use the USDA's James Duke Database online to think about using minerals to beat cancer
- The very common food additive that leaches minerals from your body

Essential Fat-Soluble Vitamins, Cholesterol, Trans-Esterified Fats, and Heart Disease
Nora Gedgaudas, CNS, CNT
What You Will Discover

- The vital roles of cholesterol, including protecting essential fatty acids from oxidation
- The true cause of most heart attacks (it's the opposite of what you think)
- Why Nora doesn't trust most Vitamin K2 supplements

Primal Ketosis, Digestion, and Restoring Foundational Health
Nora Gedgaudas, CNS, CNT
What You Will Discover

- Why Nora is not a fan of ketogenic supplements

- The lab that Nora trusts for definitively identifying food sensitivities
- Why Nora does not recommend liver-gallbladder flushes for detoxification

How Healthy Soil Puts Nutrients in Food and Protects Us from Heavy Metals
Walter Jehne
<u>What You Will Discover</u>

- How beneficial fungal organisms in the soil are ultimately responsible for your mineral nutrition
- How the same "transpiration stream" that plays a major role in climate dynamics also plays a role in your nutrition
- The "Velcro" like substance in soil that stabilizes climate and stores minerals for your plants

How to Choose a Juicer
John Kohler
<u>What You Will Discover</u>

- Why your choice of a juicer can make a 250% difference in the nutrients retained in your juices or smoothies
- Which type of food is best juiced with an "auger" style juicer
- Why you might want to make, or purchase, a vacuum-sealed blender
- How John makes super fluffy nut butters that retain more nutrients than regular nut butters
- John's coupon codes for you to save up to 30 on a juicer from him

Fat For Fuel: Live Long and Healthy with Mitochondrial Metabolic Therapy (Part 2)
Joseph Mercola, DO
<u>What You Will Discover</u>

- The dark secret of restaurant food that you need to know
- The problems with the "oxidative stress" theory of aging
- Why it can be counter-productive to take excess anti-oxidants

Minerals, Microbes, and Reversing Climate Change in a Golden Era For Food (Part 2)
Graeme Sait
<u>What You Will Discover</u>

- A tip for using foliar spraying for 12x more efficient delivery of nutrients to your plants
- The inexpensive device you can use to test the nutritional density of plants and plant foods
- The inspiring "1.6%" solution we can all take part in, plus food-growing tips about foliar sprays for your plants and humates for your soil

Food Solutions to Climate Change from Project Drawdown (Part 2)
Eric Toensmeier
What You Will Discover

- The exciting agricultural methods Project Drawdown call "coming attractions"
- "Leaf protein concentrate", the breakthrough new regenerative vegan food
- Oily fruits that could be the next wave of regenerative superfoods

Pleomorphism and Dark Field Microscopy
Kelly Kennedy
What You Will Discover

- The strange phenomenon of "endobiont" organisms that appear spontaneously in the human body and morph into various forms
- The three natural processes that cause an "endobionic flush"
- Why emotional trauma can cause lymphatic stagnation
- How dark field microscopy can quickly reveal things about your body's internal "terrain"

Zach Bush Second Interview

How to Transitioning to a More Plant-Based Diet, Microbiome Balance, Transmutation, Chernoble, and Fukushima

Brendan [00:00:00]: Welcome to the Eat4Earth event. We're exploring how you can heal yourself, your loved ones, and the earth with food. This is Brendan Moorehead and I am very excited to have Dr. Zach Bush back with us for a second conversation. Dr. Bush is a medical doctor and researcher, and he's one of the few triple board-certified physicians in the country with expertise in internal medicine, endocrinology and metabolism, and hospice palliative care. The breakthrough science that Dr. Bush and his colleagues have developed offers profound new insights into human health and longevity. In 2012, he discovered a family of carbon-based redox molecules made by bacteria. He and his team subsequently demonstrated that this cellular communication network functions to compensate for glyphosate and many other dietary, chemical, and pharmaceutical toxins that disrupt our body's natural defense systems. This science has resulted in a revolutionary class of dietary supplements including the product RESTORE™ (now called "ION* Gut Health"). Dr. Bush's education efforts provide a grassroots foundation from which we can launch change in our legislative decisions, ultimately upshifting consumer behavior to bring about a radical change in the mega industries of Big Farming, Big Pharma, and Western medicine at large. Dr. Bush, welcome back to the Eat4Earth event.

Dr. Bush [00:01:20]: Brendan, thank you so much for having me, and thank you for the kind introduction. That was a mouthful, so thank you.

Brendan [00:01:24]: Well, you're doing so much. There's a lot to talk about, a lot to say. So, Dr. Bush, I'd like to start today by summarizing some of what we covered in our previous conversation to bring everybody up to speed in case they haven't had a chance to catch that. You explained how beneficial bacteria produce complex signaling molecules, called redox molecules, that regulate pretty much everything in our bodies down to the DNA and also the lining of our gut. Yet, we're actively killing these beneficial bacteria and other beneficial organisms in our bodies with antibiotics, glyphosate, the glyphosate containing herbicide, Roundup, that's being applied at 2 billion kilograms, or I guess about 4.4 billion pounds, per year around the world, and without a healthy microbiome we can't properly "compost", as you put it, food in our guts into the signaling molecules that would properly regulate our genes, our genome, the gut lining, other membranes in our body. So, we get chronic systemic inflammation, the immune system gets overwhelmed, we can't detox and metabolize, our cells can't hydrate and can't produce normal proteins, and nutrients can't get delivered to the all-important mitochondria in our cells for cell repair. Also, glyphosate takes out the shikimate pathway in plants and bacteria that they use to produce certain amino acids and also phytonutrients that are the medicine that we're supposed to get from food. And all of this is being generated at the "foundation of life", as you put it, which is the soil in our bodies that is our microbiome, the soil outside of our bodies, which would normally supply much of the bacteria for a microbiome and support the crops that feed us. You also went into details about how this works and how the RESTORE™ (now called "ION* Gut Health") product can help rebuild and rebalance our microbiome. And I'd say that listening to that conversation over and over is a must for anybody that's committed to health and, before I go into my first actual question in this conversation, did I get all of that more or less right?

Dr. Bush [00:03:37]: Yeah, you just summarized the last 24 years of my life in about four minutes, so that's pretty impressive.

Brendan [00:03:43]: My pleasure.

Dr. Bush [00:03:46]: Yeah, outstanding overview.

Brendan [00:03:49]: So, Dr. Bush, you mentioned that plant lectins may be playing an important role in nutrient delivery by opening the tight junctions, which is a very different way of looking at them I would say, but obviously glyphosate has disturbed the balance between the opening and sealing of the tight junctions in the gut membrane. So now we seem to have an epidemic of lectin sensitivity, of which gluten sensitivity is just one example. Many people want to move to a more plant-based diet, myself included, either to heal a health condition, to reduce the ecological footprint of our diets, or because perhaps we don't want to want animals to die to feed us, but some of us are having a hard time making this shift. I tried for eight years in my 20s and I'm making another go of it in my 40s. You said that in 2010 you were seeing that about half of your patients were getting inflamed by the healthiest foods and I'm wondering what kind of foods were those? Were they things like beans, nuts, and seeds, and did restoring the microbiome correct that issue?

Dr. Bush [00:04:58]: Yeah, you're absolutely right. So, it turns out that we can be sensitive to just about any food that we put in our mouth and the more complex that food is the more likely that a leaky gut is going to have an initial kind of inflammatory reaction to it. So, the most monotonous foods that we eat, which are refined carbohydrates, you know, the white flour products, everything else—these are extremely monotonous foods that we get trained into as an American consumer. So, our gut gets used to that kind of insult environment and so as we make that big transition from kind of the processed food environment, and when I say processed food I actually mean meat. too, because meat is ultimately tons and tons of crop and chemical crops and water that's been now processed through the animal's system into a finished product of a very monotonous protein, such as beef which is L-carnitine, or salmon which is also L-carnitine. So, it doesn't matter if you're eating on the fish side or the beef side, you're getting the same protein structure and it's very monotonous - very little variability in the micronutrient content of that food, etc. So, what you're going to find when you participate in the, you know, kind of normal ecology of today your gut is inherently leaking. You have a permeable gut because of the lack of the nutrient quality of the food, the soil that you talked about ... because the food's lacking the medicinal quality, the protein content and everything else that we would seize from a complex diet is lacking and so we start to lose the bacteria. Glyphosate, as you mentioned, is doing a lot of things to our food chain but more than anything perhaps it's an antibiotic and kills the bacteria. And so that antibacterial effect of our food chain, the antibacterial effect of all the antibiotics that we pour into our meat production, dairy production, etc., all these antibiotics are trickling back down into our gut and suppressing biodiversity here. So, as a consumer you can bet that you've got a narrowed ecosystem that's dealing with a narrow bunch of nutrients that you're used to dealing with. So, that might be your steamed vegetable next to a piece of white meat, like your chicken, next to a starch. That's a very monotonous quality if you contrast that now to your classic Mediterranean diet, which has a lot of legumes and nuts and seeds and then the complex dark greens and the tomatoes and the eggplants—that's an incredibly wide nutrient profile. So, when people switch to a Mediterranean diet there's nothing magical about the fish that's in that diet. What's magical is the breadth of that diet. If you look at a traditional Indian cuisine, again, you've got massive amounts of different protein sources in a typical Indian cuisine but you also have an amazing amount of medicinal herbs, and so you've got all the spices and herbs that are creating a much more beneficial biologic effect but obviously a lot more pleasure in the experience of the food. You then turn your attention over to an Asian cuisine—again, you get a lot of unique structures that we don't typically get in the Western diet, things like the mung bean. Mung beans are super high in a lot of alkaloids and unique medicinals. They need to be cooked and not eaten raw because the alkaloids are so high in those mung beans. You know, there are things like that. Or, of course, the tropical fruits that you're getting in the Asian or more tropical diets that you would get down in Central America and things like that—so mango, papaya—these things have incredibly broad nutrient sources. The root vegetables, underrepresented in the American diet, the beets, kohlrabi, the daikon radish being a really great one, and jicama is a huge one there. So, these are unique nutrient sources that are just underrepresented. So, you mentioned you tackled a plant-based diet, and many of my patients have been making that transition for almost a decade now, trying to go from your kind of American monotonous protein diet to complex carbohydrates, nutrient dense, nutrient variety foods and, inevitably, if they're leaking they're going to develop discomfort – bloating, fatigue, brain fog, a sense of poor grounding. So they think "oh, I need the protein to be grounded", when in reality their body is just overwhelmed by the nutrient variety they have and that's the challenge. So, back in the day when I first started my clinic, to answer your question regarding did you fix the microbiome and it got better, ultimately, yes. Fixing the microbiome is a critical piece in tolerating more foods, but step one ends up being shutting those tight junctions. So, in getting that membrane to be coherent you get an intelligent gut back immediately. So, even if you don't have the microbiome yet to handle a diverse complex carbohydrate environment, where you're getting complex protein and carbohydrate mixes like you would with the beans and legumes and all these things that you mentioned, even if you can't digest those yet as long as your tight junctions are tight and you've got a solid membrane, a barrier system between your food environment and your immune system, it's not going to cause you any problems. Where you'll get inflammation from your diet, whether you're going plant-based or paleo or whatever you're doing, if you're experiencing bloating and gas pain and distension, inflammation after meals, you can bet that not only do you not have the microbiome there to break down those things effectively, you're now leaking those undigested peptides into the immune system and having to mount a food fight.

Brendan [00:10:35]: Oh, a food fight—that's a good term for it. So, I wonder if a fecal transplant from somebody who is totally adjusted to a plant-based diet, let's say a vegan who was eating a broad variety...I mean because you've got different types of vegans and some of them are just eating a lot of refined grains perhaps, some sugars and this and that, and that might not be the best vegan diet especially for a diverse microbiome and so forth, but if somebody is eating a very broad diet and they're plant-based, and a fecal transplant was done to an omnivore that was having trouble converting, I'm just curious—what would you predict and has there actually been any research on that showing what happens?

Dr. Bush [00:11:25]: Yeah, so I think you're spot-on. I think there's been, well, first of all paucity research. There's so little head-to-head data on plant-based diet versus paleo diet versus whatever other thing you pick, the bulletproof high-fat diet. Head-to-head data is impossible to come by so instead we have to, I think, keep turning to the individual's experience rather than try to figure out a population statistic. Ultimately your individual experience as somebody who's trying to transform your diet is way more important than any book you read or any study out there. So, while there's a paucity of data, the good news is this is a one-on-one experience. So I think you're exactly right in that you can have a profoundly unhealthy or narrow nutrient profile in a vegan or vegetarian diet and so, you know, you've got to be eating for diversity. But, if you have a leaky gut the ones that are going to be most difficult for you will be the raw vegetables that are high in alkaloids. So, those would be things like your nightshade vegetables. I'll be things like your high-fiber-content compounds like your kale. Too many people are just going out thinking they can get healthy by eating lots of kale salads. Well that's actually not good for your gut, to be overwhelmed constantly by a superfood like kale. You're going to actually have such a high alkaloid content that it's going to be difficult for a microbiome that's diminished and a leaking gut to deal with that level of alkaloid. So, that's where steaming and cooking your vegetables on the front end is really important. The ethnic foods are so fascinating. I mean these are recipes that have developed for thousands of years versus the American diet, where ten years ago do you remember seeing a kale salad on the menu at your local restaurant?

Brendan [00:13:05]: I don't think so.

Dr. Bush [00:13:07]: I don't think it was there. Now you can go to any restaurant—I'm pretty sure McDonald's is going to come out with a kale hamburger at any moment—like it is so overwhelmingly ridiculously overemphasized in our environment and yet it's really not any secret health ingredient. Kale is an important superfood but it should be eaten in small amounts and really, especially for a challenged gut, should be cooked. So, if you look at the Indian cuisine or you look at the Asian cuisine they cook all of their vegetables, which reduces the alkaloid content. Now this works very well if you've got fresh vegetables that are being harvested near you and then cooked fresh, you're going to have the right alkaloid and enzyme balance in that food. Where we screw things up in the Western world is we ship unripe material, unripe crops from Chile and Puerto Rico or wherever, in the wintertime. We ship that to our local grocery store, ripen it under ethylene gas infusion in our shipping containers, and so now you've got an abnormally represented vegetable or fruit that was picked unripe, has an imbalance in the enzyme content, an imbalance in the sugar to fiber content, and we force ripen it under ethylene gas and then deliver it to the grocery store. It looks pretty; it looks like it should be healthy for us, and yet we get nutrient imbalance from it. So, by and large if you're switching over to a plant-based diet, I would say go to steamed veggies and you don't need to steam these into oblivion. If you're going to saute, a water saute or steam is really fast. So you may saute vegetables for no more than two minutes in a pan, but in doing so that flash steaming of it will help break down and reduce some of the potent alkaloids to get the alkaloid:enzyme ratio right so that you can use that compound as a medicinal rather than as kind of getting this big drug effect and overwhelm inflammation. So, we want to balance those out. So, if you're having trouble switching over to a plant-based diet, steam those veggies, especially your cruciferous vegetables and the dense ones, so kale, cauliflower, broccoli—don't be eating those raw. Those are going to cause some bloating and other things. Seeds—sprout those seeds overnight and nuts as well. So, if you soak your nuts overnight you're going to have a lot less issues; you're going to off-gas those nuts. Beans are extremely obvious; so, a can of beans that you pick up the grocery store—this is what most people do switching over to a plant-based diet-- you get three cans of beans and then your bloated for a few days and you're like "well, I must not tolerate beans". Well, the beans that are prepared in a can at the grocery store go from dried beans to canned beans in seven to eight minutes. They're prepared under an intense pressure-cooker environment, so they go under very high pressure, intense heat to take that dry bean to a soft can bean in minutes. Well, now it's a soft bean; it feels like it was done just like anybody would have done traditionally with a bean but the gas and the protein content and the enzymes in there are all off, and they can screw you up until you get your gut used to it. Once you get your gut really resilient with a rich microbiome and the tight junctions, you're going to even resent ... you'll be able to tolerate canned beans without a problem. But in the short run when you're making these nutritional changes, especially if you have a leaky gut, you're going to be prone to gas from those things. But now if you soak your own dry beans you're going to get a totally different experience than the canned bean. It's pretty astounding; if you've never soaked black beans or pinto beans, I encourage you to do it if for no other reason, even if you don't eat it, look at how much gas comes off those dried beans. So, all you do is fill up a crock on your countertop; fill it with water and then dump in your dried beans. Let it soak overnight with a lid on it or a towel over it, whatever it is, a little bit of lemon juice I often add or lime juice. That lime juice will help break down some of that and the phytonutrients even more effectively, so a teaspoon of lime juice or half a lime and lemon squeezed in there. The next morning you've got this...it's literally bubbling—you've got bubbles of foam coming off the top of this thing. I've seen some of my beans that I've prepared, I've seen it fill the whole crock with bubbles and so you just have like foam sitting on top of the water. So that's the 24-hour off-gassing process. Now if you cook those beans you're going to do a slow cook on those beans because even after 24 hours of soaking they're still pretty hard. So now you're going to cook those in a crockpot for six or eight hours and they're going to continue to autodigest, break down the phytonutrients and get prepared for being a much easier compound on your gut. Again, if you look to the Central American or Mexican cuisine that uses a lot of beans, they do a lot of triple preparation of their beans. They'll soak them, then they will boil them, and then they'll crush them down and then sauté them again into like a refried bean and they'll add some fat into that. The fat:protein ratio helps reduce gas and metabolism of those as well. So there's so many different steps to making beans that are going to be really easy on your gut. We don't do that as an American consumer, so then we blame the legume or we blame the bean or we blame the nut or we blame the kale. Food isn't the problem—it's our preparation of those compounds that's really gotten lost from any sort of intelligent system. So, give your gut a break by steaming those vegetables, by soaking the beans or nuts and seeds overnight before consumption. That will really ease that transition.

Brendan [00:18:38]: I'm curious to know what you might think of the distinction that Dr. Steven Gundry makes in his book, *The Plant Paradox*, between "Old World" and "New World" plants and plant lectins. He's basically saying that New World plants, like peppers, many of the beans, nightshades...I don't mean those classes of foods entirely but many representatives in there—tomatoes and so forth, and potatoes coming from the new world and that our microbiome hasn't had a long time to adjust to these and learn to digest these. Of course, if we're nuking our microbiome then, you know, our ancestral microbiome may not be there to do anything anyway, but I'm just curious what your thoughts are about that - that idea?

Dr. Bush [00:19:30]: There's no question; again, you're right on the topic. So, the potato that you mentioned is probably one of the best examples that we have in the United States. We think of a potato as a russet potato, you know, the big white potato, long growth. We developed the russet potato to make good French fries. Literally that thing was bioengineered through breeding to create a long French fry that would be a bouquet out of the McDonald's thing. That was what drove the development of the russet potato, was we need French fries that aren't lost in the bottom, although that might be your favorite French fries—those crunchy ones down in the bottom there. But, what they were going for is let's get a long French fry, let's get that whole long thing, so we need a long potato and so they developed them from baby potatoes. They kept breeding and breeding until we got that big oblong russet potato. So, now we have a very high starch content, very low micronutrient content, and then we skin it, which removes some 99% of the micronutrient from a potato, and cook it into a French fry. In contrast if you're going down to Peru, which is the birthplace of the potato, they have over a thousand variants and species of potatoes. None of them look like a russet potato. There are big, gnarly yellow ones, there are big purple ones, there are black potatoes. I mean it's ridiculous diversity. So, if you go to a street market in Peru, you're going to see things that they call a potato and it looks nothing like anything you've seen – big, contorted, weird external shells on them and you cut them open and they have all this variation in color and everything else. So, you're going to have a completely different experience if you go back to these heirloom sources that we just bred into oblivion until we ended up with this white starch container that we call a potato today. Tomatoes, similarly; absolutely we've changed through a hybridization the tomato over the years. If you go to an heirloom tomato at your farmers' market, you already know what it looks like in your head if you've been to a farmers' market ever, is they look abnormal. They're not like the big, red, perfect apple-shaped tomato that you see at the grocery store. They're flattened or they look kind of like a doughnut where they're almost pinched through in the middle or they've got green and yellow stripes on them. They're just a totally different fruit than you would expect from that red tomato at the grocery store. So, again, heirloom is bred for biodiversity, micronutrient diversity, unbelievable nutrient pack. We breed those out of just consumer behavior into these very monotonous foods that we know today. I think that overall that the root vegetables are a little bit of a savior here. The beets have not changed much over time, the turnip has not been bred into any change, and the daikon radish is another good example of this, and the colorful carrots. So, now you're starting to see these at Whole Foods and I think even Trader Joe's I saw it recently where they started to have the mixed color carrots, where you'll have the yellow, the purple, and the orange carrots in a single bag—that was carrot life. Carrots aren't just orange little things that look like baby fingers that have been plucked off, those "carrot sticks" that we'd get bags of and you see all the kids in elementary school carrying around these little baggies, skinned perfectly. I mean, there's not even a ridge on them let alone dirt. It doesn't look like a carrot, yet in their mind this is a carrot. Now you've got a very monotonous, high-sugar content orange little thing with a lot of the micronutrients removed because it's been skinned down to this little brutal stub of what used to be a nutrient delivery system of a carrot. So, I think that you're exactly right. We're falling apart on so many avenues towards what should be a nutritious diet.

Brendan [00:23:12]: You know, speaking of potatoes and heirloom potatoes, it occurred to me...I wonder if the heirloom potatoes have a higher resistant starch content? Do you happen to know?

Dr. Bush [00:23:23]: Oh yeah, for sure.

Brendan [00:23:25]: They do. So, they're going to help feed our friendly bacteria much better than a hybridized, you know, russet or something?

Dr. Bush [00:23:32]: Absolutely. And they're going to have a bunch of phytonutrients that can fight cancer in there too. So, you've got all these...anything with color tends to have a phytonutrient in there, that's anti-cancer. So in the tomato, for example, it's lycopene and lycopene is the big cancer killer. In a potato it's going to come from the purples in those purple potatoes. Even the Yukon Gold that you can still find is a better nutrient source than your white russet. So any color you can get into that vegetable or fruit is going to be beneficial. But just because the color is there doesn't necessarily mean those anti-cancer effects are there. So, one of the good examples of this, again, let's go back to the tomato. I mentioned lycopene a few seconds ago. In the 1940s the typical tomato coming out of the backyard victory garden, which was growing 45% of our food chain, had loads of lycopene in it, to the degree that I think most prostate cancer was being prevented by tomatoes we were growing in our own backyard. And so lycopene is very potent on prostate cancer in particular. The other thing that's extremely potent for prostate cancer is the nutrients in Brussels sprouts. A really recent clinical study was done on Brussels sprout consumption in men; men who consume Brussels sprouts twice a week, had one serving of Brussels sprouts twice a week, had a 45% reduction in prostate cancer. That's an insane public health statistic. I mean, like can it really be that easy for us to turn this tide on cancer? Right now 50% of American males are getting cancer before we die, one in two. That is an epidemic of cancer, and if we could reduce prostate cancer in half by just introducing Brussels sprouts a couple times a week is a ridiculous statistic. Brussels sprouts, I think, were used in that study because, again, lycopene is becoming pretty rare in tomatoes. So, the tomatoes that you're getting at the grocery store for sure are lacking lycopene largely because they weren't grown in soil. They were grown in the hydroponic systems. And when the hydroponic growing of the tomatoes kicked in we saw a really rapid drop in that lycopene content. I think that the hydroponics are going to improve over the coming years; I think we've already seen some improvement in the nutrients that are delivered through our hydroponic systems. But I remain concerned that if we're going to start really mass producing our food that never touches soil, we're going to inherently be lacking nutrients, phytonutrients, fiber, all kinds of stuff in that food that we should have. So, the lycopene in tomatoes is, especially at the grocery store, almost non-existent now. So even though the tomato looks red— you would think it should have the lycopene in there—it's lacking it. So, you want an anti-cancer regimen in your life? Shop at your farmers' market. It's that simple. Get as close to the farmer as possible and shop as many heirloom breeds as you can.

Brendan [00:26:17]: And, on the topic of tomatoes, just briefly it would probably be good to mention that lycopene is far more bioavailable when the tomatoes are cooked, as I understand it. Is that correct?

Dr. Bush [00:26:29]: That's correct, and that's the case with a lot of the alkaloids. So, a lot of people feel like they are sensitive to the nightshades. The nightshades are the ones that have all of the most important alkaloid medicinals in them, but they become bioavailable and less noxious to us when they're cooked. So your peppers and your eggplant you definitely want to have those cooked thoroughly before consumption.

Brendan [00:26:54]: Okay. Now, back to what we were discussing in regards to shifting towards a plant-based diet. It occurred to me that the shikimate pathway, which you said is the chemical pathway that glyphosate takes out, and it exists in plants and bacteria, and it produces certain essential amino acids like tyrosine, tryptophan, and phenylalanine, which happen to be important in producing neurotransmitters in our bodies, among other things ... and it occurs to me because my own personal experience with plant-based proteins when I am used to animal-based proteins is that I feel mentally foggy. And it could be anything generating that, right?

Dr. Bush [00:27:37]: Yep.

Brendan [00:27:38]: But it did occur to me that maybe I'm missing the high doses of certain amino acids that I get from meats, and my body hasn't adjusted either to the lower doses or I don't have the microbiome that would produce those amino acids from plant foods for me. I'm just curious what your perspective is on that. Are plant-based diets with a good microbiome ... is a lot of the production of those particular amino acids happening in the gut? **Dr. Bush [00:28:07]:** Absolutely, yeah. So, you've got 26 amino acids that build over 200,000 proteins in your body. This is very much like the 26 letters of our alphabet that build hundreds of thousands of words. The essential amino acids are the eight that we can't make within our body. The vast majority of amino acids, 18 of those 26, are made within the human cells. So the human cell, at the liver especially, is able to generate amino acid production from just about anything. We can produce these in amazing fashion, but the eight essentials we can't produce within the human cell. They are produced by the bacteria, fungi, and the plants themselves through, like you said, the shikimate pathway. So the essential ... well not all of them, some of them rely on different enzyme pathways than the shikimate ... three of the eight are essential to the shikimate, but nonetheless you've got these enzyme pathways and bacteria and in the plants themselves that will make the other eight essential amino acids. So, it's fascinating that, like you say, we've got a chemical environment to our food where our food chain, both at the bacteria level and at the plant level, is lacking the ability to make these eight essential amino acids that go on to build a healthy human body. Imagine our alphabet minus the vowels. If you remove the vowels, or just a few of the vowels, like you said three amino acids from the shikimate pathway...if you remove three vowels from the alphabet, those being your essential amino acids, now what kind of body can you build? You're going to build a truncated protein structure. You're going to bring in substitute amino acids. Where you should be using alanine you'll use glutamine or something like this. And so you're rebuilding abnormal proteins by using substitutions. It's as if we started spelling every word that had an O in it and throw in a U instead. You might still be able to work out what the word is but it's not going to be correctly spelled. That's happening in our protein structure. We're literally misspelling protein structure throughout the body as we subtract out the nutrients from our food in these essential amino acids. So, it's a very powerful and frightening effect of our food chain there.

Brendan [00:30:21]: And also in the shikimate pathway, another question I have about that is that because it does in plants produce phytonutrients, do bacteria also produce phytonutrients and do they do it in our gut, in the soils? What's your view on that?

Dr. Bush [00:30:38]: Absolutely. I think that we will likely find out that the vast majority of phytonutrients, anti-cancer compounds, etc. are made by bacteria and fungi. There are 5 million (5,000,000) species of fungi—it's an insane number – 5 million (5,000,000) species, and the genomic information there is just completely mind-blowing. So, the human genome is 20 thousands (20,000) genes. The bacterial genome is around 1 to 2 million (1,000,000 to 2,000,000) genes. The parasite genome is around 2 billion (2,000,000,000) genes. The fungal genome is around 100 trillion (100, 000,000,000,000) genes. So, we have so much genetic variety when you get into the fungi and the bacteria. Such an insane amount of genetic information there. And that genetic information is building the proteins that will become our nutrients. Imagine what 100 trillion genes can produce in our food chain. I guarantee you we don't know one-thousandth of 1% of that. I mean, we know nothing about nutrient in the end. Here I have a nutrition clinic, and I study nutrition all the time—and that's my whole life and business—and I can guarantee you I know nothing about nutrition, because we are just barely scratching the surface of understanding this wealth of genomic information in the microbiome and what it's producing for our bodies. What I do know is that because of the destruction of that microbiome through our farming practices, the herbicides, the pesticides, the antibiotics in our animals, blah, blah, blah, we have destroyed that unknown, untapped resource of nutrient and protein diversity and we are seeing the public health consequences of it—1 in 40 children with autism versus 1 in 5,000 thirty years ago. We're heading towards 1 in 3 children with autism within the next 16 to 18 years at our current rate. So this level of collapse of public health is evidence of what we've lost, but we don't even know what we've lost. And so, we're literally causing mass extinction of, I think, many bacterial and fungal populations right now that we will probably never recover and we will never know what we lost.

Brendan [00:32:55]: Yeah, the fungal kingdom is pretty awe-inspiring if you look into the work of Paul Stamets.

Dr. Bush [00:33:04]: Yes, hats off to Paul.

Brendan [00:33:06]: And, yeah, you know one of the most important species to us all as humans and anybody that eats on land really is the mycorrhizal fungal organism that that associates with lots of plants—not all of them, but it makes nutrients available to them directly and overall fungal organisms were instrumental in generating what we now call soil on the planet. You know, back in the day, billions of years ago, they started it all, and they're still a key player.

Dr. Bush [00:33:40]: Absolutely still a key player. One interesting thing, and I think of it just because I took a hydrating drink there, but there are so many things that will shift the biome that we don't think of as nutrient. I'm a huge fan of tea, and some great studies have recently been done on black tea and green teas that show that these create a fundamental shift in our microbiome towards Bacteroides. So, let me digress for a moment and completely way oversimplify the gut for you for a moment. It's way more complicated than what I'm about to describe, but this is a good framework for us to understand healthy gut versus kind of unhealthy, fermenting, acidic gut. The Bacteroides is a huge genus; it used to be called the Bacteroidetes. But, Bacteroides is a huge family of bacteria and some of those have the potential to have pathogenic effects. They can be pro-inflammatory. They can cause issues if they're imbalanced or we have too many of some Bacteroides species than others. But, as a huge genus, or big family of bacteria, the Bacteroides again and again correlate with better gut health, lower inflammation scores, longevity, better hydration, etc. So, Bacteroides as a big genus is a friendly type. The other huge genus is the Firmicutes. The Firmicutes, when they get overrepresented in the gut and they start to outstrip the populations of Bacteroides, we see a huge production of acidity in the gut, we see a breakdown in immune function, we see increased permeability of the gut lining, etc. And, as it stands right now, most Americans have more Firmicutes than Bacteroides. We are eating far too much protein, especially dense animal proteins which will emphasize the Firmicutes. So, the recent studies in the teas are really interesting because you think, oh tea at zero calories it's maybe a little bit of leaf in there to give it a little bit of flavor, but in reality there are phytonutrients in those tea leaves that are preparing that black or green tea to increase Bacteroides and burn fat. When you have a high B:F ratio, Bacteroides to Firmicutes, you tend to have a fast metabolism and burn fat very effectively. High Firmicutes you tend to store fat in the liver and develop fatty liver, diabetes, etc., and so a really cool thing to realize, wow, these age-old medicinals—tea goes back to the very beginning of medicine. I mean, this is probably the very first medicine that was ever given; it was a tea, right? Boil some water with a couple of herbs and roots in there and give it to your patient—oldest therapies on earth, and we know the power of ginger, garlic, all these root things, and then you combine that with a leaf and you get all kinds of fantastic medicinal qualities. So, it's just fun to see what our pretty basic modern genomic studies are starting to bear out; oh my gosh, just a glass of black tea can change that whole B:F ratio, reduce inflammation in your body, etc. There's a huge fad of the bulletproof coffee right now and there's some interesting data around the anti-inflammatory stuff, having fat first thing in the morning and all these things. I don't think it has anything magic to do with it, and I would encourage you to think about at least varying that up. Monotony is never good for the diet, so if you're doing bulletproof coffee think about starting some of your days with a green tea or black tea, a lot less acid on your gut and it's going to change the B:F ratio much more effectively than the cup of bulletproof coffee will. So, just switch that up a little bit, and think about that microbiome before you ever worry about vegetable, fruit, legume, nut, seed. It's fun to start to bring in some of these tools that can adjust that population even before you take a bite of food.

Brendan [00:37:28]: It's interesting you should say that because I just started drinking green tea every morning a couple of weeks ago for the first time in my life, and it wasn't for that reason actually. But then I started to think about it and I said, "Okay I'm consuming more polyphenols", because that seems to be the key phytonutrient in these teas, also in coffee. And it just so happens that in the plant and soil relationships if you have plants representing five different families, the cereals, the grasses, the brassicas, chenopods, and legumes, I believe, and certain very progressive farmers when they use a cover crop species mix that includes all five or, you know, usually they have more than five species, but all five families are represented—what happens is the plants start sending phenolic compounds down into the soil and the subsoil life goes crazy. It just goes to another level of productivity, I guess. So, the whole system takes off, and that seems to be a universal effect across many different types of cells. And, of course, we have mitochondria that are very much like bacteria in our own cells, and then we've got our being outnumbered 10 to 1, isn't it, as far as the bacteria in our bodies versus our own cells? So, we're prominently bacterial and bacteria respond to these phenolic compounds.

Dr. Bush [00:39:07]: Yeah, and then you add the fungi into that environment and we're just so grossly outnumbered—it's out of control.

Brendan [00:39:15]: Yeah, we're outnumbered 100 to 1 at least with the genes, the genome.

Dr. Bush [00:39:19]: Yep, absolutely. Yeah, and at the genomic level it's probably 1,000,000 to 1 as far as the microbiome genes to us, so it's just a ridiculous outnumbering and one of the ways in which to get this back into your life is obviously the fermented foods. So, fermenting some food in your home is such a rich experience. Number one, you save yourself a lot of money. A really good wild fermented sauerkraut right now at one of your health food stores, you can pay 12 bucks for a little Ziploc bag of sauerkraut—it's ridiculous. It costs less than five cents to make that at home. Sauerkraut is simply water and salt, you mix that into a saltwater brine, and then a chopped cabbage. You buy the cabbage for a dollar, and you throw that in and once it's chopped and everything else you have a whole crock of sauerkraut for less than a dollar, and you've got yourself two weeks of prep time, something like that, and then you've got yourself a tablespoon or two of that sauerkraut with each meal, especially your midday meal. You're going to change the microbiome. You're going to get that biodiversity back into the diet. Historically we had a couple bites of fermented food with every single meal, and that was just routine until we developed refrigeration in the 1950s. And with widespread refrigeration in our homes we got lazy. We stopped fermenting foods and canning and everything else, and we just started sticking things in the fridge. We lost our nutrient density at that point. Fermentation is a more advanced way than cooking your food to get the nutrients bioavailable. Let the bacteria start to digest all those micronutrients before you ever put it in your mouth. Now if you're lacking microbiome because you've been exposed to antibiotics, etc., the food is being predigested for you by the bacteria. They're liberating the micronutrients, the phytonutrients, etc. from that food. So, when you eat the pre-prepared sauerkraut from your home wild ferment you're going to get a great response. Now if you don't do a wild ferment and you're getting something that's just prepared in the grocery store, this will be a cheaper product at the grocery store. It's oftentimes on a shelf rather than in the refrigerated section. Your wild ferments are always going to be stored in the refrigerated section in something like a Ziploc bag or a Ball jar kind of thing. In contrast you might find a can of organic sauerkraut or something like that on the shelf that will have been by and large prepared through a probiotic rather than through wild fermentation. The probiotic they just throw in one or three species of bacteria into the stew and let that digest the cabbage and turn that into it.

That's going to be a narrow micronutrient thing prepared by one bacteria. Whereas if you do a wild air ferment, where you let the bacteria from the air come into that crock for the first day or two, now you're going to have a much different result. You've got hundreds of species if not thousands of species that are now digesting that food for you and preparing it for your gut to receive both the nutrient as well as the microbial life.

Brendan [00:42:19]: Is that wild open-air ferment...I've always done mine sealed, so do you actually have the lid open?

Dr. Bush [00:42:26]: Yes. So, classic ferment for the first day you throw it into a crock or if you're doing it in jars just leave the jar open and put a towel over it. So, the towel will not be occlusive to the bacteria and so you can keep dust out of it and stuff like that with the towel. But the bacteria will be filtering through into your stew there with your ferment into the brine and introduce that. It's the same way you make Kombucha. To get the mother of the Kombucha to develop, you've got to leave that to a longstanding air ferment to get that mother built. Then once it's built, you can do it pretty much sealed. But to develop that that microbiome for either something like a Kombucha, which is more of a fungal ferment, or bacterial ferment that you will get with the sauerkraut brines and things like that, you're going to air ferment. Leave it in open air for anywhere from 24 to 48 hours and then you can cap them and let them continue to ferment under a capped environment. It's not unusual with an air ferment to get a little bit of accumulation of like a little rim of fungal material on top of the water. This is a good sign, not a bad sign. You just skim that with a spoon, take that off once a day and then go ahead and bottle it when it's done. So, you can air ferment for the full two weeks of a fermentation process, you just have to skim the water frequently. If you don't want to skim the water, then I would say 24 hours to 48 hours of air fermentation and then screw your Ball lids on. Remember, don't keep those tight unless you have an airlock release in those. To do that you just drill a hole in the middle of your Ball jar tabs and use one of the airlock systems that you can get at any brewing mart or something like that in your local environment. It is a little double plastic container that has a little water float in it so it lets the air bubble pass that but it keeps material from passing back through down into your ferment. So, you can keep that on the on the countertop for a week or two and then place that in the refrigerator for long-term fermentation at a slowed process. Kimchi is one of my favorites to prepare. Kimchi has just got ridiculous phytonutrient quality because you got all the spice in there. Those peppers under long-term influence of the bacteria have a bunch of very unique anti-inflammatory compounds in there. I think the Koreans for all centuries have been giving a couple tablespoons of that kimchi before each meal. The pre-digestion effect on the digestive enzymes and everything else is profound and has led to real longevity benefits to that Korean diet with that advent or that startup of the ferment before the meal.

Brendan [00:45:13]: Thank you. Those are some great tips. I appreciate that and definitely learned something there. So, we've been discussing how glyphosate and plant lectins and so forth interact with the gut lining. How about other membranes in the body? Are there other membranes in the body that are affected that also have tight junctions?

Dr. Bush [00:45:32]: Yeah, and this has really been supported by Monsanto and the chemical companies in spades. So, they keep pronouncing this as good news but it's a pretty scary omen. Monsanto has been justifying to the EPA that this is a safe compound because the main target is not in humans, the main target is the shikimate pathway, which only exists in bacteria and fungi. Never mind that that then eliminates the essential amino acid production from our food chain, but they've been arguing that it's safe because of that. Well our lab ... if you haven't seen our science at RESTORE™ (now called "ION* Gut Health" at IONBiome.com), you can go to that website and see a bunch of the science there ... but we've shown that glyphosate does indeed have a direct target toxin and target at the tight junction and cause that leaky gut permeability thing. And we're actually publishing a paper in the next few weeks. We already demonstrated that glyphosate sensitizes to gluten sensitivity, and now we're ready to publish in the next couple months the exact mechanism by which Roundup, or glyphosate, is causing a sensitization on the entire intestinal lining to gluten. I believe that we didn't have any gluten sensitivity in the true sense of the word until about 1992, and that's when we started spraying wheat with Roundup. And at that moment we let the canary in the coal mine die, and we just ignored it and marched on and now every year we've had 30-50% increase in worldwide acreage sprayed on wheat with Roundup ever since then. So much of our wheat worldwide is being sprayed with Roundup and Roundup is causing a hypoxic injury, a lack of oxygen, in the gut lining. That hypoxic injury upregulates the receptor for gliadin, which is the breakdown product of gluten that then causes permeability of the gut lining. So, a big story there unfolding. But to answer your question, that's just the beginning of the injury. So, as mentioned, Monsanto has been saying, "Hey, look, the targets aren't in humans; it's a totally safe chemical and, look, when you eat glyphosate you pee it out at the same rate you eat it." This is profoundly bad news when you find out that it damages membranes. Because to move from your mouth to your urine it has to cross so many membranes on the way through. The first one is your gut membrane, and I think that's probably where 80 -90% of the injury happens. When you start to see tight junctions fall apart, there's typically a compound called zonulin involved. Zonulin is actually produced by our human intestines to open tight junctions. Tight junctions should open and close naturally in response to zonulin. So, zonulin regulates the absorption of large macronutrients and big fiber and other things that need to pass through the gut lining. But if you have an injury that overemphasizes this dump of zonulin, zonulin starts to break down tight junctions all over the body. So, you're going to loosen the membranes not just at the gut but at the blood vessels. Your blood vessels are a different cell type than your gut lining. Your gut lining is called epithelium, your blood vessel lining is called endothelium. But it doesn't matter if it's epithelium or endothelium, it's still the same Velcro proteins that hold those cells together to create coherent macro membranes that would be an entire blood vessel tree, arterial tree, venous tree, lymphatic systems, or this entire gut system or the blood-brain barrier, the barrier between the blood itself and a peripheral nerve or the blood itself and your cranial nerves in your brain, all of these things. So the central and peripheral nervous system all the way to the kidney, again, tied together with tight junctions. So, as we start to say, "Oh, wow, we have a water-soluble toxin"—not a fat-soluble like most toxins that can be sequestered away in the body in fat cells—we have a water-soluble toxin in glyphosate that moves through the body readily into every single water compartment, and so it's going to be intracellular, it's going to be extracellular, it's going to move through membranes very easily. And what it's going to do on the way through is both through a zonulin injury at the gut as well as direct injury to tight junctions all the way through we're going to see damage to each of these cell types. So, what ends up happening is you get leaky sieve on the front end—you've got glyphosate giving you that permeability of the gut, and then you have abnormal filtration through the whole body. So, now the next blood vessels that have to handle that chemical load are the veins that run from your gut to your liver. So, you're already leaking and causing a leaky syndrome where toxins that should be processed and cleaned up in the liver are already leaking out into tissue before they ever get to the liver. Now in the liver, this is supposed to be the ultimate filter right? Your liver is your big filter system to protect you from whatever is coming in the gut. The liver is supposed to repackage everything, clean out the toxins and only send good nutrients, micronutrients and macro fuel nutrients, to the body. If the liver is now leaking, you've lost a barrier system. There should be a complete cellular barrier, just like your gut wall, at the liver. The hepatocytes, or the liver cells, are bound together by tight junctions and create a barrier and every nutrient that comes in your body has to now go between the cells to sneak in and now has to cross a liver cell, and the liver cell then packages things—source out the cholesterol, source out the micronutrients, gets all that repackaging. It can make glucose out of protein; about 85-90% of the protein that Americans eat gets turned into sugar at the liver because we eat too much protein. All of this beauty is happening in the hepatocyte. But, if you have glyphosate injury across that liver barrier, now stuff is leaking past the liver cell and just getting into your bloodstream unfiltered, un-repackaged, unrefined for your body. So, now you're getting all of that dumped into the bloodstream and now as it travels through your body it can get it into the brain, it can get into tissue, and then ultimately it hits the kidney tubules, which, again, are starting to leak, and you're starting to have a hard time managing electrolyte ratios of the kidney. We have the number one chronic disease in the entire world right now, chronic kidney disease. So, we're just slaughtering our kidneys through this, you know, leaking and just dumping of toxin into the system. The kidneys are just absolutely being tortured. And so we can't clear the toxin on the back end through our kidney clearance system. So, we're a sieve on the front end, can't clear from the back end, and our bodies are turning into sponges for toxin.

Brendan [00:51:52]: Wow, it's worse than we thought I guess—this sort of repeated chemical shotgun blast to our to our membranes and so many structures. On the topic of grains there's another question I have. There's a sugar, apparently called Neu5Ac, on our epithelial linings of our guts and blood vessels, and grains have lectins that bind to this sugar, I believe. So, the question I have is, is this sugar handled normally by a healthy biome so that it presents no issue, or fermentation if we pre-ferment grains or sprout them, or is it something that's an inherent risk in grain consumption? I'm just kind of curious if you know.

Dr. Bush [00:52:54]: Yeah, I think if you have a healthy microbiome, there's no such thing as a toxin. Your bacteria and fungi transmute everything. Transmutation is this incredible phenomenon that happens in the body. It's not well studied over much of the decades. It got studied very aggressively in the 1940s to 1960s in Russia and in parts of Europe and in the U.S., a lot of exciting science proving that single elements—and now we are talking about the periodic table, like you think of something like manganese or selenium or potassium—these fundamental elements that in the Newtonian model of how atoms work we believe that potassium is always potassium. Well, in transmutation potassium can combine with hydrogen; you can take the protons from those two compounds, add those protons into a single nucleus and get a different element.

Brendan [00:53:48]: Oh my gosh.

Dr. Bush [00:53:50]: That's transmutation in the true sense. So, we're finding through strict studies in sweat output and food intake that there's no way the body is keeping sodium/potassium balance true to itself and it's starting to look like potassium and hydrogen can combine to become calcium. So, we're getting a possibility that most the bone calcium is actually done by transmutation across cell membranes of potassium and hydrogen. So, we are building the periodic table inside our body through the microbiome and through the human cell potential of transmutation. So, when you start to take in that possibility, now all bets are off and it starts to make some sense. I spent a lot of time in the Philippines, and I've been down to Central America at times. And if you've been to any developing country where they have been hit with famine it is striking how resilient the human body is to such an incredibly chronic low-grade amount of nutrient. So, in Sub-Saharan Africa it's all white rice and maybe one little handful of steamed vegetables a day in these camps, and yet you see the kids running around and laughing and certainly with starvation you can get to the point where you're listless and you're dying and there's no question this is dangerous. But I'm constantly stunned at how little nutrient has to go into the body to fuel health, and certainly I saw this in the Philippines. These kids growing up in the squats of the Philippines for years under-nutrient delivered, and yet they seem to be thriving. In fact, they have lower levels of chronic disease than our American children counterparts. So it's a fascinating reality that given the opportunity to any nutrient the microbiome and your body are going to figure out ways to transmute those into nutrients that your body needs. You may need manganese that your body can't get, and I really believe that you're able to create manganese from nothing, if you will, from the other elements that are in that food that can be transmuted through your microbiome and everything else. That's an extraordinary science. And just the disclaimer is there's still, I'd say, 99% of the biochemists on Earth still don't believe that. But, if you look back through all of the literature in the 1950s and 1960s it was proven out in big clinical trials. Some of the best ones were done in Sub-Saharan Africa actually on European and American oil rig workers that were working the oil rigs in in Africa. It was a very controlled environment to study because you had guys that never would leave this this 24 x 24-foot platform, and all of their food was controlled for. So, their beverages and food were controlled for, and they would measure every day every drop of sweat by swiping the skin to measure sodium chloride and other micronutrients coming off through the skin and then all of their urine and stool output. They were showing clearly that there was an excess amount of sodium chloride going in through their diet and they were excreting tons of potassium, even though there was almost no potassium in their diet. They would follow these guys for a year, and at no point would they show any potassium or sodium deficiency. So they were transmuting all these nutrients within the body and putting this out. Now that we're starting to see the microbiome come into play, it's starting to make sense how this can be done. Because the microbiome has these incredible factories within them, these plant plastids, these little guys that are within the plant cells. The best ones known are the ones that have the chlorophyll in them—the chlorophyll are made in these little plastids—and these little things look like mitochondria but they live inside a bacteria or fungi and plant themselves. These guys are, I think, where a lot of that transmutation happens. They have very unique enzymatic environments, and they have a huge amount of electricity. And so the mitochondria and these plant plastids that look like mitochondria are literally solar events. So the mitochondria, for example, to give you a sense of how much energy is here and this is what it takes to transmute elements, to take potassium and hydrogen and combine those into a single element, there's so much energy involved in that. That's why the physicists or the biochemists will say, "Oh no, it's impossible to transmute anything in the periodic table—it takes too much energy." Well, let's take a look at how much energy is in a mitochondria. So, if you had a cubic centimeter of mitochondria and a cubic centimeter of the atomic environment of the surface of the sun in our solar system, you'd be creating about 10,000 times more energy from your mitochondria than the surface of the sun. So the amount of energy coming out of mitochondria, cubic centimeter per cubic centimeter, is 10,000 times more powerful than the surface of the sun. We believe we got elements through solar fusion and fission events, and that's where all these elements were able to break down into all these different variants. When you have fusion-fission capacity down at the cellular level within these mitochondria and everything else, there's so much energy packed into these things that I think we're able to produce nutrient from within the body. Now that's a big, huge, kind of like left-hand turn it feels like in our conversation, but I want a WOW factor in here to encourage you guys that, you know, so much of what I lecture on all the time sounds dismal, sounds hopeless like "We're screwed, we're screwed. We've taken all the medicine out of our food. It's all chemical. We've destroyed the microbiome. What the heck are we going to do?" I am convinced that, while we're just starting to come to terms with the damage that we've done to our own bodies and to our ecosystems, we also have not even begun to untangle the miracle that remains in nature and our bodies to heal everything. We can heal everything. We can transmute away the toxins. We can rebuild the microbiome. We can birth new species. We can do all kind of amazing growth down in this microbiome, but we have to stop our behavior. We have to stop spraying antibiotic all over this planet in the form of weed killers. We have to stop these practices immediately and give Nature a chance. But, if we do, we're going to see transmutation happen.

Brendan [01:00:17]: That is the most good news ever, and biology is beautiful. And thank you for taking that turn down a very illuminating path. That was ... I ... I'm just speechless.

Dr. Bush [01:00:33]: Let me give you one more piece while your jaw is on the ground there. I mean, it is a jaw-drop moment, and it continues to be for me. I've been studying this stuff for years, and it continues to just give me goosebumps every time I talk about it. But, one of my favorite examples of the power of this nature to detox our environment is Chernobyl. Chernobyl's arguably the largest environmental disaster we had right up until Fukushima, and now I think Fukushima so far outstrips Chernobyl, it's ridiculous, and Fukushima is still not getting any attention. Why don't you Google Fukushima's output right now. Like you can see it on online ... you can see—and I think it's somewhere around millions of gallons a day still—there are millions of gallons of seawater that are contaminated by that radioactive material that are still being pumped into Fukushima and right back out into the Pacific Ocean, millions of gallons of radioactive material being dumped back into our ocean from Fukushima today. How many years out are we from that event? Chernobyl, now, Chernobyl was in the 1970s, so we're 35 years out or something from Chernobyl. Well let's take some hope out of the story of the microbiome and biology's ability to transmute toxin. And so, if we look at Chernobyl the highest contamination obviously happened in the soil right at Chernobyl. So, as those radioactive elements went into the air and water systems they filtered right back down, very heavy isotopes;

they filtered into the soil. Living in the soil of Chernobyl, like many other ecosystems in the world, are voles. If you don't live around voles—like I grew up in Colorado and we don't have voles there. Now I live in Virginia, and they're the most ridiculously cute, bizarre little animal. It's kind of a cross between a mole and a small mouse—tiny little guys. But, they're blind, and they got these little funny whiskers, almost fleshy little whiskers on their face. Look up vole online images, and just laugh at how sweet these little guys are. But these voles thrive in in the soils of the Chernobyl ecosystem. Then the nuclear event happens; we dumped a bunch of radioactive material. And the voles are tunneling in radioactive material, in fact eating and consuming their micronutrient from that soil. If today, some 35 years later, you take a Geiger counter and hold it next to one of these voles you'll see they're radioactive. They have a huge radioactive signal still coming out of the soils and out of the voles themselves. Yet here we are, a couple hundred generations of voles since the Chernobyl event, and there haven't been any reported cases of birth defects in those vole populations. In fact, their litter size seems to have increased. They are thriving as a population. So, here they are radioactive for 50 or 100 generations and there have been no measurable deficits in their reproductive capacity, in their genomic capacity, even though they are today still radioactive. The ecosystem that lives off those voles are the Siberian wolves, and so the Siberian wolves around Chernobyl have, again, increased their population, increased the number of pups per litter, no cancer, no anything, and they are transmuting their main food supply, which is radioactive, into nutrient for their body without any measurable harm to their genomics or anything else from the radioactive material. I think the radioactive material is doing damage but their healing rate is so fast and so accelerated by their normal natural ecosystem and the bacteria and microbiome around them that they're transmuting it out. Pseudomonas is a very unique bacteria. We fear this guy in the hospital. Pseudomonas infections in the hospital are horrendous, especially in burn units. We have huge problems with Pseudomonas in hospital burn units, and yet that bacteria that we think of as a terrible bad bacteria can digest radioactive uranium. It can break it down into nonradioactive isotopes. So, unbelievable capacity of the microbiome to take even radioactive fallout and diminish it. So, as horrendous as Fukushima has been and as horrendous as Chernobyl has been, if we are able to get back in touch with our inherent microbiome, we as humans don't need to suffer, and the microbiome of the coral reefs and everything else and the fish, I think, can recover from that if we give it the opportunity. You know, the interesting reality of Chernobyl was we saw the highest rates of thyroid cancer in history in the humans that were exposed to that event. It just goes to show that the humans in the 1970s were already deficient in their contact with the natural world that's allowing those vole populations and the wolves to survive and thrive. We're suffering cancer because of the same radioactive material event because we're disconnected from our natural healing capacity. That's the mission of my clinic, and the clinic is the M Clinic if you want to see more information about the clinical care we're trying to bring out. It goes far beyond the gut. We're trying to figure out how do we reiterate humanity into our nature because if we do disease will cease to exist.

Brendan [01:05:36]: I could speak to you for hours, and I really want to thank you for leaving us on such a positive, inspiring, hopeful note and really for elucidating all the causes for so much hope.

Dr. Bush [01:05:55]: Awesome.

Brendan [01:05:56]: ... because you are you are really at the vanguard, if anybody.

Dr. Bush [01:06:02]: Well thank you. Brendan, it has been a pleasure. I love what you're doing and, you know, obviously as a physician and a scientist it is exciting to build knowledge and exciting to teach, but without an audience it's extremely frustrating and so I just recognize and celebrate what you're doing with Eat4Earth, and it's just very exciting to see you really tackling this public education effort so well. Without many warriors in this battle we're not going to have time to recover. Our children are suffering, and I want each of you as listeners to remember that you now have a bit of a responsibility to carry on this trajectory that Brendan's setting you on. By bringing you this information, Brendan's empowering you to become a little epicenter of change in your family, community at large, globe at large. So get passionate about something—maybe it's the fermentation, maybe it's the mushrooms, maybe it's some element of the heirloom tomatoes—get passionate about some sector of what we're talking about and if you're not passionate about it then get passionate about the people that are passionate about it. So, find your local farmers, so the CSAs, the farmers' markets, and get engaged. Get passionate about those people. Get passionate about what they're bringing into your community for your children, your grandchildren, etc., etc.

Brendan [01:07:17]: Thanks again Dr. Bush. On behalf of myself and the Eat4Earth community, thanks for being here with us again.

Dr. Bush [01:07:26]: All right, enjoy. Eat4Earth. Love It!

Brendan [01:07:29]: Dr. Bush has such an extraordinary mind. I've listened to this interview several times and I could listen to many more times. He really brings out the vast and mysterious and even magical potential of biology in our lives and our world at large. And this is so needed at this time, perhaps more than anything else, as the means for solving so many of our challenges both personally and globally.

Joseph Pizzorno, ND Interview 2

The Toxin Solution: Essential Keys to Safe and Complete Detoxification (Interview 2)

Brendan [00:00:00]: Welcome to the Eat4Earth event. We're exploring how you can heal yourself, your loved ones, and the planet, with food. This is Brendan Moorehead and we're blessed to have Dr. Joseph Pizzorno back for a second conversation. Dr. Joseph Pizzorno is a world-leading authority on science-based natural medicine, a term that he coined when founding Bastyr University in 1978. A naturopathic physician, educator, researcher and expert spokesman, he's Editor-in-Chief of PubMed-indexed Integrative Medicine: A Clinician's Journal, Treasurer of the Board of the Institute for Functional Medicine, board member of American Herbal Pharmacopoeia, and a member of the Science Boards of the Hecht Foundation, Gateway for Cancer Research, and Bioclinic Naturals. He is licensed in Washington State and the recipient of numerous awards and honors, such as the Linus Pauling Award, the American Holistic Medical Association's Holistic Medicine Pioneer, and the American Association of Naturopathic Physician's Naturopathic Physician of the Year. He has been an intellectual and academic leader in medicine for four decades, was appointed by Presidents Clinton and Bush to two prestigious commissions advising the government on how to integrate natural medicine into the healthcare system and is the author or co-author of five text books and seven consumer books. Dr. Pizzorno, it's so great to have you back with us again.

Dr. Pizzorno [00:01:24]: Well, thanks for the invitation. I enjoyed our conversation and delighted we have the opportunity to continue this effort to understand why people are sick and how to become healthy.

Brendan [00:01:33]: Yeah. So, in our first conversation, you mentioned that individuals can have up to a thousand-fold variability in Phase 1 liver detoxification and a ten-fold variability in Phase 2 liver detoxification. This is just one example of genetic differences that can have an effect on a person's detoxification processes. This is basically a new area of study in medicine that looks at genetic variations among individuals that affect many areas of health and, given how much we're discovering lately about the pervasive influence of toxins on disease, this is pretty important. Can you provide an overview of this arena and these things called "single-nucleotide polymorphisms" or SNPs, for short?

Dr. Pizzorno [00:02:19]: Yeah, great question. So, we all know that we're all biochemically unique. You look at a person and there you have these different genders, different ethnic backgrounds, different heights, and all these differences and it's all based on genetics. And the way this happens is through what are called single-nucleotide polymorphisms, or SNPs for short, in changes and how our DNA makes the proteins that form the foundation of our enzymes. So, you're looking at an enzyme. An enzyme is composed of two parts, what's called an apoenzyme, which is the protein that's determined by our genetics, and then a co-factor, which is typically a vitamin or a mineral that is necessary to convert that inner protein into an active enzyme. So, it turns out that we have huge variations in how we make these proteins and how they're made has a big impact on how well those enzymes work. And, it's not just the enzymes but, of course, you have to make sure that the nutrients necessary for the enzymes to work are there, which is why food is so important. But, equally important, the way that many of the toxins work is actually by poisoning the enzymes by displacing the co-factors. So, instead of, for example, there being selenium in an enzyme that metabolizes the T4 to T3 in the thyroid to make it more active, well, if there's mercury around or if there's cadmium around, it'll displace the selenium from the enzyme so you can't make a conversion of the T4 to the three-times-more-active T3. So, when we talk about detoxification, there's so many examples, and I'll use a personal one. So, I'll just use my wife as the counter example. So, I'm the kind of person that, if I drink a cup of coffee later than noon, I cannot sleep at night. Conversely, my wife can drink two cups of coffee with dinner and it has no impact on her sleep whatsoever. And that's because caffeine is detoxified by the enzyme called cytochromee P450 1A2 that's in the liver. And it turns out that there's a huge genetic variation in how that enzyme is made and that results in an 8-fold difference in how fast people detoxify caffeine. So, look at someone like me. The half-life of caffeine is about 8 hours, okay? So, if I drink a cup of coffee at noon, by the time I go to sleep at ten, I've only broken down a little more than half the caffeine. So it's harder for me to get to sleep. Conversely, with my wife, hers works eight times faster, which means her half-life is one hour. So, say you have dinner at 6:00 at night and you have two cups of coffee. Well, within four hours, she's pretty much gotten rid of all the caffeine, okay? Whereas for me, I'd be awake for another day or two. So, there's lots of examples. So, because of that lowered activity of that enzyme, it means I'm more susceptible to all the chemical toxins that are detoxified by that enzyme. It's a long answer to your question but, hopefully, that lays it out properly.

Brendan [00:05:27]: It's very interesting that you mentioned caffeine because I just heard something, and it related to that caffeine detoxification process. People that detoxify more slowly are, apparently, more at risk of having caffeine be a negative influence on their health, such as, apparently, on heart disease risk ...

Dr. Pizzorno [00:05:46]: Yes.

Brendan [00:05:47]: ... whereas, people who are fast metabolizers of caffeine are actually getting the benefit of the polyphenols but not the negative affects of, I guess, having caffeine move too slowly through their system and maybe over-revving them or whatever the influence is that increases heart disease risk from slow metabolism of caffeine.

Dr. Pizzorno [00:06:12]: Yes, great example. Great example.

Brendan [00:06:15]: So, lets talk about some other SNPs. Anything related to detoxification processes? Methylation, sulfation ...

Dr. Pizzorno [00:06:23]: Oh, tons and tons and tons! I mean, seriously, as we talked about, I've been working on this artificial intelligence system to help people interpret what those SNPs mean. So, first they can go to 23AndMe. They can download our technology and it will tell you what it means. So ... examples. So, let's go through some of the more important examples. Let's talk about the enzymes that are so critical for detoxifying arsenic. So, it turns out that as we've evolved as a species we're pretty good at getting rid of arsenic, and the reason I make that determination is, half-life of arsenic in the body is between two and four days. So, as long as a person's metabolism is working properly, which is true for the vast majority of the population, and as long as you are not being regularly re-exposed to arsenic, you can get rid of it. But if you are regularly being exposed to arsenic, it doesn't matter whether your arsenic systems are working fine or not, because if you are getting exposed to it all the time, then it's always there. So, it turns out, the way that we get rid of arsenic is through a double-methylation step. And, so, one methylation step converts arsenic into what's called monomethyl-arsenic and that is actually eight times more toxic than the regular arsenic, which is why we then very quickly do a second methylation to something that is called DMA or diemethyl arsenic and that, then, is four hundred times less toxic than arsenic. So basically, we go through this process where, temporarily, it is more toxic, and then we get rid of it. Well, it turns out that there's some people where the first enzyme works just fine, but the second enzyme does not work very well. And so these people are much, much more susceptible to toxicity from arsenic. In addition, I mentioned this two-step methylation process. So, if a person's having trouble producing methyl groups, it's going to be more difficult for them to break down arsenic, and what kind of people have that? Well, we know that. People that have high homocysteine levels typically have methylation problems. So you have a person with genetic susceptibility to not be able to produce methyl groups as well as they could, who have a genetic susceptibility to not be able to break down arsenic from the second, more toxic form very well, and you put them in an environment where there's arsenic in the water and, lo and behold, you've got pancreatic cancer. You've got prostate cancer. You've got stroke. You've got heart disease. All these things happening because the arsenic is causing damage because they can't protect themselves. So, genetics has a huge impact.

Brendan [00:08:48]: Yeah, and apparently there's a fair amount ... rice can often have high levels of ... I don't know whether "high" is the right term, but rice can be a carrier for arsenic into our food supply. And I'm curious, is this two-step methylation process ... is this an example of Phase 1 and Phase 2 being out of balance or is it just a two-step mechanism?

Dr. Pizzorno [00:09:08]: Right, that's a two-step methylation process. Now, the other one you talked about, the Phase 1 and Phase 2, is, of course, very, very significant. So, when we're detoxifying chemicals, they're typically detoxified through the liver, and the liver basically breaks them down in essentially two ways. Number one is, it can directly break down the chemical. That's what happens with caffeine and cytochrome P4501A2. And cytochrome P450 is the one we call the Phase 1 detox system in the liver. So some toxins are detoxed that way. We also, then, have Phase 2, and I'll talk about Phase 2 in a moment. But there are also some toxins that are detoxified by Phase 2 directly, an example being acetaminophen. You take it in Tylenol. So, one of the ways we get rid of acetaminophen is through Phase 2 detoxification. It's not the main way but it is one of the ways that it happens. But the vast majority of chemicals, particularly carcinogens and such, are detoxified in the two-step process. You have Phase 1, which converts it into what's called an activated intermediate which is actually much, much more toxic. Then you have Phase 2, which then goes through a process called conjugation, which means, basically, you bind the activated intermediate to another molecule that either neutralizes it or makes it water-soluble so it can be excreted out through the kidneys. Okay. So, people run into trouble when those two systems aren't working in balance. So, of course, we want Phase 1 to be getting rid of toxins as quickly as possible because you want to get them out of your body because they break things. They damage the body. But, if you have a good Phase 1 but Phase 2's not working very well, you actually get more toxicity because you can't get rid of the activated intermediates as quickly. And, so, we get a situation where we see people who are, what I call, the yellow canary. So, you may recall the yellow canary from when we used to have coal miners down in the coal mines, and they'd have these yellow canaries down there because the yellow canaries were really sensitive to carbon monoxide. And, rather than the miners dying from carbon monoxide, not knowing it because they can't smell stuff, they watched the yellow canaries, and as soon as the yellow canaries start to fall over, they know it's time to get out of the mine as quickly as possible. So, the yellow canaries, you might say, are the ones who are most sensitive to environmental toxicity. So a typical patient I would see like this ... I'll describe a woman I just saw a while ago who is always sick, and there's no reason for it. And she comes in a room where people have been doing a lot of spraying or some may have on some real strong perfume and she says, "It knocks me out." Okay? It just knocks her down and she just gets so sick she has to go home and leave the work environment, typically. So, what's happened with her is that her Phase 1 gets rid of those [unintelligible], and she has all greens in all her Phase 1 genetics. So everything's working fine there. But looking at her Phase 2s, we have all yellows and reds. So, reds mean you've got the slowest working version of the enzyme. Yellow means you've got kind of the halfway version of the enzyme. So, she's got all greens in Phase 1 and all yellows and reds in Phase 2. So, whenever she's exposed to chemicals, she gets really more toxic.

Brendan [00:12:19]: And these colors, yellow, red, green. Are these colors within your system like color coding the specific SNP variations in your system platform ... okay.

Dr. Pizzorno [00:12:29]: Yeah, we have about 350 SNPs right now, 75 of which are around detoxification.

Brendan [00:12:34]: Okay, wow. And what's the ... the name of the platform, I believe is IQYou, right?

Dr. Pizzorno [00:12:28]: Right. It's called IQYouhealth.com. Now, we're still in the beta testing phase, but it is working and anybody who wants to use it, now's the time 'cause it's free right now. Try it out and you will be amazed at what you see. It is so helpful. But I also want to be clear, it's not just your genetics, okay? You may have the greatest genetics but if the vitamins and minerals aren't there in your food, your enzymes aren't going to work properly and, conversely, you may have great genetics but if you're constantly exposed to toxins, it takes time—it takes metabolic energy—to get the toxins out to protect you from the toxins. So, I want to be real clear. Not many people have the genetics where you can start smoking at age five and live to 100 years old and not get lung cancer. (Laugh) Not many people have those genetics, okay? Everybody else, if you're exposed to toxins, you want to get rid of them as quickly as possible.

Brendan [00:13:31]: Yeah. And what are some of the things that we can do with our information about our individual SNPs?

Dr. Pizzorno [00:13:38]: Yes, that's what's really promising about this 'cause I always try to tell people we are not preordained to get disease but we have susceptibilities that we need to be aware of. So, for example, if a person's having trouble with methylation, making it harder for them to get rid of the arsenic, well there are multiple things you can do to improve your ability to produce methyl groups. So you can use, for example, pre-activated methyl groups and that will help your physiology work properly. Or you may happen to be a person who is Phase 1 'well-active' and in Phase 2, 'poor activity', and that means that particular person has got to be extremely careful to avoid toxins and, if you are exposed to toxins, then you need to do everything you can to make sure Phase 2 is functioning just as optimally as possible.

Brendan [00:14:29]: And, maybe what are some other examples of things we can do to enhance Phase 2, if we find out that we're slow in that regard.

Dr. Pizzorno [00:14:39]: Right. So, it turns out that many of the Phase 2 activities are limited not only by the activity of the enzyme but also by the availability of the conjugating molecules being used. And one of the most important ones is glutathione. So it turns out that, when I was mentioning, for example, the acetaminophen detoxification, most of acetaminophen is detoxified by Phase 1 and then conjugated with glutathione in Phase 2, and that keeps acetaminophen from being too toxic. But, for example, if you are using up your glutathione, then you can't detoxify the activated intermediate from Phase 1 from the acetaminophen, and it actually becomes very, very toxic. As a matter of fact, there is some pretty solid research suggesting that the kidney failure epidemic we're now seeing in the U.S. is due to toxicity from molecules like acetaminophen because people can't break it down properly because of their genetics. Okay. So, for people like that, a very good strategy is to increase the amount of glutathione in your body, and a good way to do that is by taking a nutritional supplement called N-Acetyl Cysteine or NAC for short. So taking just 500 mg of NAC will increase glutathione levels by about 30 percent.

Brendan [00:15:54]: I'm curious to know, do you know if glyphosate is one of the toxins that reduces the reserves of glutathione?

Dr. Pizzorno [00:16:06]: I would assume that's the case but, off the top of my head, I don't recall research on that. But that's probably true. Sorry, I don't recall.

Brendan [00:16:16]: We know that, at least, a voluntary toxin called alcohol reduces glutathione which, if you're drinking alcohol and taking acetaminophen, which there are probably plenty of people unwittingly doing, that is ... that's serious danger.

Dr. Pizzorno [00:16:30]: Big, big mistake and I'm glad you brought that up because I was going to bring it up next. (Laugh) And that is, indeed, that if you're going to take acetaminophen ... and, by the way, I think acetaminophen is one of the worst over-the-counter drugs available ... if you're going to take acetaminophen, don't drink alcohol because you're going to make the acetaminophen way, way more toxic. I mean, there's a bunch of really simple things people need to be doing and they're not aware of, and they have such a big effect on our health.

Brendan [00:16:59]: Yeah, so, another area that you might be familiar with ... obviously, there's so many SNPs and probably nobody knows them all (laugh) off the top of their head, or something. But the CBS relating to sulfation? I suspect that that's one of mine. I haven't actually looked at my own results. I have the 23AndMe but I haven't actually plugged it through your system yet. But, I'm curious, because I believe you've mentioned that. What can you tell us about that SNP?

Dr. Pizzorno [00:17:32]: Yes, I think that that's very, very important because it turns out that sulfation is a very important Phase 2 conjugation enzyme, and it's involved in detoxification of multiple toxins. And what's interesting about it is that researchers have also been looking at various SNPs to see if there are disease correlations, and it turns out that if a person has trouble with their sulfation reactions, they have more rheumatoid arthritis, and they have more Alzheimer's disease. That was a little surprising to me and a little worrisome because that happens to be one of the ones that I have. So, it's one of the things that I have to be really, really cognizant of and very careful about.

Brendan [00:18:10]: Is there anything that we can do about that particular one, as far as diet and lifestyle and so forth to …?

Dr. Pizzorno [00:18:15]: So, it turns out that most of the enzymes involved in sulfur metabolism are dependent upon molybdenum, the trace mineral molybdenum. So, what I found, and I actually use it myself … [laughing] One of the fun things about doing this medicine is that, not only do I get to help patients and give lectures to doctors to help other patients, but I apply it to myself as well. And I found, personally, that by working really hard to get my molybdenum levels up, I'm much less sensitive to sulfur compounds and to toxins that need to be detoxified by sulfur conjugation.

Brendan [00:18:50]: That makes sense. I'm working on the molybdenum supplementation myself, or getting it through foods. Now, I'm curious. There's so many areas of health besides detoxification that we can learn about for ourselves and can impact things that most people are attuned to like optimal weight and healthy heart and so forth. I was wondering if there are any particular SNPs that you're familiar with that are not detoxification-related but might be of interest to the average person.

Dr. Pizzorno [00:19:26]: Great question and it turns out there are actually a number of very interesting examples. And let me go through one that I was quite intrigued by. About two years ago I was invited by a group that was helping promote the health of our military by doing wellness strategies. And, one of the big areas this had been happening in was with post-traumatic stress syndrome, PTSD, which everybody knows is really bad for our brave veterans coming back from fighting wars for us. So, they're talking about how to deal with these people and, of course, this group is primarily focused on psychological interventions and things like that, which are fine. But I decided to take a different approach and say, "You know, we can probably determine which people are most sensitive to stressful events, like being shot at, by their genetics." So, it turns out that one of the key enzymes involved in detoxifying the stress hormones is called COMT. Now you may recall that COMT is also involved in methylation, as well, but the main one here is the COMT and the COMT breaks down mainly stress hormones. So it turns out that there are SNPs involved in how well the COMT works. So, if you look at the SNPs of returning veterans, you then look at the … so, you look at the COMT SNPs for the returning veterans. You then plot an axis where you are looking at on an axis the number of stressful events they had -- the number of times the guys got shot at -- guys and gals, I should say -- the number of times they have been shot at -- and then look at the measures of PTSD, and what you find is a direct correlation. The more you're shot at, the more PTSD you have. However, if you then break the group down by their ability of their COMT to break down stress hormones, it turns out that there's about a two-fold variation in how well they break down the stress hormones and, as you might expect then, the people with the slow version of COMT have about three times as much PTSD as people who don't have the slow version. This is one example of many. So, it turns out I'm now using this with my patients, the ones who are complaining a lot about, you know, "This stress really just knocks me out." I say, "Well, let's check your COMT and see if your COMT is slow," because it turns out, it is often a slow COMT. And the good news is that you can do something about it because you give these people SAM-e, that's adenosylmethianine, that then provides the molecule that helps the COMT work better to get rid of the stress hormones more effectively.

Brendan [00:21:58]: Wow! That is really important information. I hope that that gets into the military soon …

Dr. Pizzorno [00:22:03]: I planted the seed! We'll see if anything happens. [laughing]

Brendan [00:22:07]: Right, great! You know, a friend of mine mentioned to me recently that her health's great but she stays on a blood pressure regulation medicine because of, you know, genetic predisposition to high blood pressure, and I was sort of wondering if there's any SNP you're aware of related to that. Maybe it's salt metabolism? Just curious if you have any ideas about that one.

Dr. Pizzorno [00:22:36]: So, my gentle comment to your friend would be, "Please don't do that!" [laughing] I can be stronger! [laughing] Okay. Almost certainly she has a SNP that … I can't say which one it is because I haven't looked at her. I'd have to look at her particular situation. But, indeed, I should mention, there are very significant SNPs that are involved with things like how well we get rid of salt and the average person consumes way too much salt, and a lot of people have this quote, "Well, you're just genetically predisposed to get high blood pressure." Well, what it means is they have to be a little more careful about what they are exposing their body to. I'm going to be politically incorrect here. Or, maybe I should say, I'm getting more radical! I've been doing medicine for half a century. I'm getting more radical because I've just seen this stuff! In class with my students, one of the questions I always ask them is, "What's the difference between a nutrient and a toxin?" I get all these interesting answers, which are great, but then I'll say, "But, you know, it's actually very simple. Nutrients make our enzyme systems work. Chemical toxins poison our enzyme systems. And what are drugs? Drugs are chemical toxins that poison our enzyme systems." So, poisoning your enzyme system, for one, the enzymes involved in blood pressure regulation is not a good strategy because, typically, those enzymes do more than one thing and the drugs are poisonous, and the body has to detoxify. So you're depleting your glutathione every time you take a drug. I want to be clear. I'm not against prescription drugs and sometimes they are the appropriate strategy. But we use them way too much, and way too often we use a drug instead of dealing with the underlying cause of why the person is sick.

Brendan [00:24:31]: You know, and I believe also, with regard to salt, that some people excrete too much or something like. Isn't it also true that some people actually, perhaps, need to get more sodium? I'm just curious ...

Dr. Pizzorno [00:24:44]: So, okay ...

Brendan [00:24:46]: I think I'm one of those.

Dr. Pizzorno [00:24:47]: Okay. Now, it does happen. And pretty much the only cases I've seen that in are people who are what are called extreme vegetarians. So, the people who are vegan, not eating any animal products. Animal products are a pretty significant source of salt. But being a very strict vegan and also being very careful with not consuming any salt, I've actually run into people who have low salt. But that's so unusual. I mean, you're talking about 95% of the population is consuming too much salt.

Brendan [00:25:15]: You know, a minute ago you mentioned that ... you know, what the difference is between a nutrient and a toxin, a toxin being the one that poisons the enzyme system and a nutrient being the one that powers them. And there is an old idea that still prevalent, I believe, in toxicology that goes something like, "The dose makes the poison" and that companies like Monsanto, and so forth, you know, in justifying this so-called safety of products, like glyphosate, are basically just saying that, "Hey, at this level the it's not toxic." One of the things we're seeing now, and I've mentioned before in our previous conversation, is this sort of cocktail affect and we're getting this onslaught of 80,000 chemicals, only maybe 200 of which have ever been tested and, of course, they're only tested for acute toxicity under the "dose makes the poison" model. But, basically, we've got so many of these things and there seems to be a synergistic effect of poisoning enzyme systems. And, perhaps, multiple toxins can poison the same enzyme system so you get tiny, tiny parts per million or per billion of one toxin plus another plus another plus another. And it can take out your health even though you didn't get exposed to anything higher than something that's less than the EPA detectable level or something like that.

Dr. Pizzorno [00:26:37]: Right. And you're exactly right because these things are all tested in isolation, okay? So you look at one toxin by itself and it may not be too bad but, not having looked at a ton of research, I can tell you nobody's exposed to just one toxin. Trying to find a control group to compare those people who are exposed or those who are not exposed, you end up having to make compromises because everybody is exposed and toxicity is just a huge, ongoing problem. So, don't trust that. [unintelligible]

Brendan [00:27:11]: And, of course, we've got this genetic variability. Some people are canaries, and some people can smoke until they are 100. So we just need to re-examine the precautionary principle and what it tells us.

Dr. Pizzorno [00:27:28]: Very good. Exactly.

Brendan [00:27:31]: You know, a big theme of this event, and we're talking about it, is genetic variability. We're all biochemically unique and... just curious if there's anything else you might say that's interesting about how this affects the individual diet in terms of who does better on what types of food. Are there people that do better on low protein? Are there people that need more protein? Do some people need to avoid red meat more than others? I'm just curious if you have any insights there.

Dr. Pizzorno [00:28:03]: Yeah. Another excellent question and I think there are some important things here that can indeed have an impact on what diet is healthiest for them. And, frankly, I think we're early enough in the process that I'm hesitant to say anything strongly about that but can give some ideas about where we might go. So, for example, someone eating a high-meat diet is going to have a whole lot more ammonia to detoxify than somebody who is on a strictly vegetarian-type diet. Okay? So, if they're having troubles with their SNPs involved in the detoxification of ammonia, then they're the kind of people who, when they eat a heavy meat meal, aren't going to feel very good. And they're the ones who want to try being a vegetarian for a little while and then they'll find out, "Oh, you know, I'm actually feeling better as a vegetarian." So, you can see things of that nature. Conversely, you can look at somebody who may be a strict vegetarian. Well, one of the problems with being a vegan ... one of the advantages of eating animal products is that they do have some pre-made molecules in there that are useful for us. And the one everyone always thinks about is vitamin B12. And the reality is that, if you're a strict vegan and there's no B12 in your diet, you've gotta get B12 from somewhere. So there are just lots of examples where people with genetic susceptibility ... going back to the B12 example, some people ... maybe just the B12 they're getting from bacterial contamination of the food supply ... maybe they're so good at metabolizing and utilizing B12 that they can be a strict vegetarian, but that's really, really unusual that a person would have that kind of genetics.

Brendan [00:29:37]: Well, what about our microbiome-producing vitamin B12. If somebody has a healthy microbiome, and they're a vegetarian or vegan, would they potentially get enough B12? I know it tends to be a risk factor for everybody that's vegan or vegetarian, but can they possibly get enough from their microbiome?

Dr. Pizzorno [00:29:55]: Yeah, and the big challenge there is that their absorption sites for the B12 are before where the B12 is made in the colon. So, again, yeah, sure, there may be some diffusion. They may get some that way but it's a really tough one for us. And there's a reason why we store it so very, very well. You can have a person who has really good B12 stores and stop giving him B12 and it'll be five to ten years before they actually start showing B12 deficiency. So we're extremely good at storing B12 but if you're not getting it in, you eventually will run out.

Brendan [00:30:30]: Wow! I had no idea we stored it that long. That's fascinating! That might explain why a lot of people that go vegetarian or vegan, the negative effects, if it's going to be negative impact for them, are way down the line. First, they're thriving on the fact that they are so many more phytonutrients and fiber it's no longer taking up a portion of their plate. Another issue, with regard to diets with or without animal-based nutrients ... we've got ... you mentioned vitamin D ... well, you didn't mention vitamin D ... well, I'm thinking of fat-soluble vitamins, like vitamin A, D, and K2. I don't know if K1 or K2 are fat soluble. Yeah, I believe K2 is fat soluble and K2 is very important for vitamin D metabolism and, in general, only comes from the fat of animals eating their normal diet, such as grass. Basically, herbivores instead of grains, and that can be a significant source of that. For vegetarians or vegans, they may not be getting that. Although I had heard, also, that certain microbes can be in the microbiome and can produce K12. And I've also heard that maybe we can convert vitamin K1 to K2 but not a lot of it. I'm just curious what you might have to say because vitamin K2 is a very important and not many people talking about it.

Dr. Pizzorno [00:31:58]: Well, and I'm glad you are. So, you brought up a bunch of great topics. Let's focus on vitamin A and vitamin K2. So, one of the big concerns that I and my wife Laura have ... you know we do a lot of writing and lecturing on natural medicine ... is that people assume and assert equivalency between beta-carotene consumption and vitamin A consumption, not realizing that between 1/4 and 1/3 of people, because of their genetics, cannot convert, or convert very poorly, beta-carotene into vitamin A. So we see a problem, then with people who are strict vegans not having enough vitamin A levels, but they think they're fine because they have all this beta-carotene. As a matter of fact, I've had some interesting patients along those lines, but I won't get into that right now. But, anyway, so that's another example of a nutrient where, genetically, if you can't convert your beta-carotene into vitamin A, you've got to get it into your diet because there's just no other way of getting it. Another area where a vegetarian can run into trouble. Let me be real clear. I'm not anti-vegetarian. I've been vegetarian and I've been vegan for significant portions of my life. Right now I do, unfortunately, eat fish about once a week for health purposes but, if I had my druthers, I'd be eating no animal products whatsoever. But that's more philosophical and spiritual than biochemical. Anyway, so if I may, actually I think it's a bigger problem than people realize. And, you always need vitamin K2, to answer to your questions there. And, indeed, if you have the right bacteria in your gut, you will convert some of the vitamin K1 in the diet into vitamin K2. And there's some very, very slow enzymes in the body that will convert vitamin K1 into vitamin K2. But your comment about natural sources of vitamin K2, when you grass feed animals, cows, and you consume their products like dairy products and such, there will be vitamin K2 in there if they've been eating grass. If they've been eating corn, they're not going to have the vitamin K2.

Brendan [00:33:57]: Right. And do you know, with regard to vitamin A and beta-carotene conversion, from what I understand, fat needs to be present with the beta-carotene in order for the conversion to occur within our bodies. Now, does that mean ...

Dr. Pizzorno [00:34:13]: For the absorption to occur.

Brendan [00:34:14]: For the absorption to occur.

Dr. Pizzorno [00:34:15]: Just need to change that a little bit.

Brendan [00:34:17]: Gotcha. So, if people are on a very low-fat, vegan diet or vegetarian diet, could that be an issue if they are not putting enough fat? Or is it just a small, tiny amount of fat that's required that they should have for absorption of the beta-carotene?**Dr. Pizzorno [00:34:33]:** Oh, it's actually quite a significant factor. Let's look at eating raw carrots versus carrots that have been sauteed in oil, okay? Or steamed first or sauteed in oil. So, it turns out if you look at the amount of beta-carotene consumed from raw carrots versus beta-carotene consumed from carrots that have been cooked in oil, it's like five times higher absorption from the ones that have been cooked in oil. So, two things are happening. One is, you break down cell walls so that the beta-carotene in the cells is released. Then, having that extra oil greatly improves the absorption of that beta-carotene.

Brendan [00:35:08]: That's fascinating! You know, I believe that some people have a sensitivity to raw carrots. I feel like I do. I know that I have issues with my gut and too much raw vegetation irritates it. So I still haven't fixed the microbiome, I believe, that would fix all the cellulose or whatever it is.

Dr. Pizzorno [00:35:26]: Well, you're not going to digest the cellulose (laugh)

Brendan [00:35:30]: My bacteria might! (laugh)

Dr. Pizzorno [00:35:33]: Bacteria, well, yes, it might. But remember, cows have four stomachs, okay? So, breaking down cellulose is fairly difficult to do. So I don't think we should depend upon that for our nutritional status.

Brendan [00:35:46]: Okay, so if somebody is eating raw carrots what if they have them in a salad with salad dressing?

Dr. Pizzorno [00:35:55]: Let me be clear! You still get nutrients out of them. I'm not saying, "Don't eat raw carrots!" Okay? Because you do get nutrients out of them. But if you're really worried about your beta-carotene, cooking them in oil will dramatically increase them.

Brendan [00:36:07]: And it will be far better than carrots in a salad with salad dressing with the good quality oil? Still, it would be better?

Dr. Pizzorno [00:36:12]: So, the more you shave ... you break up the cell structure. Yeah, you shave the carrots, you'll release more of the beta-carotenes so they're easier to absorb. One reason why juicing is so helpful is because you've broken up a lot of cell walls so now more of the nutrients within the cells are available. Because, for the nutrients that are in the cell, and the cell walls are cellulose, whatever is in that cellulose cell you're not going to get because you can't break down the cellulose. So, the more you break down the cell's structure through mechanical means, the more you're going to absorb.

Brendan [00:36:45]: So, if you drink a juice that contains carrots in it, are you gonna get some of that beta carotene even though there are no fats added to the juice?

Dr. Pizzorno [00:36:52]: Sure, you're gonna get beta carotene, yes. But you'll get more if there's fat.

Brendan [00:36:56]: So, if you added in some high-quality walnut oil or something like that into your juice, including the carrots and other sources of beta-carotene ... I mean there are many green, leafy vegetables, like kale, that have beta-carotene. So, would that addition of some oil to a juice help further to assimilate that beta-carotene?

Dr. Pizzorno [00:37:15]: Absolutely! And, also, we talk a lot about beta-carotene and I think, in many ways, that's an historic artifact. So, in the past, we only thought beta-carotene was important because it's one of the very few carotenoids that's broken down to vitamin A. The assumption is that beta-carotene is the only thing that's important, and it's only important because it breaks down the vitamin A. Well, we now know that there are several hundred carotenoids in food, and many of those other carotenoids have hugely important roles in the body. So, yes, we say that about beta-carotenes. But look at, for example, at tomatoes. Tomatoes are high in lycopene, and lycopene is critically important for prostate health in men. You can look at lutein, that's in things like tomatoes, for example, and it's great for helping protect the retina of the eye from oxidative damage from sunlight and ultraviolet light and things of this nature. So these carotenoids are really, really important. And one of the challenges with this unnatural focus on beta-carotene is that when people start supplementing with beta-carotene by itself, it then competes with other carotenoids for absorption so, while your beta-carotene levels may go way up, all the other carotenoids actually go down in the blood when you consume huge amounts of beta-carotene. It always comes back to, "Eat real food!" Okay? Because real food has all the nutrients we need in it. And sometimes we do need high doses of a specific nutrient because of genetic needs. But make sure you know what you're doing because any time you consume a high amount of one particular nutrient, all other nutrients that need to be absorbed through the same pathway will now have difficulty getting into the body.

Brendan [00:39:00]: And would having our SNPs analyzed through your platform help us get those insights into, you know, "Okay. This nutrient maybe I should get more of but, barring that, I'm not going to take any random steps just because it showed up in an article in *Vogue* or something."

Dr. Pizzorno [00:39:15]: Yeah, so, we have that in the system, and we continue to grow it. So, we have the 350 most important SNPs in the system right now, but there are, like, two million of these things. And, in many instances, researchers don't even know what they do yet. So, this is an ongoing process of continuing evolution. So, we've picked much of the low-hanging fruit. We've picked the most important ones and we continue to add them to be able to answer that exact question that you asked, "What nutrients do I need to be particularly careful about?" And we're getting better and better at answering that question.

Brendan [00:39:48]: I'm curious, are there any differences between your platform and ... there's a growing number of platforms out there that [unintelligible] to analyze their 23AndMe results.

Dr. Pizzorno [00:39:57]: Yeah, so, what ours does, which I think is great, is ... and, again, as I said before, you can't just look at genetics. You must look at nutritional status. You must look at toxic load. You must look at epigenetic modification. What I mean by that is, based on a person's lifestyle, environment, etc., they will turn on and turn off some genes. So, you have to look at what symptoms does this person already have? What diseases do they already have? You have to look at the whole picture, and that's what we do. We're looking at the whole picture, not just the SNPs. So, we have right now in our system 2000 inputs into our system, 350 of which are SNPs. But the other 1600 are all the other factors you have to consider.

Brendan [00:40:40]: So, if somebody has entered their symptoms they are experiencing or outright illnesses they have, then that would be cross-referenced to particular SNPS, and you would say, "Okay, it would appear that this SNP is active and it would appear that you don't have to worry about this one because you're not exhibiting those symptoms."

Dr. Pizzorno [00:40:55]: Right, that's what we do. As you might expect, when you start looking into a person's biochemistry, there are 5000 enzymes in the body. So it gets really complex. What we try to do is say, "Okay. Sure, there's a lot going on. Here's the three most important things that you need to do. If you want to do more, just click on the little button, and it'll tell you other things to do." But I find, with most people, you need to start with the three most important things. And, if you do the three most important things, it's amazing how big an impact it has, doing the most important things first. You don't have to do everything. If you do the important things, you get great results.

Brendan [00:41:28]: That's really important because, you know, so often you take a random step, but we really need to be applying the 80/20 rule or 90/10 rule and ...

Dr. Pizzorno [00:41:36]: Exactly!

Brendan [00:41:37]: ... and just getting the biggest bang for our time and effort and expense, if we're going to be buying supplements or something.

Dr. Pizzorno [00:41:44]: Right.

Brendan [00:41:45]: So ...

Dr. Pizzorno [00:41:46]: The rule of thumb I have for my students, I say to them, "If you're going to a lecture and somebody is talking to you about all of these various things that are going to help patient's health ..." which, of course, you should be doing ... you always have to keep learning ... but then you start getting into extremes. You don't have to be so extreme about this and extreme about that, etc, etc, etc, and it gets more and more complex. When I see that, I say to them, "You know, what's happening is you're actually missing something that's quite important here. Because if you have to go to a lot of complexity, most likely you're missing something that's important."

Brendan [00:42:17]: Yeah, that's really good insight. So, you have a particular step-by-step strategy in the system for detoxifying safely and effectively?

Dr. Pizzorno [00:42:28]: Yes.

Brendan [00:42:29]: I wonder if ... Let me just take a look and see ... We've got a few more minutes ...

Dr. Pizzorno [00:42:35:]: Okay.

Brendan [00:42:37]: I wonder if you could tell us about the strategy and how you designed it and why you designed it the way you did.

Dr. Pizzorno [00:42:43]: Thank you for asking that question. I think it's important. There are a lot of people now promoting detoxification, which I think is great. But I think it is critical for people to realize that almost everybody now has a really heavy toxic load. And, of course, that level of toxic load depends upon how careful they've been over long periods of time. And, if you start on a detox protocol that causes release of these toxins where they've been stored in the tissues before you've prepared your body to get rid of them, you're actually risking getting sicker. That's one reason why, for example, people who have a lot of excess fat and who are obese start to lose weight, they feel really terrible as they're losing weight because their fat cells are breaking down and releasing all these chemical toxins into the body, and if your liver and kidneys can't deal with them, you're going to be even sicker. So I say to people, in my book, *The Toxic Solution*, I say, "Here's an 8-week program." Now, you say, "Well, two months!" And I say, "Yeah, it's going to take you two months. But do you want to be healthy or do you just want to pretend and hope that things will work out okay?" I've seen so many people now, I kind of know what's going on. So, what I say for the first two weeks is, "Let's stop the toxins coming into your body. There's no point in going into a detox program if you keep on letting toxins come into your body. So, let's stop the toxins coming in." So I say, "Here's where the toxins are coming from: water, food, air, health and beauty aids, etc. Stop them coming in." You'll spend two weeks doing that. Just after doing this for two weeks will start to result in some improvement in health. The next step, as I say, is spending two weeks cleaning up your gut because you have 10 times as many bacteria in your gut as you have cells in your body, and those bacteria are metabolically active, producing lots of molecules. Some molecules are good for us, like the B vitamins, for example. But a lot of those molecules are really toxic for us like the indoles and skatoles. So, I say, "Let's stop. Let's get the gut healthy. Let's get the toxic bacteria out of the gut, and let's get the health bacteria into the gut because, not only are those molecules that are getting into your body causing trouble, but your liver has to detoxify those things that are coming from the gut, which means it's just going to have less metabolic reserve left to get rid of the other toxins that you're being exposed to. So, let's clean up the gut." Then we spend two weeks cleaning up the liver. Let's get the liver functioning properly. Let's get the bile flowing properly. Let's make sure all the nutrients necessary for liver function are there. And then we spend two weeks cleaning up the kidneys. Now, this is a new strategy for me. I didn't worry about this before because we didn't see all of these kidney problems before. But now, with all the toxins we have in the environment ... all the over-the-counter drugs people can take like acetaminophen, which used to be a prescription drug, which has lots of toxicity ... so now we're now causing a lot of damage to the kidneys. So we go through a program to improve the function of the kidneys. Once you've done all that, now we can start detoxifying because your body can get rid of the toxins as they're released from the tissues.

Brendan [00:45:51]: You know, overall, I keep hearing over and over from you and every other speaker just how important it is to minimize toxins and maximize nutrients in our food. And every day we have the opportunity to build health for ourselves and, it turns out, for the planet at large just by learning how our food is grown. Just going to the next level and beyond saying, "Well, there are GMOs in this," which is very important to know. Are there pesticides in this, and this is very important to know. But also asking, "How is it grown?" Because how the soil is doing is going to affect how much of the micronutrients are in the food to power our enzymes and ...

Dr. Pizzorno [00:46:36]: Exactly.

Brendan [00:46:37]: ... that's a really key piece that I want people to take away from these kinds of conversations. And we can change the food system if we all pull together, ask for what we want, vote with our purchases. We've been doing that. Those of us who are conscious eaters, we've been doing that. With the organic food, with local food. We don't want GMOs in it or, at least, we want to know if they're in there. We want them labeled so we can make a decision. And now we've got some labels coming out for regeneratively-grown foods and that's gonna tell us that the soils are being treated well, which is gonna make sure that there are higher nutrient levels. I'm not sure that I can point to any particular piece of research right now, but there's ample evidence that that's the case. And, aside from the effect on our bodies with having more minerals and phytonutrients in our food, and taking organic to the next level and so forth, it's gonna have a big impact on our planet if we're growing soils instead of depleting them, and we're getting more carbon into our soils and back into the atmosphere. And other speakers are speaking more in depth on that, but we may be able to stabilize the health of our planet while we're stabilizing the health of our bodies just by rebuilding the soil. So I really appreciate you bringing in this kind of education with this level of detail about the detoxification process because so many of us understand detoxification is important to our health, but we can do it more scientifically and avoid the hazards of random, one-size-fits-all detoxification. You've got a great service there, and I want everybody to take advantage of it. And, once again, what's the URL for the platform?

Dr. Pizzorno [00:48:35]: IQYouhealth.com

Brendan [00:48:41]: Great. That's gonna help many of us restoring and guarding our full potential as human beings because we've gotta have our brains working well, and everything working well, to really, really thrive. And thank you.

Dr. Pizzorno [00:48:57]: Well, thank you for doing this program. I think it's fantastic. You know, health begins with what we eat, and there's just no substitute for eating real food. So, I think I mentioned before the website I and my team helped create called "The World's Healthiest Foods." It's a free website to promote eating real food and we have tens of thousands of letters from people who had this, that, and the other problem who said, "I started eating real food and my disease went away, and I started losing all this excess weight just from eating real food!" So, thank you for what you're doing.

Brendan [00:49:28]: Imagine that!

Dr. Pizzorno [00:49:29]: Health begins with the food we eat. It's just so foundational, and yet we've gotten so far from it as a society.

Brendan [00:49:38]: Yep. Well, thank you once again. It's just so great to have this level of detailed insight and the nuances so that we can all work to get it right just for our own specific individuality.

Dr. Pizzorno [00:49:50]: Great!

Brendan [00:49:51]: I hope you enjoyed that bonus interview with Dr. Joseph Pizzorno and, if it rang a bell with you, please leave a comment in the Facebook comments area at the bottom of the page. Let me know what you think.

Robert Van Risseghem Informal Bonus Interview
Identifying and Resolving Mineral Deficiencies with Food

Robert [00:00:00]: Morning, how are you?

Brendan [00:00:01]: Hey good morning, I'm good, how are you?

Robert [00:00:04]: I'm good.

Brendan [00:00:06]: In our previous interview, I think we covered all the questions that I had. I was wondering if there were others, if there are, I don't know, deeper layers that might be worth covering, other minerals that we didn't fully get to or something. Just curious what else there might be.

Robert [00:00:22]: I think an important factor to cover is identifying mineral deficiencies. And you know, It's a very easy way to take … let me tell you how I would look at it, and we'll just take prostate cancer. If I were to do a google search on mineral deficiencies associated with prostate cancer it will give me probably selenium, and maybe boron if, depending on what list I look on, and probably iodine. And then an easy way to validate the deficiency if that is indeed what you are deficient on, is to look at symptoms associated with selenium deficiency, and then it will give you a list of other conditions or deficiencies that are associated with that mineral deficiency. And usually somebody at the same table, you know if you had 20 years with the family before you moved out or your spouse, if they're eating the same thing you are, they might show a different sign of that deficiency. The problem with these deficiencies is that we don't recognize them for what they are, and usually we're just treating the symptoms. And that's the best way to both identify the deficiency and then validate it.

Brendan [00:02:06]: How do we validate them?

Robert [00:02:08]: You'd validate it by seeing if someone who is eating the same diet as you or eating from the same table as you or showing signs of that deficiency in a different form.

Brendan [00:02:20]: And how would you know definitively that that is actually from a deficiency. Would you recommend certain kinds of testing for it, or … and sometimes symptoms can be from so many, many different things that maybe a certain symptom that seems like a deficiency could be something other than that.

Robert [00:02:47]: It's an excellent question, but I would take the deficiencies for what they are. I mean look, about diabetes, we can run with a low chromium level for probably all the way up to 7 to 10 years before we start seeing the signs of deficiency. The body is changing out cells every 7 years. Symptoms won't really show until the deficiency has been over such a long period of time that it starts manifesting itself into symptoms. You know, I'll give you an example. I have tinnitus, and it's been going on for probably 5 years now. But it got extremely loud last month, so I went in, and I just did a google search on mineral deficiencies associated with tinnitus, and it was 2 of them. It was zinc and B12. So, if I got on the zinc I'm showing some of the other symptoms of a zinc deficiency, the skin disorders, weakened immune system. There are so many things that are associated with zinc deficiency, even depression, that I could identify. I started taking supplements, and within 2 days the tone of the tinnitus had dropped by 2 thirds. In fact I don't even recognize it

Brendan [00:04:30]: Are there particular sources that you use for looking up symptoms?

Robert [00:04:35]: The Doctor Duke's database has … because they are a .gov site they will say, rather than say Parkinson's is associated with a selenium deficiency, they will say selenium is an anti-Parkinson's mineral because they are government, and they are very crafty on their words because they expect everyone else to be. I hate referencing Dr Wallach's book because he doesn't cite his sources. That's originally how I got started on this, was looking at his stuff, and then I couldn't quote his stuff because he doesn't cite his sources to validate. Dr. Duke's database, they cite all of their sources and findings, and so I can go back to read the original articles and validate it that way. And not all … Dr. Duke's database is 30 years old now, identifying mineral deficiencies have come a long way. Dr. Peter Star … he's not a doctor … he's a film director … Peter Star, he's worked on men's prostate cancer non-profit for many years, and so when I talk to him he's talking to some of the most advanced researchers on prostate cancer, and he'll tell you selenium, iodine and boron, but I also know zinc from other sources, that zinc deficiency is a huge concern over prostate. There are many, many sources out there to identify it. If I was … if I could …

Brendan [00:06:58]: Hold on a second. I just can't believe I just walked away from … I've been burning my pots and pans lately because I've been so hyper-focused, and so I'm in like a hyper-focused workaholic mode, and I'm too impatient to put something on the stove on a low setting. And then I'll forget to turn timers on, or I think I have and I haven't, and so anyway, I've just burned a bunch of … so I just went running back because I was just about to burn my last pot. Its running dry, in other words. That's the thing I'm incorrigible about. I just can't set can't remember to set an alarm. Or like this morning I thought I did, and my finger touched the word "Start" on the timer on my phone … it didn't take, and I didn't notice that it didn't take. It just didn't catch my finger tap. And so anyway I was just reading about metal leaching from pots and pans and so forth, and my concern is if I burn a stainless steel pot, is it going to start leaching more nickel or something. I'm curious to know what your thoughts are about that kind of thing, and what your thoughts are about safe cookware.

Robert [00:08:15]: Oh, I think a lot of the … it's a tough question without testing. Most of our health issues come from over-cooking. If we were to boil our foods rather than fry them … even Neach (sp?) which is a great study that was done in … Oh, it's in … I'm going to grab it so I can … it's in Rodale's book Complete Book of Composting. I think it's in chapter 14. It was a study that was done on comparing diets. A lot of it was the way they prepared food, not so much the way they ate it.

Brendan [00:09:10]: I'm noticing that the heated water out of the pot that I just burned and scrubbed smells different than the heated water that I just heated in a pot that has never been burned or been burned dry. So that to me is a smoking gun.

Robert [00:08:15]: If you have salt in it, salt will definitely …

Brendan [00:09:35]: Corrode?

Robert [00:09:36]: Yeah, it will go to a chloride state. Refining metals, I have a process which I use a tremendous amount of salt. What the salt does, at red temperatures, it makes different minerals go into solution, but then all the minerals will not form a salt until a much higher temperature, where your irons and your nickels and your cadmiums will convert to salt at very low temperatures, in fact.

Brendan [00:10:11]: What are the … I don't think I've heard the list of noble metals. What is the actual list? Because when I asked you, "Oh, is ruthenium a noble metal," you said, "No it's not", so I actually don't even know which the noble metals are.

Robert [00:10:28]: When they come up with the word noble metals, the test that it requires is that it cannot be dissolved by one organic acid, and those noble metals are gold, and then you get the platinum group which is platinum, palladium, ruthenium, osmium, iridium and rhodium. And then silver is considered a noble metal, but at the time silver wasn't soluble in one acid, but at the time that definition had come out before we had this refined nitric acid to the levels that we have. They used to dissolve silver or make it into a chloride using sulfuric and adding salt.

Brendan [00:11:30]: Ok. Could you repeat them one more time? I got from the platinum group platinum, palladium, iridium …

Robert [00:11:40]: Ruthenium, osmium and palladium. There should be 6 of them.

Brendan [00:11:47]: I have 5. I have platinum, palladium, iridium, ruthenium, osmium

Robert [00:11:53]: Rhodium

Brendan [00:11:54]: Rhodium. R h o d l u m. Ok. And silver and gold.

Robert [00:12:03]: And out of those, there are people that think palladium is great on cancer treatments, but it's a very, very poisonous mineral. You know, platinum we find in our bodies.

Brendan [00:12:23]: Is that what they implant in like a prostate cancer, to kill it? There's something that they implanted in my, a long time ago—I think it was '85 or something—implanted something in my grandfather's prostate. He had pre-metastatic prostate cancer, and they implanted something and gave him over 20 years more life. And then it came back, and he took too much Lupron the second time around. He had a Lupron-crazy doctor who just had him on so much Lupron that that's what killed him. He died of kidney failure, I believe. It was either kidney failure or heart failure. He had no testosterone to maintain his body.

Robert [00:13:15]: Yeah, so many people that have done so many different treatments you know, and now I think the prostate cancer is more irradiation.

Brendan [00:13:30]: It could have been that. They could have put in a radioactive implant. It might have been that, but anyway, go ahead.

Robert [00:13:35]: Yeah, that's ... you know, the history of the different treatments on cancer ... it's barbaric when you look at it. I mean, they went through so many different poisons, thinking that they could find the ideal poison to kill the cancer, but your body would still live. And it's just a barbaric treatment. I mean they come about their treatments with that one main approach, "What can we find that will kill the cancer but not kill the carrier."

Brendan [00:14:16]: Right.

Robert [00:14:18]: And it's all the more reason why nutrition should be a part of any cancer treatment regardless how barbaric it is because if you are killing good tissue you need to rebuild that tissue, and these minerals are part of our DNA. And if you receive the cancer because of deficiency, then you have to overcome the deficiency to build new tissue. But now you've killed so many other cells in your body that you have to overcome all of those deficiencies

Brendan [00:14:59]: Yeah, so a little while ago you were about to say something, and you started to say, "It's so easy," or something like that, but I interrupted you. Do you remember what you were about to say? It was in the context of detecting or identifying deficiencies. Maybe you were just going to say it's just so easy to, stare at a list of symptoms, I don't know.

Robert [00:15:26]: If you just do a simple Google search, regardless what your illness is, just a simple Google search to look at the mineral deficiencies associated with it, I mean that's ...

Brendan [00:15:40]: I think the challenge with any kind of symptomatic approach, is that a symptom, a particular symptom can be caused by so many things, so a lot of practitioners, let's say someone has ... I don't know if I can come up with a good example because I'm not a practitioner, but I think I've heard example though where, although symptoms are super important if you get a comprehensive symptom survey it's an invaluable first step and ongoing monitoring for any practitioner. You've got to look at the constellation of symptoms, and then the particular constellation will give you clues, and like you said it's also highly individual. So I guess if one is using a symptom approach, the proof is in the results that you get from supplementing. So if it looks like this kind of looks like zinc deficiency, and you start taking zinc and notice a difference in the symptoms then bang!

Robert [00:16:51]: The reason why people don't use that approach, because it is very simplistic, is most of the time... Let's just look at a magnesium deficiency. Magnesium is one of the macronutrients. It's hard to believe ... even in our foods we still have enough magnesium in it. Why are we not absorbing it? Why are we ...

Brendan [00:17:17]: Oh so we do tend to have enough in the foods?

Robert [00:17:22]: On magnesium there should be enough in there, but the problem is why we don't retain it is we may not have enough boron in our food. And boron and calcium and magnesium are like a three--legged stool. You need all 3 legs. If you are lacking one then you won't retain the three in a proper fashion. The other problem with the simplistic approach by looking at symptoms is supplements in most cases, not all but most cases, the absorbability of these supplements are not even tested. So if I went down ... if it said a B12 deficiency, and I went down and bought the cheapest version of B12 I could find which would be a cyanide-based B12, and I'm not taking it with foods, what am I gaining, if the body doesn't recognize it as foods? That's the whole reason why I started the work that I did was we had the Doctor Duke's database that would not just tell us what the symptoms and what deficiencies, it would actually tell you the dose through a food, that we could never ensure that we were achieving those levels in our food. And now, with what we are able to do, by addressing the mineral deficiencies in our soils, that we can measure in the foods, now we have that missing link to nutrition to be able to go back now and look at a symptom of a deficiency and actually treat that symptom with food that we know is carrying these minerals.

Brendan [00:19:29]: Did you say that there's a ... I'm not sure if I caught everything that you just said ... but in this conversation or in another conversation have you said that there's a way that people can test their food?

Robert [00:19:41]: Yes.

Brendan [00:19:42]: So you have a lab service or you are a lab service or something where you just send I seem to recall now you said you basically take a sample and send it in. Is that for your service or somebody else's you're recommending?

Robert [00:19:55]: That's through a certified lab up in Canada, and I meant to give you that link and I'm sorry I didn't do my follow up from the last one. But those testing protocols are based upon green leaf tissue testing or ash testing, but they are all certified with securities and exchange certificates. They only run about $50 a sample. And so if a farmer was testing his fields it's not that expensive to do. It's actually just as cheap as any soil sample.

Brendan [00:20:38]: So maybe a little expensive for the home gardener, but then again what's your health worth? Is that green leaf or ash test from a single sample ... let's say you pick broccoli or something from the garden ... is that going to give you the full range of minerals is that going to tell you everything about 23 minerals or 45, or what's it going to tell you?

Robert [00:21:00]: It will give you about 60 minerals.

Brendan [00:21:03]: 60, nice. That's sufficient, I think.

Robert [00:21:08]: You know it won't do some of ... it won't give you a sulfur number. It won't give you an iodine number, which I wish it could. But it will give you all of the ... and then it's about $160 more, and then they'll do the noble metals, also with that. But for the $50 you'll get the gold and the silver.

Brendan [00:21:38]: Ok, now does that $160 more for the noble metals also include things like sulfur and iodine?

Robert [00:21:45]: No.

Brendan [00:21:50]: So they just don't test it. Interesting.

Robert [00:21:51]: Their test protocol probably because they're doing a sulfur nitric digestion that ... it would take a different testing standard to get those numbers.

Brendan [00:22:06]: You mentioned—numerous speakers have mentioned—sort of the obvious, that minerals are co-factors. A lot of vitamins don't work without them. Enzymes don't work without them. They are the actual catalytic part of many enzymes. I'm pretty sure you mentioned in the interview, or that you mentioned earlier in this conversation, the issue of just building tissue which obviously has many processes involved with that, probably transcribing DNA correctly and things like that ... just curious if there are other things that we should know about minerals in human physiology, in human biochemistry.

Robert [00:22:42]: Well, the biochemistry link on it, you don't see that link until you get to the DNA structure because it—we talked about it in the last interview—the particle size was so critical in the ability for the plant to deliver that particle size which gives it the absorbability through food where the other supplements are just too large a particle size to recognize if they are in a chemical compound. And I don't know if you want to go this route on this summit, but I want to tell you just a little motivation that I have on what I see in the future for the research that I'm doing. You go back to the Garden of Eden the lifespan was 900 years. And a lot of that was because we didn't have erosion since that water came from the earth up. We never had rain until the flood. There was a mist in the garden. And if you want to validate the healing power of these minerals, that's the best validation that I can see in the longevity that it gives and the health that it gives. And Isaiah 65 talks about the New Jerusalem, and it says it we will live that length again. We'll all tend our own gardens. We'll all build our own houses. But when we see that we will tend our own gardens, as we see and identify our nutritional requirements and what our deficiencies are, we'll be motivated to address our own deficiencies and never buy food like we buy foods right now that comes from all over the world. And we are basically ... have no control over what our deficiencies are and what our health symptoms are because of what we ate.

Brendan [00:25:04]: This brings up one of the central tensions I would say, in myself around the issue of who's growing the food because yes, the ultimate solution is be hands-on, grow your own food, and so forth. And a lot of the people in this event talk about that. They're basically saying that's the only real solution, or know your farmer very well so you know that's a little bit of outsourcing, but at least you've got a better eye and maybe even some influence on what is happening in the growth of your food. But then when I look at ... so my biggest motivation however, for creating this event is to change the food system because ... first of all, it would take a very long time for everybody to get to the point where they're growing their own food. There's many systemic issues that make it a little bit challenging for people, one being that the majority of people are stuck in the work-for-the-corporation model that has them "just over broke" with their j-o-b. And so it's very hard for them to find the time and a little bit of resources to invest if we are talking about, you know, balcony gardening and indoor gardening and stuff. But see all of those things, they don't address the systemic planetary issue that is oh-so-urgent and that is so driven by our agricultural … basically our food system in general. So much of the planetary destruction is being driven at the landscape management level and at the level like you said … you get these centralized food systems where food is being shipped around the world so the entire footprint of global agriculture includes all that transportation, includes all the chemical petroleum-based fertilizers and inputs or at least petroleum-intensive mechanization, all that stuff, in addition to how it's liberating greenhouse gasses from the soil and also turning the soil into a dry, hot, radiant body instead of … so, it's multiplying the main driver of the warming of the planet which is proportional to the 4th power of temperature and the Stefan-Boltzmann constant of a black body radiator, so we have to turn our soils back into moist covered soils, and doing that basically only happens by taking some of the carbon out of the atmosphere and putting it there in the soil and also then stemming the tide of nitric oxide being released from agricultural processes and so forth and restoring normal agroecosystems that will also handle any concerns about methane, likely anyway that that's the case. So my focus is on, we've got to change this big system, and then we can focus more on fine tuning with growing our own food. If we don't … if a certain percentage of us change our … grow our own food and stuff and divest from the big system, the big system is still going to lumber on for a long time. And a lot of people are still going to be caught up in it, and we're all going to … we're not all going to make it through this century. It's likely that very few of us will make it, if any, if we don't turn around the momentum in the system. And I don't think that the leverage point for that is everybody grows their own food because it's so unrealistic for that to happen, in a time frame that we need it to happen. I think it's more realistic to apply so much pressure to the food systems of the world from the bottom up and the top down and all sides that it shifts. And you know we've seen that we can shift the food system. It's been very slow, but if there is enough education, maybe then it can shift. And of course, the people who want to go further will grow their own food. But I think the focus should be on let's change the system because that will kill us no matter, pretty much almost no matter how many of us grow our own food. Let's say half of us grew our own food, a high improbability, we're still going down as a collective if we don't change the main system.

Robert [00:29:55]: I'm going to send you one of the director's information for the Rodale Institute. He's Mr. Smith, I can't remember his first name, and I'm looking here for a card.

Brendan [00:30:20]: I've got a card of someone there too. Let me just check and see if it's the same guy but go ahead, keep going.

Robert [00:30:26]: Anyway, him and I had a great conversation because we were on the same page of Rodale's book in a conversation and, what you are describing, and what we have to correct, was identified back in a study … This was Tenet C. Beeson from the Bureau of Plant Industry. It was part of the US Department of Agriculture. His miscellaneous publication number 369, it was put out in March of 1941. And Rodale had talked about this in his book, saying what this article had described in the health conditions and the degradation of health that we would see because we weren't addressing our soils and the minerals back into our soils. And what you're describing, and what we need to correct, is exactly what was identified in this publication. When this publication came out, remember this was at a time that people like Rockefeller and Carnage knew that what was in this report, and they capitalized on it by investing into pharmaceutical because they knew we couldn't correct this problem at the time that this publication came out. We can correct this problem now, because now we have everything, all the tools, to correct it. We have implements, most importantly. We have the analysis.

Brendan [00:32:25]: How do you mean "implements"? I'm just curious when you're saying "implements" … I'm just curious of you could say what it is, if you could specify what you mean by what we have available now versus then. And you mentioned "implements" as the first one. I'm just curious what you mean by "Implements".

Robert [00:32:43]: We have large enough tractors and the ability to put … we're hauling around anhydrous ammonia tanks and pumping that into the ground at the same time we're pumping seed into the ground, which is basically a full chemistry delivery system back in the soil. The work that I'm doing, by putting these minerals back in the soil … if you were to do it on a large scale would require that I build a piece of equipment that can do a chemical reaction at the time it's being administered into the soil, and that's completely possible. It was impossible … let me go back through the list, the implements, the chemistry, and the ability to test plant tissue for its outcome. You know what we've done for the last hundred years is NPK, which made it a greener plant, and then we did genetic modification which made taller bigger plants and uniform plants, but we never went back and corrected the mineral deficiencies in the plants that was described in this article, and the whole reason why we're seeing pharmaceutical industry explode, and why we are seeing symptoms of that industry. But if you go back to all of these symptoms that Dr. Duke talks about that are addressed by 23 different minerals … you know, there are a list of 260 different symptoms that are all associated with mineral deficiencies which are all associated back to the food, and back to the soil.

Brendan [00:34:45]: I'm curious what … oh, go ahead.
Robert [00:34:47]: Go ahead.

Brendan [00:34:49]: Well, so my, so I'm curious about what you think … this is another one of the central issues that I see come up in these discussions, and I haven't fully teased it … I haven't fully brought it front and center in my interviews, but I have touched upon it, and that is that some people, let's say someone like Elaine Ingham … their experience leads them … her experience leads her—and not just her experience but also global surveys of soils and so forth—leads her to believe that most soils contain plenty of the nutrients needed. It's merely a deficiency of functional biodiverse life in the soil and that when we fix that the minerals become available. The soil transforms its character in so many ways and then begins delivering the minerals to the plants. You've mentioned that there are some key leverage points by application of minerals. There are various things that can kick off that bacterial microbial process. You mentioned cobalt, and there are actually inventions out there for introducing blends of I believe it's ozone and hydrogen peroxide—they call it "peroxone" or something like that—and injecting that into the soil fires up the microbial activity and basically turns a compacted anoxic soil, anaerobic soil, into an aerobic nicely flocculated aggregated soil, and so forth. So there are certainly inputs that accelerate the process, but what I'm wondering is, is your approach to it we need to add back a lot of minerals and do it at a scale and so forth or are you basically saying well at scale we could add back cobalt and that would be one of the ways we could fire up the whole biology? Because my perspective has been heavily influenced by things that have been said by the two soil scientists that I know and respect the most which are Elaine Ingham and Christine Jones from Australia. And they are both basically saying, "Look, the Earth's crust has a lot of minerals in it." And soil and dirt, dirt being soil without biological life, are basically a mix of eroded crust …. and of course the closer you get to the surface the more leaching has occurred, and obviously there is going to be less mineral available there if there has been leaching and so forth … however, biology once established reaches down with roots and pulls up the minerals back to the surface into the topsoil and some of these roots can go down dozens of feet and so forth. And that's what they do, basically mine the Earth's crust. The whole system does. It's not just one thing, one plant, one organism. It's the whole system. Just curious about what your thoughts are about that, you know, the difference between those two ideas is that, "Hey we got to add minerals back" versus "No, we just have to restore the biology."

Robert [00:38:34]: It's twofold on that. I always thought we had to add the minerals back. When I hit the cobalt and seeing that the plants, and just like cobalt, manufactured a leaching agent in the rhizome area of the roots then it allowed all these minerals to come up. When you look at what anhydrous ammonia does. Anhydrous ammonia will—it's so corrosive—but it will etch all the minerals in the soil and even without biological activity. Now you have some nutrient level that can go back up into that plant without … you know, it's a dead soil. I mean it's a chemically dead NPK soil, but they increase some nutrient content because of putting in something so corrosive as anhydrous ammonia into the soil, and it allows access to mineral nutrients. Those are two different approaches that we see right now. In a water treatment plant when we're growing colonies, it requires food mass for these microbes to eat. And the chemical compounds out there are too toxic for the microbes to actually utilize. The approach that I use in my formulas is we bond everything to nutrient, and we make it food for the microbes in the soil. And eventually the microbes in the soil have something that they consume. And as they consume it, they're consuming these micronutrients that are bonded to it, and then they excrete these nutrients in a bioavailable size for the plant uptake. But you know to use all of these in an equation or to take just one part of it is wrong. It takes every bit of what all of the other people are talking about, including what I see. And what I'm looking at is basically the results from the testing of this lab up in Canada.

Brendan [00:41:06]: Okay.

Robert [00:41:07]: Maybe one of the doctors up in that lab up in Canada can shed some light on it. But I tell you they see amazing things up there. When that NSP certification for supplements had come out, the new requirements on those were so stringent, and it caused me to seek and find different carbon sources. But I asked them, I says, "Tell me a source out there that I could use for a carbon source, you know, a food source for my microbes that meets these ranges …" and he says "Good luck. We're having an impossible time seeing it." And it wasn't until I dug into some of the books and figured out how you get rid of arsenic and cadmium and mercury that I realized, well I've got to go to an ethanol plant and get something that's been fermented. It's a path that is very, very tough to say what is the correct path, but we've been eating with blinders on. Without being able to test with the plant tissue testing, I couldn't do the work that I'm doing, anybody couldn't validate that the minerals are up into the plants. And this testing is relatively new on the micronutrients. It's been out there for a while on the macronutrients and also some of the vital ones like chromium and stuff that they could easily see. Well, if I had all the answers I would …

Brendan [00:43:08]: ... be God.

Robert [00:43:11]: Yeah. You know when we talk about the soil, well maybe we're trying to clean up something that's so toxic that we need to start over and containerize systems you have complete control over. I mean like a greenhouse, I have complete control over what I'm doing.

Brendan [00:43:40]: I doubt that that would be necessary. The reason I mentioned it is there is a lot of evidence that I hear about—I haven't gone down the rabbit hole with it and checked sources and all that—but I do hear a bit here and there of about biology's ability to transform and sequester things and one of those things is toxic metals. And so you've got the work of Paul Stamets, you know who he is? Or Stamets. And with fungal organisms he's been able to clean up a lot of things I believe including sequestering heavy metals from toxic sites. And then Zack Bush in a conversation I had with him mentioned something along the lines of biology's ability to transmute. This is something that is not mainstream at all. The guy is brilliant though. I trust his mind just in general. He's a medical researcher, triple board-certified and, you know, even by mentioning the word transmutation I think he takes a risk, so I don't think he does it lightly. I also think he's a very spiritual man, and that he is connected to something. I think he's getting information at some level ... but whatever he's looking at he's talking about scientific stuff. He basically said that there is evidence coming out about transmutation of elements, and it's happening in our bodies. There's actually studies on humans showing, you know, at least strongly suggesting, that the body itself is transmuting elements, and we're constructing the periodic table in our body. This can only happen though when the mitochondria are working very well, and he said if you look at the energy density—I'm not sure if that's the right term—but I think it was of the surface of mitochondrial membranes, and compared it to the Sun it's 10,000 times the energy per cubic or square unit of space, at the mitochondrial membrane or something like that, compared to the surface of the Sun where we believe that there's fission and fusion and transmutation of elements. And so he says, you know, there's all this evidence pointing to not only the possibility of it, but also in these studies with men on oil platforms given a certain diet, everything was measured—every drop of sweat, everything they ingested, and what they were peeing out and so forth—and it basically suggested that they were turning, you know, potassium and hydrogen into calcium, or something like that, and perhaps other types of things. So I think that there's vast potential to not have to go to like container gardening for the human race. I think that we don't nearly need to go there, and one of the things another speaker mentioned, Walter Jehne, he said, you know, when you restore the biology ... see plants if they don't have their normal microbial buddies and fungal buddies and so forth they have a very unselective uptake of minerals and metals. So they'll just take whatever is in the transpiration stream. But when they're in their normal association with let's say mycorrhizal fungi, these organisms are selectively delivering nutrients and excluding toxic metals to those plants. So that's another mechanism by which ... okay, sure, alright we introduced a lot of cadmium to the soil from decades of application of rock phosphate fertilizers, but if we restore biology we can potentially protect the plants and ourselves from taking on so much of this cadmium, and there may be other processes by which that cadmium can be extracted or sequestered or be turned somewhat inert in the soil through biology.

Robert [00:48:22:]: I completely agree, even with the possibility of transmutating it could only happen in the DNA and the amino acids because ... well, how I'd ...

Brendan [00:48:40]: You'd have a healthy enough system to start with basically you know, you have to have a high-energy machine, biomachine happening here, I think.

Robert [00:48:50]: Well, the Pauling system …

Brendan [00:48:51]: Pauling as in Linus Pauling kind of thing?

Robert [00:48:54]: Yeah, he came up with a Pauling scale which measures the intensity of chemical bonds by elemental bonds, but chemical bonds. Sulfur has the … everybody says "Ah there's all this gold in the ocean," and there is, but that bond is with a sulfur compound, not a salt water but a sulfur, a thiol sulphate compound. The Pauling scale on that is through the charts.

Brendan [00:49:36]: Could you define it for me again the Pauling scale? What is the Pauling scale? I didn't catch it. I haven't eaten, and I'm hungry and I didn't sleep enough so my mind … you probably explained this just a moment ago, and I didn't catch it because my mind is a little "wandery".

Robert [00:49:50]: The Pauling scale is a measurement of the strength of a chemical bond.

Brendan [00:49:56]: Okay.

Robert [00:49:58]: A sulfur platinum bond is off-the-charts. A sulfur gold bond is off the charts. But even if you were looking at nitric acid or nitrates, you know, that oxygen bond to the nitrogen is extremely strong. The microorganisms in a water treatment plant, you can grow colonies of microbes that will actually eat that oxygen when you run, they are in an anoxic state. And we measure this through ORP meters, oxygen-reduction potential. And we know if we hit a certain point we can break that bond. We do the same thing, bond chemically, when we're putting in a sodium metabisulphite and hexavalent chrome, and we want to make it trivalent. We bring the pH down, add the sodium metabisulphite that the chemical reaction bond to the sodium metabisulphite will then reduce from a hexavalent to trivalent state of the chromium. We see all of these different reactions happen within the body. We see, you know, there are points in our body where we're in an anoxic state. We see for instance our body where we are making amino acids in different organs, but by manufacturing that amino acids we're releasing oxygen which allows oxygen to get to the different tendons in our bodies which have no blood flow. What I'm getting at is when you see how complex life is we can end up with, yeah, transmutation was probably more than possible. It's a matter of the body utilizing what it needs and taking what it needs in a different state. I want to go back to one of the people that you have talked to that said we have all the minerals we need in the crust of the Earth, and you know Richard Olree who wrote *Minerals for the Genetic Code* in his *Amish Handbook of Nutrition*, he comes to that same conclusion. Well, all you got to eat is this food because it's … take these minerals, and we see these minerals all across the face of the Earth. Well, most of those minerals are bound up.

Brendan [00:53:03]: Yeah, they're not bioavailable until you do something different with how you manage that. It's a question the biology versus also adding in amendments.

Robert [00:53:18]: Into life. Yes ... we see all of these different factors in our soil. We see the different factors in the minerals in our soil. The reality is what's in the food we are eating? What did all of those different components in the soil and in, you know, the minerals in the soil, what the fungi of the soil has produced, what the rhizome has created what's the outcome? What's in our food? What are the mineral content and the value of our food, because that will tell you if everything is in order and we're going to recover a product that Nature has created that can provide healing to us.

Brendan [00:54:18]: Yeah, and you know I'm curious. Go ahead.

Robert [00:54:27]: Go ahead.

Brendan [00:54:18]: Oh I was going to say, so in order for me to better understand what your products typically include, what I believe I've seen is and heard you describe is it has for different conditions, you're providing a mix of minerals, and I would guess cobalt might be like the basic first ingredient of any of those mixes because it makes so many others more available, and then maybe you have other minerals that are key you want to make sure they're in that top layer of the soil so that the vegetables growing in that very first season have everything they need to deliver a powerful medicine as opposed to, well, let's do the you know the cobalt, and adding life, and then you know a season or two later then we get up to the luxury levels of nutrients that will provide medicinal food ongoingly. I'm just curious is that kind of what yours does is you basically provide it, and you have these minerals in very bioavailable forms, you complex them with certain proteins I think you said, and that this basically jump-starts the system, the life in the soil, but also delivers everything right there so that the very first crop of radish, broccoli, or whatever is a super medicine. Is that kind of what your model is?

Robert [00:55:53]: In all of our testing we've tested the very first harvest.

Brendan [00:55:58]: Yeah.

Robert [00:55:59]: And we're measuring that increase compared to a control non-treated soil, and so we're measuring the increase of the uptake. What we also do is a maintenance harvest, you know, every fourth harvest we'll add more of the mineral nutrient to it, and what we're looking for there when we're harvesting a year later you know—it might be seven eight harvests later; I think we get 11 harvests of wheatgrass a year— but every fourth harvest we amend the soil, same soil, just added these minerals, but then after one year we tested to see if the plants were actually loading higher levels of minerals or depleting at a larger rate. And we found the consistency there pretty good except on lithium. Lithium, once we've seen almost a three-fold increase in lithium from the first harvest to the 11th, and what we see in that lithium is probably because of the toxic state of the lithium. Lithium as you know, there's a balance that we have to come up with a. Are we sterilizing the soil? Are we providing proper nutrients, or is the plant utilizing it right? And lithium, I think it has to be broke down a little bit more from the microbes for it to become bioavailable, but those microbes are just seeing this kind of stunted effect. But eventually the level of microbes come into the soil that can actually break it down, if that makes sense. It's just like in a water treatment plant you can't just turn on a water treatment plant and expect it to function, you have to have colonies growing in that water treatment plant for that to actually do BOD (biochemical oxygen demand) reductions of the nitrate reductions and different things that you're looking for. The same in the soil. You know, just saying where we're going to convert to … this is the biggest joke out there is transitional organic, when we haven't done anything. The only thing we did was stopped adding glyphosate or pesticides to the soil, and we're thinking that it's going to become a better soil. Um it doesn't. You need to …

Brendan [00:58:52]: Yeah, you know I wonder that transitional organic, headed up by Kashi, if that's what you're referring to, you know theoretically —maybe you've looked at it in depth —they could be addressing soil quality, they could be adding the things that are not really … well, one of the things I have not done, is I have not really read the US National Organic Standards myself to see if it's a matter of omission that those standards do not basically say you have to be doing these kinds of things for your soils. It should literally say, your soil organic matter should be growing up to a certain point, and it's going to hit maybe an asymptotic limit or something where it doesn't really get any better after 5, 8, 11 percent 17 depending on the soil. I mean 17 sounds really high, but Elaine Ingham mentioned a place where that happened relatively quickly from 2% or something at the end of 10 years and went from something to 17, but maybe was 20. But what I'm wondering is, do the organic standards currently have any prescriptions for soil health practices? I believe there's some, but they might not be adequate. And then the other question is, "But are they being enforced?" And so this came up in a personal conversation with Andre Leu the Director—either former Director or soon-to-be former Director because he's stepping down to do other things—but he's been leading up the International Federation of Organic Agriculture movements IFOAM, and he said, "Look, it's in the standards. It's just not being enforced." All they're enforcing is pesticide use, or lack of it. They're not enforcing the soil health measures. And of course not using toxic chemicals is a soil health measure in itself, but it's not sufficient to really build life in the soil and keep the minerals available. So anyway, that's just an aside on that. Maybe you know the answer to that. Do you know how it is in the National Organic standards?

Robert [1:01:19]: Yeah, I've tried to get my products organically certified, and one of the main reasons why my products are not organically certified are—well, there's two now—but the main reason was I use an oxidized sulfur. I use a thiosulfate as a carrier and a food for the microbes. Now that's on a banned list because it's a synthetic chemical that they use for pesticides, and they also use it as a preservative so on organics you cannot use that chemical for those reasons. But to use it as food for microbes, it shouldn't be banned. But it's on the list so it's banned. Okay, so then I thought well, and I work with a large organic wheat exporter. In fact, I work closely with him. Goes to the same church. The guy who sold a half million dollars' worth of transitional organic wheat to Kashi's just lives ten miles from me here. We've had this conversation. The three of us have sat down and had this conversation about organics, and we come to the conclusion, "Well, Bob the transition time is three years. Bring in all your soils. Do all your treatment on the soils. And start your certification." So I did that. I brought in all 400 yards of manure and under my facility put it in a pile with the intention of putting these additives into it and storing it. And then I could sell this as organic soil after three years.
Brendan [1:03:23]: Mm-hmmm.

Robert [1:03:24]: The organic certification people come out and says, "No you can't do this." I says "Well why not?" "You can't add something to the soil unless the test shows that you need to add it." And I said, "So tell me a test."

Brendan [1:03:37]: Okay, that's really bad. Yeah go ahead.

Robert [1:03:42]: So tell me a test to show that, and none of the tests would tell you to test for chromium and when you're below a certain level. And that's why down at the Regenerative Earth when they had that sustainable ... I've got the paper right here ... this regenerative organic certification. I think I sent you my comments on that.

Brendan [1:04:08]: Yep.

Robert [1:04:09]: To put on that fourth pillar.

Brendan [1:04:16]: I believe I quickly read your fourth pillar, and I had intended to go back and read it in greater depth and have not yet. I apologize, just this one-man show is overtaxed, but what I recall from it is both that we should require that the plants that we produce and call organics should have at least a ... maybe meet the fiftieth percentile or it should at least provide a certain amount of minerals in them, and then maybe I think what I'm hearing you're saying is that there's also another part in there that I didn't recall which is that it should also allow us to add things to enhance the soil without having to meet some kind of test of is it required, or at least okay well there should be a pathway for determining that it is required so that you can add it and still be organic. Is that also in there?

Robert [1:05:22]: Yes.

Brendan [1:05:24]: Okay and so a question ... go ahead.

Robert [1:05:27]: And I added specifically with minerals that I use, to be added to that list so you're not prohibited based upon just a list. You can do what's common-sense required.

Brendan [1:05:44]: Yeah go ahead, you're going to say something else.

Robert [1:05:47]: Well, if you look at organics ... when you go down to Trader Joe's or you go down to Whole Foods and you're buying all organic certified produce, why do you need to go down to that supplement and vitamin aisle now?

Brendan [1:06:11]: Right, it's ludicrous.

Robert [1:06:13]: What I'm saying is by doing proper testing you'll know whether or not you need to go through that supplement aisle.

Brendan [1:06:20]: I think what we need is grades of organic because ... I don't think this is an original thought on my part, it's just occurring to me right now in the context of this conversation, but to me it makes sense that okay we shouldn't have an all-or-nothing standard that basically says you're either perfect or you're not organic. I think there should be something where it's like grades of organic, where it's like okay this is organic. It doesn't have toxic pesticides—well, it still does; it just depends on how you define toxic. They'll allow you to introduce natural toxic pesticides in organic. But to me there should be at least two levels to it—one that doesn't require certain levels of mineralization because that can take extra time and expense, and then nobody would ever get there and not nobody but very few organic growers would get there. As it is, it's costly enough and time-intensive enough to transition to organic that it discourages the vast majority of people that might go in that direction. And so to my mind the threshold of entry should not get more difficult, but we absolutely need some kinds of standards and certifications that say well this food is actually also meeting some defined standard of nutrient delivery to your body, or at least in your food, whether your body assimilates it or not is up to your microbiome and the health of your whole lifestyle and everything. But what do you think of that idea?

Robert [1:08:09]: I completely agree, and it goes right …

Brendan [1:08:12]: That might make your suggestion more palatable and approachable … if it's not already in there, if you added that sort of caveat, say "I think this needs to be in there as in the organic level two" or something like that, I don't know. Just thinking of regenerative organic level two or maybe regenerated organic does include that, but what I don't think we should try to do is make the basic organic certification any more onerous, but maybe for regenerative organic it really should have that and regenerative organic will essentially be 2.0. However, I'm thinking maybe there need to be three levels because regenerative organic involves so much more as they're defining it now without your suggestions than regular organic that that's a big step right there, and then regenerative organic level two would be … "and this is certified to provide a certain minimum standard of nutrient delivery."

Robert [1:09:17]: Going all the way back to the beginning of our conversation when we talked about growing our own gardens or growing the need. And if you look at the different wheatgrasses that I market right now, one of them can have a thousand times stronger amount of cobalt than one of the other formulas. Same plant using it for delivery. When we look at the organics in all foods, regardless of organics, when we don't know what's in it, all's we're eating is a plant. It could be hydroponically grown, and that's the other problem with organics. They've approved the hydroponic certification. Nothing's in there. Why are we eating something that has nothing?

Brendan [1:10:12:00]: Yeah. I have heard that maybe some hydroponic are starting to get better Brix values and so forth because they're putting more into the water and so forth, but yeah normally hydroponics produce … so this is what Graeme Sait told me two years ago I believe when I was with him in Australia at his course … he basically said, or maybe he said it to the whole room … and they work in dozens of countries around the world … the guy visits 33 countries a year, and so they have not found a single example—he and his agronomist at Nutri-tech Solutions—have not found a single example of a hydroponically produced item of produce that had a Brix value higher than about 1.5. That is so exceedingly low that it is basically probably a burden on the body more than anything else. Maybe not, it's still going to deliver exclusion zone water, you know, more hydrating water, it's still going to deliver some fiber it's going to deliver some vitamins and nutrients, some minerals, but maybe too much nitrate or something. But yeah, you do raise a good point. So hydroponics ... where were we going with hydroponics when I interrupted?

Robert [1:11:24]: Well, if the problem is when we go to hydroponics and we see that organic certification ... and you talked about some people, just like would look at the soil, who's adding more to the soil, who's making it a better value? A farmer is still motivated by how cheap he can get something to market.

Brendan [1:11:50]: Right.

Robert [1:11:51]: There's nothing out there that is forcing a farmer to get ... well, he's not getting paid for value-added. If I was a hydroponic grower you know, I would be contacting somebody, a company like myself and saying, can I make this in a tea form that we can feed into the plants? Nobody's calling. Nobody's doing that, they're only doing what it takes just to make a better looking plant just like NPK will make a better looking corn or a higher yield, but nothing's in it.

Brendan [1:12:30]: Well, part of this partly comes down to, largely perhaps comes down to consumers need to understand, be educated, and then care enough to demand it, so that there's at least a vocal demand signal, and then it's also got to be backed up by spending. Because right now most people don't realize that a tomato is not a tomato is not a tomato. They don't realize that. Our whole culture has been indoctrinated into commodity-based thinking, and so, you know, we look at every single item of produce as a freaking commodity. In general, I'm speaking of general population obviously. There's those of us who buy organic for a reason. We know that we don't look at each food item as a commodity. It's either an asset or a liability, like you said. And it's a continuum of extreme liability to extreme asset and everything in between. And so part of that is the toxin level, and part of is the nutrient level and so forth. But then of course there's the fair trade and the socio-economic implications of how the food was produced. But yeah, right now, you're right, most farmers whether they don't care about anything except money, or they're just basically saying, "Well, I'd like to do more, but you've got to pay me because I ain't going to survive if I put all these inputs in and put all this effort extra effort to make my system really hum ecologically or whatever it is nutritionally, but I'm still getting what a subsidized conventional farmer's getting. That ain't going to work out. I won't be able to do it."

Robert [1:14:16]: That's where on the testing foods, and that fourth pillar, has a value, because ... let's say if you didn't even add it, but you had something in your soil that brings up a higher selenium level than in the soil two states away people will buy that. People buy higher protein levels in wheat. They pay based upon the protein levels. So you know, there's a motivation there for bringing in the quality because they're after a higher pay check or higher return. That's the whole thing on my comments on Regenerative Earth was to address the quality of food not just how it's handled but also what's in it so people can recognize the value for what it is. And that would set it above a hydroponic organic certification. The first part of that was testing for toxic levels within the food, the cadmium, mercury, arsenic, and lead. That was the first part of that, even if they weren't adding more, at least making sure that we weren't delivering crib paint in a tomato plant. That's where I come from on this here. And it isn't that I'm a specialist in nutrition or even identifying deficiencies. I just know how to address those deficiencies.

Brendan [1:16:12]: I have a question for you, going back to something you said a little earlier. You said the organic standard says you can't add something to soil unless it's needed. And what I'm wondering is, does that only apply to inorganic nutrients such as metals, minerals and other compounds, salts and various sorts, or does it apply to anything? I would imagine it doesn't apply to anything. I would imagine you're probably allowed to add compost, compost tea, which is something you're adding and you don't have a test showing that, well I need 20 tons of compost per hectare here or something. So just curious which things, which categories of things, have to be proven required in order to add them.

Robert [1:16:55]: The only thing I could say to that is call OneCert. OneCert was the one that I had contacted, and they basically said I couldn't become certified because of that requirement. It brings up a whole group of problems, especially like you say, how do you add something to water and hydroponics now. Look, what gives you the approval to do that ... if you can't add it to the soil?

Brendan [1:17:30]: So that would be the ultimate irony ... pardon me for interrupting ... but is the ultimate irony that if somebody goes certified organic hydroponic they can no longer add extra nutrients that they might have added to their hydroponic operation, if it weren't organic?

Robert [1:17:50]: That's a great question. At the time that they come up with their response to me they were under the impression that hydroponics was just going to go away off from organic certification because for six seven months there it was on the chopping block, and it only was approved when we were down there and the day before that conference started where we met.

Brendan [1:18:30]: Wow.

Robert [1:18:50]: And so just so you know why where I come from on this and what I've been told ... remember that lady that was talking that she worked for the Department of Agriculture, and she was a scientist and studying a different compound that the roots were putting out into the soils, and she did all this work, and her funding was cut. I don't know if you remember her talk.

Brendan [1:19:06]: Oh, she got a bit emotional up there because she had worked at it, and then she was basically silenced, I think. Yes, yeah.

Robert [1:19:17]: You silence people by not giving them funding. When I tried to get this approved or to get a government grant I was flat told that, "You increase the quality of life, people live longer, and our country goes broke, and so no we won't fund you for the work you're doing."

Brendan [1:19:41]: Who told you this? Somebody told you this flat out?

Robert [1:19:42]: Yes, yes.

Brendan [1:19:43]: A government agency employee or something is that what you said?

Robert [1:19:45]: Yep.

Brendan [1:19:46]: Oh … my … God.

Robert [1:19:49:00]: So when you look at, yeah when you look at organic certification … let me go all the way through this … when you look at organic certification the referee for that, and the ones that put out the fine, are the USDA.

Brendan [1:20:06]: Mm-hmm.

Robert [1:20:07]: And the USDA is a governing factor over that. Trust me, they're okay with the quality of food not improving. And you always have to keep that in mind and why something is the way it is. Why hydroponics was approved as an organic certification.

Brendan [1:20:30]: Yeah, it sounds like they're very okay with it. In fact, like you said they literally have a Malthusian perspective that if people live longer we all die. And I think that there's evidence that that is false. Especially like if you educate women they don't have as many children. If you empower women in general, not just education, they have fewer children. It seems like the more educated people in the United States unfortunately don't procreate at all, and so we're going to end up with the scenario humorously depicted in the movie *Idiocracy* perhaps. Have you seen that? Well, it's hilarious. It's basically only cretins are breeding kind of thing taken to the extreme. It goes out to the year 2505 or something like that.

Robert [1:21:33]: I didn't mean to go negative on the USDA, but if you don't believe that …

Brendan [1:21:40]: Oh, you've got to be realistic. It's not being negative. It's just having eyes wide open. We can't be running around … just like you said we can't be eating blind. Well, guess who's determining what we're basically allowed to get access to … it's the USDA. Well, we're eating blind because they're trying to keep us blind and keep us disempowered in terms of food quality. I think that the USDA can potentially … they do get behind soil conservation to a degree, right? And I think that they're potentially going to get behind soil conservation practices as a climate change policy, climate mitigation policy.

Robert [1:22:30]: What is their main goal? Their main goal is that we don't have starvation because if we have famines the government becomes unstable. And so that's their main goal. For hydroponic tomatoes to be served at McDonald's because then the dollar menu can still stay down to a dollar. Even though it has nothing in it, people are getting fed. They don't realize that their brains aren't getting fed, or their Parkinson's are getting fed, or their diabetes is going rampant because it doesn't have any chromium in it. But that's the whole problem right there. Our food should be our medicine. And if we're not building our medicine plants, which is our farms, you know the pharmacy of our food, then you know we're doomed. We're absolutely doomed if we're going to rely on drugs to crutch the farm industry. And it goes right back to that report back in 1941 where they predicted exactly what we're living through right now. We have not had the ability to correct it until right now. That's basically what we need to focus on is that report. How can we correct it. The same guy that I asked for this grant, who said why I couldn't get a grant … I said, "You can't give me a grant … can you get this type of equipment the high resolution ICP-Mass Spec back into every university, because there's only a handful of them in the world." And he knew about it because he says, "Well, that takes a special permit" because the work that can produce, the reports that that can produce, open your eyes to seeing the world because now you can truly measure the mineral content of just about everything or the contamination of just about everything. If we tested, and this is my fear, and their fear I'm sure … if we tested all of our crops and our farmland and found out that half of it was unfit because of lead contamination from leaded gasoline or arsenic contamination or mercury contamination from fossil fuel burning and coal plants, what type of crisis does that generate to the general public?

Brendan [1:25:32]: Right, right. Yeah, and like you said I think the main, one of the main sort of overriding guiding principles of our government, and probably many governments, is like you said maintain stability. So that's like their overriding mandate for themselves is basically, look we don't want starvation because that makes people and makes us and makes the system unstable. We don't want people living longer because then we'd have overpopulation, and that would destabilize things. Although all this deserves more questioning. But maybe what they're not looking at is … if we allow health to deteriorate on the track that it's on right now, by 2040 … I heard this is in a book I read by Mark Hyman … which book was it … I think it was *Eat Fat Get Thin* … and he basically said by 2040 our entire federal budget will be for health care, just a little over a few decades from now. So, that means basically, a massive increase is predicted, continued increase of chronic illness. Now, what if we did live longer? I didn't really … the first thought that came to mind was, well when you empower women they have fewer children. Well, that doesn't address the living longer part. That just addresses the rate of growth of the population of, the new humans, but it doesn't address the older humans. So just curious what you think would happen if we were all living longer. First of all, this planet under a regenerative management can produce many times more food than it does currently, so there is no issue really up to a point with food production. That is total nonsense. I think it was Dan Kittredge in my conversation with him says that—and this is research-based, or at least based on his conversations with plant geneticists and presumably they're speaking from research—that the plants we're using in our systems right now because of various things are only producing at five to fifteen percent of their genetic potential. Largely, that's because they're just not getting the nutrients they need. Which is far more than a fivefold potential increase in productivity if we do everything right in agricultural systems. And now of course genetic potential, I don't know if he meant literally production potential, or if that was sort of a term that also might include nutrient density, phytonutrient content and so forth. I'm not sure. But if all that fivefold difference applies to production potential as well as nutrient density, then yeah, all bets are off. We don't need to worry about food scarcity and population up to a point. But of course population has other impacts and footprints besides agricultural production. So what I'm wondering is what would you envision, what would happen if people are living longer? Is that going to … at first thought it does seem like something to be concerned about as far as overpopulation, but I just wonder what you think would happen if we were all living 120 or 900 years, or something in between.

Robert [1:29:13]: I talked with Dan and we talked specifically about the plant potential and stuff, and I've shared my results with him, and we truly believe that yes indeed, the plants are not giving the strength that they were designed originally to give us. And that's because of erosion and depletion. I'm going to go back to when Cain killed Abel. That's when God said because the Earth has opened up and took your brother's blood the plants won't yield their strength. Well, measuring the strength is measuring the nutrient content, and that's what this lab equipment does up in Canada. We can see the content of it. You know that curse on the

Earth didn't say that the plants will all die, and you will have no food. It's just the plants won't yield their strength. And what we've seen …

Brendan [1:30:16]: I apologize for my Biblical ignorance because I'm just not a Bible person even though I'm passionately connected to Christ, but I'm not at all a Bible reader or even necessarily what you might call a devotee of the Bible, but I am fascinated every time I hear something like this where basically what was said what was predicted makes all the sense in the world and I'm like, "Wow." So, what was the curse when Cain killed Abel? There was a curse on our agriculture?

Robert [1:30:52]: Yes. Yeah, it's in Genesis chapter 3. And what it is is because Cain killed Abel, and it said because the Earth had opened up and took your brother's blood, you'll till the Earth, but the plants won't yield their strength.

Brendan [1:31:21]: Oh my goodness.

Robert [1:31:52]: And trust me when I read something like that I have 12 other versions of Bible so I read each different version to get a full flavor of what it says, because if you if you open up some Bibles you know you'll only get one version of it. Open up five or six, do an internet search on it, but you'll see that. Somebody once said to me, "Well, Bob, if God cursed the Earth what makes you think you can change it?" And I had a problem with that, but it's just like you say believe in Jesus Christ, well he died for all of our sins, including that one. And our ability to convert that or to change that has happened in our lifetime, to change back the curse and wild plants to carry more nutrients. When you talk to Dan you know that's validation that says these plants are capable of doing that all. All you need to do is give them the right nutrition, or the soil, to give them the right bioavailable nutrients in it. And that's the work that I'm doing. What I see … we can see kale with a tenfold increase in 22 different minerals. We can make a super superfood now. Kale by itself even if you get it organically or hydroponically grown doesn't carry these nutrients, but you can load them up, they can be the carrier of your medicine into your diet. Now to go to the longevity side, I
have a longevity formula we don't market it, we've tested it. There are eight minerals that have been identified as extending life in lab testing these minerals have shown an increase of 100 percent increase in different lab testing settings. To deliver those in a bio nutrient form, those are more than capable … the difference that we will see when we utilize that is that those aren't the same minerals that we need for quality of life, and so what I'm working on before I'd ever introduced a longevity formula is to increase the quality of life. That's why my six formulas affect the six major conditions that we see in our diet, without addressing cancer because by addressing cancer I'd make myself too big of a target. But we do address cancer in a roundabout way with these same minerals. And then to say, "What would the world be like with people living a thousand years?" Well, for one, if we're following what Isaiah prophesies, which I believe, our main focus will be just on our own personal quality. What do we need? If we're having issues with mental illness, and we can type in you know mineral deficiencies with schizophrenia, and we can treat that by adding a supplement to the food we grow, why not? If we're having Parkinson's, and we can address our own Parkinson's by adding a supplement to the food we grow. And we don't have to grow a specific food; we can grow the food we like. We know that that food is capable of delivering these nutrients. We can then make a better world for ourselves. But if we thought living a thousand years with HIV and cancer and diabetes and everything else, all we're going to do is suffer

longer. We need to take care of our health and the health conditions before we look at how much longer we want to live.

Brendan [1:35:43]: But how, yeah exactly, I mean I totally agree. However, the question still remains, how would we tolerate ... how would the Earth handle a population if suddenly—it won't happen suddenly—but just as a thought experiment, if suddenly everybody was living 900 years? Can you imagine how many billions of people there would be in in 800 years and everybody is still alive. Eight hundred years of exponential growth rate of humans. I think that that is untenable. The Earth certainly has a higher human carrying capacity than morbid Malthusians would predict, but ultimately I think there is a limit for sure and that Malthusian considerations are not invalid by any means, so I'm just curious. It's just we underestimate the power of Nature, especially combined with human ingenuity. So just curious what would happen ... what in the world is practical about a population of seven billion people suddenly being able to live hundreds of years? Would we automatically see a massive reduction in procreation? I don't think so. Because it would have to go to zero for eight hundred years. Not necessarily zero but it would have to ... so that whatever the carrying capacity, at least a comfortable one, of the Earth, does not get exceeded. And I think that's what you know, well-meaning governments and bureaucrats and so forth, they're like basically looking at it from the fifty-thousand-foot elevation. They're looking down on what's happening, they're like, "Well, population is growing; it seems to be one of the major drivers of it all, of the problems we have, so we've got to control that," and then they become kind of Machiavellian as well as Malthusian.

Robert [1:37:52]: And that's probably why in Isaiah in the present it says we won't remember things as they were. And I think we need when that's prophesized and talked about ... I believe our knowledge base on plants is one thing, but our societal structure will be drastically changed. If we went back to ... if we were placed on this Earth ... God put us on this Earth to tend to a garden, and that was an only function ...

Brendan [1:38:27]: Then we'd all be Permaculturists!

Robert [1:38:30]: That's exactly it. That's why it says we won't go to work. We will grow our own foods and build our own houses. And that's all it says about it.

Brendan [1:38:41]: And we'll get a lots of vitamin C.

Robert [1:38:43]: And it says we won't remember ... Pardon?

Brendan [1:38:45]: Never mind go ahead. I'm just imagining a hammock lifestyle if I could afford it. Love it.

Robert [1:38:50]: But well, that's exactly what I'm working at. I'm thinking you know, if my house, and I knew I was going to live a thousand years, I would just start building a house and a garden to do that because I wouldn't need a job if I owned my house and my garden. Everybody's after ... you know, back in the 60s we all looked at communes and thinking that that was the right way as a society to live. Now, what were we designed for? We weren't designed for making the newest iPhone. We weren't designed for making the newest car, or being able to afford whatever that TV sells us that we cannot sustain life without.

Brendan [1:39:37]: So you saying ... yeah go ahead.

Robert [1:39:42]: Good quality food

Brendan [1:39:44]: Mm-hmm.

Robert [1:39:46]: Well it's ... go ahead.

Brendan [1:39:47]: Sorry, I'm such a such an interrupter today. This is a good conversation. So you were saying that we won't remember how it was, and I assume that what that means is we won't remember that we live differently, that we lived and that we were intended to live, in a garden, tending a garden and so forth, is that right? Is that what that means?

Robert [1:40:19]: You know that's the interpretation that I see out of the Bible. When we look at that and what a prophecy said ... trust me, I have people that come up to me that see the quality of what these foods can produce, and they're all over me saying, "Well, you know we need to get this into an Amazon type structure, need to do pyramid marketing, we need to do this ... honestly, my whole plate is full of that type of marketing people. That's what they see in marketing. And for me I see this as a change of lifestyle. I just think that if people did just that simplistically ... because I challenge anybody other than an accident or an outside toxic effect like exposure to radiation ... to identify any deficiency or any illness where the symptoms do not come from a deficiency.

Brendan [1:41:41]: Yeah, and I think that's the main thing, that's been sort of been hidden from us or we're hiding from ourselves, or we're just not recognizing it, is literally we have a machine, and it's built to perform our biological ... our body that houses our spirit and so forth ... you know it's built to perform, built to do amazing things, to heal constantly and so forth and live a lot longer than it generally does and age a lot slower and so forth. And so basically okay what's happening? Inadequate nutrients, excess toxins. That's it. Toxins of various forms. There's toxic light. There's electromagnetic toxins and of course there's the chemical toxins that we think of as chemical toxins. There's toxic thoughts. There's toxic emotions. There's toxic belief systems. All kinds of things and they're all affecting our ... both our biology and other aspects of our humanity.

Robert [1:42:44]: Yeah. And as a society just like we see symptoms of deficiencies that manifest themselves into full-blown diseases or deformities ... and I don't know how long it will take to change ... they say GMO seed will revert back to its natural form within two generations.

Brendan [1.43:14]: Oh, interesting. Oh-ho. I love it! So there's some vulnerability to Monsanto's model. That's great.

Robert [1:44:21]: Yes there is.

Brendan [1:43:22]: So, in fact you know what's interesting, when I was reading *The Source Field Investigations*, actually listening to an audio book ... have you ever heard of that book, *The Source Field Investigations*?

Robert [1:43:30]: No.

Brendan [1.43:31]: Oh, my goodness. So David Hancock, I think it is … this guy's been fascinated for three decades ever since he was a teenager in science and esoteric science. And so he never got educated as a scientist or physicist, but he studied a lot of the advanced and alternative, let's say, forms of evidence and hypotheses and theories about our physical world. And some of them are so wild, and he brings them out in that book. And so one of the things he mentions in it is—and all of it backed up by evidence, although it's not necessarily what would be considered peer-reviewed evidence, right—so some of it is published in like let's say published Russian scientists, and some of it's just like, just bizarre anecdotal evidence that did make it to newspapers. In other words, there were people looking at it and said "Well, this did happen" Or, these people, all these people, all these independent reports, they're reporting the same kind of thing where people are going, "What is that orange glow in the sky that looks like …" I'm not going to go any further than that because you have to read the whole thing, and then it starts to make some sense. So one of the things he looked at was pyramids. And he gives a plausible, I guess, explanation of through the lens of some of these alternative physical theories of what a pyramid does. And basically one of the effects that was I guess documented in some research, was that it would reverse the genetic changes in a GMO organism seed or plant. I think might have been the seed. So you put a seed in there, in a pyramid structure, and he talks about different ways people have built pyramid structures, simple things, essentially kind of refract incoming frequencies … they come into our planet from the Sun whatever … I don't know if that's the exact mechanism or if it might have been a more subtle form of energy than the ones we can currently measure … but at least that was the hypothesis of what was generating the changes that would occur in things when you put them in a pyramid. And one of the things it does, it seems to … if I'm interpreting correctly … it sort of sets biology back at its factory blueprint after being deranged in some way. And I went, "Oh, my God." And I'm calling it factory blueprint. You might call that Creators design right, or whatever. That's just fascinating to me though, that it automatically reverts, you're saying in a few generations.

Robert [1:46:27]: Yeah. Yeah, it's well you know the DNA is amazing. Selenium protects the DNA. Selenium is … your friend with prostate cancer … I can't say enough on taking selenium and make sure he buys a yeast-free selenium.

Brendan [1:46:50]: Yes, I remember that from your previous conversation. I looked at the selenium I just bought, and it's …. I didn't notice it's a yeast bound one. I'm like, "Oh great!" So I better see if I can return it opened. I've taken one pill. Probably won't kill me.

Robert [1:47:05]: You know, selenium … it's amazing because, well broccoli has a high level of selenium, mainly because the part of the broccoli that you eat is the seed. It's the bloom.

Brendan [1:47:19]: Oh okay.

Robert [1:47:21]: But you'll find that …

Brendan [1:47:23]: Must be why I love broccoli and Brazil nuts. I must really need selenium.

Robert [1:47:28]: It protects the DNA so well, and that's why when men have sexual intercourse the number one mineral that we become depleted on is selenium and zinc. If he has white spots on his fingernails that's a zinc deficiency, and that can still come from over sexual activity. And it's very easy to identify. And that's why I say if you identify a deficiency and then look at the other symptoms you can pretty much nail down that you're deficient in something by looking at the whole list of deficiencies. And if you have one or two symptoms of that deficiency or somebody in your family, it's very easy to identify.

Brendan [1:48:20]: And back to how we do that, are you basically saying go to the James Duke database it'll indicate things like white spots on fingernails for zinc.

Robert [1:48:32]: No, no that won't go to that level. You just have to …

Brendan [1:48:38]: So the James Duke database would tell you zinc is anti- … zinc and selenium are anti-prostate cancer or whatever, but you'd have to go elsewhere to find symptoms of zinc and selenium deficiency or something.

Robert [1:48:53]: Yeah, yeah, and Google is a great place to do that.

Brendan [1:48:57]: Okay.

Robert [1:48:58]: Because Google gives you all these different sources, whether or not they're a good source or not … What the James Duke database will give you is actually the dose for a different condition.

Brendan [1:49:09]: Okay it gives you the dose.

Robert [1:49:10]: If you have prostate cancer it'll tell you the selenium dosage need you know, but that database like I say it's now 30 years old. It's very goo,d but there are nutritionists out there … nobody will tell you that molybdenum is great for liver cancer. I just found that out because we did bioavailable molybdenum, and you cannot find a constant molybdenum source in a natural product store. There's a couple molybdenum sulphates or sulphites or something like that that out there, but trust me your body isn't recognizing that otherwise they would be seeing these healing effects that molybdenum can do.

Brendan [1:50:04]: The form that I'm taking is a glycinate, I just took some in this very conversation. I hope you didn't hear me, but I was taking molybdenum glycinate. What do you think of that form?

Robert [1:50:21]: The glycinates are made on amino acid, glycine.

Brendan [1:50:26]: Glycinate tends be a good form. I think it's a magnesium form that's often recommended it's easy on the gut. I certainly feel it. There is no question in my mind that this is getting into my body because of its metabolic effects. I'll say I'm an amateur student of metabolic typing so to speak. That's not quite the right word—the "typing" part of it—but there are people who've elucidated the effects of minerals on basically

Krebs cycle and other parts of our energy metabolism. And so various nutrients, and not just minerals ... minerals, amino acids and that ... so I can change almost on a dime what kind of protein I'm going to want in my next meal by which minerals, amino acids, and so forth I take because it will set me up to either want something light or heavy, let's say, red meat with nice marbled with fat or something, but grass-fed of course, and lots of fat in that meal. That's one mode, metabolic mode. Another mode if I take the right minerals will have me wanting very little protein or maybe only some fish, maybe light fish, that is, not like salmon which is more on that oily heavier side, not tuna. So it will have me wanting like some tilapia, whereas tilapia will just be revolting to me when I'm in my meat monster mode as I call it. So it's these two polar extremes, and it's totally modifiable by minerals and other things. And molybdenum is one of the things that nudges me away from wanting the heavier proteins and more of them and more fat, to wanting ... potentially being able to fast on a totally vegan diet for the day. And it wouldn't necessarily be a fast. Like yesterday I just really did not want a protein. It's been like this for a few days because I've been taking a lot of molybdenum and calcium and so forth that nudge the metabolism in that direction. But then it can swing out of it pretty fast, and then I'll be like, "Oh my God now I want meat." But I can push it right back if I want to. It's not that I'm saying meat is bad. Meat is phenomenal food from good sourcing, but it does have a more of a metabolic burden let's say than the vegetables. If there's vegetables that one tolerates well, that's some of the most healing food in the world. It's not necessarily the most building food in the world. So if you want to build, and I'm thinking organ meats, things like that. But anyway that was a long aside. Go ahead.

Robert [1:53:20]: So we went to meat because we weren't getting value out of our foods anymore. And meats were a way of those storing a massive amounts of mineral nutrients that we're not getting out of ...

Brendan [1:53:34]: That's a really good point. Are you saying basically that humans are meant to be more vegetarian and even vegan, and that because of maybe the curse and just in general what we've done to soils over the last 10,000 years—or you might have a different timeline because obviously there's differences of perspective between Biblical scholars and archaeological scholars and so forth—but is that what you're saying basically is we're not meant to eat so much meat, but we're doing it because the nutrient density has effectively been lost from our plant foods because of the soil, but animals are still concentrating them to the degree that they can, plus we actually give supplements to our livestock. Otherwise they would die. So our livestock are getting supplemented even though many of us are not. So meat is currently one of the more nutrient-dense foods especially when it comes to iron and zinc and selenium and things, but is that what you were basically ...

Robert [1:54:35]: And cobalt.

Brendan [1:54:36]: Okay. Very important.

Robert [1:54:38]: I know we're going all over the board, but that goes back to what I've been able to see. And cobalt going back into food is ... there's a company that is one of the main suppliers ... I think it's called nutraceutical or something like that ... one of the main suppliers of raw products for the supplement and vitamin companies ... and that was at Expo West last year. And they had all of their different augers and stuff and they had a wheatgrass. And I pulled the wheatgrass card out, and it said contrary to popular belief wheatgrass is not a good source of cobalt.

Brendan [1:55:23]: Hmm.

Robert [1:55:25]: And so I took that card, and I scanned it and sent a salesman an analysis and says, "Yeah you're absolutely right unless the cobalt is in the soil. And here's our wheatgrasses that we can produce with this higher level of cobalt." And it was through the roof. This is one-hundred-eighty-time factor of cobalt.

Brendan [1:55:52]: This is in your product or somebody else's?
Robert [1:55:55]: That was my product that I grew. And my whole intention is … and I talked to John Kohler about this … is if you put cobalt back into our gardens vegetarians wouldn't have to supplement themselves with B12 because we can see that high enough … that's one where vegetarians absolutely either have to take that supplement or eat meat.

Brendan [1:56:22]: Let me ask you, where would they get … so this brings up something mentioned by one of the other people I interviewed. He said reasons vegetarians have to take a supplement, or vegans at least, is that the location in the human digestive tract where vitamin B12 can be synthesized by bacteria in our gut is lower down than the point in the digestive tract where we actually assimilate B12. So I'm just curious how would the vitamin B12 end up in our bodies through plant food only. You were saying the cobalt would get in … is the vitamin B12 then being produced somehow in the plants when there's more cobalt available, or is it happening … you're saying it's going to happen in our guts when we have adequate cobalt in our diet? But then that brings up the question of is this other person correct that the location of bacterial synthesis of vitamin B12 is more downstream in the gut than where the assimilation sites are.

Robert [1:57:28]: Not to say either one of us are right or wrong. For the B12 to be manufactured it requires the proper pH balance. So the HCL level of your gut is important also. And so that's why Prilosec will interfere with that. It changes your pH of your stomach, and so you become basically B12 deficient even if you had the proper levels of cobalt. So, for cobalt to make B12 it requires a stomach acid environment. And that stomach acid environment like the gentleman said, or whoever said it, is probably lower in your stomach because that's … when your bacteria in your small intestine … your pH from your food when you consume that … when the beneficial bacteria in your stomach runs out of food they start eating themselves, and that's when they start going septic and then you have the lower pH.

Brendan [1:58:48]: Well, we're supposed to have a low pH in our stomachs though. We're supposed to have a low a low pH in our stomachs. It's supposed to be acidic in there, very acidic. Go ahead.

Robert [1:59:04]: No go ahead because I think I know what you're going to ask, and so I'd rather respond.

Brendan [1:59:08]: Okay. First of all, were you saying that we need to have a sufficiently acid environment for B12 synthesis or that we need an environment …

Robert [1:59:17]: Yes.

Brendan [1:59:18]: Okay so it needs to be sufficiently … and certainly that's the case for assimilation and so, so that part makes sense as far as assimilation. I think we're all agreed that B12 assimilation requires an acid environment, but if B12 synthesis also requires an acid environment but he's saying that B12 synthesis occurs further down than the acidic region where absorption occurs then that would seem to suggest that he's saying B12 synthesis occurs in a less acidic environment because everything south of the stomach is less acidic. Basically, it goes from somewhere between let's say 1.5 and 3.5 in the stomach or even lower than the 1.5 during active strong digestion, down to you know maybe 8, I think? It gets a bit more alkaline in the small intestine, and then it goes more slightly more acidic or more kind of neutral in the large intestine, maybe around 7 or 6, is that correct? And where are you saying, and at what pH range, would you say, are you saying, the bacterial synthesis of B12 would occur?

Robert [2:00:33]: Well, I couldn't answer that directly. All's I know that just from what I read you know the acidic environment and how that environment was disrupted by different drugs. That's my main source.
Brendan [2:00:51]: Certainly, that's going to interfere with assimilation. I'm just wondering how B12 gets into a vegan's body in a world where we have super nutrient dense plant foods, what's the source of the B12 going to be? Obviously, the source of the cobalt is there if you have plants that are delivering a lot of cobalt, but what's going to be … what and where is that B12 being generated? That's essentially my question.

Robert [2:01:18]: The B12 is being generated in, when the cobalt makes it into the stomach in the proper acid environment, then the carbon and nitrogen from the food will bond to that cobalt, and that is a molecule or the vitamin B12.

Brendan [2:01:40]: So you're saying it won't even require bacterial synthesis? Are you saying that with adequate nutrients and with adequate acidity in the stomach that B12 will synthesis will occur just naturally. It'll occur.

Robert [2:01:56]: That's the way it was always intended to occur.

Brendan [2:02:01]: Is there science indicating that that actually does happen, with a certain pH and a certain concentration of the substrates of carbon, nitrogen and cobalt.

Robert [2:02:10]: You know, where I first was introduced to it was Dr. Olree's book

Brendan [2:02:14]: Okay.

Robert [2:02:16]: That's the only source that I could tell you, but I wouldn't have any reason to believe that …

Brendan [2:02:23]: I'm going to check that out because that's ground-breaking … that's game-changing, and there may be other examples of it in the sense that maybe we've been fed a misperception or an intentional lie, I don't know, because I do sometimes suspect politicization of some of the nutritional dogma and doctrines. And maybe one of them is "B12 only occurs in animal foods and from bacterial synthesis." But if that's not true, and something else is occurring either because we didn't know, or only Dr. Olree and very few others had known it, that would be really quite interesting to say the least. Is that if we literally can get … if you're saying that Dr. Olree asserts, and he's no slouch, that this just happens … you will get vitamin B12 in a stomach that's sufficiently acidic and has sufficient concentration of the element nutrients.

Robert [2:03:32]: Yeah, if you have the proper mineral building blocks and that's, that was his whole *Minerals for the Genetic Code* and how he looked at, how the different balances of these different minerals and how they interact and how they are utilized. The only difference between Dr. Olree's beliefs and mine are he believes that all plants have sufficient minerals. And when he looks to Dr. Dukes database he only takes the high number not the low and says well if you need selenium eat Brazil nuts. Well Brazil nuts … it all depends where you buy them from.

Brendan [2:04:23]: Yeah. Given that slight blind spot that he has, I would really want to parse out and maybe I'll just contact him.

Robert [2:04:35]: I'll send you his phone number.

Brendan [2:04:37]: Yeah I want to ask him, so are you saying this and you know that carbon plus nitrogen plus cobalt plus sufficient acidity in the stomach yield vitamin B12 without bacteria or, does it mean you're going to have particular types of acid-loving bacteria in your stomach and then maybe it becomes an issue of well a lot of us have had our microbiomes destroyed and one of the areas that a microbiome can exist is the stomach, but maybe just as in large intestines our microbiomes of our stomachs may also be destroyed to certain degree.

Robert [2:05:21]: Well, he's the same reason why I have yttrium in my memory formulas is his book and the way it described the extra … yttrium is one of longevity minerals, but because it's not in our diet we age twice as fast … not that we can live twice as long on it … we're aging twice as fast because we're lacking it, and our body has to go through synthesis to compensate for the lack of that mineral in our body. And what that mineral basically does is feed microbes, our gut, probiotics in our gut, to be able to metabolize things in a different way that doesn't happen if we don't have it in our system.

Brendan [2:06:23]: Wow.

Robert [2:06:25]: His work is fascinating, and some of it is way over my head. He is on my advisory board, although he hasn't showed up to the meeting in six months. We just do internet conference calls, but I think he's a little bit turned off by the fact that I just don't buy into the Organic certifications as much as he does. And he definitely is at war with glyphosate. And then he doesn't like making himself a target on the cancer because he is Amish, and he works with the Amish community heavily, and he's watched the Amish get put into prison for making some elixir juice or whatever they've made for years. But they started selling it, and the FDA came after him and put this guy in prison.

Brendan [2:07:26]: Oh wow. What is the nature of Dr. Olree's research and his credentials and experience. Is he an agronomist? Was he with USDA? Is he a chemist?

Robert [2:07:40]: He's actually a chiropractor. He was very good friends with Charles Walters from Acres USA. They met at a conference and hit it off. And Dr. Olree's work with the periodic table and the human body is what he developed, showing how it's not just these minerals; it's the valence of the minerals that are important for the different functions. And in his book *Minerals for the Genetic Code*—which Charles Walter produced, but it's based upon his work—Doctor Olree had produced a biological periodic chart.

Brendan [2:08:38]: Did he actually do original research, and was it published, or was it just his own research that he did with plants and documented to some degree? Just curious did he have original research or was he digging in other older texts and basically piecing things together and then forming theories around it and maybe ...

Robert [2:09:04]: I guess some ... oh I didn't realize this until you asked that question ... the Olree biological periodic chart ... Walter Russell from 1926 was the one that that they have copyrighted permission to use. So, apparently this is Walter Russell's work, the original one. Then what Dr. Olree had done was break out each mineral and show how its function works and how many times you find it in the DNA. He has a certain twist to it, and a lot of that is based upon the chiropractic handbooks which I don't understand or get into. And then that's the location of the spinal segments he has written on there. But what I mainly look at, when I'm reading the book, is the proper balance in how it interacts with the different amino acids, and how it interacts with the absorbability of other minerals. That's why when I do a mineral package it's not just addressing the deficiencies with diabetes it's also addressing how our body can utilize those minerals in the other building blocks for absorbability, if that makes sense.

Brendan [2:10:47]: I think I'd have to read the book.

Robert [2:10:52]: Yeah, yeah. I've got your address, so I'll send you a copy of the book.

Brendan [2:10:55]: I'm gonna have to have somebody reading into an audio book I have no time to like read extra things. So I'm going to figure out a solution where every book that only exists in text form is somehow going to get ... I suppose it's probably real obvious solution. There's probably some software that will read it into a voice, and you choose female or male British Australian or US accent or something like that. It's got to exist, and I'll find it.

Robert [2:11:20]: What I would do is just give you the books that I have all my tabs in and just read the tab.

Brendan [2:11:25]: Oh, okay.

Robert [2:11:28]: Because I've got that around, but you know this book I had that around for almost a year and because I pick it up and just too hard to wrap my head around it. And then finally I found that one chapter where it was just five pages, read that, and then I understood the whole thing, but you don't hit that chapter until page 176 to 181. Then after that it all clicked. But it's an interesting book because it's Olree's work, but most of it is Charles Walters editing and walking you through why Walters found it intriguing.

Brendan [2:12:14]: Right. Okay. You know I look forward to that, and gosh we've been talking for well over two hours. I should let you go, and I've got an interview coming up later I got to get prepared for I suppose this suffices perhaps as our second interview, right? I mean we went deep and wide. This has been fantastic maybe just to sort of wrap this up, summarize for anybody listening to this ... so maybe you can summarize for us what are the various ways that people can interface with your company or companies and what they would get from that. What are the entry points and what are the pathways they can go with your products and so forth.

Robert [2:12:58]: I think the easiest way to identify whether or not we have products that would assist somebody's either health condition or symptoms associated with the deficiencies ... to go through a Google search on minerals associated with his specific symptom, say Parkinson's, just minerals associated with Parkinson's disease, or mineral deficiencies associated. Validate that that is a deficiency, and then we have most of the 23 minerals identified through bioavailable form we can see through plant uptake in our products.

Brendan [2:13:46]: And these are soil amendment products not human supplements, right? These are things you add to the soil, and then they become available in the plants.

Robert [2:13:55]: Yep. Our soil solutions will allow you to grow your own mineral supplements naturally through food, and that's kind of our slogan. We also grow foods and sell them. Our wheatgrass formulas are grown in the same soils, and they're marketed to a company called Naturally Noble, which for a lot of people that don't go gardens or their symptoms are so severe that they want to see if a whole foods mineral supplement can address the deficiencies in a faster rate, we have those available also.

Brendan [2:14:35]: So you're saying you do have food supplements as well?

Robert [2:14:39]: Yes, we do, but there are a hundred percent whole foods they're not supplements in the same way that the FDA would look at them

Brendan [2:14:46]: Exactly. I got to check that for. I don't know if I had fully realized that. So I've got to check into that because I believe there are many people who are in situations like you said where they're not going to be able to realistically grow their own food right now, and they need a fast solution. And many of us are just plain busy even if we could grow our own stuff because we're well enough and we have a garden or patch of ground or something. But I'm one that avails myself of various types of supplements. I do have a food based one, a zinc, it seems to work quite well, and so I'm looking forward to checking out yours as well because obviously ... and these are, these supplements are pretty much essentially food-based multis—is that right—for different purposes memory, immune system, liver health, or something like that where basically they're going to have a variety of nutrients. Go ahead.

Robert [2:15:43]: If you go to the products page which our ecommerce site is—Heaven Hope natural products—if you go to the product page on that you will actually see the testing and the comparative testing.

There's even some links to the Dr. Duke's database on those on the drop-down menus. The problem is when most people find a need for the deficiencies they already have the symptom. They're in a hurry to overcome the deficiency.

Brendan [2:16:20]: Yeah.

Robert [2:16:21]: And I think a proper balance of maintaining a garden is still the right way to go.

Brendan [2:16:28]: Yeah, and do your food based supplements actually indicate the quantities available? So for example, they'll know how much lithium, how much gold, how much the yttrium, whatever's in there, how much magnesium, zinc, coppers they got.

Robert [2:16:48]: On our nutritional panel the mineral content and the nutritional panel does reflect the actual testing that we're seeing. And if it doesn't have … let's say … one of the products that we harvest but we don't grow in our soils but the roots go down so deep is the bind weed. Our entire lab analyticals, all sixty some elements, are on the drop-down menus. So let's say for example somebody says, "Well I'm looking for something high in germanium," which we don't have a germanium product that we're marketing, just as a high food level. But they can see the different products we have and see which products have the highest germanium level. It's more versatile than just what we're marketing for. We market our GTF formula as a blood glucose formula, but if you were to look at mineral deficiency formulas you'll see that the chromium levels in vanadium are actually an energy formula, but we don't market it to that because we're marketing to assist people with mineral deficiencies that are associated with symptoms. And all's we can say is we're addressing the deficiencies. We're not treating a symptom. We're hoping that the symptoms of subsides because the deficiency's addressed.

Brendan [2:18:19]: Right.

Robert [2:18:20]: If that makes sense.

Brendan [2:18:22]: Totally. Ok great. Well, I can't wait to try some of your products. And so, NaturallyNoble.com is where people get the food source food-based human supplements. And then what's the place where they go to get the soil amendments? Is that a separate site, or Heavens Help, is that what it was?

Robert [2:18:47]: Naturally Noble will bring you to Heavens Hope. On the Heavens Hope page you'll see those soil supplements. The soil supplements by themselves are on WesternEnvironmentalServices.com, all one word. That will get you to the soil page. You'll see all of our testing and everything else is on that. The most information is on Heaven's Hope nutritional products.

Brendan [2:19:15]: Okay great. Fantastic. Again, thank you very much for all this information, all your dedication. Gosh, I can't wait for more people to get this stuff. Hardly anybody knows about this. Hardly anybody knows about you. And that's got to change. The human body has so much more potential. That's what I'm present to right now is just realizing if we start getting all this stuff right we're going to go to an entirely different level of access to, as Dan Kittredge refers to it, "our higher nature", and that's going to reverberate throughout so many things and obviously just happiness and joy, and so forth, but also creativity, connection with our source, and athletic performance I think can go to a different level. So looking forward to the coming Golden Age basically!

Robert [2:20:25]: Yeah absolutely.

Brendan [2:20:27]: Okay, all right, I'll talk to you later.

Robert [2:20:31]: All right have a great day.

Brendan [2:20:32]: Thank you, you too, God bless.

Nora Gedgaudas Interview 2
Essential Fat-Soluble Vitamins, Cholesterol, Trans-Esterified Fats, and Heart Disease

Brendan [00:00:01]: Welcome to the Eat4Earth event. This is Brendan Moorehead, and together we're exploring how food can heal you, your loved ones, and the planet. Our next guest, Nora Gedgaudas, as is a widely recognized expert on what is popularly referred to as the Paleo Diet. She is the author of the international best-selling book *Primal Body, Primal Mind: Beyond the Paleo Diet for Total Health* and Longer Life. She's also the author of the bestselling ebook, *Rethinking Fatigue: What Your Adrenals are Really Telling You and What You Can Do About It*, or latest book, *Primal Fat Burner: Live Longer, Slow Aging, Super-Power Your Brain, and Save Your Life where the High-Fat, Low-Carb Paleo Diet* is now one of my most recent favorite books. Nora is an experienced board-certified nutritional consultant and clinical neuro-feedback specialist, speaker and educator, widely interviewed on national and international radio, popular podcasts, online summits, television and film. Nora, it's so great to have you here. Thank you for all that you bring to this movement and to the health of humanity.

Nora [00:01:07]: Thank you, Brendan. It's, it's very much an honor to be here and I, you know, I'm, I'm very grateful for that, very generous introduction. Your check's in the mail [laughing].

Brendan [00:01:18]: Nora, you know, you and I have had a couple of in-depth conversations and in our past conversation, you and I spoke about diet, the dietary influences on human evolution and the role that animal fats, especially DHA and arachidonic acid and so forth, played in the evolution of our brains and the importance of fat soluble vitamins that either exist only in animal foods for are very difficult to gain in a sufficient quantities from plant foods. And, whenever the topic of animal foods are discussed, it seems like there's also a question about whether their saturated fat and cholesterol are healthy, but I think for the moment that topic has been sufficiently addressed in this event and will continue to be perhaps by additional speakers. So we'll table that one for the moment. And we're probably regardless, never all gonna agree on whether humans should eat animals and so forth.

Brendan [00:02:15]: But all of us definitely need to pay attention to fat soluble vitamins, however we obtained them. So let's dive into that a little bit so that people of all, dietary persuasions can better understand just how important these are. and then they can choose how they're going to obtain them, whether from animal sources, plant sources, or supplements. So, in terms of Vitamins D3, K2, E, and A, and maybe something I'm forgetting, of course there's many forms of K2, why are these so important as nutrients, and what do they do for us? It's a long question to unpack, so I apologize for dumping a big one on you.

Nora [00:02:55]: Well, you can't really exactly lump them altogether into doing the same thing. Individual nutrients have a variety of, of actions in the human body, but the ones that we typically make the most important use of in the most essential, uh, that are the most essential, I think for, for human health are the sources of these fat-soluble nutrients that are found in animal source foods. For instance, vitamin A, a lot of people think it's synonymous with beta carotene. It isn't. Beta carotene is a carotenoid. It is a pro vitamin, a substance that requires quite a complex process of conversion and anywhere from six to 20 units of beta carotene are needed in order to produce a single unit of retinol, which is true Vitamin A. True vitamin A, retinol, can only be gotten, only be gotten from animal source foods. It's richest of course in things like liver, but it is absolutely critical for the health of your immune system.

Nora [00:04:10]: In fact, prior to the discovery of antibiotics and that sort of thing, vitamin A was the focus, the focus of anti-infective therapy. That your vitamin A status is good, your immune function is going to be a gosh darn sight better. You need it for the health of your lungs, for the health of your brain, for the health of so many things. It does tend to be stored in its richest amounts in the liver. With respect to beta carotene, there is a very complex process that needs to take place in order to try to manufacture vitamin A, and it is a laborious process, and it's one that requires that your thyroid be working perfectly, your liver be working perfectly, and a whole plethora of nutrients need to be kind of in place and the whole process in order for that whole process to occur at all.

Nora [00:05:15]: And there's no possible way that you could actually meet your true Vitamin A requirements using beta carotene, even under optimal circumstances. And young kids can't make those conversions at all by the way. They really do need.

Brendan [00:05:30]: Oh, really? Is there a certain age before which they don't have certain enzymes?

Nora [00:05:35]: Yeah, at around age six or so they start being able to do that a little bit more. But prior to that, they're fully dependent on the formed versions of this. We're designed to consume an animal source food diet. We have a hydrochloric acid digestive system for that very purpose. And we have an ample gallbladder for that very purpose. And if you know a Vitamin K2 … Vitamin K1, which is found in plant-based foods, mainly is involved with blood clotting, and it has limited range of roles that it plays. It doesn't store very well.

Nora [00:06:19]: And the form of Vitamin K2 that has that has far and away much more important role to play is the form that is found in animal source foods. Now some people are going to say, "Well, no, it comes from from bacteria too." Yes, there are certain fermented foods in which a certain form of vitamin K2 to known as MK7 that … and of course it's the darling of the supplement industry right now because that's the cheapest way for the supplement industry to give us Vitamin K2 supplements. But the form that we evolved consuming, and the only form that's actually found in the brain at all, is the MK4 form of vitamin K2, which is exclusively found in animal source foods where the animals have been fed upon nothing but pasture, nothing but natural forage. In other words, if you're eating feed lot meat, which nobody should be doing, then chances are you're probably not getting any. It really takes a lot of fresh pasture and forage and that sort of a thing to help ruminant animals synthesize a K2 in the form that we are designed to consume it. And I know that there are arguments that, "Well, we produce a certain amount of K2 in our colons." Well, our colon makes up maybe 20 percent of our digestive tract as opposed to even our closest primate relatives, the chimpanzee which has … the fermentative portion of the chimps gut makes up about 52 percent of its system. That's a big fermentation vat. We don't have that big a fermentation vat. And the bacterial synthesis that occurs in the colon, where the bacteria are synthesizing things like K2 and B12, whatever. They're synthesizing those nutrients for themselves. They're not sharing with us. We really have to get that directly from our diet if we want it in amounts, that's actually better actually going to make any kind of measurable difference in your health at all. And with Vitamin K2 works together. Oh, it has a huge role, a variety of roles to play with respect to controlling inflammation. And it has functions in the brain, functions with your heart, all of these things. But it also is designed to work very closely with Vitamin D3. Vitamin D3 within the food supply can only be gotten from animal source foods. Now there are plant-based sources of vitamin D that has to be converted through the action of sunlight into the form of Vitamin D3, cholecalciferol, that your body actually uses.

Nora [00:09:32]: And the problem is that if you wear clothing, you live in a more northerly, northern latitude for instance, where they just don't get a whole lot of (light) right now. We just have, we're supposed to be at peak sunlight today, and it's still kind of dark out. You certainly wouldn't want to take my (sic) clothes off out there because I'd catch a chill. It's freezing cold temperatures, and where our ice age ancestors got their Vitamin D3 was from eating fat from animal source foods. And the richest natural source, actually a Vitamin D3 ironically is in fully pastured pork, which admittedly is hard to come by, but it's out there to be gotten. You can go places like EatWild.com and what have you. And try to find farmers actually producing pork. That is, that is fully pastured and in not feedlot fed.

Brendan [00:10:44]: Does that mean that if they're fully pastured, they're not getting any grain supplement, supplemental feeding? Are they just eating hazelnuts …

Nora [00:10:54]: It is so hard to find. Even the pastured producers that don't do any grains, but the good ones make it fully supplemental and not a part of, not a major part of, their daily diet. And will let the pigs out into the field. They get food scraps from wherever they get. They get to nosh on whatever is out there. Pigs will eat just about anything. And yeah, eating acorns and eating nuts or whatever that they're given as forage. I do know one pork producer that, a farm that's not far from me, that exclusively feeds their hogs basically food stuffs and, and they don't include any grains at all. There are no grains at all. Then I feel very fortunate to have him close by. But yeah, you have to do your homework.

Nora [00:11:49]: That's the thing. And nowadays it's increasingly hard for us to find real food. And particularly if you're relying on what you can buy at the grocery stores, you're going to be … you're going to be compromised. There's no way not to be compromised through grocery store foods, even the food stores that supposedly specialize in completely natural organic kinds of foods. We have to realize that the way the industry works is designed to favor the industry itself more than us, that if we're demanding organic foods, well, in order for industry to profit off of that demand, they find ways of manipulating the laws to broaden the definition of what it means to be organic. They just incorporated hydroponics into that which is, which is not supposed to be part of the legal definition of organics. But it brings a whole other range of, of manufacturers into the organic fold, charging organic prices. Organics is supposed to be based on soil. And it's supposed to be based on improving the quality of the soil, which hydroponics don't do at all. And you get a much more sophisticated array of nutrients from anything grown in soil than you ever could with hydroponics. But, but there we have it. Again, we're being told a lot of what we want to hear, and that is driving a lot of what goes on in the stores. But we shouldn't confuse that with industry giving us what we want. Industry is going to give us what is most profitable for industry to give us, and they will tell us anything to get us to buy it. So we have to be savvy. We have to be savvy consumers. We have to learn how to ask a lot of good questions, which I try to when I go to meat markets and things like that.

Nora [00:13:58]: I try as much as possible to have a firsthand knowing of where my food comes from. And whether it is through friends that have gone hunting where I've been able to kind of know, get some elk and get some good stuff that way … or I guess a person fishing in clean water, but that's a dubious prospect nowadays … or growing your own or raising your own or going to farmers markets and getting to know the farmers. Taking field trips out to the farms and taking a firsthand look at how those animals are being raised and how the food is being raised, developing that first knowing is the best defense we have against industry-sponsored degradation of our food supply. I don't know how else to put it. We've got to be on top of it. If we're going to be passive about it, good luck with what you get.

Brendan [00:15:00]: So are there any … you mentioned that industry, at least industrialized … there's chemical, industrial agriculture, and then there's industrialized organic. Are there any producers that you do trust for … obviously you trust the farmer you met locally … ultimately, as another speaker here says … this is Reginaldo Haslett-Marroquin … and he says …

Nora (00:15:31): That just rolls right off the tongue. Doesn't it? Almost as good as my name. [laughing]

Brendan (00:15:37): So he says that, ultimately how we know something is regenerative is we buy locally, and we go and check things out. And so the future of food is largely, I think decentralized and transparent and connected to the community, and there's so much joy in that you can't get from the supermarket and so much more nutrition. As long as the producers are doing what will produce the most nutritious food and just so happens that that often produces a greater bounty and greater profit margins for them and so forth. But I'm curious, are there any particular brands you trust that we would find in a store?

Nora [00:16:20]: Oh, that's a good question.

Brendan (00:16:22): I think you've mentioned Fat Works before.

Nora [00:16:24]: I have mentioned that. That was going to roll right off my tongue David Cole and his wife Mieke have gone to great pains to try to do the right things in the right way for the right reasons. And I enjoy giving my money to people who are working hard on my behalf to do the right thing. And, and of course they have to make a profit too, which means in the case of that product, you're going to pay a little more than you will for certain competing product, but you're not getting anywhere near the same thing. And, there's a product line out there, and I won't name names, although I'm tempted to because they tick me off so much, that have engaged in predatory marketing practices and have attempted to create a very similar product. They're attempting to mimic the same product, but of course they're charging less money for it. Let's just say that I wouldn't trust it.

Brendan [00:17:27]: One the benefits that I heard you calling attention to in your book … where if you can get fully pastured pork lard that's a good vitamin D source … is probably very counter-intuitive for a lot of people thinking … even those of us who accept that now that saturated fat, animal fat … well, animal fat is not pure saturated fat … but there's so much confusion in the research that vilified fat, and many of us still have this legacy load of distrust of animal fats, let's say, and rightfully so when it comes from the factory farm system where it just gets bastardized and toxin-laden and so forth … but I'm curious with the pork lard … and I have to have an aside here .. I saw on a rancher's farmhouse it had this a 50s era or 40s era poster of a happy family, and it literally said, and I think this is authentic, I don't know for sure … "They're happy because they eat lard." Isn't that funny?

Nora [00:18:45]: Yeah, up until the early 1900s. I mean, that's what everybody cooked with was lard and butter …

Brendan [00:18:53]: (and very little) cancer and heart attacks.

Nora [00:18:55]: … and long before what we call the diseases of modern civilization became such a prevailing concern, prior to that we see more animal source foods. We consumed more animal source foods. We consumed more saturated fat. Actually we're consuming less saturated fat than ever. And, you know, rates of heart disease are not going down, but we are eating a diet that is predominated by carbohydrates and also refined vegetable oils that are either partially hydrogenated, a super highly processed, interesterified, which is what is replacing the hydrogenation process. You see something that says "Trans Fat Free" on the label of a tub of what's obviously margarine, what they're not telling you is that they have swapped out the trans-fat process because that's fallen out of favor now. And the laws are going to make the majority of those foods go away this next year, and they're replacing it with an old standby called interesterification, which leads to a product that is just as bad for you, if not worse than trans fats. But the labeling laws are such that they're not required to disclose it on the label.

Brendan [00:20:15]: So yeah, we're going to have another food movement just to label …

Nora [00:20:19]: Well, that's the thing. we were crawling through broken glass on our arms or elbows and whatever struggling to try to make these changes to the food supply. We fought against the trans fats. We finally, supposedly won. Everybody's slapping themselves on the back and patting themselves on the back for that, and industry just turns around and finds another way of doing it. And again, the laws favor industry. They learned their lesson with trans fats. The way the laws are set up now, they're not forced to label inter-esterified fats. Most palm oil by the way is inter-esterified, but they do this with a lot of other fats too. And it's a way of improving shelf life by, by transforming some of the fatty acids that are likely to rancidify, usually the omega three fats on the plant-based omega three fatty acids, which don't do us much good anyway, and they go rancid really, really fast once they're out of the seed or the nut or whatever. But in any case, if you pick up a box of microwave popping corn, you might see zero trans-fat on the label. But if you look at the actual ingredients, if you actually take the next step because you're like, oh, well, you're feeling good. "Hey, no trans-fat in this. Great." But if you look at the ingredient list, you see partially hydrogenated soybean oil or canola oil, all of which is partially hydrogenated or inter-esterified as part of it's the deodorization process. Right now, the number one source of fat calories in the United States is partially hydrogenated soybean oil.

Brendan [00:22:06]: Yeah, there can be, there really should be no mystery about the epidemic of disease. That right there is a big part.

Nora [00:22:08]: Then number one, source of actual calories is like high-fructose corn syrup. Yeah. Is it any wonder that we're in trouble?

Brendan [00:22:14]: I think obviously the bottom line is ... the shortcut to having good food and keeping it simple is just to keep it simple. Just whole foods. You don't need to learn how to read every label necessarily because you shouldn't be eating out of boxes and plastic. If you're doing that, there's no way that is ever going to not have some adulterated ingredients. [inaudible] decay. I mean that's just the bottom line. Now, in terms of fats, I wanted to also ask you about duck fat because that was something that I hadn't ever thought of and it was

Nora [00:22:50]: You haven't lived. [laughing]

Brendan [00:22:52]: Yeah, I guess it's been so long since I've actually had pork lard actually because I used to cook bacon and then cooked my eggs in it ... this is from when I was a kid. I loved that and I haven't gotten back to it yet. And now I'm actually thinking, well, hey, you know I eat eggs. I always loved pork. I'm going to find me a great local producer, but in the meantime at least I can go out and try some of the Fat Works pork lard or duck fat. Tell us about duck fat. What are the distinctions with regard to that fat?

Nora [00:23:25]: Well, duck fat, poultry fat contains, I believe it's myristic acid. It has some anti microbial, some marvelous antimicrobial properties. We've heard of schmaltz, of course, chicken fat, and how people call chicken soup Jewish penicillin. It has to do with the fat. If you have fat free chicken broth, you're not going to get the Jewish penicillin ineffective. Poultry fats have higher amounts of anti-microbial fatty acids in them, which can be helpful to support your immune system. They're also, they also do tend to be a bit higher in monounsaturates and more polyunsaturated fats, which means you've got to just take really good care when you cook with them that you don't cook over low to low medium heat. I don't cook anything in a temperature other than boiling water ...

Brendan [00:24:26]: What about pressure cooking?

Nora [00:24:27]: ... more than about 260 degrees. Yeah, I think pressure cooking is a way of seemingly preserving nutrients. Everybody has those, what are they called, the instant pots now?

Brendan [00:24:40]: Yeah, mine is a little bit old school. It's not electric, but it's ...

Nora [00:24:43]: Yeah, I hear ya. I don't do a lot of that kind of cooking. I'm either using a rotisserie, the oven, or the stove for the most part.

Brendan [00:24:55]: I like to use a pressure cooker for bone broth. If I get some backs, necks, and feet or something, which is kind of hard to find. I have to order it online maybe to get it or find a local producer to get it from a great source. But then it's, oh my God, the best bone broth.

Nora [00:25:10]: Yeah, yeah, yeah, for sure. So yeah, there, there are a variety of … Yeah. So. Oh, duck fat. OK. I will tell you that duck fat is probably what I use more than anything else, mainly because it tastes so amazing and it makes everything you cook it in taste absolutely amazing. My favorite, favorite fat is goose fat, but that's also the hardest to come by. Fat Works makes that one available to some degree, but it's expensive.

Brendan [00:25:48]: Yeah, I saw one of their labels that said wild boar fat, and there was something unique about it. I don't recall what it was. I think it had a pretty decent concentration of a long chain of essential fatty acids. So, you know, EPA, I don't recall if it mentioned DHA, but 400 and something milligrams per something.

Nora [00:26:12]: Yeah. So you know, again, when you're talking about wild boar fat, yeah, you're talking about a superior form. If you want to get something that's fully pastured that's it.

Brendan [00:26:20]: Of course you get all the Vitamin D with it too because it's a …

Nora [00:26:23]: Right, you have an animal that, see pigs basically have, they don't have as much fur as a lot of other animals. And so because they have a lot of skin like we do when they go out into the sun, they produce Vitamin D just like we would being out in the sun. And if they're living out in fresh air and sunshine, and they're allowed to kind of naturally forage for the majority of what they eat, then it allows them to synthesize a lot of Vitamin D. And so Vitamin D is not stored in the liver. You know, people think of cod liver oil, which is actually a rather poor source of Vitamin D naturally.

Brendan [00:27:08]: It's more for Vitamin A, right?

Nora [00:27:09]: It's, yeah, it's mainly a Vitamin A source. There's a smidgen of omega threes in with it, and frankly most of the processing methods associated with fish oils lately … I wouldn't touch fermented fish oil with a 10-foot pole if you paid me. I refuse to have anything to do with it. It's really all rancid frankly. But even non-fermented fish oils and cod liver oils and things like that are … the processing methods are a little bit questionable, distillation. Also the sources of the fish are questionable.

Brendan [00:27:46]: Yeah, they have to do this kind of molecular distillation because otherwise they're going to carry this heavy metal burden, I suppose, right? I think we need to look at the the impact on the marine ecosystems that are already so stretched and so if we're going to like go out and eat fish oil, the catch and the by-catch where you're catching all these other larger fish and animals while you're going through the target species is tragic. Devastating.

Nora [00:28:18]: Right. Just this whole seafood thing you could do a whole podcast just on that. It's a sketchy subject. And um, I actually … go ahead.

Brendan [00:28:30]: And to have just a quick reference point, one of the other speakers in this event, I believe it was Reese Halter, who's, he's got his finger on the pulse of the ocean, the trees, the bees, everything, trees, bees and seas.

Nora [00:28:42]: That's a tiny little pulse on those bees. [laughing]

Brendan [00:28:47]: [laughing] He … it was either him or somebody else said that recently in the last 10 years, the sardine stocks on the Pacific coast of the United States are down like 85 percent. And that's just one example.

Nora [00:28:59]: And there could be a lot of different reasons for that. It may not be all due to overfishing, you know, we know that what happened at Fukushima meltdown.

Brendan [00:29:08]: And there's also the warming of the ocean. There's acidification affecting the whole food chain, the increasing acidification.

Nora [00:29:17]: Lots of going on that are compromising these. I haven't consumed anything out of the Pacific Ocean or the Gulf of Mexico or the Atlantic Ocean since 2011.

Brendan [00:29:27]: In any case, I think where we were going is that we've got animal sources, terrestrial sources, that may be safer, less expensive, and they don't need to be molecularly distilled and stretch these marine populations.

Nora [00:29:43]: There is one source of supplemental fish oil of that isn't molecularly distilled. It's the only one I'm still inclined to recommend if somebody really wants to take fish oil. But it's made by a healthcare practitioner company called Biotics Research. And what they do is they obtain their own raw materials, and it's from tiny little sardine like fish swimming in relatively cleaner waters in the southern hemisphere off the coast of Chile. The southern hemisphere is starting to be affected now by Fukushima too, so that's going to be a dicey thing in the years to come. But what they do is they bring those fish in and then they obtain the oil and then they test that raw. They test that oil for the presence of any contaminants at all. They don't molecularly distill it. They just basically get the stuff from the cleanest possible water. They test to make sure that it's not contaminated with PCBs and the mercury and whatever else. And it's sold as, I think it's called there Biomega-3 product. If somebody wants fish oil

Brendan [00:31:00]: Biomega-3? How do we know it's being sustainably sourced?

Nora [00:31:05]: Again, they're getting the oils from these tiny little sardine like fish, right? Things that are low on the food chain. And so they're going about it that way.

Brendan [00:31:16]: I think there's still questions about how we net it and so forth, and whether the by-catch is known.

Nora [00:31:26]: I don't actually take fish oil anymore, and you know …

Brendan [00:31:30]: I haven't taken any in a while either. That's why I'm happy to hear more from your content about the benefits of regenerative really raised land-based animals because there's really very little limits. In fact, we need to raise more of those to regenerate the dead grasslands around the world, and so we can actually restore the planet and produce more healthy essential fatty acid sources, and sources of fat-soluble vitamins for animal (unintelligible) people, but …

Nora [00:32:08]: It's primarily where our prehistoric ancestors got their omega-3's was from the meat and the fat of the animals that, the land animals, that they hunted.

Brendan [00:32:16]: Well, let's say I'm a vegetarian or vegan. What choices do you envision for me? I mean, I'll mention a few that I'm aware of and what are the pros and cons? I mean, let's just say I'm committed. I'm not going to eat animals. Where can I get? So I'm aware of, uh, there's algae that has DHA in it.

Nora [00:32:36]: Fairly questionable.

Brendan [00:32:38]: Hopefully my liver converts a lot of ALA, Alpha-linolenic acid that we can get from flax oil and hope that I have a way higher than average conversion ratio to get enough EPA out of that. Eicosapentaenoic acid.

Nora [00:32:52]: The best you could hope for is a six percent conversion ratio, conversion.

Brendan [00:32:58]: What about the idea that if you know, maybe that number came out of research where people are unhealthy livers. I mean, if there was an average population …

Nora [00:33:07]: Well, that's just it. There are so many things that are required for that conversion process to take place. But if you are a northern European descent or you are of, of Celtic or native descent, you can't make that conversion at all. Doesn't matter how healthy our livers are. There is an enzyme called Delta-6 desaturates that's required for the first step of that conversion process. And people that fit the ethnic criteria I just gave don't have that enzyme at all. So they can't make those conversions. They're absolutely dependent on animal source foods in order to obtain these essential fatty acids. Now, there is the algae form of DHA. Of course, there's no EPA in with that. And you know, algae is not traditionally a food source for humans, right? And you have to question the sourcing. You also have to question the processing methods because very often there are there are harsh chemicals that are used in those extraction methods.

Nora [00:34:15]: And there's a whole lot of controversy around that sort of algae based DHA. It's an alternative. I'm not sure it's the best one. It's certainly not a better one. Animal source foods are far and away the best and most reliable source … well, animal source food from animals that have been feeding on nothing but fresh green forage, right? Have been allowed to live in fresh air and sunshine and eat what's natural for them to eat. They're far and away the most reliable source of EPA and DHA. There are lots and lots of, you know, yes, your liver has to be functioning in a pristine way. Your thyroid has to be functioning in a pristine way for these conversions to occur, and it's a complex elongation process. There are many, many, many steps leading to EPA and DHA. On paper it looks like, "Oh look, well look, there's a chemical process that allows for that conversion."

Nora [00:35:20]: In reality, it happens poorly if at all, in almost anyone. And if somebody isn't from the ethnic backgrounds I mentioned, and their liver and their thyroid are aces, which if you're vegan good luck with that after a while, then ultimately you're going to be lucky to be able to convert maybe up to six percent of that ALA, that parent form of plant based in omega-3, and they won't make DHA at all.

Brendan [00:36:00]: Yeah, I was taking a product, probably created for vegetarians. I tried several of them where it was a combination of flax and some other things. Maybe fortunately they had something in there like a rosemary extract that seemed to control the oxidation. That didn't seem at all rancid. It had some algae oil and so forth. I did notice an improvement in my skin and my mood. One thing I think is with that will you actually ended up taking more of it and then so maybe you got a lower conversion ratio, but I think it was having a noticeable impact. It wasn't entirely trivial when added up the numbers and like, OK yeah, I am taking a large amount of that, so if I only convert five percent it still roughly was adding up to maybe a fish oil capsule a day or something like that.

Nora [00:36:45]: The human body will use ALA too, but guess what you can get every fatty acid that your body requires can be gotten from these animal source foods, and it's present in their insufficient quantities to meet the needs. There's nothing present in those plant-based foods that is essential for, for human health, and the problem is that the polyunsaturated levels are so high.

Brendan [00:37:10]: Yeah, that's where we had to balance it. It's gotta be one of these balanced oils like Udos or Seven Source.

Nora [00:37:14]: Yeah, but it's not balanced because it's still ... I mean they have some monounsaturates and things like that. Look, nobody has an essential requirement for these omega-9s or whatever, and oleic acid. I mean it's, you know, it's not how great for you it is. It's how bad for you it isn't right? But, but the thing is, is that you're getting the majority of what you're getting in those vegetable things are polyunsaturated at best mono and some mono unsaturated, mostly poly-unsaturated, which it isn't just about the rate of oxidation that those promote, which you're there are much more likely to get rapidly oxidized in your body. You have to realize 80 percent of what clogs arteries isn't saturated fat or cholesterol at all. The vast majority of what actually comprises those plaques are oxidized unsaturated fats.

Brendan [00:38:07]: Really?!

Nora [00:38:08]: Yep. You don't see ... If you do fried foods, and you're frying your saturated fats at high temperatures and you know, you're getting oxidized cholesterol from that and whatever else they are from like age meats and stuff. Oxidized anything isn't good for anyone. But in terms of naturally occurring saturated fat in animal source foods and cholesterol, that's not what clogging people's arteries. And I have a peer reviewed study were plaques were analyzed, and there really wasn't any evidence of saturated fat and cholesterol causing those plaques. It was all this other stuff. And you know, if you have like a bottle of vegetable oil on the counter and they're like dripping drips that go down the side, what you end up seeing is that they turn brown and real sticky, right? That's what's happening in your arteries, is that oxidative stress process.

Brendan [00:39:14]: Basically it's really changing the physical nature of that fat.

Nora [00:39:19]: Right. You're also changing the physical characteristics of your cell membranes in a way that's not beneficial. You know, we're designed to get a certain percentage of our diet, as you know, unsaturated fats. It's not the absolute number of any one type of fat that we would get in our diet that is problematic. It's the relative balance of these things, right? We've always consumed saturated fat forever and ever. We've always consumed cholesterol. We have many feedback loops in our body that are designed to manage our cholesterol levels naturally without having to be worried about whether we're going to overdo it in our diet or not.

Brendan [00:40:05]: And some of the recent research. I'm sorry were you completing …

Nora [00:40:07]: Well, I always have more, but go ahead.

Brendan [00:40:10]: There's a piece research that I think was raised by a Dr Mercola in my conversations with him, and I think I've heard it elsewhere, which is that there's some evidence that saturated fat from [unintelligible] sources actually improves the ratio of beneficial cholesterol to unhealthy cholesterol. So it increases HCL, I think, and it lowers the small particle of LDL. Is that correct?

Nora [00:40:33]: Well, OK, so the point I want to make very quickly is that there is no such thing as good cholesterol, bad cholesterol, unless you're talking about oxidized cholesterol being bad.

Nora [00:40:41]: Now there's only one form of cholesterol, right? Now, what you're talking about are high density lipoproteins and low density lipoproteins. The word cholesterol isn't in there anywhere. What those are … Ok, cholesterol is not soluble in the bloodstream, so it has to be carried by lipoprotein, by a lipoprotein carrier. And it's carted around. Low density lipoproteins are produced in the liver and they carry with them not just cholesterol, but also fat-soluble nutrients and essential fatty acids. And it takes them out of the liver, it for transport around the body to do all the things it does. When it's kind of spent and whatever else, then it's HDL, high density Lipoproteins recycle that back to the liver. It's interesting. It's not taking whatever cholesterol is on the LDL and trying to dump it somehow by bringing it to your intestines or your kidneys or something to excrete. It's bringing it back to your liver so it can be recycled again. This is a precious substance. You know, your body, every cell in your body has a means of manufacturing it's own supply. We produce a couple of thousand milligrams a day, and your body will regulate.

Brendan [00:41:56]: How could so many cells be wrong, right? [laughing]

Nora [00:41:59]: Well, exactly. It's not like your body is saying, "You know, I think I want a plaque our arteries. Let's start producing cholesterol." Cholesterol is needed for so many different things in the human body. It just is not even funny. There is not a single cell in your body that can live without cholesterol, and cholesterol makes up a good portion of your cellular membranes and saturated fats too, in order to give the cell membrane some stiffness, some integrity, and allow more of a semi permeability so that nutrients and waste products are kind of selectively moving across the membranes in a way that can help maintain the health of the cells and also maintain the cellular integrity. When you start over consuming polyunsaturated fats, as with some of these vegan source oils and things like that, you actually create much too much membrane fluidity and what you end up with are cellular membranes that start kind of collapsing.

Nora [00:42:58]: And this is one reason why those polyunsaturated fats tend to lower serum cholesterol. You have to realize that what's getting measured in the bloodstream is only what's in the bloodstream. There's cholesterol in every cell in your body everywhere, but only the serum cholesterol is what gets measured. It's not necessarily reflect reflection of your total pool. And what happens if you you have those compromised cell membranes is that cholesterol ends up getting shunted out of the bloodstream and other places to those cells to shore them up. So that's why it disappears from the serum. And everyone's like, oh, isn't this beneficial? It's lowering my cholesterol. Well, again, we have to be careful not to read too much into blood chemistry markers, right? Because cholesterol is not a disease. Cholesterol is an essential substance in the human body we cannot live without. We have always consumed it. We're designed to consume it. We are very well designed to consume and make healthy use of it from quality sources, animal source foods, exclusively. But if you see cholesterol levels that are kind of edging up to 250 to 260 whatever it's not time to panic about cholesterol. What the time is, is to say, OK, what is cholesterol trying to tell me? Because ... well, the first thing it's telling you is that there's something going on for which cholesterol is needed. Cholesterol functions like an antioxidant in the body. It's an acute phase reactant. We generate more cholesterol, and levels will tend to elevate, in the presence of inflammatory conditions, free radical processes, like cancer. And in fact, if there is extreme chronic inflammation or if there is a serious free radical process going on, sometimes what you will find is not cholesterol levels that are too high but cholesterol levels that are too low. And again, we need to ask ourselves, what is it trying to tell us? Cholesterol is an indicator. It's an intermediate indicator and going in and trying to take cholesterol-lowering medications to artificially lower cholesterol as if, you know, just getting lower numbers better somehow, isn't asking the right questions for starters, but it's the equivalent of getting rid of the firemen that have come to put out the fire and blaming them for the fire. Cholesterol lowering medications aren't ... excuse me, cholesterol is no more the cause of heart disease, I should say, than gray hair is the cause of old age. It's an associated thing in some cases, but we also know that up to three fourths of people that have coronary events have perfectly low, or even are perfectly normal or even low cholesterol, serum cholesterol levels.

Brendan [00:46:07]: I heard a statistic, I can't remember if I heard it or read it so I probably won't quote it exactly right, but it said something like 75 percent of heart attacks were in people ... those people had I think total cholesterol of 150 or lower or something like that.

Nora [00:46:26]: Yeah.

Brendan [00:46:27]: That's considered very, you know, quote unquote healthy or you'd have to ...

Nora [00:46:34]: Yeah, I am much more concerned when I see cholesterol levels that are too low and I consider anything too low like below like 180.

Brendan [00:46:42]: 25 percent of those heart attacks were like under a hundred or something. So it's almost like you've got to wonder like, are they having heart attacks because of the cholesterol is too low?

Nora [00:46:50]: Well, and that's entirely possible too, right? Again, we require cholesterol for the health of every cell in the human body. And cholesterol has a protective role to play with our health. It's also a source of a steroidal hormones, for instance. I mean, you can't make steroidal hormones without cholesterol. You can't make your own Vitamin D without cholesterol. And you can't make stress hormones without cholesterol, and all of those things certainly are going to also a role to play in the quality of your cardiovascular and your immune function and a whole bunch of other things. And so, we put way too much importance on that cholesterol number. And increasingly now they're looking to try to lower the threshold of what's acceptable because that brings ... that allows them to write more prescriptions. I mean, it's as simple as that has nothing whatever to do with promoting human health. And what's really terrifying is that where the future of cholesterol lowering is going now is actually a vaccination. They're developing a vaccine that will actually have an effect of modifying your genes and whatever else too, so that you make less cholesterol.

Brendan [00:48:14]: There is no limit to how misguided the intellect can be, the human intellect. The rabbit hole of reductionistic thinking or whatever. Whatever has generated that idea.

Nora [00:48:26]: Well what has generated that idea is the inclination towards profit, right? You kinda, they, I mean, you just, you really have to follow the money here to know why they're doing this. If they were so concerned about human health than they would be eliminating things like glyphosate from food production and they would be responding to our demands to clean up the preservatives and all additives and all of that crap that go into our food supply and all the processing and all of the ...

Brendan [00:49:04]: You know one of the things ... you brought up Vitamin D again just recently. Let's go back to Vitamin D because there are relationships between Vitamin D and Vitamin K2 and Vitamin A I think are interesting to understand. Is that something you can give a little bit about?

Nora [00:49:19]: Well, I don't want to go into it in too much depth. I mean, suffice it to say that these fat soluble nutrients in their fully formed, in other words in there fully activated forms, retinol, you know, animal source of Vitamin A, Vitamin K2 , which is found exclusively -- the MK4 variety from animal source foods -- unfortunately, MK4 supplements, I'll just say really quick, are nearly all synthetic and they do not function in the same manner as the naturally occurring MK4 in animal source foods. The only, and I just happened to have this, the only really high natural source of MK4 for that I've ever found in a supplement form is in this particular a brand and genetic strain of emu oil and Walk About Health Products. They have a fabulous supplement that is like the highest natural source of Vitamin K2 that you can find pretty much anywhere. So it's really, really good. But and I don't have any financial ties to them at all by the way. I love what they're trying to do actually. That's, that's really literally all there is to it. I don't make money from, from them selling the product at all. and then of course, Vitamin D3, which is so necessary for the absorption of so many important minerals. But just using calcium as an example, which is an extremely abundant mineral in our food supply by the way. It's just very abundant.

Nora [00:50:58]: But in order to absorb that calcium, for starters, you have to have sufficient hydrochloric acid for it to become properly ionized. And then Vitamin D3 takes and also aids in the absorption and utilization of that calcium. Unfortunately though, if you're taking lots of Vitamin D pills and you're not getting sufficient Vitamin K2 either from pastured fat of animals or from some supplemental source, then, and there's really only one non-synthetic supplemental source that I'm aware of, then what you're doing, you're probably calcifying things that were never meant to be calcified. You're calcifying your arteries, your calcifying, your joints, and your calcifying, your brain and nervous system, um, in ways that aren't supposed to happen. And so really it takes these three fat-soluble nutrients working together for everything to function properly. And that's just the way Nature designed us, and it designed us that way because that's what our evolutionary antecedents consumed. I mean the Diet that they consumed for about 2.6 million years, um, helped to establish not just our physiological makeup but our most basic nutritional requirements.

Brendan [00:52:24]: What about the idea … the only vegetarian source of Vitamin D I know of, and there's maybe others, but you put a shitake mushrooms in sunlight and then they convert the D, the vitamins …

Nora [00:52:37]: Yeah, good luck meeting your Vitamin D needs with that is all I have to say.

Brendan [00:52:41]: You'd have to eat a lot, huh?

Nora [00:52:43]: I'm not, I'm not convinced that that occurs that effectively.

Brendan [00:52:47]: Oh, OK. Alright. You mentioned digestion. Obviously very important if we're going to get, if we're going to access our minerals we gotta have hydrochloric acid. If we're going to digest proteins, whether animals source or a vegetable source, gotta have good hydrochloric acid. and if we're going to simulate the all-important fatty acids, uh, excuse me, yeah, fatty acids and fat soluble vitamins we've got to have good fat digestion, which in large part is, is dependent on, on liver and gallbladder function. I, for one had been somebody who had a very congested gallbladder and liver for a long time. I'm still cleaning out the junk from overeating. I was an emotional eater. I didn't gain a lot of weight from it. I was also a carb … I ate a lot of carbs when I was younger. I was not eating enough fats. So I was not stimulating a lot of bile perhaps to keep the flow going. So what are some of the factors that influence our ability to produce sufficient hydrochloric acid and have good bile flow?

Nora [00:53:47]: Well, the first thing we need to understand is that digestion is a north to south process, and it actually where it starts is in the brain, right? It's in a … you have to … your brain has to be … your nervous system has to be in a calm, relaxed, parasympathetic state in order for the process to even start to occur. In other words, if you are in a sympathetic overdrive, you're in fight or flight because you're stressed out over your job or you're late, you know, for this or that, or you're watching car chases and explosions on TV while you're trying to eat and your sympathetic, nervous system is more activated digestion just isn't happening for you. Your body is prioritizing fight or flight. It's prioritizing survival. It's not prioritizing, "Well, let's put our, all our energy into digestion now that her life is threatened," you know, kind of thing.

Nora [00:54:39]: And so that's first and foremost, you've got to be in that focused state. You've got to sit down, do your meal and focus on that meal and not on the TV or on, or with your head spinning with whatever happened to work today at work today or whatever else. Also, we need to take in the aromas, right? Because through the olfactory input, those aromas also helped to stimulate the production of gastric juices and all of that. Also you need a healthy functioning thyroid, because when we consume protein from concentrated sources like animal source foods, which is how we're designed to consume it, it's that that triggers well gastrin production for starters, which is the impetus for the secretion of hydrochloric acid, and that hydrochloric acid in our stomachs. And our stomachs are acid organs. They're designed to handle near pure acid, like, point eight (pH of 0.8) is roughly the pH of your stomach when it's digesting food. That's nearly pure acid.

Brendan [00:55:49]: Oh, I thought it was like 1.5 to 3.5? Are you saying ...

Nora [00:55:52]: No, no, that's at the stomach maybe at rest, but no at 3.5 you are not digesting. But you could get, you could certainly have GERD, you and you could experience a lot of uncomfortable burning.

Brendan [00:56:03]: That's like esophageal reflux disease.

Nora [00:56:06]: Uh huh. Because what happens if the pH isn't low enough ... your stomach is an acid organ, you know ... it's designed to handle that. It's happy as heck when it's being bathed in acid. And it's that pH signaling that actually helps to trigger the rest of the signaling process all way down the rest of the digestive process. So it isn't until the pH reaches a certain level that for instance, the whole pyloric sphincter opens up and allows this stuff from your stomach to actually enter into your small intestine where then a bicarbonate and other things are secreted in order to neutralize that acid and then allow the next phase of digestion, the slightly more alkaline process that then brings in the pancreatic enzymes that break things down into smaller size. And also that signaling process is also necessary for the appropriate biliary signaling.

Nora [00:57:09]: I mean everything is dependent on this pH signaling process. And if your pH isn't low enough, so say instead of point eight, you know, your stomach acid is that 3.5, I think you were saying, well that's still pretty acid, but it's not as acidic enough to rapidly digest proteins. And if you've consumed a lot of carbohydrates, you know, like starchy carbohydrates and things like that, with that protein, well, starches tend to prefer a more alkaline environment for their digestion. And you know, if you remember your acids and bases from high school chemistry class, you know, when you combine an acid and base it, they kind of neutralize each other. So your body is kind of struggling to try to do what it needs to do. Now, the other thing that happens, and I sometimes talk about this blender test ... If you take a blender and you throw, say a burger and fries in there and dump a Coca Cola into it and um, and then, uh, you know, you blend it up and spit in it and then put it out on your countertop where it's 98 point six degrees, you know, on a hot, on a hot, humid day with no air conditioning.

Nora [00:58:22]: You see what kinda happens after a couple of hours, right? What's going to happen is that the protein starts to putrefy. But the carbohydrates in there, the sugars and starches and whatever else kind of start to ferment. And that begins producing lots of little gas bubbles. And you're that pyloric sphincter at the base of your stomach is very, very fussy about what it allows into the next phase of digestion. It wants to make sure that the chyme that you have chewed, and hopefully digested is thoroughly digested before it releases it into your small intestine for the next phase to take place. And if it isn't, or there's just a bunch of toxic fermenting glop, you know, the proper signaling isn't occurring, and it's not going to be eager to let that in.

Nora [00:59:18]: So what happens is that the stuff sits in your stomach, and it just kind of starts to ferment. And the, the, you know, the, you know, the sphincter at the top of your stomach, it's sometimes called the cardiac sphincter is … if the gas is start to build … it will allow that food, that kind of undigested glop at three point five, to back up into your esophagus, which has, you know, no defense really against acidity. And it's going to burn. It's going to be uncomfortable. And so people are taking antacids for this, when the exact opposite is probably what's necessary. Gastroesophageal reflux occurs not as a result of too much acid but not enough acid.

Brendan [01:00:13]: So people should be downing betaine HCL with pepsin or something.

Nora [01:00:17]: Well, yeah, now if you basically, if this has been going on for a while and you have just an inflamed esophagus, you don't want to throw acid on top of that, right?

Nora [01:00:26]: You're going to have to do things to try to bring down that inflammation if you have, or if you have H. pylori overgrowth in your stomach and the stomach endothelium has sort of been infiltrated by H. pylori overgrowth and the stomach lining is sort of weakened as a result of that and inflamed, you're going to be very uncomfortable taking hydrochloric acid. You've got to address that. In other words, first you've got to do some things to try to heal that first. But for the average person that just isn't digesting well, you know, they feel really full for a couple of hours after meals. They get, they get indigestion or they start burping a lot, that kind of thing. Hydrochloric acid supplementation is oftentimes a good way to go to counter that and improve things. A poor man's version of that, but it's not as effective, but sometimes people, if it's super mild, that hydrochloric acid deficiency is, super mild, like raw cider vinegar added to a little bit of water, sipped with the meal as you consume it. That some people find a little bit helpful for calming down those indigestion kinds of symptoms.

Brendan [01:01:47]: That's because it adds a little bit of acidity. To move the pH down a little bit.

Nora [01:01:52]: Yeah, move it down a little bit.

Brendan [01:01:54]: Closer to where it should be without, without too much hazard to a very endangered, let's say already inflamed esophagus.

Nora [01:02:01]: Right. Sometimes it's kind of a tasty after dinner drink with a little cider vinegar in water. But I don't have any illusions about that necessarily being sufficient to correct a severe hydrochloric acid deficiency. But if you're under a lot of stress or you have thyroid problems or you know, you're over consuming carbohydrates or not consuming sufficient concentrated animal source protein that is going to trigger hydrochloric acid production, or maybe you're producing parietal cell antibodies, which is not actually that uncommon, which is more of an autoimmune process …

Brendan [01:02:34]: Parietal cells are the cells of the stomach that …

Nora [01:02:36]: which are the cells in the stomach that produce the hydrochloric acid. Yes, sorry about that. I should've clarified that. That's the case in some. You would probably … it would show up in blood work as what looks like pernicious anemia actually because that tends to also coincide with very, very poor absorption of Vitamin B12 and that kind of thing. But at any case, there are nutrients like zinc that you need in ample amounts in order to manufacture hydrochloric acid. But the irony is that you also require hydrochloric acid in order to be able to properly ionized and absorbs zinc. So it becomes a catch 22. So for those people, ionic zinc supplements are probably the way to go to replenish zinc levels. Because if you're taking zinc pills and you don't have sufficient hydrochloric acid to begin with, good luck with absorbing it.

Brendan [01:03:35]: I've been taking a fermented product. I heard that like taking a mineral with some sauerkraut can help the assimilation.

Nora [01:03:46]: Nah, I wouldn't rely on that. Yeah, I wouldn't rely on that.

Brendan [01:03:52]: What I love about you is you've got such a breadth and depth at the same time. It's like nothing escapes you. There's no simple answers because there aren't.

Nora [01:04:00]: Well, right. There's so many conditions. It's like, it depends, right? You know. Yeah.

Brendan [01:04:05]: I mean, the simplicity is simply eating, eating whole foods that are raised in ways that are natural for those animals. If it's animals or plants, a combination in alignment with our genetic and evolutionary heritage, as you put it. And the last point I'll make is obviously people listening to this … I hope we had enough information in this for people who aren't going to eat animal products no matter what. But ultimately we don't have to agree on everything. We're going to go our separate pattern, unique paths. I hope everybody finds their health and their joy in their food. The one thing that we have to do is we do have to come together and shift the food system so that whatever we're growing, whether it's grains or animals or vegetables or nuts, that it's restoring the planet, not destroying it.

Nora [01:05:01]: Right. Absolutely. And we should not be willing to compromise the quality of our food. Absolutely not. Just because it might seem cheaper, you know, the…

Brendan [01:05:11]: And it's not cheaper! Your *Primal Tightwad* you did it, you know, your ebook, you hired somebody to...

Nora [01:05:18]: Well, I didn't hire her. I suggested that she write the book because she was so knowledgeable about how to make this way of eating economical that I just, I got on bended knee and said, "Please write this book, and please call it *Primal Tightwad*. And she's like, 'OK.'" So she did. And she actually found that if you do it right, it can not only be cheaper to eat this way, to eat the right way, but it can actually work out to be something like $1,500 per person per year less expensive than the standard American diet that everybody seems to think is all they can afford. Look, processed food really expensive. Yeah. You know, I will also point out there is that same person that actually is producing pork that isn't grain fed at all. Has a farm here locally in Portland is called Heart 2 Heart Farms.

Nora [01:06:07]: Actually, you might actually want to interview this guy, his name's Tyler Boggs. He's, he's trying to change the way food is produced and the way food is distributed and to make the highest quality food available, accessible to everybody. So if you go to his farm, and your family is on food stamps and you're like, "Look, you know, we understand the value of really high quality grass fed meats and pastured eggs and all this other stuff. We get it, but we can't afford to pay in a retail prices for that stuff in all the places you know, the fancy grocery stores and things, but we'd like to buy some meat from you." He's like, "Hey, no problem. What can you do?" And you know, you can talk about your skill sets and things like that, but he'll put you to work doing whatever for a couple of days and you go home with a huge box full of meat that can feed your family for a good while.

Nora [01:07:10]: And he also finds ways of ... this guy is actually found ways of raising completely organic and pastured sources of food and wild cut sources of food for families in need in Oregon. He's done more of that than the Oregon Food Bank. He's raised something like 500,000 pounds of food last year alone. It's unbelievable what this guy is doing to feed families that otherwise can't afford to eat. And with the best quality food that money can buy.

Brendan [01:07:41]: That's awesome! You said his name is Tyler, Tyler Bogs, Bogs. And what's the name of his farm? Heart 2 Heart Farms.

Nora [01:07:45]: Heart 2 Heart Farms. The word Heart, numeral 2, Heart 2 Heart Farms. And he's just a few miles up the road from me here. And he and his wife started out wanting to raise food in the right way for themselves and their family. And then they realized that there was a real community need. And part of what they do is they go out to places where there is like, you know, there's excess extra produce or produce that maybe isn't as pretty, that didn't make the cut for the for the organic market that was just going to be thrown into a landfill, and it's like he goes and he rescues those, those foods and then makes them available to families in need at essentially no cost to them. It's crazy. It's crazy how brilliant it is. And what I love is that there is another way of making this affordable if more farmers and ranchers want to adopt this model because frankly there is more than enough high quality food being produced. It's just the distribution is skewed.

Brendan [01:08:56]: Exactly. That's what I was kind of getting at. You know, true abundance is a mindset. Instead of thinking that there's a scarcity, if you just know that there's enough, and you start to realize that intellectually when you actually look at how things are really working in natural systems and then go, "Oh my God, there's so much untapped abundance." And he's going out and just kind of capturing some of the excess. There's all this production that's happening. Like I said, I mean it's like 40 percent food waste, and you're just talking about one of the many sources that [inaudible] massive number. I mean, we can almost double the food supply by not wasting anymore.

Nora [01:09:27]: There's, there's no excuse for anyone in this country to go home hungry, go to bed hungry. There's plenty of food being produced, and there's plenty of high-quality food being produced. It's just because of the way it's distributed because of the way the system is sort of set up, a huge percentage goes to waste. And what Tyler is figuring out how to do is to repurpose that food that would otherwise go to waste and get it to families that otherwise wouldn't have an opportunity to eat quality food.

Brendan [01:09:56]: Yeah, I definitely want to speak with him.

Nora [01:09:57]: You totally do.

Brendan [01:09:59]: And thank you for being here with us in the EatEarth community and sharing your deeply nuanced knowledge and wisdom. Thank you so much,

Nora [01:10:10]: Brendan. It's an honor and a pleasure, and a hey, anytime.

Nora Gedgaudas Interview 3
Primal Ketosis, Digestion, and Restoring Foundational Health

Brendan [00:02]: So people … Obviously, the reason people are attracted to the ketogenic thing is energy, mental function …

Nora [00:07]: So there are about as many different versions of being ketogenic almost as there are people claiming to practice it, and not all forms of adopting a ketogenic metabolism are necessarily...or adopting ketosis … are all necessarily created equal. There are some that I think are actually downright problematic. And so, I'm very careful to define what I do, to distinguish it from the way others are perhaps approaching it. And what I'm advocating for is a fat-based, dietary fat-based, including the fats from animal source foods, not just coconuts and olive oil. ketogenic approach that is low, very low in carbohydrates, no more than about maybe 50 grams of utilizable carbohydrate in a given day. That is eating foods of absolutely uncompromising quality in alignment with our evolutionary and genetic heritage. I advocate for the moderation of protein intake and we talked about that at some length in our previous interview and all of the important reasons there are for doing that. And then also I'm inclined to recommend against the use of a dairy fats, which tend to be a little over-represented in the ketogenic genre. I'm also not a big fan of exogenous ketone supplements or overdoing things like MCT oil. Coconut oil is fine for a lot of things. You actually don't generate a ton of ketones, but you're going to generate more ketones from coconut oil than you would from a lot of other sources of fat. The whole idea is to eat a very wide variety of fats that can meet your essential fatty acid needs and a whole variety of purposes in the human body and not just one or two sources of fat. The point is not more ketones are better. The point to all of this is to develop a metabolism that relies on fat as your primary source of fuel and only secondarily, only as an auxiliary source of fuel using glucose as absolutely needed under very specific circumstances; either emergencies or extreme exertion. We need a very minute amount of glucose to fuel our red blood cells, to fuel the retina of the eye. There's a smattering of cells inside the Adrenal Medulla that rely on glucose that have a more glycolytic metabolism. Just because they don't … these are cells that don't have mitochondria. But anything that contains mitochondria will work better on fat, on free fatty acids and ketones than it will on glucose. Ketones are like a super fuel. They more efficiently produce ATP than glucose or free fatty acids. But the human brain is unique among all mammalian species, among all species in the world that it can actually run full time, non-stop on almost nothing but ketones. There are some animals that can do ketosis in a very limited way, but we humans are by far the best designed to make the most efficient use of ketones.

Brendan [04:01]: I suppose we should take a hint from that.

Nora [04:05]: Well I think that we need to. I mean, we're born literally in a state of effective ketosis where ketones become, in the infant's brain, the major fuel for brain development and we don't start craving sugars until adults start feeding it to kids. Kids don't start craving carbohydrate foods and start relying on carbohydrate foods until adults start feeding it to them. They're born. We're born as human beings. As natural born fat burners.

Brendan [04:45]: This makes so much sense to me personally because as I ... and I'm definitely not transitioned totally to a fat burning metabolism, but each time I start to get into that before I screw it up with not enough sleep or something. What I've noticed, my taste for sugar goes down and my taste for fat goes up, and then if I eat sugar, even though I didn't really have a taste for it ... I'm like just whatever, then the craving for sugar comes back.

Nora [05:11]: Right. And sometimes we have those cravings for sugar because we have come to our reliance on sugar as a primary source of fuel. Which is a very volatile and unreliable source of fuel and it requires constant replenishment. Fabulous for the food industry, for big agribusiness, for as big agribusinesses is the primary customer for big oil. And it's great for pharmaceutical profits. It's great for the chemical industries that supply all the pesticides and herbicides. It's great for the pesticide industry that's basically strip mining phosphorus out of the ground in places to create artificial fertilizers. Great for the biotech industry that's doing GMOS. Everybody's making out like bandits except for the people actually eating that diet. And I call it a form of metabolic enslavement. There isn't any incentive to change dietary recommendations to promoting a fat based metabolism.

Brendan [6:13]: There's too many [unintelligible] that are depending on us eating that way.

Nora [06:17]: This is politics and economics, folks. It doesn't have to do with human health. Doesn't it make sense that even the thinnest person watching this probably has anywhere from a 100 to 150 calories or kilocalories of fat on their body at any given time that they could be drawing from as a source of ongoing energy even in the absence of regular meals. You don't get these big swings of energy up and down and your mood up and down and all of that. Brain fog up and down.

Brendan [07:00]: It's like you said in your book one of the benefits, this is like a definitely a big favorite benefit for me, is that if I'm in a situation where I don't really have my good food with me and there isn't good food, really good food available I don't have to compromise because I'm not going to fall off a cliff of mental and physical function if I just get a little bit hungry. I don't have to stop at a 7-Eleven and prop myself up in some way for the next 10 minutes before I crash again.

Nora [07:24]: I'm constantly grateful for that because I travel a lot and where I live here in Portland, Oregon I'm spoiled. I have access to lots of really high quality source of food here. That's real food. But when I travel it can become quite challenging, and if I'm not able to find ... I mean I always travel with some little things that I know I can eat, bring things along. But if I go to ... there's a sponsored dinner somewhere or something like that, and they're putting stuff in front of me, and I don't know what it is I'm not going to eat it. And I'm ok not eating it. I mean, I might be bummed because I like to eat, but I'm not going to be brain fog. I'm not going to be irritable. I'm not going to be ... my energy isn't going to be in the toilet and all that kind of a thing. I'm going to be fine. Clear-headed and fine. And in fact, I actually have yet to eat my first meal of the day yet today because I've just been kind of going, going, going all morning.

Brendan [08:37]: All I've had ... I've had food. I was getting pretty hungry, but I've gotten by and I'm a little bit hungry now, but I've actually gotten by on basically almost vegan today cause I ate enough protein yesterday. That's another thing that's great is like when I have the appetite for protein I'll eat it, but I don't have to have this balance between glucagon and insulin secretion. When I'm in a sugar burning mode, I've got to balance those just right or I don't feel right after a meal, but right now I don't mind my protein assimilation or at least metabolism is more efficient and I'm not relying on that for my energy when all my body needs is more calories than I have it from nutritious fat and good fiber to keep the bacteria happy and polyphenols. So my breakfast, which was brunch, was basically a salad. I started with just olives, a scoop of ghee and I'm like, wow, I should have some vegetables with this because it always everything digest better with vegetables. Plus they taste good. So I made a simple salad, I dumped some pre mixed olive oil and lemon juice and just dump some of that on there, radish. Really simple. And then I steamed up, or sauteed some bok choy with some spices and some rain forest safe palm oil. What else? That's all I've had. I've had almost no carbohydrate; basically the amount of carbohydrate and protein in fibers, vegetables. That's it.

Nora [10:16]: Something else I want to point out that it characterizes my dietary approach, which I'm starting to refer to ... I've just decided to give myself my own genre. I'm calling it "primal genic" because then I know I've got certain ... everything is just sort of automatically implied in that term and I'm not having to try to explain constantly.

Brendan [10:16]: That you're not Atkins with too much protein.

Nora [10:42]: Right. It's like, "No, I'm not Atkins." And you know, Paleo and ketogenic diets have become so highly commercialized now, and there's so many things compromising those dietary approaches that I just really kind of want to separate myself out from all of that because I really take a fairly uncompromising approach. But one of the things I failed to mention when I was describing the qualities that characterize the dietary approach I advocate is that even though I advocate for very small amounts of utilizable carbohydrates in the forms of sugars and starches and that includes limiting fruit and that includes starchy vegetables and things. I just don't consume much of that at all ever. But, I have an enormous amount of fibrous vegetables and greens in the diet that I eat and from as diverse a variety of sources and also prepared in different ways because there's some advantages to eating vegetables cooked and there's some advantages to eating vegetables raw. There are pluses and minuses to all those things. Obviously cultured vegetables are far more nutritious. So I say, yes, do a little of all three. And so I get all of the benefits of vegetarianism without any of the potential risks or downsides associated with that. I probably eat more vegetables than most vegetarians.

Brendan [12:11]: Mark Sisson said the same thing. I think the same thing is true of many of us that we're actually eating more vegetables we're in one respect more vegetarian than vegetarians or at least vegans because so much of the space on their plate is going to legumes and grains. Not every vegetarian or vegan, but many of them. So it's pushing some of the vegetables off the plate.

Nora [12:36]: Or meat substitutes are highly processed stuff. Vegetarian diets of necessity have very high antigenic diet. It's going to be very high in lectins that are foreign to our immune systems and in the era where autoimmune disease now is probably exceeding everything else in terms of the global health burden in a way that is completely unappreciated by certainly allopathic medicine, but also even natural medicine. There are more than a hundred autoimmune diseases that have been identified now and at least another 40 or 50 that are thought to have an autoimmune component. And we know that dietary antigens are a major impetus for the initiation and development of those autoimmune diseases. And grains and legumes are near the top of the list and dairy products, which is one reason why I don't actually promote dairy in my dietary approach. I think that unless you've been able to test with Cyrex labs and Cyrex says, no you don't have any kind of immune reactivity to dairy. Well then I hate you because I miss cheese. But frankly, I'd say probably more people are better off without it. And it's certainly not required by anybody. And casein for instance, which is the ... it's a very, very large complicated molecule found in dairy protein. It's not the only dairy protein that's potentially problematic, but it's very similar in its molecular structure to gluten and actually has a very strong cross-reactivity with gluten. And half of everyone with gluten immune reactivity has dairy as a cross-reactive thing. In other words, certain sensitive immune systems simply cannot tell the difference between the two. And unless you have ferreted this out with a lot of testing and you know what is or isn't a source of immune reactivity for you what I recommend is that people just stay away from it. Casein also is the animal protein to which humans are the least well adapted. We've been consuming that for the least amount of time of any other animal source food. And you know, T. Colin Campbell, who of course wrote the China Study, what he relied on is the facto source of animal protein that he continually referred to as detrimental throughout his book was casein. Well, duh.

Brendan [15:17]: I'm not too familiar with how he constructed his research or his analysis and so on. Did he basically malign all animal protein by picking the one most antigenic?

Nora [15:26]: That's basically what he did. Yes. The science in that book is so poor, and it's actually been debunked many times over now. But, that was what he wrote. It was a piece of propaganda. It wasn't a study. The China Study makes it sound like it was a peer reviewed study that they put into a readable form. No, it wasn't a study, it's a book by that title. Just sorta like Federal Reserve isn't any more federal than Federal Express.

Brendan [16:07]: So you have a program. You have a year-long program and I am dying to hear what I would get out of that if I were to take that program. I'll throw in a couple of questions that you might answer in the process of introducing me to that. Just because it kind of ties into the theme of this event. I am curious, what are the things that make it easier or more difficult for individuals to make this transition? I have a operating hypothesis that this ties into your commitment to uncompromising commitment to quality. I think that maybe part of the problem with people who have so called broken metabolisms don't transition so well to keto, ketogenetic metabolism. Some people do it in 24 hours. They already start noticing a difference and they're not having headaches and stuff. And some people days and weeks and even longer before they really start to feel comfortable minimizing carbohydrates. And I'm wondering is it magnesium deficiency or other nutrient deficiencies? Is it like a pesticide load that's causing inflammatory situations that dampen basically all metabolic processes?

Nora [17:19]: There are a lot of things that can factor into the ease or difficulty of adopting a fat based ketogenic metabolism. I would argue that it is the normal metabolic state of humankind.

Brendan [17:36]: It can't be other than that. Some people argue that we emerged on starches. And I just don't see how that was going to work during that time.

Nora [17:43]: There is literally no evidence for that anywhere in the human fossil record anywhere in the decades of stabilized isotopic analysis.

Brendan [17:50]: We really start to see it a hundred thousand years ago, but that's long after our brains evolved.

Nora [17:52]: Long after our brains were developed. The amylase enzyme, amylase genes or whatever that allow us some relative degree of capacity to digest and make use of starchy foods is highly variable in different people groups. We had had some people may only have 2 pair. Some may have as many as 16 pairs.

Brendan [18:17]: The reason some people do ok, some people seem to do great on vegetarian and vegan diets. Whereas I can't do that.

Nora [18:25]: For a while. I would argue that it is virtually impossible to be optimally healthy with that dietary approach and I can provide a lot of different reasons why and that would take a whole other podcast, but I could really go on and on about that. The fact of the matter is that there's no question that we have a hydrochloric acid based digestive system. Ours is not a fermentative based digestive system as is characteristic of obligate herbivores. We can consume a certain amount of plant based foods, but we're not designed to make optimal or complete use of plant based foods. There could be a lot of minerals and nutrients encased in, kind of locked up in the cellulose of plants, but that doesn't necessarily mean that those nutrients are available to us. That we're going to be able to optimally digest and absorb. And again, the way herbivores do it is through bacterial fermentation. We don't have vats and vats and vats of bacteria in our stomachs. We don't have four stomachs to do this, and a rumen. We don't have a large fermentative gut. Our large intestine, which is the fermentative part of our gut, makes up only 20 percent of our total digestive tract. And the nutrients that are generated there are largely generated for the bacteria that live there. Again, they're not really sharing with us. There's no question that we have a much longer small intestine, much shorter large intestine than other primates. We actually have a digestive system that is much more reminiscent of carnivores than herbivores. It's closer. But, plant based foods can supply us with certain types of antioxidants and phytonutrients that I think give us an added advantage today that may not have been as essential or as necessary or as whatever is needed by our prehistoric ancestors that lived in a much more pristine environment. We're exposed to so much toxicity and so much compromise to our health that I think these phytonutrients certainly have clearly beneficial effects. And the fiber adds extra bulk, which if you're not overeating, if you're not over consuming protein the extra bulk kind of gives you more of a feeling of fullness.

Which is kind of nice. And also you're providing more fodder for our poor beleaguered and embattled internal wildlife that is sometimes how I refer to the microbiome. It is a way of getting diverse types of food to the microbiome, which in turn leads to greater microbial diversity. We can actually ferment the fibers found in meats and connective tissue and that sort of thing.

Brendan [18:25]: I never knew there were fibers in meats. That's interesting.

Nora [21:55]: It's meat fiber, it's not like cellulose. But they're usable. They're usable as a fermentable substrate by our gastrointestinal bacteria and that's very well established.

Brendan [22:13]: The idea that there is no fiber in meat is not entirely correct. It's just not cellulose fiber.

Nora [22:17]: It's not cellulose fiber, but there are fermentable elements in animal source foods that our gut can use to make perfectly healthy bacteria and prebiotic substrates and all those kinds of things. Now that said, the greater the diversity of your diet and of your fermentable sources of food the greater the diversity of your bacteria. And that bacterial diversity is really, really helpful for the health of your immune system. You want healthy bacterial diversity. And so fibers, vegetables and greens also supply us with the ability to diversify in that regard. The things that feed them.

Brendan [23:06]: There's the idea that's been advanced with some evidence whether it's good evidence or not, whether it's good studies or not that the microbiome of animal eating-humans turns carnitine and choline into TMAO which is associated with [unintelligible] cancer risk. Just curious. And then vegetarians when you hand them a steak or vegans anyway, their microbiome does not turn those nutritional compounds into pro carcinogenic [unintelligible].

Nora [23:38]: Because they probably won't be able to digest the meat at all. It's probably going to be their problem. And we need choline and l-carnitine is one the most important nutrients for the heart and for the functioning of the mitochondria that there is. So you're not going to have something that is inherently ... that we need with a certain degree of abundance in our diets that is going to, also in turn, kill you. It has to do with the makeup of number one your capacity to properly digest what you consume. You can be eating the best quality diet in the world ... if you can't digest it then at best you're not getting anything out of it. At worst, you're making things worse for yourself. But that particular bit of research, it was certain bacteria that were present that were responsible for those unhealthy conversions. And look, there are a lot of potential things in our diet and in our environment. Well, for starters, the problem isn't choline. The problem isn't the carnitine. The problem is the type of bacteria present that are converting those substances into less desirable substance. So you can't blame animal source foods for this. You have to blame what would probably be defined as a certain type of dysbiosis that is making unhealthy conversions of those substances. What we do know is that, again, we've eaten meat as an evolving species for at least 2.6 billion years and actually longer than that. And yet, cancer is a fairly new thing. In fact, cancer rates are expected to increase over 70 percent over the next 20 years according to the World Health Organization. Is it because we're eating more animal source foods than ever? No, it's not.

Brendan [25:38]: We're eating less.

Nora [25:39]: Yeah, we're eating less as time goes on. And people like Bill Gates have a corner on the, what they call the vegan meat market. You have to be a little bit suspicious of some of this so called scientific rhetoric that comes along. It doesn't make sense when you put all of this... when you shine the light of our evolutionary genetic heritage on this. When you look at how we're physiologically designed. When you look at the nature of ... well you look at the fact that there are certain essential nutrients that cannot be gotten any other way than through animal source foods. And I don't care how much flax oil you're guzzling if DHA isn't your diet it's not in your brain.

Brendan [26:41]: Let me ask you this. How does this ... You've got an antidote basically to all of the problems that erupt from eating a standard American diet. The problems that erupt from eating let's say a vegetarian or vegan diet when it's not, let's say, ideal for us. And so you've got this program, and I'm really curious what is in that program? Number one who's it for? And what does it do?

Nora [27:06]: It's a year-long educational certification program. Every single week you get a new either module or some portion of a module basically delivered to your inbox that you can view. And it's ... let's just say that I have a tendency to over deliver. So it's very, very rich with information. It's not fluff. And, I tried to put things in as understandable terms as possible. Because I would say that right now, slightly more than half of the people subscribed to the program are actually practitioners of all different kinds. Everything from nutritionists and health coaches to naturopaths and chiropractors and even the medical doctors that are part of the program. But there's also a pretty healthy representation of just sort of average people that really want to learn about nutrition in ways that they're not likely to get any other way. And so I take on subjects like blood sugar. I take on the subject of ketosis. I take on cardiovascular health and disease. I take on the whole digestive thing. There are several parts to some of these modules. The brain module is nine full weeks of just really in-depth information. But basically the kinds of people that are taking my course, there are a lot of people that have their own health challenges or challenges in their families or whatever who just want to understand all of this better. And there's a ton of information for them to make use of. It's not just educational stuff, it's also very practical, applicable, actionable information that people can really make use of. But it's also worth pointing out that this course is fully supported by the Nutritional Therapy Association and is accredited for CEU's. I'm also the process of obtaining other certificate, other CEU accreditation as well.

Brendan [29:36]: So you mentioned that this is like certification. Does that mean there's also like CEU credits or something? So somebody could actually advance their health coaching or health profession as well as be somebody who just wants to fix their body from so much [unintelligible].

Nora [30:07]: If you are a Nutritional Therapy Practitioner, you are an NTP, you are accredited as a Nutritional Therapy Practitioner by the Nutritional Therapy Association. My program will provide you with CEU's that you can use toward your meeting your recertification goals. I'm also working toward obtaining other CEU accreditation, and that's very soon to come. So in short it's not fluff. I'm not creating little fluff pieces that I can use to market all kinds of stuff to you. That's not how I operate. I'm deeply passionate about supplying people with the information they need to be empowered, to help themselves and those that are either in their care are those they love be as optimally healthy as humanly possible in our heavily compromised world. And there's a lot to know, and I'm always being interviewed for podcasts and things like that where I have to speak a little bit in soundbites. But really if you want the most actionable information it helps to understand how things are put together. It pays to understand this machine that we inhabit and not just simply entrust it's care to someone whose interests may not be in your best interest, but may instead just be in the interest of profit. And my program provides an enormous amount of bang for the buck. It's called Primal Restoration. It's all about kind of restoring your primal birth right. Restoring healthy systems, not simply learning how to take certain supplements that are going to address certain symptoms. Which is a very allopathic mindset, even among a lot of natural health care providers.

Brendan [31:57]: That's one of the big problems out there, I think. In the alternative health world, it's just like a naturalized allopathic model.

Nora [32:01]: Yeah. If somebody comes to me and says that they feel depressed, I'm not going to say, oh, that's too bad take some St John's wort that'll fix it. It's the same thing as taking a Prozac. You're basically doing something similar to try to treat a symptom rather than getting to the bottom of things. My orientation when I teach is very foundational, and it's very functional, and it is very, very based in peer reviewed evidence. And I supply that peer reviewed evidence to people so that they can see where this information actually comes from. I'm not making it up. A lot of it just makes very fundamental common sense too. With this you don't just get the well how do we better optimize our diet and our nutrition to have healthier heart or healthier brain or whatever else. But it's really about digging down to the bedrock and meeting those foundational and functional needs. There is a cohesive foundational framework upon which everything in this educational program is built.

Brendan [33:20]: Let's say that I've got challenges maintaining mental clarity. I think it's blood sugar or I think it's who knows what. And let's say I have digestive issues. Let's say kind of maybe tend a little towards constipation. Whatever it is. And my digestion's not real strong. I've tried many diets. I find some things work, some things don't work so well. Let's say that I do feel like my internal organs may be a little not working completely, whether it's my liver or something. Some symptoms of low thyroid and I don't know if it's this adrenal fatigue thing or whatever. What kinds of things might I learn and expect?

Nora [34:05]: Well what you're going to learn really quickly is that all the different symptoms that you mentioned they're going to be interrelated. One of the things that people taking my course will tell you is that it is a dot connecting course. You realize how these things interact together. You have digestive problems and you have brain problems, you better believe those two are going to be related to each other. And understanding how these relationships and the complexity of these interrelationships work is really foundational to fixing pretty much anything. I look at symptoms in large measure like points on a constellation. When people come to my office and they sit in front of me and they're going on and on about, "Oh, you know, well, I'm depressed and oh, by the way I'm anxious and oh I don't digest very well and I don't sleep very well.

And did I mention that I also kind of have ADD and my memory's kind of going south on me and that I've got all this inflammation here and I wonder what that's all about. And by the way I have asthma." Well, to me every one of those complaints is a different point on the same constellation and those things are heavily interrelated with each other. To me there's just not a problem in connecting those dots. But if you go into the average doctor's office, whether they be a natural healthcare provider or an allopathic provider, you're either gonna walk out with a half dozen prescriptions, or you're going to walk out with a shopping bag full of supplements. And you're not necessarily going to have answers as to what is the underlying thing here. And I'm very frustrated on behalf of people struggling with their health everywhere and suffering everywhere because even where there are, I'm not saying that all of these practitioners are kind of secretly trying to gouge people. They're conditioned to think about what they do in a certain way that it's supposed to be profitable for their industry. And even if they aren't thinking in terms of profit, the way they've been taught automatically kind of moves things in that direction. But look, we've been in a Newtonian mindset now for the last few hundred years which kind of teaches us that everything is sort of compartmentalized from everything else. Everything's about physical objects. Western medicine is kind of largely based on a Newtonian construct. Where you have your psychiatrist over here and your gastroenterologist over there and your cardiologist over here, your pediatrician over there and you're gerontologist back there and whatever. As if all these different things weren't somehow interrelated in some way. All these different systems are going to relate to each other in really meaningful ways. And unfortunately the way medicine operates is in a fairly compartmentalized fashion. A person's gastrointestinal problem might have everything to do with their neurological symptoms for instance. But a neurologist isn't going to see it that way. They're going to say nope, nope. When you learn to think in very foundational and functional terms and you take into account the complexity of the interrelationships between our different organs and systems, and understand that there needs to be a cohesive foundational framework in which to understand the operations of all those things.

Brendan [38:03]: Does it lead to a framework for diagnosis?

Nora [38:06]: I shy away from claiming that anything I do diagnosis or treats anything because they're huge liabilities associated with that. But people are going to have a really good handle on where to look and how to think about. They're going to recognize themselves in a lot of the descriptions that come up and they're going to say, "Oh my God, I never realized before that was me, you know, that's me. That's how it is for me." And people will be able to kind of ferret out the parts that apply to them or apply to whoever their patient or client might happen to be or whatever else. And it's going to provide with a source of information and a way of thinking about things that might be a little off the beaten path, but tends to be a lot more productive long-term in terms of creating changes in health that really last and not just going after symptoms. I'm enormously frustrated with the symptom based approaches.

Brendan [39:14]: Within your program how do the understandings translate into action or intervention or correction? I'm not sure what word to use, but...

Nora [39:19]: Well, again, with each module I supply the underlying information. I'll say here are some of the approaches. Here some new approaches you may not have even heard of before that are showing some effective ways of addressing x, y, or z. There's an autoimmune module that talks about things that I promise you're probably not going to hear about in any other autoimmune module.

Brendan [39:47]: That's the fastest growing category of diseases, right?

Nora [39:50]: Yeah, exactly. It's an area of tremendous expertise and passion for me. It has to be because I'm the only member of my entire family that does not have an autoimmune disease. And so I have to work very hard at this. This is not like ... I mean my family genetics, it certainly gave me some metrical features and it gave me a fairly decent brain, and it also just gave me every other disadvantage that you can just possibly shake a stick at. I have no wiggle room. I have almost no wiggle room for error and for indulgence. I've got to be on my toes when it comes to safeguarding my own health. And I think just having some modicum of health in today's world can be a real challenge, much less, the sort of fabled ideal of optimal health I think is an increasingly elusive thing. And very few people, frankly, have very much wiggle room, if any anymore. And so the more we can understand about this machine that we inhabit and take responsibility for it ourselves the better your odds of basically overcoming all of the things that are basically out to compromise it. And it's just more of that than there is wood work for it to seep out of. It's really up to us, and nobody will ever care more about your own health and wellbeing than you. No matter how well-meaning a practitioner might be. The more that you understand yourself for starters if you do end up having to go into, say something weird does come up and you have to go to the hospital for some reason, you're going to be far better equipped if you understand some of these foundational concepts. To basically be your own best advocate. To be a quality advocate and know how to ask the right questions in the right way so that you get the right kinds of answers that are going to better direct your care. If you don't have that some kind of advocacy in that mainstream healthcare system today, or disease management system as it should be more appropriately called, it's going to eat you alive. You know, it's a meat grinder. The best antidote to that is the kind of self-empowerment that comes with knowledge and a good foundational education. And that's what I'm trying to provide with, with my Primal Restoration program. It's about restoring health, right?

Brendan [42:43]: You mentioned that you're perhaps one of the leading experts in autoimmune conditions and what that really is that you have a unique perspective on it or brings something to the table that's a little different than what people might have been exposed to. Are there any other particular realms that you have a specific focus in that kind of stands out?

Nora [43:14]: Part of what I bring to the table is more than 20 years of very full time clinical experience. During that 20 years I spent a great deal of my focus on the brain. And the brain and nervous system and all of the ways in which that brain and nervous system also influenced a lot of other aspects of our health. I bring a lot of expertise to kind of the brain and cognitive and kind of mental, emotional health aspect of what it is that I am able to teach. And that's an area of enormous strength for me because it was just such an area of ... And that's the other thing, the fact that I have based so much of what I do on more than two decades of working with real people with very real problems with whom I was able to get very real results. So I'm not just an arm chair researcher of some sort or somebody who understands the theories behind biochemistry or whatever else that can talk about that in some kind of educational capacity. I'm interested in how do we apply this in a very real way? What works and what doesn't? I have a good deal of clinical experience I'm able to bring to the table when it comes to applying not just a bunch of loose theories and whatever, but I mean, just solid information.

Brendan [45:04]: You know I'm curious because one of the topics that is of interest to many people and it has been one that I've needed to learn a bit about it in my own process is detoxification.

Nora [45:14]: I have a whole detoxification module. It's actually, I think there are three or four parts to it, went for a whole month I think. Again, a lot of information people aren't likely to find any place else. You're going to be hearing things in that detox module that are going to be ... some things are may overlap a little bit with some of what you've heard before. I promise some of it is stuff that you haven't heard before and that's really, really, really effective and safe and there's a lot of things that people do to detoxify themselves that I don't necessarily see as safe and effective. So, I address that too.

Brendan [45:58]: People sometimes, they go too fast or they don't have the supports.

Nora [46:01]: Or they're trying to do a chelation therapy; not a good idea. Or they're doing gallbladder flushes, which I'm not a fan of. Or whatever. And again, I supply the reasons and the whys and the wherefores and I substantiate everything with peer reviewed evidence so that people know it's not just Nora's opinion. She's not just blathering about what she believes to be true. It's [unintelligible] supporting evidence.

Brendan [46:31]: Could you elaborate about gallbladder flushes, just for a moment, just to satisfy my curiosity because I happen to be a fan of them.

Nora [46:34]: Yeah. Well, you've been lucky, and some people are not so lucky and there's the problem is that not all gallstones are made from the same thing. Now, cholesterol stones that the most common kinds, but they are also calcium stones and there are oxalate stones and pigments stones and things like that. They're detected differently and they're dissolved differently. Most of these gallbladder flushes are kind of designed to get at the cholesterol based stones. They're not necessarily going to do a lot for the calcium based stones or whatever else. And here's the problem. You're doing these things that are kind of helping to soften and maybe start to dissolve ... like malic acid can be really good for softening and starting to dissolve cholesterol-based stones. I'm not saying don't use malic acid. But the problem is that part of what ends up happening is that people are instructed at some point to slug down like a whole bunch of olive oil or a whole bunch of whatever. Now that is going to cause your gallbladder to contract in a pretty strong way. God forbid you have an oversized stone in there that gets squirted into your bile duct. Now you're on your way to the emergency room where you will probably be parted from your gallbladder forever. I think that these approaches ...

Brendan [48:06]: Does that happen? That was one thing I wondered about and as I was reading in the past about gallbladder flushes, I wonder has it ever harmed somebody? From what I gather there wasn't really evidence that it had. But are you saying that …

Nora [48:22]: Evidence by the people promoting these gallbladder flushes. All it takes is a stone that wasn't quite dissolved far enough or a type of stone that that gallbladder flush wasn't really addressing and you can end up in the emergency room really fast. I think that there are protocols for improving the health of your gallbladder that don't have to necessarily result in challenging it in a way that puts you at risk. I would not … I personally think it's not a smart thing to take those approaches into your own hands. Work with a healthcare provider that is knowledgeable about the restoration of gallbladder health, what it takes to restore biliary health. It takes more than apple cider vinegar and some lemon and some shred shredded beet tops and whatever else. And then slugging … washing that down with a cup of olive oil. I think that there are people out there who get themselves into real trouble with that. And there's a lot of potential for trouble with that. You really want to restore the health of your gallbladder first and foremost. And there are systematic steps for this and there are certain nutrients that are needed for this that help to supply bile. And there's some people that don't have gallbladders at all because it's already kind of past, or they've got a lot of stagnation either because they've eaten a diet overly high in carbohydrates and too low in fat. And it's kind of one of those things, if you don't use it, you might lose it. If you have compromised thyroid function, which is probably the single most common source of biliary problems, you'd better address that. You're not going to fix your gallbladder unless you have done something to address that thyroid issue. And 90 percent of all low-functioning thyroid cases are autoimmune in nature so you're going to probably have to look at some of that. Again, lots of dots to connect here. But again, the idea's restoring foundational health and not just simply treating symptoms and I consider gallbladder flushes a little bit of going about and doing this more of a symptomatic approach as opposed to a restorative approach. I know that there are people that claim to have gotten good things from that to which I say, "Whew, you were lucky." I will never recommend that approach for anybody because there's way too much liability with it. For good reason.

Brendan [51:06]: Wow. So this sounds like a very deep and nuanced well contexted course. I'm curious, if I want to go and look is there like a webpage and comprehensive view of whatever?

Nora [51:32]: Yeah primalrestoration.com is the website. They are different payment plans and things like that ways of approaching it. It's, I think, ridiculously affordable for the quality of the information people are getting, the quality and the depth of the information. I really pay attention to the feedback that I get from people who are subscribed to the program. And overwhelmingly people are just thrilled. I mean, they're just like, I can't wait. Every week I'm so excited for the next installment because it's all just kind of really interesting and engaging information that are helping people connect their own dots. And that's an exciting thing to feel those light bulbs going off and saying, "Oh my God, I never thought of it that way before. That's so cool the way that relates to this. And oh, ok, that's so neat." I do supply, I don't sell supplements, I'm not a supplement huckster per se, but I do make some recommendations, and it's different companies do different things well, and it's not like I'm just promoting one or two companies here. I'm very cautious in my recommendations about particularly... In fact there's even a module, a whole module on supplements and supplementation and how to understand how the supplement industry works and what kinds of things to look for on labels, what kinds of things to avoid. A lot of people were just shocked by the information in that one. You can see the available, the currently available course curriculum. The last couple are probably going to change as I'm in the process now completing the full 52 weeks' worth of installments. But at any rate you can see what kinds of information is available through the course. A 30 day money back guarantee and all that good stuff.

Brendan [53:46]: I look forward to checking it out myself. Thank you once again for your generous contribution of your time and helping us understand more about our bodies and how we can live better.

Nora [53:59]: Thank you so much for giving me the opportunity to share some of this information. I wish I could've condensed a lot more into the time that we had. There's never enough time. Never.

Brendan [53:59]: That requires the course. Not infinelty condensable.

Nora [54:13]: Yeah. No, it's not.

Walter Jehne Interview

How Healthy Soil Puts Nutrients in Food and Protects Us from Heavy Metals

Brendan [00:00:00]: Welcome to the Eat4Earth event. We're exploring how you can heal yourself, your loved ones, and the Earth with food. This is Brendan Moorehead and I'm very happy to welcome back our guest Walter Jehne for a second conversation. Walter is an internationally recognized soil microbiologist, climate scientist, and innovation strategist with extensive field and research experience at a national level with Australia's Common Wealth Scientific and Industrial Research Organization and at an international level with the United Nations. He recently presented at an invitation-only United Nations gathering of scientists and decision-makers to discuss including soil in the next report of the intergovernmental panel on climate change. With his diverse experience in science, government, and industry, he is an expert at transforming challenges into opportunities. Walter has developed a new paradigm that connects Earth's ecological and atmospheric systems to provide powerful solutions for stabilizing climate, cooling the planet, and even restoring high levels of nutrition to our food supply. Walter, it's so good to have you back with your earth-shaking revelations with us once again.

Walter [00:01:10]: Well, look, thank you, thank you Brendan, and it's not me, of course. Mother Nature has been there all that time with all those processes and understandings, and I think we are just jointly trying to explore them and, of course, say how do we use them for our future.

Brendan [00:01:27]: What I want to do first is kind of summarize our first conversation and then dive into this one. So, in our previous conversation you explained how carbon and water control both the heating and cooling of the planet, and that it's merely a question of reestablishing the natural balance between heating and cooling, a balance that we have the power to influence through ten key natural processes. Perhaps most important of those ten processes and essentially the foundation for all the others is building carbon-rich soil. And healthy carbon-rich soils are also very important to our personal health. The first thing I want to dive into is what is the first thing we need to know in order to understand why healthy carbon-rich soils are so important to our health?

Walter [00:02:19]: Right. Thank you, Brendan. And yes, there's a whole connection between soil and health. Perhaps it's easiest to explain if we go a little bit back and then we go back 420-million years ago when the whole planet simply had ocean and rock; there was no life on land. Basically, what happened is a process called pedogenesis happened, right? So, this is the formation of soils. And soils were formed when minerals or detritus and rock was broken down by fungi and then plants and actually created soil structure, right? So, the mineral particles were separated, and you created the Earth's soil carbon sponge. So, think of mineral particles held apart by literal carbon springs, little carbon detritus, and that created this loose, soft, spongy soil matrix. And it's that soil matrix which holds the water, which governs the whole hydrology, which then is governed to cooling and climate temperature regulation of the planet. It's that matrix of soft carbon spongy materials, plus all the voids and all the surfaces in that soil carbon sponge, which is, of course, also the site where all the nutrients are. All the nutrients that we rely on on this whole planet actually come from stardust, 4.6 billion years ago when the whole solar system was formed. And those mineral nutrients and then they're on these surfaces. So here are surfaces in that soil for those nutrients to be absorbed off for use in life. The organic matter, the carbon, is a bit like Velcro. It's got massive numbers of negative charges on it, and those negative charges can hold all those cations, all those essential nutrients. And so basically it creates a cation exchange capacity of the soil, which is really the inherent nutritional fertility and availability of those nutrients. So you can see that soil through that carbon matrix becomes both massive surface areas holding nutrients and then also these organic surfaces again holding more nutrients. And so the whole availability of nutrients depends on this carbon matrix. It's again very important and not radical, it's quite real, but over 90% of the fertility of any soil is governed by the availability of these nutrients to plants. It's not how many nutrients in a soil if they're locked up and unavailable, but it's how available they are. So it's the soil carbon sponge, these surfaces that make those nutrients available. And of course ...

Brendan [00:05:39]: I want to ask you a quick question, just for a definition. So a cation is a positively charged mineral nutrient such as calcium, zinc, magnesium ...

Walter [00:05:51]: Precisely. Magnesium, manganese, yes exactly, and so they're absorbed onto those negative charges, but they're available to the fungi; they're available to the plants. But because they're absorbed onto those charges, they're not leached out of that soil and lost into the oceans so that makes them again extra available. It's very, very critical. The nutrients were initially unavailable, they were part of the mineral matrix of the sand mineral particles, but then of course, the fungi have solubilized them as part of pedogenesis and, in a sense, left them on these Velcro hooks to make them available. A fertile soil is really a soil teaming with available nutrients on these surfaces and on this carbon matrix.

Now, coming back to the question about soil and health and this is really fundamental, we are, of course, an animal. We run on biochemical processes and those chemical processes are all driven by enzymes. Enzymes are protein molecules that mostly have a mineral cofactor, which is the essential part of that functioning of that enzyme and so our biochemical health and activity depends entirely on the availability - have we got enough of these essential nutrients for our health for our biochemical function. There are about 96 natural elements in the whole solar system, but over 50 are used biologically and we know of over 30 essential mineral nutrients for our health. Our health fundamentally depends on have we got enough of these nutrients in the right forms, concentration, ratios, and balances to keep our biochemical systems and processes healthy. Linus Pauling back in the 50s, four Nobel prizes and what have you, lead in saying look, it is actually the nutrition that governs over 90% of our preventative health that is fundamental to that health. The nutritional integrity of our food, which is really the only place we get these nutrients from, becomes critical to our preventative health. Therefore, that whole soil-food process is really the foundation of health. The Greeks way back 3,000 years ago made that point, 'let thy food be thy medicine'. It's just so fundamental. We are what we eat.

Brendan [00:08:42]: So when we're farming here in the 21st century, we've been doing a certain type of mass farming for decades, and the soils are not getting better, they're getting worse. Many scientists tell us we have somewhere between 40 to 60 harvests left and that's because we've depleted the soil carbon, correct? We've depleted this organic matter, is that correct?

Walter [00:09:08]: Right.

Brendan [00:09:11]: And so obviously this is partly from tilling, partly from applying certain types of fertilizers that actually accelerate the rate of the bacterial activity in the soil, such as applying chemical nitrogen fertilizer in excess. It can still be used in moderate amounts, but what I want to get to is, we have maybe an oversimplified system where we apply three nutrients, nitrogen, phosphorus, and potassium and this kind of came out of the whole law of the minimum approach. I'm curious if you can say something about that. Where did that come from and why does that not give us nutrient-dense, healthy soils and instead it gives us the opposite now?

Walter [00:09:57]: Brendan, just to go back a little bit further because you raised the thing about what we've done. All through the evolution of life on Earth for those 420-million years, every living organism, every plant, fungus, bacteria, animal has depended on those nutrients and those nutrient uptake processes. It's really these fungi solubilizing, taking out nutrients from these surfaces, transferring them to the plant, and then, of course, we are eating those nutrients in the food that we eat. Up to the Second World War, basically all of human nutrition was based on this natural nutrient uptake process. All our food was effectively grown naturally organically right? After the Second World War, we, of course, had a major food crisis. Populations were growing, but we also had the industrial capacity and then we said, okay on a mass basis, we have to go into industrial agriculture, massive cultivations, fertilization, irrigation, biocides, the whole pesticide story, and we went into a massive sort of industrial agriculture system that was really the "Green Revolution". Of course, we're breeding plants to exploit that capacity, and we have fundamentally changed since the Second World War how plants take up nutrients because rather than taking them up through these biological processes, we've now sort of said, "Look, we can add these nutrients", basically from chemical fertilizers, and, as you say, we're adding basically nitrogen, phosphorus, potassium, NPK. We sometimes add some other trace elements, but these are three of the key nutrients, no question about it, but as we said before there are over 30 essential nutrients that we need for our biochemical health. And often our food now in our agriculture system doesn't make all these 30+ essential nutrients available and certainly not in the right forms, concentration, ratios, and balances. Why that's happened is because with this industrial agriculture, as you rightly say, we've effectively been oxidizing that organic matter, that carbon from our soils. Soils that used to have above 5% carbon now often have less than 0.5% carbon and by that oxidation we've collapsed the soils, but also we've destroyed that cation exchange capacity, all those negative charges holding, as you said, all the zinc, the calcium, the magnesium, the manganese, etc., etc., right? So we've basically compromised the capacity of that soil to hold nutrients. We've compromised its moisture-holding capacity. We've compromised its rootability, the capacity for roots to proliferate through it and, really, that is the whole systemic degradation of agricultural soils. And, as you rightly say, yes, we may have 30, 40, or whatever harvests left, but we are seriously mining, degrading soils, and we are completely compromising the fertility, the natural fertility, and we can't replace that by just adding fertilizer.

Now coming to the point about limiting returns, and it's a very complex, but important process. Back in the 1840s, scientist Liebig basically was understanding chemistry of soils and stuff who said, look here all these nutrients and is saying, look, plants need these 33+ nutrients and basically, yes, if I just add these nutrients then I can grow plants and you can because that's what hydroponics does, right? You've basically got just a liquid solution water and if you add the 33 nutrients in the right concentration and forms then yes, you can grow plants. The capacity for plants to grow in healthy ways depends on what nutrient of those 33 is a limiting nutrient, and the growth of the plant is limited by whatever that limiting nutrient is. So you can have an abundance of 32 of those nutrients, but if the selenium, for example, or cobalt or a couple or one of these trace elements was missing or deficient, that would limit the growth of the plant. We have beautiful case studies in the field exactly of that, where there's a trace nutrient deficiency and nothing grow. And so the answer was this whole "more-on" attitude to farming where we're adding nutrients to try and overcome different limiting factors, but in a sense you can't do that just by adding NPK because they're just three of the 33+ and those…

Brendan [00:15:32]: Did that come about, pardon me for interrupting, the NPK, did that come about because those were most frequently the limiting nutrients?

Walter [00:15:40]: No question, they're the dominant nutrients. Plants need those in bigger quantities, no question, and certainly you get the biggest mass response to the growth of plants. And often you can grow a plant, you know the plant will grow, but that does not mean it has the nutritional integrity. It doesn't mean it has the complements of nutrients. And this is really where we are now, 2017, 50 years after the Green Revolution, where our industrial food now has, we can still grow it, it's still big, it still looks good, but it often has less than 1/3 of the nutrients that it did pre-World War II. We often have to eat three times more wheat or corn or whatever, three times the volume to get the nutrients that we need. We see that, for example, with cravings. A pregnant lady will have a craving, and her body may need zinc. And she's gonna eat lettuce or something which gives her that zinc. And her body will say look, I need that zinc, I am craving for it. We are really walking around with gross systemic nutrient deficiencies because we eat a lot of food, but its just salt, starch, water, sugars. It's not giving us the essential nutrients we need.

Brendan [00:17:17]: So, what is it gonna take for us to start getting high nutrient levels available in soils and then into plants and into our bodies?

Walter [00:17:27]: It's really understanding that narrative that we've just gone through and saying, right, we depend, our health depends on those essential nutrients in that total balance. We evolved through this natural process, which provided them. We can't replicate that chemically because, certainly not with NPK, but even if we tried hydroponically, we have no idea what nutrients are needed at what concentration and what forms and balance when. I mean it's just too complicated to work out. Really all we can do and all we need to do is actually, say, well look, Mother Nature worked that all out 420-million years ago. All we have to do is to say if we grow our food through that same natural process, right, then we can rely on these processes giving us that nutritional integrity. So, you go back to your case study of Elizabeth to say, yes, I've increased the carbon in my soil, I'm growing healthy food. That food, because of how it's grown, has that nutritional integrity; therefore, it has that health value and that quality and we can then simply say look, yes, I can trust Nature because that's what we are; that's how we evolved.

Brendan [00:19:02]: So, when you're consulting with farmers, what are you telling them to grow their soils? How does this happen? How are we restoring Nature to the farming system?

Walter [00:19:16]: Okay, yes very important because we'll go to a farmer and, yes, we've degraded soils of less than half, and of course the first thing you have to do is you have to restore the health of that soil. You've got to restore that soil carbon sponge, put that carbon back. The only way that we can do it is exactly what nature did 420-million years ago. We grow a plant in it, but then we make sure as much of that carbon from the plant gets turned into organic matter and gets turned into stable soil carbon rather than oxidized off of CO_2. That organic matter builds that sponge, builds that Velcro, builds that cation exchange capacity, builds that water-holding capacity, and then very rapidly, progressively, we can actually move up and actually create and improve the fertility of that soil without adding nutrients. We do that because as we increase the carbon in that soil then the natural fungi and bacteria are solubilizing those nutrients from minerals and making them available in that and increasing the fertility of that soil. The fertility is not the "more-on" thing -- how much have I added -- it's how available the natural nutrients are and how efficiently are the natural solubilization, fixation, access, uptake, and cycling processes. And all of those are microbial. All of those are actually driven by these microbial processes that we are restoring and enhancing by building the carbon in the soil.

Brendan [00:21:08]: So, in other words, we're gonna have healthy soils and available minerals from the parent material of the soil, the sand, silt, and clay, as long as we're supporting microbial life, is that correct?

Walter [00:21:22]: Right. Absolutely.

Brendan [00:21:23]: So we gotta stop chopping them up with a plow and stop scorching them with harsh chemical fertilizers and pesticides and fungicides.

Walter [00:21:33]: Exactly.

Brendan [00:21:34]: But a lot of people will say, well how are we gonna grow crops without pesticides? You know you've got lots of pests and so forth and what would be your answer to that because we have pest problems on these fields. How are we going to handle it? If I were answering the question, I have my answer, but I'd love to know what yours is.

Walter [00:22:02]: Well look, it's again very simple. In Nature, there's no such thing as a pest. There's no such thing as disease. There are just simple organisms that accelerate the recycling of plants and animals when they've become moribund or at the end of their life. And they recycle them because those nutrients get returned back into that available pool to enhance the fertility, right? So, when you start thinking of cycles, there's no such thing as pests and disease. There are just recycling agents. The whole point is, if you've got a healthy plant that's growing vigorously with enough nutrients, it is effectively immune from pests and diseases, right? It's the same as a human. When a healthy, young, fit person doesn't get the colds, doesn't get the flu, is generally speaking healthy. And so it's actually the health of that organism that gives you the resistance to disease. Again, there's a whole lot of sophisticated biochemical processes that we understand, our whole immunity and our whole antagonism to the organisms, there's a whole microflora in our gut and on our bodies and on the plants that resist these pathogens and so forth so really a healthy plant has got enough chemical defenses, enough immunity to resist that disease. A healthy plant also, in a sense, gives off signals that tell, for example, a pest, don't even try to eat me because if you try to eat me, I am so toxic or unpalatable, or I will zap you. So, an insect will fly over a field, leave all the healthy plants alone and wait for a stressed, weakened plant to appear below it, and then land on that to grow its eggs.

Brendan [00:24:09]: I've heard that the way that happens is that healthy plants emit a steady, strong infrared signal or something, some kind of form of light, I guess. Plants, I guess, do emit photons just like they're absorbing from the sun, and they're reemitting them in another form and that the weaker plants are emitting an irregular signal and that's how an insect knows, "Oh, that's a weak plant. I've got an easy meal there because its not gonna have the immune system responses. It may have thinner cell walls so I'm not gonna wear out my mandibles chewing on it," that kind of thing.

Walter [00:24:49]: Absolutely. Look, Brendan, and it's ultraviolet. An insect's eyesight and its brain is working on ultraviolet light, and it sees colors differently from what we see them, but absolutely, it's picking up these things exquisitely and yes, it's just like us looking through foods and saying, "Hey that looks ripe and that doesn't look ripe" and we pick it up on that basis. The other thing is, why it doesn't land on those other foods, is because often they'll have toxic materials or acidities or otherwise that will be completely unpalatable to that insect.

Brendan [00:25:25]: So, you know, I've also heard that when we apply too much nitrate fertilizer that plants absorb it and they swell up with water, it's effectively a salt, and they swell up with water. They become dilute bags of water relative to a plant that's not got too much of that going on, and so then it can't really absorb as many of the trace minerals and therefore can't build a healthy structure and immune system, is that correct?

Walter [00:25:57]: Absolutely. This is why this balance of nutrients is so critical. It's not just NPK, but it's this right balance of nutrients, the 33, at different stages of the lifecycle. If we give a plant excess nitrogen, which is basically what all our agriculture is based on, and we're using massive quantities, 150% of the natural nitrogen that plants use we're now adding as ammonium nitrate fertilizers in our industrial agriculture. If we give a plant excess nitrogen, things happen very quickly. First of all, it induces auxins, which is a plant hormone that encourages more green shoot growth. So, we get this explosion of extra green shoot growth and it really looks very green and luxuriant, but the plant does that growth at the expense of the root system because more of the sugars are going to the shoot rather than the root. So we again unbalance straight away that root-shoot ratio. So we're preordaining that plant to subsequent drought stress because, hey, the roots are needed for nutrients and water uptake. So, we've got this softer, greener plant, but also because it's a faster growing plant, you've got bigger cells with thinner walls and most of those cells are filled with water vacuoles, so they're big sacs, membrane-bound sacs of water and relatively little cytoplasm proportionally in each of the cells. And, of course, these soft, watery, cells are extremely vulnerable, not just to insects because it's just sweet and easy tucker...

Brendan [00:27:50]: Tucker is like food, right? (laughing)

Walter [00:27:53]: Tucker is food in Australia. Sorry! Right, mate! Yeah, yeah, you got it; you got it (laughing). Anyway, the score is so even things like frost and so you'll see, for example, you have even a mild frost and here in this fertilized field and everything comes down and it's dead because the minute an ice crystal breaks a membrane on that water sac, you're back down to just soup. The whole thing's dead. And yet, here's other plants that haven't been fertilized and they're quite resistant to that frost and the same goes with insects and the same goes disease. We are just creating soft, vulnerable, unbalanced plants. Now obviously they become, by definition, vulnerable to insects and disease because these insects and disease, they're smart. They say, look, here's an easy feed, soft, green junk food tissue whereas if I try to take that natural plant, it would basically be tougher, but also it would have its own resistance against my eating it, you know, basically phenolics or other resistance factors. So, we're really encouraging disease through the way we grow plants and, of course, then we say, hey, we've got to stop this disease so let's put on a biocide or one of these pesticides. Then, when we add the biocide, we've got worse because we kill all the natural organisms, the natural organisms, that we know are so critical in their nutrient uptake processes. So we've not just unbalanced it, now we've starved it because we changed the root-shoot ratio, but we've starved them because we've killed all the microbial interface between the soil and that root so it can't take up nutrients. It can't solubilize, it can't fix, it can't access, it can't uptake, it can't cycle. And so now we've got a hydroponically dependent, vulnerable, soft plant. And we have to add more nutrients.

Brendan [00:30:05]: Right. So it's kind of like we've become chemical addicted in our farming so we get a quick blush of growth from NPK, but over the long term it's creating vulnerability and no nutrient density and ultimately a sick population; at least not as robust a population as we would have and did have just decades ago.

Walter [00:30:32]: And we've compromised, totally compromised a plant's capacity to grow without those dependencies, "more-on" nutrient dependency. That plant invariably, because it's soft, has 1/3 or less of the nutrient density that we need for our food and often has zero of the essential trace elements we need for our health because those trace elements can only be taken up by these fungal and microbial processes. Again, this is another major factor. There are fundamentally differences in how a natural plant takes up nutrients from how a hydroponic, industrial agricultural plant takes up nutrients, fundamentally different. Ninety-eight percent of the nutrients that plants took up in Nature, they took up through these microbial membrane interfaces, you know, the interfaces between the soil, the microbes, the plants. Plants naturally, yes, they've got roots, but they're pretty limited physical structures and plants naturally, 98% of plants, form mycorrhizal associations with these fungi. These are the fungi that first created soils 420-million years ago. There's vast networks of mycorrhizal fungal hyphae that proliferate from the roots throughout the soil system interfacing with that soil and doing all that solubilization. We're both sitting down, but we're measured 25,000 kilometers of fungal hyphae per cubic meter of healthy soils.

Brendan [00:32:27]: Oh my God!

Walter [00:32:29]: So the membrane interface – you know, πr^2 – the membrane interface across that link is just enormous. And that membrane interface is selectively, intelligently absorbing, concentrating essential nutrients and excluding toxins. So, we have this 25,000 kilometer of quality control membrane interface between the often toxic mineral soil and the plants that derive the food we eat. When we go into industrial agriculture, we kill all of that because we kill all of those fungi interfaces, and now the nutrition of that industrial hydroponic plant is dependent on whatever nutrients are in the soil solution. They can't access any of those nutrients on those cation exchange absorption sites readily anymore. They're really dependent on the soluble ions in the soil solution. They are the N, the P, the K, the sodium; in acid soils the aluminum, the cadmium, the lead. And these plants are indiscriminately sucking up this soil solution, but have no means to do any quality control. So the plant will be getting those nutrients like N, P, K, cadmium, lead, salt as it is in the salt solution. And so you can see we've got a fundamentally different nutritional integrity over a naturally grown plant compared to a hydroponic plant. And it as fundamentally different health consequences.

Brendan [00:34:25]: So you're referring to fungal organisms like mycorrhizal fungi that set up associations with plants, and the plants actually allow the fungal organisms to put a little drill bit, I don't know what else to call it, you probably got a technical term for it, but a hyphae lets say, put it into the plant root. Is that correct? Is that what you're referring to as the membrane interface? And then the fungal organism has this 25,000 kilometers of hyphae going down into the soil and mining the soil selectively for minerals and delivering them to the plant because the plant is feeding it sugar, and it's basically a take-out and delivery service.

Walter [00:35:08]: Yes. So we've got this interface, we've got this fungal intersect, but I'm going to take it a little bit further. It's a bit hard for us humans to do because these are fungi, but in fact, they were the primary organism, life on land. It was fungi that colonized land. The fungi are effectively protoanimals. They are closer to us phylogenetically then any other living life form. They're effectively animals, us. And it's actually the fungi that nurture these plants because the fungi can do pretty well in that soil, but what they can't do is they can't fix sugars. So the fungi are farming these plants, these photosynthetic sugar factories above the ground to feed them sugars. And the fungi effectively, in Nature, are basically supplying nutrients to these plants for the plants that keep feeding them sugars. So really, the fungi are in charge of this game, but let's not get competitive about this. It's a symbiotic association, a marriage, and yet Nature works through these cooperative symbiotic relationships. Ninety-eight percent of plants in Nature have these mycorrhizal associations, and well over 99% of the nutrition of plants and life is governed by the nutrient uptake processes of these microorganisms, these fungal membrane quality control systems. So Nature operates through these selective intelligent membrane interfaces. If we go esoteric, we go right back to 3.8-billion years ago, the first living cell, and it evolved only because exactly of that same membrane interface. The first cell was just a little liquid droplet surrounded by a lipid membrane that could concentrate essential nutrients, exclude toxins. Life is really, that's all it is, it's just a chemical soup inside the cell with different biochemistry because of that selective membrane. And these fungi are just an extension of that, and our life and our health is just an extension of that.

Brendan [00:37:37]: And so, when we kill them, we get unselective uptake by the plants of the minerals so they're not getting the specific trace minerals that they need like zinc and selenium and that we need in our food. Instead, they're just pulling up whatever comes through the water column, or the transpiration stream … so it could be all kind of stuff that's not being …

Walter [00:38:02]: And it's the toxins that are important, you see, because then, because we have lost the quality control system through those intelligent membranes, we are taking up the lead, the calcium, the aluminum, the sodium, all of which are toxic and we might as well be back in the dead chemical soup from 3.9-billion years ago.

Brendan [00:38:25]: Isn't it also the case that, let's say if zinc is not very available in the soil because the particular soil organism is not out there mining it for the plants because we've killed that soil organism with nitrate or chemical or pesticides, then cadmium substitutes for zinc and then lead for calcium and just different substitutes. So if we're not having the soil organisms making sure that the nutritional minerals are available, we're gonna get the toxic substitutes that have, I guess similar valences, charges, and atomic weight so they can substitute in, sort of, for certain processes.

Walter [00:39:04]: Yes. And, in our biochemistry, Brendan, it's a ratio that balances. It's very sophisticated, but exactly that. These nutrients or these minerals, all of them are toxic in excess, all of them are toxic if they're not balanced, right? And it's this very sophisticated yet diverse mixture at the right concentration, forms, and balances at the right time. And any of those going wrong can create ill health.

Brendan [00:39:39]: You know, on the topic of calcium (meant to say cadmium not calcium), I heard recently that it's basically the cause of 25% of heart attacks - I had no idea - and a big influence on osteoporosis. It's a very toxic metal and we're actually dumping more cadmium into the soil every time we bring in rock phosphate from various sources. Is that correct? We're bringing in cadmium because we're dumping so much NPK, the phosphorous, which, if we had mycorrhizal fungi in abundance in the soil, they'd be making all the phosphorous available and excluding the cadmium.

Walter [00:40:25]: Take it this way, look, the Earth formed 4.6-billion years ago from stardust. We've got all those toxic minerals, all those beneficial minerals, they this is Earth, they're still here. None of them left the planet, right? But life depends, as we said, on this right concentration, formed, ratios, etc., and so the whole life depends on what is the quality control system in this toxic mixed diverse stardust world, and if we mute that quality control system, we're exposed to that whole mess. So not that any one ion is good or bad, what's bad is losing the quality control system that gives us those essential balances for health. So, this is trouble, and you can't fix his with one mineral nutrient and this is where Liebig and the limiting nutrient levels are so misleading. It's not just one nutrient; it's that whole balance of nutrient, and it's health consequences and therefore our whole biochemistry. So it's not just a matter, yeah, you gotta take a zinc pill because too many zinc pills will do just as much damage as not enough zinc.

Brendan [00:41:52]: So I'm curious, what would you say the average person can do to make sure that they're getting nutrient-rich food, that they're food choices are helping to influence the food system that hopefully will heal the Earth?

Walter [00:42:09]: Okay, now look, and this is a key point. To get away from all this complexity, which it is, but really it's very, very simple and very natural, and very, very safe, is simply to eat food that you are confident has been grown through these natural processes. It's that simple because if you're saying, look, we are an organism, we are part of Nature, this is how we evolved. If I rely on these selective intelligent quality control systems that allowed us to evolve, if I have food that's grown in that manner, I'm sweet. I don't have to worry. You're still gonna die, but what I'm saying is you're giving your body, your biochemistry, your genetics the very, very best chance through the food you eat for a healthy life for as long as you've got. It's simply a matter of can I select the food based on my confidence on how it was grown and this comes back to just simple local stuff. Elizabeth that you mentioned. Here is a local farmer, we know they're growing food that way. We're confident that the fungi that are naturally in charge and naturally doing their quality control would've given that nutrient and that plant, whatever it is, or that food, whatever it is, that balance of nutrients.

Brendan [00:43:48]: Just to give people a reference point because I mentioned Elizabeth Kaiser outside of this conversation, yeah, with Singing Frogs Farm she's also in this event and doing amazing things with her soil. So basically, what it comes down to, if I hear you correctly, is people just need to know how there is being grown and I'm hoping that people will pick up on one of the questions to ask. I suppose maybe you could tell us, what are the questions people should ask to see how their food is being grown?

Walter [00:44:27]: Well, it's simply grown in these natural ways through these organic or these natural processes without the excesses, cultivation, biocides, fertilizer, all that industrial thing, but also you've got confidence, yes, I know that Farmer Mary or Joe is growing it that way so it's almost re-localization of food. It's coming back into the whole farmer's market, but it doesn't have to be a farmer's market. If I know this food comes from farmers who are growing it in this way, I can have that confidence. We don't have to be so scared about it because we still have the same microbiome in our gut. And so we can take in a lot of food, and our gut microbiome, as long as we keep those membranes, exactly the same process, as long as we keep those quality control membranes in our gut healthy, they will select what we need and exclude what we don't need and excrete it. As long as we know where our food is grown, how it is grown, go more to local, naturally grown food, it doesn't have to have an organic label on it per say, just that it's grown in these ways, we can be confident. Then we can rely on our gut microbiome to say that yes, here's our secondary quality control system that can make sure that what we get inside our cells has that nutritional integrity has that preventative health value.

Brendan [00:46:15]: So three questions come to mind for me as far as what I would ask people at a farmer's market to see if they're growing in a way that is supporting the soil health, the nutrient availability for the plants and for me. The first one would be, "Are you tilling, or are you not tilling? And if you're tilling, is it conservation tillage," which just means minimal tilling. So I'd want to know that because if they're constantly plowing it over or plowing the soil every season or several times a season then that's going to keep the soil struggling to survive, like keep the organisms constantly exposed to the light and too much of the elements in breaking up those fungal networks that are so important to the soil. Number two, I guess I would ask, "Do you have biodiversity in your planting, and do you have hedgerows?" Elizabeth and Paul Kaiser, they use hedgerows with perennial plants that are specifically selected because they're favorites of the predatory insects that keep the pest insects in check so they're using integrated pest management in that way. Another question I would ask is, "Are you keeping the soil covered at all times" because even if you're not tilling, if you're growing vegetables, you're putting crops in, you're taking them out, putting them in, taking them out so the soil is getting exposed. How they do it is they use a lot of mulch so they're constantly keeping the soil covered with straw or woodchips, things like that, which, of course, the soil organisms love, especially a certain fungal and bacterial species, turning that stuff into wonderful soil, but also they'll do companion planting with a fast growing lettuce in combination with a slower growing brassica like broccoli and so the lettuce quickly covers the soil area, and then it gets harvested at some point perhaps before the broccoli is mature, but now the broccoli is covering more of the soil. So, little things like that, but you know, I think I'll put together a list of questions after speaking to enough people so that people can have a concise list to go and be able to ask questions in a friendly manner of their farmers to see, you know, how are you doing this? (I) love your vegetables and how're you growing them. Chances are, though, that the number one thing is the taste test. If they taste amazing then those farmers are doing something right.

Walter [00:48:58]: Yes. Look Brendan, you're absolutely right except I don't think we need to always go and do the questionnaire. I think it's very much once farmers get it, once they say yes I see the biological or the natural organic way of growing and they're on that page, then automatically they'll say, yes, okay how do I do less damage; how do I do less oxidation disturbance. I suppose a big thing is biocides and all our industrial biocides, fungicides, pesticides, all that stuff are really dangerous and damaging things so the first thing is, get rid of those things. Get rid of excess high salt processed fertilizers, like the actual NPK out of the bag, but there's nothing wrong, this is very important to stress, there's nothing wrong with putting on recycling nutrients. Say if you're putting on mulches or manures or rock dust or whatever because these are natural forms and the fungi will use what it wants and not use what it doesn't want until it wants it. So again, you're not killing the system, and it's just there as a resource. It's actually very important because over half of us already live in cities, these urban concentration camps, and over the next 30 to 50 years, 80% of us will be in cities. Basically, we've got this very dangerous and silly export mining of nutrients from the land, from agriculture, going as food into the cities and, of course, that's going into their effluents and polluting their water and just setting up the next pandemic. And, of course, we've got to get those nutrients out of those effluents and away from that pandemic back onto the land. And so this idea of building a nutrient cycle between city and agriculture is critical and we can do it, there's whole very elegant, beautiful safe, natural ways of doing that. So there's nothing wrong with adding nutrients to land, but add them in these organic or in these natural forms as sort of mulch and what have you. You don't have to, as you said before this, addicted heroin, more-on industrial agriculture, we don't need to add them as an addicted soluble salt. We can just add them as a raw material and then let the organisms break them down and use them naturally.

The answer, as far as talking to a farmer or going to the farmer's market, yes, look if they're at the farmers market most of them are already going to be in that biological mind space. Talk to other people because you don't necessarily want to go out there and say, have they got a hedgerow or haven't they got a hedgerow, but basically if they're in that space, if they're going that way, yes, you can reinforce that. Then, I suppose the other thing is, it's a bit harsh here, but say, look, these are simple local natural foods. If they come in processed boxes from an industrial process with a lot of labels on the box or whatever you're getting them in, you've already got to be suspect to say, "Hang on, is this food or is this industrial product?' So, you know, how far down the natural raw material food chain do I move over my foods rather than in this stuff, right?

Brendan [00:52:58]: Yes and I think to an extent we can interact with our food supply more directly further up the chain, fresher foods and in also talking to farmers. I think what it really comes down to, as far as consumers, is just enthusiastically chatting with farmers about what they're doing and maybe sharing stories. What I'd like to see is a resource, maybe an online resource, where consumers can turn their farmers onto it, like, hey check this stuff out. These guys are exceeding the county and state revenue averages per acre. That's what Paul and Elizabeth Kaiser are doing. They've got six times the highest, not just the average, but six times the highest revenues of organic systems. It's phenomenal. They're getting $105,000 per acre versus $17,000 versus 14 versus 11 versus 35 versus $2,000, $2,000 being at the rock bottom, if I'm remembering the numbers correctly. It's astonishing what the potential is, and I would think we could get a lot of farmers excited about that, if the people that were buying food from them just talked to them about it. Looking forward to seeing some kind of resource available to just point forward and show that there is a way because a lot of farmers don't want to be exposed to these chemicals. They don't want to have to use them.

Walter [00:54:46]: Clearly, we all don't. There is also some powerful market factors that can help you in this. The first thing is, yes, you're at a farmer's market or whatever or you've talked to people and if there's no product left, if those organic potatoes are sold out, they must be bloody good, right? Because there's a demand driver giving you a signal whereas somebody else has sort of brought these other things in and people say, "Hey, I don't want those, I'd rather have those so let the market speak, right?" So talk with friends. You've got your local communities. You can get enormous powerful feedback because if somebody's got bad product or suspect product, just talk to people and hey, that information comes out.

The other fundamental market thing, and this is so important, we live in democracies and we have a democracy and every time we spend a dollar we are voting and we vote in a capitalist democracy with our dollars. Forget about the politicians every five years or whatever, right? It's when we spend our money, we are voting. So basically, use that power of the market, of voting with our dollars, and you can very rapidly at a regional level turn that food system around because basically people will be demanding nutrient integrity. They'll work out which are the ones that are supplying it. And the ones that aren't supplying it, hey, they're not viable. They can't compete in this because the people aren't that dumb. So then you go with, here are nutrient integrity health values, naturally grown food values, and very quickly that demand driver will drive the change and give you the comfort and assurance that, hey, we're going in the right way.

Brendan [00:56:50]: And that's why, you know, things like Organics is growing so fast, but we can even, I believe, encourage conventional farmers to, without even having to go organic, they can do so much better for themselves and there are lots of them that are. There are lots of regenerative farmers that are not technically organic, are not certified organic, but they're doing great things and so, yes, just voting with our dollars and being very committed to our own health and very committed to the planet's health and just saying, yes, this is what I stand for. This is what I'm buying. And that demand signal, the stronger it grows, the more of us do that, the faster we're going to see the kind of change we want to see.

Walter [00:57:34]: And we also have to be very wary that, you know, we're in a capitalistic jungle and so that people don't just appropriate brands like organic. You see organic is set up a brand, but [inaudible] we don't use fertilizer, we don't use biocide, you'll find some industrial port will move into that and say, oh look, I'm gonna call my stuff organic but still be selling compromised food so we may have to go beyond organic. We might have to reinforce our values beyond just the brand name. It's just the reality of the marketplace, always be aware, always at the local community level be astute and discriminate.

Brendan [00:58:22]: That's a very good point because we're seeing that the big players and even the government are getting involved with trying to water down organic standards. And, like you said, the big companies coming in, and they're not in it with their heart necessarily as much as the smaller organic producers typically are. And so we can't necessarily just rely on the organic label or some other thing, we have to really know, I think, and I'm looking forward to more transparency throughout the food system, but how really were these soils treated, how was the system managed so that there's a high mineral content and low, if not totally absent toxin content in our food.

Walter [00:59:14]: Totally. And so this whole discussion is moving beyond organics and into this whole nutrient integrity space. Can we have assurances about the nutritional integrity and you get that by how the thing was grown. Has it had these intelligent selective microbial interfaces, these animals doing their quality control for us? When I say animals, fungi, you know, have we used that natural system to give us that quality control or are we dependent on the more-on agriculture with an organic label brand stuck onto it. I think that's the discrimination that the whole debate is moving into, beyond organics into nutritional integrity, preventative health, and just that localized, re-empowering localized food systems.

Brendan [01:00:21]: Well said. And I will say this much though … I don't want people to think that organic is no longer meaningful or that we're jettisoning organic because that has been our only refuge. And yes, it's been a little bit tainted, but we can get it back. We can get the organic standard strengthened again. In fact, we can go to regenerative organic, and there's a label in the works by that name.

Walter [01:00:51]: And we are going higher up the ladder to higher quality. You see, that's the point. We're not going back, but we're rebuilding, re-enforcing organic to go higher up the ladder to re-enforce integrity.

Brendan [01:01:06]: And really get back to the roots of organic because organic, that term refers to carbon in the soil. That's where the whole thing came from, and it's just been watered down since then, so just bringing organic back to its roots and also providing, I believe, a path for farmers who don't necessarily want to call themselves organic or get certified organic to also produce high quality food because once they're actually tending to the soil it's going to look a lot like organic anyway, the way organic is supposed to look. And really the best thing that most organic producers can do if they're not already doing it to get to the highest level of their game is stop tilling.

Walter [01:01:47]: Yes, and it's a little bit what we started this discussion with, Brendan, it's going back to pedogenesis, you know. Here we had rock and ocean. It was these fungi that created the soil, that's created the whole terrestrial biosystem, our whole hydrology, our whole climate. And so we've just gotta go back to those same principles, that microbial interface between the soil and the plant doing their quality control, giving us nutritional integrity, giving us health, giving us our future.

Brendan [01:02:19]: Yes. Thank you, Walter. As always, it's been fascinating and enlightening to speak with you. I'm very excited that the United Nations, again, I said this before, is paying attention to what you have to say and also that you're working on some high-level financing mechanisms for investing in large scale projects for regenerative agriculture and eco-restoration. That could be for another conversation. (I) would love to dive into that, but for now, thank you for your brilliance and energetic contributions in the world and here with us in the Eat4Earth community.

Walter [01:02:55]: Thank you very much, Brendan, and all of the very best for everybody. And yeah, let's go for it.

John Kohler Interview 2
How to Choose a Juicer That Doesn't Destroy Nutrients

Brendan [00:00:00]: We're back with John Kohler with YouTube channels Okraw, GrowingYourGreens, and DiscountJuicers. And we're going to chat about why juice at all, what's the best juicer to get, under what circumstances to juice or blend. So, John, what's the first question to address in that realm?

John [00:00:27]: The question probably is "Should somebody even be juicing?" Some people might hear that "Hey, when you juice fruit, you're concentrating all the sugars, and that's junk food now" or something like that. And in my opinion there's a lot of confusion about juicing unfortunately. Probably the first thing I would say is that when you juice, unlike blending... which these are two different functions... when you put things in a blender ... basically whatever you put in the blender gets ground up into whatever it is but just a smaller particle size. Some blender companies would like you to believe that you're making a "total juice" because it contains the fiber and all. But there are inherent challenges with blending, the biggest of which in my opinion is that when you blend, the blender runs at extremely high speed. Some of the higher power blenders like the Vitamix run in excess of 20 000 RPM, some of the newer high power blenders run in excess of 30 000 RPMs. RPM stands for revolutions per minute, that's how fast the blade is spinning around inside there and when you're running the blender. I mean you could see down in the blender, you see that little vortex. If you just run water in your blender that vortex would kind of look like a tornado coming to Kansas and coming to tear up all the houses and the roofs off of Walmart and destroy things. That's exactly what you're doing inside the blender when you have that vortex running at 20 000 RPMs. Basically the blender blades are cutting open all the cell walls to basically turn the nutrients inside out and expose all the nutrients so that we could get better digestion of them.

That being said, at the same time it's blown open the cell walls and now the antioxidants are revealed from inside the cell walls and have no protection, and because it's happening at a high speed with the air being injected, it's oxidizing some of the nutrients. There's a study that I've seen showing that there's actually less of some of the antioxidants when you blend broccoli for example vs. when you use a slow juicer in order to create broccoli juice.

The other thing that I have with blending ... I think blending is way better if it allows you to get more fruits and vegetables in you than not. So don't say "John says blending is no good", I actually blended tonight but I use a special blender that I'll talk about in a minute. But the thing is, when you blend, whatever you put in there you get a one for one ratio. If you put a pound of carrots in, you get a pound of carrots out. And in this day and age, from my research and what I've learned, it's very important to maximize the amounts of fruits and vegetables and especially the leafy greens in a person's diet. These are the most healing foods on the entire planet, and it's unfortunate that most Americans simply do not eat enough vegetables specifically, but even more specifically leafy green vegetables.

I think the per capita consumption of kale is maybe like a quarter pound and that's not a day, a month -- that's a year.

Brendan [00:03:34]: Oh my God. I'm trying to make up for ten people or so. I had a whole big old bunch of kale yesterday, it was actually too much. I was like "Oh, I'm detoxing".

John [00:03:49]: My goal every day is to actually eat two pounds of greens -- kale or otherwise, every day. I don't always meet that goal, but that's my goal. But normally I get to eat about a pound pretty easily unless I'm traveling. Today I had a whole big head of lettuce for dinner.

But the thing is with the blender, once again, a one to one ratio. You put one pound of kale in, you get one pound of kale out. And you know, a pound of kale ... that takes a lot of volume in your stomach in addition now because you put it in a blender at high speed, and it's oxidized some of the nutrients in the kale. But the thing is if you take a pound of kale and put it through one of these slow juicers... these slow juicers are very efficient at the leafy greens ... you'll get about only one cup of juice, which is 8 ounces of juice, which is basically now you're concentrating the nutrients in the kale. You're removing some of the fiber... and the juicer... there's two spouts in the juicer. The juice comes out one spout, like on this vertical juicer, it comes out the front, and the pulp comes out the side over here. But what people don't remember, or fail to realize, is that when the machine is working, the pulp that's coming out over on this side is actually one type of fiber, primarily. And, you know, it's a little bit wet depending on the juicer you're using as well. But the fiber that you're actually losing is the insoluble fiber. Because all the fiber that is soluble in the produce is actually coming out with the juice because it's soluble, or it dissolves in water.

For example even if you juice carrots. Carrots are approximately 50-50 soluble to insoluble fiber. I think it's actually like 48% to 52% based on some documentation I've seen. So even when you're juicing carrots, you're getting approximately 50% of the fiber. But by the same token you juice the pound of carrots, now you've got 8 ounces of juice. I can sit there and easily juice five pounds of carrots in one sitting, and make five cups of juice which then ... I could now get the nutrients of five pounds of carrots in me. But I couldn't in my right mind unless somebody held a gun to my head, eat five pounds of carrots. Especially with the degraded food system that you've talked about or many other people on this conference talk about. It's important especially if you're not growing your own food like I am, to maximize some of the phytochemicals, antioxidants, vitamins, and more importantly the minerals in the food. And that's why I really love juicing so much. In addition this runs at a low RPM. This runs at 43 revolutions per minute so that's really slow, I mean I could turn it on. It just runs really slow. It's not like 20.000 or 30.000 RPMs like one of those high speed blenders. This means you're going to maximize the nutrition. I do not actually recommend the high speed juicers because once again, like the high speed blender, that also tends to oxidize more nutrients than the low speed juicer. But that being said, I'd rather have somebody make a high speed juice than to drink a coke, or a soda, or eat at McDonalds, or some other kind of food that is even worse for them.

Brendan [00:06:50]: That makes a lot of sense. I'm just curious, what's the brand on that, Omega?

John [00:06:57]: Yeah so this is called The Omega VSJ843, and this is my favorite juicer actually. This is the one that sits on my counter day in, day out. I like it because it takes me about three minutes to clean. It's the most versatile. If you said "Hey John, I want to juice a little bit of everything, I want to juice fruit, I want to juice hard vegetables, I want to juice leafy greens, I want to juice some wheatgrass sometimes" This machine will basically handle them all and do a fair job at all those different items. Plus actually, for a vertical juicers which are notorious for putting out a bit more pulp in the juice, this one actually puts the least pulp in a juice that I've tested, and tends to have less problems with clogging or jamming up.

That being said, when using any juicer, there are certain procedures that you should follow when juicing, like pre-cutting produce properly and all this kind of stuff. I have a video on YouTube called "Juice Like a Pro in any Vertical Slow Juicer" where I go over my tips so somebody could have a really easy time juicing and not really get frustrated, and not have a bad experience.

Brendan [00:07:59]: Okay, and is there a particular model number on that or are there several choices?

John [00:08:03]: So this is the Omega VSJ843, and that is the model number. The choices are... actually they have it in... this is the square version. I like the square version because the on and off switch is in the front. Then you have a rounded version that actually cuts off all this, so you just see kind of this part, and it's a little bit fatter in the back, and there are switches in the back. But those are the main two options.
The only other option is that it comes in silver and it comes in red, depending on what color better matches your kitchen or your lifestyle.

Brendan [00:08:37]: What do those usually cost?

John [00:08:38]: These ones run right now at this time at $399 on the website, and if any of the viewers today use a special coupon code "SAVE30", S-A-V-E that's all capitals, no space, 30 -- that will give them thirty dollars off, so it's $369.99. We pay for the shipping at Discountjuicers.com unless you live in the state of Nevada, we don't charge you sales tax or collect sales tax either.

Brendan [00:09:02]: Okay, cool. And what's this other juicer that also says Omega? It's entirely different style. It's a horizontal juicer. Is that for like wheatgrass or?

John [00:09:14]: Right yeah, this is the Omega. This model is the Omega NC800, and this is called the horizontal auger juicer. This style is if somebody wants to do straight leafy greens and wheatgrass and do a lot of them. This style is going to handle the leafy greens a lot more effectively than this guy [VSJ843] because it doesn't tend to jam or clog. One of the coolest things I get to use this machine for is okra. If I grow okra in my garden, I like to pick the okra young when it's nice and tender and not as fibrous and I'll eat it fresh and raw out of my garden. But sometimes I'm traveling and I come back and the okra has gotten really long -- it gets really fibrous and gnarly, and most people would probably just compost it at that point. But actually, I learned that if I took that and put it through this machine [NC800] without even cutting it up... I put it in this machine, and it will juice hard mature okra, squeeze out all the fibers out the front and give me a really nice, delicious... I call it okra slime. Actually I have a really fun video where I actually juice my mature okra and made that slime stuff like when you were a kid, and I was trying to drink it and it's so thick and slimy I almost choked. And to eat it I had to dehydrate it into like okra juice...

Brendan [00:10:34]: Chips?

John [00:10:35]: Like yeah, chips. I guess it was kind of like chips but I'd say it's like brittle, okra juice brittle. And then eat it, and I got the nutrients out of my mature okra that I otherwise wouldn't have eaten.

Brendan [00:10:49]: Me being a Californian boy... I think okra is sort of a southern food, I don't know if that's accurate, but okra has never been a thing that I have been attracted to. What are the nutritional attributes of okra?

John [00:11:05]: Oh jeez, so ... I haven't looked at that specifically but I know it's one of those mucilaginous food and in general mucilaginous foods are good for your intestinal tract, the lining in the intestinal tract. I'm sure it's full of vitamins and minerals and all kinds of other stuff. Plus I always encourage people to get diversity into their diet. I know people get used to eating their green salad every night, they have this for breakfast every single day. I always encourage them to get something new and different because there may be some phytonutrients in that food that you may need to prevent and ward off disease or even cancer in your life. My favorite okra is actually a red okra. It comes in green normally and then you could also get the red, it's kind of reddish-purple and that has lots of anthocyanin pigments which are really good for us.

Brendan [00:11:52]: Yeah, anything purple. I try to ... every time I see purple lettuce I get it. I get purple cabbage, I make purple cabbage sauerkraut. What's the price on that one [NC800] and why would somebody get one vs. the other if they had to choose just one?

John [00:12:12]: So the price on this one currently is $329.99, this is a little bit less expensive, like 70 dollars cheaper than this guy over here. Actually both these Omega products have the longest warranty in the juicing industry, they're actually both 15 years long. You can imagine if your iPhone had a 15 year long warranty, or your computer. You could just buy one now and for the next fifteen years you wouldn't actually have to buy another computer. Luckily juicers don't get outdated as fast as computers or iPhones because basically they do the same thing, and while they are making minor and small improvements every year -- there's no major advances. None have happened actually in the last five to ten years that I've seen anyways.

The main reason why you'd want to get this one [NC800] is ... I know there's a lot of people that don't like to clean their juicer, I mean to me, this one [VSJ843] takes three minutes, it's a breeze, there's less nooks and crannies than other vertical juicers on the market. This guy [NC800] is actually the easiest juicer to clean that I've ever found in the entire world. I actually have a video on it "The Fastest Juicer to Clean in The World" that's the video title. I just timed it on my iPhone as I'm cleaning it. You see me cleaning it, I explain it, my iPhone's stop watch is running to be 80 seconds.

Brendan [00:13:23]: Oh wow.

John [00:13:25]: That being said, cleaning is easy. But then because on this machine [NC800] you actually have to put the item in there and then push it in to the machine, each item you put in, you have to push in so it's probably going to take longer to use. Whereas on this machine [VSJ843] actually I don't use the pusher nor do

I recommend using the pusher because with this one you just take the produce and you must chop your greens and celery or just drop in carrots whole, or pieces of apple, or whatever. This one auto feeds. So this one will basically will run through the produce a little bit faster, but this one [NC800] is actually easier on the cleaning. This one [NC800] is more efficient on the greens. This one [VSJ843] is actually more efficient and juices fruits better.

And especially I want to address that, people think "John if you juice fruits you're just getting the fruit sugar, and sugar is bad"... because I know people are into keto diets and all these different things. All I'm going to say is this: If juicing a pineapple allows you to juice or drink some kale with your pineapple because if you just make straight kale juice ... I'm sorry, it tastes pretty strong, especially if you get kale from the store that's already old and bitter. But if you juice a pineapple and you juice some kale with it and now you're able to drink that kale because of the pineapple—in my opinion that's a good thing, especially when you're not eating the kale in the first place. And furthermore people are still sitting there slugging down soda and then they're complaining "Oh, fruit juice has too much sugar". The fact of the matter is ... although fruit juice has sugar in it, the fact of the matter is fruit juice has a lot of other things besides just the sugar.

Brendan [00:14:55]: Of course.

John [00:14:56]: Fruit juice has the filtered water, better than the freaking tap water they're using to make your soda. This is filtered water by the plant. It's structured water. It also contains vitamins and minerals and phytochemicals. Especially pineapple juice contains bromelain which is an enzyme that may be good for anti-inflammatory uses. I mean there's a lot of things in there besides just the sugar. And yes, the sugar is in there, it removes some of the fiber although it does keep the soluble fiber. The soluble fiber based on my research is the one that actually helps to regulate the blood sugar. In addition, according to research, documented, scientific studies out there, there are properties in fruits ... not all fruit, but some fruits that actually slow down the digestion. So that slows down the absorption of the sugars in the fruits. I'm talking about fresh fruit juice you make in the juicer, I'm not talking about these processed juices that you don't know how the heck they're made, what the heck they're doing to it or what they're adding to it. If it's reconstituted that is not the same thing as a fresh made juice full of life and enzymes and structured water.

Brendan [00:16:01]: Yeah, that structured water is really key. A professor ... I think his last name is Pollack, he calls it "exclusion zone water" but it's the same kind of idea as what we've been calling structured water for quite a while. But basically yes, it's just a more hydrating water that gets into your cells, as opposed to tap water which has a very hard time ... your body has to actually kind of energize it to sort of break up the adhesions among the water molecules so that it can become a more hydrating water.

John [00:16:42]: Not to mention ... somebody who's still drinking the tap water... it has the chlorine, and the fluoride ... Actually, I saw a thing on my local news here and they're saying our water source here in Las Vegas actually has ... they tested it and it actually has ... what is it ... birth control drugs in the water supply. I mean I would much rather drink some celery cucumber water... or juice in the morning to get my structured water that has already been filtered by the plants, and I don't have to worry about all of those toxins in the water.

Brendan [00:17:14]: Yeah. And with the fruit sugar content ... I personally am somebody who's very sensitive to sugar in general, including food sugar, beet sugar, carrot sugar. I have to dilute it. When I did kale juice yesterday morning, I did just kale and celery.

John [00:17:32]: That's hardcore man.

Brendan [00:17:34]: Yeah, I mean it was a bitter drink, don't get me wrong. Actually, there's a lot to be said for going after bitter taste, from an Ayurvedic perspective it will get your liver kicking -- and it did. It got my liver detoxing. But the liver likes sweet taste as well, so add whatever amount is appropriate for your constitution. I want to ask you this ... so I've got a Blendtec blender, a high-speed blender as you know. How would you rate that? Is that one of these obscenely high-speed blenders you're concerned about?

John [00:18:11]: Absolutely. I mean any ... basically 99% of all blenders out there, whether it's a Vitamix, or Blendtec, the KitchenAid, the Breville ... basically any blender out there that you could buy is a standard high-speed blender that I'm not a fan of personally. Once again I like to teach good-better-best. If a blender, whether it's a Vitamix, or Blendtec, or just a 29 dollar one you got at Walmart, allows you to get more fruits and vegetables—that's a good thing in my book. But once again I'm not looking for good in my life, I'm looking for optimal, or the best. So I actually prefer juicing ... number one because I could concentrate the nutrients to also get the higher level of nutrition. But now actually, just this year earlier this year, the first vacuum blender was released into the USA, it's actually called the Tribest vacuum blender or Dynapro blender. This is a little bit different than a standard blender because this blender blends under a vacuum. This technology was invented in Japan in the early 1990s that now this company in Korea is making. The vacuum blender works a little differently, pretty much it works like a ... you know they sell those food savers at Costco and then you buy big things in bulk, if you've got the food savers you could suck out the air when you're storing your cheeses, or meats, or fruits, and vegetables, and then they just basically last longer. That's because now whatever you're food saving and removing the excess air out of, the air is not in the packaging to cause oxidizing damage, to break down that food faster. And that's exactly what happens when you put your blender under vacuum and then you blend. You're removing all the excess oxygen. So now when you blend, you're not blending in there... and it still does create that vortex because now you're under vacuum. There's not all the oxygen or not the high quantity of oxygen molecules bumping around in there.

I've done demonstrations where I'll blend apples and water in a non-vacuum and a vacuum blender and you'll see the notable difference in the color of the blend after it's done, but even more impressive five or ten minutes after you're done blending. The one that you've already done the oxidative damage to continues to oxidize and get even worse. Meanwhile the one that you vacuum blended it literally stopped it in time and how it comes out is pretty much how it's going to look for a good period of time afterwards because it's just massively done less oxidative damage.

A testing in Japan showed that say when you blend blueberries for example in a high-speed blender, whether that's a Vitamix, or Blendtec, or probably just any other blender vs. a vacuum blender, you're going to get 2.5 times more of a certain polyphenol antioxidant that they tested for in the vacuum blender. Basically when you're blending things in the standard blender you're losing a significance of some of the most important nutrients in my opinion, and some of the antioxidants. Now, I'm sure minerals are minimally affected and some other nutrients are affected. Vitamins could be affected. Vitamin A could be decreased by three times. And this depends of course on the food. This is just based on testing I've seen on certain foods. And of course they could be cherry-picking for all I know. But what I can tell you is this—when I've blended in a vacuum blender vs. blending in a standard blender, the same exact mixture—number one, you see the difference in color. The one in the vacuum blender is a lot more vibrant. Number two, the one in the vacuum blender will stay fresher longer and it won't oxidize as bad.

I mean I've made banana smoothies in like a Vitamix or a Blendtec, and you make a big smoothie and then your eyes are bigger than your stomach, you make so much and then you drink almost all of it except you leave that much in the blender. And then you put it aside or you're working on the computer, you drink all of it except that much and then you put it aside. You come back after about three hours to go drink it again, and you drink it, and you're like "Ugh, this is nasty". That's because it's oxidized so much. But in the vacuum blender, after you vacuum blended it, you can let it sit three hours and it's going to have barely any taste change.

Also ... the other thing when you vacuum blend. When you do taste the mixture, the smoothie or whatever you're making, it has a better flavor profile. You taste the flavors more. If you're blending mint, you don't have to put as much mint to get the same minty flavor as you did with the standard blender, because the standard blenders are oxidizing the nutrients, and the nutrients are what makes the flavors. Those are some of the benefits of the vacuum blender. It's amazing technology, probably by the time this is out there'll be maybe two maybe three of the vacuum blenders on the market, and for those of you guys out there that don't want to spend $550 or $650 dollars to buy a new vacuum blender, which in my opinion, depending on the model you get is worth it. I do have a video on YouTube on how to basically hack your NutriBullet for twenty bucks and a drill to make your own vacuum blender out of your NutriBullet.

Brendan [00:23:18]: No way! [laughs]

John [00:23:19]: Yeah, and I only did that because I learned about vacuum blending, and once I learned about vacuum blending at the trade show, I wanted the vacuum blender like yesterday. [inaudible] "John you've been on your diet for twenty years now and you've been blending in a standard blender, think about if you had a vacuum blender twenty years ago how much healthier you would be now, because you'd have two to three times more of certain phytonutrients and nutrients in the blended mixture". So then I had to figure out "How can I make the vacuum blender now because the vacuum blenders aren't out," and I feel bad anytime I blend without vacuum now, I know I'm losing nutrients.

Brendan [00:23:51]: And you're wasting money.

John [00:23:52]: You're wasting money, you're wasting nutrients, and you could be compromising your health. If the extra polyphenols in the blueberries or the whatever you need in the kale is lowered and just that twice as much is what you need to keep you healthy. Especially if you're immunocompromised or have health challenges. It can make a big difference in my opinion.

Brendan [00:24:14]: Yeah, I'm definitely going to check out that video. I don't know if you have one for turning a Blendtec into a vacuum blender.

John [00:24:23]: I tried that already, and if you're a little bit handy and you could make like a nice top with a nice gasket and just put like basically one-way valve on the top, you could turn any blender into a vacuum blender. I tried to do it really easily and it wasn't quite successful. You will need to probably use a 3D printer and make your own top, and there are some people out there doing this and hopefully they'll come to market soon and have tops for Vitamixes and Blenstecs so that people could easily turn their standard blender into a vacuum blender. That being said a standard blender is not designed to be a vacuum blender. If you put it under vacuum it may blow out the seals or something down below next to the bearings prematurely, but I think that'd be worth it.

Brendan [00:25:08]: You're a diehard purist, but it makes sense. I mean I've noticed it myself when I've left a mixture, because my eyes often are bigger than my stomach ... I used to fill up my Blendtec with so much stuff, I couldn't down it all, and it would turn brown pretty fast.

John [00:25:30]: Yeah.

Brendan [00:25:32]: But I haven't been doing anything like I was doing. I was going at it pretty hard core in 2012 I think it was. Now it's far more occasional, and I think I'm doing more juicing than blending these days. You gave a bit of a description of the differences between juicing and blending, is there anything else that we should know? I mean I saw ... I think I saw somewhere that certain nutrients are more preserved by blending and some are more preserved because of the fiber being present, and obviously you can only handle so much fiber in a day, so juicing is good if you want to concentrate down a lot of kale ... and kale is actually pretty hard to handle as a blended drink. That's the kind of thing you definitely want to juice. So just curious if there are certain nutrients that tend to be better extracted by juicing and other nutrients that are better retained by blending.

John [00:26:42]: Yeah, I have seen some studies that show depending... once again, nothing is ever clear black and white ... "juicing is always better with all the nutrients than blending" ... there may be nutrients sometimes and blending gets more nutrients than juicing. That's why actually in my life I don't just juice exclusively or blend exclusively. I do both.
And in addition to that I use the best juicer and blender in the entire world that all of us were given free, and that's our teeth. We just have to remember to chew our food into a mush, and that's all we could give babies -- baby food because they don't have teeth. But if we chewed all our food into a mush we would get the optimal digestion out of that. Except for the fact that a lot of people these days especially after eating a non-proper diet all these years ... their bodies aren't used to high volumes of fiber. They don't have the beneficial probiotics in their gut to help them digest that fiber, for that reason I think especially if somebody's new in getting into health, juicing should be your first stop before blending, because blending could be a little bit more challenging for digestive purposes.

Brendan [00:27:49]: Okay, yeah. I'm a big fan of chewing my way through a lot of vegetables, I like huge salads. I'll have anywhere from two to four of them a day, and often two in one meal … because I like the flavor, and having each bite tastes a little bit different as opposed to throwing a bunch of brazil nuts and pecans and olives and avocado. As you could tell I love the fatty foods, and the romaine red leaf, the daikon radish, carrots and all that. So if you throw it all in one thing then you kind of lose all the distinctive flavors, it's just blended into an average something. That's why I just stick with salads more when I'm going for the whole vegetable. And I don't do as much blending lately. Also I don't do a lot of fruit, otherwise I'd probably be doing more blending. Putting some spinach in with fruit or something like that, and some nuts. That's really nice actually, throwing in some nuts with fruit and a green…

John [00:28:58]: And actually I do recommend to people to actually eat their fruits whole or blend them instead of juicing them. I think that's far better. But once again, it's not like my rule to never juice fruits. If I have some watermelon that's actually not as ripe as it should be and it's really not sweet, I'm eating it and I don't enjoy it through eating… I'm not going to throw it out or just put it into my compost. I'm actually going to juice it, so at least I could have the good water content and even if it's not super sweet, it's better going through me as water instead and I'll enjoy it more than actually eating an unripe fruit. That being said, if it takes some fruit to get you to get more greens or vegetables in you, once again that's also a good thing in my book. But yeah, I like to eat my fruits whole and ripe preferably. I vacuum blend them if I don't eat them whole and ripe, and I like to juice my leafy green vegetables predominantly. And also I like to juice my vegetables, my hard vegetables like carrots and beets and things. In addition every night my main meal every day is like a salad or a nice big soup made with a juice. One of my favorite soups is actually a pepper soup. I juice a bunch of peppers, I could get like 32 ounces of pepper juice, I'll take that and put it in a vacuum…

Brendan [00:30:20]: 32 ounces?

John [00:30:22]: Yeah, yeah.

Brendan [00:30:23]: That's a lot!

John [00:30:25]: 32 ounces … maybe it might be 16, it depends because usually I'll make a double batch. I'll put that juice in the blender with Brazil nuts, mushroom powder, some flax seeds, different kinds of nuts, sauerkraut, seaweed … I don't think I've said that, maybe a little bit of miso. And then I'll blend that up into a nice thick … it's not quite a sauce because it's still watery. And then I'll cut greens from my garden in there, I'll put some natto maybe some unpasteurized tempeh in there sometimes, some additional soaked sea weed in there, shredded carrots, chopped up onions -- whatever. It's basically like a super thick dressing for my salad that I've actually put in there. It's a nice hardy soup and the base is the pepper juice which is probably one of the highest antioxidant, especially vitamin C, non-sweet fruits out there.

Brendan [00:31:21]: What kind of pepper are we talking about?

John [00:31:23]: Sweet pepper. I mean I like to use red pepper predominantly but if I can't get red then I'll use orange or yellow, but I don't use green.

Brendan [00:31:30]: Yeah, love those. They're kind of expensive though. Are you growing them yourself to get 16 ounces?

John [00:31:36]: Yeah so I do grow my own peppers. Actually I'm going to do one more harvest tomorrow and then we're going to get a freeze. And then also I go to the wholesale produce terminal down in LA, so I get peppers for really cheap. I got 11 pounds of organic peppers hothouse grown, for 8 bucks.

Brendan [00:31:56]: Wow, 11 pounds for 8 bucks. Nice. You're making me hungry just thinking about it. My mother makes the best salads, everybody's mother makes the best food.

John [00:32:12]: My mom don't. [laughs]

Brendan [00:32:13]: Not your mom? My mother is big into salads, and she's always got some sweet peppers in there, and I love it. I just don't seem to buy them myself. That was an intriguing soup recipe, I've got to say. That was all raw, is that correct? None of that is cooked.

John [00:32:35]: Right, it's all fresh, all raw, it's not heated. I mean I blend it in the vacuum blender as a first step, after juicing it I blend it with the nuts to kind of emulsify the nuts and make it a creamy kind of sauce. I might add some hot peppers in there to make it hot but not actually hot, or I could add some ginger in there, or garlic also.

Brendan [00:33:00]: What's your experience of the soup, how would you describe it?

John [00:33:04]: I mean I've never tasted anything like it, I've never been anywhere that makes anything like it because I've been raw now for 22 years and I just try to maximize my nutritional intake. To me that's like a salad with a really thick sauce that it's just swimming in ... And a lot of different ingredients in there that makes the texture. I mean I could also put like zucchini noodles in there too. There's a lot of cool textures in there and it's just savory. I could put taco seasoning in there one night. I could put curry season the next night. I could put a pizza seasoning to make it go Italian. I could maybe do more like Asian spices and stuff in there for an Asian flare. I always make it different.

Brendan [00:33:49]: That sounds fun, I've never tried raw soups where you're getting creative on the seasoning and so forth. You've got a recipe you could share with us? Is that posted on YouTube?

John [00:34:02]: I do have a video actually on making raw soups on my YouTube channel. Actually instead of just giving you a recipe, I teach you the concepts behind how I made that recipe and how you could make your own recipes, not based around peppers but sometimes I have a lot of cucumber or I have a lot of celery, or I have a lot of carrots and then I make my soup base around that vegetable instead of peppers that some times of the year I can't get them for super cheap so I'm using carrots because they're a lot less expensive.

Brendan [00:34:30]: Wild. Back to these juicers here, on the horizontal Omega juicer, is there also any coupon on that as well ... or what was it, is it $329 or $229?

John [00:34:46]: This [NC800] is $329 over on this side yeah...

Brendan [00:34:49]: And the other one was?

John [00:34:51]: $399. So for this guy [NC800] you could use a coupon code "YOUTUBE" all capitals, that's good for 15 dollars off.

Brendan [00:35:00]: Okay. So those are the two main juicers that you offer, or are there any others that we should ...

John [00:35:09]: I sell all the main brands that have good customer service. I mean another one I could pull out here ... I have it right here...

Brendan [00:35:18]: That's a beast.

John [00:35:19]: Yeah, this is if you want the top of the line juicer out there, this is the one you're going to want to get. When somebody asks John "I want to get the juicer that makes the highest yield on root vegetables and leafy greens when juicing them together, and I want to get the highest nutritional quality juice". This is actually called The Green Star Pro, it's actually similar to the Green Star Elite. But the Pro model has actually all stainless steel gears and unlike an auger juicer... this [VSJ843] is a vertical auger, this [NC800] is a horizontal auger. This [Green Star Pro] is actually a twin gear juicer. If you take this apart here you can see this is like really worth the money right here. These are two twin gears and they basically just run around in the machine, kind of like gears in a transmission and you're putting the produce into these and it's grating it up, it grinds it up a little and then the second and third step is it actually mixes and then presses or squeezes out the juice. This by far is the most efficient, I mean I own this machine, but I don't regularly use it because it actually does take longer to use, and it does have more parts to clean. But some people ... I'm a really busy guy, I've got lots of things. I mean I planted out a 108 lettuce starts in my garden, half of which were red and half were green, and I had to prepare soil and make soil to amend my beds and I had to do this call, and I have to work my business, and I have to do a lot of other stuff, make my food. So I don't have the time to do this. I either do this [VSJ843] or I wouldn't do it at all because it's a lot easier.

But some people just want to get the maximum. Some people might live in South Florida. I was just out in South Florida actually recently, but produce prices down there are insane. I got really good produce prices here in the West Coast, but if I lived in South Florida I'd probably take the time to use this machine [Green Star Pro] because the produce prices are ... I wouldn't say not quite double, but it's getting quite expensive down there. I was really amazed, but yeah this one will get a higher yield, so you're not going to be ... basically your pulp is going to come out drier and you're going to have a higher quality juice with more nutrition overall based on testing I've seen.

Brendan [00:37:32]: Is the reason that the produce prices are so high there ... is that because of the storms? Did they wipe out a lot of production this year, or is it just ... that's how it is in Florida?

John [00:37:43]: I mean every time I go to Florida it's more expensive. For example Costco... this is my benchmark. Costco here in West Coast ... 10 pounds of organic carrots is $4.99, and 10 pounds of the same brand carrots in South Florida were $7.99. Like three dollars more for driving the truck across the country. And in other places I've been ... like Chicago it might be $5.49 or something like that, but $7.99 that's insane. Maybe they just charge people more because they know they can because it's all the rich New Yorkers that go down there, South Florida. I don't know.

Brendan [00:38:24]: I guess I'm sold on ... I like that one [Green Star Pro]. I would love to get one of those. I'm not going to be able to buy one tonight, but I like the idea of squeezing it dry and having it be a process that preserves all the nutrients. It's not overheating it. I'm curious, when you say "auger" what does that mean exactly... is that a...?

John [00:38:54]: So this [NC100] is an auger juicer here, the Omega. This is just racially a single auger, you can see this auger is just plastic. So this plastic auger... basically you put the produce in here, and this is kind of like an old fashioned meat grinder. It goes in there, and this is rotating around, and as it rotates around... the space between the auger gets smaller and smaller so that it's crushed and then squeezed up and then the juice comes out during this last stage here. So that's a single auger.

But then on this guy [Green Star Pro], this is actually a dual gear, so it's a bit different than the auger. Unlike the auger, what's basically grinding things up... this gear, right when you put it in there, the produce literally goes between these two gears, and that's another con of this juicer, if you try to push a carrot in here, you do need to have some downward force. And so people that are elderly or old, or are getting arthritis and don't have good strength -- it might be more difficult to use this machine. But this basically just grinds up the produce in between the gear, and because it's grinding up the produce it's a bit more efficient in grinding it up and opening all the cell walls. Whereas the auger doesn't quite do as an effective job and the pulp will be maybe a little bit larger particle size **[00:40:00]** and not get as much juice out of them.

Brendan [00:40:03]: What's the cost of that Green Star Pro?

John [00:40:05]: So this Green Star Pro... this is a commercial model actually, with commercial electric certification. It's pending commercial NSF equivalent certification. This was actually $795. This is probably one of the most expensive juicers. But it also comes with a fifteen year warranty so you just don't have to worry about it.

But if you want to get the model that's like this, it's actually called The Green Star Elite. It looks identical. The gears instead of being all stainless, are stainless here and then plastic on the bottom. That model would be only $549. And basically the yield would be the same. There's about ten things that are different with this commercial one than with the household one. But I really like the stainless steel gears because one of the challenges I've seen with the gears over time... my friend has owned one of these for I don't know ... fifteen years, and the plastic on the gears will tend to get worn, chipped, cracked overtime, but that would never happen with this guy.

Brendan [00:41:03]: Okay, that makes sense.

John [00:41:05]: And I do have a video showing the ten things that are different with this one rather than the home version, the Elite model. But that thing's like 250 dollars less. I mean if you've got money, if you're going to get a juicer and it's going to be like one of those one-time investment things, I would get the right one the first time. This one actually has an improved motor cooling over the standard unit, but otherwise all the parts, even the gears are actually interchangeable. If you want to get the gears to upgrade your Elite, the gear set alone is about 200 dollars, that pretty much makes up the difference.

Brendan [00:41:43]: Is there any price break on that one right now?

John [00:41:46]: Yeah I mean, you could also use the coupon code "SAVE30" for the thirty dollar discount on this guy also.

Brendan [00:41:54]: Got it. So let's review those coupon codes, for the vertical auger Omega [VSJ843] what was the coupon code to get 30 dollars off of that?

John [00:42:04]: Yeah this is "SAVE30" and that's the same coupon code you could use for the Green Star Pro or the Green Star Elite. And then the 15 dollar off coupon code for the Omega NC800 is "YOUTUBE" all capitals.

Brendan [00:42:23]: Okay, I'll just write "YOUTUBE". Okay, awesome. Thank you John, thank you for this introduction. And now I'm hungry, I'm going to make some ... I don't know if I have anything quite as exciting as all that, but I do have some soy miso. It's that ... I don't know how to pronounce it... it starts with a "D", do you know what I'm talking about? I just got introduced to this recently, it's supposed to be a great probiotic. Dargene something. I don't know. So I've got that, I've got some scallions, I like the green parts raw.

John [00:43:12]: Oh yeah.

Brendan [00:43:13]: And what else do I have? Prompt me here. What do I need to look for? I do have an onion, I think though that with yellow and white onions I do much better if they're cooked, they're a little harsh for me raw. Anyway, I'll figure something out. Blend it up with some nuts in my overly fast Blendtec, which is better than not eating anything.

John [00:43:39]: It'd probably be better to juice some cucumbers, celery, or carrots to make the juice and then use that and then stir in the miso. Mix all the miso in but it will kind of dissolve so now you'll have a miso-base soup with your vegetable juice as the base, and then chop up your scallions and put other chopped up vegetables in there for like a nice little raw soup without blending.

Brendan [00:44:04]: Yeah, if I want it to be creamy with nuts... say I throw in some Brazil nuts, pecans, whatever, macadamia nuts ... that's what I've got on me now. I would throw those in at what point?

John [00:44:16]: Yeah, so if you want to do that, then you'd actually... what I would do is I would only blend half of the juice you made with all the nuts, and then I would actually blend that really well and once it's blended I would pour in the rest of the juice and mix it up by hand so that you're not oxidizing half the juice at least, because you don't have a vacuum blender yet. The other thing you could do that's really smart is you could actually make a nut butter first with your nuts. Turn it into a nice butter and once you've got the butter you could take the butter and mix it into the juice by hand. It might take a little bit of mixing power, but once you have it into a nut butter it's going to mix up easier into the juice so that you actually don't have to blend the juice and lose some of the viable phytonutrients from the juice. But then you're blending the nuts at high speed which then may cause some fast oxidizing. So that's why I only like vacuum blending, and it's worthwhile to look into it and invest in one if you have the money.

Brendan [00:45:09]: What do you think is the best way to create nut butter? Are there any slow nut butter grinders maybe that specialize in that, it seems to me that would be the way to go if you can.

John [00:45:18]: So two things: number one, I actually do have a video where I use one of the vacuum blenders to make the nut butter. It turned out amazing, because the thing is that when you blend fat... this is the other thing I didn't talk about... when you blend fats in the vacuum blender, it makes it more fluffy. I made amazing ... basically it was cacao, honey, avocado, coconut water, coconut meat, vanilla meat and dates, like a mousse in a standard blender and I did it in a vacuum blender. And the vacuum blender came out like really fluffy, it was amazing. But any fats you blend in the vacuum blender will be a lot more fluffy and better, and plus because you're blending it in a virtually oxygen free environment, you're not going to get the problems with rancidity and oxidizing some of the fats or the nutrients in the nuts.

That being said, all of these machines here... actually the slow juicers will make nut butters. Roasted peanuts are easy, put the roasted peanuts in, you get basically peanut butter out. Now if you're doing raw nuts that can be more challenging because in raw nuts there's two factors working against you. One is that they don't generally have as high of a fat content, because if they're roasting the nuts, generally they roast them in oil and when they roast them in some oil, the nuts absorb more oil. So when you put them through the machine they come out more creamy and they stick together better, they solidify better or whatever. And the other thing is when they roast them, that takes down the moisture level even lower, so when you do raw nuts, it has a higher moisture level and not as much fat.

So if I put raw almonds through here, this will make a nut flour, which is still good. And then actually if you just keep putting that nut flour through about a couple of five times, it'll finally start to congeal together but it won't look like that nut butter you get at the store. If you want to get it to look like that nut butter, they you're going to add some additional oil to your nut butter. I personally don't like to do that, I would just... pretty much usually if I use nuts, I end up blending the nuts anyways, so I just put those in my vacuum blender when I blend whole nuts because it's a lot cheaper to buy whole nuts than premade nut butter. And they're probably made at high temperature, high speed, when they're doing whatever they do to make the nut butter, when you buy it from the store.

Brendan [00:47:33]: Have you heard of the Philosopher's Stoneground nut butters?

John [00:47:38]: Some of the best stuff. I love those guys. I interviewed them at the Heirloom expo.

Brendan [00:47:42]: How cool.

John [00:47:43]: Yeah, and that's awesome because what they do actually... they take it to the next level. They actually soak the nuts, start to sprout them, they dehydrate them, then they're down to a low moisture content, then they turn them into nut butter. That stuff is so tasty, so delicious.

Brendan [00:47:57]: Yeah it is.

John [00:47:58]: It's just so expensive too.

Brendan [00:48:00]: Fortunately every time I see Tim at a conference he gives me some samples. [Laughs]

John [00:48:05]: That's great.

Brendan [00:48:06]: That's awesome. I don't know if you've ever tried this but I put some of his nut butter on some sauerkraut.

John [00:48:16]: Oh wow, I have to try that one.

Brendan [00:48:17]: It's awesome!

John [00:48:18]: Oh my God, I've never tried nut butter and sauerkraut. Except to the extent that I actually put sauerkraut and nuts in my blended soup, make a little batter, and then it's all congealed together with other flavors, but not just those two.

Brendan [00:48:33]: Yeah, it was quite interesting because almonds are sweet, and then the tangy from the sauerkraut. Anyway. Right on. Thank you so much this has been an inspiration and an education and thanks for the coupons. For anybody watching this, is there a time limit on these coupons, or is it just sort of anybody that happens to hear it, they can use it for themselves?

John [00:49:05]: Yeah those are ongoing coupons at this time, but they may expire at any time so use them as soon as possible.

Brendan [00:49:12]: Exactly. Okay, very good. Thanks again John, have a great night. I really appreciate your time and your talents and wisdom.

John [00:49:20]: Great, thank you.

Joseph Mercola, DO
Fat for Fuel: Live Long and Healthy with Mitochondrial Metabolic Therapy (Part 2)

Brendan [00:03]: Dr. Mercola, one of the other questions I've been wanting to ask you is about fat from meat. You know, there's the saturated fat issue and others, and there's labeling. We've got grass-fed meat, we've got what they call grass-finished, and what's the difference?

Dr. Mercola [00:23]: Well, ideally the certification for grass-fed should signify or represent what pastured animals have done historically, which is just eat pasture, grass and that's it. Nothing else. They were never designed to be given these grains which change the composition of the fats in their body and also diminish their health. I don't know if most people watching this are aware, but when I've visited some of these farms, like Will Harris's farm, most of these CAFO cattle that are raised, I mean they have life expectancies of literally a few years, four, five, six years, that's it. That's how long they live and they die when they're given these types of diets, and when the normal life expectancy of a cow is like closer to 20 or 30 years.

Brendan [01:20]: I had no idea.

Dr. Mercola [01:22]: Yeah, it radically reduces their lifespan, and it's just, it's almost criminal what they're doing, but they're getting away with it, and it does work. I mean, it creates meat that you can eat. It's not necessarily healthy, but it does create meat, and people seem to enjoy it. So, it's a bastardization, really, of the labeling system to call it grass-fed. And I'm not sure what the exact status of the labeling laws are now, but I believe it's still legal to deceptively label a meat as grass-fed even if it was given grass anytime in their life. And almost all calves are raised on grass. I mean, that's just natural. Even CAFO cattle, they're raised on grass. So the problem becomes when they finish them, they put them to the slaughterhouses and the feeding lots, and they give them all these grains that are, literally, industrial. They're contaminated with herbicides and they're given, of course, growth hormones, typically, and antibiotics and pesticides. And of course most people know that 80% of the antibiotics used in the United States are used in animals, they're not used in humans. So that's likely where you're going to get a dose of antibiotics. Not only antibiotics, but more importantly antibiotic-resistant bacteria, which are a significant source of food poisoning in the United States every year. So you've got to be careful. That's a real good incentive to eat clean and be really diligent in your process of identifying healthy meats. I personally don't think, unless you absolutely know the owner and the infrastructure behind the restaurant, that it's wise to ever eat meat at a restaurant, unless you're sure. And it's, "So what am I going to do?" Well, it's easy. You can still have animal protein. It's so simple. And I travel a lot. I travel at least once or twice a month. And they make these things called sardines.

Dr. Mercola [03:36]: You can put them in your luggage. Now if you put them in your carry-on, I just want to warn you that you will be screened. You'll be patted down. So you have to proactively take the sardines out because they'll think it's a bomb or something. So, instead they let this run through the scanner, and they'll do that separately. But this way you don't get slowed down. But you can bring your sardines. Like I'm traveling to Boston tomorrow. I'll be bringing two cans of sardines. I'll put them in the tray before and they'll check that, and everything will be fine. And I have a source of protein, clean healthy protein, and, even better, DHA. So you get both of those, and it's a lot less expensive, too. So I've got my protein source right there. Healthiest protein you can get. So you don't have to … you know, I think that's where most people screw up, they screw up in the restaurants. And it's just that, "Well, I mean, now, we're celebrating, you know, I can have …" No, you can't! You know, you're not someone special. I'm not someone special. Biology doesn't respect any—if it's bad for you, it's bad for you, whether it's in a restaurant or in your home. So don't be deluded into thinking just because it's in a restaurant, you're okay to eat it. You're not. I was lecturing in New Jersey last month, and, with a bunch of the speakers, we went out for dinners afterwards. And one of the other speakers was reflecting on the menu and said, "Oh, organic salmon!" And I saw that, about laughed out loud. I said, "Organic salmon. Organic salmon!" So I asked the waiter, "How are they going to get that salmon organic?" And he said, "I don't know." "So then, ask your manager." He goes in the back, asks the manager, and the manager says, "Oh, it's farm-raised."

Dr. Mercola [05:15]: Which brings up another point. There's no law. There's no regulations that require restaurants to be honest. They can lie to you, and they will never have any repercussions. You can't trust what's on there. Now I'm not saying this is true for all restaurants, but certainly for a significant percentage, especially when it comes to seafood. They can blatantly, outright lie. There's a lot of substitution. There's a great book called *Real Food, Fake Food* by Larry Olmsted which goes into this in great detail. The more expensive the fish, the more likely it is to be substituted, and completely different from what they said, some inferior, less expensive primarily, potentially even more toxic. It certainly was the case for the salmon. They were using cheap, farm-raised salmon and selling it as organic salmon. So that was probably the worst thing on the menu for most people, and people thought it was the best.

Brendan [05:15]: Right.

Dr. Mercola [06:12]: So, and that just makes me livid because most people want to do the right thing. They want to eat healthy, they want to do … but you've got to dive deep and know the details, otherwise you're going to make bad choices, and not intentionally.

Brendan [06:29]: Right. You know, we've got all this junk meat in our food supply and junk oils and so forth. And how did all this come about? Because if you look back, if food is the cause of so many of our ailments, and if you look back 100 years, so many of our illnesses, cancer, heart disease, diabetes and so forth, obesity, were rare. And so, was our food supply different? Then what changed? What changed our food supply?

Dr. Mercola [07:02]: Well, it's the industrialization of the food supply which started pretty much at the beginning of the 20th century, probably a little bit before then, but that's when most of it started. The ability to inexpensively process foods in large quantities to lower the price and make it less expensive and more affordable and more convenient for individuals. And then of course to deliver it, the infrastructure to do that, so now we can have food that we were never designed to eat out of season, which you can have pretty much any day of the year. So that's another part of the problem is to eat seasonally, because your body doesn't understand that. I don't think you should ever eat fruit that's really grown out of season, or rarely ever eat it. I think fruit can be a real problem. Gundry has a problem with it in his Plant Paradox, especially for people initially.

Dr. Mercola [07:48]: And I think it should be avoided for most, until you're metabolically flexible, and then even be careful with it. But if you're going to eat it, it needs to be ideally picked from your backyard. And most people live in a climate—even if it's, like in Chicago—you can get fruit maybe two, three months out of the year out there. You know I live in Florida, so I pretty much have fruit at least nine months out of the year, I can harvest it. But it's a seasonally appropriate fruit. It's only grown when the climate allows it to so that it's in synchronization with my biology, so it's less likely to cause metabolic harm and damage. And of course if it's grown here on my property it's not contaminated with some of these typical pesticides.

Dr. Mercola [08:48]: Although people make an argument about geoengineering and spraying aluminum silicates down on everything in the rain and glyphosate being deposited, too. But, you know, there are strategies that we talked about in the other episode that you can do with, like Biosil, which is sort of a silicic acid which helps remove some of the aluminum. And if you're eating clean, I eat a lot of food from my yard, and I still check myself for glyphosate. I have no glyphosate. So I know there's glyphosate in the rain and it's kind of hard. Unless you're growing in a greenhouse, you're going to have some exposure, but it's relatively limited, and your body, if you're healthy, can compensate for that.

Brendan [09:20]: But wasn't there also a shift? I mean, there was a shift in macronutrient ratios in our diets, and the food pyramid has been something that played a role, didn't it? How did that come about?

Dr. Mercola [09:34]: Well, Ancel Keys started the process in the middle of the 20th century and started the low fat diet myth, which was a result of observation of the epidemic of heart disease in the first half of the 20th century. And he vilified saturated fat, when in fact the villain was industrially processed vegetable oils and trans-fat that was causing the damage, not the saturated fat. So saturated fat got eliminated, which meant a reduction in the animal products, which in some cases was good because people were eating too much meat, especially industrial processed meat. But they substituted these vegetable oils and carbohydrates. Not just carbohydrates, but industrially processed carbohydrates—they're even worse. So it was a prescription for disaster, and the results were absolutely predictable, and we're still experiencing a good portion of those results.

Dr. Mercola [10:23]: When you make these substitutions, you veer away from naturally optimized food choices, you're going to have metabolic aberrations that result in the pathology that you're seeing, this massive epidemic of chronic degenerative diseases. So, no surprise. And the beautiful thing is that when you shift your diet back to something like we discuss in *Fat for Fuel* or *The Plant Paradox*, which are pretty similar, which, also *The Plant Paradox* integrates the complexity of eliminating lectin exposure, which if you're following *Fat for Fuel*, you're pretty much doing. Just pay a little careful attention to some minor plant aberrations like cucumbers, which have seeds and lectins, and chia seeds, which have lectins. But for the most part *Fat for Fuel* and his book are pretty similar. But it's a really powerful strategy. When you do this and you optimize the food that you're designed—the fuel that your body's going to run on, you just get healthy.

Dr. Mercola [11:24]: That's what your body wants to do. You give it the right fuel, stay away from toxins—and that includes electromagnetic toxins and photobiological toxins—and essentially get enough sleep and movement—not exercise, but movement. Then your body goes in one direction. Almost invariably, it goes to health, because you're giving it what it needs, the fundamental building blocks of health. You're not going to go to disease, because you can't have both. You can't have disease and health at the same time. You're going to either be healthy, or you're going to be diseased. So when you move towards health, the disease disappears. So if your goal is health, you don't even have to worry about preventing disease because you're doing it. You're optimizing these systems that will essentially eliminate almost all the risks for these degenerative diseases. People concerned. "Well, I've got the genetic risk factor for cancer or breast cancer. " Well, it's not the genes that are the issue, it's the expression of the genes. And the expression of genes are epigenetically regulated largely by lifestyle and diet. 90% of the human genome was previously classified as junk DNA, which is actually microRNA and these long non-coding RNA sections, which are epigenetic regulators of the genes.

Dr. Mercola [12:39]: So it's the genetic expression that's the issue. It's not the gene. And you can do that with your lives. You can turn your whole life around by optimizing the food you're eating and paying attention to these mitochondrial biohacks which improve mitochondrial function and optimize your health.

Brendan [12:55]: A lot of us are taking supplements to try to make up for what's not in our food or at least in our diet. You mentioned antioxidants in your book, something that's kind of counterintuitive about them. I'm curious if you can say more about that.

Dr. Mercola [13:15]: Denham Harman literally 50 years ago developed this oxidative stress theory of aging. And that's excessive oxidative exposure to our environment that catalyzes the aging process. And that was well-accepted for a long time. As a result of that, there was an embracing of the concept that—well, oxidation, so yes, let's take a lot of antioxidants like vitamin C and Vitamin E and lipoic acid and a whole variety of others. So the problem with that is, that theory has been revised over time, and now it's come to ... the subtlety is that it's not oxidative stress that's the problem. It's excessive oxidative stress because you need some oxidative stress. Just like exercise, right? Or hormetic stresses from these polyphenols. You need some stress. It actually is healthy for you, and without the stress you'd be dead. So you need some. It's when you have excessive stress that it's a problem. And how do you get excessive reactive oxygen species? Well, you burn the wrong fuel as your primary fuel. Most people burn glucose, and that's far more inefficient, somewhere between 30-50% more inefficient. By inefficient, I mean that when you burn it, you generate these artifacts—pollution, essentially—called reactive oxygen species, and you make 30-50% more when you're burning glucose than you do from these water-soluble fats called ketones. And when you have excess reactive oxygen species, that causes a free radical, which is a molecule with an unpaired electron, which decimates mitochondrial and nuclear cell membranes, proteins and DNA, which causes mitochondrial dysfunction, genetic abnormalities, and really the source of why we get sick.

Dr. Mercola [15:07]: So you want to make sure that's optimized. You can actually be counterproductive to take excessive antioxidants. Not that they're bad, or they can't be used targeted like a rifle. I certainly use them. But it's important to know that supplements are just that—they're supplements. They're not a magic bullet. They're an addition to a sound dietary strategy and lifestyle practice.

Brendan [15:36]: Got it. So, we want to take in healthy fats, and we want to eliminate unhealthy fats as much as possible. One of my favorite fats is avocados, and it gets expensive, especially if I'm eating several a day. I'm just curious, any thoughts on ways to make high quality fat more affordable? I mean, granted it does have a high calorie density, so actually, as a food, it's probably the least expensive, I'm guessing, to put more of in your diet overall, but I don't know.

Dr. Mercola [16:07]: Well, I don't know. It can be pricy. I was just in an interview with an Australian blogger last week, and she was telling me organic avocados are like $8 apiece. So that's really …

Brendan [16:07]: Where? Australia?

Dr. Mercola [16:18]: Australia, yeah. So let me tell you, first of all, the basics here to cut your costs down significantly because, avocados—I couldn't agree more, they're probably one of the healthiest foods I know of. Probably avocados, egg yolks, sardines would be the top three health foods that I know of. I mean foods— a source of nourishment. The big thing for avocados is they have lots of potassium, much more than bananas, and they will optimize your sodium-to-potassium ratio in the right direction.

Dr. Mercola [16:55]: I typically have one to three avocados a day. First of all, it's important to know, you don't need to buy organic avocados. We've done the tests. We've sent them out to the labs. There's no difference in pesticide content between organic and non-organic avocados, so that will save you a bundle. Secondly, you wait until they go on sale. Most grocery stores put them on sale as a loss leader. And then once they're on sale you buy as many as you're going to need for the next month, which could be 30 to 50 to 70, you know, you figure it out. And the key is to buy them rock hard and green. Really rock—I mean, you've got to be able to throw it at a window and it'd break. But then when you bring it home, put it in the refrigerator. And the key here is to take it out three days before you're going to use it because it takes about that long for it to ripen outside of the refrigerator. But it will last about a month in your refrigerator. So it's a really good key to optimize your budget on healthy foods.

Brendan [18:00]: Excellent. Can you share any other really hot tips on how to how to go ketogenic or how to make this all work?

Dr. Mercola [18:09]: Well, one of the other snack foods because people obviously like snacks, and I think it's an important part of the diet. Well, intermittent fasting is another useful tool, too, so try to limit your window of eating to 6 or 8 hours a day, so that would mean for 16 to 18 hours you're not eating. You're fasting. It's called intermittent fasting, and I pretty much do that on a daily basis. I think it's a rational strategy, meaning, you don't have to do it every day, but most every day it's a pretty sound challenge, especially when you're optimized weight, because it's really hard to go do a regular fast for much longer without losing weight.

Dr. Mercola [18:48]: You don't want to lose weight when you're at optimal weight, or optimal lean body mass would be more accurate. So macadamia nuts are really useful. The challenge there, of course, they're pricey. They can be about $20 a pound. The key here is that usually if you're doing the *Fat for Fuel* approach, likely and hopefully it's not just you, it's someone you know, a relative or a friend or several people, and if that's the case it's even better because you can pitch in and you go to nuts.com and you can find macadamia that you buy, for five pounds it's like $20 a pound or $19 a pound, but if you buy them in 25 pounds, it goes down to $13 a pound. So you're saving … that's a pretty significant reduction. And it's not like you're not going to go through them. I literally order 25 pounds every few months.

Dr. Mercola [19:42]: I mean I order at least four times a year, maybe five or six times a year. Probably every two months I order it, and I'm just eating it for myself. So I have a lot of macadamia nuts. I enjoy them. In fact, that reminds me, I haven't eaten some today because I'm in a different location. For those of you who are watching and not used to seeing this background in my house, it's because my desktop computer broke, and I'm coming to you through my notebook computer. And that's where my macadamia nuts are, in my desk in my office. So I forgot about it today. But that's a good tip, macadamia nuts, because that could be a significant … that can actually be up to half your calorie intake.

Brendan [19:42]: Just from, you mean, from macadamias alone, is that what you're saying?

Dr. Mercola [20:31]: Yeah. Yeah, and it's a healthy source. It's the healthiest nut. Why? Because it has relatively low carbohydrates. It's the lowest carbohydrate nut on the market. Well, one of the lowest. There's some exotic ones that cost twice as much that are even better, but not much. And then you've got— it's the lowest protein, too. Remember, the high protein is not something you want to go. And then it also has the highest fat and the fat is really beneficial. The primary fatty acid is oleic acid, which is the beneficial fat in olive oil, so it's a high monounsaturated fat. You got a little bit of omega-3 and omega-6 in there, but it's primarily monounsaturates. So it's a healthy, healthy source of fat. Most people I know like macadamia nuts. I would not get them roasted, which is a process, and I would not get them salted. Just get them raw—raw macadamia nuts.

Brendan [21:26]: How are they on phytates and lectins?

Dr. Mercola [21:26]: They're virtually lectin-free.

Brendan [21:32]: Oh Wow. Cause that's rare for a nut, isn't it?

Dr. Mercola [21:41]: Some nuts. No, there's actually … most of the nuts are okay. Some are better than others, but macadamias and pecans are fine. They're absolutely not a problem in *The Plant Paradox* lectin approach. The nut that is really not a nut, but it's a legume, which are lectin-loaded would be peanuts. So you can stay away from peanuts. And a common one that many, many health people don't get is cashews. Cashews are the worst, cashews and peanuts. So stay away from those. Those are lectin-loaded. Some of these lectins in legumes you can destroy by using a pressure cooker. I don't know that you can do that with the nuts.

Brendan [21:41]: How about Brazil nuts?

Dr. Mercola [22:23]: Brazil nuts are okay in small amounts. No, no. You shouldn't have like more than two or three a day anyway.

Brendan [22:23]: Oh yeah? And why is that?

Dr. Mercola [22:31]: That's all you need. That probably gives you the RDA for selenium, if those Brazil nuts were grown in healthy soil. That's probably why you want to get organic Brazil nuts, because if they were industrially grown and the soil was selenium-depleted, there's not going to be a lot of selenium in there. But most clinicians who are testing for selenium find that people who are getting Brazil nuts are on a sound foundation. Selenium is really important. I mean, you really need to eat Brazil nuts pretty much every day, two or three. or take a supplement. You know, I take a supplement just because it's easier. You definitely need selenium. Almost everyone watching this needs selenium in some form—food form or a supplement.

Brendan [23:16]: Well, thank you for making this approach more accessible and giving us some tips and spending this time with us today.

Dr. Mercola [23:24]: I'm happy to do that and give people some tools and resources they can use to stay healthy because that's what it's all about. You know, identifying simple strategies that don't cost a lot, that can literally turn your life and your health around. So thanks for the opportunity.

Graeme Sait Bonus Conversation
Minerals, Microbes, and Reversing Climate Change in a Golden Era for Food
(Conversation After Interview)

Brendan (00.00.00): So, you mentioned that you are doing a multi-enterprise farm, or two farms. You've got fifty enterprises. Tell me a little bit about them, like what are you growing with fifty enterprises? I guess these are all economically producing, enterprise different crops and so forth?

Graeme (00.00.17): Yes, what I'm trying to demonstrate is that what I am seeing globally, is a move away from this model of getting bigger or get out. Because, you know what we see if people get more and more efficient, you can't get any more efficient, and they're are still not making money, and they're still not having fun in the most important of all professions. So, what we are seeing is this model, and part of it has been driven by the phenomenon in farmers' markets and in my little region here, there are 400 000 people on the Sunshine Coast, there are 69 farmers' markets, some of which attract like 10 000 people on a four-hour period. So, that's a chance for people to put a face to their food, and as you said the hugely important things of making choices, your wallet becomes one of the most expensive change tools, because wherever you put your money, interest flows. If you buy food from people that are doing it right others farmers say, "Well why are they going to this store? Well, I better change the way I do things!" And you've inspired that change. And that's why that whole argument of yours is so hugely important in that context.

But back to the farms, so I want to demonstrate on these two farms. So I've got one that is three and a half hours from the Sunshine cost where I am based, up in the only area where it gets really cold, because most of the world has four seasons, and the subtropics down here doesn't. And so it snows up in this area called Stanthorpe, and it is 1500m up. So that's perfect because I can demonstrate all of these models in a temperate climate and in a subtropical climate. But the concept is to have many eggs in your basket, and it makes it much more fun. You know we've got to bring back some young people. We've got to get them passionate about growing. And young people don't get, aren't going to get passionate about monoculture and chemicals, that whole model. The current age of farmers in your country is 65, and in our country is 62, who is going to produce the food if we can't bring passion back into our food production? When you start getting involved in direct marketing, you've got a sense of responsibility because you are responsible for the health of all those people you're selling to, you've got a sense of pride in the quality of what you produce, and it's not being just chucked in with everyone else's rubbish. And on the farm you want to have lots of interrelated enterprises. It's kind of like a permaculture, which permaculture is actually Australia's greatest intellectual export, and we are applying those principles through to farming. Saying, "OK this will dovetail with this, which will dovetail with this."

So, on this farm where I'm sitting at the moment in the office, we've got bees, quite a number of beehives. We've got commercial scale greenhouse where we are producing all sorts of plants including the seedlings for our various herbs and vegetables and fruit trees and so forth, that we are producing here. We've got worm composting. We teach people this whole new way to make their own worm composting units very inexpensively, and they are wonderfully effective. We've got lots of them. We've got conventional composting. We've got anaerobic composting. We've got a dragon fruit farm, really neat fruit high in antioxidants, delicious. And we've developed this technique where you put red lights around them and it triggers the flowering. And you can actually get three crops of this wonderful antioxidant food, and they grow at a hell of a pace down here at the tropics, subtropics. So we've got dragon fruits. We've got pawpaw. And you want to have crops with multiple earning potential, like papaws. You call them papayas. I mean you get crop virtually two crops a year. The leaf ... you know, listen, we talked about multiple income streams from one crop. The leaf is actually really very valuable because it is used as an anti-cancer tea now that many people are seeking. So you can sell just the leaf if you choose. Then the green fruit which takes half the time to ripen and actually has a higher dollar value than the red fruit, well the yellow fruit in your case. We like the red papaws over here. But the reason for the importance of that green fruit, and again there is another value-adding trick that I can add in here, but the greent fruit ... you know there is a whole theory of longevity and health based upon enzymes. The theory that comes from Professor Edward Howell is that we are born with a certain capacity to produce enzymes in our lifetime. So we have, we have you know digestive enzymes and metabolic enzymes. So enzymes, particularly the metabolic enzymes, govern everything we do. Every breath, every thought we make, every breath we take, sounds like a Sting song coming up. But you know our lymphatic system, our circulatory system, everything is governed by enzyme reactions, metabolic enzymes. And then we've got the most energy intensive process in the human body, which is digestion, governed by digestive enzymes. And so we have our liver and our pancreas particularly producing, you know protease and cellulase and amylase and lipase and so forth to digest fats and proteins and sugars and so forth. But, the finding is that we've got a limited capacity and it's actually genetically inherited, we've only got a certain bank account we can draw from. And if we start running out, this is Howell's theory, basically if we start running out, say because we cook all our meat, we run out of protease, and that will vary because of your genetic inheritance, on when you're gonna run out of it, but when you do there is all sorts of issues most commonly linked to inflammation, and inflammation is linked to every major disease, so that's a major major player.

So the deal if you go to Thailand and you eat a protein dish ... you eat fish, chicken or meat, or beef or whatever, you will always have or most commonly have a green papaya salad. And the reason for that is that papaw contains papain, and papain is more powerful as a protein digesting enzyme then protease. And so if you can take a food that's rich in something that's going to digest your cooked meat, then you're not going to draw from your own bank account and you're gonna live longer, 'cause how it works is that once you've exhausted protease, or cellulase or whatever, then you, because you can't, for that digestion nothing works, your metabolic enzymes are doing everything else can multitask so they come down and do digestion. But, whatever they were doing is not been done anymore. And that's when the wheels start falling off. Until enough wheels … and that's called degenerative illness according to Howell. It's a really compelling and quite well-supported theory. And so part of the reason you eat lacto-fermented foods, is that it contains the enzymes, so you're not going to draw from your own bank account. Part of the reason that raw food is such an amazing thing is that all food contains the enzymes, and the raw form contains the enzymes to help digest it.

So coleslaw contains enzymes to help digest it, whereas cooked cabbage doesn't, for example. So, the more cooked food you eat, the more enzymes you need to supplement with. And that's why eating fermented food gives you a little bit of that supplementation. Or, traditional wisdom. Why do the Asians eat green papaya salad? Because it's got 40 times, the green papaw has 40 times more papain than the ripe papaw. So, you just grate it up with a little bit of chilli and a little bit of coriander and a few other things with it. Delicious! Green papaya salad. And you don't draw from your own bank account, and you live longer. You don't suck your own protease. So it makes perfect sense. And that's why it's worth more money, because people are waking up to so many of these concepts.

So you got the green papaw, then you got the red papaw, which is delicious and sells in this country for $6 a kilo. You get two crops a year, so you don't wait around for 5 years for your fruit crop, you got it first season. Then, you can slice them, dehydrate it really simply, and it's really sought after because it's a delicious dry papaw which is now magnified. If it's the red one, it's got lycopene, which is now 4 times concentrated in the dry papaw, so it's kinda medicine for your prostate, lycopene is one of the most powerful nutrients for prostate health. And there it is in the red papaw, and not in the yellow, that's why we like the red one.

So you've got that income stream, which is real simple, a dehydrator, nothing to it, it's pretty easy to slice up a papaw. Then you've got the seeds, you've got hundreds of seeds in each plant, that you can so easily dry them in the sun and take 3 seeds, put them in a pot, you get three plants. Two of them will probably gonna be males, and then you take the one that is the least vigorous, which will be the female, a couple of months after you've put them in the ground, then you kill the two males, and leave your female, and that's how you plant papaws. You always have three plants together, but you can take from each fruit, and you get 50 fruit on a plant twice, from each fruit, you can make 300 seedlings for arguments sake, 200, 200 groups of seedlings which sell for $3. So do the sums. That's $600 per fruit. You know the income streams are limitless. You got 6 income streams on one plant that you can get the first yield on within 8 months. So that's, we've got a whole papaw plantation for example. Then we've got herbs. We've got these yacon, on the large scale. We've got berries. We've got up at the top farm, I've got almost every conceivable form of stone fruit. I've got a lot of garlic; we're growing garlic here. We've got a ginger plantation. We've got a turmeric plantation. Turmeric is just the most amazing thing. And if you grow it well, then the active ingredient curcumin, which is the most powerful anti-inflammatory yet discovered, is much more powerful ...

The thing is, you can say, "Oh blueberries are great. You know, I'm getting all these anthocyanins, and all these other beneficial compounds," but, the way you grow it, you can actually, some research in the UK, about 4 years ago, they actually found oranges, that they researched that had zero vitamin C. You think, I'm eating an orange. I am getting plenty. Well, maybe you are, maybe you're not. It depends on how that orange was grown. It depends on how the farmer produced that food. If you just chuck a bit of nitrogen in there, and that goes in with water, and dilutes everything, you can actually produce food that has no medicinal value. And that's why it's so important. We are what we eat, and what we eat comes from the soil. We need to change that soil, and we change the health of all of us. That's the bottom line.

Brendan (00.09.54): I can't wait to go out on the land myself, start growing. I don't have any land at the moment. But, you know, when we're growing our own food, typically we're not using nitrate fertilizer, and there's something that you talked about in the nutrition course, regarding nitrate fertilizer and what it does in the plants, and therefore what it does to our nutrition from those plants. I thought it was pretty profound.

Graeme (00.10.22): Yeah, it's not so much that nitrates are poison; it's just the balance. There are two forms of nitrogen. The ammonium form of nitrogen and the nitrate form. And the way that we fertilize in large chunks, you know with nitrogen in large amounts at one time, and so forth, much more than what the plant requires at that time. You're far better off for example to foliar spray nitrogen, than you are in many instances in particular urea and calcium nitrate are wonderful foliar sprays, particularly if you put some fulvic acid with them, to increase their uptake and improve their effect. But foliar fertilizing is 12 times more efficient. So you don't have to have all the leaching of nitrates and the outgassing of nitrous oxide, which is 310 times more thickening of the blankets. So it's a huge issue. Agriculture produces 80% of the nitrous oxide that thickens the blankets, traps the heat and changes our world. So, we can do that better. And that involves nitrogen management and understanding that, well a really important thing is the balance between those two forms of nitrogen within the plant. Not the soil, in the soil they need to be at equal parts per million. In the plant you need 3 parts ammonium to 1 part nitrate. And most foods that you buy, you buy cabbage at the supermarket and test it. It's 3 parts nitrate to 1 part ammonium, and that's 'cause of the way that we fertilize. Because we want to pump it up quick, and we put a whole heap of nitrates on there. We only got 50 cents for the cabbage and the supermarket sold it for $4. So we sort of, from consumers' point of view, we kind of, because we support that model, we kind of got what we deserve. We got a piece of toxic crap, because there is no debates about the link between nitrates and cancer. Professor Otto Walberg, won his Nobel Prize for identifying the root cause of cancer. And that hasn't changed. The root cause of cancer according to Otto is called anaerobism, and it's about the blood's incapacity to carry enough oxygen to satisfy the oxygen requirements of all of our cells. Now, what is nitrate? What's nitrate poisoning in animals, or what is nitrate poisoning in humans? Why are nitrates proven carcinogens? Because they reduce the blood's capacity to carry oxygen. And now everywhere, every waterway is filled with nitrates. Most plants you're eating have got far too high a nitrate component because we mismanage the fertilizer.

But the serious part from a nutrient density and medicinal point of view is that the nitrate form of nitrogen, if we've mismanaged it, doesn't mean we can't use it, but we've used it wrong most of the time. The nitrate form enters the plant with water, always, so high nitrates in a plant, which is almost every plant you test, if it is intensively grown, high nitrates means low everything else because the water that always carries nitrate nitrogen into the plant, dilutes everything else within the plant. Now what we use in the field, and I didn't answer your question because you touched upon it earlier, very, very simple little tool called a refractometer. Little sawn off telescope where you squeeze in a little bit of plant sap with a garlic crusher onto the sloping screen of this little sawn off telescope. And then the sun refracts through the dissolved solids that are found in the plant sap. You're measuring nutrient density. You're measuring dissolved solids. You are literally measuring your skills as a food producer, and it's called Brix levels. Now people are familiar with the testing the fruit and so forth, but we are talking here about the refractive index, it's called, of the leaf. It's about the plant itself, not its end product, because sometimes they don't even correlate. So Brix levels are referred to as not equivalent to Brix levels of the plant of the leaf, so, you can buy these tools for 50 or 60 dollars on eBay, and every home gardener should have one. You should be testing, simply, just taking one leaf at the markets and find out who is a good grower and who is not, who has high Brix levels 'cause high Brix levels are high nutrient density, which means the food is much more medicinal.

The higher the Brix level, the lower the need for chemical intervention there would not have been the same requirements for sprays with high Brix levels because that's how it works. The higher the Brix, the less insect pressure, the less disease pressure, the less chemical contamination of that food. So, it's just a simple way to say, what can I do to lift the Brix levels, to lift the quality, improve the resilience, reduce the chemical requirement and increase the medicinal quality and the shelf life and the flavor. See, the thing that amazes me that supermarkets have not more widely caught on … Woolworths in South Africa … I've trained all of their growers … and they launched something called "Farming for the Future", which is all about adopting these Nutrition Farming principles and producing this food. Well what Woolworths noted within the first 6 months was this huge increase in shelf life of their food. Because flavor and people flooding to the supermarkets to find food with forgotten flavors. People want some flavor back in their foods. And flavor, shelf life, the need for chemical intervention, the whole quality of the plant, all of that is the same thing. Basically, the better it tastes, the better it is for you. Your tastebuds are the perfect tool to govern, the sweeter it is and the better flavor, the more intense flavor. That's how you differentiate that junk celery, compared they look the same, one of them was pumped up with nitrogen and watered down, and the other one will have that intense flavor, and you'll know as soon as you taste them, there will be just this massive difference. And the flavor is nutrition, and nutrition is your health. And the best way you'll ever get healthy is to eat plants. If you got a vegetable garden, why I say that a vegetable garden is actually, without any argument at all, the most important wellness tool, everyone's got to have one ... is not just that you can grow it, you understand with the humus and the minerals, so you got this very very healthy produce, but more importantly, and this is actually a fact, more importantly you harvest directly before you're gonna eat. There is so little understanding of how much is lost during storage. You take a snow pea overnight, so you've picked it on the night, and it reached the supermarket the next day, which takes longer than that in actual fact, and it stores on the shelf much longer than a day, but overnight 50% of the vitamin C is gone. There is a tremendous loss of nutrition, as I say with shelf life, and you've got all the chemicals, 'cause, I know, I mean I work with growers all over the world. Tomatoes, you know, it's actually our favorite fruit, 'cause spaghetti has just been listed as Australia's favorite food. So we are using this tomato concentrate to make our spaghettis, of course. Tomatoes have three famous Australian pesticides, every three days, from the time they go in, till the time you push them over at the end. There's no way of knowing if that spaghetti is not horrifically contaminated, and no one's measuring it.

So, but if you've got your own garden, you can grow all of that stuff yourself without the chemicals with the nutrient density. But most importantly, you'd never pick it and leave it in the fridge and eat it the next day, you pick it 5 minutes before you're gonna eat it. I come home, drive up my drive, there's all these vegetable and herbs, and I pick what I'm gonna eat that night and take it up and eat it 10 to 15 minutes later. And that is nutrient density at its champagne level.

That is, that's the real joy of a garden. You taste food like you've never tasted it, fresh and at its most nutrient dense, and at its most medicinal. Then you've got a serious wellness tool in your home vegetable production.

Brendan (00.17.27): Wow. So let's say somebody has a patch of land, and they are gonna grow food, grow soil. They implement the best practices. They've got five species present from chenopods, grasses, cereals, legumes, brassicas. Did I miss one? Did I repeat one? Somewhere in there are 5. And so they are building soil ... what's the calculation, I don't know if there is calculation in there to call out, but how much soil might somebody, or rather how much carbon might somebody expect to capture in their soil and maybe store long-term? Like how many tons of carbon?

Graeme (00.18.10): Well, If you were to, if you were to say, put in some green manure crops whenever there is an opportunity. Add some compost into your programs. Maybe add one of these natural acids that are actually ... you make when you make compost, which are called humic and fulvic acid. But you can also extract them from brown coal, and they're just an incredibly powerful humus building tool and a soil life stimulant. They're probably the hottest things in agriculture, but the home gardeners have not yet discovered them. But if you were to bring in those sorts of practices, you know, reduce the amount of cultivation whenever you can, because every time you open the soil you lose some carbon. You can build 1%. You know it's not hard to build 1% a year. And we only need to, we only need to build 1.6 % globally. I understand how doable this is. 1.6% reverses climate change. So ...

Brendan (00.19.07): 1.6 % over how many billions of hectares? I just wanted to ...

Graeme (00.19.11): That's the whole, that's the global, we have to build … you know, we've gone from 5% down to 1.5% organic matter globally. That's the average, so we've got to build 1.6%. So say we're going to go to 3. If we can make 3% the global average, which is doable, and really, if you really, really got into it, and brought the army into it, and every person got into it, you can do it in 2 or 3 years. You can actually reverse the entire scenario.

Brendan (00.19.38): All of agricultural land worldwide, if everybody just got …

Graeme (00.19.39): Yes everybody, every park, every football field, every, you know all the potential for urban agriculture as Kiss the Ground and so forth are doing. You're taking vacant blocks and building humus on them. Even in pots on your veranda you could be building humus and sequestering humus. So it's a really, it's a neat equation. But we all can get involved, you know. And it's such a win-win scenario. 'Cause not only are you saving the day for this beautiful planet, but you are also contributing this amazing amount to your own health, so it's kind of the ultimate win-win scenario.

Brendan (00.20.11): Totally!

Graeme (00.20.14): Yeah. I'd better go and do some work now.

Brendan (20.15): Thank you so much for all your time. I really appreciate it. Thank you.

Graeme (20.18): Ok, it's a great pleasure. Talk to you again sometime.

Brendan (00.20.23): Yep, talk to you soon. Bye.

Graeme (00.20.24): Later buddy.

Eric Toensmeier Extended Conversation
Food Solutions to Climate Change from Project Drawdown
(Conversation After Presentation)

Brendan [00:00:00]: So, one of the first things sort of to give this all a context, there were three numbers you kept referring to for each solution. One was the model input, and that was tons of carbon per hectare, right?

Eric [00:00:17]: Yes, yes. Sequestration, measured in tons of carbon per hectare per year. Yep.

Brendan [00:00:19]: That was in the upper right. And then down below that, lower right, were three different scenarios, and that was gigatons of carbon sequestered in the 30-year period between 2020 and 2050.

Eric [00:00:36]: Yep. And also the million hectares of new adoption of the solution in each of those scenarios over that 30-year period.

Brendan [00:00:44]: Okay.

Eric [00:00:46]: I took another one out. I had another one in there that was the annual rate of sequestration in 2050, which is often what scientists will actually use to compare these to each other. They'll say, "Well, what's the annual…" Is it going to give me at least a gigaton a year by 2050? But it just makes it … Visually, it makes it even more crowded on those slides, so I took it out. I figured this is not the crowd that's going to yell at me if I don't have that in there. So, keep the visual part as uncrowded as possible was my goal for communication.

Brendan [00:01:27]: Okay, and could you…

Eric [00:00:46]: [inaudible] … on the Drawdown website and we also compare those projections… We compare our projections to benchmarks.

Brendan [00:01:35]: Okay.

Eric [00:01:36]: So, how does our managed grazing compare to the IPCC? Well, we're actually right in the … We're in it, but we're at the high end of it and so on. And those are usually based on the annual emissions reduction or sequestration.

Brendan [00:01:53]: Okay. And so, those numbers, those gigatons in those 30-year periods, we saw a lot in the teens to twenties of gigatons. And to give that perspective, we're at 402 and, of course, you've got to translate from tons of carbon to parts per million of carbon dioxide. So, if we're going to say we want to go … Let's say we want to go below 350 and below 300 even in parts per million of … And the reason I'm saying that is there's plenty of people who are very bullish about regenerative agriculture's potential to say, "Hey, we can go back to pre-industrial atmospheric carbon," which means below 300 and even a little further than that. But if we got below 300, we're probably going to be okay, but we have to do it fast. And the question is, okay, so that's between 300 and 402 … or 404, 405, where are we?

Eric [002:49]: It goes up and down. Yeah, we're a little over 400. It goes up and down with the season.

Brendan [00:02:53]: Yeah, okay. So, let's just say 402. So, we want to take down 100 parts per million in carbon dioxide. What does that translate to in gigatons of carbon …

Eric [003:07]: The challenge is it partly depends on what you think is happening with the rest of all those emissions. Are they continuing to increase? Are they going up or down? So, it turns out to be a complex question. Each part per million is equivalent to roughly two billion tons of carbon, and each ton of carbon is equivalent to 3.67 tons of carbon dioxide. So, you're looking at, what, maybe seven billion tons, seven gigatons of carbon dioxide per part per million. But it doesn't quite work as … some of them get absorbed by the ocean. There is also the natural emissions that come out of the land and ocean every year, which vary enormously from year to year. So, all of those are very complex and over my head. We have some folks on our team who understand that better than I do. Suffice it to say that I would be thrilled to see us achieve 350 parts per million. I'm skeptical about going back to 280 or 300 or whatever, reason being that we have a lot of land that's in things like buildings and roads and parking lots right now. So, if 280 parts per million is where we were before the dawn of agriculture and if we consider how much carbon there was then the maximum achievable, which is arguable but is what most people think… most scientists think, then we would somehow have to get back to a world that would look from space like the world did before agriculture in order to achieve that level, which would be difficult.

[004:57]: If, however, we can figure out some ways to hack saturation with practices like biochar, with building with wood, and so on, then maybe. Then maybe. I'm very open to those possibilities. I would love to see those things happen, but my personal take on things is probably, if we can achieve 350 parts per million, we would have done something absolutely phenomenal and we can pat ourselves on the back real well. If we can manage to do that, it would be a feat unprecedented in all of human history, a level of coordination never before seen by humanity. That's a plenty good goal for me, let's put it that way. I'm personally satisfied with that. I don't know what Drawdown would say, but that's my personal approach. And Drawdown found that by 2050, we're getting that impact on many of our solutions continue through 2100 and beyond. So, it's not as though that level is the only amount you're ever going to get, like solar will continue to go for a long, long, long time. Forest protection will continue to matter and so on, but… Some of the agricultural solutions will start to slow down at some point as the original land that was converted in 2020 starts to hit saturation after… we assume 30 years for saturation. So… But as new land continues to go to those … or really, as you upgrade. You start with conservation ag, you move to regenerative ag, then you start to add some whatever, you know, some agroforestry elements in there, and then you're going to start to integrate your livestock in. I think we can ratchet each piece of land up piece by piece over time. And we see people do that all the time. We see practitioners do that all the time. They continue to add more regenerative elements to their operation over time.

[006:54]: Just can we get enough people to do that fast enough is the real question. And that's where issues of finance come in, and policy issues come in, and the question of how do we assist farmers to make that transition is a very juicy question. I've spent a lot of time thinking about it, but a lot of people have spent a lot of time thinking about it, and there's a lot of things to show what does and doesn't work. If farmers are renting their land, then there's no incentive for them to do these things because to pay-off period ... You're really looking at three to four years before, let's say, managed grazing or regenerative ag or conservation ag start to bring you back to the level where you were when you started. And agroforestry perennial cropping solutions are more like seven to eight years as global average. So, we need to assist farmers to make that leap. We need to assist farmers to get through ... to get over that hump so they come out the other side and are, in fact, as profitable or more than when they started. But I've never met farmers anywhere in the world who have money to burn like that, who have money even to invest in production like that. So, it's on us as consumers and governments and buyers of those products, corporate buyers of those products and so on, to figure out how to assist people with the finance, with the learning, with access to the tools and equipment, and seeds they need to do these things, whether it's different breeds of livestock or solar-powered fencing or cover crop seed or no-till drills or whatever. There's all different kinds of things people need to get their hands on to do these things, figuring out the right species and the right spacing for silvopasture to make sense and so on.

[00:08:44]: There's many, many, many ways in which we need to organize civilizations to assist farmers to make this transition. Because even if we reduce emissions to zero tomorrow, like stop burning all fossil fuels and basically all civilizations stop tomorrow, we're still over the 350, which is the safe line at where to be for parts per million. So, we're still toast even if all emissions stop tomorrow. We can't get to where we want to be without drawing down that extra carbon and sequestering it. It can't be done. It can't be done without that. And there isn't enough land to reforest and still have food. We have to do it on land. We can't do it without farmers. We can't mitigate climate change without agriculture. Only agriculture isn't enough to do it, but we can't do it without it. It's an essential part of the balanced breakfast of climate change mitigation.

Brendan [00:09:38]: Yeah. I mean, you made a couple of really good points. And so Graeme Sait, Nutri-Tech Solutions in Australia, the person whose course started Ryland Engelhart and Finian Makepeace on their journey with this incredible organization called Kiss the Ground. And then, you know, I visited Graeme and took his course in 2015. It was amazing! And you know what he repeatedly says is farmers are the most important people in the world. They are. They always have been. So, that's how he puts it, and we need to really get that that is important, and that's true in so many ways. And why not become a farmer, because farmers ... you know, another person says something about farmers. Jonathan Lundgren, a fabulous entomologist formerly with the ... what is it? The Agricultural Research Service, I think it is. Anyway, he suspects farmers were like the original scientists, you know, they're observing, observing, observing what's happening in my fields, figuring things out. Unfortunately, we did not get agriculture right in many cases. And so, the net trend was it's put us in a predicament.

[00:11:01]: Another thing about that is that the whole draw down, you know, drawing down carbon... There's another speaker in his event, Walter Jehne, he makes a point that I think is oh, so critical that nobody's been talking about in the world except him, as far as I know, maybe one other person, and now more people are talking about it. He's got the attention of the IPCC, and this is what he's saying. Drawing down carbon into soils, yes, it's important to reduce atmospheric carbon, but not so much for... It is very important, especially for the oceans, because the oceans are absorbing so much carbon dioxide, they're acidifying. And if they acidify sufficiently, which is what will happen very soon if trends don't reverse very quickly, we are potentially all toast, but...

Eric [00:12:00]: Very bad news. Very bad news.

Brendan [00:12:02]: Yes, very bad news. The oceans issue is the number one issue of our time, and it's intimately linked to our agriculture and our soils, because only agriculture can draw down enough carbon to spare the oceans and the rest of everything that depends on enough oxygen, and then that [unintelligible] ... because oceans produce almost two-thirds of our oxygen. But the point he makes is that soil is a water sponge, right? And that in its capacity as a water sponge, when it's healthy - the higher the organic matter, that the more water it holds - it's a massive part, a predominant part, of the climate regulation system that regulates how all these atmospheric processes involving water ... transpiration from the soils up through the plants and into the atmosphere, and then what happens to it up there ... is it greenhouse gas or is it high albedo clouds that are reflecting incoming solar radiation? And also, are these clouds persistent or do they rain periodically? And he basically says rain is a heat window, creates a heat window in the atmosphere, and that's how a lot of the heat escapes. But with fewer areas of healthy soils and healthy forests generating ... and of course, clouds are being generated off shore in the oceans, but a lot of them are also being generated over forests. And the key thing is, with forests, you've got these hygroscopic bacteria that are more prevalent above forests than anywhere else, and they are the predominant precipitator of rain in our atmosphere. So, we don't have forests, we don't have as much rain, we don't have as much heat escaping the planet. And then the other thing about soils, if they're retaining water, they're staying cool. They're only retaining water if they're under plants. And the bigger the plant party, the more fertile the soil, the higher the carb and the higher water sequestration.

[00:14:26]: On the other hand, by letting our soils get degraded, and then we have bare soil that doesn't grow anything, it gets heated up more by the sun. And the amount of heat being re-radiated from the Earth's surface is an exponential ... there's an exponential relationship between how much heat is reradiated and the temperature of the soil. So, the temperature of the soil, a hot, dry, bare soil compared to a covered, cool, wet soil is quite vast. And then give that an exponential factor, and you've got an exponential driver of the heat input into the atmosphere and the whole climate system. So, water is the key regulator of the climate system. And we always thought we couldn't even influence it, so we didn't model it. So, our model is based on something we knew we were influencing, which is carbon dioxide, but our biggest leverage point is rebuilding the soil. So, we draw down carbon, because that's how you build soil.

[00:15:32]: But the actual influence on climate is two-fold. It's drawing down a greenhouse gas, a very important greenhouse gas called carbon dioxide. And greenhouse gases are actually, according to him a small

… and he says this is Climate 101, and that basically, the greenhouse gases are a smaller part of the picture than some of these hydrological processes and of the greenhouse gases, water is the most important one. And we thought we couldn't affect it, but how we affect it is soil.

Eric [00:16:06]: Well, it's tricky, because water vapor is a climate forcer. It does cause warming, but it itself is a symptom of climate change, that's causing [unintelligible] the gases…

Brendan [00:12:02]: Yeah, as opposed to getting clouds, you get what he calls humid hazes, which is a combination of what you're saying, plus aerosol, you know, dust particles from soil, from diesel exhaust, from…

Eric [00:16:30]: The black carbon gets up in there and stuff, too, yeah. We looked at modeling a rainwater harvesting solution as well, because … well, 'cause it's cool and because harvesting of rainwater allows more water to be available. And you need water for photosynthesis, and photosynthesis is what makes carbon sequestration happen. So, where you can capture more rainwater, you can increase your carbon sequestration. And often, that's part of reversing this process of degradation of landscapes. Rainwater harvesting infrastructure is often a first step towards bringing a landscape back to life, or is one of the first steps you can take in many climates. We just were able to get like no data on how widely it is practiced. Nobody seems to know. We were able to find some sequestration rates of around one ton per hectare per year, but it's so variable. It just wasn't a model-able, but it remains one of my highest priorities. And certainly, if you live in a place where it's dry, it's pretty darn important, whether for agricultural systems or just for ecosystem restoration. There are various kinds of things people do for ecosystem restoration, where they're not going to eat stuff. where they're capturing water to help a degraded and barren landscape revegetate itself. So, there's a whole toolkit out there. It's quite fascinating.

Brendan [00:18:02]: You mentioned a few coming attractions. Are there any others you had mentioned that are exciting to you?

Eric [00:18:07]: Sure, I mean, lots and lots of them. The one that I'm really excited about right at the moment is various kinds of marine aquaculture. So, farming seaweed, for example, feeding seaweed to livestock is great for reducing emissions. Seaweed is great fertilizer. It's great food for people. It's great feedstock for biofuel and for bioplastic. There isn't enough land for us to have liquid biofuel be a really significant part of the puzzle for energy. There just is not enough land to do that. It can't be done… unless everyone was vegan, and I don't know that a lot of people… I think the global potential for everyone to be vegan is fairly low.

Brendan [00:18:51]: Well, yeah, and some people would argue that it just doesn't work for certain bodies.

Eric [00:19:01]: Mine among them. Mine among them. So, anyway, the seaweed gives us the potential to do that, but it also reduces ocean acidity locally around where you're farming it. So, it can be potentially used, for example, to protect coral reefs.

Brendan [00:19:17]: Oh, wow!

Eric [00:19:21]: Because it removes the CO2 from the water via photosynthesis and reduces acidity.

Brendan [00:19:23]: Right! Hadn't thought of that.

Eric [00:19:25]: So, that's very cool. But even better are these - They're calling them marine permaculture - essentially big floating farms that would be in the open ocean, not in the shallow water, with the wave action powering a pump to bring up nutrients from deep below. So, you'd have nutrient-rich water at the surface. And then you're farming like, let's say, fish. And then the fish waste is used to raise like mussels and seaweed, and then the remaining waste and the mussel waste and so on goes to sea cucumbers and sea urchins. So, these kind of very integrated, cyclic, wave-powered ocean farming systems are extremely exciting, extremely exciting. They're very much a new... I mean, seaweed farming is practiced pretty widely. There's around 20 million hectares of seaweed farming. But in terms of this more sophisticated system, it's very much a new notion. I mean, there are some traditional systems that it looks like, but basically, it's kind of a new idea, and it seems like it could really be another very, very, very promising... I don't know that I want to be out on one of those during a hurricane particularly. As weather gets more and more challenging, that may be one barrier to them, but that seems really promising, for example. And also, I really liked the ... We modeled the protection of coastal wetlands, like seagrass beds and mangroves and salt marshes, but also, I think the restoration of those is really big. Coastal wetlands and peatlands are really unique in that they don't have saturation. They can continue to sequester carbon, even if the rate isn't that great. They can do it for thousands and thousands of years. That's where fossil fuels come from. They can just keep going forever, at one or two tons per hectare per year, but for millennia. And that's a very, very exciting thing. And there are some... So, first of all, restoration production [unintelligible] is critical, but there are some farming systems that are based on or modeled on those systems that I think have a lot of potential. There's a grass called nipa, which is a perennial salt marsh grass. Salt marshes are one of these coastal wetlands. This thing is yielding pretty well. It tastes good.

Brendan [00:22:00]: So, it's a grass. It's like ... you eat it.

Eric [00:22:03]: It's a perennial grass. You eat the grain. It makes like a short grain brown rice. And that has some ... there's a lot of enthusiasm about that moving forward. There are also some mangrove agroforestry type systems. There are people doing agroforestry on deforested peatlands. And it's an open question. Will that enable the sort of like perpetual growth there again? That's a really ... Those are things that just tickle my fancy these days, anyway. And it's a big enough field, you can't actually keep up with all of it. There's so many different things happening. And the livestock integration, which I wrote about in my *Carbon Farming* book, but we weren't able to get any numbers really to work with for Drawdown. People only did livestock integration wherever there were livestock until the sudden wide availability of petroleum-powered fertilizer production. You just couldn't... How would you not integrate livestock? It couldn't be done. And a return to that in some of these very new sophisticated kinds of livestock integration are deeply exciting, like grazing orchards or integrating livestock in multi-strata systems and so on. These are all very, very interesting solutions that I think are certainly on my radar as up-and-coming things from the Gabe Browns of the world to the folks grazing cattle under coconuts … which actually increases the yield of coconuts, because you can find all of the coconuts when the grass is shorter.

Brendan [00:23:53] Okay! [laughing]

Eric [00:23:56]: All right, great! And there are a lot of very sophisticated ways livestock can be integrated in all the systems we were talking about today, like people raising fish and ducks with rice in low methane rice systems and so on that are all really awesome, unexplored things. The more systems you add, the more layers you add, the more complex the modeling gets, but those are very, very important systems. I practice those to the best of my ability here in my garden. I do aquaponics … Aquaponics is another one where you're integrating fish production with … Hydroponic vegetables grown in the fish waste, which then cleans the fish water, so the fish water can re-circulate. And the nitrous oxide from fish manure is a pretty big problem of emissions from the global aquaculture industry, which is on its way to being half of all the world's fish very soon and on its way to being way the majority of the fish that we eat. So, aquaponics basically can remove a lot of that nitrous oxide, what would become nitrous oxide, and use it as fertilizer for those plants before it is emitted. So, that's really…

Brendan [00:25:22] Yeah, so I mean I guess a lot of the aquaculture … How much of it is like freshwater and contained versus in saltwater and where you might not have … Well, I suppose you could combine these sort of …

Eric [00:25:38]: The seaweed farming systems are basically aquaponics in the sea, as far as I can tell.

Brendan [00:25:44]: Are they growing fish there, too? So, you get the aqu a…

Eric [00:25:48]: They are, they are. And they're also indoor saltwater …

Brendan [00:25:51]: I guess that's the definition of aquaponics. So, you kind of answered that in a word, yeah.

Eric [00:25:55]: Well, yeah, I mean there are other people, some people use ducks instead of fish and so on, but mostly they're using using fish. I think all those things are really very, very promising…very, very promising. Some of the traditional fish farming systems from China are also very promising and are still very much in production today. They mostly produce carp, and I don't know how to make carp into a good dinner.

Brendan [00:26:20]: Yeah, I've never been a fan. I tried it once, and I just could not make it good.

Eric [00:26:24]: And it's pretty much illegal through all of the United States to raise carp. So here, that's not going to be our solution for fish production.

Brendan [00:26:30]: Well, yeah. It's an invasive species here and it's a problem.

Eric [00:26:34]: So, we're not advocating …

Brendan [00:26:35]: I think it's invasive …

Eric [00:26:37]: Well, certainly some of those carp are really not very popular here. However, in China, where they are native, it makes every bit of sense to continue and expand those kinds of farming systems. So, there's so many different ways all this can go. There's really … Like I say, we don't want to just focus on organic or just focus on grazing, because there's a huge constellation, such a diversity in practices, we need to be looking at all of them. And really, to have a global food system that works and mitigates climate change, we have to …

Brendan [00:27:10]: Yeah, instead of transplanting the same system like, "Oh, this is it," and then trying to take it everywhere, you know? It's a problem.

Eric [00:27:15]: This is it here, but if we export what works here somewhere else that's what got us to where we are now is we took Europe's farming system with lots of plowing and annual grains, and we exported it to parts of the world where that was extremely ill-advised and mandated that everyone farm that way there. And that's a lot of what has resulted in so much degradation around the tropics, is the exportation of what worked in one place to a place where it didn't, the forced exportation and imposition of those practices. So, yeah, we need to let a thousand flowers bloom, and we need to let every valley figure out what's the right practice for that, or suite of practices for that place. It's not as easy as saying everybody must do just like me, but I think there's a more accurate and likely-to-succeed kind of approach or system. It's just a murkier message.

Brendan [00:28:09]: Right.

Eric [00:28:11]: I haven't worked that out yet. That's why my book is 500 pages long, and Paul will sell eight million more copies than I will—Drawdown— because it boils it down a message. He's much better at messaging than I am. I want all the details in there, and it can confuse the message sometimes if we do that. So, I think between us, we got a good distillation. We have enough practices that you can see a lot of diversity within and they embody a lot of diversity. But hey, here's a rank of the 80 of them, and here's the number. If you're really a reductionist person, you can just go and look for that, too. That's really important, because a lot of people think that way. So …

Brendan [00:28:54]: You know, just sort of tie it back into food real quick. So, you said that we couldn't have enough land for, let's say, producing liquid biomass fuels (liquid biofuels). Now I'm curious, is that based on the assumption of non-vegan foods right now coming from conventional systems where it's heavily grain based, and you've got to grow all this grain to then get, you know, a 1-5 or 10, or 1-to-20, I don't know, yield… You've taken all this land and then you produce just a little bit of meat out of it because of that model, instead of…

Eric [00:29:34]: Right.

Brendan [00:29:35]: Yeah, so I'm just wondering if that's the assumption that goes into it versus … well, in certain… you know, if you put the cattle and the chickens and the pork into systems where it's a stacked enterprise and it's actually facilitating the overall, let's say, silvopasture agroforestry system….

Eric [00:29:51]: Yeah. That's the version I like. That's called livestock on leftovers. So, the everyone's vegan model, the thing is feeding livestock takes more land. Whether they're grain fed or grass fed, the number of people you can feed per hectare is greater with plant-based food than it is with livestock-based food. So, in the vegan's scenario, a lot of land is available for reforestation and whatnot, but actually, you can feed more people in a vegetarian scenario because livestock can use land that people can't. They can eat grass, we can't. They can … you know, and so on.

Brendan [00:30:35]: Vegetarian in the sense that …

Eric [00:30:37]: Well, you'd be eating a lot of dairy and stuff and …

Brendan [00:30:44]: Wouldn't there also be some meat? I mean, obviously these animals …

Eric [00:30:47]: They die and you eat them at the end of life. And they make boy cows that don't make milk, and you eat them, and so on. Right? So, the scenario called "livestock on leftovers" is where livestock consume only things that people cannot eat. The cropland grows crops for people to eat, and land that can't grow crops is used to produce livestock, and livestock are also fed food waste and crop residues, whether that's corn stalks or stuff that's left in the field or … a lot of it is actually like when you press peanut oil or soybean oil, you get this press cake left. You press all the oil out and you're left with all the stuff that's really high in protein. So, you can feed that to chickens and pigs that can't eat that much grass. Ten percent of their diet or something can come from grass. They need to eat more like us. They're more like us. We can't get all our diet from lettuce. We need to eat other things, too. They basically have the same digestive system that we do. So, if you fed livestock only on, let's say, land that's too steep or that's already in grassland or whatever … land where you can't really grow or it's too remote to grow annual vegetables, like it's in the middle of the Siberian taiga or something, let's say, it's remote, remote …

Brendan [00:32:06]: Yeah. I mean you can't do irrigation in a seasonally dry grassland, and that's where the Holistic Management idea …

Eric [00:32:13]: Sure. That's a good place for grazing, really good place for grazing. Absolutely. Then in those scenarios, we can't feed in this livestock on leftovers … the numbers … the couple studies that came out last year show that you can't feed everyone … to eat the amount of meat that the average American eats, you would have to eat about a third. If everyone in the world got to eat the same amount of livestock products, which is what we would ideally like. Everyone who wants them should be able to eat some. We won't make vegans eat them, and we won't make Hindus eat meat and whatever. We won't make Muslims eat pork. You get about a third the amount of animal protein that Americans eat. So, you don't get to eat a steak every day in that world, in that livestock on leftovers world, with the current numbers. Now, intensive silvopasture and some other things might, you know, up those numbers a little bit. But fundamentally, not everybody gets to like an American. We can't waste all that food, and we can't all eat a steak every day. Maybe if you live in Montana, you can eat a steak every day, because that's where steak is from.

Brendan [00:33:30]: But again, that's not necessarily the best health choice …

Eric [00:33:32]: No, it's not the diet that's good for you, anyway, and the way to achieve adoption of that, Drawdown basically thinks, is to advocate for healthy diet, not to advocate for everybody to be vegan, but to say that if everybody ate a healthy amount of meat, that would have a huge impact. And that's a good goal, anyway, is for everybody to eat a healthy amount of meat and dairy. The other game changer, I'll just say, is that there's a product called leaf protein concentrate. And this is not a Drawdown one. This as an Eric one here. Leaf protein concentrate is like a tofu or cheese that's made from leaves. You can make it from grass. You can make it from poplar leaves. You can make it from all kinds of stuff, all kinds of stuff. Not everything, but many plants, you can make it from. Basically, to make it at home, you run the stuff through a juicer and then you simmer the juice and you skim off the protein kurds, just like if you're making milk or soy milk or making cheese or Tofu, right? A very similar process, and the amount of protein per hectare that you get from this is higher than any other kind of food production that we have.

Brendan [00:34:50]: Really?

Eric [00:34:51]: It's the most protein per hectare of any kind of food production there is. It's also the grossest tasting protein that there is. It tastes a lot like wheat grass juice, which is to say, I don't want to sit down to a steak that tastes like wheat grass juice or … I like wheat grass juice, but what you do with this as you mix it. So, I'd mix it with avocado.

Brendan [00:35:13]: Interesting!

Eric [00:35:14]: And it makes an awesome, very bright green guacamole, or you mix it in with tortillas and you get green tortillas that are incredibly high in protein and all the vitamins and stuff that are in those leaves. So, it's not so much a food that you're going to eat on your own as something that gets mixed into other things, that gets baked into bread, that gets mixed into other things that you're eating. It has enormous potential. It can be made from all kinds of perennials, including these perennial biomass grasses they want to use for energy. As you make your energy pellets, you can remove the protein and have high-quality protein as a byproduct of energy production.

Brendan [00:35:50]: Woah! Talk about stacking!

Eric [00:35:53]: So, there's some stacking. And also, you can … basically, you can just take grasslands that exist today, grass and clover, and you can make leaf protein concentrate out of grass and clover. So, that would actually be a more productive use of that land than grazing it, in terms of the yield per hectare of food. But I don't think we're gonna get everybody to switch to eating that. We can feed it to pigs. We can feed it to chickens instead of the soy beans that we're making now. We can mix it into foods, to some degree, for people. And that would be a piece of the puzzle, right? There's people who want that to be the only silver bullet, and I'm not going to eat only that. It's gross, you know, but how much can we lean into that? To what degree could that be a part of the solution? I think it can be part of the solution, and the IPCC is getting excited about it, actually, as a livestock feed, as a livestock feed, not as a people feed, but that would be great. They don't care. A pig doesn't care. They're not real picky. Chickens aren't real picky about what they eat. And if we could stop growing soybeans for them, it would be a really huge ... A third of all cropland is growing feed for livestock. It's obscene!

Brendan [00:37:12]: Yeah, it's just crazy. And you know, in terms of soy, I actually love to have some of my protein from vegetable sources. And my body also loves and seems to need ... because I've tried so many times to go vegan, and it just does not work, you know, for me ... so, my body wants the animal source proteins and the very good quality fatty acids that come from those animals ...

Eric [00:37:44]: Absolutely! But you don't have to eat meat at every meal, right?

Brendan [00:37:47]: Clearly not, and what's amazing to me, and this is at least touched on in multiple talks in this event. We're going into what happens when you reduce your protein consumption, increase your fat consumption, and reduce your carbohydrate consumption? You get into a ketogenic type of metabolism, and your need for protein plummets, because you're not burning it. You're not on a sugar metabolism rollercoaster, anymore, where when your sugars get low, your body says, well, the only other place for sugar quickly enough is my muscle tissue. So, then you reduce your, you know... so it's going catabolic, anabolic, catabolic, anabolic. You're breaking tissue down to supply blood sugar, if you're on a sugar burning roller coaster. If you shift and you're burning ... getting a lot more of your energy from fat, then it's sparing your protein. Your appetite for protein just drops. Actually, to get there, you have to drop your protein consumption, but it's not a difficult transition. You just add... You're adding in all this delicious high-quality fat, which is going to satisfy you more than a lot of things.

Eric [00:38:56]: There are a lot of perennial crops that produce really good fats, too, just so many tree-based fats, so many tree-based fats that are delicious. Many of them are really, really, truly...

Brendan [00:39:12]: Yeah, we only hear about avocado, and then you mention this lemon lime avocado from Africa. And what else you got? Are there any other quick favorites?

Eric [00:39:19]: Oh, well, there's seaberry, which is one that grows in northern climates even all the way up to like where it's 40 degrees below zero. Seaberry is a... it fixes nitrogen, also. It has all kinds of applications as livestock feed and in agroforestry. It makes a little sour fruit that kind of tastes like sour passion fruit that is very high in oils of exceptional quality. And the yield is actually... The oil yield right now is comparable to sunflower seed oil in terms of how much oil do you get in a hectare. So, that's very promising. Seaberry, I think, is the only fruit I found for cold climates that's really loaded with oil. Well, there's all kinds of palms, so many different kinds of palms, that produce oils. There's a lot of very interesting fruits. We have ... from the Amazon, there's a bunch of large, fleshy fruits that have a really oily flesh. Often, you have to cook them a little bit and then you eat them and they're like a savory oily flesh, kind of like eating a kalamata olive or something, but on a grapefruit-sized fruit in the grocery. So...

Brendan [00:40:37]: So, instead of eating six avocados a day, I'd just need two of those.

Eric [00:40:41]: You might just need two of those, or, you know, mix it up in a really killer fruit salad or something. Yeah, there are ... caryocar is one of the gender of those. The Amazon and then also the Cerrado, which is a Brazilian savanna area, are like especially high in these really oily fruits for whatever reason. They're loaded with oily fruits and nuts and oily palm fruits that have a huge, huge potential, I think.

Brendan [00:41:12]: Let's celebrate the Cerrado for a minute... And I hope I'm pronouncing it right. That sounded more Spanish and Portuguese, but...

Eric [00:40:41]: Yeah, I'm no good at Portuguese.

Brendan [00:41:12]: Cerrado ... I think that's how they pronounce it in Portuguese. It's been a while, and I actually don't remember even using the word while I was down there, because we were just in the region. I was in the Pantanal region, which is adjacent ... I did venture into some Cerrado areas where it's much drier. What an interesting foliage! It's so different. It's such a different ... it's a different planet in a way. Then again, I mean, I've only been ... there may be similar environments in other places, but it's just extraordinary. Unfortunately, it's so very threatened, as much as the Amazon is, from soy cultivation.

Eric [00:42:02]: Big hotspot for land use change, even though it's a source of so many amazing perennial crops, and it's kind of a natural silvopasture already, in that there's trees and grass, right?

Brendan [00:42:12]: But it's not like dense forest. It's sort of more ... it's a little more savanna like.

Eric [00:42:17]: Open forest and savanna, yeah. Yeah, it's really not a place that we want to see converted to agriculture. We want to ... what's there, maybe you can develop some agricultures based on what's there, because of these amazing wild plants that are already growing there and amazing wax palms and all different kinds of amazing industrial crops and fruit crops that are there. It's a marvelous place that really needs to be, you know, preserved and managed properly instead of just clear cut and plowed up and planted out to soybeans and whatever. It's a disaster. Absolutely. Savanna, as an ecosystem, is really undervalued for its ecological benefits, and is the model for silvopasture. Silvopasture is basically just a human created savanna. That's basically ...

Brendan [00:43:15]: Yeah, you know, as far as savannas, I met ... at the Permaculture Voices conference in 2015, I met somebody who was like a savanna evangelist. So, maybe he's a "savangelist."

Eric [00:43:26]: There's quite a few of those these days. Mark Shepard is one of them. There's a Savanna Institute now that's pushing this savanna-based agriculture. Again, that's another one of these likely very high carbon systems that's just germinating now, just really getting started that I'm very enthusiastic about.

Brendan [00:43:46]: Well, I want to thank you for...

Eric [00:43:47]: This was a delight, absolute delight.

Brendan [00:43:49]: [inaudible] these conversations. And your book, I assume these extraordinary plant species are cataloged in your book.

Eric [00:43:58]: In great detail!

Brendan [00:44:02]: Yeah. What's the name of the book again?

Eric [00:44:04]: It's called *The Carbon Farming Solution.*

Brendan [00:44:06]: But also, isn't there the one about the tree crops?

Eric [00:44:10]: Oh, sure. We had that one incorporates all the tree crops in it. It has six chapters on perennial staple crops and six chapters on perennial industrial crops for materials, chemicals, and energy to replace all the other junk that we do. And then there's a whole encyclopedia of the practices like we talked about today, all these different kinds of carbon farming practices. And then there's a piece on the... how do we get from here to there in terms of implementation and farmer training and finance and policy and all those kinds of things as well, so ... It's 500 pages long. It's a beast, but it does cover a lot of ... It covers a lot of ground.

Brendan [00:44:49]: Cool. Well, thank you. Thank you once again for being with us here in the Eat4Earth community.

Eric [00:44:55]: Absolutely.

Kelly Kennedy Extended Interview
Pleomorphism, Dark Field Microscopy

Brendan (00:00): So Kelly, I want to jump into one of your other areas of specialty, which is pleomorphism, the microbiome, dark field microscopy. Again, stuff that, you know, it's firmly in the realm of biological medicine but a lot of people haven't really been exposed to it and don't realize just how profound it is. So I'm not sure where to start in there, but let's dive into that a bit.

Kelly (00:26): So I think, yeah, the place to start that comes to me is the place that started for me when I saw a dark field. So I got introduced to this concept of biological medicine through Dr. Thomas Rau and the classes he was teaching at the time about 20 years ago. And the first class, he did two things. He did contact regulation thermography, and he did live blood analysis. And these were quantitative assessments of the milieu, or of the terrain. And when he put the microscope up and put it up on the screen, I was like a kid in a candy store because years ago... So my story is that I was pre-med at Cornell. I was in a horrible car accident. A month later, I started having ovarian cysts. A few weeks after that my father had a stroke. Five months later, he had a second stroke.

Kelly (01:15): Five months after that, he was dead. In 12 months, I was in a car accident, had ovarian cysts, and my father had two strokes and died. It was a rough year. 1993 was for me real rough. And when I went to my guidance counselor and said, "I want out of this industry" 'cause I wanted to be a doctor because my father had Hodgkin's disease. And it was a selfish endeavor, in all honesty. I didn't want to get cancer. Nobody could tell me if I could get cancer, if it was genetic. Nobody could tell me how to not get cancer. So my own little brain went, "Wow. If you can become a doctor, maybe you can figure it out."

Kelly (01:47): So I set on that journey and I wanted to help people not live like I lived. I lived in a home that it felt like a lot of people are living in today with Coronavirus that they feel like they don't know how they can get it, how they don't get it. They don't know how to protect themselves from it. And if they get it, are they going to die? It's a horrible way to live. Can we all agree? And that is the house I grew up in. And I wanted to protect myself and others from living that way. And here we are, 23 years later, I'm now living on a planet that everybody is feeling like I did growing up, and all I want to do a shout from the top of the mountain go, "No it's terrain theory, not germ theory. You guys are so confused. You don't know how your body works. I felt just like you did and so felt like a victim, didn't know how my body works, and was taught all this germ theory." Right? This is Louis Pasteur and the concept that germs outside our body make us sick. And that's where antibiotics come from. This whole concept.

Kelly (02:46): In Europe they talked about the environment in which the cells live in. And it's all about the terrain. And it's all about the milieu, which is a French word that means terrain. So we're going to call it terrain 'cause Kelly doesn't say that "m" word (milieu) very well. So the terrain of which the cells live in, and it made a lot of sense to me because I knew that there was more lymph fluid than there was blood. I knew that there was more spaces between the cells than there were cells. I just knew that from anatomy and physiology. So as I started, as he put the microscope up ... and he uses a phase microscope, or not a phase but a dark field microscope. So it's a different condenser. Like back in the day, when you know, you're in high school microbiology or high school biology, you look at your microscope.

Kelly (03:33): It's just like a regular condenser that throws up light. And you can look at red blood cells. Well, this is a type of condenser that traps the light from being up through the microscope so that when you use oil, an immersion oil, it shines on the spaces between the cells. And you get to see this entire environment, this microbiome that everybody discusses, you get to see it in the microscope. It's the coolest thing ever. It looks like the universe. It looks like the constellations. And you get to see the red blood cells, nice little circles floating around, moving cause it's live blood moving like little creek. Then you see the endobionic field, the endobionic load, which is the funguses. You know, we are more fungus, bacteria, and virus than we are cells. I'm a big bag of bacteria and virus, fungus, and mold with some Kelly Kennedy cells thrown in there. So the concept of knowing that we are more non-pathogenic, non-disease bacteria and virus and fungus than we are anything else is the first understanding we need to have of the body. You know, the fungus of which all of life is, you know. I don't know a lot about mushrooms and fungus, but I can put you in contact with somebody that does. And funguses and mushrooms are so incredibly interesting.

Brendan (04:58): They really are.

Kelly (04:58): They have the entire network. Every mushroom on the planet is connected to every other mushroom on the planet. And they have an entire communication system that makes fiber optics look like paper cups and strings, like when we were kids. Like it's a joke compared to WiFi, we think 5G, blah. The mushrooms have it all over us. Trust me. They've got it all over us. But we are more fungus than we are anything else. There's three funguses that live in our body from a pleomorphic understanding. This is two different doctors, Dr. Wilhelm Reich---Professor [Gunther] Enderlein and Wilhelm Reich were the two scientists, doctors, both in the 1950s that discovered under a dark field microscope this whole terrain. They both had their own schools of thought of language of what they called it because they had to make up words. Nobody had ever seen this before. So they had to make up their own words. So there's kind of two schools of thought in this world.

Kelly (05:57): But they created, but they both call them protetes or symbi protetes [symbiproteins?]. And the three funguses are mucoraceous, *Aspergillus niger*---black mold, and *Penicillium forte*. So when somebody comes in and goes, I'm allergic to penicillin, I go, "Uh, are you allergic to water too? 'Cause that's like being allergic to yourself." You can't, you can't be allergic to penicillin. You might be allergic to the manmade penicillin that's made outside your body, but your body is more *Penicillium*, muc [short for mucoraceous fungi], and Aspergillus than it is anything else. And it's those endobionts that come from nothing in a sterile field.

These will start to show up because from nothing comes something, and this is the dark field problem. This is the issue with live blood that people go, "Whoa".

Kelly (06:44): First of all, I can prick your finger, a phlebotomist can prick your finger, look at your blood under the microscope, and in five minutes, know what the environment is. It's not a diagnostic' it's an assessment tool because you and I can have exact same thing looking in our microscope, in our blood. You might have no symptoms, and I've got stage four cancer, but our blood looked exactly the same. So it's not a diagnostic. It's what our body's up against. Maybe we both have a lot of metal. Maybe we both have a lot of acid. Maybe we both have a lot of fungus outgrowing as a pathology. The difference is your constitution is maybe stronger than mine. Your lifestyle's a little more conducive to health than mine. And so that blood for me and you changes and morphs quicker than mine to degeneration and your blood changes and morphs into regeneration because of how you live. Because blood is not stagnant. Life is not stagnant. Nothing is stagnant. All of life can be defined. I steal this definition from a good colleague of mine, but as "Life is change in motion".

Brendan (08:00): Like always a flux. You're always moving in one direction or another. It's not just stagnant. It's a flux.

Kelly (08:07): Yeah. I arrived. I'm healthy. I'm here. Okay. You're healthy now, but what are you going to make ... what's the next decision you're gonna make? What are you going to put past your lips? What thoughts are you going to think? What are you going to listen to? What are you going to look at that's going to re-instill health or degenerate because the body only goes towards regeneration or towards degeneration. That's it. Those are the options all day long every day. And the goal is, can we get the toxins out faster than they can come in? And the goal is, can we go in regeneration more than we go in degeneration?

Brendan (08:38): So how is this tied to lymphatic drainage? Is it that you're essentially ... when you keep the lymphatics flowing you're creating the conditions for regeneration versus degeneration, or what really, what exactly happens? How is it related to these endobionts?

Kelly (08:57): In the spaces between the cells is where the lymphatic lives and the lymphatics is a network of blind-ended capillaries that move in one direction that are collector tubes that collect all the fluid that's surrounding the cells, pulls it into the lymphatic, identifies it through the lymph nodes, and identifies it. Is this a bacteria? Is this an immune challenge? Is this a metal? Is this a chemical? Is this a nutritional? Is this a mineral? Is this a vitamin, a mineral. So it determines that. And then the body will circulate it through the cardiovascular system, will excrete out by peeing, pooping, sweat, and bleeding and will hold on. And proper functions will take over through our liver, our kidney, and all the other organs of the body.

Kelly (09:42): So how it relates is in every single way because that space between the cells, if that space is full of acids from improper foods or improper thoughts, or if that space is full of immune challenges, Lyme spirochetes, or Epstein-Barr virus spirochetes, or if that background is full of metals, because they're a landscaper and they use RoundUp all day long, or they're a beautician that uses harsh chemicals on people's hair and skin, or they're an esthetician that uses that, or they work at a water chemical plant, or maybe they work at a machine factory, or maybe they work at a computer lab, and they're in a cold room all day long, and they're exposed to high amounts of radiation, WiFi type radiation. And those were just off the top of my head.

Kelly (10:33): That's all affecting the lymph because the lymph is our antenna system in addition to our heart as the conductor. The lymph is the filter. The lymph is in our environment, filtering everything and what our lymph can't filter, it holds onto. And what we hold onto is the problem. Whether that's emotional or physical, we need to let that sh_t go, literally and figuratively. All of it. I wanted to for the holidays ... I got a friend of mine a little candle. I thought it was a big candle, but when it came, it was literally this big, and it was a woman sitting in Lotus that just says, "Let that sh_t go". And I just thought it was cute because it's all about that. The lymph is about letting it go physically and emotionally. And traumas and dramas and emotions are 90% of all Illness.

Kelly (11:27): So go back to those two microscopes, yours and mine. If you're an optimist, obviously you mentioned it early and I would agree. And I think I'm pretty optimistic as well, but let's just say I wasn't. Let's say I was a pessimist. "Ugh. It's going to be cold outside today. Ugh, I got to get my kid on the school bus tomorrow. Ugh, I gotta make dinner tonight". My body is to feel that vibration, and that's going to create acid in my body. Versus, "Oh my gosh, it's beautiful out today. It's sunny. It's 22 degrees, but it's sunny. I get to go home and make dinner, be with my family because I don't have to work too late. I get to actually have dinner with my family tonight. Oh, I'm so excited about that. I can't wait to make dinner. I'm not psyched about really making it, but I'm excited about eating it. I can't wait to eat my dinner. I love eating." I can focus on those good things in that vibration that gives my body is very different, and that's going to change the physiology in my body. And we could spend five hours just on that subject. But the emotional body translates everything that happens to us physically and everything that emotionally happens to us is translated physically. So it's constantly going back and forth between the two sides and the lymph is about letting all of it go.

Kelly (12:42): So when---I'll throw my brother under the bus---so when my brother was a jerk to me growing up and never use my name for like seven years of my life and called me "it". [Brendan: Oh, God.] Oh yeah, yeah. Let's just throw Michael right under the bus. Hear this, my girls listen to my podcast sometimes my nieces, his girls. So I'm doing this just for them. 'Cause I recently heard that they listened to my podcast. So let's throw Michael Ryan under the bus. So that could have created a lot of acid. And I would tell you, Brendan for surety in my developing years, from 10 to 20, it definitely created a lot of acid in my body. Now, I love it because I know that he made me a stronger person. And I did a lot of emotional work to overcome that, but it made me a stronger person because of it. Now I love when he says the word "it", because it just brings it up for me and him. And it makes him feel bad; it makes me feel good.

Kelly (13:34): And I don't want to make him feel bad. I want him to face what he did, and why he maybe shouldn't do that to young women or anybody for that matter. But the emotional components, I chose to change that at some point in my life. So that history doesn't make a sour pill for me anymore. That history is now my golden history, that because of who he is, he intimidated me more than anybody ever has in my life. Now there's nobody that can ever intimidate me because of who my brother was in my life. Thank God for him because there's nobody that intimidates me. And in the position that I find myself in now, that's a really good thing. Would you not agree?

Brendan (14:14): Especially if you're talking about pleomorphism, [Kelly: Exactly.] especially in the current environment.

Kelly (14:23): You read between the lines. I grew up in an environment that made me tough. And while I was growing up, I had a sour feeling about it, and it made a lot of acid in my body. And when I did the emotional work, and I was able to see that I love my brother and there could be no two better brothers than the two that I have for me and my life. No two better brothers. They're the perfect brothers for me. But growing up, I hated both of them. Now. I love them, both for what they give me in my life. And I know that because of them and because of my growing up that's who I am today. So that same sour pill I changed, but I had to do that work to shift that. So my body changed that same experience, and I filter it now a different way. So I had to let it go for a long time. I don't have to let it go anymore. It's not a thing, but we just played a relative insanity card game at the holiday party. And something came up about it. And we were laughing so hard through that whole experience that it became like this thing that we can commune and over versus this thing that's negative in our past. That's true healing. And that's done on the emotion components and through the lymphatics. I mean, that was a big, round ...

Brendan (15:36): [unintelligible], so we can use the lymphatics to actually access all the stuck stuff, the emotional stuff that has physical counterparts in our body, that's stuck with it. And so we can ... so you're saying that working with the lymph can help us work with the emotions and the trauma that's been there for so long.

Kelly (15:55): Just like the metals and chemicals are stored in there, the traumas are stored in there. So we've got to let all of that go to really release to create the room and the space, so that cell, that intracellular space, can dump into that extracellular space, which is where the lymphatics is, which is what we looked at the dark field, which is where those three funguses live. And how that all relates to the lymph is if that environment and the lymph is full of acids and full of improper foods and full of metals and chemicals, then those funguses that are non-pathogenic are going to morph and change and grow into pathogenic bacteria and viruses and cause problems. And as we get healthier, as we change the environment, as we drain the lymph, as we change our emotional state, as we get rid of the silver fillings in our mouth properly with a biological dentist, and we remediate that and we properly detoxify it, we change that environment.

Kelly (16:47): And now those same funguses that were non-pathogenic that outgrew into pathogy [pathology] can change back down to nonpathogenic fungus in our bodies as true life forces as our endobionic load because of the environment change. and then they were able to change. And this is the concept that one thing isn't one thing, that pleomorphism occurs, that things morph and change all the time. And it's evidenced by our coronavirus this year. Everybody's "Oh, there's a new strain." Is there a new strain or did it morph? This virus has continued to morph over the last 15 months since we've been watching it because it wants to survive. It's not even a living organism, and it wants to survive because it wants to upgrade our DNA, and it wants to help make us a stronger human being. You can't do that unless the human being gets uncomfortable. Under signs of comfort does not a human being expand and grow. No, no, no. Humans, Homo sapiens, expand and grow because we are uncomfortable at times that allows us to expand and grow. It doesn't have to be painful; just can be a little uncomfortable.

Brendan (18:00): Can you say more about this idea that this virus and maybe other viruses, serve to upgrade our DNA? That's something I've heard Zach Bush say, but I've never heard any in-depth explanation or evidence for it, as opposed to just like an idea.

Kelly (18:20): I stole that from Zach Bush, too. Honestly, I don't ... I want to give him credit because when he said it, I realized I heard him say it about, I don't know, four months ago. And I was like, "Oh my God, that's basically what I've been saying, but not in those exact words. And I appreciate his words because he also understands terrain. And I don't want to put words in his mouth. I'm not any part of his speaking platform or anything, but what he said made a thousand percent sense to me as a scientist because all of life is information. Everything on the planet is vibration. We are emotional beings. Having a physical experience. Our DNA is the footprint is the blueprint. I'm sorry, it's the blueprint that tells our body what could happen. Based upon the environment we either allow that DNA to be expressed fully or to be under-expressed.

Kelly (19:15): Some of those DNA scripts, some of the coding is for our benefit. And some of the coding in our DNA is for our detriment, right? So we want all the things in our DNA that help us thrive. Well, bacteria, virus, and funguses, they are here to help us do just that, to help us grow and help us morph and change to allow this ecosystem to continue to thrive in the environment as these other entities are growing and changing around us because it is a codependent relationship that we are in completely in this ecosystem. We cannot think that killing a bacteria or a virus or a fungus outside our body is not going to affect us because it's all connected. And it's all related from the perspective that you cannot say, "Where do I end, and where do you begin?" If we were in the same room, even, that would be hard to determine because your energy field is seeping outside of you.

Kelly (20:23): Whether you can see it with your physical eyes or not is the question, but your energy body is much bigger than your physical body and emanates outside of you anywhere from two and a half to three feet. And if I'm standing three feet, and you're standing three feet, or let's say we're standing six feet apart, the three feet in the middle, they're still touching, right? And those molecules are having all sorts of interactions. And those molecules are, are communicating and reflecting back on each other. And that own individual ecosystem is now compensating or lacking compensation for this information. And whether that can compensate or not is [the] concept of regulation. And the concept of regulation is the concept of regenerative and regenerating. And the concept that that's how the body works. The body's always self-healing and regenerating until it can't because it's overwhelmed by the input or it's aged so much from a toxic load or exposures, or functional obsolescence, or it's only designed to live 120 years or so.

Kelly (21:39): It's just gotten to the point where it no longer can create that ecosystem, can no longer create those enzymes to break down all that food. So we've got to take a little enzymes by the time we're 40 or 50. There's not as many enzymes as we had when we were 10, but you can also ... the best anti-ager area you got is right here [gesturing to the head, shoulders, and heart area]. It's not sticking Botox in my skin. It's not sticking collagen in my skin, and it's not using all these anti-aging creams and lotions. It's about moving my lymph, getting rid of the wrinkles. I'm 46 years old and have hardly any makeup on at this hour of the day. I'm not saying I don't have wrinkles. My son comments about my wrinkles all the time, but I don't have the crow's feet. And I don't have the common wrinkles that 46 year old women usually have because I move my lymph a lot.

Kelly (22:29): And I make sure my lymph is moving to make sure that my body's not up against the toxic load, because what I know about aging is we are up against acids, and we're up against toxins. And if you can get the acids and toxins out, or you can stop putting them in, then you will age gracefully and mature, like a fine wine and get better with age, get smarter, wiser, more efficient, more effective, and happier, more joyful, and like a kid in a candy store. Right? Welcome to my world. Come and join me. Do your lymph. Move your lymph. Let that go, and watch your body thrive, and regenerate instead of degenerate and get older.

Brendan (23:22): I'm curious how you use, or how anybody would use, dark field microscopy to get, you know, practically speaking, so you look at what your blood is doing, and what can you do with that information? You know, as a practitioner---I guess you're a practitioner of that---what do you do with that? And how does it help somebody?

Kelly (23:43): So when I look at somebody's live blood I'm looking for the top two to three things that are the gross things that are showing up. Like I can get lost in somebody's blood and look at it for five, six hours, but that doesn't do me any good. I want to know what is the majority of the top two to three things they're dealing with? Uh, you have a lot of congestion in your blood. All your cells are stacked on top of each other. Well, that's 'cause you know, it's highly acidic. Well, is that nutritionally based? Is that emotionally based? So we're going to figure out why. Where does it come from? And we're going to ... so first is we're going to go, okay, assess one of the top three things we're dealing with. Then is where are those top three things coming from? Is that exposure, or is that leaking, or is that lifestyle?

Kelly (24:23): And then what do we do to change those things? You know, maybe it's emotions. Maybe I've got a poisonous, you know, past trauma history, you know. Maybe something horrible happened to me as a kid, and I just can't let it go. And it's now my whole entity is, you know, I was, you know, abused by my father when I was three. And now that's my story and I'm 47 years old, and it's still my story. Well, then we've got to move through that. We've got, you know ... or I was cheated on by my first husband and left me with two kids to raise on my own 20 years ago. I mean, it sucks. It does. There's no ... either one of those scenarios they suck, but ... and the reality is that's your life, so accept it, and move on, and let that go, and stop acting like the victim and move that through your system so that you can thrive and stop blaming somebody.

Kelly (25:10): There's two, always two people to tango. I, you know, my best friend is an Argentinian tango instructor, and she was my maid of honor. And she taught me, it takes two to tango, and it takes somebody leaning and somebody holding to make a beautiful tango. And so you don't get in through a divorce. You don't get through anything in life without two people bringing it, even abuse. I hate to say it, but it's true. So we've got to allow ourselves the opportunity to go, okay, what was I supposed to learn from that? What was I supposed to get from that? And let that move through my system. I know you had another question, but I got off on a tangent.

Brendan (25:46): Well, I'm sort of thinking in terms of the dark field microscopy, what do you do with what you see? So you can start to see what's going on. Okay. There's acidity. The red blood cells are stacking in a rouleaux kind of formation where they're, you know, like lifesavers that you, you know, pull them out of the package and they're all stuck together.

Kelly (26:06): He knows a little bit about live blood 'cause he said a word I hadn't used yet. Very good. Yes, that's [unintelligible].

Brendan (26:11): I've had somebody look at my blood once, and they were showing me how much rouleaux there was. And then they did a treatment on me. I forgot what the nature of it was. And we looked again, and that one treatment helped to reduce the rouleaux effect.

Kelly (26:24): And that's why I use it as well. One is I want to see what's the effectiveness of the therapy I'm doing, number one. Number two, I look at it for ... if I've been working with somebody for two or three months and clinically, they seem better maybe, but I want to see it quantitatively then I'll look at it there. And I want to see how long it stays changed. So like for instance, you did your live blood, you do a therapy, and then you do another live blood. That's great. It changed it for that time period. But next day, does your blood still say changed. Two weeks late does your blood still ... or how quickly does it go back into rouleaux patterns? Right? So it tells me the efficacy of therapy, but also is a quick snapshot in regards to ... like I do another test called contact regulation, thermography, which is the 119 points of the body of temperature.

Kelly (27:13): And then you cool off. And then I take the 119 points of temperature again, or one of my staff does. It's a German test. You have to do it in the morning. You have to do before noon. You can't shower before you take it. You can't have any lotions on your body. You know, if you're a man, you gotta be fully shaven, and it takes an hour to administer. And you have to stand in the room naked for 10 minutes. That's a whole heck of a lot of variables and everything else versus can you avoid food and caffeine for an hour? I'm going to prick your finger, or you're going to prick your finger. We're going to look at your blood on the microscope, and we're going to have a snapshot of what's going on, and what's been going on since the last time I saw you.

Kelly (27:47): I don't do it at every visit by any stretch, but I do it maybe in the beginning of a case that's a little more complicated. I can't really see what I'm fighting. Like I had a young woman who we've known since about 10 years. We've worked with her father. We've worked with our mother. We've worked with her brother and for different things throughout the year. Dad had---I feel like it was dizziness or something---but it was from his silver fillings. Dad got his silver fillings out; started to detoxify. Dad started to feel better. Sent mom in for something years later; handled that. Sent [his] son in for something years later; handled that. Now daughter's coming in with anxiety, 17 years old. Looking at her, she looks like a typical, beautiful average teenager, no symptoms, other than anxiety, no silver fillings in her mouth.

Kelly (28:35): No nothing. So my husband worked with her for a few weeks. Did some emotional work. No real difference. We're not used to that. We're not used to not getting a difference in a few weeks. So my husband's like, "Oh, what's going on for her. How about you do a live blood and see what the hell's going on? I'm suspect[ing] she has a lot of mercury from her mom and maybe her lymph is really stagnant. I was like, "All right." Pricked her finger. Sure enough verified exactly what he thought to be true. So we're not doctors, but we call ourselves medical intuitive biological investigators. So there's a perfect example. My husband was very intuitive about what was going on, but he wanted me to biologically investigate to verify his intuition. We verified it. We said, yeah, sure enough, you got a hundred percent target cells. Pretty much every cells full of a metal.

Kelly (29:19): Your lymph is really, really stagnant. So all the emotional work he wants to do is great. But your body's preloaded with mom's toxic load. So how about we move your lymph a little bit, and then we'll get your body to drain and we'll let the detox take over by itself. The next six to eight months, we might add something for detox, but probably not just open up your lymph. Opened up her lymph the first session doing FLOWPresso. She commented back to me the next day and said, "Oh, my anxiety was a little bit up during the session, but I pooped as soon as the session was over, just like you said, I would. And I feel really excited about doing my next session. Now I'll know what to expect. And I don't think I'll be as anxious as I lay there."

Brendan (30:00): Interesting. What did you say? You said she had a hundred percent something. It sounded like toxics ... "target cells".

Kelly (30:08): Which is an indication of heavy metal toxicity. It can be dehydration at times as well.

Brendan (30:15): What as a target cell?

Kelly (30:17): A target cell looks like it has a donut in the middle. It looks like it has a hole. And so it can be different colors. And so you can see that it's a metal. You don't know what metal it is, but you can identify it's a metal. You'd have to do a different assay, a different analysis, whether that was a urine challenge or a challenge under a blood test or a hair mineral analysis, to determine what metals. Again, it's not a diagnostic. It's an assessment of what the body's up against and how much is it up against? And what are the major three things it's up against? And then as a biological investigator and through their history and some other assessments, we can determine why the body's up against that. Is this lifestyle? Is this emotion? Is this some chronic thing that you've been dealing with?

Kelly (31:00): Is this a leak from the mouth? Why? And then address whatever that situation is. Okay, well maybe we need to find you a good biological dentist, while maybe you need to move out of your moldy house while maybe you need to have a conversation with your toxic person that's in your life that. Or maybe you need to not have that conversation. Maybe you just need to radically forgive them and work through that. Maybe whatever. But it's a combination thereof because it's never one thing that causes one thing. But throughout the whole thing---lymph, lymph, lymph. In the middle, in the beginning, at the end to let it go to let it drain out because whatever that is, that my body's holding onto isn't allowing my own physiology to take over its natural function, because all that stuff is interrupting. I need to get rid of all that that's impeding my body from doing its proper functioning to allow it to do its job. Anything that I've given it, that's manmade, it's just screwing it up.

Brendan (32:00): Well, this has been really helpful. I really appreciate being able to dive into this because, um, the standard, let's say functional medicine approach, I think sometimes leaves a few things to be desired because it's kind of like just an ... it ends up being like an herbal allopathy. Or instead of using pharmaceutical poison and poisons to kill microbes or pharmaceutical drugs to manipulate symptoms, sometimes we're using herbs to kill microbes and herbs to manipulate symptoms. And maybe that has its place. For example, I think adaptogenic herbs are great because they're facilitating the regulatory balance. Depending on where you are in dysregulation, it'll move you back towards center, these tonic herbs. And where the jury's kind of out for me is when you're dealing with the microbiome, is there more value than harm in using herbs to kill off what's perceived ... what's like a pathogenic organism, a pathogenic form, when maybe there's other ways to just shift the system back to where it via the pleomorphic shifts that organism no longer shows up in that form. And it goes back to another form that's beneficial or commensal or whatever to the overall human superorganism. So I'm kind of curious if you've seen these specific ... I assume that's kind of your approach.

Kelly (33:36): It's a hundred percent. You're spot on because the goal is that we want to get the body to heal, right? And so we, we do that by not forcing the body to do something that it's not ready to do with herbals or pharmacy. We do it with information, whether that's vibrational, homeopathic orthomolecular after the blockade, see healing or remove, which is scar influences in dental influences. So you remove the blockades to healing, then you get the body to upregulate and that upregulation down-regulates the pathogen, the pathogens. So you upregulate the healing capacities and you down-regulate the pathogens and you allow the body to beat all the non-pathogenic because Zach Bush and many of the others, Dr. Zach Bush, and many of the others have commented that it's not good bacteria, bad bacteria. It's bacteria behaving badly because of the environment they're in. Bacteria are not bad.

Kelly (34:30): Fungus aren't bad. This is just a concept we've been sold that black and white and good and bad. And it's not like that. It's all gray, and it's all good. And you need light to have dark, and you need dark to have light. Whoa, hello. We can't appreciate the moon unless we have the sun. I can't appreciate the heat of the summer, unless it's 21 degrees outside in January in Philadelphia. Then when it's 90 in August, I'm super happy, right? So you have to have both sides of it to have the middle. That's how you get the middle. So you got to have all the bacteria and the viruses and the fungus, but behaving as they should because of the environment they live in is appropriate biologically, meaning there aren't chemicals or manmade things, or woman-made, in here that are allowing the body to go, "I don't understand what that is. That's something that I don't recognize." That's a vibration that's not natural because the body only sees frequencies and vibrations, and you cannot escape frequencies and vibrations. And when they're naturally occurring frequencies and vibrations, we have a complete affinity for it. And when they're not, it creates disharmony and illness. And what we're looking for is harmony all the time.

Brendan (35:51): Amen. [Kelly: Amen.] One last question. I have in my notes from a past conversation, something called an endobionic flush, and is that just sort of a kind of paraphrasing what a lymphatic flush is, or is it something else? 'Cause I don't remember what that was in reference to. Endobionic flush. So we've been talking about the endobionts, these organisms ...

Kelly (36:19): I have no idea what we were talking about.

Kelly (36:23): Oh, well, we could maybe ... how you get ... so there's three ways to create endobionts in your life. This could be why. One is time in Nature without your cell phone. Time in Nature.

Brendan (36:34): So endobionts ... let's actually define that formally real quick. So endobionts are what?

Kelly (36:39): It's your life force? It's your natural chi. It's where from nothing comes something. Okay? And it's these three funguses, and it's what pleomorphism, the science of pleomorphism, is based in knowing that we are these three funguses: *Aspergillus*, muc [mucoraceous], and note [*Penicillium*?].

Brendan (36:56): Yeah, we did cover that. Okay, cool.

Kelly (36:57): Yep. So that's what endobionts are. Okay? How do they get created is the question? How do we get them? Three ways, time in Nature without your cell phone because cell phones kill it. So time in Nature. They'll be naturally assimilated into your body. Eating organic food, which is time in Nature, basically again. By eating organic live food, not organic food that's then been microwaved because that kills it again. But organic live food---and it doesn't have to be raw---but just live. And [the] third one is orgasms. So Wilhelm Reich was one of the scientists that realized all this, and he was a student of Freud. And they fell apart because Freud said it was all about the orgasm, and Wilhelm Reich said, "No, it's all about orgone." And orgasm creates orgone.

Kelly (37:54): And it creates a huge endobionic flush, if you will. And let me ask you this, for those listening, when are you more enthusiastic ever in your life than right after an orgasm? You're the most enthusiastic. And if you break down the word enthusiastic, it comes from Greek meaning entheos, meaning God within. God within is our own healing capacity. It's the self-healing nature. It's this innate intelligence. The God within is what we get to humbly look at when we're looking at a dark field microscope. We get to see the spaces between the cells. We get to see this amazing healing regulatory capacity of the body that's not tangible but ever-moving and ever-changing and ever-healing and absolutely amazing. And I will shout it from the rooftops if they let me because this is what we've got going on. This is the real medicine is inside of us.

Kelly (38:52): This is the real healing is love. And the fact that we are all connected through the God part of us, and we need to have faith in that and have faith that God is doing all of this, and that the upgrade that's happening is for a good reason. And yes, some of the weak are not surviving through it because they need to wake up and realize that they're weak because 88% of our population is walking around with a metabolic disorder, thinking they're strong, and they are weak. And that's the real wake-up call of Coronavirus. Realize how strong you are, but that you are not maybe right now because you're taking your mass [meds?] down to put your McDonald's in it after you take your cholesterol pill and thinking that it's all okay, and that's not how the organism works. You need fresh air. You need love. You need connection. And you need shelter, fresh air, and fresh water. That's it.

Kelly (39:47): We need more air than we do food. We need more connection and love than we do food. This is the reality because we are emotional beings having a physical experience. And when I was at Cornell University, this was not what I thought at all. This was not what I walked into Cornell going, "I'm going to become a doctor because I know the etherical body is where it's all at. Not at all. I was forced into this world with a horrible car accident and a horrible death of my father leaving me at such an early age, forcing me to want to find another way to heal. And I was so blessed to find this man who is now my husband. When I came to his office, he tapped my back, gave me some Chinese herbs, and in less than a month, I started getting rid of my pain and was like, "How the hell did you do this?

Kelly (40:31): I don't understand." And he goes, "Energy!" And I go, "What? What's 'energy'?" He goes, "Energy! Cool, huh?!" "No! What the hell is energy? And how do I get some? And how do I make sure this never comes back?" And that's what you're looking at the dark field microscope. You're looking at the energy. That's what you're testing when you're looking at heart rate variability, when you're looking at computerized regulation thermography. You're looking at that healing energy in the body, and it's quantitative. We can assess it now because we can take all of that ancient wisdom we have with this amazing technology that we have and brand them to braid them together. And we get to see the energy that's healing inside all of us. And it doesn't wait for the blood to show up a problem. It happens way more subtly in the subtle energies of the body, not in the gross anatomy of the body.

Brendan (41:21): I got like chills and was tearing up with part of what you were talking about as far as the, um, I don't remember what it was exactly, but thank you for that, and really connecting us back into the source of life, the sources of life. And it kind of reminds me ... I was also in a pre-med program at an Ivy league type school. And I recall a graduate---I think it was a graduate student---and he was kind of poo-pooing this idea of vitalism because some people in biology believe in vitalism, and that's kind of what we're talking about [Kelly: Absolutely.] as opposed to "No, we're just simply physiochemical machines." In fact, the physics part is actually often left out of most biologists' worldview. And they just think it's all chemistry. Even back then, I was like, "Why is this guy ... he's taken more courses than we have, but he doesn't get this. There were some of us younger biology students, and we kind of had an intuition for this. And this guy was like, "Psssh" about this vitalism, and I'm like, "What else do you think moves the chemistry? I mean, the chemistry doesn't move itself, believe it or not, you know. They come up with explanations about how somehow chemistry is the alpha and omega of life. {Kelly: Of all of it, yeah.] And it really just the signals of what's happening. It's kind of like ... it actually follows.

Kelly (42:52): Right. It's false vitalism. It's the note that vitalism is leaving for you. It's like the post-its that they're leaving. That's a really good way to look at it. [Brendan: Yeah.] That's a really good one.

Brendan (43:05): Before we conclude, I wondered if you could ... I mean, I would imagine if I was hearing this for the first time, I might want to kind of investigate further, look deeper, you know. Are there any books, anything you would suggest to people? I think I had something in my notes here about *Biological Medicine*, *The Swiss Secret*, *Say Yes To Life*, something like that. The book, *Get Off Your Acid* by Darryl Gioffre.

Kelly (43:33): So there's the Biological Medicine books from Dr. Thomas Rau. I don't have Dr. Geoffre's books out here, but Dr. Darryl Gioffre has written two books. One is *Get Off Your Acid*, and it just came out. The second one is, *Get Off Your Sugar*. {Brendan: Okay.] And then Say Yes To Life by Dr. Ralf Oettmeier, O E T. *Say Yes To Life*. And Dr. Joseph Fitzkelly. They're from the option clinic in Switzerland. These are Dr. Thomas Rau's books from Switzerland. These are what's going to explain in today's terms, layman terms, about pleomorphism, and the understanding of pleomorphism. Those six books. There is another book about the lymphatic system, but if you're not very scientific-y, it's going to bore the crap out of you. But if you're a practitioner and listening to this, it got translated about seven, eight years ago into English. It's a German book.

Kelly (44:26): Hold on. I can see it. It's black ... it's blue and red. And the title is, um, the ground substance. I'll get you the title, Brendan. I can't remember that. I like know it, the book, but I can't tell you the title. It's like the extracellular matrix, the ground healing substance of all of life, the biological healing of ... it's like it's got such a comprehensive title. And it's something about extracellular matrix and the biological healing of the body [possibly referring to *The Extracellular Matrix and Ground Regulation: Basis for a Holistic Biological Medicine*] because it really teaches you all about the ground substance, which is the extracellular matrix, which is the spaces between the cell, which is where the lymph lives. There's not a lot of books on the lymph. I'm writing one. There's a really thick book called *Science Waves*. But it's like, if you want to be a lymph therapist to read it. Outside of that ... [gestures gagging herself]

Kelly (45:21): So I'm trying ... I'm writing right now like a 101, like lymph 101. It's going to be like 15 pages. And then my friend, colleague, Desiree, and I are writing a bit longer of a book, a little bit more comprehensive for the practitioners 'cause there's not really great books out there about the lymph because it's a subject that not a lot of people have talked about in regards to pleomorphism. Most of them are just written by professor Andrew Lane and Dr. Wilhelm Reich, which again, very heady, very science-y, very microbiology type books,. But Bruce Lipton's book, *The Biology of Belief*, which I'm very sure you're familiar with is a great place to start. If you don't know anything about anything we talked about today, go read Biology of Belief. Or he has a two-hour lecture on YouTube, which kind of broad-scopes all his concepts of biology of belief. But it's exactly what Brendan had said earlier that you can't look at the cells without understanding how the cells are being signaled and the signal of the cells coming in from outside the cell. So it kind of throws the whole germ theory kind of out the window because where's all the information coming from? Don't we want to like figure that out so we can signal the cell to behave properly?

Brendan (46:33): And along those lines too, somewhat related, is Candace Pert's book, *Molecules of Emotion*.

Kelly (46:41): Yeah. [*The*] *Emotion Code* is another one. And *Feelings Buried Alive Never Die* is another one. *Who Switched Off My Brain*, Dr. Caroline Leaf. These are all incredible books that teach about the emotional components to health. And Caroline Leaf proved that 90% of all illness is emotional. And she proved it from the DNA and how the DNA changes. And then Joe Dispenza's books, you know, *The Placebo* [*You Are The Placebo*] and *How to Break the Habit of Being You* [*Yourself*]. He takes it a little bit further into understanding how to create the neural programming to reeducate your DNA so that it outputs what you want it to output.

Brendan (47:26): Yeah. That's good stuff too.

Kelly (47:30): It's a magic carpet ride [unintelligible] [Brendan: I have three of his books.] Yeah, they're great. They're great.

Brendan (47:37): Thank you so much for bringing these elements, these crucial aspects of the whole journey, into the Eat4Earth conversation and community. Thanks for being here with that.

Kelly (47:47): My absolute pleasure. Thank you for all the work you're doing, and thank you all for listening. Have a great, great day, and get some sunshine.

Conclusion

The experts interviewed for Eat4Earth included popular and respected educators, as well as little-known innovators that are paving the way for food to regain its rightful place as our first medicine and an essential foundation of human potential.

How we grow our food has emerged a dominant influence on planetary health, with healthy soil and beneficial soil organisms now being recognized as the "medicine" that could rescue our oceans and stabilize climate, in addition to restoring high levels of nutrition to our food.

The stakes are high for our bodies and for the Earth. Fortunately, we are discovering the under-appreciated power of Nature to heal virtually anything if we work with her instead of against her.

Now more than ever, it is time to Eat for Earth.

It is time to seize our power as citizens, consumers, and entrepreneurs to influence the food system from one that destroys soils to one that restores them.

We can start to do that right now with our daily food choices and our conversations about them.

Let us forget our differences and unite around common values of food quality, planetary stewardship, and humane treatment of animals. We don't need to agree on everything. We simply need to restore global soils.

Made in USA - North Chelmsford, MA
1170461_9798640736991
10.20.2021 1810